C000212581

Genetic Diseases of the Eye

OXFORD MONOGRAPHS ON MEDICAL GENETICS

1. R. B. McConnell: *The genetics of gastrointestinal disorders*
2. A. C. Kopeć: *The distribution of the blood groups in the United Kingdom*
3. E. Slater and V. A. Cowie: *The genetics of mental disorders*
4. C. O. Carter and T. J. Fairbank: *The genetics of locomotor disorders*
5. A. E. Mourant, A. C. Kopeć, and K. Domaniewska-Sobezak: *The distribution of the human blood groups and other polymorphisms*
6. A. E. Mourant, A. C. Kopeć, and K. Domaniewska-Sobezak: *Blood groups and diseases*
7. A. G. Steinbert and C. E. Cook: *The distribution of the human immunoglobulin allotypes*
8. D. Tills, A. C. Kopeć, and R. E. Tills: *The distribution of the human blood groups and other polymorphisms: Supplement I*
10. D. Z. Loesch: *Quantitative dermatoglyphics: classification, genetics, and pathology*
11. D. J. Bond and A. C. Chandley: *Aneuploidy*
12. P. F. Benson and A. H. Fensom: *Genetic biochemical disorders*
13. G. R. Sutherland and F. Hecht: *Fragile sites on human chromosomes*
14. M. d'A Crawfurd: *The genetics of renal tract disorders*
16. C. R. Scriver and B. Childs: *Garrod's inborn factors in disease*
18. M. Baraitser: *The genetics of neurological disorders*
19. R. J. Gorlin, M. M. Cohen, Jr., and L. S. Levin: *Syndromes of the head and neck, third edition*
20. R. A. King, J. I. Rotter, and A. G. Motulsky: *The genetics basis of common diseases*
21. D. Warburton, J. Byrne, and N. Canki: *Chromosome anomalies and prenatal development: an atlas*
22. J. J. Nora, K. Berg, and A. H. Nora: *Cardiovascular diseases: genetics, epidemiology, and prevention*
24. A.E.H. Emery: *Duchenne muscular dystrophy, second edition*
25. E.G.D. Tuddenham and D. N. Cooper: *The molecular genetics of haemostasis and its inherited disorders*
26. A. Boué: *Fetal medicine*
27. R. E. Stevenson, J. G. Hall, and R. M. Goodman: *Human malformations*
28. R. J. Gorlin, H. V. Toriello, and M. M. Cohen, Jr.: *Hereditary hearing loss and its syndromes*
29. R.J.M. Gardner and G. R. Sutherland: *Chromosome abnormalities and genetic counseling, second edition*
30. A. S. Teebi and T. I. Farag: *Genetic disorders among Arab populations*
31. M. Michael Cohen, Jr.: *The child with multiple birth defects*
32. W. W. Weber: *Pharmacogenetics*
33. V. P. Sybert: *Genetic skin disorders*
34. M. Baraitser: *Genetics of neurological disorders, third edition*
35. H. Ostrer: *Non-mendelian genetics in humans*
36. E. Traboulsi: *Genetic diseases of the eye*
37. G. Semenza: *Transcription factors and human disease*

OXFORD MONOGRAPHS ON MEDICAL GENETICS NO. 36

GENETIC DISEASES OF THE EYE

Edited by
ELIAS I. TRABOULSI, M.D.
The Center for Genetic Eye Diseases
The Cleveland Clinic Foundation
Eye Institute

Consulting Editors
Irene H. Maumenee, M.D.
A. Linn Murphree, M.D.

New York Oxford
OXFORD UNIVERSITY PRESS
1998

Oxford University Press

Oxford New York
Athens Auckland Bangkok Bogotá Buenos Aires Calcutta
Cape Town Chennai Dar es Salaam Delhi Florence Hong Kong Istanbul
Karachi Kuala Lumpur Madrid Melbourne Mexico City Mumbai
Nairobi Paris São Paulo Singapore Taipei Tokyo Toronto Warsaw

and associated companies in
Berlin Ibadan

Published by Oxford University Press, Inc.
198 Madison Avenue, New York, New York 10016

Oxford is a registered trademark of Oxford University Press

Library of Congress Cataloging-in-Publication Data
Genetic diseases of the eye / edited by Elias I. Traboulsi.
p. cm.—(Oxford monographs on medical genetics ; no. 36)
Includes bibliographical references and index.
ISBN 0-19-509676-2
1. Eye—Diseases—Genetic aspects.
2. Eye–Abnormalities.
I. Traboulsi, Elias I.
II. Series.
[DNLM: 1. Eye Diseases, Hereditary.
WW 140 G3275 1998] RE906.G39 1998
617.7′042—DC21 DNLM/DLC for Library of Congress 97-34011

9 8 7 6 5 4 3 2 1

Printed in Hong Kong
on acid-free paper

Foreword

VICTOR A. McKUSICK

Ophthalmologists have always been at the forefront in the clinical delineation of genetic disorders. Like dermatologists, with whom they share that priority, they have enjoyed the advantage of accessibility of the phenotype. Pioneers in ophthalmologic genetics who come to mind include Falls, Franceschetti, François, Horner, Leber, Nettleship, Sorsby, Tay, Usher, Waardenburg, and many others of earlier generations, as well as many who are still contributing.

Furthermore, disorders of the eye have been important in the definition of basic principles of genetics. These include the characteristic X-linked recessive pedigree pattern described for colorblindness by Zürich ophthalmologist, Horner, in 1876; cytoplasmic (now called mitochondrial) inheritance, pointed to in 1936 by Imai and Moriwaki for Leber optic atrophy; the single active X chromosome (Lyon hypothesis), giving a mosaic pigmentary pattern of the fundus in females heterozygous for ocular albinism, as pointed out by Mary Lyon in 1961; the two-hit hypothesis of the development of hereditary cancers worked out first on the basis of retinoblastoma by Knudson in 1971; digenic inheritance, demonstrated by Dryja's group (1994) for a form of retinitis pigmentosa that developed only when a mutation was present in each of two separate genes, and many more.

The eye has always provided a diagnostic window on the central nervous system and indeed on the entire patient. The cherry-red spot, retinal hemangioma, and angioid streaks; iridescent lens opacities and lens subluxation; lattice corneal dystrophy and whorl-like corneal opacities; and oculomotor apraxia and ptosis are some of the ocular features useful for diagnosis of disorders that are wider in their effects than the eye alone. This broader value for diagnosis is based on one of the cardinal principles of clinical genetics: pleiotropism (multiple phenotypic effects of a single gene mutation).

The eye also provides many examples of a second principle of clinical genetics: genetic heterogeneity (what appears to be the same disorder is in fact fundamentally distinct). For example, the differentiation of Hurler syndrome and Hunter syndrome was possible on the basis of presence or absence of corneal clouding; Marfan syndrome and homocystinuria, on the basis of upward or downward displacement of the lenses, respectively; and so on.

In recent times, molecular genetics has contributed much to ophthalmologic genetics (or genetic ophthalmology), just as it has contributed much to all branches of medicine. It has thrown light on the basic molecular changes in classic ocular traits such as colorblindness and in classic genetic disorders of the eye such as retinoblastoma. It has helped in refining the phenotypic limits of particular disorders with the redefinition of seemingly identical conditions: heterogeneity at the level of different mutations in the same gene (allelic heterogeneity) and at the level of different loci (locus heterogeneity). In other cases it has demonstrated that some disorders considered separate on the basis of clinical characteristics have proved to be the same disorder.

One can expect that ophthalmology will continue to lead in its contributions to medical genetics. It is possible that some of the earliest examples of successful gene therapy will be achieved in the case of hereditary diseases, for example.

It is extraordinarily timely to have this comprehensive treatise on the eye from a large group of clinical investigators now actively studying these disorders.

Preface

Physicians thrive on the resolution of their patients' ailments. The reward of observing the joy of the patient whose cataracts have been removed and who can now see is incomparable. Restoring sight is what ophthalmology is all about. Unfortunately, most genetic ocular diseases are not "cureable" because of our poor understanding of pathogenesis or lack of therapeutic methods.

During my visits to the Middle East in recent years I was distressed to see numerous children blind from autosomal recessive diseases such as congenital glaucoma and Leber congenital amaurosis. The high rate of consanguineous marriages, the large number of offspring, and the lack of genetic counseling and prenatal diagnosis contribute to the high prevalence of these diseases and the tremendous impact on families and society. I examined a family in the United Arab Emirates where two of three children were blind from Leber congenital amaurosis. The parents suspected that a genetic cause was involved and quickly understood my explanation of autosomal recessive inheritance. When I advised non-consanguineous marriages for their children in the future and for other family members at any time, the children's uncle was quick to point out to me that in one of his preachings ("Hadeeth") the prophet Mohammad states: "Marry from far and you shall be healthy." The advent of easy communication and transportation, as well as the recognition of genetic diseases as such, combined with molecular genetic testing and prenatal diagnosis, will undoubtedly minimize if not eradicate some of these disorders.

The authors of this book have summarized current knowledge on the clinical manifestations, etiology and management of genetic diseases of the eye. The project started about twenty years ago when Doctors Linn Murphree and Irene Maunemee became aware of the lack of a concise yet authoritative source of information on genetic eye diseases. They wrote the draft of a text for a catalogue/atlas of these diseases and gathered illustrations from the large collection of the Johns Hopkins Center for Hereditary Eye Diseases and the Johns Hopkins Hospital. Some of these beautiful photographs are included in this text. The exponential growth in the field of medical genetics and molecular biology in the 1980s and 1990s became a major hindrance to progress on the Atlas and the concept of an edited text became more appealing. I proposed to serve as editor of the text with advice from Doctors Maumenee and Murphree. An outline was developed and colleagues were asked to contribute chapters in their areas of interest. Some chapters could be written as a synthesis of their subject matter while others had to cover numerous disease entries. The resulting book is not intended to be an encyclopedia of genetic diseases of the eye and of the ocular manifestations of inherited disorders, but rather a useful reference on most genetic eye diseases and their management.

The recognition of genetic diseases as a leading cause of blindness in adults and in children, the extraordinary efforts to determine the underlying defects, the development of diagnostic and therapeutic molecular genetic tools, and the campaign to educate ophthalmologists and primary care physicians about these diseases will foster the prevention and treatment of genetic blindness.

This book is dedicated to my wonderful wife Mayya and my children Alex and Nadeem who continue to tolerate my long working hours, and to my parents Alexandre and Renee from whom I was forcefully separated by an unfortunate and unnecessary war. I am very grateful to the continued support of my first teacher of medical genetics, Vazken Der Kaloustian, now at Montreal Children's Hospital, without whose encouragement I would not have been able to proceed with and finish this project. I thank Irene H. Maumenee for her guidance, advice and for teaching me ophthalmic genetics. I thank all the authors for their superb work and for their patience during the editorial and production phases of this project.

This work would not have been completed without the assistance of Scott Proctor, Susan Hannan, and my wife, Mayya Traboulsi. I thank Oxford University Press and Jeff House in particular for giving me the opportunity to present this information to the medical community.

Cleveland, Ohio E.I.T.
March 1998

Contents

III RETINAL DYSTROPHIES AND DEGENERATION

IV DISORDERS OF OCULAR MOTILITY

V OCULAR MANIFESTATIONS OF INHERITED SYSTEMIC DISEASES

VI TUMORS

VII MANAGEMENT

Contributors

LISA S. ABRAMS, M.D.
Parris-Castoro Eye Care Center
Bel Air, Maryland

MARYAM AROICHANE, M.D.
Hôpital Ste. Justine
McGill University
Montreal, Quebec, Canada

DIMITRI AZAR, M.D.
Massachusetts Eye and Ear Infirmary
Boston, Massachusetts

J. BRONWYN BATEMAN, M.D.
University of Colorado Health Science Center
Denver, Colorado

ALAN C. BIRD, M.D.
Institute of Ophthalmology
Moorfields Eye Hospital
London, England

SHU WUN CHANG, M.D.
Chang-Gung Memorial Hospital
Tiwan, Republic of China

JOSEPH L. DEROSE, O.D.
The Cleveland Clinic Eye Institute
Cleveland Clinic Foundation
Cleveland, Ohio

SAMIR S. DEEB, PH.D.
Departments of Genetics and Medicine
University of Washington
Seattle, Washington

ARLENE V. DRACK, M.D.
Emory Eye Institute
Emory University School of Medicine
Atlanta, Georgia

ELIZABETH C. ENGLE, M.D.
Department of Neurology
Children's Hospital
Harvard Medical School
Boston, Massachusetts

MORTON F. GOLDBERG, M.D.
The Wilmer Eye Institute
The Johns Hopkins University
School of Medicine
Baltimore, Maryland

MICHAEL B. GORIN, M.D., PH.D.
The Eye and Ear Institute
University of Pittsburgh
Pittsburgh, Pennsylvania

JOHN HECKENLIVELY, M.D.
Jules Stein Eye Institute
University of California at Los Angeles
School of Medicine
Los Angeles, California

KATRINKA L. HEHER, M.D.
Children's Hospital of Philadelphia
University of Pennsylvania
Philadelphia, Pennsylvania

MICHAEL HUMAYUN, M.D.
Department of Ophthalmology
Washington Hospital Center
Washington, D.C.

ETHYLIN WANG JABS, M.D.
Department of Pediatrics and Center for Craniofacial Development and Disorders
Center for Medical Genetics
The Johns Hopkins Hospital
Baltimore, Maryland

JAMES A. KATOWITZ, M.D.
Children's Hospital of Philadelphia
University of Pennsylvania
Philadelphia, Pennsylvania

JOHN B. KERRISON, M.D.
The Wilmer Eye Institute
Johns Hopkins University
School of Medicine
Baltimore, Maryland

ROBERT K. KOENEKOOP, M.D., PH.D.
Department of Ophthalmology
Montreal Children's Hospital
McGill University
Montreal, Quebec, Canada

ALEX V. LEVIN, M.D.
Hospital for Sick Children
University of Toronto
Toronto, Ontario, Canada

AMY FELDMAN LEWANDA, M.D.
Johns Hopkins University
Baltimore, Maryland

IAN M. MACDONALD, M.D.
Department of Ophthalmology and Ocular Genetics Laboratory
University of Alberta
Edmonton, Alberta, Canada

DAVID MACKEY, M.D.
Department of Ophthalmology
Royal Children's Hospital
University of Melbourne
Melbourne, Victoria, Australia

IRENE H. MAUMENEE, M.D. (CONSULTING EDITOR)
The Wilmer Eye Institute
Johns Hopkins University
School of Medicine
Baltimore, Maryland

VICTOR MCKUSICK, M.D.
Johns Hopkins University
Baltimore, Maryland

ARNO G. MOTULSKY, M.D.
Department of Medical Genetics
University of Washington
Seattle, Washington

A. LINN MURPHREE, M.D. (CONSULTING EDITOR)
Children's Hospital
University of Southern California
Los Angeles, California

LARA PALINCSAR, M.S.
Georgetown University
Washington, D.C.

ANTHONY G. QUINN, M.D.
Hospital for Sick Children
University of Toronto
Toronto, Ontario, Canada

YARON S. RABINOWITZ, M.D.
Jules Stein Eye Institute
University of California at Los Angeles
School of Medicine
Los Angeles, California

NICOLA K. RAGGE, M.D.
Department of Ophthalmology
Hospital for Sick Children
London, England

DANIEL F. ROSBERGER, M.D., PH.D.
Cornell University Medical College
New York, New York

HESHAM SALAMA, M.D.
El-Maghrabi Eye and Ear Hospital
Jeddah, Saudi Arabia

ARTURO SANTOS, M.D.
CUCS–Universidad de Guadalajara
Guadalajara, Jalisco, Mexico

PAUL A. SIEVING, M.D., PH.D.
Department of Ophthalmology
University of Michigan
Ann Arbor, Michigan

ARUN D. SINGH, M.D.
Department of Ophthalmology
University of Florida
Gainesville, Florida

SUSHANT K. SINHA, D.O.
Macon County Eye Center
Southern Illinois University
Decatur, Illinois

KENT W. SMALL, M.D.
Jules Stein Eye Institute
University of California at Los Angeles
School of Medicine
Los Angeles, California

OLOF SUNDIN, PH.D.
The Wilmer Eye Institute
Johns Hopkins University
School of Medicine
Baltimore, Maryland

JANET S. SUNNESS, M.D.
Visual Function Services
The Wilmer Eye Institute
Johns Hopkins University
School of Medicine
Baltimore, Maryland

JOANNE SUTHERLAND, Ms.C.
Department of Genetic Counseling
Hospital for Sick Children
Toronto, Ontario, Canada

ELIAS I. TRABOULSI, M.D. (EDITOR)
The Cleveland Clinic Eye Institute
Cleveland Clinic Foundation
Cleveland, Ohio

SUHAS TULI, M.D.
Johns Hopkins University
Baltimore, Maryland

DAVID S. WALTON, M.D.
Harvard Medical School
Boston, Massachusetts

RICHARD G. WELEBER, M.D.
Departments of Ophthalmology and Molecular and Medical Genetics
Casey Eye Institute
Oregon Health Sciences University
Portland, Oregon

JANEY L. WIGGS, M.D., PH.D.
New England Eye Center
Tufts University
Boston, Massachusetts

DANPING ZHU, M.D.
The Wilmer Eye Institute
Johns Hopkins University
School of Medicine
Baltimore, Maryland

I.

Developmental Abnormalities

1

Embryology of the Eye and the Role of Developmental Genes

OLOF SUNDIN

This chapter introduces the reader to molecules and cellular processes that take part in the formation of the eye. The basic question of embryology is how a single cell, the fertilized egg, gives rise to a complex organism. Classical embryology has provided an important framework for the anatomical description of this process and identified some of its component events. More recently, the application of genetic and biochemical methods has begun to uncover many of the molecular mechanisms that guide development.

THE EMBRYO DEVELOPS AS A COMMUNITY OF CELLS

Some key concepts and their associated terminology are essential to the discussion of current embryology and are summarized as follows:

1. Cells grow and divide in a highly controlled manner to build the multicellular embryo.
2. Individual cells acquire specialized functions, process known as *differentiation*.
3. When and where the processes of growth and differentiation take place are carefully controlled.
4. The DNA in each cell of an organism, known as its genome, contains all the information required to direct development of the embryo and to make its structural components. Genomic DNA directs the synthesis of RNA which, in turn, makes protein molecules. Nearly all 3 billion DNA base pairs and the estimated 100,000 genes of the human genome are in the cell's nucleus; there is also a small, maternally inherited genome in the mitochondrion.
5. Many different kinds of protein molecules regulate RNA synthesis. These *transcription factors* determine which genes will be used as DNA templates to make mRNA. The selective production of mRNA by transcription is a major factor determining which genes will be functionally active (expressed) and which will be inactive.
6. The genes that are expressed in a cell collectively determine its primary features: its potential to grow and divide, its shape, it capacity for movement, and specific metabolic functions. In addition, the expressed genes determine what signals the cell can send to other cells, what signals it can receive, and how it will respond.
7. Inductive interactions involve the production of signaling molecules by certain cells

and their recognition by receptor molecules on other cells. These signals can alter the developmental fate of the responding cells. In addition to timing developmental events, inductive signaling provides the geometric measuring tools that are essential for establishing patterns, both in the ordered organization of cells within tissues and in the body plan of the embryo.[33,43]

In summary, development is a complicated process that relies heavily upon the storage and transfer of information to regulate cell fate and structures. There are many points at which gene mutations can disrupt or alter the formation of a human embryo.

DEVELOPMENTAL PROCESSES ARE ANCIENT AND CONSERVED

Within the past decade, tens of thousands of genes and their products have been cloned by recombinant DNA technology and characterized at the molecular level. In addition to human genes, many are from a variety of experimental organisms, including the nematode *Caenurhabditis elegans,* the fly *Drosophila melanogaster,* the zebrafish,[42] the frog, the chicken, and the mouse.[52] An extremely important generalization to emerge from these genetic studies is that the molecules and networks of gene interactions that direct development have been highly conserved during evolution.

One example of the evolutionary conservation of gene structure and function is the Hox class of homeobox genes (reviewed by Gehring;[27] Krumlauf;[49] in the eye: Beebe[6]), which encode a family of transcription factors. These genes, originally identified and characterized in the fly *Drosophila,* act to regulate the expression of mRNA by other genes. Because of the highly conserved structure of these genes, DNA hybridization techniques were used to isolate their counterparts from a great variety of vertebrates and invertebrates,[44] where they serve to specify the positional identity of cells along the craniocaudal body axis.[59] Metazoan animals share a molecular code for "head" and "tail" that has been preserved for over 600 million years.

As with the general body plan, it is now clear that genes regulating formation of the eye have also been highly conserved.[36] One of these is the human *PAX6* gene, which is mutant in the ocular disorder *aniridia.*[29,85] Like the Hox genes, *PAX6* functions as a transcription factor and plays an essential role in the developing eye. The sequence of the 422 amino acids of the human PAX6 protein is identical to that of the mouse[89] and has 97% identity to fish Pax6.[72] Mutations in the mouse *Pax6* gene, known as *Small eye,* cause iris hypoplasia and other defects that are very similar to human aniridia.[28,39] The *Drosophilia eyeless* gene, which is the fly counterpart of human *PAX6,* is also essential for eye development.[73] The *eyeless* gene has the very special ability to initiate the whole process of eye formation. When expression of *eyeless* protein is genetically engineered to take place at specific sites in the larval precursors of legs and wings, the *eyeless* gene has the amazing ability to direct the formation of small, perfectly formed eyes at these sites on the legs and wings of the adult fly.[37] As with much of *Drosophila* genetics, this result has yet to be fully assimilated into our understanding of what role *Pax6* plays in vertebrate eye development. We do know, however, that when the mouse *Pax6* gene is similarly introduced into the fly embryo and expressed at these same sites, it also causes the formation of eyes on the legs and wings.[37] This is dramatic proof that the biochemical functions of *Pax6* have remained fundamentally unchanged over an enormous span of time. It is possible that the vertebrate counterparts of *sine oculis, eyes absent,* and other genes known to be required for development of the *Drosophila* eye[36] may also have important roles in human eye development and disease.

GENOME PROJECTS AND HUMAN GENETICS

The Connection from Animal to Man

The human genome is estimated to contain 100,000 distinct genes, and as many as half of these have been at least partially characterized at the sequence level.[52,80] Before the end of the century it is expected that mRNA sequences and chromosomal map positions will be available for most human genes, and within a decade the complete genome sequence will be publicly available. The challenge will be to identify which of these genes are associated with known genetic disorders and to understand their function.

Unfortunately, the vast body of mRNA sequence data available from randomly sequenced human cDNA clones is usually not accompanied by an understanding of where these genes are expressed and how they function during development. However, by comparing their sequences to well-studied genes in model organisms such as the mouse, fish, *Drosophila,* or *C. elegans,* it is usually possible to guess the general biochemical function of the gene, and sometimes what it does during development. Again, the validity of making such connections between organisms rests on the highly conserved nature of embryonic development and the fact that genes usually exist in large families that encode proteins sharing basic biochemical mechanisms.[25]

In addition to the great numbers of mutant genes studied in *C. elegans* and *Drosophila,* there is currently a major effort to identify mutations affecting development of the zebrafish.[42] Mutations defining hundreds of novel genes affecting fish eye development have already been identified. In the mouse, many of the classic mutations have been isolated and characterized at the level of DNA sequence, and the new technology of targeted mutagenesis ("gene knockout") has already yielded mutations in several hundred genes (Table 1.1).

Table 1.1. Summary of Essential Information About Some of the Genes Involved in Vertebrate Eye Development

Gene	Type	Gene Family	Key Sites of Activity	Mouse Mutations	Human Disease
BMP7	GF	TGF-β	Optic primordium, kidney skeleton	Knockout—microphthalmia polydactyly	None yet
Brn3B	TF	POU domain	Retinal ganglion cells	Knockout—optic nerve hypoplasia	None yet
Chx10	TF	Homeobox	Retina, brain	*Ocular retardation* microphthalmia	None yet
γ-crystallin	ST	$\beta\gamma$-crystallins	Lens nucleus	*Eye lens obsolescence* (*Elo*)	Coppock cataract
Mi	TF	Basic HLH-zip	Retinal pigment epithelium, pigment cells	*Microphthalmia*	Waardenburg syndrome type II
ocrl-1	EN	Inositol phosphatase	Lens, brain, kidney function	None yet	Lowe syndrome
Otx1	TF	Homeobox	Iris and ciliary epithelium, ocular surface	Knockout—brain seizures lacrimal gland missing	None yet
Otx2	TF	Homeobox	Retinal pigment epithelium, optic nerve	Knockout—dies in early development	None yet
Pax2	TF	Homeobox	Early optic nerve, kidney defects	Knockout—eye, kidney	Oculorenal syndrome
Pax6	TF	Homeobox	Lens, retina, nose, brain	Small-eye	Aniridia, anophthalmia, brain, nose defects, Peters' anomaly

The headings are explained as follows: **genes,** gene abbreviation, using terminology for mouse, which is usually shared for other animal species; type, functionality class of gene: EN = enzyme, GF = growth factor, inductive signaling molecule ON = oncogene or tumor suppressor, ST = structural component, TF = transcription factor, (TF) = transcription factor associated; **gene family,** the biochemical family, designated by founding member, or protein structural motif; **key sites of activity,** sites of gene expression of special note or relevance to genetic defects; **mouse mutations,** k.o.: knockout mutations have been made by targeted mutagenesis technology, followed by phenotypic effects; *italics:* descriptive name of mouse gene, as defined classically by mutation. **Human disease,** name or description.

Candidate Genes and Human Genetics

The "positional candidate" approach has become the dominant method of cloning new disease genes.[15] When genetic linkage data are available for a rare disorder, it is usually not possible to identify the gene purely on the basis of its position on the genetic and physical maps of a chromosome. Often linkage data will narrow the initial field of 100,000 human genes to a chromosomal subregion containing hundreds of genes. With today's technology, it is still impractical to screen these for mutations by sequence analysis. Projects are also underway to integrate existing information and to map the patterns of expression systematically for all genes in the mouse embryo.[52] Knowledge of gene expression patterns and the function of related genes in model organisms is a valuable tool for narrowing the candidate pool to a number of likely suspects.

It is also possible to go in the other direction, to begin with a gene known to be involved in vertebrate eye development and search for a human disorder caused by mutations in that gene. Making mutations to order for a particular gene in the mouse by targeted mutagenesis[74] provides a mouse model for the disease. The phenotype exhibited by these mutant mice thus can then be used to search the clinical literature for individuals with a similar disorder. As the mouse "gene knockout" technology becomes more routine, this will be an increasingly important route to identifying genes underlying human disorders. Because many common human diseases are suspected to result from mutations in multiple genes,[52] the mouse will become an increasingly important experimental system in which to test how combinations of mutations affect development and adult function.

THE BIOCHEMICAL NATURE OF GENES REQUIRED FOR DEVELOPMENT

Functional Classes of Genes

Structural genes constitute the architectural components of the embryo and the specialized machinery required for the function of its differentiated cells. At the most basic level are the "housekeeping" genes, which carry out the biochemical functions required in nearly all cells. There are also specialized proteins that endow different cells in the body with unique physical properties and functions. For example, the strength of tendons and other connective tissues is dependent upon cytoskeletal genes, including the many distinct collagens and intermediate filament proteins that are expressed in the connective tissues. Function of the photoreceptor requires specialized transducing proteins and enzymes that belong to the phototransduction cascade.[2,62]

Regulatory genes primarily determine when and where in the embryo (and adult) other genes will be expressed.[12] This class includes transcription factors, as well as regulators of intracellular metabolism such as the protein kinases, and the extracellular signaling molecules and their receptors that mediate inductive interactions between cells in the embryo.[43] Regulatory genes are involved in storing, transmitting, and acting on information, directing the construction of an embryo from the building blocks encoded by the structural genes.

Gene Families

The similarities of proteins encoded by different genes in an organism usually reflect their shared ancestral relationship. Gene families are thought to have arisen during the course of evolution through the duplication of chromosomal segments within the genome, followed by the gradual mutation of these duplicated genes in these regions so that each performs related, but unique, functions.[44] The existence of gene families allows the daunting number of 100,000 individual genes to be divided into a much smaller number of prototypes, with the members of each gene family representing variations of a basic structural theme.[52]

Transcription Factors

Transcription factors act as molecular switches that regulate the production of mRNA by other genes, and are highly specialized for this purpose. The majority of identified transcription factors bind directly to promoters, specific

DNA sites in the genes that the factors regulate. There are, however, examples of proteins that regulate mRNA synthesis by binding to other transcription factors. One important feature of transcription factors is that their function is confined to the cell where they are expressed. Here they determine what genes will be activated or inactivated in the cell, and are key determinants of the *identity* of the cell. Genes encoding DNA binding transcription factors are very numerous, and most can be grouped into several large families based on the structure of the DNA binding domains that are part of the protein. A few examples are described in the paragraphs that follow.

Homeobox Genes

The prototypes of the family of homeobox genes are the *Drosophila* genes *antennapedia* and *bithorax*. They were originally called *homeotic* genes because mutations caused an interchange of identity between embryologically homologous structures such as legs and antennae.[27,59] A 180-base pair DNA sequence motif was found to be extremely conserved between the several known fly homeotic genes, as well as with previously unknown genes in vertebrates. This motif is the homeobox, which encodes a 60-amino acid DNA binding element of the protein (the homeodomain), which in turn determines target gene specificity for the transcription factor.[27] Structurally, the homeodomain consists of three alpha helices folded together into a compact structure that likely shares an ancient common ancestor with lambda repressor and other bacterial transcriptional regulators. Several hundred homeobox genes have now been isolated in a variety of organisms ranging from yeasts and plants to humans.[44] As with other transcription factors, they are involved in a very wide range of developmental functions, but frequently are involved in determination of regional identity in the embryo or individual cell fate and differentiation.

Other transcription factors have DNA binding domains that are distantly related to the classic homeodomain, notably the *paired* domain, originally identified in the *Drosophila paired* gene. This larger DNA binding domain contains the structural remnants of two homeobox-type motifs. Members of this family often have a paired and a homeobox domain. The paired, or PAX family is exemplified by *Pax6* and *Pax2* (reviewed by Chalepakis et al.[12]). Another variant is the *POU* domain, a DNA binding structure that is closely associated with a homeodomain element. The name is derived from the prototype genes, *pit-1*, a transcription factor required for pituitary gene expression, *unc-86*, a nematode cell lineage gene, and *oct-1*, a nearly ubiquitous mammalian transcription factor. *Brn3B* is a mouse *POU*-domain gene that is expressed in ganglion cells of the eye. Targeted mutations in *Brn3B* cause a decrease in the number of ganglion cells and result in optic nerve hypoplasia.[26]

Zinc Finger Genes

This DNA binding motif consists of a small loop of amino acids held together at their base by a zinc atom coordinated to a group of histidines and cysteines. These small loops are often clustered in a modular manner to build up a DNA binding domain with considerable DNA sequence specificity.[47] Although this is perhaps the most abundant family of transcription factors and includes developmentally important genes, relatively few have yet been associated with eye disorders. One example is the nuclear receptor family (reviewed in Mangelsdorf et al.[56]), which includes genes for the retinoic acid receptors *RAR* and *RXR*. These are a family of nuclear proteins that are regulated by the direct binding of the vitamin A derivative retinoic acid. Mutations in some of these receptors have been found to disrupt normal development of the eye.[45]

Helix-Loop Helix Genes

The helix-loop helix genes constitute another large gene family that includes the oncogenes *myc*, *jun*, and *fos*. Their essential structure is a dimer of helical DNA binding domains held together by an extended dimerization domain known as a "leucine zipper." In *Drosophila*, the *scute* and *achaete* genes regulate development of sensory bristles and other neural structures. A key feature of this family is that different genes can exchange subunits and form heterodimers, which appear to have distinct regulatory properties. The mouse microphthalmia and human Waardenburg syndrome genes are examples of this class,[40] and the mammalian counterparts of *scute* and *achaete*, and *Mash* gene family, are expressed during the formation of neurons in the central nervous system and retina.[84]

Signaling Molecules and Their Receptors

In its essentials, embryonic induction involves the production of a signaling molecule by a cell, followed by the binding of this molecule to a receptor on or in another cell.[43] This binding to the receptor then activates the internal signal transduction machinery of the responding cell. The result may be changes in cell metabolism, structure, and the activity of transcription factors. Ultimately, the signal changes the developmental fate of the cell. Studies in *Drosophila* and nematodes[33,91] indicate that inductive iteractions between cells are not mediated by a single class of mechanism or molecule but by a wide variety of signaling molecules, many of which also have functions in the adult. A sample of these signaling molecules and their receptors is presented in the paragraphs that follow.

Small Organic Molecules

The simplest pathway from signaling molecule to the regulation of gene expression is provided by small molecules. The best known of this family are the retinoic acids, steroids, and thyroid hormones, which are synthesized by specialized enzyme pathways. Because of their small size and hydrophobic nature, these molecules can diffuse through cells and their membranes without need of special channels or transport mechanisms. In the case of thyroid hormone and steroids, they may be distributed throughout the embryo by the circulatory system. Retinoic acid and its isomers are thought to form gradients in which higher concentrations of the signaling molecule are found near the site of synthesis. The action of such retinoic acid gradients acting on the expression of *Hox* genes is thought to determine positional identity along the anteriorposterior body axis.[59,83]

Retinoids, steroids, and thyroid hormones all bind directly to specific transcription factors in the cell that belongs to the nuclear receptor superfamily.[56] These molecules contain a transcription activator/regulatory domain, a zinc-finger DNA binding domain, and a ligand binding domain. When the ligand binding domain binds the signaling molecule, this alters the DNA binding and gene activation properties of the receptor. This in turn causes the activation of suppression of transcription in specific target genes.

Secreted Proteins and Membrane-Bound Ligands

A more common pathway involves the synthesis and secretion of protein signaling molecules by a cell, and the detection of these signaling molecules by receptor molecules on the surface of a responding cell. The best known of these are the "growth factors." One is IGF-2, an insulinlike growth factor that promotes lens fiber cell differentiation and establishes the asymmetry of the lens.[5] Also important are the several fibroblast growth factors (FGFs), which are expressed in the eye and at many other sites during development.[43] One of the largest families is the transforming growth factor-beta (TGF-β) superfamily, which is generally involved in altering cell fate and promoting differentiation. An important subfamily of these are the bone morphogenetic proteins (BMPs), which are involved in an extremely diverse set of developmental processes, including eye development.[23,55]

Most of the receptors for these secreted signaling proteins are single polypeptides that are anchored in and span the cell membrane. They have an external ligand binding domain and a signal transduction domain inside the cell. Binding of the signaling molecule induces receptor dimerization or other structural changes that are transmitted to the intracellular domain.[33] This signal is relayed further to other proteins in the cell's cytoplasm. The most common is the protein kinase domain, an enzyme that uses nucleotide substrates to add single phosphates of the hydroxyl group to tyrosine residues in a specific set of target proteins.[46] Other classes of receptors contain a protein phosphatase that can specifically reverse this modification. In addition to intracellular protein kinases, transcription factors, metabolic enzymes, and cytoskeletal proteins are among the cellular components that have functions known to be regulated by phosphorylation. In the case of the large TGF-β family of signaling molecules, the specific effects of individual factors are reflected in the altered function of transcription factors belonging to the *Mad* family.[65]

Another means of signal transduction is the G protein–coupled receptor. G proteins are small cytoplasmic proteins that bind to a specific site on the intracellular domain of the receptor. The receptor may have several transmembrane domains, as in the case of rhodopsin. These proteins use the binding and hydrolysis of the nucleotide guanosine triphosphate (GTP) to cycle between activated and inactivated protein conformations, transmitting conformational changes of a single receptor into the activation of many other molecules, such as kinases. They also regulate the metabolism of intracellular second messenger molecules, such as cyclic AMP (adenosine monophosphate), cyclic GMP (guanosine monophosphate, or the inositol phosphates. Second messengers are very important in determining whether cells will exercise certain basic options, such as whether to proliferate, differentiate, or die, as well as physiological responses such as the release of secretory granules by secretory cells or nerve terminals.

Some signaling molecules are proteins that remain tethered to the cell surface at their site of synthesis. The signal is received only by cells that make direct contact with the signaling cell. One example is the *Drosophila Delta* gene, which encodes a membrane-bound signaling molecule that interacts with the *Notch* transmembrane receptor to ensure that the responding group of cells make only a single r8 photoreceptor. The *Delta* gene is essential for assembling the precisely defined photoreceptor array in the compound eye of insects.[4,91] Vertebrate homologues of these genes, suitably named Notch and Delta, also appear involved in determining neuronal cell fate in the central nervous system[84] and retina. In another example, posttranslational cleavage of the *sonic hedgehog* signaling protein is accompanied by its coupling to *cholesterol*.[71] This is apparently essential to its normal function of establishing midline structures of the embryo.[13,76] Cholesterol is thought to act by anchoring the signaling molecule in the cell membrane. Even the secreted protein growth factors may have limited ranges of action; many are known to bind very strongly to the extracellular matrix, and are in principle almost immobilized after their secretion by the cell.[43]

It is important to keep in mind that our molecular understanding of embryonic induction is still very incomplete. In principle, inductive signals allow the construction of spatial structure in the body because they provide a means of measuring distance. This is analogous to using a compass to draw circles of defined radius around initial reference points and following simple instructions to build this into a well-defined geometric structure. The radius of such circles might vary. Inductive signals known to act primarily on adjacent cells might involve molecules that remain tethered to the cell. Readily diffusible small molecules or secreted proteins could mediate longer-range interactions. It is also possible that longer distances can be spanned by successive waves of short-range interactions.

AN OUTLINE OF EYE DEVELOPMENT

Overview

Optic Primordia

The vertebrate eye is a composite structure, which arises from the joining of two different types of primordia. One of these, the optic vesicle, arises from the forebrain region of the anterior neural plate. The other primordium is the lens placode, which originates in the surface ectoderm of the head. These arise independently and are then brought into close contact, an event that begins a series of inductive interactions that shape the eye. The portion of the optic vesicle that faces the lens placode becomes specialized to generate retina, while the surrounding tissue becomes pigment epithelium, and the stalk of the optic vesicle folds to become the optic nerve. The retina, in turn, provides inductive signals that regulate the growth and orientation of the lens. At this optic cup stage, the eye has already formed its basic pattern elements. A vitreous cavity forms between the lens and the retina, and the iris and ciliary body arise from the margin of the optic cup.

Recruitment of Mesoderm and Neural Crest

During later development, other tissues contribute to this structural nucleus of the eye. Neural crest cells migrate into the space between the lens and corneal ectoderm to build the stromal and endodermal layers of the cornea. Neural crest mesenchyme also migrates into close contact with the pigment epithelium to form the sclera. Muscles of the eye, however, arise from the paraxial mesoderm of the early embryo. Innervation of these muscles takes place by extension of motoneuron and sensory fibers from the hindbrain.

Connections to the Brain

The eye makes extensive connections with the brain in order to transmit the information collected by its photoreceptors neurons. Nerve fibers from ganglion cells in the retina project their growth cones into the ventral face of the optic stalk and build up an axonal fiber tract known as the *optic nerve*. To relay visual information, these fibers eventually make topographically selective connections with sites in the lateral geniculate of the thalamus and the superior colliculus of the midbrain. Neurons based in the hindbrain and cranial ganglia extend connections to the extraocular muscles and iris in order to control their movement.

Early Development: Primordia of the Eye Derive from Surface Ectoderm and the Central Nervous System

Eye development begins in the gastrula stage with the establishment of cells that have acquired the tendency to develop ocular tissues and cell types when excised and grown in isolation from their normal site in the embryo. At this stage, the embryo consists of a primitive ectoderm known as the *epiblast*. Portions of this epiblast are undergoing transformation into endoderm and mesoderm as a result of their ventral movement through the primitive streak. At the anterior end of the primitive streak is a structure known as *Hensen's node*, and anterior to this is a special type of mesoderm known as the *prechordal plate*. Epiblast near the prechordal plate is fated to contribute to the forebrain and eyes, and it is this centrally located region, the eye field, which has acquired the potential to develop as ocular tissue.[1,14] Inductively active mesodermal cells of the midline (prechordal plate, notochord) are necessary to divide the eye field along the midline to generate two separate eye fields. A key inductive signal in this process is the *sonic hedgehog* gene. Failure of midline formation results in *cyclopia*, a deformity in which midline structures are missing, producing a single, centrally located eye. Homozygous mutants in the mouse *sonic hedgehog* generated by targeted mutagenesis result in multiple embryonic defects, including severe cyclopia.[13] Although the mouse heterozygotes show no abnormalities, human patients with cyclopia or holoprosencephaly have been shown to carry heterozygous mutations in the *Sonic hedgehog* gene.[76] Interestingly, there is variation in severity within a single family ranging from mild to extreme, suggesting that environmental or other genetic factors are important in functioning of the human gene. As noted earlier, activity of Sonic hedgehog protein is dependent on its coupling to cholesterol,[71] and it is possible that cholesterol deficiency is the variable contributing factor.

By the neural plate stage embryo, lens primordia and the bilaterally arranged optic primordia are fully established (Fig. 1.1). The lens primordium is a strip of the head ectoderm located outside the neural plate. The optic primordium is located within the neural plate, and it later forms the optic vesicle, and outgrowth of the developing forebrain. It is important to note that *lens and optic primordia arise independently*. Classic studies by Spemann[82] (1938) and others early in this century suggested that contact with the optic vesicle could cause any

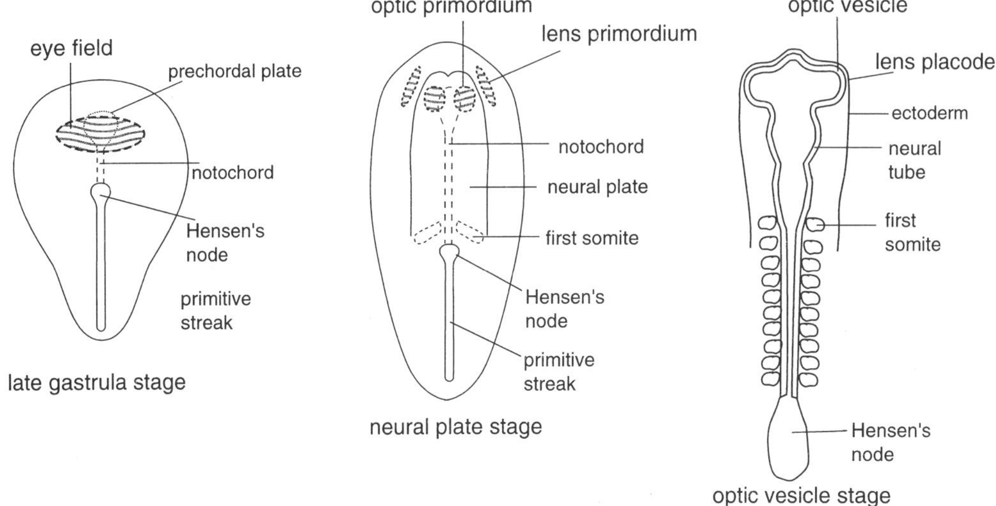

Figure 1.1. Early eye development. Origin of the eye primordia in the chick embryo is depicted at the late gastrula neural plate and optic vesicle stages. Embryo diagrams are drawn as if viewed from above (dorsal face), with underlying structures indicated in dashed lines. Anterior is up. The last gastrula embryo is approximately 3 mm long, and roughly reflects the size and configuration of a human embryo. **Late gastrula stage:** The dorsal surface of the paddle shaped area pellucida consists of primitive ectoderm. The shaded oval area indicates the approximate extent of the eye field in the primitive ectoderm. Underneath this is the prechordal plate mesoderm. **Neural plate stage:** The primitive ectoderm becomes divided into a central neural plate, and the surrounding rim of epithelium that will generate the surface ectoderm. Location of the pair of optic primordia, fated to become the optic vesicle and its derivatives is indicated. Approximate boundaries of the lens primordia are also indicated. At this stage and earlier, the primordia are not visible morphologically; their locations are defined experimentally. **Optic vesicle stage:** The neural epithelium is configured as a tube that extends from the anterior to near the caudal end of the embryo. The optic vesicles are outgrowths of the forebrain at the anterior end of this tube. Lens placodes develop from lens primordia in the head ectoderm that are brought into contact with the optic vesicle.

region of embryonic surface ectoderm to generate a lens. This work was extremely important to the field of embryology, as it established the concept of embryonic induction. However, it has recently been shown that these earlier experiments were flawed[78] and that lenses can in fact only develop from the head ectoderm. In the complete absence of the optic vesicles, head ectoderm is in fact able to generate properly located lens placodes, thickened regions of head ectoderm that are precursors to the lens. Full development and growth of the lens, however, does require association with the optic vesicle and optic cup. Similarly, although the optic vesicle can arise independently of the lens placode, close contact of the optic vesicle with the lens placode is required for its further development into an optic cup,[18] but the molecular nature of these inductive interactions has yet to be determined. Interference with the establishment of these primordia or their inductive interactions may cause *anophthalmia* or *microphthalmia*, disorders in which the orbits and outer facial features form, but eyes are either absent or reduced in size.

The Optic Cup Stage: Basic Body Plan of the Eye

Once the optic vesicle and the lens primordium make contact, the head ectoderm thickens dramatically to generate the lens placode, and the optic vesicle flattens into a paddlelike structure (Fig. 1.2). The layer of neural epithelium facing the placodal ectoderm proliferates and thickens, a first indication of its commitment to forming the neural retina. The thinner portion of the optic vesicle, which faces away from the

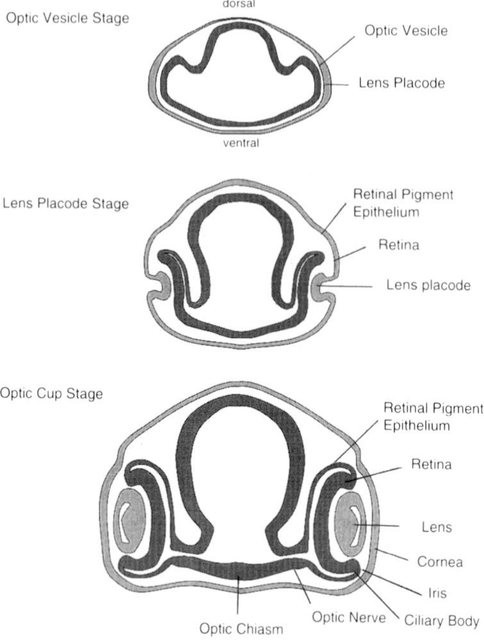

Figure 1.2. Formation of the optic cup. Diagram showing key stages in the transformation of optic cup and lens placode into the optic cup and lens vesicle. Embryos are depicted as transverse sections through optic structures of the head. Depicted are the neural tube epithelium (inner tissue layer) and the surface ectoderm (outer layer). **Optic vesicle stage:** This is a transverse section through the optic vesicles at the third stage shown in Figure 1.1. **Lens placode stage:** Showing collapse of the optic vesicle into a paddle-shaped structure joined to the ventral forebrain, and invagination of the lens placode to form a lens pit. **Optic cup stage:** Embryonic tissues are labeled with the adult structures that they will later generate: The retinal epithelium, which has thickened markedly, consists almost entirely of precursor cells. A thinner layer tissue on the other side of the optic cup will generate the pigment epithelium. The lens vesicle has pinched off from the surface to become a hollow ball of epithelium, and the portion facing the retina has begun to differentiate into lens fiber cells. The entire rim of the optic cup (only one edge is indicated) will form the iris, and the zone just inside of this will generate the ciliary body. The transverse section has been made just posterior to the choroid fissure. Similar sections passing through the choroid fissure are depicted in Figures 1.4 and 1.5.

lens, generates the retinal pigment epithelium. The center of the lens placode then invaginates and closes off its connection with the surface, forming the lens vesicle. The portion of the lens placode that remains on the surface will generate the corneal epithelium and conjunctiva. In the malformation known as Peters' anomaly, lens and corneal epithelium are still connected by a bridge of tissue, an apparent interference with the separation process.[57]

The ventral rim of the optic vesicle and the optic stalk are fated to generate the ventral half of the eye and nerve fiber path of the optic nerve. This takes place by formation of the choroid fissure, a furrow running along the ventral face of the optic stalk and including the ventral edges of the optic cup. The joining of these edges generates the choroid fissure, a nearly invisible seam in the adult eye. Inherited malformations known as *colobomas* represent a failure of the choroid fissure to close properly, giving rise to breaks in the ventral eye, most conspicuously in the ventral retina and iris.[57] Normally, the developmental stitching together of the ventral eye is successful in constructing a nearly radially symmetrical structure from a very *asymmetric* embryonic rudiment.

At this stage the lens provides inductive signals that direct the margins of the optic cup to develop specialized structures including the ciliary body and iris. The localized expression of several homeobox genes suggests that these future territories are already determined at the optic cup stage.[6,32] Aniridia, an inherited disorder caused by heterozygous mutations of the *PAX6* homeobox gene, causes nearly complete absence of the iris.[63] Studies of mice heterozygous for mutations in the mouse *Pax6* gene (*Small eye*), indicate that the iris initially forms.[34] *Pax6* is in fact expressed strongly along the margins of the cup, the region that will give rise to the iris. This suggests a role for Pax6 in establishing pattern prior to the differentiation of cells in the iris. *Pax6* is also expressed prominently in the lens epithelium,[53,89] and an alternate hypothesis is that a decrease in Pax6 expression caused by the mutation affects the level of inductive signals released by the lens.

An interesting feature of aniridia is that it can be considered a panocular disorder.[63] This may reflect the fact that *Pax6* is expressed in several different ocular tissues during their development. With regard to tissues originating from the head ectoderm, Pax6 expression appears to define the boundaries of the early lens primordium[53] and is expressed in all nucleated cells of the mature lens, cornea, and conjunctiva.[48] In this regard it is of interest that mutations in PAX6 have been associated with defects in the corneal epithelium[60] and in Peters' anomaly.[38] Aniridia patients are also missing the fovea, a retinal specialization that may have its origin in the optic cup stage. In mice homozygous for *Pax6* mutations, eyes are completely absent. The earliest defect appears to be the complete failure of lens placode formation. In these mutants, the optic vesicle forms but fails to grow further and form an optic cup, possibly because the optic vesicle does not receive signaling molecules from the lens placode.

From the Head Ectoderm: Lens, Cornea, Conjunctiva, and Adnexa

The lens vesicle is initially a spherically symmetric epithelial structure. However, growth factors released by the optic cup induce cells on the inner face to elongate and begin differentiation into lens fiber cells. The cells facing the corneal surface remain as a thin layer of epithelial stem cells that contribute new fiber cells during growth of the lens. The inductive origin of this asymmetry can be demonstrated by reimplanting the lens in an opposite orientation, followed by the reprogramming of cellular development to generate a correctly oriented lens.[18] During growth, new fibers are added and accrue in an "onionskin" manner outside layers of earlier fibers. As they differentiate, lens fiber cells accumulate huge amounts of crystallins, specialized proteins that confer a high refractive index and transparency upon the lens.[19] Developmental regulation of crystallin gene expression generates a gradient of decreasing refractive index as one proceeds from the center of the lens to its periphery; this design leads to a lens of better optical quality than one of uniform refractive index. In addition, the differentiation of lens fibers also involves the programmed elimination of all nuclei and mitochondria. These are obstructions to transparency and, amazingly, are not required by the cell. The lens fiber cell can enjoy a "life" of several decades as it is sustained via an extensive set of intercellular gap junctions. Interference with the delicate biochemical equilibrium of the lens fiber cell might lead to cataracts, a common disorder in which lens crystallins aggregate in a disorderly fashion, scattering light and rendering the lens opaque.[16]

In the early optic cup stage, the lens vesicle releases signals that induce the overlying surface ectoderm to differentiate into corneal epithelium B,[16] the basal surface of which releases extracellular matrix proteins (collagen I, II, and X: primary stroma), which promote the migration of cranial neural crest into this area. This neural crest gives rise to an internal cell layer known as the *corneal endothelium*. The epithelium, endothelium, and fibroblast crest cells secrete additional collagen, forming the secondary stroma of the embryonic cornea, which is sandwiched between these layers. This embryonic cornea is at first translucent rather than transparent. As the thyroid gland matures, increased thyroxine in the circulation stimulates the corneal endothelium to pump sodium out of the stroma, resulting in dehydration and increase in transparency. In addition, high levels of crystallin-like molecules expressed in the corneal epithelium decrease light scattering at the corneal surface. The shape of the cornea makes a major contribution to refractive properties of the eye, and its malformation may lead to disorders such as astigmatism.

Peripheral to the corneal epithelium, the remaining portion of the lens placode develops as the conjunctiva, an epithelial layer that covers the ocular surface and the inside of the eyelids. It contains a large number of secretory goblet cells that help maintain a lubricating mucous layer. The lacrimal glands develop as ingrowths of this conjunctival epithelium. During development, the eyelids form as ridges on the dorsal and ventral edges of the eye. The inner face of the eyelid, the palpebral conjunctiva, is continuous with the bulbar conjunctiva that covers the globe. Beyond the edge of the eyelid begins the skin. The eyelids grow until they meet and then fuse at their edges, sealing the conjunctiva and cornea into a vesicle.[24] The fused eyelids again open prior to birth. In disorders involving cryptophthalmos, in which the skin of the forehead passes in an unbroken manner over the eyes and into the cheek, it appears that the lids either fail to form or degenerate, and that the ocular surface is transformed into skin. This condition can exist on its own or in conjunction with other malformations, such as in Fraser's syndrome.

From the Central Nervous System: Retina, Iris, Ciliary Body, Pigment Epithelium, and Optic Nerve

Organization of the Optic Cup

The internal neuroepithelium of the optic cup gives rise to the retina, while the closely apposed outer cell sheet forms the pigment epithelium. The space between these two cell layers is continuous with the ventricular cavities of the brain. One consequence of this basic organization is that dividing precursor cells of the neural retina will undergo mitosis near the ventricular surface, as they do throughout the central nervous system. The other consequence is that ciliated cells develop along the ventricular face. Retinal photoreceptors contain a ciliated process known as the outer segment, which protrudes into this space and is in close contact with the pigment epithelial cells on the other face of the ventricular cavity.[2] Although this interaction is crucial for the functional maintenance of photoreceptors, it is interesting that the association is not a strong one, and injury can readily tear apart the two layers leading to retinal detachment. Because the apical face of the developing neural retina faces the pigment epithelium, the other face secretes a special basal extracellular matrix consisting primarily of collagen type II and hyaluronic acid. These form a large gel mass, the vitreous. Neural crest mesenchyme entering the optic cup differentiates into hyalocytes, specialized cells that also secrete glycoprotein components of the vitreous. Growth of the vitreous apparently is crucial to maintaining early growth of the eye, serving much like the inflation of a balloon.[16]

Retina and Optic Nerve

Development of the retina and its cell types proceeds in a highly regulated manner.[2] The first cells to differentiate are the ganglion cells, which appear near the vitreal face of the pseudostratified epithelium and send axonal fibers just under its surface. This tract passes into the furrow of the optic nerve tract, through the optic chiasm, and into the brain. During ganglion cell differentiation, most retinal cells remain undifferentiated precursors. Later, amacrine cells, bipolar cells, horizontal cells, photoreceptors, and Müller gial cells are formed and make synaptic connections to complete the layered retinal structure. Photoreceptors come in four types: rods, which are sensitive to low light and comprise most receptors in the human retina, and the red, green, and blue cone cells, which require higher levels of light but respond more rapidly and can discriminate colors. In the human and primate eye, the fovea is an area at the posterior pole specialized for high acuity color vision. It contains an extremely dense array of cones, and appears to be absent in individuals with aniridia (Pax6) or ocular albinism.[57,63] Why mutations in these genes have this effect on foveal specialization during retinal development is not yet understood.

The origin of retinal cell types is apparently *not* determined by an invariant cell lineage (Fig. 1.3). Studies in which retinal precursors were labeled by infection with a retrovirus marker demonstrated that individual precursors could give rise to a variable assortment of neural and glial cell types.[88] This suggests that local environmental cues within the embryonic retina are important in determining cell fates. Experiments with cultured retinal precursor cells suggest that the primary, default pathway for retinal development is the photoreceptor, and that signaling molecules from other cells are required to induce the formation of other neurons and glia.

Iris and Ciliary Body

The edges of the optic cup develop specialized structures under the inductive influence of the lens. The most marginal of these, the iris, arises from the neural retina and pigment epithelial layers of the optic cup. This is perhaps the only place in the body where muscle tissue is derived directly from the central nervous system. The sphincter pupillae, which closes the iris opening, arises from the inner, neural retina layer, while the opposing dilator pupillae arises from

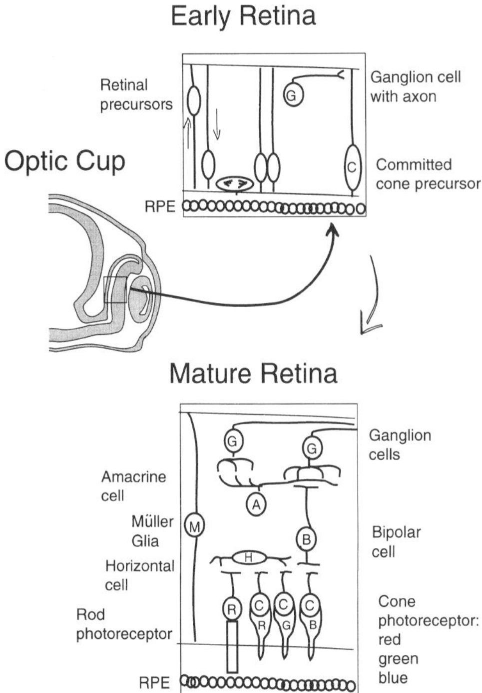

Figure 1.3. Origin of retinal cell types. **Early retina:** Highly schematized diagram of optic cup stage retinal epithelium. The retina and retinal pigment epithelium (RPE) are shown in cross section, with the vitreous up, and in contact with the inner face of the retina. Retinal precursor cells are long, spindle shaped neuroepithelial cells that span the cell layer, remaining attached to both inner and outer faces of the retina. During the cell cycle the cell bodies (ovals, containing the nucleus), migrate away from and then back toward the ventricular surface, which faces the RPE. Mitosis takes place when the cell body is near this surface. Differentiation of ganglion cells has just begun, as indicated by the outgrowth of axons toward the optic nerve and chiasm. Cone cells also cease division and are committed to their cell fate relatively early during development, although this occurs later than ganglion cells. The cone cells wait until late development before they fully differentiate. **Mature retina:** As the retina matures, other cell types are recruited from the precursor pool and differentiate into their adult forms. These are the amacrine cells, bipolar, horizontal, and finally the rod photoreceptors and Müller glia. The synaptic connections form in distinct layers, the inner and outer plexiform layers. Ganglion cell axons travel between the ganglion cell body layer and the vitreal surface of the retina.

the outer, pigment epithelial layer of the optic cup.[16] Innervation of these is also from distinct sources: the sphincter is innervated by acetylcholine-secreting nerve fibers originating in the ciliary ganglion, whereas the dilator is innervated by a norepinephrine-secreting nerve originating in the superior cervical ganglion. Also derived from the optic cup, adjacent to the iris, is the ciliary body, an epithelial organ that secretes the aqueous fluid of the anterior chamber.

Mesoderm and Neural Crest: Vasculature, Sclera, and Extraocular Muscles

Origin of Tissues

The vitreal, retinal, and choroidal vasculature, as well as the sclera that surround the retina, are derived from a complicated mix of cells originating in the head mesoderm and the migratory neural crest mesenchyme. In general, vascular endothelial cells are always derived from mesoderm, but the surrounding smooth muscle and connective tissue originates from the neural crest. The sclera surrounding the eye is derived from the neural crest and mesoderm. Outside the sclera are the extraocular muscles, which attach to the sclera and control movement of the globe. These muscles are of purely mesodermal origin.[68]

Vitreal Retinal Vasculature

In the early optic cup stage embryo, neural crest and mesodermal cells migrate into the choroid fissure and establish the hyaloid artery, which occupies the center of the optic nerve and early vitreous, and provides a vascular bed to sustain the lens during its development.[24] The portion of the hyaloid artery that passes through the vitreous is a transient embryonic structure, and normally degenerates before birth in order to leave a clear light path. Persistance of some hyaloid vasculature occurs in 3% of full-term infants and a majority of premature infants. In the congenital defect known as persistent hyperplastic vitreous (PHPV), a dense remnant associated with this artery is left in place. The retinal blood vessels arise primarily by budding from primitive retinal veins associated with the hyaloid artery and invade the neural epithelium. The level of oxygen is known to play an important role in this process and is thought to guide formation of the vascular network. Interference with this developmental process in premature infants by excessive oxygenation followed by the withdrawal of oxygen can have severe consequences, resulting in the excessive and abnormal growth of vascular tissue that leads to retinopathy of prematurity.[16]

Choroid and Sclera

The early optic cup is surrounded mostly by mesenchymal tissue of neural crest and mesodermal origin. The embryonic retinal pigment epithelium (RPE) releases inductive signals that cause this neighboring mesenchyme to differentiate into the tough, protective sclera. Between the sclera and the pigment epithelium develops the choroid, a dense vascular bed. As with other vasculature in the eye, the endothelial cells of the choroid are derived entirely from the head mesoderm, whereas the other vascular and connective tissue is of neural crest origin.[68] The congenital ocular disorder nanophthalmos is accompanied by an excessive thickening of the sclera that is associated with an ocular globe that is hyperopic and smaller than normal.

Extraocular Muscles

The six muscles that move the globes are all derived from head mesoderm in the orbit surrounding the eye. The muscle masses develop from two mesodermal complexes, one superior and another inferior. Myoblast fusion and differentiation happen evenly along the length of these complexes, and the muscles appear fully formed, along with their connections to the orbit and the sclera of the globe.[81] Many of the congenital defects involving eye movement appear to reside in the central nervous system. There are, however, examples of inherited defects that involve the muscles. Among these is a group of inherited disorders involving ptosis, the inability to retract the upper eyelid. This is caused by absence of the levator palpebrae superioris muscle. Sometimes ptosis occurs alone, but it is usually associated with the absence of the superior rectus muscle. During development the levator palpebrae superioris arises from the muscle primordium of the superior rectus.[57] A developmental defect of unknown origin apparently prevents formation of the common precursor of these two muscles.

Innervation of the Eye

The Optic Chiasm

Beginning in the optic cup stage embryo, retinal ganglion cells send their axons toward the brain through the optic nerve and toward the optic chiasm, which is located at the ventral midline of the forebrain (Fig. 1.4). The chiasm is a decision point at which the growing ganglion cell axons are routed to either the same or opposite sides of the brain. In most vertebrates, which have no binocular vision, all fibers cross the midline, while in primates and mammalian carnivores, fibers arising from the lateral retina are selectively prevented from crossing over. This achieves

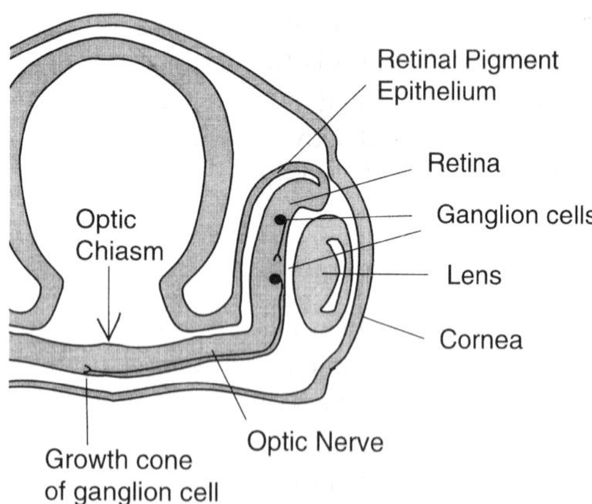

Figure 1.4. Pathway of ganglion cell axons. Cross section of an optic cup stage embryo, with the plane of section passing through the choroid fissure. This view illustrates the topographical relationship of the retina and optic stalk, and the path of ganglion cell axons. At this stage, relatively few ganglion cells have differentiated and begun to project axons toward and across the optic chiasm. Once reaching the chiasm, most fibers either cross (as shown) and follow a more caudal path toward the midbrain (colliculus) or thalamic nuclei (lateral geniculate, suprachiasmatic nucleus) on the opposite side of the embryo. Alternatively, fibers can turn back and connect to these structures on the same side.

a coherent representation of the visual field in the brain when both eyes face forward. In humans and animals with ocular albinism, control of this process is abnormal, leading to too many fibers crossing the midline, and improper visual representations in the brain. The reason for this remains unknown.[64]

Connections in the Brain

Most retinal ganglion cells make connections with the lateral geniculate, a structure in the thalamus that is organized in several layers. Each layer is specific for rod or cone vision. Information is then relayed to the visual cortex for further processing. A smaller set of ganglion cells connects with the superior colliculus, which mediates rapid responses to visual stimuli.[22] At each step, visual information is transmitted by means of a topographically ordered connection of ganglion cells to synaptic targets in the brain. Although the process is not yet understood, the initial topography seems to be accomplished primarily through gradients of molecular cues that guide the paths of axonal growth cones. Additional sharpening of the topographic projection is thought to be accomplished by a "learning" process dependent on endogenous neural activity in the embryo and on postnatal visual stimuli.[64]

Eye Movement

The innervation of extraocular muscles is achieved by hindbrain motor neurons that send their processes to the eye via a complicated assortment of cranial ganglia and nerves. The nerves reach muscle precursors early in development, and become part of a neural mechanism that regulates eye movement in the context of visual input. A disorder of general interest, congenital nystagmus, is usually related to abnormalities in the brain.[57] In the cases of aniridia and ocular albinism, nystagmus results from the fact that the retina develops without a fovea.[63]

In the zebrafish, a number of mutations have been isolated that specifically affect connections between retinal ganglion cells and their targets in the brain, as well as eye movements.[42] Once identified, the affected genes could provide important insight into neurological disorders affecting vision.

GENE EXPRESSION AND FUNCTION IN THE DEVELOPING EYE: SELECTED EXAMPLES

PAX6: Mouse Small Eye, Human Aniridia

The *Pax* gene family was originally isolated from the mouse on the basis of homology to the *Drosophila paired* gene, and has been an unusually rich source of dominant genetic disorders.[12] *Pax6* was originally shown to be selectively expressed in the developing eye[89] and, shortly afterward, the dominant ocular disorder aniridia was found to result from mutations in human *PAX6*.[29,85] In addition to a congenital hypoplasia or agenesis of the iris, aniridia usually involves several very different ocular structures.[63] In the retina, the fovea fails to form, resulting in poor visual acuity and nystagmus. In later life, individuals with aniridia develop an abnormal opacity and vascularization of the corneal surface known as a pannus. They often have cataracts by middle age and are at a high risk for glaucoma.[31] Although the effects on the eye are progressive and eventually severe, aniridia is highly specific for the eye and usually is not accompanied by any other bodily or mental disorders. Individuals with pure aniridia have mutations that destroy the function of one copy of the *PAX6* gene, so that the disorder is a result of haploinsufficiency rather than true dominance. As with other members of the PAX family, the levels of *PAX6* expression are important to its function.[30] A significant subset of aniridia patients have the WAGR syndrome, in which aniridia is associated with Wilms' tumor, mental retardation, and genitourinary disorders. This syndrome is caused by a large heterozygous deletion within chromosome 11 that includes the aniridia gene.

In the mouse, heterozygous mutations in *Pax6* (Small eye) also cause an aniridia-like phenotype (Fig. 1.5).[39,41] The mutations range from deletions to point mutations within the highly conserved protein. As with human aniridia, the heterozygote phenotype is not a true dominant,

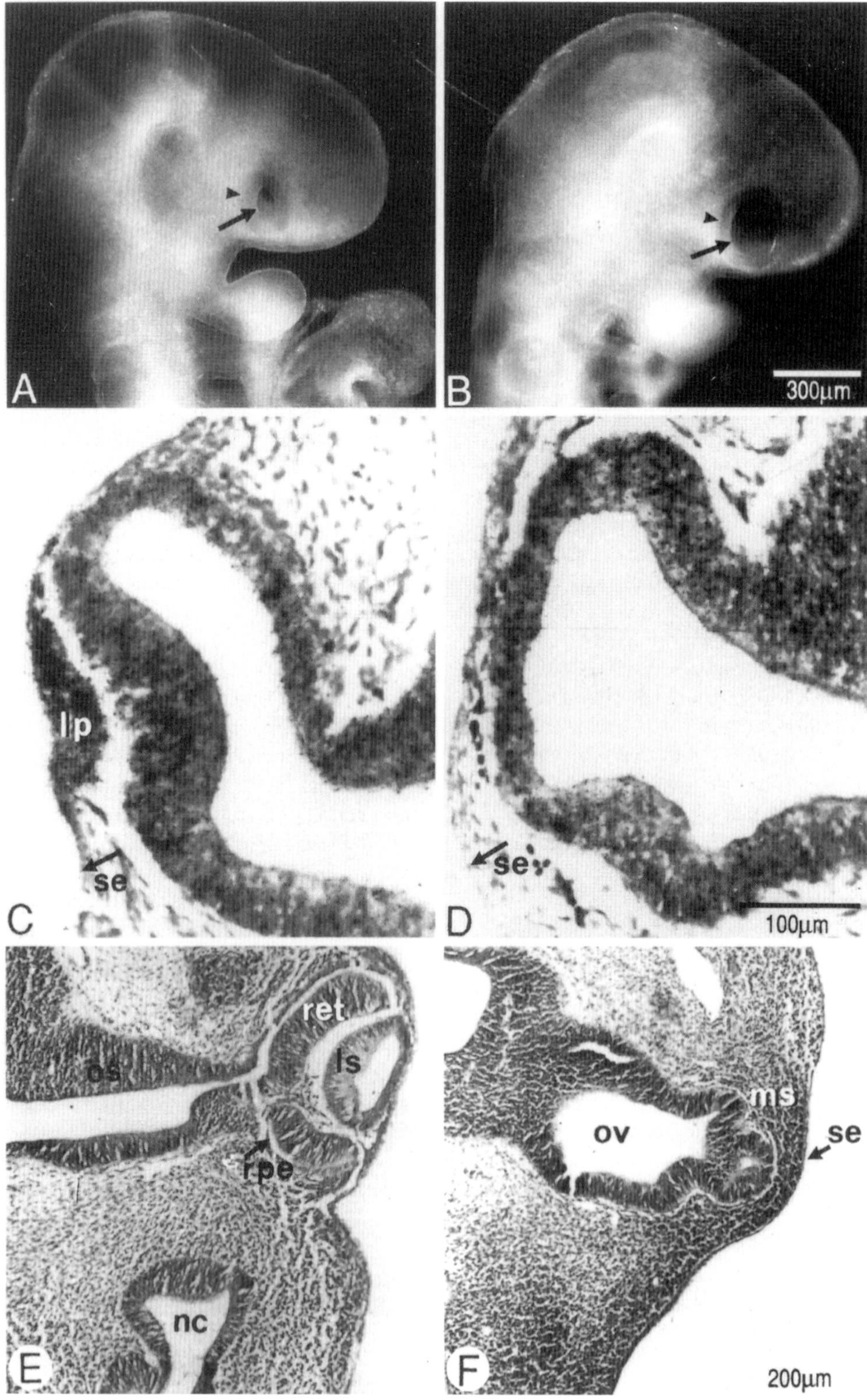

Figure 1.5. The lens placode and optic cup fail to develop in mouse embryos homozygous for a mutation in *Pax6*. Early phenotype of *Sey/Sey* embryos. Characteristic appearance of the eye at E9.5 of (**A**) wild-type embryo and (**B**) *Sey/Sey* embryo. *Sey/Sey* optic vesicle is broader than normal and has failed to constrict

but haploinsufficient. The iris is small or absent, and the animals develop cataracts. In the mouse it is readily demonstrated that Sey (*Pax6*) is an essential gene for eye development as well as survival. Homozygous mice are born anophthalmic, without nasal epithelia and with deficiencies in brain development, and they die shortly after birth. Homozygous Small eye mouse embryos appear to develop normally until the optic vesicle stage without the benefit of functional *Pax6* protein. The first visible defect is the failure of the lens placode to thicken,[34,41] and this is related to a requirement for *Pax6* expression in these cells. Although the first defect is in the lens, at birth the mutant mice are not simply missing a lens, but the whole eye. The reason for this is that the optic vesicle becomes arrested in its development and does not form the optic cup. It is possible that this is due to the absence of a lens placode, which normally provides signals essential to optic cup development.[18] *Pax6* expression may also be required in the optic vesicle neural epithelium. From the aniridia phenotype it can be inferred that formation of the iris is sensitive to the level of Pax6 protein in cells at the margin of the early optic cup, where the gene is transiently expressed at high levels.[34] *Pax6* expression may be important in directing these cells toward differentiation into the iris, as opposed to the ciliary body and retina.

Pax6 is expressed prominently throughout the retina prior to cell differentiation and becomes restricted to the emerging amacrine and ganglion cell layers.[7] The gene continues to be expressed in adult amacrine and ganglion cell layers, suggesting that *Pax6* may also be required for the maintenance of cell-type specializations in the adult. In humans, there is also evidence that the development of regional specialization in the central retina is dependent on the expression of *PAX6*. In human aniridia, the cone-rich fovea fails to develop.[63] This phenotype is very similar to that observed in ocular albinism, and it is possible that the effect is due to some special requirement for *PAX6* in the pigment epithelium, which also expresses the gene during early development. Unfortunately, the problem is not readily studied in the mouse, which lacks a fovea.

As described earlier, establishment of the lens placode in the early mouse embryo is completely dependent on the function of *Pax6*. The gene also continues to be expressed in the derivatives of this tissue throughout development and into adulthood. Pax6 protein is detected in the anterior lens epithelium during development, and it is possible that it is required for lens fiber differentiation.[48] Binding sites for the paired domain of the transcription factor have been identified in the promoters of lens crystallins, the major structural proteins of the lens.[19] Alteration in the expression of these proteins is important to the integrity of fiber cells and lens development. It is possible that the high incidence of cataracts observed in human aniridia is due to altered regulatory activity of Pax6 in the lens epithelium.

It has recently been observed that Pax6 protein is normally present throughout the adult corneal, limbal, and conjunctival epithelium of the mouse, all of which are directly descended from the lens placode.[48] The domain of expression extends from the central cornea to the very edge of the palpebral conjunctiva. As such, the pattern of *Pax6* expression supports the notion that these surface epithelia are uniquely ocular and closely related at the molecular level. Conjunctival epithelium is able to undergo a dra-

proximally. *Arrows* = proximal restriction of optic vesicles. *Arrowheads* = extent of the eye region. Histology of the eye at (**C**, **D**) E9.75 and (**E**, **F**) E11.5. At E9.75, the lens placode (lp), a prominent thickening of the surface ectoderm (se), is present in the littermate (**C**) but absent from the *Sey/Sey* embryo (**D**). Later *Sey/Sey* embryo, at 11.5 (**F**) lacks the developing lens (ls) and nasal cavity (nc), present in littermate (**E**). Normal littermate optic vesicle has produced an optic stalk (os) and optic cup with distinct retina (ret), and pigmented retinal epithelium (rpe). *Sey/Sey* optic vesicle (ov), is broader than normal, distorted at the distal end and separated from surface ectoderm (se) by intervening mesenchymallike cells (ms). (Reprinted with permission from Grindley, Davidson, and Hill.[34])

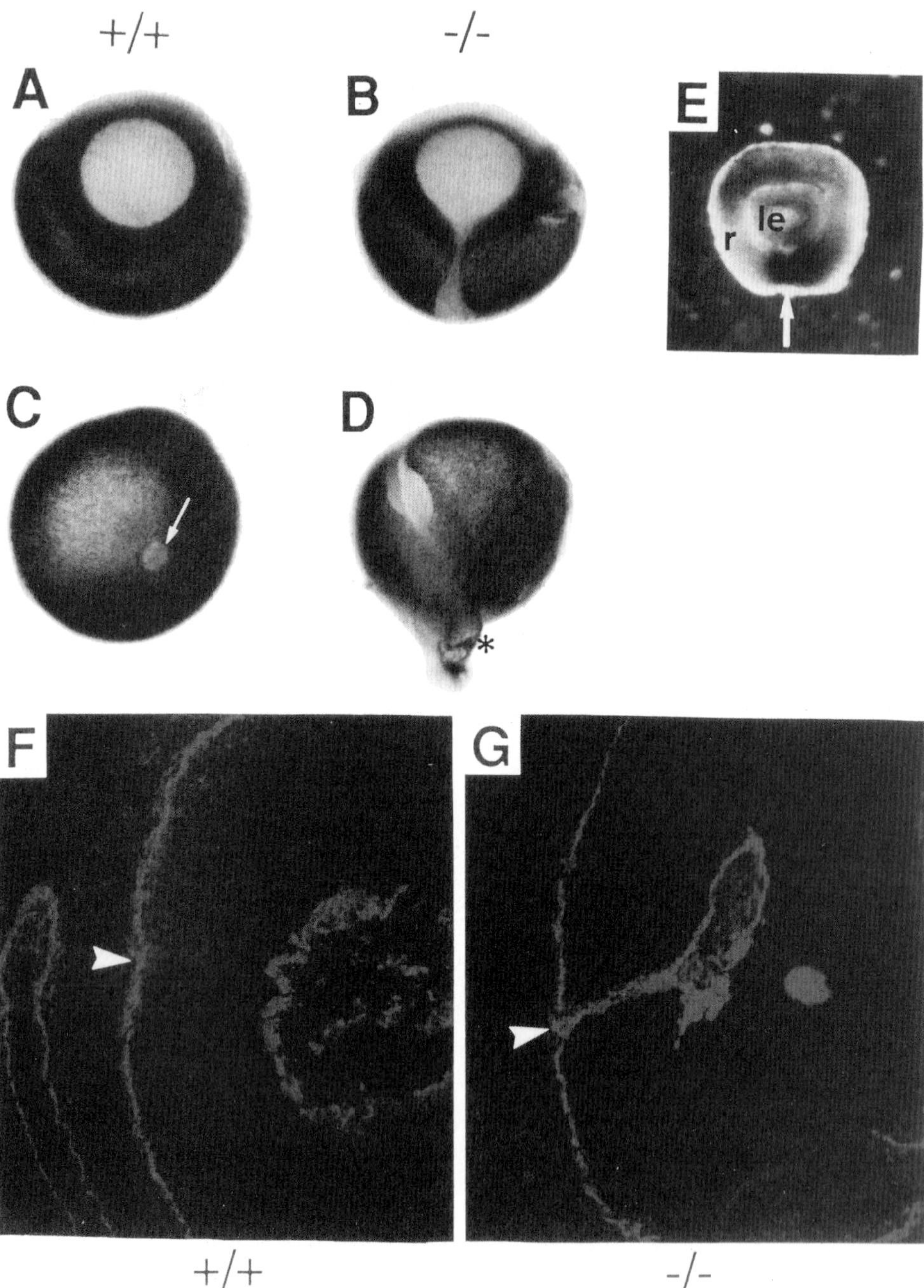

Figure 1.6. The choroid fissure fails to close in mice lacking *Pax2*. *Pax2* is required for the closure of the optic fissure (**A–D**): Whole-mount eyes dissected from an E17 fetus (**A**) and (**B**): Front views of, respectively, wild-type and mutant embryonic eyes. (**C**) and (**D**): Back views of the same eyes. Note the open optic fissure in the mutant and the absence of a defined boundary (arrow in (**C**) and asterisk in (**D**) limiting the pigmented retina at the back of the eye. (**E**) Front view of a whole-mount dissected eye hybridized with a *Pax2* probe at E11.5, when the closure of the optic fissure starts. Note that *Pax2* transcripts at this stage are restricted to the converging lips (arrow) of the retina on both sides of the optic fissure. (**F**) Detection of laminin by immunofluorescence to identify basal lamina in sagittal sections of a wild-type E13 embryo. Note how basal lamina has dissolved in the contact regions of the converging lips of the prospective retina at the former optic fissure (arrowhead) so that it is now continuous around the lens. At a similar stage, the mutant eye shows persistence of the basal lamina as judged by the presence of laminin (shown in (**G**), even though the converging lips seem to contact each other. R = retina; le = lens. (Reprinted with permission from Torres, Gomez-Pardo, and Gruss.[87])

matic structural transformation into a tissue very similar to corneal epithelium when it migrates onto the corneal stroma.[50] Aniridia is often accompanied by corneal pannus formation, a phenomenon involving opacification of the corneal epithelium and localized vascularization. It has been suggested that the corneal defects in aniridia result from stem cell deficiency, which leds to conjunctival cells invading the corneal epithelium.[67] *Pax6* expression has been shown to promote cell proliferation, very much like an oncogene,[58] and it is possible that high levels of *Pax6* expression are required for effective maintenance of precursors of the corneal epithelium.

PAX2: Optic Nerve Hypoplasia and Renal Defects

The *PAX2* gene belongs to the same family as *Pax6*. As with *Pax6* the gene dosage of *PAX2* is very important for function, and heterozygous null mutations have distinctive phenotypes, while homozygotes are lethal.[12] The expression pattern of *Pax2* in the mouse embryo has provided a guide to function of the gene and linking the gene to a human disease. *Pax2* is expressed in both the ureteric bud and surrounding mesenchyme of mouse embryos. In the eye, *Pax2* is expressed in the ventral optic stalk, the portion of the optic vesicle that will generate the optic nerve, and in the optic nerve head. During subsequent formation of the optic nerve, the gene continues to be expressed in this tissue. Knockout mice with a null mutation in the *Pax2* gene have been constructed, and they are completely defective in the development of the kidney. Heterozygotes have smaller kidneys.[86] These mice also develop with exencephaly due to the failure of the anterior neural tube to close properly. Similarly, the choroid fissure of the eye and optic nerve also fail to close. In addition, there are abnormalities in the path finding of retinal ganglion cell axons, which do not cross at the chiasm, and instead project to the same side of the brain. *Pax2* is also expressed in the developing otic vesicle, and the homozygous mutant mice show agenesis of the cochlea and spiral ganglion.[87]

Studies of the mouse *Pax2* gene have been extremely helpful in identifying a human disease associated with *PAX2* (Fig. 1.6).[79] The DNA sequence of *PAX2* was determined for a family of patients in which impaired vision and severe deficiency of kidney function were inherited in a dominant manner. This analysis uncovered a frameshift mutation in *PAX2* which causes loss of the carboxy terminal half of the protein. These patients had very poor visual acuity, and fundus photographs revealed bilaterial optic colobomas. There is also a deficiency of retinal pigment epithelium and choroid in a region surrounding the nerve. As the optic nerve and associated regions are primary sites for *PAX2* expression, the results suggest that optic nerve development requires a full level of *PAX2* activity to undergo closure and organize retinal structure around the nerve head.

CHX10: Microphthalmia and Retinal Bipolar Cell Deficit in the Mouse

The human *CHX10* gene was originally isolated from a cDNA library on the basis of its conservation between mammals and its preferential expression in the adult retina.[54] *CHX10* is a homeobox gene that encodes a transcription factor related to the *ceh10* gene of the nematode, *C. elegans*, and is highly conserved throughout the vertebrates. The homeobox has similarities to the homeobox of *Pax6*, but the Chx10 protein does not contain a paired domain. Expression of the mouse *Chx10* gene begins in the early optic vesicle, specifically in the region that will give rise to the retina. Expression is also found at a variety of sites throughout the central nervous system, but the greatest concentration is in the eye. In the undifferentiated neural retina, *Chx10* is distributed in all cell layers, but as differentiation proceeds, expression becomes localized to the inner nucleus layer, and finally the bipolar cells, which continue to express the gene in the adult.[7]

A human genetic disorder has yet to be associated with mutations in *CHX10*. However, in the mouse, a spontaneous null mutation in *Chx10* is the basis of the microphthalmic *ocular retardation* mouse (*or*) (Fig. 1.7). The homozygous *or* mutant is severely microphthalmic, with apparently no other abnormalities else-

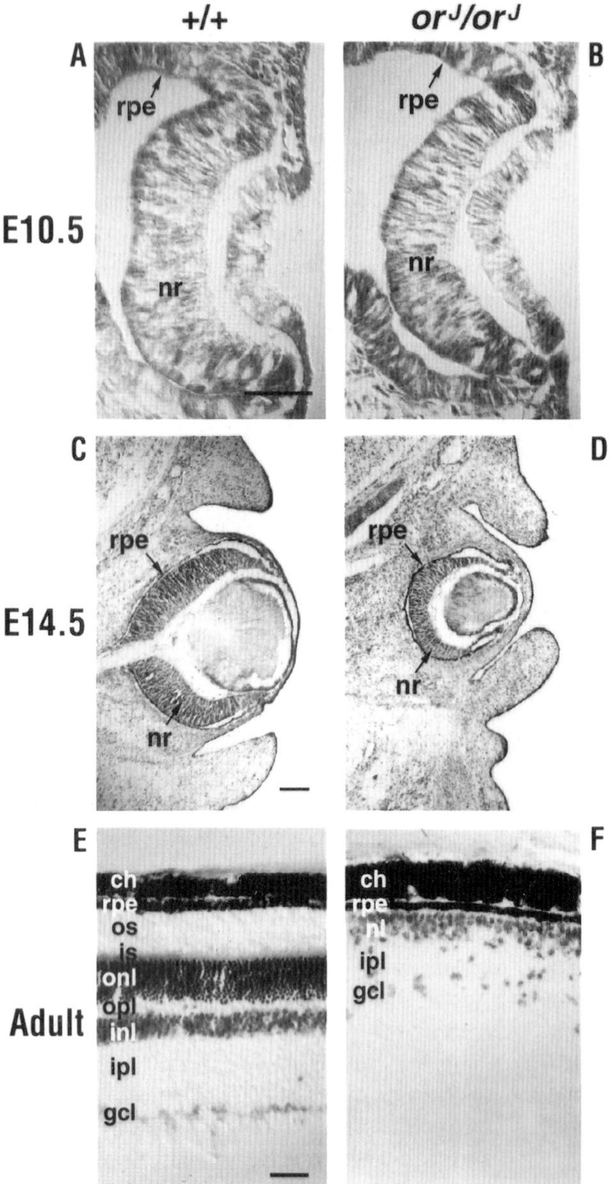

Figure 1.7. Mutation in the *Chx10* gene causes microphthalmia and absence of bipolar cells. Retinal morphology of wild-type 129/Sv (+/+) and mutant ocular retardation 129/Sv-or^J (or^J/or^J) mice in Nissl-stained sections. In the developing eye at E10.5, the morphology of the neural retina (nr) and retinal pigment epithelium (rpe) is similar in wild-type (**A**) and mutant (**B**). By E14.5 (**C, D**), the reduced size of the mutant eye and its neural retina are apparent, and the mutant eye has no optic nerve. In the normal adult retina (**E**), three cell layers—the ganglion cell (gcl) and the inner nuclear (inl) and outer nuclear layers (onl)—are separated by inner and outer plexiform layers (ipl and opl, respectively). In the mutant adult retina (**F**), lamination is poor, with a weakly defined ganglion cell layer separated from another morphologically unidentifiable nuclear layer (nl) by an ipl of variable size. Inner and outer segments of rod photoreceptors = is and os, respectively. Retinal pigment epithelium = rpe. Choroid = ch. Scale bar: (**A**) and (**B**): 50 μm; (**C**) and (**D**): 100 μm; (**E**) and (**F**): 50 μm. (Reprinted with permission from Burmeister et al.[10])

where in the body. Development proceeds normally until the early optic pit stage (day 10.5), but once the optic cup is well formed (day 14.5) it is apparent that the whole eye is much smaller than normal *Chx10* function may be required to promote growth of the retinal precursors, but this hypothesis has yet to be properly tested. The lens in these mice is also much smaller than normal, even though *Chx10* is not expressed in the lens. This may reflect the fact that lens growth depends on inductive factors provided by the retina.[5,18,82] During later development, the homozygous mutant retina generates all cell types, with the exception of bipolar cells. It appears likely that the bipolar cells initially fail to develop, and not that they are lost through degeneration. It is reasonable to consider that *Chx10* is required to specify how a retinal precursor chooses a bipolar cell fate rather than that of an alternate cell type. *Chx10* activity may also maintain functions specific to the adult bipolar cell. An especially interesting feature of the *or* mouse is that it fails to generate an optic nerve. This is especially puzzling because neither the retinal ganglion cells nor the optic stalk appear to express the gene.

BMP7: Microphthalmia, Renal, and Skeletal Defects in the Mouse

The transforming growth factor beta (TGF-β) superfamily comprises a number of signaling molecules that are secreted by cells that mediate inductive interactions during development.[43] Among these are the bone morphogenetic proteins (BMP). The prototype BMP genes were originally isolated on the basis of their biological activity in promoting the development of cartilage and bone,[90] but additional family members with diverse functions have been isolated and are designated as BMP genes largely on the basis of structural similarity. For example, BMP2 and BMP4 genes are required for gastrulation.

BMP7 is expressed in a wide variety of tissues during development, including the embryonic mesonephric mesenchyme and derived tissues in the urogenital system. Mice lacking *BMP7* have recently been generated by targeted mutagenesis, and are initially viable but are severely deficient in kidney development. This defect results from a failure of mesonephric mesenchyme to condense and begin the development of renal glomeruli. The expression of *Pax2* is not activated, suggesting that *BMP7* functions as an inductive signaling molecule required to turn on the *Pax2* transcription factor.

Eye phenotype in the *BMP7* homozygous null mutants[23,25] is visibly abnormal and variable in penetrance, with 60% of eyes being anophthalmic, and 40% microphthalmic (Fig. 1.8). Differences from normal development are observed at very early stages. Formation of the optic vesicle and thickening of the lens placode at first appear to proceed normally. After this point, various defects are observed in development of the lens, in which the lens placode fails to fold inward to make a lens vesicle. In some cases, the optic vesicle fails to generate a normal optic cup, and there is early degeneration of the eye rudiment. In other cases the lens placode invaginates but fails to do so completely. These more mildly affected structures eventually develop into microphthalmic eyes, which are approximately half normal size. Because *BMP7* mRNA is expressed in both optic vesicle and lens placode ectoderm, it is possible that this signaling molecule is secreted by and regulates the development of each of these tissues. Because the earliest abnormality appears in the lens, it is possible that BMP7 is one of the lens inducing factors released by the optic vesicle, and that the variable defects in optic cup development are the result of improper lens growth or lack of close contact with the lens.

Mouse mutants have distinctive features that could be of value in identifying disorders caused by mutations in human *BMP7,* which maps to chromosome 20.[35] Mice lacking the *BMP7* gene have extra digits and multiple skeletal abnormalities, including the misalignment of rib pairs and rib fusion. The skull and face are reasonably normal but also show distinctive abnormalities.[23,25] Although mutations in the human *BMP7* gene have not yet been associated with clinical genetic disorders, the knockout mice, which exhibit microphthalmia, anophthalmia, polydactyly, and renal agenesis provide striking clues. It is important to consider that the unexpected association of optic and renal defects is likely to have its roots not only in the highly conserved nature of the genes themselves but also in their functional partnerships. Both *BMP7* and *Pax2* have been reutilized in these two very different developmental processes, and evolution apparently has chosen not to reinvent the wheel for a different tissue. But which came first, the kidney or the eye?

γE-Crystallin: Lens Defects in Mouse and Human Congenital Cataract

The defects in eye development described in the preceding examples are all the result of mutations in regulatory molecules. Mutations in structural genes generally affect adult structures, the best known examples being retinal degenerations caused by mutations in photoreceptor architectural components such as peripherin, and in the phototransduction machin-

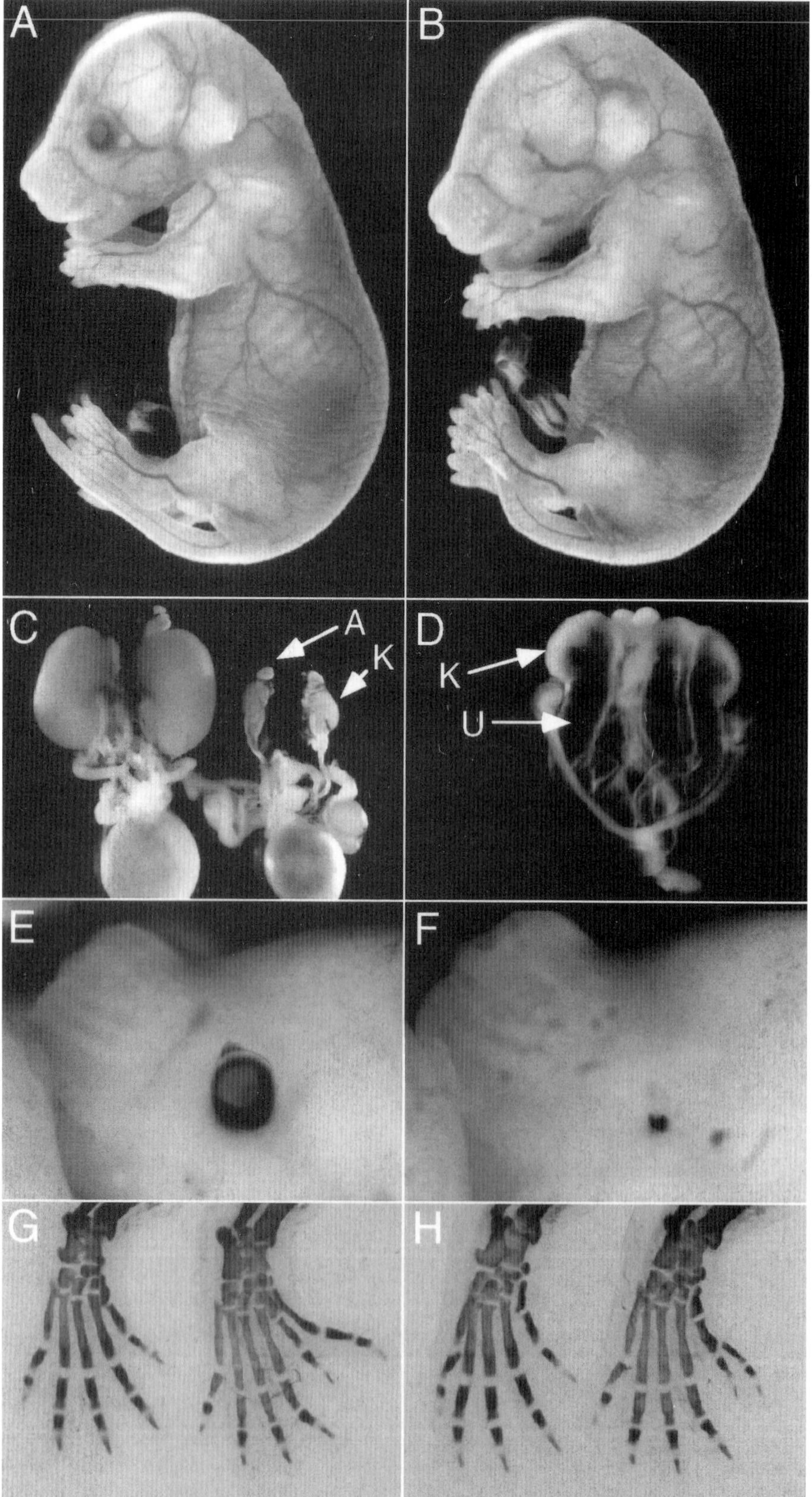

Figure 1.8.

ery.[8,77] In principle, however, developmental defects can also be caused by mutations in structural genes selectively expressed by an embryonic tissue.

Formation of the lens proceeds by the progressive addition of lens fiber cell layers. As described earlier, new fibers arise from proliferating cells in the lens epithelium and are layered on the surface of a preexisting "lens nucleus" that consists of earlier fibers.[19,57] The *eye lens obsolescence* (*Elo*) mutation of the mouse is a dominant allele that interferes with formation of the lens nucleus and causes abnormal lens development and microphthalmia.[69] It has been shown that *Elo* results from a mutation affecting the C-terminal portion of the *γE-crystallin* gene, which is expressed in the fibers that form the central lens nucleus.[11] Crystallin proteins typically accumulate in massive amounts during the differentiation of lens fiber cells, and their physical properties are responsible for the transparency and refractive qualities of the lens. The effect of *Elo* is first seen when the fiber cells have just begun to differentiate within the lens vesicle. These fibers at first elongate less than normal and later begin to die, resulting in massive disorganization of the lens nucleus. It should be noted that the anterior lens epithelium remains normal in appearance, and that the defect is confined to differentiating fiber cells, where the γE-crystallin gene is expressed.[69]

In the mouse genome there are six embryonic gamma crystallins γA through γF, located within a 50 kb cluster. It remains unclear why a mutation in one crystallin out of the several normally expressed should have such a drastic dominant effect. One might expect that refractile properties or size of the lens might be slightly altered if one of these crystallins is lost by mutation. In the corresponding *γ-crystallin* cluster on human chromosome 2q33-35,[9] only γA through γD appear functional, while γE and γF are inactive pseudogenes. Therefore γE is not even required in another mammal. It seems likely that the *Elo* mutation is a true dominant mutation. The *Elo* mutation is a frameshift that causes loss of the C-terminal portion of the protein, and it may be significant that the mutation substitutes novel, functionally irrelevant amino acids in its place. One theory is that expression of this abnormal protein disrupts the normally orderly packing of highly concentrated crystallins within the cell, altering osmoregulation or some other physiological process. By an unknown mechanism, this eventually causes the embryonic lens fiber cells to die. Absence of the initial lens nucleus results in the disorganization of later lens fibers. In turn, this disorganized lens fails to contribute the normal amounts of inductive factors required for growth of the optic cup.[18] The result is a microphthalmic eye.

A human genetic disorder, the Coppock-like hereditary cataract[57] maps to the γ-crystallin locus.[9] This disorder causes a cogenital cataract of the embryonic nucleus. In comparison with the *Elo* mutation of the mouse, the defect is very mild and nonprogressive, as later development of the lens proceeds normally. However, the Coppock cataract again involves the γE gene, which in the human genome usually appears as a pseudogene. Normally, ψγE contains a stop codon in the second intron, removing the C-terminus. In addition, the promoter of the ψγE pseudogene normally functions at a

Figure 1.8. Gross morphological analysis of BMP7 mutant embryos. Adjacent panels photographed at the same magnification showing heterozygous (**A**) and homozygous mutant (**B**) littermates at 17 days p.c. (**C**) At 19 days p.c., kidneys (K) from *BMP7* mutant embryos (right) are significantly smaller than those from a heterozygous littermate (left). The remainder of the urogenital tract and adrenals (K) are morphologically normal. (K) Kidney. (**D**) Acute hydroureter phenotype displayed by the majority of *BMP7* mutants at birth. A small mass of kidney tissue remains (K), whereas the renal pelvis (R) and ureter (U) are extremely distended. (**E, F**) High magnification views of eyes at 13.5 days p.c. The wild-type embryo (**E**) shows a well-developed pigmented retinal epithelium, whereas the *BMP7* mutant embryo (**F**) has only a residual mass of pigmented retinal epithelial cells (**G, H**) Preaxial polydactyly of the hind limbs. Whole-mount preparations comparing the cartilaginous structures present in wild-type (left) and BMP7 mutant (right) limbs are shown. (Reprinted with permission from Dudley, Lyons, and Robertson.[23])

low level. In individuals with Coppock cataract; however, there are mutations in the $\psi\gamma$E promoter that restore the optimal TATA box promoter sequence and result in a ten-fold increase in the expression of $\psi\gamma$E-crystallin expression when the promoter expression is assayed in cultured lens fibroblasts. The hypothesis is that overexpression of the truncated pseudogene disorganizes the crystallins in the fibers of the lens nucleus, which are the primary site of γ-crystallin expression. The proposed mechanism for the disorder involves the same gene and is strikingly similar to that of *Elo*, but for unknown reasons, the effect is much less severe. This may be due to other differences between mouse and human lens development, or to differences between the two truncated proteins.

CONCLUSION

In the case of inherited birth defects, it is important to keep in mind that the primary site of the defect is the gene. Genes are often expressed at diverse and seemingly arbitrary sites in the embryo. This provides a straightforward explanation for the fact that many inherited disorders affect distant and apparently unrelated tissues in the body. The association of optic nerve colobomas and kidney disease with mutations in the *PAX2* gene is a prime example of this phenomenon. The example of *PAX2* also illustrates how knowledge of embryonic gene expression pattern and function in an animal model can provide valuable clues to the molecular basis of human genetic disorders.

REFERENCES

1. Adelmann HB. Experimental studies on the development of the eye. II. The eye forming potencies of the median portions of the urodelan neural plate. *J Exp Zool* 1929;54:291–371.
2. Adler R, Farber D. *The Retina:* A Model for Cell Biology Studies. New York: Academic Press, 1986.
3. Adler R, Hatlee M. Plasticity and differentiation of embryonic retinal cells after terminal mitosis. *Science* 1989;243:391–393.
4. Baker NE, Yu S, Han D. Evolution of proneural axonal expression during distinct regulatory phases in the developing Drosophila eye. *Current Biol* 1996;6:1290–1301.
5. Beebe DC, Silver MH, Belcher KS, Van Wyk JJ, Svoboda ME, Zelenka PS. Lentropin, a protein that controls lens fiber formation, is related functionally and immunologically to the insulin-like growth factors. *Proc Natl. Acad Sci* 1991; 84:2327–2330.
6. Beebe DC. Homeobox genes and vertebrate eye development. *Invest Ophthalmol Vis Sci* 1994; 35:2897–2900.
7. Belecky-Adams T, Tomarev S, Li H-S, Ploder L, McInnes R, Sundin O, Adler R. Prox-1, Pax-6 and CHX10 homeobox gene expression correlate with phenotypic fate of retinal precursor cells. *Invest Ophthalmol Vis Sci* 1997;38:1293–1303.
8. Berson EL. Retinitis pigmentosa. The Friedenwald Lecture. *Invest Ophthalmol Vis Sci* 1993;34:1659–1676.
9. Brakenhoff RU, Henskens HAM, VanRossum MWPC, Lubsen NH, Schoenmakers JGG. Activation of the gE-crystallin pseudogene in the human hereditary Coppock-like cataract. *Hum Mol Genet* 1994;3:279–283.
10. Burmeister M, Novak J, Liang M-Y, Basu S, Ploder L, Hawes NL, Vigden D, Hoover F, Goldman D, Kalnins VI, Roderick TH, Taylor BA, Hankin MR, McInnes RR. Ocular retardation mouse caused by Chx10 homeobox null allele: Impaired retinal progenitor proliferation and bipolar cell differentiation. *Nature Genet* 1996;12:376–383.
11. Cartier M, Breitman ML, Tsui L-C. A frameshift mutation in the gamma E-crystallin gene of the Elo mouse. *Nature Genet* 1992;2:42–45.
12. Chalepakis G, Stoykova A, Wijnholds J, Tremblay, P, Gruss P. Pax: Gene regulators in the developing nervous system (review). *J Neurobiol* 1993;24:1367–1384.
13. Chiang C, Litingtung Y, Lee E, Young KE, Corden JL, Westphal H, Beachy PA. Cyclopia and defective axial patterning in mice lacking the *Sonic hedgehog* gene function. *Nature* 1996; 383:407–413.
14. Clarke LF. Regional differences in eye-forming capacity of the early chick blastoderm, as studied in chorio-allantoic grafts. *Physiol Zool* 1936;9: 102–128.
15. Collins F. Positional cloning moves from perditional to traditional. *Nature Genet* 1995;9:347–350.
16. Cook CS, Ozanics V, Jakobiec FA. Prenatal development of the eye and its adnexa. In *Duane's Foundations of Clinical Ophthalmol-*

ogy, W. Tasman and E. Jaeger, eds. Philadelphia: Lippincott, 1994.

17. Cotsarelis G, Cheng S-Z, Dong G, Sun T-T, Lavker RM. Evidence of slow-cycling limbal epithelial basal cells that can be preferentially stimulated to proliferate: implications for epithelial stem cells. *Cell* 1989;57:201–209.
18. Coulombre AJ. Regulation of ocular morphogenesis. *Invest Ophthalmol Vis Sci* 1969;8:26–31.
19. Cvekl A, Piatigorsky J. Lens development and crystallin gene expression: Many roles for Pax-6. *Bio Essays* 1996;18:621–630.
20. Cvekl A, Sax CM, Li X, McDermott JB, Piatigorsky J. Pax-6 and lens-specific transcription of the chicken delta 1-crystallin gene. *Proc Natl Acad Sci USA* 1995;92:4681–4685.
21. Dorsky RI, Chang WS, Rapaport DH, Harris WA. Regulation of neuronal diversity in the xenopus retina by delta signalling. *Nature* 1997; 385:67–70.
22. Dowling JE. The retina, an approachable part of the brain. Cambridge, MA: Belknap Press, 1987.
23. Dudley AT, Lyons KM, Robertson EJ. A requirement for bone morphogenetic protein-7 during development of the mammalian kidney and eye. *Genes Dev* 1995;9:2795–2807.
24. Duke-Elder S, Cook C. Normal and abnormal development. *System of Ophthalmology*, Vol. III. St. Louis: C.V. Mosby, 1963.
25. Epstein CJ. The new dysmorphology: application of insights from basic developmental biology to the understanding of human birth defects. *Proc Natl. Acad Sci. USA* 1995;92:8566–8573.
26. Gan L, Xiang M, Zhou L, Wagner DS, Klein W. POU domain factor Brn-3b is required for the development of a large set of retinal ganglion cells. *Proc Natl Acad Sci USA* 1996;93:3920–3925.
27. Gehring WJ. Homeoboxes in the study of development. *Science* 1987;236:1245–1252.
28. Glaser T, Lane J, Housman D. A mouse model for the aniridia-Wilms tumor deletion syndrome. *Science* 1990;250:823–827.
29. Glaser T, Walton DS, Maas RL. Genomic structure, evolutionary conservation and aniridia mutations in the human PAX6 gene. *Nature Genet* 1992;2:232–239.
30. Glaser T, Jepeal L, Edwards JG, Young SR, Favor J, Maas RL. PAX-6 gene dosage effect in a family with congenital cataracts, aniridia, anophthalmia and central nervous system defects. *Nature Genet* 1994;7:463–471.
31. Grant WM, Walton DS. Progressive changes in the angle in congenital aniridia, with the development of glaucoma. *Am J Ophthalmol* 1974;78: 842–847.
32. Graw J. Genetic aspects of embryonic eye development in vertebrates. *Dev Genet* 1996;18:181–197.
33. Greenwald I, Rubin GM. Making a difference: the role of cell-cell interactions in establishing separate identities for equivalent cells. *Cell* 1992;68:271–281.
34. Grindley JC, Davidson DR, Hill RE. The role of Pax-6 in eye and nasal development. *Development* 1995;121:1433–1442.
35. Hahn GV, Cohen RB, Wozney JM, Levitz CL, Shore EM, Zasloff MA, Kaplan FS. A bone morphogenetic protein subfamily: Chromosomal location of human genes for BMP5, BMP6, BMP7, *Genomics* 1992;14:759–762.
36. Halder G, Callaerts P, Gehring, WJ. Induction of ectopic eyes by targeted expression of the eyeless gene in *Drosophila. Science* 1995;267: 1788–1792.
37. Halder G, Callaerts P, Gehring W. New perspectives on eye evolution. *Current Biol* 1995; 5:602–609.
38. Hanson IM, Fletcher JM, Jordan T, Brown A, Taylor D, Adams RJ, Punnett HH, van Heyningen V. Mutations in the PAX6 locus are found in heterogeneous anterior segment malformations including Peter's anomaly. *Nature Genet* 1994;6:168–173.
39. Hill RE, Favor J, Hogan BLM, Ton C, Saunders GF, Hanson IM, Prosser J, Jordan T, Hastie ND, van Heyningen, V. Mouse Small eye results from mutations in a paired-like homeobox-containing gene. *Nature* 1991;354:522–525.
40. Hodgkinson CA, Moore KJ, Nakayama A, Steingrimsson E, Copeland NG, Jenkins NA, Arnheiter H. Mutations at the mouse microphthalmia locus are associated with defects in a gene encoding a novel basic-helix-loop-helix-zipper protein. *Cell* 1993;74:395–404.
41. Hogan BLM, Horsburgh G, Cohen J, Hetherington CM, Fisher C, Lyon MF. Small eyes (Sey): A homozygous lethal mutation on chromosome 2 which affects the differentiation of both lens and nasal placodes in the mouse. *J Embryol Exp Morphol* 1986;97:95–110.
42. Holder N, McMahon A. Genes from zebrafish screens. Nature 1996;384:515–516.
43. Jessell TM, Melton DA. Diffusible factors in vertebrate embryonic induction. *Cell* 1992; 68:257–70.
44. Kappen C, Schugart K, Ruddle FH. Early evolutionary origin of major homeodomain sequence classes. *Genomics* 1993;18:54–70.

45. Kastner P, Grondona JM, Mark M, Gansmuller A, LeMeur M, Decimo D, Vonesch JL, Dolle P, Chambon P. Genetic analysis of RXR alpha developmental function: Convergence of RXR and RAR signaling pathways in heart and eye morphogenesis. *Cell* 1994;78:987–1003.
46. Kazlauskas A. Receptor tyrosine kinases and their targets. *Curr Opinion Genet Dev* 1994; 4:5–14.
47. Klug A, Rhodes D. Zinc fingers: A novel protein fold for nucleic acid recognition. *Cold Spring Harbor Symp Quant Biol* 1987;52:473–482.
48. Koroma BM, Yang J-M, Sundin O. The Pax-6 homeobox gene is expressed throughout the corneal and conjunctival epithelia. *Invest Ophthalmol Vis Sci* 1997;38:108–120.
49. Krumlauf R. Hox genes in vertebrate development. *Cell* 1994;78:191–201.
50. Kruse FE. Stem cells and corneal epithelial regeneration. *Eye* 1994;8:170–183.
51. Lai E, Clark KL, Burley SK, Darnell JE. Hepatocyte nuclear factor 3/fork head or winged helix proteins—A family of transcription factors of diverse biologic function. *Proc Natl Acad Sci USA* 1993;90:10421–10423.
52. Lander ES. The new genomics: Global views of biology. *Science* 1996;274:536–539.
53. Li HS, Yang JM, Jacobson RD, Pasko D, Sundin O. Pax-6 is first expressed in a region of ectoderm anterior to the early neural plate: Implications for stepwise determination of the lens. *Dev Biol.* 1994;162:181–194.
54. Liu IS, Chen JD, Ploder L, Vidgen D, van der Kooy D, Kalnins VI, McInnes RR. Developmental expression of a noval murine homeobox gene, Chx10: Evidence for roles in determination of the neuroretina and inner nuclear layer. *Neuron* 1994;13:377–393.
55. Luo G, Hofmann C, Bronckers ALJJ, Sohocki M, Bradley A, Karsenty G. BMP-7 is an inducer of nephrogenesis, and is also required for eye development and skeletal patterning. *Genes Dev* 1995;9:2808–2820.
56. Mangelsdorf DJ, Thummel C, Beato M, Herrlich P, Schutz G, Umesono K, Blumberg B, Kastner P, Mark M, Chambon P. The nuclear receptor superfamily: the second decade. *Cell* 1995;83:835–839.
57. Mann I. Developmental abnormalities of the eye. Philadelphia: Lippincott, 1957.
58. Maulbecker CC, Gruss P. The oncogenic potential of Pax genes. *EMBO J.* 1993;12:2361–2367.
59. McGinnis W, Krumlauf R. Homeobox genes and axial patterning. *Cell* 1992;68:283–302.
60. Mirzayans F, Pearce WG, Macdonald IM, Walter MA. Mutations of the PAX6 gene in patients with autosomal dominant keratitis. *Am J Hum Genet* 1995;57:539–548.
61. Morse DE, McCann PS. Neuroectoderm of the early embryonic rat eye: Scanning electron microscopy. *Invest Ophthalmol Vis Sci* 1984; 25:899–907.
62. Nathans J, Merbs SL, Sung CH, Weitz CJ, Wang Y. Molecular genetics of human visual pigments. *Annu Rev Genet* 1992;26:403–424.
63. Nelson LB, Spaeth GL, Nowinski TS, Margao CE, Jackson L. Aniridia, A review. *Surv Ophthalmol* 1984;28:621–642.
64. Nicholls JG, Martin AR, Wallace BG. From neuron to brain: A cellular and molecular approach to the function of the nervous system. Sunderland, MA: Sinauer Associates, 1992.
65. Niehrs C. Mad connection to the nucleus. *Nature* 1996;381:561–562.
66. Nieuwkoop PD. Inductive interactions in early amphibian development and their general nature (suppl). *J Embryol Exp Morphol* 1985; 89:333–347.
67. Nishida K, Kinoshita S, Ohashi Y, Kuwayama Y, Yamamoto S. Ocular surface abnormalities in aniridia. *Am J Ophthalmol* 1995;120:368–375.
68. Noden DM. Periocular mesenchyme: Neural crest and mesodermal interactions. In *Duane's Foundations of Clinical Ophthalmology*, W. Tasman, E. Jaeger, eds. Philadelphia: Lippincott, 1994.
69. Oda S-I, Watanabe K, Fujisawa, H, Kameyama Y. Impaired development of lens fibers in genetic microphthalmia, eye lens obsolescence, *Elo*, of the mouse. *Exp Eye Res* 1980;31: 673–681.
70. Piatigorsky J. Lens crystallins and their genes: diversity and tissue-specific expression. *FASEB J* 1989;3:1933–1940.
71. Porter JA, Ekker SC, Park WJ, von Kessler DP, Young KE, Chen CH, Ma Y, Woods AS, Cotter RJ, Koonin EV, Beachy PA. *Hedgehog* patterning activity: Role of a lipophilic modification mediated by the carboxy-terminal autoprocessing domain. *Cell* 1996;86(1):21–34.
72. Püschel A, Gruss P, Westerfield M. Sequence and expression of pax-6 are highly conserved between zebrafish and mice. *Development* 1992;114:643–651.
73. Quiring R, Walldorf U, Kloter U, Gehring WJ. Homology of the eyeless gene of *Drosophila* to the *Small eye* in mice and *Aniridia* in humans. *Science* 1994;265:785–789.

74. Ramirez-solis R, Davis AC, Bradley A. Gene targeting in embryonic stem cells. *Meth Enzymol* 1993;225:855–877.
75. Rodbell M. Nobel lecture: Signal transduction: evolution of an idea. *Biosci Rep* 1995;15: 117–133.
76. Roessler E, Belloni E, Gaudenz K, Jay P, Berta P, Scherer SW, Tsui LC, Muenke M. Mutations in the human sonic hedgehog gene cause holoprosencephaly. *Nature Genet* 1996;14:357–360.
77. Rosenfeld PJ, McKusick VA, Amberger, JS, Dryja, TP. Recent advances in the gene map of inherited eye disorders: primary hereditary diseases of the retina, choroid and vitreous. *J Med Genet* 1994;31:903–915.
78. Saha MS, Spann CL, Grainger RM. Embryonic lens induction: More than meets the optic vesicle. *Cell Diff Dev* 1989;28:53–172.
79. Sanyanusin P, Schimmenti LA, McNoe LA, Ward TA, Pierpoint MEM, Sullivan MJ, Dobyns WB, Eccles MR. Mutation of the PAX2 gene in a family with optic nerve colobomas, renal anomalies and vesicoureteral reflux. *Nature Genet* 1995;9:358–364.
80. Schuler GD, Boguski MS, Stewart LD, et al. A gene map of the human genome. *Science* 1996;274:540–546.
81. Sevel DA. A reappraisal of the origin of human extraocular muscles. *Ophthalmology* 1981;88: 1330–1338.
82. Spemann H. *Embryonic Development and Induction.* New Haven: Yale University Press, 1938.
83. Sundin OH, Eichele G. An early marker of axial pattern in the chick embryo and its respecification by retinoic acid. *Development* 1992;114: 841–852.
84. Tanabe Y, Jessell TM. Diversity and pattern in the developing spinal cord. *Science* 1996; 274:1115–1122.
85. Ton CC, Hirvonen H, Miwa H, Weil MM, Monaghan P, Jordan T, van Heyningen V, Hastie ND, Meijers-Heijboer H, Drechsler M. Positional cloning and characterization of a paired-box and homeobox-containing gene from the aniridia region. *Cell* 1991;67:1059–1074.
86. Torres M, Gomez-Pardo E, Dressler GR, Gruss P. Pax-2 controls multiple steps in urogenital development. *Development* 1995;121:4057–4065.
87. Torres M, Gomez-Pardo E, Gruss P. Pax2 contributes to inner ear patterning and optic nerve trajectory. *Development* 1996;122:3381–3391.
88. Turner DL, Cepko CL. A common progenitor for neurons and glia persists in rat retina late in development. *Nature* 1987;328:131–136.
89. Walther C, Gruss P. Pax-6, a murine paired-box gene, is expressed in the developing CNS. *Development* 1991;113:1435–1449.
90. Wozney JM, Rosen V, Celeste AJ, Mitsock LM, Whitters MJ, Kriz RW, Hewick RM, Wang E. Novel regulators of bone formation: Molecular clones and activities. *Science* 1988;242:1528–1534.
91. Yamamoto D. Positive and negative signalling mechanisms in the regulation of photoreceptor induction in the developing *Drosophila* retina. *Genetica* 1993;88:153–164.

2

Malformations of the Ocular Adnexae

ELIAS I. TRABOULSI

HYPERTELORISM AND TELECANTHUS

Hypertelorism is a clinicoradiologic diagnostic term that refers to increased distance between the two orbits and an increase in the angle between the axes of the orbits. This angle normally measures 71° at birth and 68° in adults. The interorbital distance can be estimated from an increase in the interpupillary distance and from clinical appearance (Fig. 2.1). Hypertelorism results from an arrest of the forward migration of the orbits in embryonic development. It is present in a large number of malformation syndromes such as Waardenburg and Crouzon syndromes. Hypertelorism may be associated with agenesis of the corpus callosum or other midline brain defects, basal encephalocele, and a number of optic nerve head malformations such as the morning glory disk anomaly, optic nerve hypoplasia, or optic nerve dysplasia (see also Chapter 7).

Telecanthus refers to increased distance between the inner canthi relative to interpupillary or interorbital distance. True hypertelorism may or may not coexist. The interpupillary and hence the interorbital distance are normal. The term *secondary telecanthus* may be used if it is the result of true hypertelorism. The ratio between the inter–inner canthal distance and the inter–outer canthal distance is approximately 1:3. Telecanthus is believed to result from overgrowth in width of the frontonasal process. Telecanthus can be measured in terms of the Mustarde index, which is calculated as the inter–inner canthal distance divided by the interpupillary distance. Normal values of this index for infants, children, and adults are around 0.50. Values over 0.55 indicate the presence of telecanthus. Telecanthus is also present in a number of multisystem malformation syndromes.[44]

COLOBOMA OF THE EYELID

Lid colobomas are full-thickness notch defects of the lid margin. They may be triangular or quadrilateral in shape (Fig. 2.2). Upper eyelid defects (the majority of colobomatous lid defects) are usually nasal and occur between the inner and middle third of the lid. In the lower eyelid colobomas are temporal and are located between the middle and outer thirds.[21] Lashes and tarsus are missing in the area of the lid defect. Colobomas of the lid may be due to failure of the mesodermal folds to fuse completely during development. The developing lids may fail to fuse by the second month of gestation or may prematurely separate before the fifth to seventh month of gestation, interfering with lid margin, tarsal, and eyelash differentiation.

Colobomas of the upper eyelids are seen in some patients with Goldenhar syndrome,

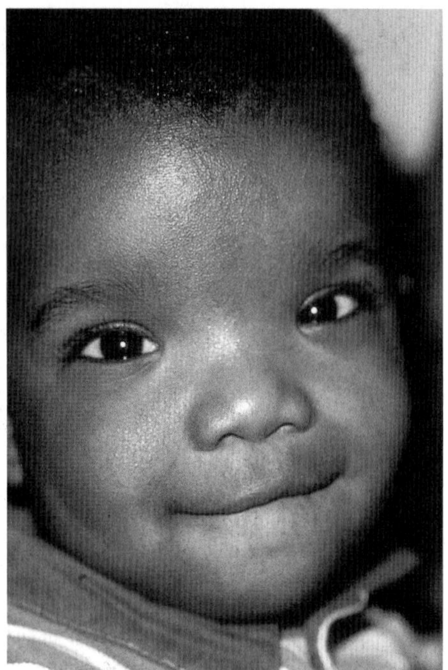

Figure 2.1. Patient with hypertelorism-hypospadias syndrome.

a variant of the oculo-auriculo-vertebral sequence; the coloboma usually overlies an epibulbar dermoid, and patients may have preauricular skin tags, microtia, deafness, facial asymmetry, macrostomia, microstomia, and vertebral anomalies. Goldenhar syndrome results from faulty development of structures derived from the first and second branchial arches and the first branchial cleft between the sixth and eighth week of gestation.[7,23]

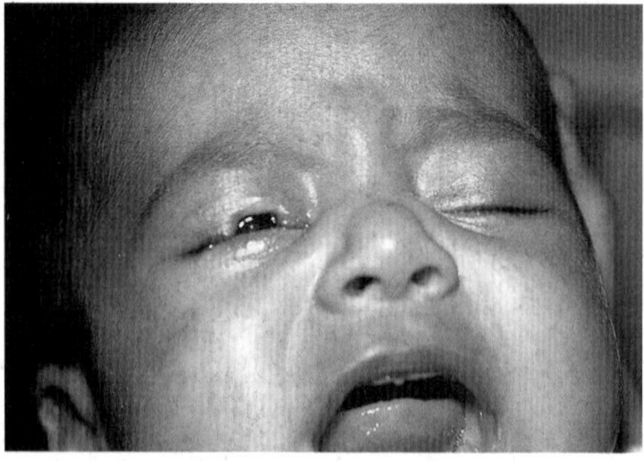

Figure 2.2. Coloboma of right upper lid involves more than one-third of lid margin. Patient was investigated extensively and did not have any associated malformations. Defect was repaired by primary approximation with excellent cosmetic and functional result.

Lower eyelid colobomas are encountered in Treacher Collins syndrome, also called mandibulofacial dysostosis or Franceschetti syndrome.[23,83,101] The primary features of this malformation syndrome are antimongoloid palpebral fissures, mandibular and malar hypoplasia, malformed external ears, and lower lid colobomas. Deafness occurs in almost half the cases. The face has been described as being "birdlike" in appearance. Most of the patients with Treacher Collins syndrome are of normal intelligence. There is a wide variance in expression of the disorder. Additional fairly common findings include a tendency toward macrostomia, malocclusion, high palate, and a high nasal root. The hair growth patterns are unusual, often showing tonguelike extensions of hair onto the cheeks. There may be grooves, clefts, or pits on the cheek between the mouth and the ear. This syndrome represents the most extensive abnormality of the first branchial arch.[84]

The ophthalmic features are among the most consistent and diagnostic in this syndrome. They include antimongoloid slanting of the lids (lateral canthi are lower than the medial canthi), lower lid colobomas in 75% of patients, with partial to total absence of the lower eyelashes. Occasionally, the coloboma may involve the upper lid. Microphthalmia and defects of the orbital rim are occasionally seen.[35,84,103]

The Hallerman-Streiff syndrome is inherited in an autosomal dominant fashion and 60% of cases are due to new mutations. When there is a positive family history, the gene is almost 100% penetrant. There is wide variability in expression of the disorder among family members. There seems to be a statistically significant increase in affected progeny of affected female versus a decrease in the affected progeny of affected males.[84] The gene was mapped to 5q31.3-q33.3 by Dixon et al.[26] and by Jabs and co-workers[55] after a clue to the location of the gene to that region was given from the finding of a girl with the syndrome and a de novo balanced translocation t(5;13)(q11;p11).[5] Treacher Collins syndrome is differentiated from the Goldenhar syndrome by the rarity of

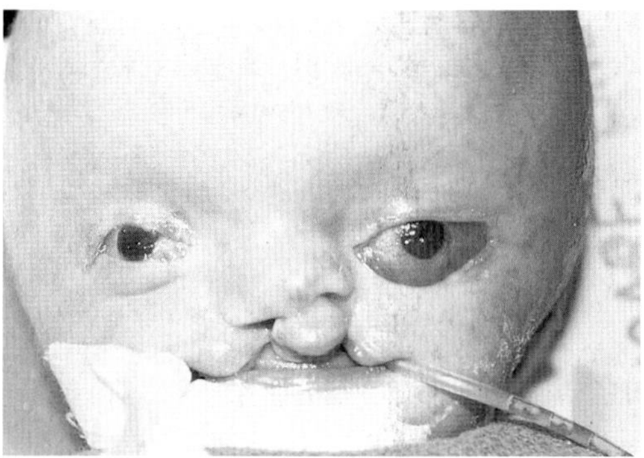

Figure 2.3. Newborn with amniotic band syndrome. Amniotic bands resulted in clefts of the lip, deformities of the nose, colobomas of the lids, and hydrocephalus.

lower lid colobomas in Goldenhar syndrome, and the absence of epibulbar dermoids in the Treacher Collins syndrome.

Upper and lower eyelid defects may also be seen in the amniotic band syndrome (Fig. 2.3).[72]

CRYPTOPHTHALMOS

In typical cryptophthalmos (hidden eye) or ablepharon (absence of the lids), skin continues from the forehead onto the cheek and there are no recognizable lid structures.[109] The eyes are usually malformed with anomalies ranging from anterior segment dysgenesis to microphthalmos.

Francois[37] divided cryptophthalmos into three types. In the first, *typical and complete form,* the eyelids are absent and skin extends continuously from the forehead to the cheek, passing in front of the orbit where it forms a small depression (Fig. 2.4). The eyebrows are poorly developed or nonexistent. The eyelashes, meibomian glands, lacrimal glands, and lacrimal punctae are absent. The eyeball can be palpated through the skin to which it is usually adherent. There is reaction to light shined through the skin with contraction of the orbicularis, but the eye is usually microphthalmic with major dysplasia, more marked in the anterior segment. There is no conjunctival sac and incision of the skin often opens directly into the eye. In the second, *incomplete, atypical, or partial form* of cryptophthalmos, there are rudimentary lid structures and a conjunctival sac may be present temporally. The eyeball is usually microphthalmic and covered with skin. In the third, *abortive form,* the upper eyelid is adherent to the eyeball, does not carry lashes, and continues over the cornea as an epidermal membrane (Fig. 2.5). The lower eyelid is nor-

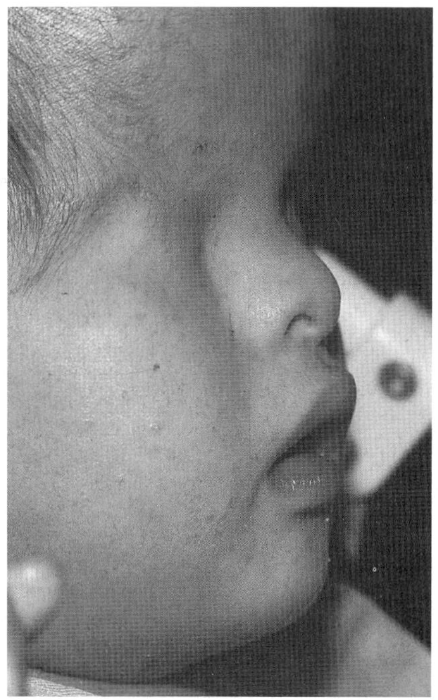

Figure 2.4. Cryptophthalmos with forehead skin continuing over globe and cheek. The hair line is displaced forward and merges with the brow. (Courtesy of Irene H. Maumenee.)

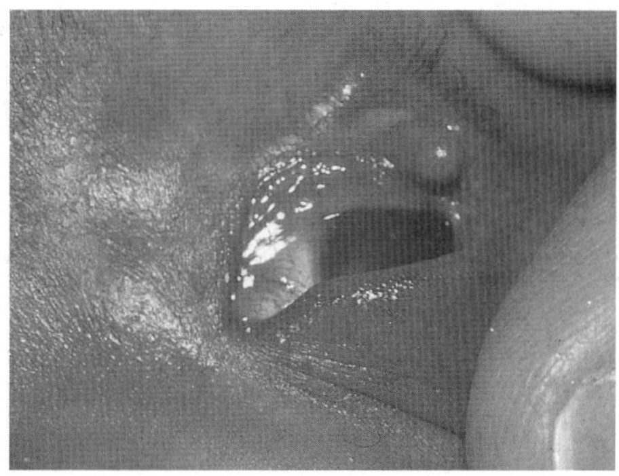

Figure 2.5. Abortive form of cryptophthalmos. Upper lid structures are adherent to the globe. There is a skin tag and corneal opacification.

mal but may lack a lacrimal punctum. The free part of the cornea may be vascularized, opaque, or keratinized. The eyeball is of normal size or may be microphthalmic. Cases such as those reported by Key[58] and Sugar[96] where there is typical cryptophthalmos on one side and abortive cryptophthalmos on the other indicate that the two anomalies are equivalent. Cases have been reported with typical cryptophthalmos on one side and a dermoid, microphthalmos, or lid coloboma on the other side. A fourth type of *isolated cryptophthalmos* exists where the lids are formed with a full complement of adnexal accessories. The lid fissure is displaced inferiorly close to the inferior orbital rim, but the conjunctival sac is rudimentary and the globe is not visible. There is a wide upper lid that adheres to the underlying malformed globe and a short lower lid. The family members reported twice by Coover[19,20] (the same family was mentioned by Magruder,[64] and the mother and daughter were reported by Saal and colleagues[85]) are examples of this apparently distinct autosomal dominant syndrome where cryptophthalmos is not accompanied by mental retardation or other congenital anomalies (Fig. 2.6).

Cryptophthalmos is most often accompanied by systemic anomalies and inherited in an autosomal recessive fashion, hence the terms cryptophthalmos syndrome, cryptophthalmos-syndactyly syndrome, syndromic cryptophthalmos, and Fraser syndrome.[3,25,38,45,54,99,105] The most prominent features of the cryptophthalmos syndrome include mental retardation; dyscephaly with skull malformations mostly in the region of the temples and forehead; anomalies of the auricles, ear canal, or inner ear; anomalies of the nose; laryngeal atresia; total or partial syndactyly of the toes and/or fingers; renal anomalies; and malformations of the genital organs, especially in females. Other less common malformations include anal atresia and umbilical hernias or a low-set umbilicus. Renal malformations such as renal agenesis or dysplasia may occur, resulting in spontaneous abortions, stillbirths, or neonatal deaths.[12,14,16,63,68] Indeed, the diagnosis of cryptophthalmos-syndactyly syndrome should be considered in the absence of cryptophthalmos if the other abnormalities are present.[60]

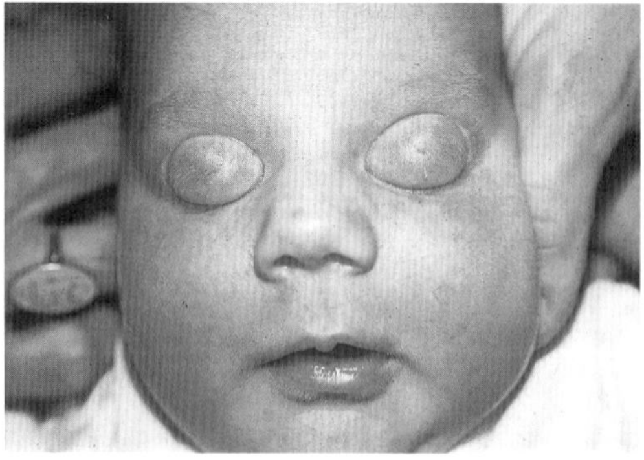

Figure 2.6. Dominant cryptophthalmos syndrome. The skin of the upper lid is elongated, adheres to the underlying globe with a dimple over the cornea, and fuses with the shortened lower lid. The lashes are intact. (Courtesy of Marshall M. Parks.)

The pathogenesis of cryptophthalmos is unclear. The association with midline[43] and renal and distal limb anomalies in the cryptophthalmos syndrome may reflect late gestational developmental field defect anomalies affecting the lid and upper facial structures that are derived from ectoderm, and the underlying anterior segment of the eye. The lid fissure forms in the sixth month of gestation after the upper and lower eyelids have developed their complements of tarsus, meibomian glands, and lashes.

Surgical incision in the area of the palpebral fissure may open directly into the anterior segment of the eye. The absence of a conjunctival sac and hence of a normal ocular surface makes the prognosis for a clear corneal graft, if it is performed, very poor. Furthermore, the globe in typical cryptophthalmos is often malformed both in its anterior and posterior segments rendering visual prognosis very guarded even if a good reaction to light is elicited through the skin covering the eyes. In partial or abortive cryptophthalmos, surgical intervention may result in cosmetic and functional improvement.[13]

EURYBLEPHARON

In this condition, the outer one-half of the lower lid appears to sag inferiorly and is not well apposed to the globe. This widens the palpebral fissure and gives the appearance of lower-lid ptosis. The skin, however is tight and shortened. Euryblepharon may be isolated and inherited in an autosomal dominant fashion or may be a feature of the Kabuki makeup syndrome.

MICROBLEPHARON

Microblepharon is an abnormality characterized by vertical shortening of the lids. An extreme form is seen in the ablepharon–macrostomia syndrome.[15] Ablepharon (no lids) should not be used synonymously with cryptophthalmos.

EPICANTHUS AND EPIBLEPHARON

There are four distinct types of epicanthus[57]: *(1)* epicanthus supraciliaris, where epicanthal folds arise from the region of the eyebrow and run toward the tear sac or the nostril; *(2)* epicanthus palpebralis where the fold arises in the upper lid above the tarsal fold and extends to the lower margin of the orbit; *(3)* epicanthus tarsalis, where the fold arises laterally above the tarsal fold and loses itself in the skin next to the inner canthus; and *(4)* epicanthus inversus, where a small fold arises in the lower lid and extends upward, partially covering the inner canthus. Epicanthus inversus is usually seen in the blepharophimosis syndrome along with ptosis and telecanthus. Epicanthus tarsalis is seen in Orientals and epicanthus tarsalis and epicanthus palpebralis are both seen in children of all races. Epiblepharon is probably an exaggerated form of epicanthus tarsalis. Epicanthus supraciliaris is common to a large number of syndromes, that will not be discussed here. All types of epicanthal folds tend to become less conspicuous with age and any cosmetic surgery should be withheld until full facial growth.

ANKYLOBLEPHARON

In internal ankyloblepharon there is union of the lids from the inner canthus outward with true connective and vascular tissue. The inner canthus is not displaced outward as in telecanthus. The lids are fused from the outer canthus inward in external ankyloblepharon which should not be confused with blepharophimosis.

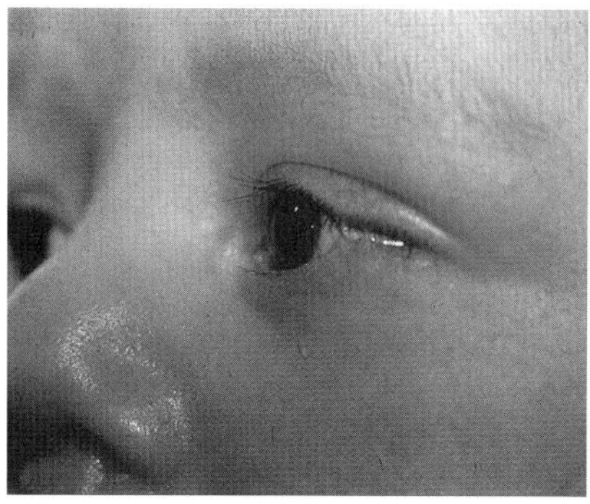

Figure 2.7. Ankyloblepharon filiforme adnatum. (Courtesy of Dr. James Katowitz.)

In ankyloblepharon filiforme adnatum, there are areas of fusion between the upper and lower lids by strands of fibrovascular tissue (Fig. 2.7).[1] These can usually be separated by traction or may require surgery.

Ankyloblepharon filiforme adnatum has been associated with trisomy 18,[4,31] the dominant syndrome of popliteal pterygium, digital and genital anomalies[34,59] and with a possibly different syndrome of cleft lip/palate paramedian mucous pits of the lower lip and popliteal pterygium, with isolated cleft lip and/or palate.[30,62] The relationship between these last two syndromes and the CHANDS syndrome (curly hair, ankyloblepharon, nail dysplasia)[6,101] is unclear. Ankyloblepharon has also been reported in a patient with congenital glaucoma and irido-gonio-dysgenesis.[87]

Hay and Wells[47] reported on seven members of four families with an autosomal dominant syndrome of ectodermal dysplasia, ankyloblepharon filiforme adnatum, hypodontia, and cleft lip/palate. Similar familial cases were described by Speigel and Colton[93] and by Seres-Santamaria et al.,[88] although the two patients reported by Seres-Santamaria et al. were siblings, indicating a recessive form of the syndrome or germinal mosaicism in one of the parents.

CONGENITAL ENTROPION

Congenital entropion of the upper eyelid is a very rare abnormality affecting mostly females and has been reported in fewer than 20 patients.[51,108] Congenital entropion is considered an ocular emergency[21] because corneal ulceration and permanent scarring can result from the associated trichiasis if surgical management is not promptly instituted.[11] This abnormality may be due to congenital levator aponeurosis disinsertion[104] or to extreme kinking of the tarsus.[11] One patient had an associated agenesis of the corpus callosum.[51] Congenital entropion of the upper or lower eyelid should be suspected in infants with atypical or persistent corneal ulceration. An examination under sedation or anesthesia prevents squeezing of the eyelids and allows the correct diagnosis. The presence of concomitant distichiasis or other congenital eyelid anomalies are helpful diagnostic clues.

CONGENITAL ECTROPION OF THE EYELID

Also called congenital eversion of the upper eyelids, this condition is more common in black infants[8] and in patients with Down syndrome.[56,94] It may also be seen in patients with lamellar ichthyosis.[27] Congenital ectropion is generally self-limited and is best managed by lubrication with or without taping of the lids together intermittently or during sleep. Persistent eversion is rare and may require surgical intervention.[2] Congenital upper eyelid eversion is thought to be due to impaired venous return from the upper lids resulting in eyelid swelling, chemosis, and eversion[95]; orbicularis spasm may also be a contributory factor.[80] Injection of hyaluronidase into the chemotic conjunctiva followed by placement of a lid suture to revert the eyelid resolves the condition in 1 or 2 days.[8]

DISTICHIASIS

This term refers to the growth of true cilia in ectopic locations and in extra rows along the lid margin and out of the orifices of meibomian glands. The accessory row(s) of lashes are usually seen on all four lids and run on the inner part of the intermarginal strip. The cilia may be soft and depigmented, or fully developed and pigmented and may rub against the globe resulting in corneal damage. Several families with autosomal dominant distichiasis have been reported in the world literature.[36]

The distichiasis-lymphedema syndrome consists of distichiasis and lymphedema causing painless swelling of the extremities, predominantly below the knee.[32,52,82] The diagnosis is based on the physical findings and the family history. Mild pitting edema may be the earliest sign of lymphedema. A lymphangiogram of the lower extremities shows hypoplastic lymph channels. Other features of the syndrome include epidural spinal cysts, vertebral anomalies,[82] partial ectropion of the lower lid, (webbed neck) and pterygium colli.[32] The lymphedema first becomes evident between 5 and 20 years of age, most commonly during adolescence. The extra row of lashes involves all four lids. They may be well developed or lanugolike. Superficial punctate keratitis and photophobia are frequent findings if the lashes rub against the cornea. Strabismus was also present in Campbell's original pedigree.[52] Partial ectropion of the lower lid gives a proptotic appearance to the eyes in some patients. An apparent deficiency of the inferior tarsus may be found on clinical examination. The disorder is inherited as an autosomal dominant trait with variable expression. In some members of a family with this disorder distichiasis or lymphedema may occur alone. Males seem to be more often affected with the full syndrome than females.[32,82] Distichiasis may be an isolated dominantly inherited disorder unrelated to lymphedema, and for this reason is frequently confused with the distichiasis-lymphedema syndrome, especially before puberty when the lymphedema usually first appears. Lymphedema may also be an isolated hereditary disease. Disability from lymphedema can be prevented with early diagnosis and treatment. If removal of lashes is absolutely necessary, they should be electrolyzed.[52]

CONGENITAL EYELID RETRACTION

This is a static condition that affects the upper or lower eyelids, or both.[17] It is diagnosed after the exclusion of other causes of lid retraction such as hyperthyroidism, trauma, proptosis, seventh-nerve palsy, and Marcus-Gunn jaw winking. Patients usually present an abnormal appearance of the eyes. Corneal exposure is a rare complication. No treatment is required except for lubrication in patients with exposure keratitis. Extensive investigation is not required if the history and clinical course are suggestive of the diagnosis. Some degree of upper eyelid retraction is a normal finding in newborns and young infants. In severe cases, eyelid retractor lengthening procedures may be performed, but the results may be unpredictable with resulting secondary ptosis.

EPIBULBAR CHORISTOMAS

Choristomas are benign tumors derived from tissue not normally present in the tumor's location. Epibulbar and orbital choristomas are the most common epibulbar and orbital tumors in children. Four histopathologic types are recognized: *(1)* dermoids, which are made of collagenous connective tissue covered with epidermis; *(2)* lipodermoids, which, in addition, contain adipose tissue; *(3)* single-tissue choristomas that consist either of dermislike tissue or of ectopic mesectodermal tissue of one origin; and *(4)* complex choristomas that contain tissues of different origins. Clinically, dermoid cysts contain one or more dermal adnexal structures and are lined by keratinizing epithelium; epidermoid cysts have no adnexal structures; teratomas contain tissues derived from all three germinal layers; and teratoid tumors are derived from only two germinal layers.[66]

Epibulbar choristomas are solid tumors of the ocular surface that occur in 1 to 3 per 10,000 live births. These tumors may be white yellow or pink and vary from small flat lesions at the limbus to large masses that cover most of the interpalpebral area. Lesions may be unilateral or bilateral and multiple tumors have also been reported. Of 82 epibulbar choristomas reported by Ash, 52% were in the bulbar conjunctiva, 29% at the limbus, 6% in the cornea, 4% in the caruncle, 4% in the canthal area, 2.5% in the fornix, and 2.5% in the palpebral conjunctiva. Associated ocular and facial abnormalities include scleral and corneal staphyloma, aniridia, congenital aphakia, cataract, miliary aneurysms of the retina, microphthalmia, osseous choristoma of the choroid, dermoid cyst of the orbit or eyelid, choristomatous malformations of the face and scalp, and preauricular tags. Epibulbar choristomas that involve the cornea may induce astigmatism, necessitating their surgical excision and the optical correction of the astigmatism to prevent amblyopia.

Epibulbar choristomas are associated with the Goldenhar syndrome[42] in the facio-auriculo-vertebral spectrum of anomalies. They may also be seen in patients with the epidermal nevus syndrome,[90] which includes skeletal, neurologic, vascular, and dermatologic abnormalities. The choristomas in the epidermal nevus syndrome are usually of the complex variety and may involve the whole ocular surface.[65] Peer and Ilsar[76] reported an epibulbar complex choristoma in a female newborn child with nevus sebaceous of Jadassohn. The mass was pedunculated and originated from the superotemporal scleral and limbal area of the left eye. The child also had two atypical chorioretinal colobomas temporal to the disc in the affected eye.

Epibulbar choristomas may be inherited, usually in an autosomal dominant fashion,[70,78] but also in an X-linked recessive[100] or autosomal recessive manner.

Episcleral osseous choristomas are rare whitish pea-sized raised lesions that occur 5–10 mm posterior to the limbus and are composed of compact bone vested by periosteum.[28] These tumors are freely movable but may adhere to sclera or to extraocular muscles.

LINEAR NEVUS SEBACEOUS OF JADASSOHN

Although the name implies a dermatologic disease, this syndrome involves multiple other systems, including the central nervous system and the eyes. At birth, striking raised hairless, yellow-orange, or tan plaque(s) with irregular margins are present on the face, scalp, neck, body, or, occasionally, the oral mucosa.[49] The lesions are initially composed of small papules but become verrucous and nodular at puberty. A congenital bald lesion is present when the nevus involves the scalp. Children with this disorder are frequently mentally retarded and often develop seizures in the first few weeks or months of life.[9,33,49] Frequently, one large nevus extends from the forehead to the tip of the nose. The nevi may be large but generally respect the midline. There is usually failure to thrive, with poor growth and development, although milestones in the first few months of life may be normal. Hypoplastic teeth and a depressed nasal bridge may be present. The sebaceous glands in the lesion may emit a putrid, foul odor.[97] The electroencephalogram may show seizure activity or diffuse encephalopathy. The EKG may be abnormal due to cardiac involvement.

The clinical findings in this syndrome may overlap with those in some of the phakomatoses and the nevus is best considered a hamartoma.[10] Malignant transformation of the nevi occurs in 15%–20% of cases.[10,107a]

The nevi may extensively involve the eyelids and a vascularized choristomatous mass may involve the lids, conjunctiva, and cornea.[107] There may be nystagmus, strabismus, ptosis,[46] scarring, and vascularization of the cornea.[46,73] In addition, iris coloboma,[67] choroidal coloboma,[73] corectopia, with an updrawn pupil,[73] limbal dermoids,[9,97] lipodermoids,[46,67] and slanting palpebral fissures have all been described in patients with this disorder. Biopsy of the conjunctival lesions demonstrates multiple choristomas with hyperplastic sebaceous glands, apocrine glands, and immature hair follicles.[73] Poor vision in the most involved eye is common.[73,107] Haslam and Wirschafter[46] reviewed the ocular findings in this disorder and described a congenital third nerve palsy associated with a dermolipoma in one patient. The limbal dermoid lesions may continue to enlarge during the first decade of life.[107] Intrascleral cartilage and bone have been documented.[107] One patient had a choroidal osseous choristoma with an overlying choroidal neovascular membrane.[61a] One patient with linear nevus sebaceous and bilateral optic nerve hypoplasia has been reported by Katz and co-workers.[57a]

The disorder is generally isolated and sporadic. Mental retardation and seizures without the nevus have been described in other family members on two occasions.[10,67] The nevi in the linear nevus sebaceous of Jadassohn are slightly elevated and should not be confused with the flat, red, blanching nevus flammeus seen in Sturge-Weber syndrome, nor with the flat, smooth-bordered cafe-au-lait spots of neurofibromatosis. The Goldenhar syndrome has several features in common with this disorder including asymmetry of the orbits, epibulbar dermoids, lipodermoids, and colobomas of the lids and irides.[7] Other conditions that are frequently considered in the differential diagnosis of this disorder in childhood include nevoxanthoendothelioma, juvenile melanoma, and scarring alopecia. At an older age, the nevus must be differentiated from nevus verrucosus, verruca vulgaris, scarring alopecia, and xanthoma.[4]

Profound mental retardation may lead to institutionalization. The seizure disorder is severe. No known treatment is available except anticonvulsant medication and supportive custodial care. Surgical repair of the choristomatous scarring of the cornea and conjunctiva is rarely beneficial. Death can occur in the first decade. Patients have lived into the second decade, however.

AGENESIS OF THE EXTRAOCULAR MUSCLES

There are two theories for the development of the extraocular muscles (EOMs). Gilbert[39] postulated that the EOMs are derived from neural crest. He stated that at 24–26 days of gestation a premandibular condensation gives rise to the muscles that are innervated by the oculomotor nerve, whereas the lateral rectus and superior oblique are derived from mesoderm. Through a series of experiments looking at histologic sections of EOMs and orbits at different stages of embryologic development, Sevel[89] concluded that the EOMs develop from in situ differentiation in the orbit. He found that the entire length of the muscle develops at the same time rather than grows from the apex of the orbit toward the sclera. According to Sevel,[89] the muscles develop from two mesodermal complexes: *(1)* a superior complex that gives rise to the superior oblique, superior rectus, and levator palpebrae superioris and *(2)* an inferior complex that gives rise to the inferior rectus and inferior oblique muscles; the medial and lateral rectus muscles are derived from both complexes.

AGENESIS OF THE SUPERIOR OBLIQUE TENDON

The largest series of patients with congenital absence of the superior oblique (SO) tendon was reported by Helveston et al.[48] A few other scattered case reports are found in the literature.[69,74,77] Patients with this condition present with a clinical fourth cranial nerve palsy with a head posture consisting of chin depression and head tilt toward the nonparetic side. Diagnosis is made if the superior aspect of the globe is explored in an attempt to tuck or shorten the tendon and no tendon is found. Computed tomography may demonstrate an absence of the tendon. Helveston et al.[48] reported an incidence of 18% (6 of 40 patients) among patients with fourth cranial nerve palsy; their experience, however, is not shared by other strabismologists who believe this figure to be a large overestimate. Pollard[77] reported 11 patients with Apert syndrome and bilateral superior oblique palsy. Of seven patients who underwent surgical exploration, five had no superior oblique tendon in either eye and the other two had small fibrous band remnants. Patients with Apert syndrome and those with other craniofacial malformation syndromes probably have a high incidence of absence of the SO tendon and other extraocular muscles.[22,24,81,92,106] Treatment of the absent SO tendon consists of weakening of the antagonist inferior oblique muscle and recession of the contralateral inferior rectus or ipsilateral superior rectus muscle.

AGENESIS OF THE INFERIOR RECTUS MUSCLE

Numerous cases of functional absence of the inferior rectus muscle have been reported.[18,40,71,74a] About 50% are bilateral. Patients have no inferior rectus muscle function, and no muscle is found on surgical exploration. Computed tomography may suggest the presence of inferior rectus muscles in the posterior orbit. Patients with bilateral affection usually have a chin-down head posture. No associated conditions have been reported. Treatment consists of disinsertion of the superior rectus muscles in bilateral cases. Muscle transposition procedures are performed in unilateral cases.

AGENESIS OF THE SUPERIOR RECTUS MUSCLE

Most patients with absent superior rectus muscle have craniofacial dysostosis.[73a] Other extraocular muscles such as the SO may also be absent or anomalous and there may be associated blepharophimosis, as in the bilateral case reported by Drummond and Keech.[29] One patient had paradoxical eye movements. Muscle transposition or union procedures, as well as free tenotomies of the inferior rectus muscles, are performed for treatment.[53,68a]

AGENESIS OF THE MEDIAL RECTUS MUSCLE

There are very few documented cases of absence of the medical rectus muscle in the modern literature.[41,75,91] Patients have a large-angle exotropia and cannot adduct the eye on the side of the agenesis beyond the midline. One patient with oculocutaneous albinism had associated uveal colobomas and myopia.[75] Treatment is in the form of muscle union procedures. Although the muscle insertion in such cases is not identifiable, rudimentary muscle structures or very posterior insertions cannot be ruled out.

AGENESIS OF THE LATERAL RECTUS MUSCLE

In one reported case of documented isolated absence of the lateral rectus muscle in a female with Axenfeld anomaly and developmental glaucoma,[86] a large esotropia was treated successfully by a muscle transposition procedure.

REFERENCES

1. Akkermans CH, Stern LM. Ankyloblepharon filiforme adnatum. *Br J Ophthalmol* 1979;63: 129–131.
2. Alvarez EV, Wakakura M, Alvarez EI. Surgical management of persistent congenital eversion of the upper eyelids. *Ann Ophthalmol* 1988;20:353–354.
3. Azevedo ES, Biondo J, Ramlho LM. The cryptophthalmos in two families from Bahia, Brazil. *J Med Genet* 1973;10:389–392.
4. Bacal DA, Nelson LB, Zacakai EH, Lavrich JB, Kousseff BG, McDonald-McGinn D. Ankyloblepharon filiforme adnatum in trisomy 18. *J. Pediatr Ophthalmol Strabismus* 1993; 30:337–339.
5. Balestrazzi P, Baeteman MA, Mattei MG, Mattei JF. Franceschetti syndrome in a child with a de novo balanced translocation (5;13)(q11;p11) and significant decrease of hexosaminidase B. *Hum Genet* 1983;64: 305–308.
6. Baughman FA. CHANDS: The curly hair-ankyloblepharon-nail dysplasia syndrome. *Birth Defects Orig Art Ser* 1971;VII(8): 100–102.
7. Baum JL, Feingold M. Ocular aspects of Goldenhar's syndrome. *Am J Ophthalmol* 1973;75:250–257.
8. Bentsi-Enchill KO. Congenital total eversion of the upper eyelids. *Br J Ophthalmol* 1981; 65:209–213.
9. Berg JM, Crome L. A possible case of atypical tuberous sclerosis. *J Ment Defic Res* 1960;4: 24–31.
10. Bianchine JW. The nevus sebaceous of Jadassohn. A neurocutaneous syndrome and potentially pre-malignant lesion. *Am J Dis Child* 1970;120:223–228.
11. Biglan AW, Buerger GF. Congenital horizontal tarsal kink. *Am J Ophthalmol* 1980;89: 522–524.
12. Boyd PA, Keeling JW, Lindenbaum RH. Fraser syndrome (cryptophthalmos-syndactyly syndrome). A review of eleven cases with postmortem findings. *Am J Med Genet* 1988; 31:159–168.
13. Brazier DJ, Hardman-Lea SJ, Collin JRO. Cryptophthalmos: Surgical treatment of the congenital symblepharon variant. *Br J Ophthalmol* 1986;70:391–395.
14. Burn W, Marwood RP. Fraser syndrome presenting as bilateral renal agenesis in three sibs. *J Med Genet* 1982;19:360–361.
15. Cesarino EJ, Pinheiro M, Freire-Maia N, et al. Brief clinical report: Lid agenesis-macrostomia-psychomotor retardation-forehead hypertrichosis—A new syndrome. *Am J Med Genet* 1988;31:299–304.
16. Codere F, Brownstein S, Chen MF. Cryptophthalmos syndrome with bilateral renal agenesis. *Am J Ophthalmol* 1981;91:737–742.
17. Collin JRO, Allen L, Castronuovo S. Congenital eyelid retraction. *Br J Ophthalmol* 1990; 74:542–544.
18. Cooper EL. Congenital absence of the inferior rectus muscle. *Arch Ophthalmol* 1971; 86:451–454.
19. Coover DH. Two cases of cryptophthalmia. *Ophthalmoscope* 1910;8:259.
20. Coover DH. Cryptophthalmia. *Ophthalmoscope* 1915;13:586.
21. Crawford JS. Congenital eyelid anomalies in children. *J Pediatr Ophthalmol Strabismus* 1984;21:140–149.
22. Cutton JM, Brazis PT, Miller MT, et al. Absence of the superior rectus muscle in Apert syndrome. *J Pediatr Ophthalmol Strabismus* 1979;16:349–354.
23. De Fries PD, Katowitz JA. Congenital craniofacial anomalies of ophthalmic importance. *Surv Ophthalmol* 1990;35:87–119.
24. Diamond GR, Katowitz JA, Whitaker LA, et al. Variation in extraocular muscle number and structure in craniofacial dysostosis. *Am J Ophthalmol* 1980;90:416–418.
25. Dinno ND, Edwards WE, Weiskopf B. The cryptophthalmos-syndactyly syndrome. *Clin Pediatr* 1974;13:219.
26. Dixon MJ, Read AP, Donnai D, Colley A, Dixon J, Williamson R. The gene for Treacher Collins syndrome maps to the long arm of chromosome 5. *Am J Hum Genet* 1991; 49:17–22.
27. Donoso LA, Eiferman RA, Magargal LE, et al. Spontaneous resolution of congenital ectropion in a collodion baby. *J Pediatr Ophthalmol Strabismus* 1981;18:23–25.
28. Dreizen NG, Schachat AP, Shields JA, et al. Epibulbar osseous choristomas. *J Pediatr Ophthalmol Strabismus* 1983;20:247–249.
29. Drummond GT, Keech RV. Absent and anomalous superior oblique and superior rectus muscles. *Can J Ophthalmol* 1989;24: 275–279.
30. Ehlers N, Jensen IK. Ankyloblepharon filiforme congenitum associated with harelip and cleft palate. *Acta Ophthalmol* 1970;48:465–467.

31. Evvans DGR, Evans ID, Donnai D, Lindenbaum RH. Ankyloblepharon filiforme adnatum in trisomy 18 Edwards syndrome. *J Med Genet* 1990;27:720–721.
32. Falls HF, Kertesz ED. A new syndrome combining pterygium colli with developmental anomalies of the eyelids and lymphatics of the lower extremities. *Trans Am Ophthalmol Soc* 1964;62:248–275.
33. Feuerstein RC, Mims LC. Linear nevus sebaceous with convulsions and mental retardation. *Am J Dis Child* 1962;104:675–679.
34. Foster-Iskenius UG. Popliteal pterygium syndrome. *J Med Genet* 1990;27:320–326.
35. Franceschetti A, Klein D. *The Mandibulofacial Dysostosis, A New Hereditary Syndrome.* Copenhagen: E. Munksgaard, 1949.
36. Francois J. Distichiasis. In *Heredity in Ophthalmology.* St. Louis: C. V. Mosby, 1961:274.
37. Francois J. Malformative syndrome with cryptophthalmia. *Int Ophthalmol Clin* 1968; 8:817–837.
38. Fraser GR. Our genetic load: A review of some aspects of genetical variation. *Ann Hum Genet* 1962;25:387–415.
39. Gilbert PW. The origin and development of the human extrinsic ocular muscles. *Contrib Embryol* 1957;36:59.
40. Giller H. Congenital absence of the inferior rectus muscle. *Arch Ophthalmol* 1962;68:182.
41. Girard LJ, Neely RA. Agenesis of the medial rectus muscle. *Arch Ophthalmol* 1958;54:337.
42. Goldenhar M. Associations malformatives de l'oeil et de l'oreille, en particulier le syndrome dermoide epibulbaire-appendices auriculaires-fistula auris congenita et ses relations avec la dysostose mandibulo-faciale. *J Genet Hum* 1952;1:243–282.
43. Goldhammer Y, Smith JL. Cryptophthalmos syndrome with basal encephaloceles. *Am J Ophthalmol* 1981;80:146–149.
44. Gorlin RJ, Cohen MM Jr, Levin LS. *Syndromes of the Head and Neck.* New York: Oxford University Press, 1990.
45. Hancheng Z. Cryptophthalmos: A report on three sibling cases. *Br J Ophthalmol* 1986; 70:72.
46. Haslam RHA, Wirschafter JD. Unilateral external oculomotor nerve palsy and nevus sebaceous of Jadassohn. *Arch Ophthalmol* 1972; 87:293–300.
47. Hay RJ, Wells RS. The syndrome of ankyloblepharon, ectodermal defects and cleft lip and palate: An autosomal dominant condition. *Br J Dermatol* 1976;94:287–289.
48. Helveston EM, Giangiacomo JG, Ellis FD. Congenital absence of the superior oblique tendon. *Trans Am Ophthalmol Soc* 1981;79: 123–135.
49. Herbst B, Cohen ME. Linear nevus sebaceous. *Arch Neurol* 1971;24:317–322.
50. Hertle RW, Quinn GE, Katowitz JA. Ocular and adnexal findings in patients with facial microsomias. *Ophthalmology* 1992;99:114–119.
51. Hiles DA, Wilder LW. Congenital entropion of the upper lids. *J Pediatr Ophthalmol* 1969; 6:157.
52. Hoover RE, Kelley JS. Distichiasis and lymphedema: A hereditary syndrome with possible multiple defects—A report of a family. *Trans Am Ophthalmol Soc* 1971;69: 293–306.
53. Hummelsheim E. Weitere Erfahrungen mit partieller Schnuberpflanzung and dem Augenmusklen. *Arch Augenheilkd* 1980;62:71.
54. Ide CH, Wollschleger PB. Multiple congenital abnormalities associated with cryptophthalmia. *Arch Ophthalmol* 1969;81:638–641.
55. Jabs EW, Li X, Coss CA, Taylor EW, Meyers DA, Weber JL. Mapping the Treacher Collins syndrome locus to 5q31.3-q33.3. *Genomics* 1991;11:193–198.
56. Johnson CC, McGowan BL. Persistent congenital ectropion of all four eyelids with megaloblepharon: Report of a case in a mongoloid child. *Am J Ophthalmol* 1969;67:252.
57. Johnson CC. Epicanthus and epiblepharon. *Arch Ophthalmol* 1978;96:1030.
57a. Katz B, et al. Optic nerve hypoplasia in the syndrome of nevus sebaceus of Jadassohn. *Ophthalmology* 1987;94:1570–1576.
58. Key SN. Report of a case of cryptophthalmia. *Am J Ophthalmol* 1920;3:684.
59. Klein D. Un curieux syndrome hereditaire: Cheilo-paltoschisis avec fistules de la levre inferieure associee a une syndactylie, une onychodysplasie particuliere, un pterygion poplite unilateral et des pieds varus equins. *J Genet Hum* 1962;11:65–71.
60. Koenig R, Spranger J. Cryptophthalmos syndactyly syndrome without cryptophthalmos. *Clin Genet* 1986;29:413–416.
61. Kolin T, Johns KJ, Wadlington WB, Butler MG, Sunalp MA, Wright KW. Hereditary lymphedema and distichiasis. *Arch Ophthalmol* 1991;109:980–981.
61a. Lambert SR, Sipperley JO, Shore JW, et al. Linear nevus sebaceous syndrome. *Ophthalmology* 1987;94:278–282.

62. Lemtis H, Neubauer H. Ankyloblepharon filiforme et membraniforme adnatum. *Klin Monatsbl Augenheilkd* 1959;135:510–516.
63. Lurie IW, Cherstvoy ED. Renal agenesis as a diagnostic feature of the cryptophthalmos-syndactyly syndrome. *Clin Genet* 1984;25:528–532.
64. Magruder AC. Cryptophthalmos. *Am J Ophthalmol* 1921;4:48.
65. Mansour AM, Laibson PD, Reinecke RD, et al. Bilateral total corneal and conjunctival choristomas associated with epidermal nevus. *Arch Ophthalmol* 1986;104:245–248.
66. Mansour AM, Barber JC, Reinecke RD, et al. Ocular choristomas. *Surv Ophthalmol* 1989;33:339–358.
67. Marden PM, Venters HD Jr. A new neurocutaneous syndrome. *Am J Dis Child* 1966;112:79–81.
68. Mashimoto H, Ikeda T, Matsuo T, et al. Cryptophthalmia syndrome with laryngeal atresia and bilateral renal agenesis: A case report and a review of the literature. *Cong Anom* 1987;27:1.
68a. Mather TR, Saunders RA. Congenital absence of the superior rectus muscle: A case report. *J Pediatr Ophthalmol Strabismus* 1987;24:291–295.
69. Matsuo T, Ohtsuki H, Sogabe Y, et al. Vertical abnormal retinal correspondence in three patients with congenital absence of the superior oblique muscle. *Am J Ophthalmol* 1988;106:337.
70. Mattos J, Contreras F, O'Donnell FE. Ring dermoid syndrome. A new syndrome of autosomal dominant inherited bilateral annular limbal dermoids with corneal and conjunctival extension. *Arch Ophthalmol* 1980;98:1059–1061.
71. Mets MB, Parks MM, Freeley DA, et al. Congenital absence of the inferior rectus muscle: A report of three cases and their management. *Binocular Vision* 1987;2:77.
72. Miller MT, Deutsch TA, Cronin C, et al. Amniotic bands as a cause of ocular abnormalities. *Am J Ophthalmol* 1987;104:270–279.
73. Monahan RH, Hill CW, Venters HD Jr. Multiple choristomas, convulsions and mental retardation as a new neurocutaneous syndrome. *Am J Ophthalmol* 1967;64(suppl):529–532.
73a. Morax S, Pascal D. Absence of the right superior rectus muscle in Apert's syndrome. *J Fr Ophthalmol* 1982;5:323–326.
74. Mumma J. Surgical procedure for congenital absence of the superior oblique. *Arch Ophthalmol* 1974;92:221–223.
74a. Munoz M. Congenital absence of the inferior rectus muscle. *Am J Ophthalmol* 1996;121:327–329.
75. Murphy BF, Annable WL. Congenital absence of the medial rectus muscle with review of previous case reports. *Binocular Vision* 1987;2:87.
76. Peer J, Ilsar M. Epibulbar complex choristoma associated with nevus sebaceous. *Arch Ophthalmol* 1995;113:1301–1304.
77. Pollard ZF. Bilateral superior oblique muscle palsy associated with Apert syndrome. *Am J Ophthalmol* 1988;106:337–340.
78. Pouliquen Y, Dhermy P, Cotinat J, et al. Dermoid bilateral héréditaire (étude clinique histologique et ultrastructurale). *J Fr Ophthalmol* 1978;1:443–450.
79. Price NJ, Pugh RE, Farndon PA, Willshaw HE. Ablepharon macrostomia syndrome. *Br J Ophthalmol* 1991;75:317–319.
80. Raab EL, Saphir RL. Congenital eyelid aversion with orbicularis spasm. *J Pediatr Ophthalmol Strabismus* 1985;22:125–128.
81. Robb RM, Boger WP III. Vertical strabismus associated with plagiocephaly. *J. Pediatr Ophthalmol Strabismus* 1983;20:58–62.
82. Robinow M, Johnson GF, Verhagen AD. Distichiasis-lymphedema: A hereditary syndrome of multiple congenital defects. *Am J Dis Child* 1970;119:343–347.
83. Rogers BO. Berry-Treacher Collins syndrome: A review of 200 cases. *Br J Plast Surg* 1964;17:109.
84. Rovin S, Dach SF, Borenstein DB, Cotter WB. Mandibulofacial dysostosis, A familial study of five generations. *J Pediatr* 1964;65:215–221.
85. Saal HM, Traboulsi EI, Gavaris P, Samango-Sprouse CA, Parks M. Dominant syndrome with isolated cryptophthalmos and ocular anomalies. *Am J Med Genet* 1992;43:785–788.
86. Sandall GS, Morrison JW. Congenital absence of lateral rectus muscle. *J. Pediatr Ophthalmol Strabismus* 1979;16:35–39.
87. Scott MH, Richard JM, Farris BK. Ankyloblepharon filiforme adnatum associated with infantile glaucoma and iridogoniodysgenesis. *J Pediatr Ophthalmol Strabismus* 1994;31:93–95.
88. Seres-Santamaria A, Arimany JL, Muniz F. Two sibs with cleft palate, ankyloblepharon, alveolar synechiae, and ectodermal defects: A

new recessive syndrome? *J Med Genet* 1993; 30:793–795.

89. Sevel D. A reappraisal of the origin of human extraocular muscles. *Ophthalmology* 1981; 88:1330–1338.
90. Shochot Y, Romano A, Berishak YR, et al. Eye findings in the linear sebaceous nevus syndrome: A possible clue to the pathogenesis. *J Craniofac Genet Dev Biol* 1982;2:289.
91. Silverman SJ, Fletcher MC. Agenesis of three extraocular muscles. *Am J Ophthalmol* 1965; 60:919.
92. Snir M, Gilad E, Ben-Sira I. An unusual extraocular muscle anomaly in a patient with Crouzon's disease. *Br J Ophthalmol* 1982; 66:253–257.
93. Speigel J, Colton A. AEC syndrome: Ankyloblepharon, ectodermal defects, and cleft lip and palate. *J Am Acad Dermatol* 1985;12: 810–815.
94. Stern EN, Campbell CH, Faulkner HW. Conservative management of congenital eversion of the eyelids. *Am J Ophthalmol* 1973;75:319.
95. Stillerman ML, Emanuel B, Padoor MP. Eversion of the eyelids in the newborn without an apparent cause. *J Pediatr* 1966;69:656.
96. Sugar HS. The cryptophthalmos-syndactyly syndrome. *Am J Ophthalmol* 1968;66:897.
97. Sugarman GI, Reed WB. Two unusual neurocutaneous disorders with facial cutaneous signs. *Arch Neurol* 1969;21:242–247.
98. Sullivan TJ, Welham RA, Collin JR. Centurion syndrome. Idiopathic anterior displacement of the medial canthus. *Ophthalmology* 1993;100:328–333.
99. Thomas IT, Frias JL, Felix V, et al. Isolated and syndromic cryptophthalmos. *Am J Med Genet* 1986;25:85–98.
100. Topilow HW, Cykiert RC, Goldman A, et al. Bilateral corneal dermis-like choristomas: A X-chromosome-linked disorder. *Arch Ophthalmol* 1981;99:1387–1391.
101. Toriello HV, Lindstrom JA, Waterman DA, Baughman FA. Re-evaluation of CHANDS. *J Med Genet* 1979;16:316–317.
102. Traboulsi E, Saal HM, Castelbaum A, Smango-Sprouse CA, Gavaris P. A new dominant cryptophthalmos syndrome with microphthalmia and Peters anomaly (abstract). *Am J Hum Genet* 1991;47(suppl):A80.
103. Treacher Collins E. Case with symmetrical congenital notches in the outer part of each lower lid and defective development of the malar bones. *Trans Ophthalmol Soc UK* 1900;20:191–192.
104. Tse DT, Anderson RL, Fratkin JD. Aponeurosis disinsertion in congenital entropion. *Arch Ophthalmol* 1983;101:436–440.
105. Waring GO, Shields JA. Partial unilateral cryptophthalmos with syndactyly brachycephaly and renal anomalies. *Am J Ophthalmol* 1975;79:437–440.
106. Weinstock FJ, Hardesty HH. Absence of superior recti in craniofacial dysostosis. *Arch Ophthalmol* 1965;74:152.
107. Wilkes SR, Campbell RJ, Waller RR. Ocular malformation in association with ipsilateral facial nevus of Jadassohn. *Am J Ophthalmol* 1981;92:344–352.

107a. Wilson-Jones EW, Heyl T. Naevus sebaceus: A report of 140 cases with special regard to the development of secondary malignant tumours. *Br J Dermatol* 1970;82:99–117.

108. Zak TA. Congenital primary upper eyelid entropion. *J Pediatr Ophthalmol Strabismus* 1984;21:69–73.
109. Zehender W. Eine Missgeburt mit hautueberwaschsenen Augen oder Kryptophthalmus. *Klin Monatsbl Augenheilkd* 1872;10:225.

3

Surgical Management of the Patient with Ocular Adnexal Malformations

KATRINKA L. HEHER
JAMES A. KATOWITZ

MICROPHTHALMIA AND ANOPHTHALMIA

Microphthalmia is a varied spectrum of conditions ranging from a small remnant of ocular tissue in the orbit to a congenitally cystic eye or to a small, well-formed eye known as nanophthalmos or pure microphthalmos. True anophthalmia is the total absence of the tissues of the eye and can only be distinguished from extreme microphthalmia by histologic examination. In this chapter we use the term *clinical anophthalmia* when referring either to cases of true anophthalmia or to extreme forms of microphthalmia where no ocular remnant is clinically visible.

The goal of treatment of clinical anophthalmia is to provide a cosmetically acceptable appearance that is symmetrical with the normal opposite side. For bilateral cases, it has been argued by some that since these patients are blind they are not bothered by the deformity and thus no treatment is indicated. It is our belief, however, that outward appearance greatly affects social interactions. For that reason, even in bilateral cases, we believe in trying to improve appearance as long as there is sufficient mental capacity.

The management of clinical anophthalmia must begin with socket expansion as early in life as possible.[1] This involves the use of progressively larger conformers. The ophthalmologist must work in close association with the ocularist, and initially the conformer may need to be changed at intervals of 1–2 weeks. By 3–4 months of age, the conformers need not be changed as frequently, and usually a cosmetic prosthesis can then be fitted. The prosthetic shell can then be progressively enlarged as the socket expands. The prosthesis will become more spherical with successful expansion, and in order to create a thinner better fitting shell with a greater ability to expand horizontally, we augment orbital volume with a dermis fat graft (Fig. 3.1). By permitting a thinner prosthesis to be fit, there is less gravitational effect on the lower lid.

Although many cases respond to this method of management, some orbits remain recalcitrant to efforts to promote growth. The use of inflatable orbital tissue expanders is being explored, but in some severe cases, as a last resort, craniofacial surgery is necessary to expand the bony orbit to permit adequate soft tissue expansion.

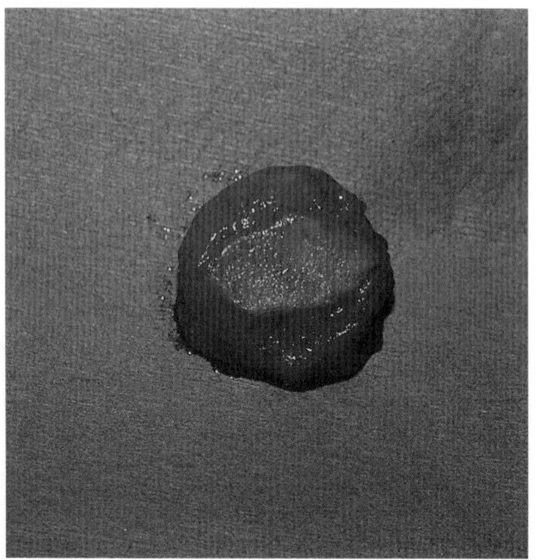

Figure 3.1*A*. Dermis fat graft.

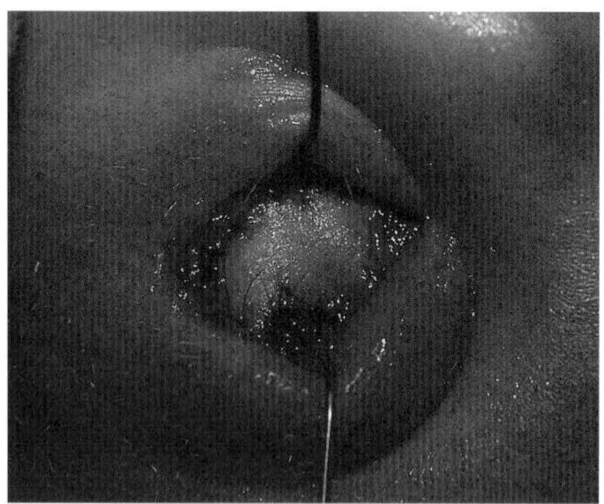

Figure 3.1*B*. Graft sutured into anophthalmic socket.

CRYPTOPHTHALMOS

Cryptophthalmos is a rare condition where the lid structures fail to differentiate. In complete or true cryptophthalmos the skin passes uninterrupted from the forehead to the cheek and is attached to the globe beneath, which is usually malformed. There can be partial forms in which the cul-de-sac is obliterated and the lid adheres to a portion of the cornea.

Management of these patients is extremely challenging. The primary goal of treatment is to secure some form of visual function. Visual potential can be estimated with the aid of ultrasound, computed tomography, magnetic resonance imaging, visual evoked response, and electroretinography. Once visual potential is demonstrated, surgery may be attempted. Procedures should be aimed at obtaining a clear visual axis in addition to creating some form of functioning lid structures. Difficulties in obtaining satisfactory results arise from the absence of conjunctiva and eyelid structures, and the severe anterior segment abnormalities. In the ideal situation, a penetrating keratoplasty would be performed in combination with the creation of a cul-de-sac and lids. Unfortunately, the corneal graft is usually doomed to fail, and to date there have been no published reports of successfully salvaged vision in the complete forms of cryptophthalmos. In the future, a keratoprosthesis may be the most viable solution for this severe deformity.

SYNDROME OF BLEPHAROPHIMOSIS, BLEPHAROPTOSIS, EPICANTHUS INVERSUS, AND TELECANTHUS

The tetrad of blepharophimosis, blepharoptosis, epicanthus inversus, and telecanthus (Kohn-Romano syndrome) commonly occurs as an isolated disorder and is inherited in an autosomal dominant fashion. The palpebral fissures are shortened both horizontally and vertically, and the ptosis is characterized by poor levator function and absent lid crease formation. Epicanthus inversus occurs in combination with telecanthus.

The surgical approach in these patients is oriented primarily toward correcting the ptosis, which is the most disabling feature of this disorder. Although some surgeons recommend delaying the repair of the epicanthus and telecanthus, as these may improve with age, in our experience this condition is fairly stable, and we find that correcting the epicanthal folds and telecanthus greatly enhances appearance. We incorporate the repair of the ptosis, epicanthus inversus, and telecanthus into one surgical stage.

A frontalis brow suspension must be used to elevate the lids since the function of the levator palpebrae superioris is poor or absent. Autologous fascia is the preferred sling material; however, for those patients who are below age 4–5 years, where an adequate length of fascia cannot be obtained, donor fascia can be utilized. Prior to elevating the lids, the telecanthus is repaired (see Canthal Deformities).

Following surgery, the children must be carefully monitored for corneal exposure. Aggressive lubricant regimens are initially used and then are slowly tapered off over the ensuing weeks.

CONGENITAL PTOSIS

Congenital ptosis is caused by a developmental deficiency of striated muscle fibers in the levator muscle. It occurs unilaterally in about 75% of cases, and is usually sporadic; however, a positive family history may be present.

The treatment of congenital ptosis is surgical. Although many surgeons prefer to postpone surgery until the patients are 4 or 5 years old, we advocate repair at a younger age to lessen psychosocial stresses. Ideally, the child should be at least 6 months old in order to avoid any increased risk of general anesthesia; however, should amblyopia develop that is unresponsive to patching, surgery can be performed sooner.

The choice of procedures is influenced by the degree of ptosis, the amount of levator function, and the lid's response to 2.5% Neosynephrine. A Fasanella-Servat operation may be elected for patients whose lid is adequately elevated 5 minutes after the instillation of 2.5% Neosynephrine into the cul-de-sac. These patients tend to have mild (2 mm) to moderate (3 mm) amounts of ptosis, and levator function is variable. A levator resection by the external approach is performed on those patients with a poor response to 2.5% Neosynephrine, who have at least a few millimeters of levator function. If the levator function is nearly absent, then a frontalis sling procedure is performed, using either Supramid (a synthetic suture), radiated donor fascia lata, or autogenous fascia lata. Autogenous fascia lata is the preferred material; however, in order to harvest an adequate length, the child must be about 4–5 years old. Supramid is usually reserved for temporizing procedures where there is total ptosis, especially unilateral, with a possibility for recovery of neurologic function, such as following trauma. The use of Supramid makes it possible to perform a "reversal" of the procedure should levator function eventually return.

COLOBOMA OF THE EYELID

Lid colobomas can occur in isolation or can be part of a clefting syndrome. The severity of the defect is variable ranging from a nearly complete absence of the lid to only a small notch in lateral aspect of the lower lid as seen in Treacher Collins syndrome. The upper lid colobomas can more frequently lead to exposure keratoconjunctivitis, whereas those defects occurring nasally on the lower lid are often associated with nasolacrimal system anomalies.

The treatment of lid colobomas depends on the size, configuration, and location of the defect.[2] Lid-sharing techniques are to be avoided as these run the risk of causing amblyopia. Sliding or rotational flaps are preferred techniques. Semicircle flaps can be fashioned to correct a variety of colobomas and can range in size from small (Tenzel) to a large cheek flap (Mustarde). In some cases the coloboma can be converted to a pentagonal defect which is then repaired in the same way as a lid margin laceration. This technique can be used to correct up to 50% of lid margin defects if combined with a canthotomy and cantholysis (Fig. 3.2).

ENTROPION

Congenital entropion can occur alone; however, it is frequently accompanied by epiblepharon. It is seen commonly in East Asians. The clinical course is often asymptomatic with spontaneous resolution. Surgery is indicated in those cases that persist or in which corneal integrity is threatened. Because the etiology of congenital entropion is usually due to disinsertion of the lower lid retractors, the recommended procedure is a tuck or advancement of the lower lid retractors usually combined with excision of a small ellipse of skin and underlying orbicularis muscle.

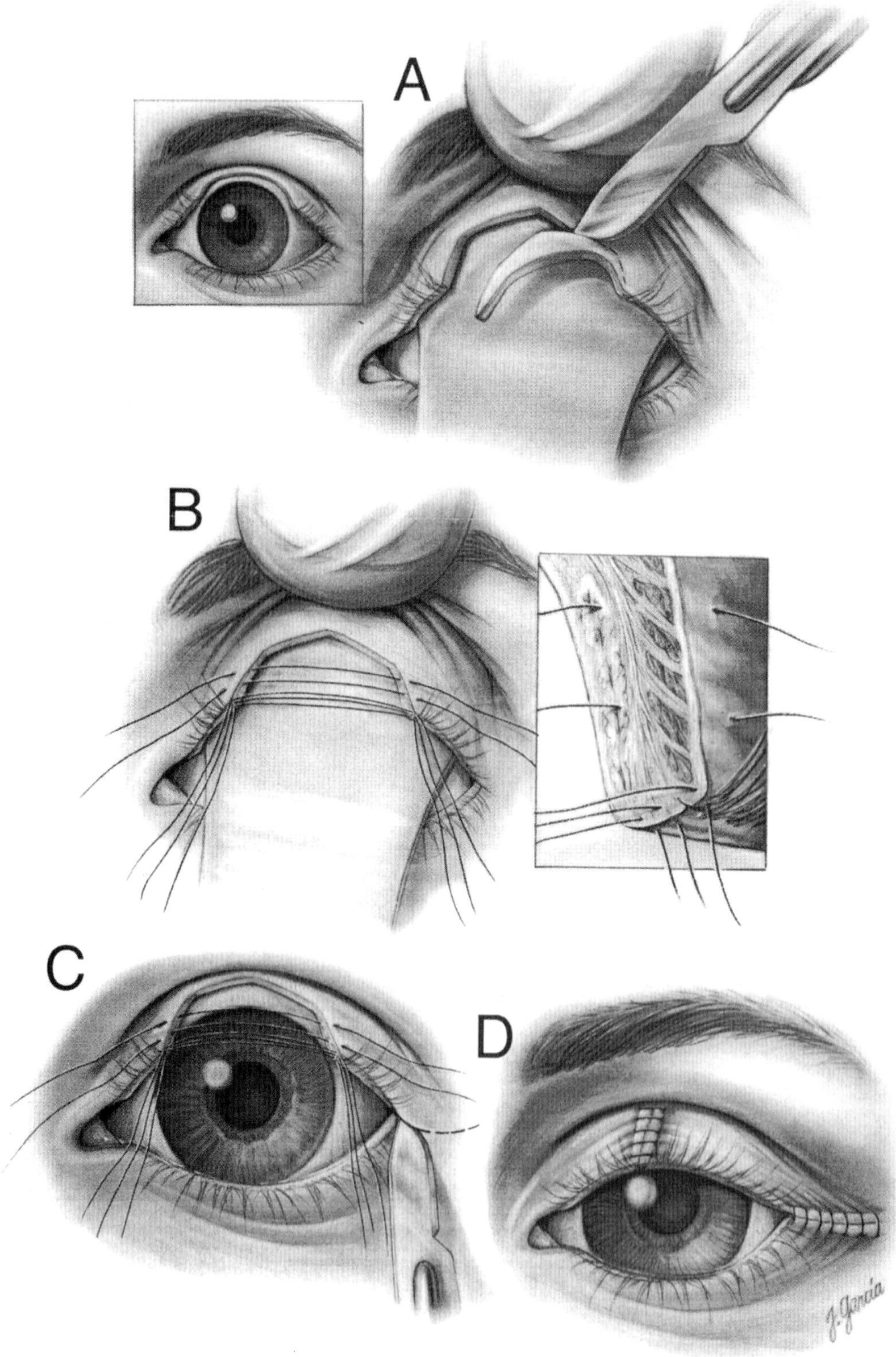

Figure 3.2. Upper lid coloboma repair. *A:* Pentagonal wedge excision around defect. *B:* Reapproximation of margin with tarsal sutures and three margin sutures. *C:* Additional horizontal laxity is obtained with lateral canthotomy and cantholysis; the incision may be extended in a semicircular flap. *D:* Sutured incision.

ECTROPION

Congenital ectropion is much less common than congenital entropion and is usually the result of vertical skin deficiency. It can cause chronic epiphora and exposure keratitis.

Treatment is directed at both tightening horizontally and lengthening vertically. In the lower lid, tightening the lid horizontally can be achieved by shortening the lateral canthal tendon. Full-thickness skin grafting is required to lengthen the anterior lamellae. In the upper lid, care must be taken to rule out chlamydial infection, which can lead to a congenital eversion. This is reversible with proper medication. If a true upper lid ectropion is present, a full-thickness wedge resection may be performed to achieve proper alignment of the lid to the globe.

EURYBLEPHARON

Euryblepharon is a horizontal widening of the palpebral fissure usually due to horizontal lengthening of the involved lids. Frequently, the palpebral fissure also has an antimongoloid slant because of an inferiorly displayed attachment of the lateral canthal tendon. Chronic tearing and exposure keratitis are common symptoms.

Surgical repair combines horizontal lid shortening with repositioning of the lateral canthus. A canthotomy with cantholysis is performed, followed by full-thickness lid shortening. A lateral canthopexy is then done with superior placement of the canthal tendon.

CANTHAL DEFORMITIES

Many of the craniofacial syndromes are associated with telecanthus and medial and lateral canthal dystopias. As with many of the lid abnormalities, epiphora and exposure keratitis are common symptoms.

Surgical correction of these deformities is usually performed at the time of craniofacial repair, as the approach for reconstruction provides excellent exposure of the medial and lateral orbital walls. However, in some cases, the canthal deformity repair is performed as a separate procedure at a later time.

Medial canthal dystopia is corrected with a canthopexy that can be performed in a number of ways depending on the severity of the problem. For milder forms, the canthal tendon can be tucked or advanced with sutures placed into the periosteum. Alternatively, if periosteum is not present, a titanium screw can be positioned behind the anterior lacrimal crest to which the canthal tendons can be attached. For more severe cases transnasal wiring is most effective (Fig. 3.3). A hole is created behind the site of insertion of the canthal tendon. The tendon is then secured with a 30-gauge stainless steel wire that is passed transnasally. For bilateral cases, the wire will exit a similarly created hole in the bone on the opposite side; for unilateral cases, the wire passes through two small holes drilled just above the opposite medial canthal tendon and lacrimal sac.[3]

Abnormal insertion of the lateral canthal tendon may be due to deficiency of the tendon itself or to a faulty position of an otherwise normal tendon. In mild cases, a lateral canthopexy can be performed by suturing the lateral tarsus to the periosteum in the region of the lateral canthal tubercle. For a lateral dystopia of moderate severity, a tarsal strip procedure must be done. In more severe cases, the lateral canthal tendon or lateral tarsal strip must be

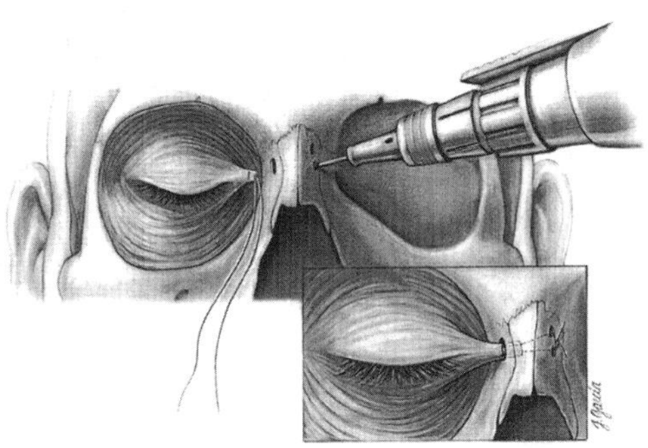

Figure 3.3. Transnasal wiring technique for medial canthopexy. The medial canthal tendon is isolated. Nasal osteotomies are drilled. The medial canthal tendon is secured with a 30-gauge wire.

secured with a stainless steel wire passed through two drilled holes positioned superiorly and directly behind the rim.

Surgical repair of telecanthus consists of separate approaches to the three soft tissue elements responsible for creating the deformity. The skin is most commonly repaired with a Y to V flap. The subcutaneous tissue and muscle are excised under direct visualization, and the medial canthal tendon is shortened by a tuck, resection, or transnasal wiring, as described previously. For larger folds, multiple Z-plasty techniques can be employed. It is important to excise the fibrous band of tissue that runs beneath the skin and muscle and contributes to the fold.

REFERENCES

1. Katowitz JA, Kropp TM. Congenital and developmental abnormalities of the orbit: Synophthalmos, anophthalmos, microphthalmos, cryptophthalmos. In *Oculoplastic, Orbital and Reconstructive Surgery*, vol 2, A. Hornblass, ed. Baltimore: Williams & Wilkins, 1990:817–825.
2. Foster JA, Katowitz JA. Embryology and anomalies of the eyelid, orbit, and lacrimal system. In *Surgery of the Eyelids, Orbit, and Lacrimal System,* vol 1, W. B. Stewart, ed. San Francisco: American Academy of Ophthalmology, 1993:100–124.
3. Katowitz JA, Hertle RW, Quinn GE. Ophthalmic management of craniofacial syndromes. In *Duane's Clinical Ophthalmology*, vol. 6, W. Tasman, ed. Philadelphia: Lippincott, 1993:1–31.

4

Colobomatous Microphthalmia, Anophthalmia, and Associated Malformation Syndromes

ELIAS I. TRABOULSI

Colobomatous malformations of the eye are present in 5%–10% of blind European children and in about 2% of blind adults. In a prospective study of 50,000 pregnancies in the United States, the incidence of microphthalmia/clinical anophthalmia was 0.22 per 1000 births; the incidence of coloboma was 0.26 per 1000.[87] From 0.6%–1.9% of blind adults have microphthalmia/coloboma,[21,124] and 3.2%–11.2% of blind children are microphthalmic.[62,66] Two percent of 650 severely or profoundly retarded institutionalized adults had microphthalmia or clinical anophthalmia.[108]

COLOBOMATOUS MALFORMATIONS

Microphthalmia

In microphthalmia the volume of the eye is reduced.[15,59,145] The term *microphthalmia* applies to globes with an anteroposterior diameter of less than 20 mm in adults (normal range: 21.50–27.00 mm).[59] Weiss and co-workers[219] provided normograms for axial length and anterior segment measurements in the first 10 years of life. These authors defined simple microphthalmos as an eye that is normal except for an axial length less than 2 standard deviations below the mean age-matched control measurement. The reduction in size of the eye varies from minimal to severe. In clinical anophthalmia, e.g., remnants of optic vesicle-derived structures may only be identified on serial histologic sections of the orbit.

Uveal Coloboma

Uveal colobomata were first reported by the Danish anatomist Bartholini[13] in 1657 in the course of his description of patients with the features of trisomy 13. Bartholini[14] later described a hereditary form of iris coloboma.

Colobomata (from the Greek *koloboma*, mutilation or defect) are defects in the iris (Fig. 4.1), ciliary body, choroid (Fig. 4.2), and/or optic nerve (see Chapter 7) and are generally located in the inferior or inferonasal portion of the globe along the line of closure of the embryonic fissure. The author prefers to reserve the term "optic nerve coloboma" to defects of the optic nerve head that result from

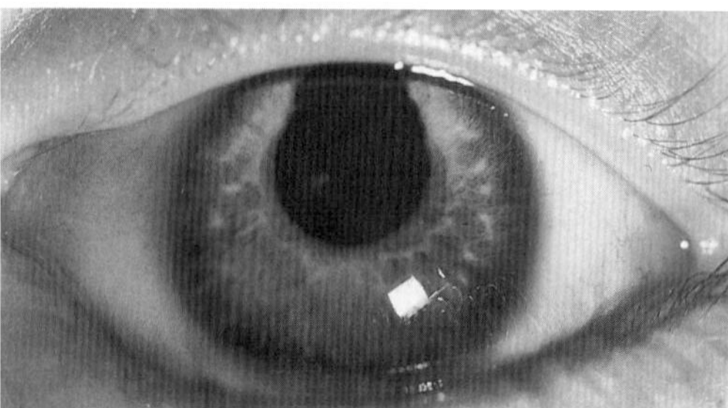

Figure 4.1. Typical iris coloboma in a patient with Lenz microphthalmia syndrome.

faulty closure of the embryonic fissure. Optic nerve colobomas are generally accompanied by colobomas of the uvea and retina (Fig. 4.3). Other more descriptive terms such as the morning glory disc anomaly, optic pit, contractile peripapillary staphyloma, and optic nerve dysplasia are used to describe the abnormalities that fit their individual diagnostic criteria.

OTHER MALFORMATIONS OF THE GLOBE

Anophthalmia

In true anophthalmia, there is complete failure of outgrowth of the primary optic vesicle[47]; or the optic vesicle has completely degenerated.

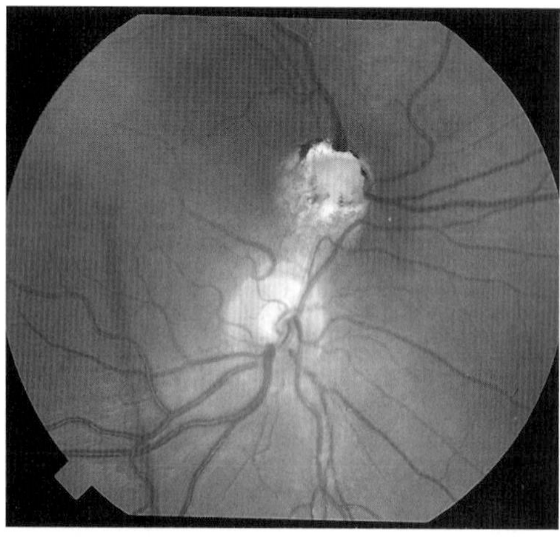

Figure 4.2. Localized typical inferior chorioretinal coloboma giving the false impression of duplication of the optic nerve head. (Courtesy of Dr. Maryam Aroichane.)

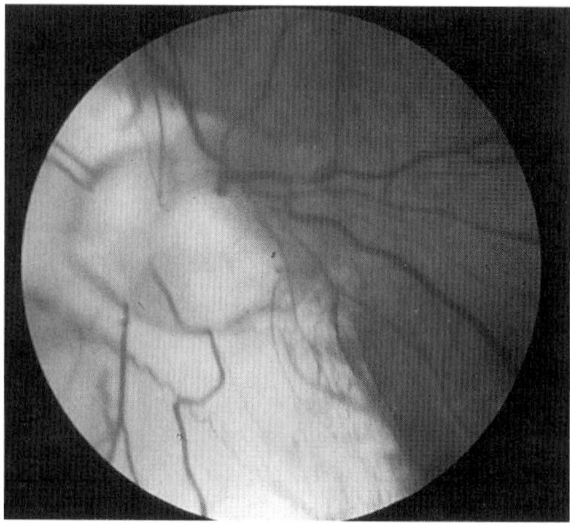

Figure 4.3. Large chorioretinal coloboma involving the optic nerve head in a patient with Lenz microphthalmia syndrome.

Cases where neural epithelial derivatives are found on histopathological examination of the orbit have been referred to as having extreme microphthalmia or clinical anophthalmia.[78] Clinical anophthalmia refers to the apparent absence of the globes in an orbit that otherwise contains normal adnexal elements (Fig. 4.4).

Nanophthalmos

In nanophthalmos (dwarfed eye) the eyes are deep set, and the palpebral fissures are narrow. There are no gross malformations of the globe. Axial length varies from 16 to 18 mm. There usually is a hyperopia of 15–20D. Nystagmus and strabismus are occasional findings.

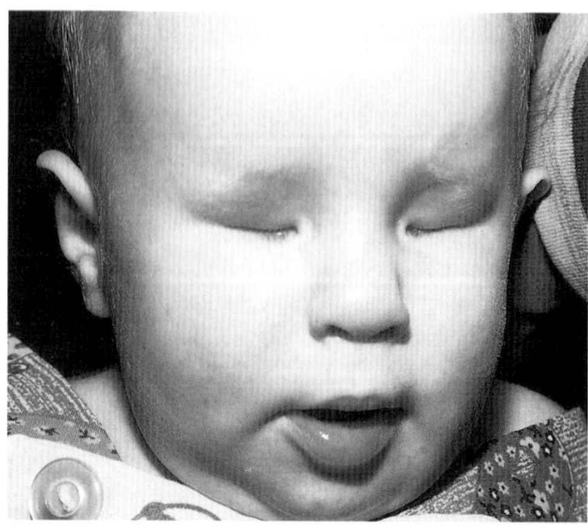

Figure 4.4. Bilateral clinical anophthalmia.

Visual acuity may be normal early in life but may be decreased if retinal complications occur. The anterior chamber is shallow and although the lens is of normal size, it is relatively large for the nanophthalmic globe. The retinal vessels may be tortuous and engorged. Some patients have poor macular development or a papillomacular fold[177] and a "heaped-up" optic nerve head. Uveal effusions can develop and subside spontaneously and lead to chorioretinal pigmentary changes and choroidal thickening. Some patients with nanophthalmos develop narrow-angle glaucoma because of the shallow antior chamber and the anterior displacement of the lens by the choroidal effusion. Brockhurst[27] advocated the use of vortex vein decompression for the treatment of nanophthalmic uveal effusions. This has been performed with variable success. Most cases are sporadic, but many are inherited in an autosomal recessive fashion[33,38,54,131,133,164,177] and rarely as dominant traits.[33,203]

Microphthalmia with Cyst

A condition closely related to typical colobomatous microphthalmia, in microphthalmia with cyst, the globe is small and there is an inferior uveoretinal coloboma. There is also a defect in the posterior aspect of the eye through which a cyst lined by neuroectodermally derived tissue protrudes into the orbit. The size of the cyst is variable: it may be small and able to be detected only on ultrasonography or orbital imaging (Fig. 4.5), or it may be large, producing a characteristic bulge in the lower lid and displacing the globe superonasally or inferotemporally. If the cyst enlarges, the proptosis may become more noticeable with time. Most cases are isolated, but familial occurrence has been reported in siblings with normal chromosomes[125,152] and in monozygous twins,[114] pointing to the genetic etiology of this likely autosomal recessive malformation syndrome. Furthermore, the malformation has been noted to be hereditary in certain stocks of laboratory animals[125] and in rabbits.[205] Unilateral and bilateral cases have been reported.[7] Fellow eyes may be normal, or microphthalmic, with or without cyst. Mann[126] attributes the development of the cyst to differential growth and differentiation of the inner and outer layers of the

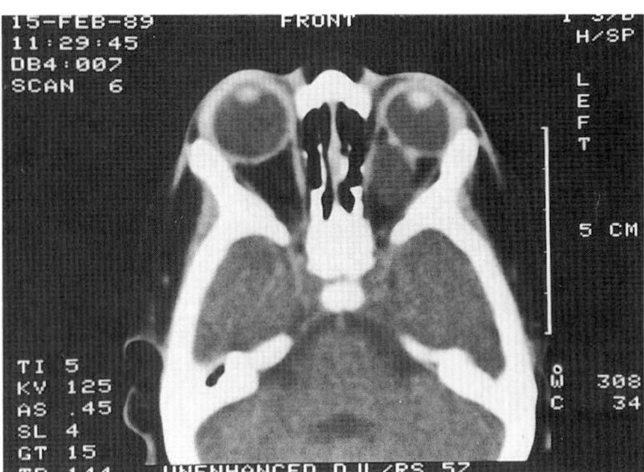

Figure 4.5. Computed tomography of the orbits in patient with left microphthalmia with cyst. There is an ophthalmoscopically visible direct communication between the microphthalmic eye and the cyst. (Courtesy of Dr. Deborah Alcorn.)

optic vesicle at the margin of the colobomatous defect. If there is eversion of the inner layer and differention into retinal tissue, a cyst is formed. Histologic studies show that the globe is malformed with thickening of the sclera and vascularization of the cornea. Anterior segment structures are undifferentiated. The retina is dysplastic with folds, neuroglial proliferation, and rosette formation. Ultrasonography and radioimaging are helpful in differentiating microphthalmia with cyst from orbital tumors, congenital cystic eye, meningocele, and orbital teratoma.[53,220,224] A number of management options exist depending on the degree of maldevelopment of the microphthalmic eye, the size of the cyst, and the cosmetic and functional status of the patient. Fluid from the cyst may be aspirated in cases where enlargement leads to significant proptosis. Excision of the cyst with or without preservation of the globe may also be performed along with the appropriate orbital and eyelid reconstruction procedures.

Congenital Cystic Eye

Congenital cystic eye should be differentiated from microphthalmos with cyst. A congenital cystic eye results from failure of invagination of the optic vesicle. The contralateral eye is usually normal[11,45,88,151,157,170] but may be microphthalmic with cyst.[216] The cyst may contain rosettes and undifferentiated retinal tissue or may simply consist of loculated cavities. The cyst may also contain lens material, and there may be upper eyelid skin tags.[45] Rice and coworkers[157] reported a child with a left cystic eye and a rudimentary limb attched to the lower lid. The cases of Dollfus et al.,[45] Rice et al., [157] and Pasquale et al.[147] all may have the oculocerebrocutaneous syndrome of Delleman.[4] Patients with this condition have intracranial cysts, agenesis of the corpus callosum, and dermal appendages associated with microphthalmia with cyst. Nonocular-associated abnormalities include agenesis of the corpus callosum[151,216] and facial clefting.[216] Goldberg and co-workers[73] reported postmortem findings in a child with midfacial clefting, basal encephalocele, and bilateral cystic eyes; serial orbital sections failed to show evidence of a microphthalmic eye. One of the cystic structures had enlarged and was excised at the age of 2 years.[111]

DIAGNOSIS AND CLINICAL FINDINGS

Microphthalmia can be unilateral (Fig. 4.6) or bilateral and may or may not be associated with uveal coloboma, hence the general classification into colobomatous and noncolobomatous categories. Asymmetric reduction in the volume of the eye is common in bilateral cases. Complicated microphthalmia refers to the association of a small eye with a variety of other ocular abnormalities such as corneal opacification, corectopia, aniridia, cataract, persistent hyperplastic primary vitreous, and retinal dysplasia.[126]

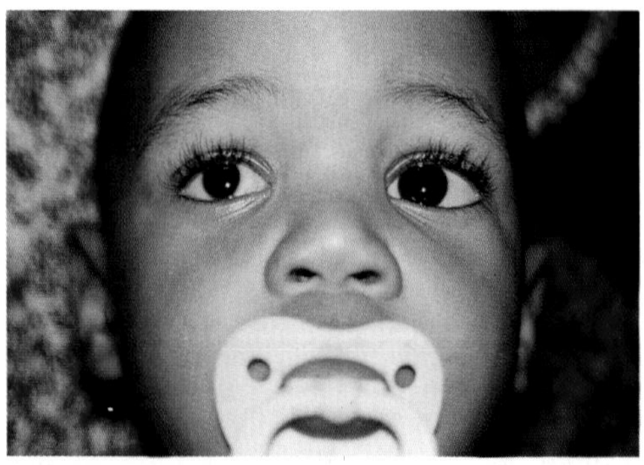

Figure 4.6. Unilateral colobomatous microphthalmia.

The diagnosis of microphthalmia can generally be made by clinical inspection. Palpating the globe through the closed lids gives an estimate of the size of the eyeball. Measurements of the anteroposterior diameter of the eye may be obtained using A-scan ultrasonography. The cornea is usually less than 10 mm in size in microphthalmic eyes but may be normal in simple microphthalmia[219] or in posterior microphthalmia.[177] Conversely, isolated microcornea can occur in the absence of microphthalmia or even with posterior macrophthalmia.[16] Weiss et al.[218] found small eyes in patients with achondroplasia, myotonic dystrophy, diabetic embryopathy, pseudo-trisomy 18, fetal alcohol syndrome, Maroteaux-Lamy syndrome, mucolipidosis III, isolated growth hormone deficiency, and mental retardation with radial ray defect. We have noted the presence of high hyperopia and crowded optic nerve heads in the mucopolysaccharidoses and in mucolipidosis III.[37,197] Weiss et al.[218] postulate that because the cornea is of near-adult size at birth, while the globe continues to enlarge, microcornea will only be found in conditions of prenatal onset such as malformation syndromes, whereas progressive postnatal diseases such as the mucopolysaccharidoses would be associated with a normal corneal diameter.

True or primary anophthalmos is extremely rare and results from failure of the optic vesicle to bud out from the cerebral vesicle; the optic nerves and tract are usually absent. In patients with secondary anophthalmos there may be associated forebrain malformations such as holoprosencephaly, and affected fetuses are usually aborted. Consecutive or degenerative anophthalmos results from regression or degeneration of the optic vesicle.

Any combination of uveal colobomatous defects may be present in the individual patient and within families. The lens may be cataractous, sometimes in the sector underlying an iris coloboma (Fig. 4.7). Familial microphthalmia and cataracts is well described in the literature[31,191,227] with either autosomal dominant, autosomal recessive, or X-linked recessive inheritance. Yokoyama and co-workers[225] reported a three-generation family with total cataracts, microphthalmia, and a translocation between chromosomes 2 and 16. These authors suggest

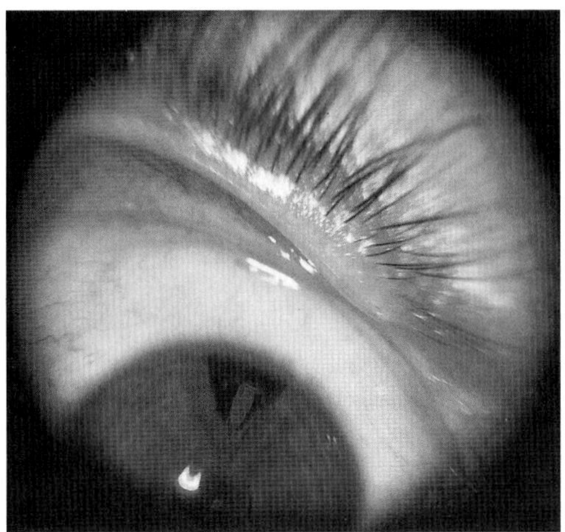

Figure 4.7. Inferonasal iris coloboma. There is a sectoral cataract in the area of the coloboma. The vision and the rest of the ocular and systemic examinations were normal.

that a gene located on 16p13.3 is reponsible for the abnormalities in this family.

Visual acuity depends on the extent of retinal involvement and on coexisting ocular pathology and amblyopia. Small iris or choroidal colobomas are compatible with excellent vision, whereas macular and optic nerve head involvement are indicative of poor visual prognosis. Microphthalmic eyes usually have high hyperopic refractive errors but are sometimes highly myopic because of staphyloma formation in the area of the coloboma. Maumenee and Mitchell[132] found that one-third of their 82 patients had visual acuity better than 20/40 in the better eye. It is wise not to make any predictions about visual acuity based on the fundus appearance in babies. Surprisingly good vision may be possible in moderately malformed globes while poor vision may be associated with unilateral, seemingly mild cases. In clinical anophthalmia the lids are structurally normal except for decreased horizontal dimension. Normal conjunctiva lines the inside of the lids and orbit and there is a functioning lacrimal gland. Rudiments of optic vesicle-derived structures and structures derived from mesoderm and/or neural crest may be found on histopathologic sectioning of the orbit in consecutive or degenerative anophthalmia but not in primary anophthalmos.[78,142,148,167] The orbit is shallow and orbital volume remains small with increasing age, apparently because of the absence of a trophic action of the globe on the orbit. Clinical anophthalmos may be unilateral or bilateral. When unilateral, there may be contralateral microphthalmia.

Large colobomata may produce a white pupillary reflex, and small round choroidal colobomas may look like white tumors, leading to diagnostic confusion with retinoblastoma in rare cases. Uncommon ocular complications of microphthalmia/coloboma include angle-closure glaucoma, subretinal neovascularization,[116] and rarely, retinal detachment.[100,132]

PATHOGENESIS

Typical (inferiorly located) colobomata result from faulty closure of the fetal fissure in the invaginated optic vesicle. The embryonic fissure begins to close at 4 weeks of gestation in the midperiphery of the developing globe and proceeds anteriorly and posteriorly. This process is usually completed by the sixth week of gestation. The inferior iris, ciliary body, choroid, and optic nerve are involved to the extent that the fissure has failed to close. A cyst may form in the area of defective closure and protrude out from the globe, leading to the microphthalmia with cyst.[120,216]

The pathogenesis of microphthalmia is unclear. A defect in the formation of the secondary vitreous has been postulated to result in a small globe because of the absence of expansive forces inside the eye.[219] Degeneration of the developing optic vesicle is also believed to be the cause of secondary or consecutive microphthalmia or anophthalmia.[126]

GENETICS AND ASSOCIATED CONDITIONS

Microphthalmia can be isolated, sporadic, or familial, or can occur in a number of single-gene, chromosomal, and embryopathic multisystem malformation syndromes (Table 4.1).[60] A specific diagnosis can be established in 20%–45% of cases.[132,168,174,211,227] Advances in chromosomal studies, the publication of rare syndromes, and the advances in the clinical

Table 4.1. A Practical Classification of Colobomatous Microphthalmia

Isolated
Microphthalmia (AD)
Colobomatous
Isolated uveoretinal coloboma
Microphthalmia with cyst
Noncolobomatous

Microphthalmia with Ocular Anomalies
Microphthalmia with cataract (AD, AR)
Microphthalmia with myopia and corectopia (AD)
Microphthalmia with ectopia lentis
Microphthalmia with congenital retinal detachment (AR)
Persistent hyperplastic primary vitreous (sporadic)
Aicardi syndrome

Microphthalmia with Mental Retardation
Microphthalmia with mental retardation (AD, AR, XR)
Microphthalmia with mental retardation and congenital spastic diplegia (Sjögren-Larsson)

Microphthalmia with Craniofacial Malformations
Facio-auriculo-vertebral sequence
Hallermann-Streiff syndrome
Amniotic band syndrome
Transverse facial cleft
Microphthalmia with cleft lip/palate
Microphthalmia with microcephaly
Microphthalmia with microcephaly and retinal folds (XR, AR)
Microphthalmia with hydrocephalus and congenital retinal nonattachment (Warburg syndrome)
Linear nevus sebaceous of Jadassohn

Microphthalmia with Malformations of the Hands and Feet
Microphthalmia with polydactyly
Waardenburg anophthalmia syndrome (AR)
Subgroup of CHARGE association (bifid thumbs)

Microphthalmia with Multiple Congenital Anomalies (Syndromes)
CHARGE association
Lenz microphthalmia syndrome (XR)
Oculo-dento-osseous dysplasia (AD, AR)
Cryptophthalmos or Frasier syndrome (AR)
Cerebro-oculo-facial syndrome or COFS (AR)
Goltz syndrome or focal dermal hypoplasia (XD)
Lowe syndrome (XR)
Meckel-Gruber syndrome (AR)
Basal cell nevus syndrome of Gorlin-Goltz (AD)
Congenital contractural arachnodactyly (AD)
Rubinstein-Taybi syndrome
Cross syndrome (AR)
Fanconi syndrome (AR)
Diamond-Blackfan syndrome (AR)
Epidermal nevus syndrome
Branchio-oculo-facial syndrome (AD)
Aicardi syndrome (XD)

Microphthalmia in Chromosomal Anomalies
Trisomy 13 (Patau)
4p− (Wolf-Hirschhorn)
18q−
18r
Trisomy 18 (Edward)
Cat-eye syndrome (marker 22)
Other chromosomal aberrations (see ref. 18)

Microphthalmia and Intrauterine Insults
Maternal drug intake: thalidomide, alcohol, isotretinoin, others
Maternal vitamin A deficiency
Maternal fever or radiation exposure
Maternal uncontrolled phenylketonuria
Intrauterine infections: CMV, EBV, varicella, herpes simplex, rubella, toxoplasmosis

AD = autosomal dominant; AR = autosomal recessive; XR = X-linked recessive; XD = X-linked dominant.

workup of patients with malformation syndromes have led to improved diagnostic precision.[211] Sjögren and Larsson[174] reviewed the medical records of 137 patients with microphthalmia. They identified three families with X-linked, four with autosomal dominant, and four with presumed autosomal recessive inheritance. In that article they proposed that the syndrome of microphthalmia, mental retardation, and spastic cerebral palsy that now bears their name was distinct. Warburg[212] studied 86 patients with mental retardation and microphthalmia and/or coloboma. Sixteen patients had prenatal infections, 6 had chromosomal abnormalities, and 36 had combinations of malformations that had been previously described.[212] Maumenee and Mitchell[132] reviewed the data on 82 patients from 69 families with colobomatous microphthalmia. Ocular complications in their series include retinal detachment in two patients and presenile cataracts in six. Identifiable syndromes were diagnosed in 28 patients. Five had chromosomal abnormalities including two cases of 4p−, two of trisomy 13 and one of XXXY. There were eight pedigrees where the mode of inheritance could be determined: five were autosomal dominant and three were presumably autosomal recessive. From their data, Maumenee and Mitchell[132] calculated an empirical risk of 9% for a subsequent child to be affected if both parents were normal and there were no affected siblings. The risk increased to 46% if one parent was affected. In a review of 1313 cases of microphthalmia/coloboma, Fujiki and co-workers[66] found that 15% were autosomal recessive, 22% were autosomal dominant, and the rest were sporadic. Diagnostic precision is generally maximized by complete family history and examination, and by ancillary laboratory testing and karyotyping.[211]

Autosomal Dominant Nonsyndromal Colobomatous Microphthalmia

Autosomal dominant microphthalmia/coloboma may be isolated or may be associated with congenital cataracts,[35] or with myopia and ectopic pupils.[201] Variable expressivity is the rule in familial cases, with some patients having severe microphthalmos and others having only small asymptomatic uveal colobomata in normal-sized eyes.[57] Hence the importance of ocular examination of all family members of seemingly isolated cases in order to establish the possible mode of inheritance. Because of incomplete penetrance, Fujiki and co-workers[66] estimated that, in families with dominant microphthalmia/coloboma, unaffected individuals have an 8.6% chance of having an affected offspring.

Autosomal Dominant Nonsyndromal Pure Microphthalmia

There are a few reports of autosomal dominant noncolobomatous or pure microphthalmia.[58,203] Vingolo and co-workers[203] described 14 affected members of a four-generation Italian family with reduced total axial length of the eye (18.4–19.7 mm) and microcornea (8.0–9.7 mm). Five patients were examined and had varying degrees of hyperopia, choroidal thickening, glaucoma, nystagmus, visual loss, and corneal opacification. Symptoms started in the first decade of life and patients lost vision from complications of glaucoma. This family appears to have a dominant form of nanophthalmos, a condition that is most often inherited in an autosomal recessive fashion.

Autosomal Recessive Nonsyndromal Microphthalmia/Anophthalmia

When inherited, isolated anophthalmos is usually autosomal recessive.[41,110] This disorder has been reported in Arab isolates,[110,189] in the Amish,[38] and in some Brazilian isolates.[41] Patients have bilateral severe microphthalmia or clinical anophthalmia in the absence of other systemic malformations. The occurrence in inbred pedigrees is highly supportive of autosomal recessive inheritance. Zlotogora and co-workers[228] reported five families with autosomal recessive colobomatous micropthalmia and stated that the gene for this condition has a high frequency among Iranian Jews.

Hereditary Posterior Microphthalmos with Papillomacular Fold and High Hyperopia

This autosomal recessive condition[177] is most likely related to, or allelic with, nanophthalmos.

X-Linked Recessive Microphthalmia

Colobomatous microphthalmia may be inherited in an X-linked recessive fashion and is frequently accompanied by mental retardation.[174] The Lenz microphthalmia syndrome[117,196] is described in more detail later in this chapter. The family reported by Hoefnagel and co-workers[92] probably has the Lenz syndrome.

CHROMOSOMAL ABNORMALITIES

A large number of chromosomal abnormalities have been associated with uveal coloboma, microphthalmia, anophthalmia, or any combination thereof. Warburg and Friedrich[215] reviewed the chromosomal abnormalities associated with microphthalmia/coloboma until 1987 and provided an extensive bibliography on the subject. Some of these chromosomal defects are more common than others and are associated with consistent phenotypes. These include trisomy 13, trisomy 22 (cat-eye syndrome), 4p− (Wolff-Hirschhorn syndrome), 11q−, 13q−, 18q−, ring 18, trisomy 18, and Klinefelter syndrome (XXY). These chromosomal syndromes are reviewed in detail in Chapter 30.

Microphthalmia with Linear Skin Defects

Al-Gazali et al.[5] described two female patients with de novo X;Y translocations and irregular linear areas of erythematous skin hypoplasia involving the head and neck. These patients had microphthalmia, corneal opacities, and orbital cysts. This syndrome was initially considered to be distinct from focal dermal hypoplasia (Goltz syndrome) (vide infra) and from incontinentia pigmenti. The breakpoint in the X chromosome was at Xp22.3 in both females. Al-Gazali et al.[5] suggested that deletion or disruption of DNA sequences in the region of Xp22.3 was responsible for the clinical manifestations of the syndrome. Temple and co-workers[190] reported a third case with a terminal deletion of Xp22.2-pter. Another patient was described by Allanson and Richter.[6] This infant died of severe respiratory distress from a diaphragmatic hernia. At autopsy there was absence of the septum pellucidum and an ectopic area of gray and white matter. The mother had an identical terminal deletion of the X chromosome with the breakpoint at Xp22.2; she was of normal intelligence but she was short and had depigmented skin patches and unerupted wisdom teeth. This X-linked dominant syndrome is presumably lethal in the hemizygous male. Happle et al.[83] proposed the name MIDAS syndrome (microphthalmia, dermal aplasia, and sclerocornea). Using cell lines from affected patients with MLS and from patients with ocular albinism, Wapenaar et al.[208] determined that MLS was proximal to OA1. These authors also pointed out that some features of MLS such as retinal lacunae, agenesis of the corpus callosum, costovertebral abnormalities, mental retardation, and seizures overlap with those of Aicardi and Goltz syndromes, suggesting that different defects in the same gene may be responsible for these three disorders.

MONOGENIC DISORDERS WITH MICROPHTHALMIA

In some of these syndromes, colobomatous microphthalmia is a major and most often constant feature of the syndrome, whereas in other syndromes the ocular malformation is an inconsistent finding and may not be required for the clinical diagnosis. Table 4.1 lists syndromes where colobomatous microphthalmia has been reported. This chapter covers only conditions where microphthalmia is a relatively common or a major diagnostic feature.

Lenz Microphthalmia Syndrome

The Lenz microphthalmia syndrome[117] is inherited in an X-linked recessive fashion and is characterized by microphthalmos or clinical anophthalmos in all patients, developmental delay in 92% of patients, abnormal ears and microcephaly in 83%, skeletal abnormalities such as a barrel chest and clavicular malformations and dental abnormalities in two-thirds of patients, urogenital anomalies and digital anomalies such as clinodactyly or duplication of the thumb in about 50% of cases, and cleft lip/palate in one-third of patients.[196] The diagnosis should be considered in boys with microphthalmia and skeletal or urogenital malformations.

X-Linked Microphthalmia and Mental Retardation

Cuendet[39] described a family with X-linked microphthalmia and mental retardation. There were no associated congenital malformations except for a cleft palate in one patient. A girl in the youngest generation had bilateral embryonal cataracts but no microphthalmia or retardation. The author postulates that the cataracts are more likely a sign of partial expression of the X-linked microphthalmia gene than a coincidental finding.

Waardenburg Recessive Anophthalmia Syndrome

Waardenburg recessive anophthalmia syndrome is characterized by mental retardation, unilateral or bilateral clinical absence of the globe, distal limb abnormalities in the form of syndactyly, camptodactyly or hypodactyly, and other inconsistently present malformations such as widely spaced nipples and genitourinary malformations.[158,199,206]

Matthew-Wood Syndrome

This autosomal recessive disease combines anophthalmia and pulmonary hypoplosia. It has been reported in isolated cases and in sibs.[168a]

Goltz Syndrome (Focal Dermal Hypoplasia)

The constellation of abnormalities that constitute this X-linked dominant syndrome was first outlined by Goltz and colleagues[74] in 1962. The characteristic focal skin lesions consist of streaks of dermal hypoplasia that appear reddish-brown and of a different hue than the surrounding skin (Fig. 4.8). Telangiectasias and nodules of herniated fat may be covered by thin strands of connective tissue. The skin lesions are usually present at birth as a generalized and erosive dermatosis of blisters and crusts. The nails may be dystrophic or absent and there is marked hypoplasia of the teeth with late eruption and irregular placement. Syndactyly of the fingers and toes, especially the third and fourth fingers, is common. Papillomatous lesions are present on the lips. Short stature, joint hypermobility, congenital heart defects, partial alopecia, digital anomalies, and microcephaly are less frequent findings. Intelligence varies from normal to severely curtailed. The variability in clinical manifestations is presumed to be the result of differential X chromosome inactivation.[217]

One of Goltz's original patients had optic atrophy, a lack of retinal pigmentation, nystagmus, and esotropia. A second patient had colobomas of the iris, choroidal sclerosis, and strabismus.[74] Seven of 12 patients reviewed by Holden and Akers[93] had microphthalmia.

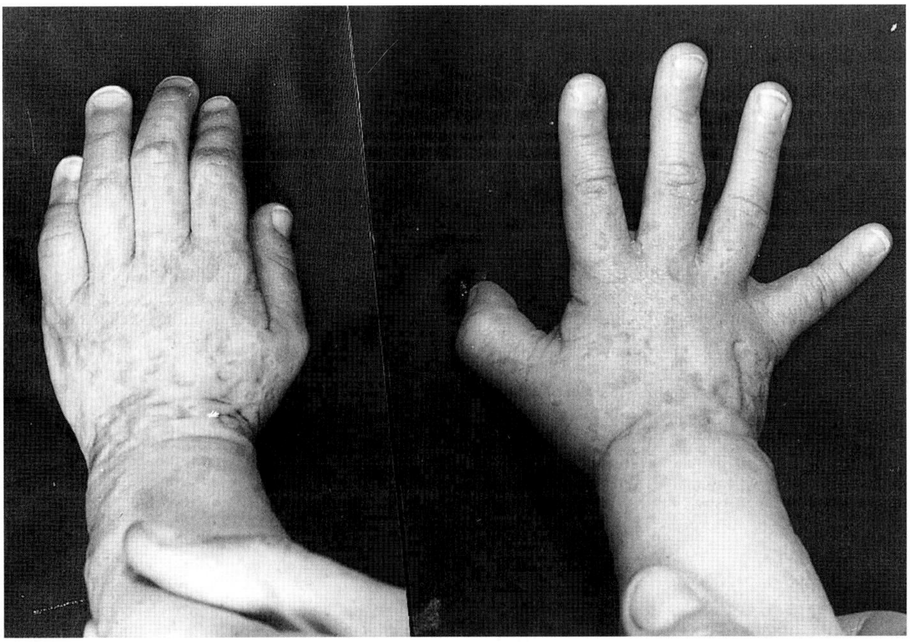

Figure 4.8. Punched-out cutaneous lesions of focal dermal hypoplasia. (Courtesy of Drs. Linn Murphree and Irene H. Maumenee.)

There are many similarities between the Gorlin-Goltz syndrome and incontinentia pigmenti but the dermal lesions are not thin in the latter disorder. Congenital poikiloderma (Thomson syndrome) is a dermatosis that eventually leaves the skin shiny and atrophic with prominent telangiectasia. Linear brown pigment may even be present in Thomson syndrome, but this is due to epidermal atrophy rather than hypoelastic collagen.

Branchio-Oculo-Facial Syndrome

This autosomal dominant malformation syndrome is characterized by the presence of pathognomonic cervical/infra-auricular skin defects. Forty-three reported patients have been reviewed by Lin and co-workers.[123] The cutaneous defects have aplastic, hemangiomatous or otherwise abnormal overlying skin, and draining sinus fistulas. The severity of clinical involvement is variable and atypical cases constitute about 10% of reported patients.[123] Renal malformations are frequent. Cardiac and central nervous system defects are rare. Developmental delay, hypotonia, and visual, hearing, and speech problems are common. There is some overlap with the branchio-oto-renal syndrome.

Microphthalmia, anophthalmia, and colobomas are present in about 50% of cases. Nasolacrimal duct obstruction with recurrent dacryocystitis occurs in 75% of patients. Two patients in the series of Lin and co-workers[123] had severe anterior segment malformations. Occasional patients have orbital dermoids.

Sjögren-Larsson Syndrome

The Sjögren-Larsson syndrome is inherited in an autosomal recessive manner. Most cases have family origin in northern Sweden but have been reported in other populations. The disease is frequent in the Haliwa triracial isolate group in North Carolina among whom intermarriage is common. In Northern Sweden the prevalence of the disease varies between 0.4 and 8.3 per 100,000 persons, and the frequency of gene carriers varies between 0.5% and 2.0%.[97]

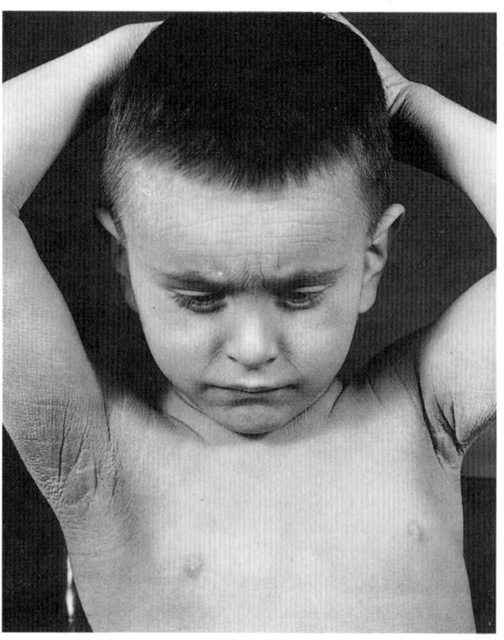

Figure 4.9. Five-year-old boy with Sjögren-Larsson syndrome. The child is mentally retarded. There is ichthyosis involving the axilla and the forehead. (Courtesy of Drs. Linn Murphree and Irene H. Maumenee.)

The syndrome has three cardinal signs: congenital ichthyosis, severe mental retardation, and spastic diplegia (Fig. 4.9).[175] Glistening macular "dots" have been observed in many cases (Fig. 4.10). At birth, the skin changes may look like congenital ichthyosiform erythroderma. There is lifelong scaling and hyperkeratosis over most of the body. Spastic diplegia is noted before the age of 3 years. The mental retardation may be severe. Jagell et al.[98] found bright glistening intraretinal dots in all 35 Swedish patients with the Sjögren-Larsson syndrome. The youngest patient was 1 year old at the time of the examination and the oldest was 57 years old. Because of the severe mental retardation, accurate visual acuity measurements were not possible. The fundus findings were identical in all 35 patients. The number of dots varied from 5 to 50 per patient; they were of irregular shape and size and were nonconfluent. The number and size of the dots are unrelated to age, severity of the retardation, or spasticity. All patients had marked photopho-

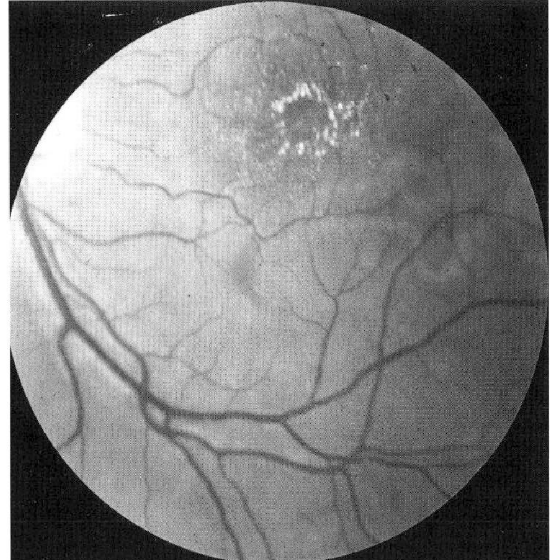

Figure 4.10. Glistening dots in the fovea of a 42-year-old man with Sjögren-Larsson syndrome. (Courtesy Dr. Jagell, reprinted with permission from Jagell et al.[98])

bia. The electrooculogram was normal in 2 patients. The electroretinogram has been also reported as normal. Gilbert et al.[69] described punched-out macular lesions in both eyes of one patient who also had glistening dots. Jagell et al.[98] found corneal changes in 16 of the 35 patients. These findings were symmetrical and varied in severity from punctate epithelial erosions to gray stromal opacities with vascularization. The corneal changes were usually in lower half of the cornea and in the anterior stroma (Fig. 4.11). Photophobia in all patients is as likely a result of punctate keratitis, as part of the generalized epithelial disease.

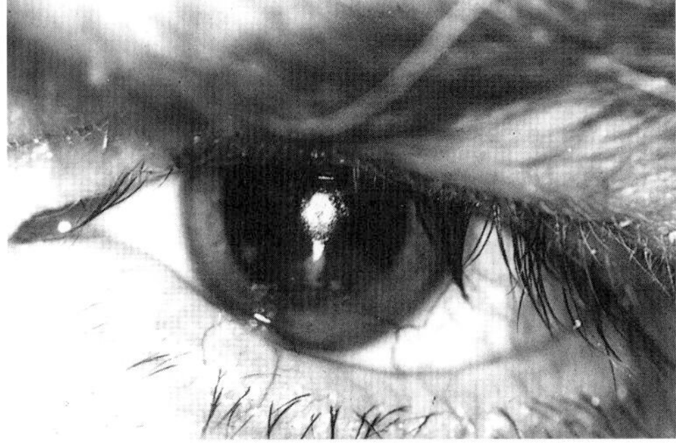

Figure 4.11. Gray corneal opacities in a 58-year-old patient with Sjögren-Larsson syndrome. There was ichthyosis around the eye and a punctate keratitis. (Courtesy Dr. Jagell, reprinted with permission from Jagell et al.[98])

The diagnosis is clinical. Neuroimaging does not assist in making the diagnosis,[153] and no specific treatment is available. The severe mental retardation and spasticity may require institutionalization. Survival into old age is not uncommon.[175]

Warburg Syndrome

Warburg[210] delineated a syndrome of congenital hydrocephalus, mental retardation, microphthalmos, and congenital retinal nonattachment or retinal dysplasia. She found 15 similar cases in the literature and suggested a genetic etiology. Numerous cases have been reported since and because of the association with a Dandy-Walker malformation of the brain in some patients, the eponym Walker-Warburg syndrome is sometimes applied to this autosomal recessive condition.

Aicardi Syndrome

About 200 cases of Aicardi syndrome are on record in the world literature. This syndrome, first described by the French radiologist Jean Aicardi in 1965 and later in 1969,[1,2] is characterized by a triad of infantile flexion spasms, structural brain abnormalities, the most consistent of which is partial or complete absence of the corpus callosum, and typical "lacunar" chorioretinal lesions.[46] A number of other congenital malformations may also be present including costovertebral defects in the form of hemivertebrae or butterfly vertebrae, absent or abnormal ribs, cleft lip and/or palate, hiatal hernia, hip dysplasia, postaxial polydactyly (personal observation), and precocious puberty. A few patients have developed tumors: choroid plexus papillomas in five, teratoma of the soft palate in one, and embryonal carcinoma of the cheek in one.[187]

Seizures develop in the first year of life and may disappear later. Flexion contracture spasms are typically seen; however, grand mal seizures, staring spells, or twitching may be the presenting neurologic symptoms. Patients may initially present because of developmental delay or even because of poor vision. Neuroimaging studies reveal partial or total absence of the corpus callosum, cortical heterotopias, abnormal ventricular system, and frequently severe posterior fossa malformations like hypoplasia of the vermis or Dandy-Walker cyst formation. Choroid plexus cysts and papillomas have been observed in a few patients with Aicardi syndrome. Characteristic electroencephalographic findings with hypsarrhythmias and dissociation between the two hemispheres are often present.

The chorioretinal lesions of Aicardi syndrome are characteristic and their presence often leads to the correct diagnosis. The lesions are round, well-defined, excavated (lacunar), with minimal pigmentation along their edges, and most frequently found around the optic nerve head and in the posterior pole (Figs. 4.12, 4.13). The lesions decrease in size and number towards the peripheral fundus. Electroretinographic studies are normal or minimally disturbed. Ocular histopathology in one case reveals abnormalities of retinal architecture with anterior displacement of retinal insertion, areas of atrophy and hyperplasia and migration of the retinal pigment epithelium, and photoreceptor rosette formation; the sensory retina may be completely absent in the "lacunae."[43] Thus the ocular findings are most consistent with a hypoplastic/dysplastic process involving the retina and retinal pigment epithelium. Other associated ocular malformations include microphthalmos, typical chorioretinal colobomata at the disc or elsewhere in the inferior fundus, gliosis at the nerve head, persistence of the hyaloid system of blood vessels, persistence of the pupillary membrane, posterior synechiae, retinal detachment, nystagmus, and sixth cranial nerve palsy.

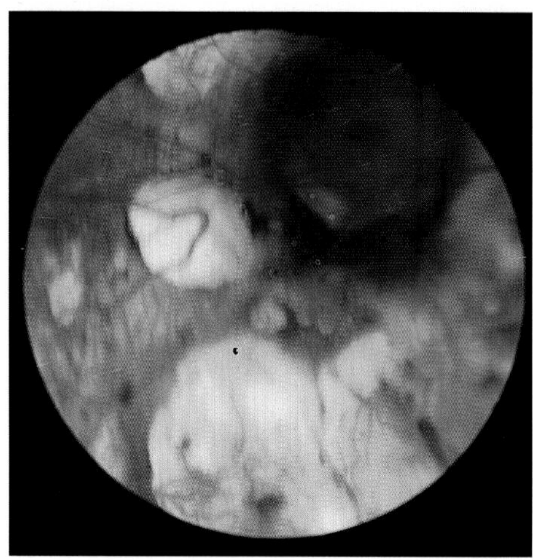

Figure 4.13. Characteristic lacunae and optic nerve head pigmentation and coloboma in a girl with Aicardi syndrome. (Courtesy of the late Dr. David Friendly.)

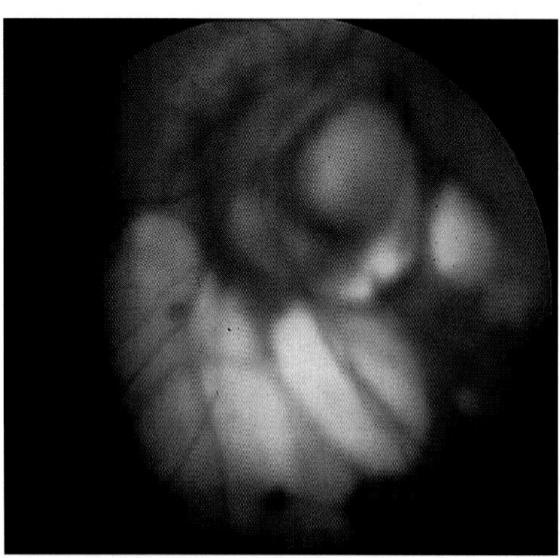

Figure 4.12. Optic nerve coloboma and retinal lacunar defects in a patient with Aicardi syndrome. (Courtesy of Dr. Irene H. Maumenee.)

Aicardi syndrome results from mutations in an X-linked dominant gene. All reported patients, except for one or two, have been females. Affected male fetuses are aborted. Only one pair of sisters have been reported; the remaining cases are thought to result from new mutations. One patient had a balanced X/3 translocation with a breakpoint at Xp22 suggesting that the Aicardi gene may be at that location.[162]

A definite diagnosis requires presence of the three major features: (*1*) infantile spasms or seizure activity, (*2*) absent corpus callosum, usually with other brain malformations, and (*3*) characteristic ocular fundus chorioretinal lacunae. Other congenital malformations may or may not be present.

The chorioretinal lesions in Aicardi syndrome may be confused with fundus lesions of congenital toxoplasmosis, prompting the search for other evidence of intrauterine infection; the absence of florid RPE hyperplasia along the margins of the lesions, their characteristic appearance and location around the disc, and the rest of the clinical and neuroradiologic findings allow differentiation between the two conditions. DeMorsier syndrome with optic nerve hypoplasia or dysplasia and absence of the septum pellucidum or corpus callosum may be confused with Aicardi syndrome; however, males and females are equally affected in DeMorsier syndrome and the brain malformations are much less severe than in Aicardi syndrome. In the Miller-Dieker syndrome, cerebral dysgenesis and type I lissencephaly (thickened cortex with four rather than six cell layers) and infantile spasms occur in association with a chromosome 17p abnormality (monosomy) in some patients. The corpus callosum may be absent. Patients with this syndrome, however, have a characteristic physiognomy with a small anteverted nose, a high forehead, and vertical forehead soft tissue ridging. The Miller-Dieker syndrome is thought to be one of the contiguous gene syndromes. Finally, the Warburg syndrome combines severe brain and eye malformations with death in the neonatal period in the majority of affected individuals. The Warburg syndrome is autosomal recessive. Brain malformations in this syndrome include agyria, pachygyria, cerebellar hypoplasia, occipital encephalocele, Dandy-Walker cyst, and hydrocephalus. Ocular abnormalities may be severe and include microphthalmia, retinal detachment with dysplasia, Peters' anomaly, cataracts, and persistent hyperplastic primary vitreous. The typical chorioretinal lacunar lesions of Aicardi syndrome are not found in either the Miller-Dieker or Warburg syndromes.

Most patients with Aicardi syndrome die in the first decade of life, usually from recurrent pneumonia and debilitation. One patient survived to 15 years of age. Treatment consists of antiepileptic medications and general supportive measures. Seizure activity is often difficult to control despite multidrug use; ACTH is probably the most effective antiepileptic agent in Aicardi syndrome.

Genetic counseling should emphasize the unlikelihood of a couple having another affected child. However, if a maternal balanced chromosomal abnormality is found, the risk of another affected female child increases to 50%.

X-Linked Microcephaly, Microphthalmia, Anterior Segment Abnormalities, and Brain and Urogenital Malformations

Duker and co-workers[48] reported a family with an X-linked recessive syndrome of severe brain malformations, microcephaly, microphthalmia, ptosis, anterior segment malformations, and urogenital defects. There was absence of the corpus callosum and ventriculomegaly. Histopathological examination of the eyes revealed retinal dysplasia, anterior segment disorganization, and cataracts. Chromosomal studies were normal. This syndrome appears to be distinct from Norrie disease (also see Chapter 38),[209] from the syndrome reported by Jarmas and coworkers[99] and by Young et al.[226] and from the autosomal recessive cerebro-oculo-facio-skeletal (COFS) syndrome.[77,149] The patients in the family reported by Siber[172] most likely have the same condition.

Microcephaly, Microphthalmos, and Retinal Folds

Jarmas and co-workers[99] described two brothers with severe microcephaly, microphthalmos, and retinal folds. Young et al.[226] described another patient with the same constellation of findings. In both families, the mothers had microcephaly and mental retardation. The sister of the patient reported by Young et al. also had mild manifestations of the disease. This could be a distinct X-linked recessive syndrome with manifesting female carriers or could be allelic with classic Norrie disease. A mutation in the Norrie disease gene has been found in the family initially reported by Godel and Goodman[71] to have X-linked recessive primary retinal dysplasia with mild findings in carrier females. Gartner[67] reported a male child born to consanguineous parents. It is more likely that this patient has the same X-linked disease. The differential diagnosis of falciform retinal folds includes retinopathy of prematurity, Norrie disease, familial exudative vitreoretinopathy, Warburg syndrome, and ocular toxocariasis.

MICROPHTHALMIA AND OCULAR DISEASES

A number of ocular phenotypes have been associated with microphthalmia, uveal coloboma, or a combination of both. These ocular syndromes are undoubtedly genetically and etiologically heterogeneous. We will discuss some of the more common ones that feature microphthalmia in a significant proportion of cases.

Persistent Hyperplastic Primary Vitreous (PHPV)

PHPV[156] is a complex malformation of the eye affecting mostly the vitreous but also the retina, ciliary body, iris, and lens. PHPV is characterized by the presence of remnants of the hyaloid system of blood vessels and by the presence of a plaque of fibrovascular tissue behind the lens.[79,223] Elongated ciliary processes converge to, and are pulled toward, the retrolental fibrovascular tissue (Fig. 4.14). The eye is variably reduced in size and a cataract may be present. Anterior and posterior varieties of PHPV have been described.[154,155] Both appear to be on the same continuum of malformations. Although some authors have included the morning glory disc anomaly (MGDA) under the general heading of PHPV[165] and other authors have erroneously labeled cases of MGDA as posterior PHPV,[36] this author believes that MGDA is a well-defined clinical entity of separate etiology that may, in some cases, have remnants of the hyaloid system of blood vessels in its center.[29,200] Congenital falciform fold of the retina may be a manifestation of a posterior form a PHPV.

PHPV is unilateral in about 90% of cases. The size of the globe varies from normal to moderately decreased, being slightly smaller than normal in the majority of cases. The cornea is clear. The anterior chamber is shallow in smaller eyes because of anterior displacement of the iris/lens diaphragm; this predisposes patients with PHPV to angle-closure glaucoma, which usually develops later in life. Some authors advocate lens extraction to prevent secondary angle-closure glaucoma. The iris may be normal but frequently shows small notches at the pupillary margins where iridohyaloidal vessels coursed in the developing eye and failed to regress with maturation of iris structures and disappearance of the tunica vasculosa lentis. Iridohyaloidal vessels persist and run over the anterior iris surface and over the pupillary margin and posterior iris surface to anastomose with vessels in the retrolental membrane (Fig. 4.15). It is thought that such iridohyaloidal vessels are extremely suggestive of PHPV[134]; their presence in a small eye with

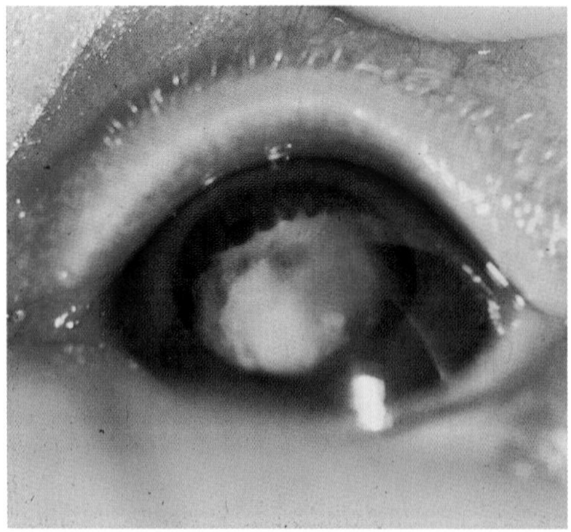

Figure 4.14. Cataract and elongated ciliary processes in a patient with persistent hyperplasia of the primary vitreous. (Courtesy of Drs. Terrence O'Brien and Morton F. Goldberg.)

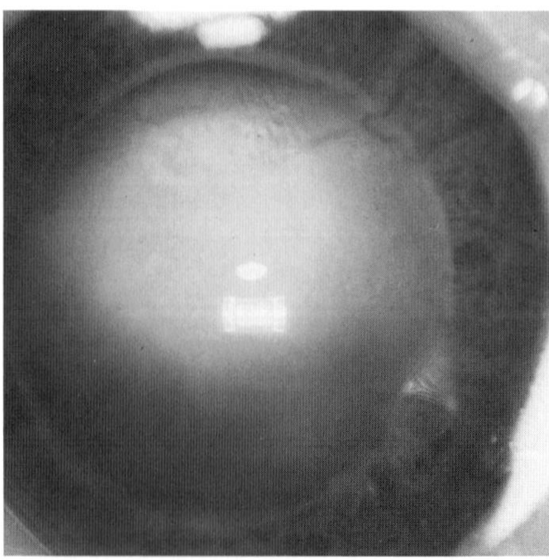

Figure 4.15. Retrolental membrane and iridohyaloidal vessels in a patient with persistent hyperplasia of the primary vitreous. (Courtesy of Drs. Terrence O'Brien and Morton F. Goldberg.)

a white pupillary reflex is diagnostic of this condition. The lens may be completely clear or may be cataractous. The fibrovascular plaque may adhere to the posterior lens capsule and vessels can invade the lens giving a clinical picture very characteristic of PHPV. The retrolental membrane may contain adipose tissue, cartilage, and smooth muscle tissue.[55] This is thought to be the result of metaplastic changes in tissue of mesenchymal origin. In a series of 47 eyes, Font et al.[55] found adipose tissue in 10 and cartilage in 1. The ciliary processes are usually elongated and attached to the retrolental membrane that seems to draw them centrally. The peripheral retina may also be drawn anteriorly into the retrolental membrane. In what has been referred to as "posterior PHPV," the retina around the disc is pulled up into the posterior vitreous and is thrown in folds that may involve the macula and lead to poor vision (Fig. 4.16). The retina may have dysplastic changes.[22] Vitreoretinal traction can lead to retinal breaks and detachment. The fellow eye in PHPV is generally normal but may have a Mittendorf dot or, rarely, one of a number of abnormalities.[10,65]

Patients with PHPV present with one of three findings: (*1*) a small eye since birth, (*2*) a white pupillary reflex because of the associated cataract or retrolental membrane, and/or (*3*) strabismus because of poor vision. Ultrasonography and computed tomography are helpful in the differentiation between PHPV and retinoblastoma in eyes with leukocoria. There is no intraocular calcification in PHPV, and the retrolental mass and/or retinal detachment can be visualized by ultrasonography and by computed tomography with contrast enhancement.[72] Retinoblastoma generally occurs in eyes of normal size but has been rarely reported in a microphthalmic eye. Additionally, PHPV and retinoblastoma have rarely coexisted in a microphthalmic eye.[96,119,141]

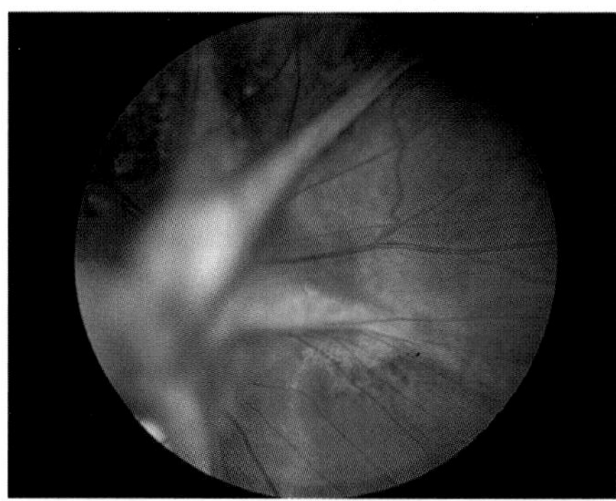

Figure 4.16. Persistent hyperplasia of the primary vitreous. Retinal folds are pulled up around the nerve into a stalk that was attached to the posterior aspect of the disc.

The incidence of PHPV is unknown, but this is not an extremely rare condition. PHPV is generally isolated and unilateral without associated congenital malformations. It has, however, been reported in a patient with oculo-dento-osseous dysplasia,[195] in one patient with protein C deficiency,[89] and in the oculo-palato-cerebral syndrome.[64] There is also one report of a family with Rieger anomaly and PHPV in two generations.[181]

PHPV may be due to a defect in formation of the secondary vitreous that is derived from the inner retinal cells starting in the ninth week of gestation. The secondary vitreous fills the developing fetal eye starting from the ocular wall region and progressing centrally. It compresses the regressing primary vitreous, which is derived from mesenchyme, and contains the hyaloid system of blood vessels that anastomoses with the tunica vasculosa lentis anteriorly. A defect in the formation of the secondary vitreous, failure of regression of the primary vitreous and of the tunica vasculosa lentis, or a combination of both mechanisms may lead to the clinical picture of PHPV. The globe remains small because its growth depends partly on the expansion of the secondary vitreous. Precipitating factors and etiologic agents leading to PHPV have not been identified yet. PHPV has been reported in dizygotic twins,[207] in two brothers,[135] and in a mother and son.[121]

Visual prognosis in eyes with PHPV is generally guarded. Associated visually significant cataracts should be extracted in the first few weeks of life and appropriate aphakic correction and amblyopia therapy instituted. Early surgery may result in relatively good visual results in selected patients.[106] If the pathology is localized to the anterior segment of the eye, the lens and retrolental membrane are removed through a limbal approach.[179] If significant midvitreal or posterior vitreal components to the PHPV are present, then a combined lensectomy-vitrectomy using a pars-plana surgical approach should be considered. Lensectomy possibly prevents the development of secondary angle-closure glaucoma, which is a source of visual loss in these patients with limited visual potential. Traction and rhegmatogenous retinal detachments have been reported in patients with PHPV and are treated as needed. Very rarely, the anterior or posterior lens capsule ruptures in PHPV and an inflammatory ocular response may be induced.[32,56,204]

Peters' Anomaly

One-fourth to one-third of patients with Peters' anomaly have microphthalmia with or without uveal coloboma.[198] Although the anterior segment may be enlarged in patients with Peters' anomaly, total axial length may be reduced. Corneal enlargement and anterior staphyloma formation result from severe anterior segment dysgenesis or associated congenital glaucoma. For a complete discussion of Peters' anomaly see Chapter 5.

Anterior Polar Cataracts

Eyes with anterior polar cataracts are frequently slightly smaller than normal. In unilateral cases, the affected eye is more hyperopic than the contralateral eye and may have a smaller corneal diameter. Clementi and coworkers[35] reported autosomal dominant inheritance of anterior polar cataracts and microphthalmia in five members of one family. Harman[84] had reported nine members of another family with the same constellation of findings. One gene for anterior polar cataracts was mapped to chromosome 13.

Retinoblastoma and 13q Deletion

The eyes of patients with retinoblastoma are characteristically of normal size and have clear lenses. Patients with deletion of the long arm of chromosome 13, however, may develop retinoblastoma in a microphthalmic eye. These patients are frequently developmentally delayed and have dysmorphic facial features and other congenital malformations.[222]

DEVELOPMENTAL GENES AND MICROPHTHALMIA

The elucidation of the molecular biology and genetics of congenital malformations has lagged behind the delineation and gene mapping of single-gene disorders because most cases are isolated, without other relatives with the same disease. Hence, the paucity of large families with individual malformations and the difficulty in performing linkage analysis and gene mapping. Isolated patients, however, lend themselves to the study of candidate genes for mutations. Candidate genes and "candidates" for the disease of interest either because they are expressed in the tissue of the affected organ, or because their protein product performs a function that is essential to the normal function or development of the tissue of interest.

Homeotic genes are responsible for the orchestration and regulation of normal development of biologic systems. The homeobox is a DNA segment, 183 base pairs long, that codes for a 60-amino acid protein that constitutes the DNA binding region or "homeodomain" of some homeotic gene products. The proteins coded for by homeobox-containing genes regulate DNA transcription by binding to downstream (toward the 3′ end of the chromosome) genes and also regulate their own production. Homeobox-containing genes are arranged in clusters on one or more chromosomes (one in *Drosophila melanogaster* and four in mice and humans). These genes regulate the development of body segments cephalad to caudad depending on their location in the gene cluster.[68,109,118] There are clear-cut boundaries and synchronized expression of proteins for homeotic genes in the developing embryo. Targeted disruption of homeotic genes results in predictably and severely malformed animals. Ton and co-workers[192] cloned and characterized a paired box- and homeobox-containing gene from the aniridia region on chromosome 11 (later identified as PAX6, or paired-box containing gene no. 6), making aniridia the first well-defined malformation demonstrated to result from the alteration of a homeotic gene. Glaser et al.,[70] Jordan et al.,[103] and numerous other investigators have found mutations of the PAX6 gene in patients with aniridia. Mutations in the PAX3 gene result in Waardenburg syndrome (hypertelorism, hypopigmentation, and deafness),[188] and mutations in the PAX2 gene cause optic nerve colobomas and renal malformations.[166] Homeobox-containing genes such as the PAX genes are hence attractive candidates for human and murine malformation syndromes. Furthermore, malformation syndromes that map to, or are associated with, deletions of chromosomes containing the homeobox gene clusters are good candidate diseases for defects in these genes.

Cataract genes are also possible candidate genes for microphthalmia because of the association of cataracts and microphthalmia, and because of the occurrence of microphthalmia in presumed homozygote carriers of autosomal dominant cataract genes.[23]

Yokoyama and co-workers[225] reported the association of autosomal dominant congenital cataract and microphthalmia with a familial t(2;16) translocation; they postulated that a gene that lies on 16p13.3 is important in ocular development and is responsible for the disorder in this family.

NONINHERITED MULTISYSTEM MALFORMATION SYNDROMES WITH COLOBOMATOUS MICROPHTHALMIA—ASSOCIATIONS AND DEFORMATIONS

Associations are defined as the nonrandom simultaneous occurrence of a number of independent, nonspecific malformations whose etiology is unknown.[178] Organs are affected if their progenitor cells are located close to each other or if these cells share a predisposition to be affected by a certain teratogen.

The associations that feature microphthalmia and colobomas are the CHARGE association, facio-oculo-auriculo-vertebral sequence or Goldenhar syndrome, and the VATER association. These three syndromes have overlapping clinical characteristics and the diagnosis of the individual patient depends on the presence of minimal diagnostic or characteristic criteria for each.

The CHARGE Association

It is estimated that 15%–30% of patients with microphthalmia/coloboma have the CHARGE association (Fig. 4.17*A*).[213] The components of this association are *c*oloboma of the uvea, congenital *h*eart disease,[40] *a*tresia of the choanae, *r*etardation of growth and mental development, *g*enital anomalies, and *e*ar malformations with hearing loss.[42,44,80,91,105,115,122,143,146,163,173,213] Four of the six major findings are generally required for diagnosis. Additional abnormalities include seventh cranial nerve palsy (Fig. 4.17*B*) in up to 45% of patients[163] and facial clefts. Most cases are sporadic, but autosomal dominant transmission has been described in a few instances.[91,105,137,139]

Russell-Eggitt and co-workers[163] reviewed the ophthalmic features of 50 patients with the CHARGE association examined at the Hospital for Sick Children in London. Males and females were equally represented. Thirteen patients died in the first year of life. One of 48 karyotypes showed a balanced translocation between chromosomes 6 and 8. Eighty-eight percent of patients had ocular abnormalities that included a typical coloboma of the iris of varying severity in 82% of cases. Two patients had nasal iris colobomas. Posterior segment colobomatous defects were present in 38 of the 50 patients and varied from large chorioretinal colobomas to subtle optic nerve colobomas and inferior small reti-

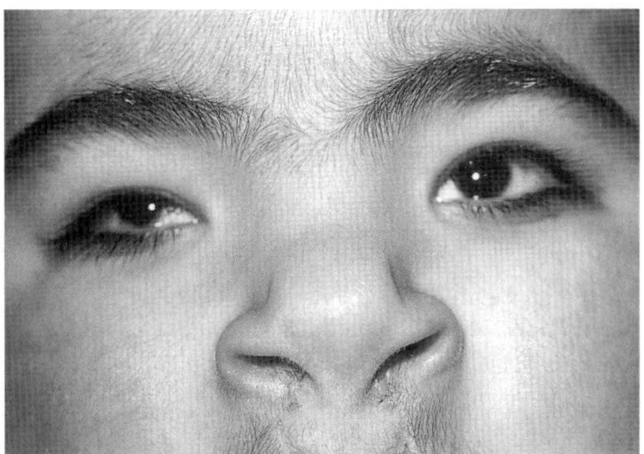

Figure 4.17*A*. Bilateral colobomatous microphthalmia in a patient with the CHARGE (coloboma, heart disease, atresia choanae, retarded growth and retarded development and/or CNS anomalies and/or deafness) association. Bilateral clefts of the lip and palate were repaired. *Figure continued on following page.*

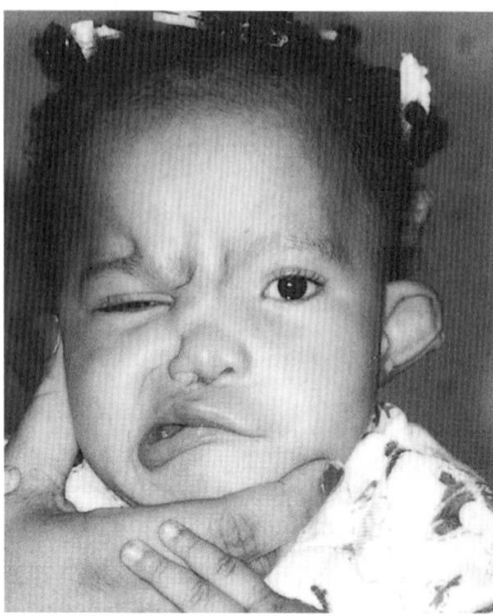

Figure 4.17*B*. One-year-old patient with most of the features of the CHARGE (coloboma, heart disease, atresia choanae, retarded growth and retarded development and/or CNS anomalies and/or deafness) association including a left congenital facial nerve palsy. The left ear is malformed and there is a right cleft lip. The patient has bilateral colobomatous microphthalmia, choanal atresia, cardiac defects, and mental retardation.

nal pigment epithelial defects. Eight patients had bilateral and 13 had unilateral microphthalmia. The reduction in size of the globe was mild in all cases. Four patients had optic nerve hypoplasia. Persistent hyperplastic primary vitreous (PHPV) was present unilaterally in two patients. Two patients had congenital cataracts and 17 had strabismus. Facial palsy was bilateral in 2 patients and unilateral in 20 One patient had Marcus-Gunn jaw winking and ptosis. Four patients had delayed visual maturation. The differential diagnosis of the CHARGE association includes the cat-eye syndrome (partial tetrasomy 22), Di George syndrome, and retinoic acid embryopathy.

Facio-Oculo-Auriculo-Vertebral (FOAV) Dysplasia, Goldenhar Syndrome, Goldenhar-Gorlin Syndrome

Patients with this association have a variety of facial anomalies including microtia, hemifacial microsomia with maxillary and sometimes mandibular hypoplasia, macrostomia, preauricular appendages and/or pits, deafness, and facial palsy.[127,159,160] Over 70% of patients are males. Diminished or absent parotid secretion and malfunction of the soft palate are common. Cleft lip and cleft palate are occasionally present. About 70% of cases have unilateral facial abnormalities, and the right side is involved more often than expected. When both sides of the face are affected, the extent of the abnormalities is markedly asymmetric. Vertebral abnormalities occur in the cervical region. Occasional and rare associated malformations include cardiac defects, tracheoesophageal fistulas, renal malformations, imperforate anus, genital defects, and limb abnormalities such as radial dysplasia and clubfoot anomalies. Mental retardation and brain malformations are rare. Ocular abnormalities include colobomas of the upper lid, Duane syndrome,[150,202] and epibulbar dermolipomas and/or limbal dermoids (Fig. 4.18). Colobomatous microphthalmia occurs in about 20% of patients of FOAV, predominantly those with epibulbar dermoids.

The cluster of developmental anomalies is the result of errors in morphogenesis of structures derived from the first and second branchial arches. The presence of epibulbar dermoids is necessary for the designation of Goldenhar syndrome.[17,51,169] Most cases are sporadic although autosomal dominant and presumed autosomal recessive[159] inheritance have

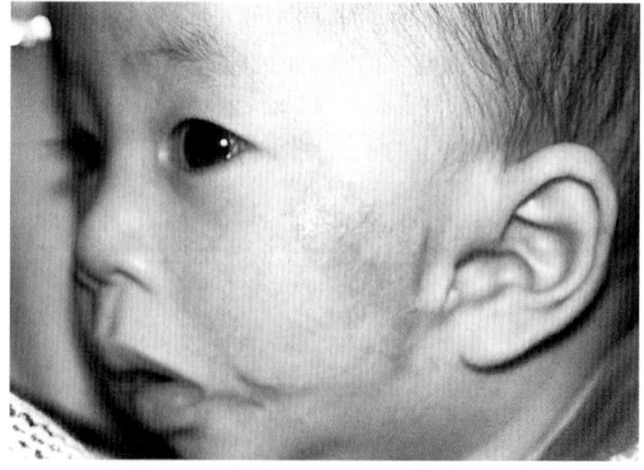

Figure 4.18. Patient with facio-oculo-auriculo-vertebral sequence. There is a left hemifacial microsomia, an abnormal auricle, Duane syndrome, and hearing loss. The patient also had duplication of his thumb.

been reported in rare instances. In a study of 12 monozygotic twins with this syndrome, only two pairs were concordant.[30]

The FOAV association should be differentiated from the Franceschetti syndrome,[185] the CHARGE association, and the VATER association.

VATER Association

The components of this association are *v*ertebral anomalies, *a*tresia of the anus, *t*racheo*e*sophageal atresia or fistula, *r*adial limb defects, and *r*enal malformations. Microphthalmia occurs more frequently in patients with hydrocephalus than in those without it.

Linear Nevus Sebaceous of Jadassohn

This nonfamilial condition is characterized by the presence at birth of yellowish-orange or tan and brownish raised linear skin lesions on the face, head and neck, or thorax. The skin lesions are usually distributed along the midline of the face and chest (Fig. 4.19). Patients frequently have convulsions and developmental delay. Histologically, the lesions are rich in sebaceous glands and immature hair follicles. The nevi become verrucous and nodular at puberty, and malignant transformation may occur in the postpubertal period in 15%–20% of cases.[20,129] Rare associated findings include hypoplastic teeth, a depressed nasal bridge, and cardiac defects.

Lid malformations and colobomatous microphthalmia have been reported in several cases (Traboulsi, personal observation).[128] The nevus may involve the eyelids extensively, and a large vascularized choristomatous mass may comprise the lids, conjunctiva, and cornea.[221] Patients may have nystagmus, strabismus, ptosis, and scarring and vascularization of the cornea. Iris and choroidal colobomas have been described,[140] as have corectopia, limbal dermoids, and lipodermoids. Conjunctival lesions are choristomas and consist of hyperplastic sebaceous glands, apocrine glands, and immature hair follicles.[140] Intrascleral cartilage and bone have been documented.[221] Visual acuity is reduced in the more severely involved eyes. The

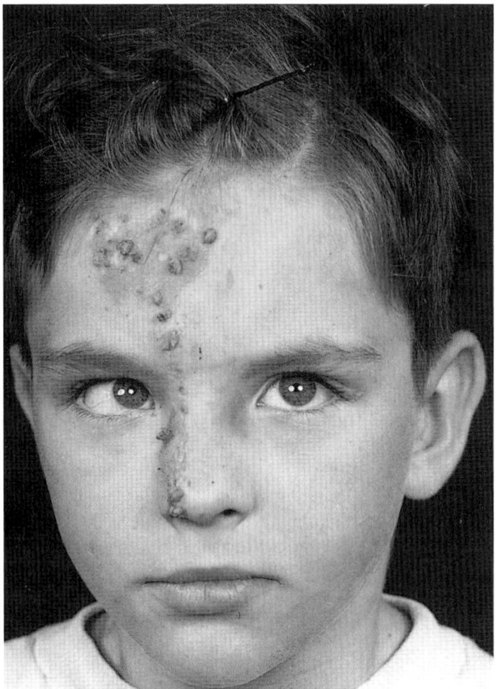

Figure 4.19. Young boy with linear nevus sebaceous and involvement of the right eye. Some of the lesions are verrucous and respect the midline. The child has esotropia. No other ocular involvement with the nevus is evident. (Courtesy of Drs. Linn Murphree and Irene H. Maumenee.)

limbal dermoids may enlarge during the first decade of life.

The differential diagnosis of linear nevus sebaceous includes tuberous sclerosis, Sturge-Weber syndrome, neurofibromatosis 1, and Goldenhar syndrome. These disorders can be differentiated by the appearance and histopathology of the cutaneous lesions and by the presence of other characteristic clinical findings. Cutaneous lesions mimicking isolated patches of nevus sebaceous include nevoxanthoendothelioma, juvenile melanoma, and scarring alopecia in children, and nevus verrucosus, verruca vulgaris, scarring alopecia, and xanthoma in adults.[20]

Anticonvulsant medication and supportive care are needed in severely affected patients whose prognosis is guarded. Surgical repair of the choristomatous scarring of the cornea and conjunctiva is difficult but may be attempted. Because of possible malignant transformation, enlarging nodules should be biopsied.

COLOBOMATOUS MICROPHTHALMIA DUE TO ABNORMAL INTRAUTERINE ENVIRONMENT

Toxic insults to the developing fetus can result in colobomatous microphthalmia or in anophthalmia. These prenatal factors include maternal metabolic disease, infections, exposure to hyperthermia or irradiation, or ingestion of toxic agents. Any of these factors may disrupt normal morphogenesis and the fetus would develop ocular or other malformations or associations of malformations.

Intrauterine Infections

Microphthalmia can result from intrauterine infection with cytomegalovirus (CMV), Epstein-Barr virus, rubella,[75] toxoplasmosis, herpes simples, and varicella.[34,184] Intrauterine infections frequently lead to other ocular abnormalities such as cataracts in rubella and chorioretinal scars in CMV, toxoplasmosis, and varicella infections. Intrauterine infection with parvovirus B19 may lead to microphthalmia, aphakia, retinal folds, and anterior segment malformations.[85]

Drugs and Environmental Toxic Agents

Maternal intake of alcohol,[183] retinoic acid (Accutane),[63,113] LSD,[130] hydantoin,[81] and other drugs[24] can lead to microphthalmia or anophthalmia in the offspring.[184] Numerous animal studies have been performed documenting the teratogenic effects of ethanol, retinoic acid, methotrexate, vincristine, vitamin A, and other medications. The shortcoming of such studies is that the doses of drugs that are administered to the laboratory animals are proportionately much larger than those to which humans are exposed, making inferences to cause and effect difficult in some human cases. Human fetuses exposed to medications have facial anomalies such as broad nasal bridge, short upturned nose, hypertelorism, low-set ears, and prominent lips. Warburg[214] stated that colobomatous microphthalmia occurs much less frequently than facial malformations in such instances.

Maternal fever, hypoxemia, and exposure to radiation have also caused microphthalmia in laboratory animals.[186] In a retrospective study of 479 patients with malformations, there was a history of maternal fever in 55 instances.[61] Five (14%) of 48 patients with microphthalmia were born to women who had had a febrile episode in the first 5 months of gestation. The causal effect of fever or of viruses or bacteria in the etiology of microphthalmia in these cases is difficult to prove.

Exposure to the fungicide benomyl results in retinal dysplasia and clinical anophthalmia in laboratory animals exposed to massive doses of this pesticide.[95] Brain malformations are invariably present and the proposed mechanism by which the teratogen produces its effect is chromosomal aneuploidy. Although there has been suspicion of clusters of human anophthalmia related to exposure to benomyl in England and in Europe, careful epidemiological studies failed to prove any association between the malformation and exposure to the pesticide.[176]

There is one report of microphthalmia, brain malformations, and cardiac defects in a child born to a woman who was exposed to the insecticide oxydemeton-methyl when she worked in a field that had been sprayed 20 hours prior with the insecticide.[161] Care should be taken not to overlook a possible genetic etiology of malformations in the cases of infants exposed to teratogens in utero. Syndrome identification and chromosomal studies should be performed.

Maternal Diabetes

Maternal diabetes may also be associated with an increased risk of colobomatous microphthalmia. Mothers with long-standing and poorly controlled insulin-dependent diabetes are at higher risk of giving birth to babies with caudal regression sequence, conotruncal cardiac defects, vertebral, ear, and CNS and renal malformations.[12,76,101]

Amniotic Band Syndrome

Amniotic band syndrome (ABS) refers to a constellation of malformations that result from entrapment of fetal parts by fibrous bands of amniotic origin.[28,182,194] ABS occurs in 1 of 5000 to 1 of 10,000 pregnancies.[82] The clinical manifestations are extremely variable and range from minor constriction bands around digits to major craniofacial and visceral abnormalities.[102,104] This variability in clinical findings makes the diagnosis difficult unless highly suspected. Even though limbs are the most commonly affected structures, craniofacial defects occur in as many as one third of patients. Cleft lip/palate abnormalities are common and result from interference with fusion of the facial processes by a strand of amnion. Clefts may be unilateral or bilateral and may be accompanied by colobomatous lid defects on the same side of the face. A proboscis can result from interference with formation of the frontonasal processes. An amniotic band coming across the flexed embryo may result in an omphalocele with deficiency of the abdominal wall. Limb abnormalities include the virtually diagnostic constriction bands around any part of the upper or lower extremities and/or amputation defects of the fingers, toes, part of, or all of a limb. In the CNS there may be agenesis of the septum pellucidum or corpus callosum, or a major malformation of the ventricular system leading to hydrocephalus. Other abnormalities include lack of a normal hair whorl pattern and an altered dermal pattern.

Ocular findings consist of corneal leukomas and eyelid colobomas, often contiguous with facial clefts.[25,138] There may be strabismus, hypertelorism, and microphthalmos. Unilateral atypical (i.e., not inferonasal in location) chorioretinal coloboma is an interesting but relatively rare finding in ABS.[18,86,138]

All cases of ABS have been isolated occurrences in otherwise normal families except for the account by Etches and co-workers[49] where there were multiple siblings with amputation defects. The etiology of amniotic band formation is only speculative.[144] Second-trimester amniocentesis,[8] LSD use,[9] oral contraceptive use, and instrumentally attempted abortions have been associated with ABS. Torpin[193] suggested that congenital defects associated with ABS are due to amniotic bands that form following rupture of the amniotic cavity; such bands cause malformation, disruption, and deformation of fetal parts. The clinical findings in most patients with ABS support Torpin's theory. For example, a straight imaginary line at a nonembryological site of closure can be drawn through a lid coloboma to a cleft lip, implying disruption and deformation of the eyelids and nasofrontal and maxillary processes by a single amniotic band. Swallowing a tethered amniotic band by the fetus has also been implicated in the formation of craniofacial anomalies. According to Higginbottom et al.,[90] amniotic rupture at 45 days of gestation results in severe craniofacial and limb anomalies, at times incompatible with life, whereas rupture after 45 days usually results in mild limb anomalies.

A diagnosis of ABS should be suspected in all newborns with facial clefts and colobomas, especially if the suggestive limb amputation or constriction defects are present. Other conditions with a similar phenotype include trisomy 13, Meckel-Gruber syndrome, and the CHARGE association.

Aggressive reconstructive surgery can lead to excellent functional results.[136] Extensive lid colobomas require emergent surgery to prevent the development of corneal ulceration and scarring.[94] Lubricating ointment is used until and after surgery. Hydrocephalus is treated by shunting. Limb defects are usually irreparable but appropriate expert consultations should be obtained. Patients with ABS require a multispecialty team management approach that often gives rewarding results.

Intrauterine Injuries

BenEzra and colleagues[19] reported one child with bilateral clinical anophthalmia and his brother with unilateral microphthalmia, central corneal scarring, and a cataract. Although the original interpretation of the clinical findings was that of variable clinical manifestations of an autosomal recessive gene, the authors believe that the unilateral microphthalmia was the result of an amniocentesis needle injury.

Orbital Encephaloceles

There are reports of microphthalmia or anophthalmia in patients with congenital encephaloceles.[50,112] Although it is postulated that the ocular abnormalities in these cases are examples of deformation of the developing eye by the encephalocele, the globe is most often normal in patients with other types of orbital masses such as orbital teratomas. Rather, it may be that the ocular and anterior brain and orbital malformations are the result of a developmental field defect.

OCULAR COMPLICATIONS OF COLOBOMATOUS MICROPHTHALMIA

Retinal Detachment

Retinal detachment is an uncommon but real complication of uveal colobomas. One patient developed a unilateral detachment and another, bilateral retinal detachments in the series of 83 consecutive patients reported by Maumenee and Mitchell.[132] Jessberg and Schepens[100] have stated that the detachment may be a coincidental finding in some patients, with retinal breaks away from the area of the colobomas, while it may be a true complication of the colobomatous defect in other cases where breaks develop at the edge of the coloboma and lead to inferior or total retinal detachment. These authors have also observed demarcation lines in four of their seven patients, indicating that the detachment was stationary for a prolonged period of time.

Subretinal Neovascularization

Leff and colleagues[116] attributed the development of neovascularization at the edge of a chorioretinal coloboma in two older individuals to defects in Bruch's membrane and the retinal pigment epithelium in that location of the abnormal fundus. This presumably allowed the ingrowth of vessels from the adjacent choroid into the subretinal space. One of the two patients had macular drusen. In another case, krypton and argon lasers were used to treat a subretinal membrane.[180]

PROGNOSIS, PREVENTION, AND TREATMENT

The treatment of microphthalmia/coloboma depends on the severity of ocular involvement. Errors of refraction should be corrected early in life, keeping in mind that high myopia may be present despite the small size of the cornea.[16] Amblyopia should be treated if its presence is suspected, especially in unilateral cases where visual acuity is not commensurate with the physical findings. Cataract extraction is performed if the lens opacity is judged to be significant. The procedure is possible even in very small eyes and visual acuity may improve significantly. Intraocular lenses can be implanted as in other children or adults. Cataract extraction in nanophthalmic eyes may be complicated by uveal effusion, and Brockhurst recommends prophylactic lamellar scleral resection 2 months or more prior to cataract surgery. Corneal transplantation should be considered if the cornea is opaque as in Peters' anomaly with microphthalmia. Feldman and co-workers[52] transplanted corneas in nine microphthalmic eyes of five patients. Axial length ranged from 12.5–16 mm. Seven corneas remained clear and vision developed in all eyes.[52]

Patients with blind small eyes may have prostheses fit over the globe for cosmetic purposes. The discussion of orbital augmentation surgery for clinical anophthalmia is beyond the scope of this chapter and is covered in Chapter 3 by Heher and Katowitz.

Genetic counseling should be provided after examination of available family members and determination of possible mode(s) of inheritance in familial cases. The risk of recurrence in a sibling varies from 2%–9% if both parents are unaffected and increases to 14%–46% if one parent is affected.[66,132]

Because of the common occurrence of other anomalies in patients with colobomatous microphthalmia, every effort should be made to identify developmental, cardiac, genitourinary, and brain malformations. A thorough physical examination and review of systems give the clues for the presence of these potentially life-threatening anomalies. Radiographic and ultrasonographic imaging studies are obtained as needed. The growth curve of children is closely monitored for signs of retardation. If height increase is not progressing as expected, or if there is any evidence of endocrinologic abnormalities, appropriate hormonal investigations should be instituted. Five of 13 patients with microphthalmia or clinical anophthalmia drawn from 650 mentally retarded adults had hypogonadotropic hypogonadism.[108] Four were male and had low testosterone levels and sexual infantilism, and one female had primary amenorrhea. All hormonal studies in these patients were normal except for low gonadotropin levels. This association had been noted previously by Al Fryh et al.[3] in a patient with anophthalmia, microcephaly, hypotonia, hypogonadism, failure to thrive, and developmental delay. Kemmann and Jones[107] reported one patient with microphthalmia and Kallmann syndrome (i.e., the association of hypogonadotropic hypogonadism with anosmia).

The yield of chromosomal studies is poor in isolated microphthalmia/coloboma but increases significantly if there is associated mental retardation and at least one other congenital malformation.[211] If the size of the eye is significantly reduced, prenatal diagnosis should be possible using high quality ultrasonographic studies.[171]

REFERENCES

1. Aicardi J, Chevrie J, Rousselie F. Le syndrome spasmes en flexion, agenesie calleuse, anomalies chorioretiniennes. *Arch Fr Pediatr* 1969;26:1103–1120.
2. Aicardi J, Lefebvre J, Lerique-Koechlin A. A new syndrome: Spasms in flexion, callosal agenesis, ocular abnormalities. *Electroencephalogr Clin Neurophysiol* 1965;19:609–610.
3. Al Fryh A, Facharzt T, Haque K. Anophthalmia, microencephaly, hypotonia, hypogonadism, failure to thrive and developmental delay. *Dysmorphol Clin Genet* 1987;1:64–66.
4. Al-Gazali L, Donnai D, Berry S, Saay B, Mueller R. The oculocerebrocutaneous (Delleman) syndrome. *J Med Genet* 1988;25:773–778.
5. Al-Gazali L, Mueller R, Caine A, Antoniou A, McCartney A, Fitchett M, et al. Two 46 XXt(XY) females with linear skin defects and congenital microphthalmia: A new syndrome. *J Med Genet* 1990;27:59–63.
6. Allanson J, Richter S. Linear skin defects and congenital microphthalmia: A new syndrome at Xp222 (letter). *J Med Genet* 1991;28:143–144.
7. Arstikaitis M. A case report of bilateral microphthalmos with cyst. *Arch Ophthalmol* 1969;82:480–482.
8. Ashkenazy M, Bornstein Z, Segal M. Constriction of the umbilical cord by an amniotic band after mid-trimester amniocentesis. *Acta Obstet Gynecol Scand* 1982;61:89–91.
9. Assemarry S, Neu R, Gardner L. Deformities in a child whose mother took LSD. *Lancet* 1970;1:1290.
10. Awan K, Humayun M. Changes in the contralateral eye in uncomplicated persistent hyperplastic primary vitreous. *Am J Ophthalmol* 1985;99:122.
11. Baghdassarian S, Tabbara K, Matta C. Congenital cystic eye. *Am J Ophthalmol* 1973;76(2):269–275.
12. Barr M, Hanson J, Currey K, Sharp S, Toriello H, Schmickel R, et al. Holoprosencephaly in infants of diabetic mothers. *J Pediatr* 1983;102:565–568.
13. Bartholini T. Historia XLVII. Monstrum sine oculis in *Historiarum anatomicarum rariorum. Centuria III & IV: Ejusdem cura accessere observationes anatomicae,* Hafniae, Sumptibus Petri Haubold, 1657:95.
14. Bartholini T. *Acta medica et philosophica Hafniensia.* Hafniae, Sumptibus Petri Haubold, 1673.
15. Bateman J. Microphthalmos. *Int Ophthalmol Clin* 1984;24(1):87–107.
16. Bateman J, Maumenee I. Colobomatous macrophthalmia with microcornea. *Ophthalmic Paediatr Genet* 1984;4:59–66.
17. Baum J. Ocular aspects of Goldenhar's syndrome. *Am J Ophthalmol* 1973;75:250–257.
18. BenEzra D, Frucht Y. Uveal coloboma associated with amniotic band syndrome. *Can J Ophthalmol* 1983;18:136.
19. BenEzra D, Sela M, Pe'er J. Bilateral anophthalmia and unilateral microphthalmia in two siblings. *Ophthalmologica* 1989;198:140–144.
20. Bianchine J. The nevus sebaceous of Jadassohn. A neurocutaneous syndrome and patentially pre-malignant lesion. *Am J Dis Child* 1970;120:223–228.
21. National Society to Prevent Blindness. *Vision Problems in the U.S.* New York: National Society to Prevent Blindness, 1980.

22. Blodi F. Preretinal glial nodules and hyperplasia of primary vitreous. *Arch Ophthalmol* 1972;87:531.
23. Bodker F, Lavery M, Mitchell T, Lovrien E, Maumenee I. Microphthalmos in the presumed homozygous offspring of a first cousin marriage and linkage analysis of a locus in a family with autosomal dominant cerulean congenital cataracts. *Am J Med Genet* 1990;37:54–59.
24. Bogdanoff B, Rorke L, Yanoff M, Warren W. Brain and eye abnormalities. Possible sequelae to prenatal use of multiple drugs including LSD. *Am J Dis Child* 1972;123: 145–148.
25. Braude L, Miller M, Cuttone J. Ocular abnormalities in the amniogenic band syndrome. *Br J Ophthalmol* 1981;65:299–303.
26. Brockhurst R. Cataract surgery in nanophthalmic eyes. *Arch Ophthalmol* 1990;108(7): 965–967.
27. Brockhurst R. Vortex vein decompression for nanophthalmic uveal effusion. *Arch Ophthalmol* 1980;98:1987–1990.
28. Broome D, Ebbin A, Jung A, et al. Aberrant tissue bands and craniofacial defects. *Birth Defects Orig Art Ser* 1976;12:65.
29. Brown G, Gonder J, Levin A. Persistence of the primary vitreous in association with the morning glory disc anomaly. *J Pediatr Ophthalmol Strabismus* 1984;21:5.
30. Burck U. Genetic aspects of hemifacial microsomia. *Hum Genet* 1983;64:291–296.
31. Capella J, Kaufman H, Lill F, et al. Hereditary cataracts and microphthalmia. *Am J Ophthalmol* 1963;56:454.
32. Caudill J, Streeten B, Tso M. Phacoanaphylactoid reaction in persistent hyperplastic primary vitreous. *Ophthalmology* 1985;92:1153.
33. Cennamo G, Magli A, Corvino C. Genetic and ultrasound study of hereditary pure microphthalmos. *Ophthalmic Paediatr Genet* 1985;6:37–42.
34. Charles N, Bennett T, Margolis S. Ocular pathology of the congenital variocella syndrome. *Arch Ophthalmol* 1977;95:2034–2037.
35. Clementi M, Rossetti A, Pesenti P, et al. Microphthalmia-congenital anterior polar cataract: An autosomal dominant syndrome. *Ophthalmic Paediatr Genet* 1985;6:189–192.
36. Cockburn D, Dwyer P. Posterior persistent hyperplastic primary vitreous. *Am J Optom Phys Optics* 1988;65:316.
37. Collins M, Traboulsi E, Maumenee I. Optic nerve head swelling and optic atrophy in the mucopolysaccharidoses. *Ophthalmology* 1990;97:1445–1449.
38. Cross H, Yoder F. Familial nanophthalmos. *Am J Ophthalmol* 1976;56:454–458.
39. Cuendet J. La microphtalmie compliquee. *Ophthalmolgica* 1961;141:380–385.
40. Cyran S, Martinez R, Daniels S, Dignan P, Kaplan S. Spectrum of congenital heart disease in CHARGE association. *J Pediatr* 1987;110:576–578.
41. Da Silva E, De Sousa S. Clinical anophthalmia. *Hum Genet* 1981;57:115–116.
42. Davenport S, Hefner M, Mitchell J. The spectrum of clinical features in CHARGE syndrome. *Clin Genet* 1986;29:298–310.
43. Del Pero R, Mets M, Tripathi R, Torczynski E. Anomalies of retinal architecture in Aicardi syndrome. *Arch Ophthalmol* 1986;104:1659–1664.
44. Dobrowski J, Grundfast K, Rosenbaum K, Zajtchuk J. Otolaryngologic manifestations of CHARGE association. *Otolaryngol Head Neck Surg* 1985;93:798–802.
45. Dollfus M, Marx P, Langlois J, Clement J, Forthomme J. Congenital cystic eyeball. *Am J Ophthalmol* 1968;66:504–509.
46. Donnenfeld A, Packer RJ, Zackai EH, Chee C, Sellinger B, Emanuel B. Clinical, cytogenetic, and pedigree findings in 18 cases of Aicardi syndrome. *Am J Med Genet* 198;32: 461–467.
47. Duke-Elder S. *System of Ophthalmology. Congenital Deformities.* London: Henry Kimpton, 1964.
48. Duker J, Weiss J, Siber M, Bieber F, Albert D. Ocular findings in a new heritable syndrome of brain eye and urogenital abnormalities. *Am J Ophthalmol* 1985;99:51–55.
49. Etches P, Stewart A, Ives E. Familial congenital amputations. *J Pediatr* 1982;101:448–449.
50. Fargueta J, Menezo J, Bordes M. Posterior orbital encephalocele with anophthalmos and other brain malformations. Case report. *J Neurosurg* 1973;38:215–217.
51. Feigold M, Baum J. Goldenhar's syndrome. *Am J Dis Child* 1978;132:135–139.
52. Feldman S, Frucht-Pery J, Brown S. Corneal transplantation in microphthalmic eyes. *Am J Ophthalmol* 1987;104:164–167.
53. Fisher Y. Microphthalmos with communications orbital cyst-ultrasonographic diagnosis. *Ophthalmology* 1978;85:1208–1211.
54. Fledelius H, Rosenberg T. Extreme hypermetropia and posterior microphthalmos in three siblings. An oculometric study. In *Ophthalmic Echography*, K. Ossoinig and M. Nijhoff, eds.

Dordrecht, The Netherlands: WJ Junk. 1987:87–91.

55. Font R, Yanoff M, Zimmerman L. Intraocular adipose tissue and persistent hyperplastic primary vitreous. *Arch Ophthalmol* 1969;82:43.
56. Ford J, Irvine A. Persistent hyperplastic primary vitreous associated with anterior rupture of the lens capsule. *Arch Ophthalmol* 1961; 66:467.
57. François J. A propos d'une famille presentant des anomalies ocularies du type colobomateux depuis le colobome unilateral de l'iris jusqu'a l'anophtalmie bilaterale associée au syndrome de Bardet-Biedl. *J Genet Hum* 1953;2:203–218.
58. François J. In *Heredity in Ophthalmology.* St. Louis: C. V. Mosby, 1961:171–175.
59. François J, Goes F. Ultrasonographic study of 100 emmetropic eyes. *Ophthalmologica* 1977;175:321.
60. François J, Pallota R, Gallenga P. Microphthalmos and malformative syndromes. *Ophthalmic Paediatr Genet* 1983;3:201–205.
61. Fraser F, Skelton J. Possible teratogenicity of maternal fever. *Lancet* 1978;ii:634.
62. Fraser G, Friedman A. *The Causes of Blindness in Childhood.* Baltimore: Johns Hopkins University Press, 1967.
63. Fraunfelder F, LaBraico J, Meyer S. Adverse ocular reactions possibly associated with isoretinoin. *Am J Ophthalmol* 1985;100:534–537.
64. Frydman M, Kauschansky A, Leshem I, et al. Oculo-palato-cerebral dwarfism: A new syndrome. *Clin Genet* 1985;27:414.
65. Fujii M, Hayasaka S, Setogawa T. Persistent hyperplastic primary vitreous in the right eye and congenital grouped pigmentation of the retina in the left eye. *Ophthalmologica* 1989;198:135.
66. Fujiki K, Nakajima A, Yasuda N, Tanabe U, Kabaswa K. Genetic analysis of microphthalmos. *Ophthalmic Paediatr Genet* 1982;1: 139–149.
67. Gartner S. Congenital retinal folds and microcephaly. *Arch Ophthalmol* 1941;25:93–100.
68. Gehring W. Homeoboxes in the study of development. Science 1987;236:1245–1252.
69. Gilbert W Jr, Smith J, Nyhan W. The Sjögren-Larsson syndrome. *Arch Ophthalmol* 1968; 80:308–316.
70. Glaser T, Walton D, Maas R. Genomic structure evolutionary conservation and aniridia mutations in the human PAX 6 gene. *Nature Genet* 1992;2:232–239.
71. Godel V, Goodman R. X-linked recessive primary retinal dysplasia: Clinical findings in affected males and carrier females. *Clin Genet* 1981;20:260–266.
72. Goldberg M, Mafee M. Computed tomography for diagnosis of persistent hyperplastic primary vitreous. *Ophthalmology* 1983;90: 442.
73. Goldberg S, Farber M, Bullock J, Crone K, Ball W. Bilateral congenital ocular cysts. *Ophthalmic Paediatr Genet* 1991;12(1):31–38.
74. Goltz R, Peterson W, Gorlin R, Ravits H. Focal dermal hypoplasia. *Arch Dermatol* 1962;86:708–717.
75. Gregg M. Congenital cataract following German measles in the mother. *Trans Ophthalmol Soc Aust* 1941;3:35–46.
76. Grix A. Malformations in infants of diabetic mothers. *Am J Med Genet* 1982;13:131–137.
77. Grizzard W, O'Donnell J, Carey J. The cerebro-oculo-facio-skeletal syndrome. *Am J Ophthalmol* 1980;89:293.
78. Guyer D, Green W. Bilateral extreme microphthalmos. *Ophthalmic Paediatr Genet* 1984;4:81–90.
79. Haddad R, Font R, Reeser F. Persistent hyperplastic primary vitreous. A clinicopathologic study of 62 cases and review of the literature. *Surv Ophthalmol* 1978;23:123.
80. Hall B. Choanal atresia and associated multiple anomalies. *J Pediatr* 1979;95:395–398.
81. Hampton G, Krepostman J. Ocular manifestations of the fetal hydantoin syndrome. *Clin Pediatr* 1981;20:475–478.
82. Hanson J, Freeman M. Aberrant tissue bands and multiple congenital defects: An epidemiologic assessment. In *New Chromosomal and Malformation Syndromes,* D. Bergsma, ed. Miami: Symposis Specialists for the National Foundation—March of Dimes, 1975:329.
83. Happle R, Daniels O, Koopman R. MIDAS syndrome (microphthalmia dermal aplasia and sclerocornea): An X-linked phenotype distinct from Goltz syndrome. *Am J Med Genet* 1993;47:710–713.
84. Harman N. Congenital cataract—A pedigree of five generations. *Trans Ophthalmol Soc UK* 1909;29:101.
85. Hartwig N, Vermeij-Keers C, Van Elsacker-Niele A, Fleuren G. Embryonic malformations in a case of parvovirus B19 infection. *Teratology* 1989;39:295–302.
86. Hashemi K, Traboulsi E, Chrousos G, Scribanu N, Chavis R. Chorioretinal lacuna in the

amniotic band syndrome. *J Pediatr Ophthalmol Strabismus* 1990;28:238–239.

87. Heimonen O, Slone D, Shapiro S. *Birth Defects and Drugs in Pregnancy.* Littleton, MA: Publishing Sciences Group, 1977.
88. Helveston E, Malone E, Lashmet M. Congenital cystic eye. *Arch Ophthalmol* 1970;84(11): 622–624.
89. Hermsen V, Conahan J, Koops B, et al. Persistent hyperplastic primary vitreous associated with protein C deficiency. *Am J Ophthalmol* 1990;109:608.
90. Higginbottom M, Jones K, et al. The amniotic band disruption complex: Timing of amniotic rupture and variable spectra of consequent defects. *J Pediatr* 1979;95:544–549.
91. Hittner H, Hirsch N, Kreh G, Rudolf A. Colobomatous microphthalmos heart disease, hearing loss and mental retardation—A syndrome. *J Pediatr Ophthalmol Strabismus* 1979;16:122–128.
92. Hoefnagel D, Keenan M, Allen F. Heredofamilial bilateral anophthalmia. *Arch Ophthalmol* 1963;69:760–764.
93. Holden JD, Akers WA. Goltz's syndrome: Focal dermal hypoplasia. A combined mesoectodermal dysplasia. *Am J Dis Child* 1967; 114:292–300.
94. Hollsten D, Katowitz J. The ophthalmic manifestations and treatment of the amniotic band syndrome. *Ophthalmol Plast Reconstr Surg* 1990;6:1–15.
95. Hoogenboom E, Ransdell J, Ellis W, Kavloch R, Zeman F. Effects on the fetal rat eye of maternal benomyl exposure. *Curr Eye Res* 1991;10(7):601–612.
96. Irvine A, Albert D, Sang D. Retinal neoplasia and dysplasia. II. Retinoblastoma occurring with persistence and hyperplasia of the primary vitreous. *Invest Ophthalmol Visual Sci* 1977;16:403.
97. Jagell S, Gustavson K, Holmgren G. Sjogren-Larsson syndrome in Sweden. A clinical, genetic and epidemiological study. *Clin Genet* 1981;19:233–256.
98. Jagell S, Polland W, Sandgren O. Specific changes in the fundus typical for the Sjogren-Larsson syndrome. *Acta Ophthalmol* 1980;58: 321–329.
99. Jarmas A, Weaver D, Ellis F, Davis A. Microcephaly microphthalmia falciform retinal folds and blindness. *Am J Dis Child* 1981; 135:930–933.
100. Jessberg D, Schepens C. Retinal detachment associated with coloboma of the choroid. *Arch Ophthalmol* 1961;65:35–45.
101. Johnson J, Fineman R. Branchial arch malformations in infants of diabetic mothers: Two case reports and a review. *Am J Med Genet* 1982;13:125–135.
102. Jones K, Smith D, Hall B, et al. A pattern of craniofacial and limb defects secondary to aberrant tissue bands. *J Pediatr* 1974;84: 90–95.
103. Jordan T, Hanson I, Zaletayev D, Hodgson S, Prosser J, Seawright A, et al. The human PAX 6 gene is mutated in two patients with aniridia. *Nature Genet* 1992;1:328–332.
104. Juan C, Graff G, et al. The amniotic band syndrome. *Obstet Gynecol* 1973;41:332–336.
105. Kaplan L. Choanal atresia and its associated anomalies. Further support for the CHARGE association. *Int J Pediatr Otorhinolaryngol* 1985;8:237–242.
106. Karr D, Scott W. Visual acuity results following treatment of persistent hyperplastic primary vitreous. *Arch Ophthalmol* 1986;104: 662.
107. Kemmann E, Jones J. Microphthalmia and olfactogenital dysplasia: A possible relationship. *Am J Obstet Gynecol* 1977;129:219–220.
108. Keppen L, Brodsky M, Michael J, Poindexter A. Hypogonadotropic hypogonadism in mentally retarded adults with microphthalmia and clinical anophthalmia. *Am J Med Genet* 1990;36:285–287.
109. Kessel M, Gruss P. Murine development control genes. *Science* 1990;249:374–379.
110. Kohn G, El-Shawwa R, El-Rayyes E. Isolated aclinical anophthalmia in an extensively affected Arab kindred. *Clin Genet* 1988;33: 321–324.
111. Kuchle H, Normann G, Lubbering J. Ein Beitrag zum kongenitalen Zystenauge. *Klin Monatsbl Augenheilkd* 1986;188:239–241.
112. Kulali A, Rahmanli O. Lateral frontal encephalocele associated with dysplasia of the orbit eyeball and eyelid. *Child Nerv Syst* 1990;6: 54–56.
113. Lammer E, Chen D, Hoar R, Agnish N, Benke P, et al. Retinoic acid embryopathy. *N Engl J Med* 1985;313:837–841.
114. Leatherbarrow B, Kwartz J, Noble J. Microphthalmos with cyst in monozygous twins. *J. Pediatr Ophthalmol Strabismus* 1990;27: 294–298.
115. Leclerc J, Fearon B. Choanal atresia and associated anomalies. *Int J Pediatr Otolaryngol* 1987;13:265–272.
116. Leff S, Britton W, Brown G, Lucier A, Brown J. Retinochoroidal coloboma associated with subretinal neovascularization. *Retina* 1985;5: 154–156.
117. Lenz W. Recessiv-geschlechtsgebundene Mi-

kroppthalmie mit multiplen Missbildungen. *Z Kinderheilkd* 1955;77:384.

118. Lewis E. Clusters of master control genes regulate the development of higher organisms. *JAMA* 1992;267:1524–1531.
119. Liang J, Augsburger J, Shields J. Diffuse infiltrating retinoblastoma associated with persistent primary vitreous. *J Pediatr Ophthalmol Strabismus* 1985;22:31.
120. Lieb W, Rochels R, Gronemeyer U. Microphthalmos with colobomatous orbital cyst: Clinical, histological, immunohistological, and electron microscopic findings. *Br J Ophthalmol* 1990;74:59–62.
121. Lin A, Biglan A, Garver K. Persistent hyperplastic primary vitreous with vertical transmission. *Ophthalmic Paediatr Genet* 1990;11: 121.
122. Lin A, Chin A, Devine W, Park S, Zackai E. The pattern of cardiovascular malformation in the CHARGE association. *Am J Dis Child* 1987;141:1010–1013.
123. Lin A, Gorlin R, Lurie I, Brunner H, van der Burgt I, Naumchik I, et al. Further delineation of the branchio-oculo-facial syndrome. *Am J Med Genet* 1995;56:42–59.
124. MacDonald A. Causes of blindness in Canada: An analysis of 24,605 cases registered with the Canadian Institute for the Blind. *Can Med Assoc J* 1965;92:264.
125. Makley T, Battles M. Microphthalmos with cyst—Report of two cases in the same family. *Surv Ophthalmol* 1969;13:200–226.
126. Mann I. *The Development of the Human Eye*. London: British Medical Association, 1964.
127. Mansour A, Wang F, Henkind P, Goldberg R, Shprintzen R. Ocular findings in the facioauriculovertebral sequence (Goldenhar-Gorlin syndrome). *Am J Ophthalmol* 1985; 100:555–559.
128. Marden P, Venters H Jr. A new neurocutaneous syndrome. *Am J Dis Child* 1966;112: 79–81.
129. Stavrianeas NG, Katoulis AC, Stratigeas NP, et al. Development of multiple tumors in a sebaceous nevus of Jadassohn. *Dermatology* 1997;195:155–158.
130. Margolis S, Martin L. Anophthalmia in an infant of parents using LSD. *Ann Ophthalmol* 1980;13:78–81.
131. Martorina M. Nanophthalmie familiale. *J Fr Ophtalmol* 1988;11:357–361.
132. Maumenee I, Mitchell T. Colobomatous malformations of the eye. *Trans Am Ophthalmol Soc* 1990;88:123–132.
133. Meire F, Leys M, Boghaert S, De Laey J. Posterior microphthalmos. *Bull Soc Belge Ophtalmol* 1982;231:101–106.
134. Meisels H, Goldberg M. Vascular anastomoses between the iris and persistent hyperplastic primary vitreous. *Am J Ophthalmol* 1979;88:179.
135. Menchini U, Pece A, Alberti M, et al. Vitré primitif hyperplasique avec persistance de l'artère hyaloide chez deux frères non jumeaux. *J Fr Ophtalmol* 1987;10:241.
136. Merriam J. Reconstruction of the lids of a child with microblepharon and multiple congenital anomalies. *Trans Am Ophthalmol Soc* 1988;86:55–86.
137. Metlay L, Smythe P, Miller M. Familial CHARGE syndrome: Clinical report with autopsy findings. *Am J Med Genet* 1987;26: 577–581.
138. Miller M, Deutsch T, Cronin C, Keys CL. Amniotic bands as a cause of ocular anomalies. *Am J Ophthalmol* 1987;104:270–279.
139. Mitchell J, Giangiacomo J, Hefner M, Thelin J, Pickens J. Dominant CHARGE association. *Ophthalmic Paediatr Genet* 1985;6:31–36.
140. Monahan R, Hill C, Venters H Jr. Multiple choristomas convulsions and mental retardation as a new neurocutaneous syndrome. *Am J Ophthalmol* 1967;64:529–532.
141. Morgan K, McLean I. Retinoblastoma and persistent hyperplastic vitreous occurring in the same patient. *Ophthalmology* 1981;88: 1087.
142. Nasr A, Tomey K. Computerized tomography and ultrasonography in unilateral congenital anophthalmos: A clinicopathologic case report. *Orbit* 1982;1:113.
143. Oley C, Baraitser M, Grant D. A reappraisal of the CHARGE association. *J Med Genet* 1988;25:147–156.
144. Ossipoff V, Hall B. Etiology factors in the amniotic band syndrome: A study of 24 patients. *Birth Defects Orig Art Ser* 1977;13:117.
145. Pagon R. Ocular coloboma. *Surv Ophthalmol* 1981;25:223.
146. Pagon R, Graham J, Zonana J, Yong S-L. Coloboma, congenital heart disease, and choanal atresia with multiple anomalies: CHARGE association. *J Pediatr* 1981;99:223–227.
147. Pasquale L, Romayananda N, et al. Congenital cystic eye with multiple ocular and intracranial anomalies. *Arch Ophthalmol* 1991; 109:985–987.
148. Pearce W, Nigam S, Rootman J. Primary anophthalmos: Histological and genetic features. *Can J Ophthalmol* 1974;9:141–145.
149. Pena S, Shokeir M. Autosomal recessive

cerebro-oculo-facio-skeletal syndrome. *Clin Genet* 1974;5:285–293.

150. Pieroni D. Goldenhar's syndrome associated with bilateral Duane's retraction syndrome. *J Pediatr Ophthalmol* 1969;6:16–18.
151. Pillai A, Sambasivan M. Congenital cystic eye—A case report with CT scan. *Indian J Ophthalmol* 1987;35:88–91.
152. Porges Y, Gershoni-Baruch R, Leibu R, Goldscher D, Zonis S, Shapira I, et al. Hereditary microphthalmia with colobomatous cyst. *Am J Ophthalmol* 1992;114(1):30–34.
153. Probst F, Jagell S, Heijbel J. Clinical CT in the Sjogren-Larsson syndrome. *Neuroradiology* 1981;21:101–105.
154. Pruett R. The pleomorphism and complications of posterior hyperplastic primary vitreous. *Am J Ophthalmol* 1975;80:625–629.
155. Pruett R, Schepens C. Posterior hyperplastic primary vitreous. *Am J Ophthalmol* 1970; 69:534–543.
156. Reese A. Persistent hyperplastic primary vitreous. *Am J Ophthalmol* 1955;40:317.
157. Rice N, Minwall S, Wania J. Case of congenital cystic eye and accessory limb of the lower eyelid. *Br J Ophthalmol* 1966;50:409–413.
158. Richieri-Costa A, Gollop T, Otto P. Autosomal recessive anophthalmia with multiple genetic abnormalities—Type Waardenburg. *Am J Med Genet* 1983;14:607–615.
159. Rollnick B, Kaye C. Hemifacial microsomia and variants: Pedigree data. *Am J Med Genet* 1983;15:233–253.
160. Rollnick B, Kaye C, Nagatoshi K, Hauck W, Martin A. Oculoauriculovertebral dysplasia and variants: Phenotypic characteristics of 294 patients. *Am J Med Genet* 1987;26:361–375.
161. Romero P, Barnett P, Midtling J. Congenital anomalies associated with maternal exposure to Oxydemeton-methyl. *Environ Res* 1989;50: 256–261.
162. Ropers H, Zuffardi O, Bianchi E, Tiepolo L. Agenesis of the corpus callosum, ocular and skeletal anomalies (X-linked dominant Aicardi's syndrome) in a girl with balanced X/3 translocation. *Hum Genet* 1982;61:367–368.
163. Russell-Eggitt I, Blake K, Taylor D, Wyse R. The eye in the CHARGE association. *Br J Ophthalmol* 1990;74:421–426.
164. Ryan E, Zwaan J, Chylack L. Nanophthalmos with uveal effusion. Clinical and embryologic considerations. *Ophthalmology* 1982;89: 1013–1017.
165. Sang D. Embryology of the vitreous. Congenital and developmental abnormalities. *Bull Soc Belge Ophtalmol* 1987;223:11–35.
166. Sanyanusin P, Schimmenti LA, et al. Mutation of the PAX2 gene in a family with optic nerve colobomas renal anomalies and vesicoureteral reflux. *Nature Genet* 1995;9:358–363.
167. Sassani J, Yanoff M. Anophthalmos in an infant with multiple congenital anomalies. *Am J Ophthalmol* 1977;83:43–48.
168. Scouras J, Catti A, Cuendet J. Les microphtalmies congenitales. *Ann Oculist (Paris)* 1970; 203:953–970.
168a. Seller MJ, Davis TB, Fear CN, Flinter FA, Ellis I, Gibson AG. Two sibs with anophthalmia and pulmonary hypoplasia (the Matthew-Wood syndrome). *Am J Med Genet* 1996; 62:227–229.
169. Shokeir M. The Goldenhar syndrome: A natural history. *Birth Defects Orig Art Ser* 1977;13/3C:67–83.
170. Shukla Y, Kulshreshta O, Bajaj K. Congenital cystic eye—A case report. *Indian J Ophthalmol* 1984;34:249–250.
171. Shulman L, Gordon P, Emerson D, Wilroy R, Elias S. Prenatal diagnosis of isolated bilateral microphthalmia with confirmation by evaluation of products of conception obtained by dilation and evacuation. *Prenatal Diagn* 1993;13(5):403–409.
172. Siber M. X-linked recessive microencephaly microphthalmia with corneal opacities spastic quadriplegia hypospadias and cryptorchidism. *Clin Genet* 1984;26:453–456.
173. Siebert J, Graham J, MacDonald C. Pathologic features of the CHARGE association: support for involvement of the neural crest. *Teratology* 1985;31:331–336.
174. Sjögren T, Larsson T. Microphthalmos and anophthalmos with or without coincident oligophrenia. *Acta Psychiatr Neurol Scand* 1949;56(suppl):1.
175. Sjögren T, Larsson T. Oligophrenia in combination with congenital ichthyosis and spastic disorders: A clinical and genetic study. *Acta Psychiatr Neurol Scand* 1957;32(suppl 113): 1–112.
176. Spagnolo A, Bianchi F, Calabro A, Calzolari E, Clementi M, Mastroiacovo P, et al. Anophthalmia and benomyl in Italy: A multicenter study based on 940,615 newborns. *Reprod Toxicol* 1994;8(5):397–403.
177. Spitznas M, Gerke E, Bateman J. Hereditary posterior microphthalmos with papillomacular fold and high hyperopia. *Arch Ophthalmol* 1983;101:413–417.

178. Spranger J, Bernirschke K, Hall J, Lenz W, Lowry R, Opitz J, et al. Errors of morphogenesis: Concepts and terms. *J Pediatr* 1982;100:160–165.
179. Stark W, Lindsey P, Fagadau W, Michels RG. Persistent hyperplastic primary vitreous. Surgical treatment. *Ophthalmology* 1983;90:452–457.
180. Steahly L. Laser treatment of a subretinal neovascular membrane associated with a retinochoroidal coloboma. *Retina* 1986;6:154–156.
181. Storimans C, Van Schoonefeld M. Rieger's eye anomaly and persistent hyperplastic primary vitreous. *Ophthalmic Paediatr Genet* 1989;10:257–262.
182. Streeter G. Focal deficiencies in fetal tissues and their relation to intrauterine amputation. *Contrib Embryol Carnegie Inst* 1930;22:1–44.
183. Strömland K. Ocular involvement in the fetal alcohol syndrome. *Surv Ophthalmol* 1987;31:277–283.
184. Strömland K, Miller M, Cook C. Ocular teratology. *Surv Ophthalmol* 1991;35:429–446.
185. Sugar S, Berman M. Relationship between the mandibulofacial dysostosis syndrome of Franceschetti and the oculo-auriculo-vertebral dysplasia of Goldenhar. *Am J Ophthalmol* 1968;66:510–514.
186. Sulik K, Cook C, Webster W. Teratogens and craniofacial malformations: Relationships to cell death. *Development* 1988;103(suppl):213–232.
187. Tagawa T, Mimaki T, Ono J, Amia K, Yabuchi H. Aicardi syndrome associated with an embryonal carcinoma. *Pediatr Neurol* 1989;5:45–47.
188. Tassabehji M, Read A, Newton V, Harris R, Balling R, Gruss P, et al. Waardenburg's syndrome patients have mutations in the human homologue of the Pax-3 paired box gene. *Nature* 1992;355:635–636.
189. Teebi A, Al-Saleh Q. Nonsyndromal microphthalmia. *Clin Genet* 1989;34:311–312.
190. Temple I, Hurst J, Hing S, Butler L, Baraitser M. De novo deletion of Xp22.2-pter in a female with linear skin lesions of the face and neck, microphthalmia, and anterior chamber eye anomalies. *J Med Genet* 1990;27:56–58.
191. Temtamy S, Shalash B. Genetic heterogeneity of the syndrome: Microphthalmia with congenital cataract. *Birth Defects Orig Art Ser* 1974;10:292–293.
192. Ton C, Hirvonen H, Miwa H, Well M, Monaghan P, Jordan T, et al. Positional cloning and characterization of a paired box- and homeobox-containing gene from the aniridia region. *Cell* 1991;67:1059–1074.
193. Torpin R. *Fetal Malformations Caused by Amniotic Rupture During Pregnancy*. Springfield, IL: Charles C Thomas, 1968.
194. Tower P. Coloboma of lower lid and choroid with facial defects and deformity of hand and forearm. *Arch Ophthalmol* 1953;50:333.
195. Traboulsi E, Faris B, Der Kaloustian V. Persistent hyperplastic primary vitreous and recessive oculo-dento-osseous dysplasia. *Am J Med Genet* 1986;24:95–100.
196. Traboulsi E, Lenz W, Gonzales-Ramos M, Siegel J, Macrae W, Maumenee I. The Lenz microphthalmia syndrome. *Am J Ophthalmol* 1988;105:40–45.
197. Traboulsi E, Maumenee I. Ocular findings in mucolipidosis III. *Am J Ophthalmol* 1986;102:592–597.
198. Traboulsi E, Maumenee I. Peters' anomaly and associated congenital malformations. *Arch Ophthalmol* 1992;110:1739–1742.
199. Traboulsi E, Nasr A, Fahd S, et al. Waardenburg's recessive anophthalmia syndrome. *Ophthalmic Paediatr Genet* 1984;4:13–18.
200. Traboulsi E, O'Neill J. The spectrum in the morphology of the so-called "morning glory" anomaly of the optic disc. *J Pediatr Ophthalmol Strabismus* 1988;25:93–98.
201. Usher C. A pedigree of microphthalmia with myopia and corectopia. *Br J Ophthalmol* 1921;5:289.
202. Velez G. Duane's retraction syndrome associated with Goldenhar's syndrome. *Am J Ophthalmol* 1970;70:945–946.
203. Vingolo E, Steidl K, Forte R, Zompatori L, Iannacone A, Sciarra A, et al. Autosomal dominant simple microphthalmos. *J Med Genet* 1994;31:721–725.
204. Von Domaru D, Rieger H, Naumann G. Recurrent iritis caused by persistent hyperplastic primary vitreous with pseudophakia lipomatosa. *Ophthalmologica* 1979;179:354.
205. Von Szily A. Die Ontogenese der idiotypischen (erbildichen) Spaltbildungen des Auges des Mikrophthalmus und der Orbitalcysten. *Z Anat* 1934;74:1–230.
206. Waardenburg P. Autosomally-recessive anophthalmia with malformations of the hands and feet. In *Genetics and Ophthalmology*, P. Waardenburg, A. Franceschetti, and D. Klein, eds. The Netherlands: Royal Van Gorcum, 1961:773.

207. Wang N, Phillips C. Persistent hyperplastic primary vitreous in non-identical twins. *Acta Ophthalmol* 1973;51:434.
208. Wapenaar M, Bassi M, Schaefer L, Grillo A, Ferrero G, Chinault A, et al. The genes for X-linked ocular albinism (OA1) and microphthalmia with linear skin defects (MLS): Cloning and characterization of the critical regions. *Hum Mol Genet* 1993;2:947–952.
209. Warburg M. Norrie disease. *Acta Ophthalmol* 1966;88(suppl):13.
210. Warburg M. Hydrocephaly congenital retinal non-attachment and congenital falciform fold. *Am J Ophthalmol* 1978;85:88–94.
211. Warburg M. Diagnostic precision in microphthalmos and coloboma of heterogeneous origin. *Ophthalmic Paediatr Genet* 1981;1:37–42.
212. Warburg M. Microphthalmos and colobomata among mentally retarded individuals. *Acta Ophthalmol* 1981;59:665.
213. Warburg M. Ocular coloboma and multiple congenital anomalies The CHARGE association. *Ophthalmic Paediatr Genet* 1983;3:189–199.
214. Warburg M. Update of sporadic microphthalmos and coloboma: Non-inherited anomalies. *Ophthalmic Paediatr Genet* 1992;13:111–122.
215. Warburg M, Friedrich U. Coloboma and microphthalmos in chromosomal aberrations. *Ophthalmic Paediatr Genet* 1987;8:105–118.
216. Waring G, Roth A, Rodrigies M. Clinicopathologic correlation of microphthalmos with cyst. *Am J Ophthalmol* 1976;82:714.
217. Wechsler M, Papa C, Haberman F, Marion R. Variable expression in focal dermal hypoplasia. An example of differential X-chromosome inactivation. *Am J Dis Child* 1988;142:297–300.
218. Weiss A, Koussef B, Ross E, Longbottom J. Complex microphthalmos. *Arch Ophthalmol* 1989;107:1619–1624.
219. Weiss A, Koussef B, Ross E, Longbottom J. Simple microphthalmos. *Arch Ophthalmol* 1989;107:1625–1630.
220. Weiss A, Martinez C, Greenwald M. Microphthalmos with cyst clinical presentations and computed tomographic findings. *J Pediatr Ophthalmol Strabismus* 1985;22:6–12.
221. Wilkes S, Campbell R, Waller R. Ocular malformation in association with ipsilateral facial nevus of Jadassohn. *Am J Ophthalmol* 1981;92:344–352.
222. Wilson W, Campochiaro P, Conway B. Deletion (13)(q141q143) in two generations: Variability of ocular manifestations and definition of the phenotype. *Am J Med Genet* 1987;28:675–683.
223. Wolter J, Flaherty N. Persistent hyperplastic vitreous. *Am J Ophthalmol* 1959;47:491.
224. Wright D, Yuh W, Thompson S, Nerad J. Bilateral microphthalmos with orbital cysts: MR findings. *J Comput Assist Tomogr* 1987;11:727–729.
225. Yokoyama Y, Narahara K, Tsuji K, Ninomiya S, Seino Y. Autosomal dominant congenital cataract and microphthalmia associated with a familial t(216) translocation. *Hum Genet* 1992;90:177–178.
226. Young I, Fielder A, Simpson K. Microcephaly microphthalmos and retinal folds: Report of a family. *J Med Genet* 1987;24:172–184.
227. Zeiter H. Congenital microphthalmos. A pedigree of four affected siblings and an additional report of forty four sporadic cases. *Am J Ophthalmol* 1963;55:910–922.
228. Zlotogora J, Legum C, Rax J, Merin S, Ben Ezra D. Autosomal recessive colobomatous microphthalmia. *Am J Med Genet* 1994;49:261–262.

5

Malformations of the Anterior Segment of the Eye

ELIAS I. TRABOULSI

This chapter covers the clinical aspects of congenital malformations of the cornea and anterior chamber angle and some of those that involve the iris and lens. This grouping is arbitrary and reflects the anatomic proximity of the structures involved rather than common pathogenetic or embryopathic mechanisms among the different anomalies. Embryology and genetics are discussed in each section.

CONGENITAL ANOMALIES OF THE CORNEA

Cornea Plana

The radius of curvature of the cornea is larger than normal in patients with cornea plana; this results in apparent continuity of the curvature of the sclera over the area of the cornea.[30–32,69] Eriksson and co-workers[28] list the following five clinical groups of signs in patients with cornea plana: (*1*) The corneoscleral limbal area is widened and there is superficial haziness of the limbus and an indistinct merge between sclera and cornea. The clear corneal diameter is small. Arcus senilis occurs at an early age. (*2*) There is a round gray central corneal zone that measures about 5 mm in diameter. The corneal stroma is thin at the margin of this area and thicker in its middle. The parenchyma of this disc-shaped central area is more opaque than the rest of the corneal stroma. (*3*) The corneal radius is larger than normal. The anterior portion of the eye is therefore less prominent or bulging than normal when visualized from the side. (*4*) The cornea is thinner than normal. (*5*) There may be mild ptosis in some patients.

The clinical findings are fairly consistent between the two eyes of one patient and among affected family members. In mild cases, visual acuity ranges from 20/25 to 20/30. In severe cases, other ocular abnormalities may be present such as malformations of the iris, a slitlike pupil, or adhesions between the iris and cornea. Absence of the lens has also been described. Eriksson et al.[28] reported 34 sibships comprising 56 cases of cornea plana. Seven patients with the dominant form of the disease were found in two families. Twenty-six patients from 13 sibships with the recessive form had common ancestors and lived in Lapland. Patients with the milder dominant form of cornea plana do not exhibit the central opacity that is typical of the recessive form. Corneal curvature deviates from normal by 5–8 diopters only in dominant cases. In the recessive form, corneal refraction (K readings) may be as low as 23 diopters and most readings are below 34 diopters. Despite the expected decrease in refractive power of the cornea, based on keratometric readings, there is no significant hyperopia in most patients; this is probably due to the increased thickness of the central portion of the cornea. The average axial length of 34 eyes was 24.1 mm (21.4–27.4 mm).[28] Some patients with long globes may even be myopic. No signs are present in the parents of patients with recessive cornea plana. Some patients develop glaucoma later in life. The gene (CNA2) for the autosomal recessive form was mapped to 12q21 by Tahvanainen and co-workers.[109]

Management of patients with cornea plana consists of correction of associated errors of refraction and the early detection and treatment of glaucoma.

Megalocornea

The cornea measures between 13.0 and 16.5 mm in diameter at birth but is otherwise normal in curvature, thickness, and endothelial cell density (Fig. 5.1).[76,103,131] In contrast, patients with congenital glaucoma have a hazy and thick cornea with decreased endothelial cell density. Patients with megalocornea may develop presenile cataracts, and with age are found to have a corneal arcus and a crocodile shagreen pattern of opacification of the corneal stroma (Fig. 5.2).[76] Carrier females do not have any corneal anomalies.

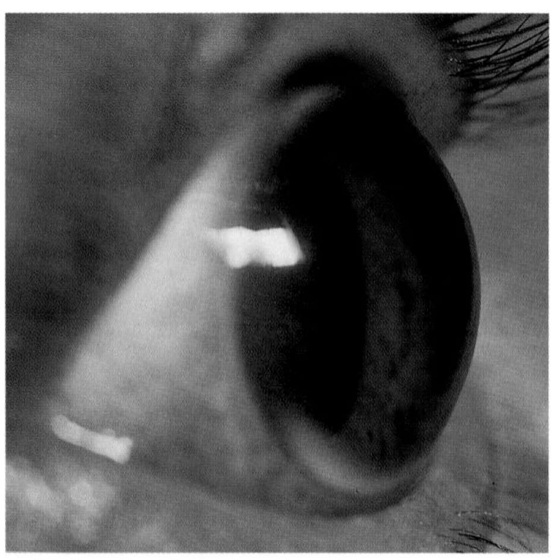

Figure 5.1. Megalocornea.

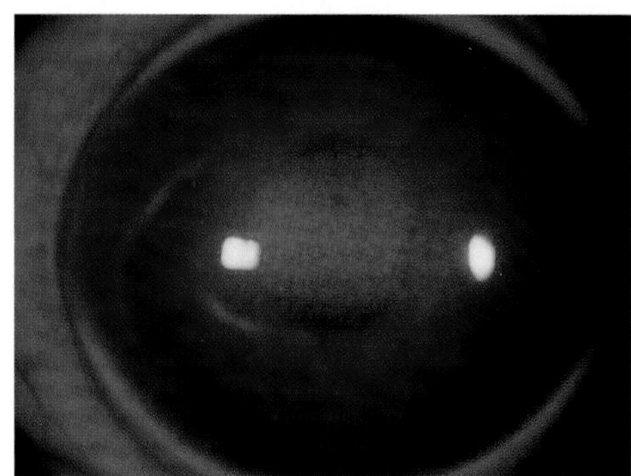

Figure 5.2. Posterior crocodile shagreen in a patient with X-linked megalocornea. (Courtesy of Dr. David Mackey.)

Megalocornea is generally inherited in an X-linked recessive fashion and the gene was mapped to Xq21.3-q22.[17,76] Megalocornea is occasionally present in patients with Marfan syndrome, Down syndrome, or Rieger syndrome. A dominant pedigree of megalocornea has been reported by Kraft and co-workers.[66] Three females in three generations had megalocornea, iris thinning, iridodonesis, but no evidence of goniodysgenesis. Kraft and co-workers[66] do not comment on the systemic evaluation of their patients to rule out the Marfan syndrome. It is also possible that the patients reported by Kraft et al.[66] have megalocornea associated with iris hypoplasia as a sign of anterior segment dysgenesis in the Axenfeld-Rieger spectrum. There is a well-recognized autosomal recessive syndrome of megalocornea and mental retardation.[85]

Management of megalocornea consists of the exclusion of congenital glaucoma, and the recognition of associated systemic disease when it is present. Older patients may require cataract extraction.

Microcornea

The corneal diameter in microcornea is less than 9 or 10 mm at birth. Ocular size as determined by ultrasonography is normal in isolated microcornea, and it is small in microphthalmia. Microcornea may be inherited in a dominant or in a recessive fashion. Microcornea with cataracts is X-linked recessive and is part of the Nance-Horan syndrome of cataracts, microcornea, and dental and ear anomalies.[71,72,121] Associated ocular anomalies include aniridia,[23] cataracts,[34,90] subluxated lenses, and glaucoma.[33] Management of patients with microcornea includes treatment of the associated glaucoma and cataract if they are present.

Sclerocornea

In sclerocornea there is congenital, nonprogressive corneal opacification that may be peripheral, sectoral, or central in location. The cornea has a flat curvature. The great majority of cases are bilateral.[27] On histologic sections, corneal collagen bundles are larger than normal in diameter and the collagen fibers and lamellae are irregularly arranged, resulting in corneal opacification. Descemet's membrane and the endothelium may be absent or abnormal.[61] A number of associated ocular anomalies have been reported and sclerocornea has occurred in well-defined malformation syndromes such as Hallerman-Streiff syndrome and Mieten syndrome.[98,124] Corneal transplantation may be required in some patients with sclerocornea and central corneal involvement.

Corneal Dermoids

Corneal dermoids may be isolated clinical findings or may be a manifestation of the Goldenhar syndrome (see also Chapter 4).

Autosomal dominant inheritance of ring corneal dermoids was reported by Mattos and coworkers in a Peruvian family.[78] None of the five affected members had extraocular abnormalities. The dermoids straddled the limbus for 360° in all patients and extended about 5 mm onto the conjunctiva.

A probable X-linked form of corneal dermoids was reported by Henkind and co-workers[50] in two cousins who had no other ocular or systemic abnormalities.

THE AXENFELD-RIEGER SPECTRUM

Definition, Morphology, and Histopathology

In the Axenfeld-Rieger spectrum there is a variety of anterior ocular segment malformations that have arisen from abnormal development of the anterior chamber angle, cornea, and iris. Terms that have been used to describe the various configurations of these anterior segment abnormalities include anterior chamber cleavage syndrome, mesodermal dysgenesis of the cornea and iris, *dysgenesis mesodermalis corneae et iridis*, primary dysgenesis mesodermalis of the iris, iridogoniodysgenesis, and Axenfeld-Rieger syndrome.[2,102,125]

Included under the heading of anterior segment dysgenesis are (*1*) posterior embryotoxon, in which there is a prominent and anteriorly displaced line of Schwalbe (the most peripheral portion of Descemet's membrane) in the peripheral cornea; (*2*) Axenfeld anomaly, in which strands of iris tissue attach to Schwalbe's line[6]; and (*3*) Rieger anomaly, where, in addition to an Axenfeld anomaly, there is clinically evident iris stromal atrophy with hole or pseudo-hole formation and corectopia.[94,95]

Anterior displacement of Schwalbe's line is present in most patients with Axenfeld-Rieger spectrum of malformations but is not a universal finding and is not necessary for the diagnosis. Prominence of the peripheral edge of Descemet's membrane or posterior embryotoxon is present in about 15% of the general adult population[15] and is accompanied by bridging iris strands (Axenfeld anomaly) in 6% of otherwise normal individuals. The incidence of Rieger anomaly is not known.

Ocular Findings

Anterior segment dysgenesis or the Axenfeld-Rieger spectrum is a bilateral, often symmetrical condition that affects males and females equally. There is a wide variation in clinical expression within families where the disease is inherited as an autosomal dominant trait. Some infants are discovered because of the abnormal appearance of the iris. Others have signs and symptoms of infantile glaucoma such as tearing, photophobia, and corneal clouding. The diagnosis in other patients is made in adolescence or early adulthood when they may present with visual loss and are found to have advanced childhood or juvenile glaucoma. Finally, patients may be identified as they are examined because of a positive family history of the disease. Nonocular abnormalities suggesting a di-

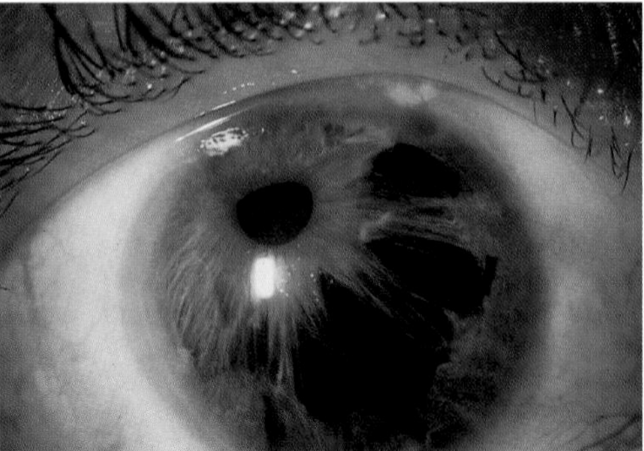

Figure 5.3. Rieger syndrome. Pupil is displaced superiorly. There are large areas of iris atrophy and a prominent and anteriorly displaced Schwalbe's line.

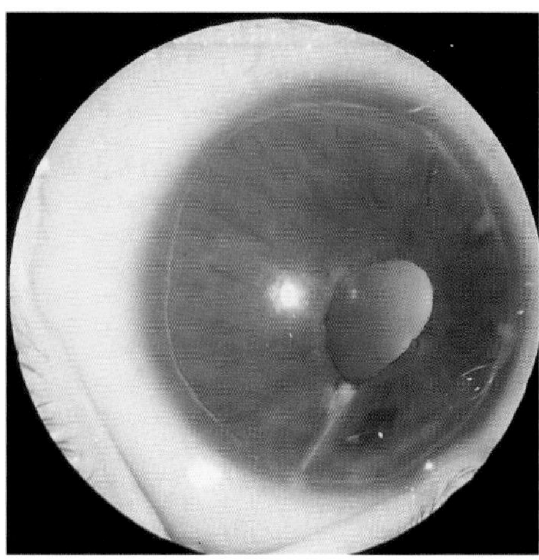

Figure 5.5. Anterior segment dysgenesis with posterior embryotoxon and fibrous band bridging the pupil to the angle.

agnosis of Rieger syndrome (vide infra) may prompt an ocular examination.

The appearance of the iris is highly polymorphic. The peripheral iridocorneal adhesions may be thick and wide, or they may be fine and lacy, occupying any segment of the circumference of the angle. The trabecular meshwork may appear normal or may be obscured by an anteriorly inserted iris. The iris stroma is usually thin and there may be extensive defects with polycoria (multiple pupils) (Fig. 5.3) or pseudopolycoria (Fig. 5.4). The pupil may be ectopic (corectopia) (Fig. 5.5), in which case iris hypoplasia is most severe in the sector of iris away from the direction of corectopia. In some patients the corectopia may simulate a typical uveal coloboma of the iris (Fig. 5.6). In contradistinction to essential iris atrophy, the iridal changes in patients with the Rieger anomaly are nonprogressive except in rare instances.[42,60,101] I observed spontaneous release of iridocorneal adhesions in an infant with this condition and restoration of a round pupil from one that was tear shaped. Megalocornea is an occasional association, but the corneal diameter is generally normal or occasionally small. Rieger's anomaly is rarely associated with other ocular abnormalities such as aniridia, blue sclerae, cornea plana, dislocated lenses, hypoplasia of the optic nerve head, macular degeneration, medullated nerve fibers, and retinal detach-

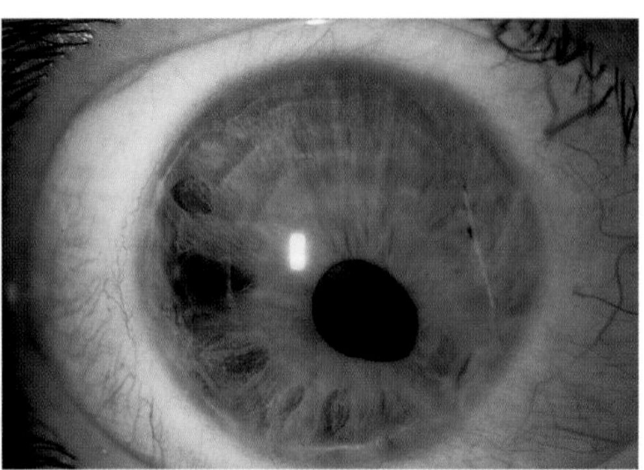

Figure 5.4. Anterior segment photograph of a patient with classic findings of Rieger syndrome.

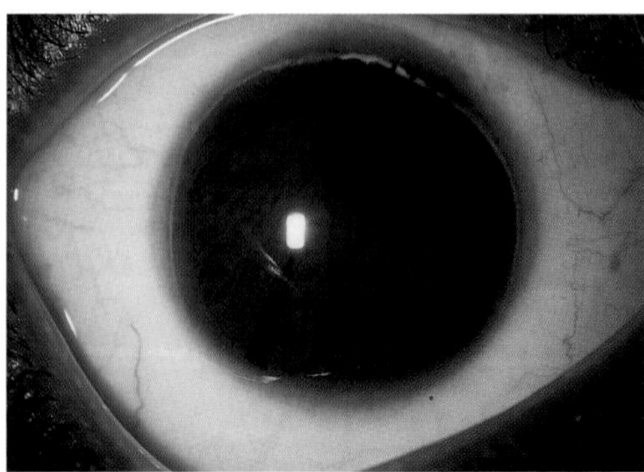

Figure 5.6. Rieger syndrome. Pupil is drawn inferiorly and attaches to a prominent and anteriorly displaced Schwalbe's line, giving the appearance of a coloboma. Patient was initially diagnosed as having typical iris coloboma.

ment.[101,104] Ectropion of the pigmented posterior layer of the iris onto the anterior surface of the iris in the region of the pupil may be present in some patients.

Congenital Ectropion of the Iris

Congenital iris ectropion (Fig. 5.7) is classified by some investigators[129] with the goniodysgenesis syndromes and is attributed to late arrest of anterior segment development with retention of primordial endothelium. Patients with congenital iris ectropion have iridotrabecular dysgenesis and are predisposed to glaucoma. In addition to the ectropion, patients have a thin iris stroma, goniodysgenesis and, occasionally, blepharoptosis. This disorder may be a separate well-defined abnormality of neural crest development and differentiation or may be a variant of the Axenfeld-Rieger spectrum of abnormalities.

Glaucoma

Glaucoma, the only vision-threatening complication, occurs in about 50% of patients with anterior segment dysgenesis by age 20 years and in 10%–15% of patients per decade thereafter. The elevation of intraocular pressure is presumed to result from poor drainage of aqueous humor through abnormally developed anterior chamber angle structures. Some authors, including Bahn et al.,[7] have included primary infantile glaucoma with the goniodysgenetic disorders because of the abnormal development of the anterior chamber angle and trabecular meshwork in this last group of patients. Primary infantile glaucoma is, however, most often inherited in an autosomal recessive fashion, and two of the causative genes have been mapped to chromosomes 2p21 and 1p36.[1a,97a] Mutations in cytochrome P4501B1 were shown to lead to the disease linked to the 2p21 locus.[105a]

Rieger Syndrome

Rieger syndrome is a multisystem autosomal dominant condition where anterior segment dysgenesis of the eye (Rieger anomaly) is accompanied by facial, dental, umbilical, and skeletal abnormalities.[2,21] Rieger syndrome is estimated to occur in 1 in 200,000 persons. The ocular findings are extremely variable between

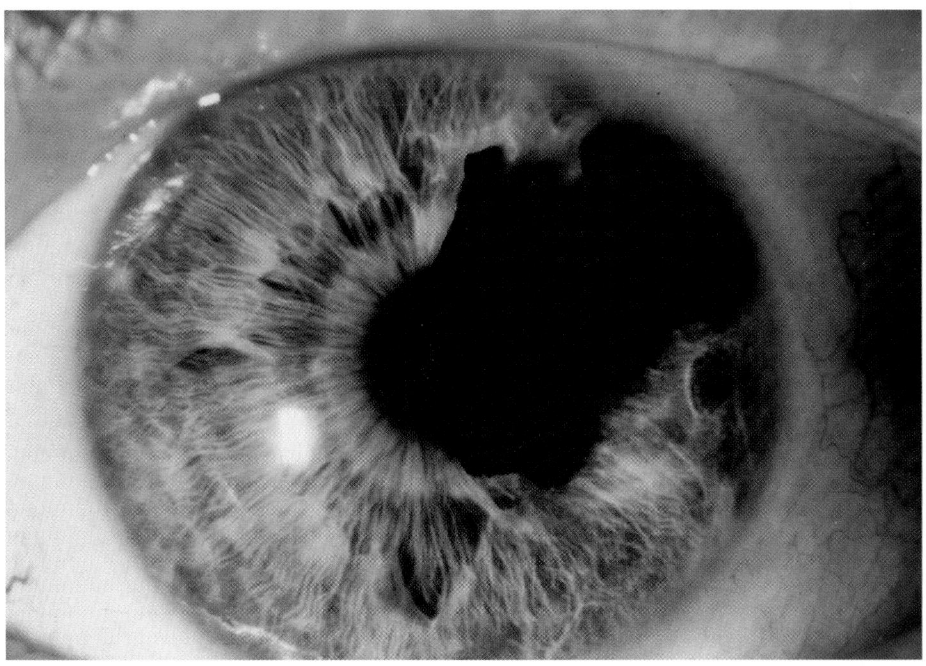

Figure 5.7. Congenital ectropion of the iris. (Courtesy of Dr. M. Edward Wilson.)

and within families with this condition. Pearce and Kerr[86] and Feingold and co-workers[29] have described large families where the variability of expression of the gene is very well illustrated. The characteristic facial features of the Rieger syndrome consist of a broad nasal root with telecanthus, maxillary hypoplasia and a prominent lower lip. Dental anomalies include hypodontia and partial anodontia, most commonly absence of the central and lateral maxillary incisors (Fig. 5.8).[59] The remaining teeth have small crowns. Failure of involution of the periumbilical skin is a cardinal feature (Fig. 5.9)[59]; the redundant skin is often mistaken for an umbilical hernia leading sometimes to unnecessary surgical procedures. The normal length of the periumbilical skin in newborns is 12.36 ± 3.23 mm cranially and 8.76 ± 3.10 mm caudally.[110] Toppare et al.[110] suggest that if the length of the periumbilical skin is more than 18.82 mm cranially (> 2 standard deviations from the mean), Rieger syndrome should be considered. Anal stenosis is a less well-recognized feature of the syndrome.[22] Four of ten affected of a family reported by Chisholm and Chudley[18] had hypospadias. Rare associated findings include empty or enlarged sella turcica,[64] growth hormone deficiency,[97] and growth hormone deficiency with congenital parasellar arachnoid cyst.[101] There is a rare association of Rieger anomaly with psychomotor retardation[24,120]; it is not clear whether this represents a separate syndrome or the fortuitous association of the two abnormalities. The mother and three children described by De Hauwere et al.[24] also had mild deafness and dilatation of the cerebral ventricles.

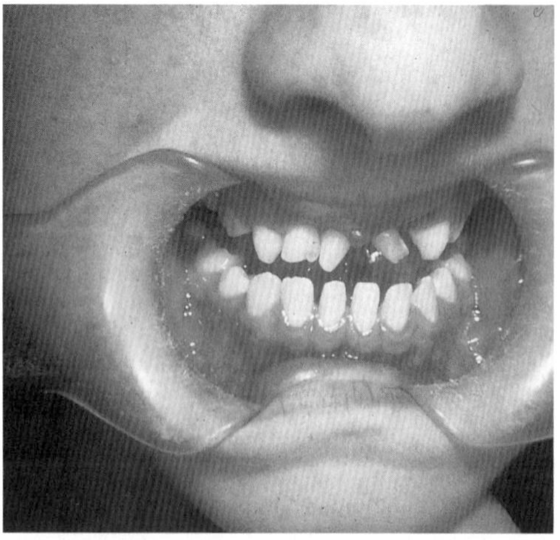

Figure 5.8. Misshaped and missing teeth in a patient with Rieger syndrome. (Patient of the late Dr. Steven Levin.)

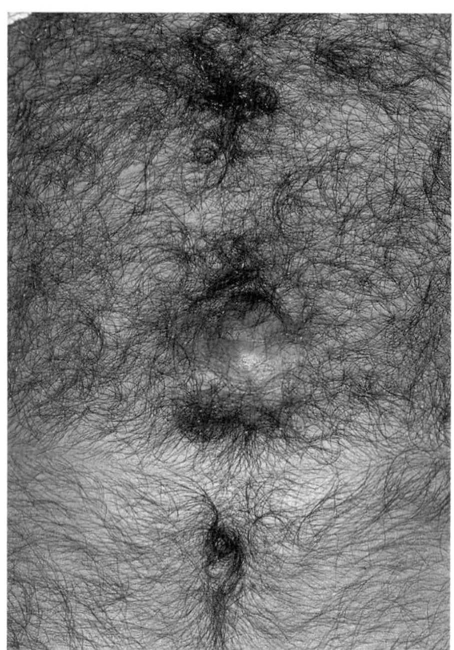

Figure 5.9. Umbilical redundant skin in an adult with Rieger syndrome.

Etiology and Genetics

The Axenfeld-Rieger spectrum of anomalies is thought to be due to an abnormality of neural crest development and/or resorption.[58,101] Shields and co-workers[101,102] have postulated that, late in gestation, a developmental arrest leads to retention of the primordial endothelium over portions of the iris and anterior chamber angle. Incomplete posterior recession of the peripheral uvea produces a high insertion of the iris. This arrest also causes the zone of differentiation between the corneal and anterior angle endothelium to be abnormally located and associated with prominence and anterior displacement of Schwalbe's line. The retained endothelial cells may bridge the angle along with a few iris strands and contract pulling the iris strands towards the center. Contraction of the primoridal endothelium also leads to corectopia and ectropion uveae. Endothelial cells will later disappear leaving the abnormal iris configuration. In Rieger syndrome, associated systemic anomalies are also due to abnormal neural crest differentiation. Neural crest-derived structures such as facial bones and cartilage, dental papillae, and the primitive periumbilical ring are affected resulting in facial dysmorphism with maxillary hypoplasia and a receding chin, hypodontia and peg-shaped teeth, and redundant periumbilical skin.

The genes for Rieger syndrome are autosomal dominant, fully penetrant, and variable in expressivity. Clues to the location of these genes came from reports of patients with anterior segment dysgenesis and chromosomal aberrations involving chromosomes 4, 6, 10, 13, 16, and 22.[1,37,48,51,105,107,128] Vaux and co-workers[117] suggested that Rieger syndrome maps to 4q25-q27 in a family with an interstitial deletion of that segment of the long arm of chromosome 4. Similarly, Fryns and Van Den Berghe[36] found a deletion of 4q25-q26 in a patient with Rieger syndrome and mental retardation. Using a set of short tandem repeat polymorphisms and linkage analysis, Murray and colleagues[83] mapped the gene for Rieger syndrome to 4q in one large family. The region of 4q25-q26 contains the gene for the epidermal growth factor, which was felt to be an excellent candidate for Rieger syndrome. Alward and Murray[3] studied several families for sequence variants in this gene and failed to find cosegregation of these variants with the disease, indicating that the epidermal growth factor gene was most likely not the Rieger syndrome gene. Motegi et al.[82] reported a girl with multiple malformations, deletion of band 4q26, and no Rieger malformation. Furthermore, Legius et al.[70] failed to show linkage to 4q markers in a three-generation family with facial and ocular, but no dental or umbilical findings of the Rieger syndrome, suggesting genetic heterogeneity. Héon and co-workers[50a] studied a family with dominantly inherited iris hypoplasia and found linkage to 4q25 markers, suggesting allelism between this form of anterior segment dysgenesis and more classical Rieger syndrome.

Evidence of genetic heterogeneity was presented by Walter and co-workers,[122] who excluded the 4q25 locus in a family with what the authors termed iridogoniodysgenesis anomaly (IGDA; i.e., anterior segment dysgenesis with iris hypoplasia, excess tissue, and anomalous vascular tissue in the angle) in the absence of nonocular features such as hypertelorism, maxillary hypoplasia, dental anomalies, umbilical hernia, and hypospadius in males. These authors[122] established linkage to the 4q25 locus in another family with the iridogoniodysgenesis syndrome (IGDS), which includes ocular and systemic abnormalities. The same group later mapped the gene for the family with iridogoniodysgenesis anomaly to 6p25.[80]

Phillips and co-workers[88] identified another locus for the Rieger syndrome on chromosome 13q14. These authors[88] studied a four-generation family with the characteristic ocular phenotype and other systemic abnormalities including, sometimes in only one family member, oligodontia, premature loss of teeth, hearing loss, maxillary hypoplasia, hydrocephalus, congenital hip malformation cryptorchidism, and congenital tricuspid valve abnormality.

Semina and co-workers[100] cloned the Rieger syndrome gene located at 4q25. This gene, *RIEG*, is a novel, *bicoid*-related homeobox transcription factor gene. Its murine homologue, *Rieg*, is expressed in periocular mesenchyme, maxillary and mandibular epithelia, the umbilicus, Rathke's pouch, vitelline vessels, and limb mesenchyme. Semina et al.[100] identified six *RIEG* mutations in families with Rieger syndrome.

Associated Syndromes

A few multisystem disorders feature anterior segment dysgenesis and a careful ophthalmologic evaluation should be part of the routine workup of patients with these syndromes. These include Alagille syndrome or arteriohepatic dysplasia, the Wolf-Hirschhorn syndrome (4p− syndrome),[128] and the Abruzzo-Erikson syndrome.[118]

Alagille syndrome is characterized by dysmorphic facial appearance and neonatal jaundice as a result of congenital absence of the bile collecting ducts in the liver.[66a] Patients may also have spine abnormalities such as butterfly vertebrae or hemivertebrae. Alagille syndrome is caused by mutations in *Jagged 1*, a gene that encodes a ligand for *Notch 1*.[73a,85b] This gene is located on chromosome region 20p12.[52,93] Many patients have a prominent posterior embryotoxon observable without the use of the slit lamp; this is not a universal finding, however.[13,127] Pigmentary changes in the fundus accompanied by choroidal atrophy are present in some patients.[92] Up to 90% of patients have unilateral optic nerve head drusen and as many as 65% have bilateral drusen.[85a] If patients have elevated serum cholesterol levels, arcus juvenilis may develop. In some patients there is marked tortuosity of the retinal vessels. Keratoconus is a rare associated finding.[112] The liver dysfunction improves with age.

An association of anterior segment dysgenesis and oculocutaneous albinism has also been reported (and three personal observations).[74] Additionally, Rieger syndrome has been reported in association with a number of chromosomal abnormalities reviewed by Stathacopoulos et al.,[105] who have reported a patient with Rieger syndrome and an interstitial deletion of chromosome 13 (q14-q31).

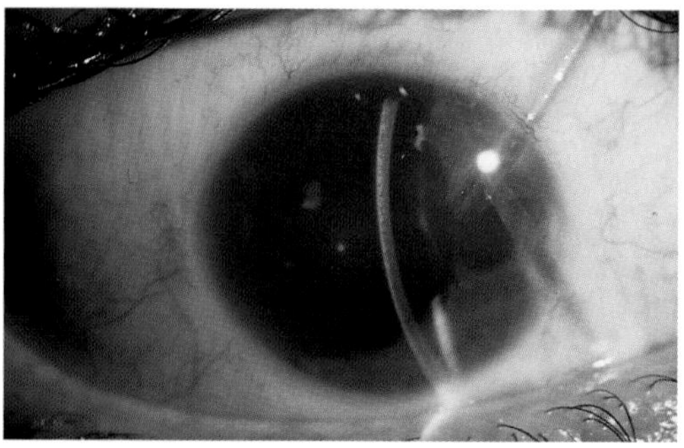

Figure 5.10. Two filtering tubes in anterior chamber of a patient with Rieger syndrome and advanced glaucoma. Most of the iris is missing from birth.

Management, Prognosis, and Prevention

The major complications of the Axenfeld-Rieger spectrum of ocular anomalies are the development of glaucoma and glaucomatous visual loss. When glaucoma presents in infancy, it is easily detected because of the associated signs and symptoms of photophobia, tearing, corneal clouding, and corneal enlargement. Early surgical intervention and postoperative visual rehabilitation result in a fair prognosis for vision in some patients. Patients who develop glaucoma in late childhood or early adulthood may not come to medical attention until field defects impinge on central vision. Such patients are first treated with topical antiglaucomatous medications but often require filtering surgery with a guarded visual outcome (Fig. 5.10). Affected siblings and children of patients with Axenfeld-Rieger anomaly should be monitored closely for the development of glaucoma before the development of visual field loss. Frequent ocular examinations (every 4–6 months) are recommended in patients with this spectrum of ocular disorders. All available family members should be examined for anterior segment malformations. Genetic counselors should take into consideration the autosomal dominant mode of inheritance of the disease, the nearly complete penetrance of the gene, and the variability of clinical presentation.

When anterior segment dysgenesis is associated with a multisystem malformation syndrome, prognosis depends on the severity of the associated congenital abnormalities and their impact on the patient's general health.

PETERS' ANOMALY

Peters' anomaly consists of a central corneal leukoma, absence of the posterior corneal stroma and Descemet's membrane, and a variable degree of iris and lenticular attachments to the central aspect of the posterior cornea.[87] Histopathologic studies are numerous and confirm the clinical diagnosis.[68,84,89,91,106,111]

The spectrum in the morphology of Peters' anomaly is very wide. There may only be a faint corneal leukoma with a small strand of iris attached to the posterior surface of the cornea and a clear lens, or the malformation may be so severe as to produce total corneal opacification, extensive iridocorneal adhesions, and a total cataract (Fig. 5.11). This author also includes some cases of sclerocornea in this spectrum because of the absence of Des-

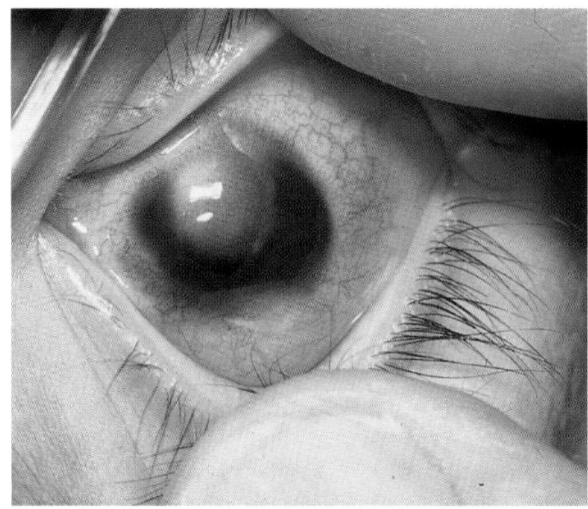

Figure 5.11. Central corneal opacification in a patient with Peters' anomaly. (Courtesy of Dr. Irene H. Maumenee.)

cemet's membrane in many cases of sclerocornea and the coexistence of sclerocornea and classic Peters' anomaly in some patients.

Genetics, Associated Malformations, and Syndromes

Peters' anomaly may be an isolated ocular abnormality or may be associated with ocular defects such as microcornea, anterior polar cataracts, glaucoma with or without buphthalmos, spontaneous corneal perforation, aniridia,[11,65] congenital aphakia,[47,53] persistence of the hyaloid system, and total posterior coloboma of the retina and choroid.[99] Traboulsi and Maumenee[113] found colobomatous microphthalmia in 7 of 29 patients.

Associated systemic congenital anomalies include short stature, abnormal ears, cleft lip/palate abnormalities, malformation of the genitourinary system, cardiovascular anomalies, defects of the extremities, and mental retardation.[4]

In the Peters-plus syndrome,[116] Peters' anomaly occurs in association with cleft lip/palate, mental retardation, and abnormal ears. Traboulsi and Maumenee[113] have shown that the spectrum of malformations in Peters-plus syndrome includes midline defects, cardiovascular and urogenital anomalies as well as the craniofacial anomalies and mental retardation. These authors reviewed the clinical findings in 29 patients and found developmental delay in 15 patients, congenital heart disease in 8, external ear abnormalities in 5, CNS structural defects in 4, genitourinary malformations in 4, cleft lip/palate in 3, hearing loss in 3, spinal defects in 2, and other less common malformations in single cases. One patient had the fetal alcohol syndrome, one had Pfeiffer syndrome, and one had short stature, ulnar hypoplasia, and joint laxity. Colobomatous microphthalmia was present in 7 patients and persistent hyperplastic primary vitreous in 3. Ten patients developed glaucoma and 3 had retinal detachment unrelated to ocular surgery. In the same series, there was no sexual predilection for the development of the anomaly. Sixty-three percent of patients had bilateral disease and 60% had associated systemic malformations or developmental delay (significant failure to achieve normal cognitive and/or motor developmental milestones). Patients with bilateral involvement were as likely to have associated systemic malformations or developmental delay (12 of 18 patients) as those with unilateral involvement (5 of 11 patients). Patients with posterior segment ocular involvement were not more likely to have associated systemic malformations than those with anterior segment malformations only. Patients with unilateral Peters' anomaly were as likely to have posterior segment involvement as those with bilateral disease.

Familial isolated Peters' anomaly is recessively inherited in the majority of cases,[5,8,12,108] and there are occasional pedigrees with autosomal dominant transmission.[25]

Peters' anomaly with multiple congenital malformations has been reported in patients with chromosomal abnormalities such as an interstitial deletion of the long arm of chromosome 11,[9] a partial deletion of the short arm of chromosome 4,[79] a deletion of the long arm of chromosome 18,[39] a ring chromosome 21,[19] and a balanced translocation between chromosomes 2 and 15.[63] The multiplicity of chromosomal deletions leading to Peters' anomaly is an indication of the genetic heterogeneity of this malformation syndrome and of the limited ability of the developing eye to demonstrate specific phenotypes in response to different genetic defects. Hence it could be argued that Peters' anomaly per se is a nonspecific ocular phenotype that may or may not accompany other congenital defects depending on the underlying genetic or teratogenic insult.

The syndrome of Peters' anomaly with brachymorphy (short stature), also known as the Kivlin-Krause syndrome, appears to be a distinct autosomal recessive condition with several reports of familial cases.[16,35,63,67,96]

More recently, Hanson and co-workers[43] described a child with Peters' anomaly and deletion of one copy of the PAX6 gene (see Chapter 6, Aniridia). The patient did not have other systemic malformations but did have a slight developmental delay. The same authors also reported affected members of a family with dominantly inherited anterior segment malformations and an R26G mutation in one copy of the PAX6 gene. This family, previously reported by Holmstrom and co-workers,[54] was comprised of a mother and daughter with iris hypoplasia and posterior embryotoxon, a son with Peters' anomaly, and another son with iris hypoplasia.

Etiology

Peters' anomaly probably results from an abnormality in the separation of the lens vesicle from the surface ectoderm, with interference in the differentiation of the central cornea and the formation of lenticulo-irido-corneal adhesions. Cook and Sulik[20] developed a mouse model of Peters' anomaly by exposing the mouse fetuses to high doses of alcohol or isotretinoin. Miller and co-workers[81] reported seven patients with Peters' anomaly and fetal alcohol syndrome. Isotretinoin intake in the first trimester of gestation can lead to the development of lenticulo-irido-corneal adhesions and a clinical picture identical to Peters' anomaly. Traboulsi and Maumenee[113] interpreted the nonrandom pattern of associated systemic congenital malformations in their series of 29 patients with Peters' anomaly as evidence for the existence of a clinical syndrome combining Peters' anomaly and other congenital anomalies (so-called Peters-plus syndrome). This is not necessarily a monogenic syndrome; genetic defects that affect organs that differentiate at the same gestational period or that rely on the products of specific genes for proper development may lead to the same broad association of malformations or syndrome. No single chromosomal abnormality has been consistently associated with Peters' anomaly or the Peters-plus syndrome, but the reported deletions or duplications provide starting points to search for a gene or a group of genes involved in ocular development.

Prognosis, Prevention, and Treatment

The visual prognosis of patients with Peters' anomaly depends on the degree of corneal opacification and on the severity of associated ocular malformations. Combined penetrating keratoplasty and cataract extraction is needed in severe cases, whereas simple separation of iridocorneal adhesions or an optical iridectomy[60] suffices in mild ones and results in significant clearing of the corneal opacification with a fair visual outcome. Unilateral cases are usually associated with deep amblyopia and the risk/benefit ratio of surgery in such cases is probably very high. Congenital or postsurgical glaucoma is a major cause of visual loss in many cases.[40] As many as 50% of patients with Peters' anomaly eventually lose all light perception.[40]

Chromosomal studies should be obtained in those patients with multiple congenital malformations and Peters' anomaly. Families with a child with isolated bilateral Peters' anomaly should be counseled as to the possible recessive mode of inheritance of this condition.

Patients with Peters' anomaly should be screened for the presence of systemic malformations, especially those involving midline body structures such as the pituitary, heart, and kidneys. Therapeutic interventions for medical problems resulting from such defects may be life-saving.

CONGENITAL APHAKIA

Absence of the crystalline lens has been divided by Manschot[77] into primary and secondary types. In primary aphakia, there is failure of induction of the surface ectoderm to form a lens placode. Primary aphakia is usually accompanied by severe ocular malformations such as colobomatous microphthalmia, anterior segment dysgenesis such as Peters' anomaly,[46] or anterior segment aplasia.[77,130] Primary aphakia has been reported in patients with trisomy 13,[46] in aborted fetuses with rubella,[119] and in those with parvovirus B19 infection.[126]

Normal PAX6 gene function has been shown to be pivotal in the induction of normal lens and ocular development.[73,123] It is conceivable that mutations in this gene could result in primary aphakia. To date mutations in the PAX6 gene have led to the development of aniridia,[38] and much less commonly to Peters' anomaly, anterior segment dysgenesis, and cataracts.[44]

In secondary aphakia, the lens develops but is later resorbed or expulsed from the developing eye. There may be associated corneal or anterior segment abnormalities, but there are no severe ocular malformations.

ANTERIOR POLAR CATARACTS

Anterior polar cataracts are dense white opacities of the central part of the anterior lens capsule. They vary from a fraction of one to a few millimeters in size. The opacities may be relatively flat, and reduplicate under the anterior lens capsule, or they may assume a pyramidal shape and protrude into the anterior chamber. Although generally considered to be of little visual significance, lenses with anterior polar opacities may opacify with time and may require surgical intervention (and personal observations).[57] Anterior polar cataracts may be accompanied by other congenital malformations of the anterior segment of the eye such as iris atrophy, anterior embryotoxon, and cornea guttata, and as such may be included under the category of anterior segment dysgenesis. Anterior polar cataracts are bilateral in two thirds of cases. Amblyopia is unlikely to develop in patients with bilateral anterior polar cataracts, but we have observed it in unilateral cases.

The syndrome of cornea guttata and anterior polar cataracts was first described in a Scandinavian family by Dohlman[26] in 1951. He postulated that a developmental defect in anterior segment formation may have resulted in both anomalies. Traboulsi and Weinberg[114] reported another family of Scandinavian descent and confirmed Dohlman's observations (Figs. 5.12, 5.13). Two loci for autosomal dominant anterior polar cataracts have been mapped to chromosomes 1p and 17p.[11a,56a]

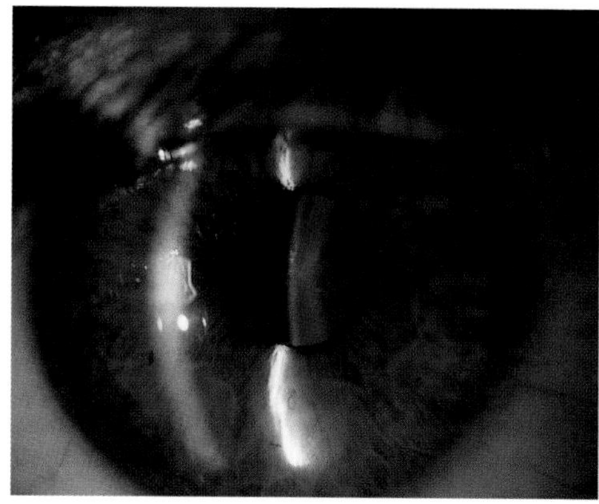

Figure 5.12. Small anterior polar opacity in a patient with dominant anterior polar cataracts and cornea guttata.

Ocular malformations associated with anterior polar cataracts include microphthalmia, aniridia, and remnants of the pupillary membrane (personal observations).[45,57] Brown and coworkers[14] described a patient with bilateral retinoblastoma and bilateral anterior polar cataracts. Green and Johnson[41] reported a family with autosomal dominant Peters' anomaly and cataracts, some of which were anterior polar. We have recorded a variety of anterior segment malformations in several patients with anterior polar cataracts. These malformations included

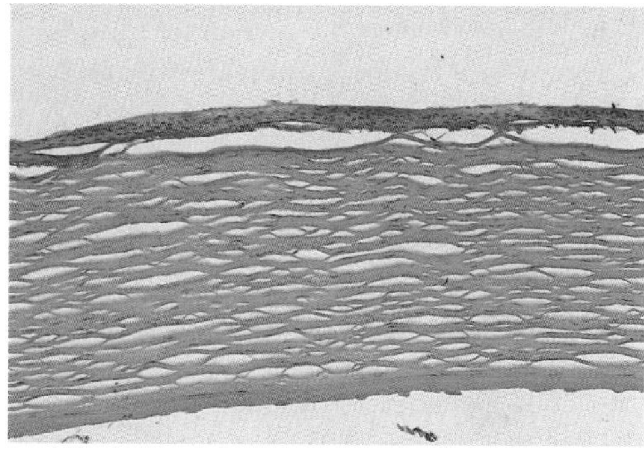

Figure 5.13. Numerous cornea guttata (excrescences of Descemet's membrane) in a patient with associated anterior polar cataracts.

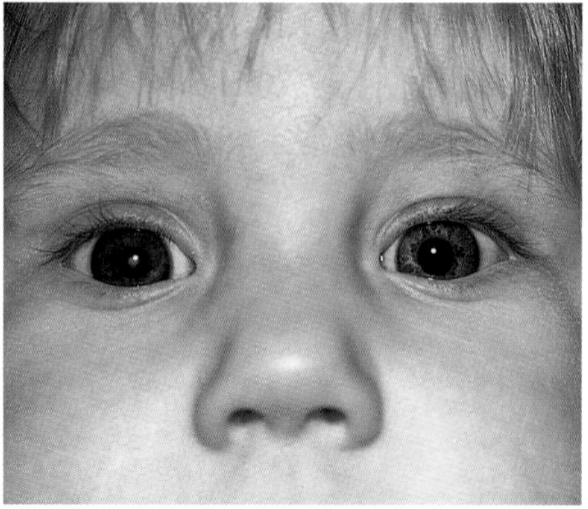

Figure 5.14. Right anterior polar cataract with hypoplastic iris. Right cornea is 0.5 mm smaller than left and there is mild hyperopia of the right eye.

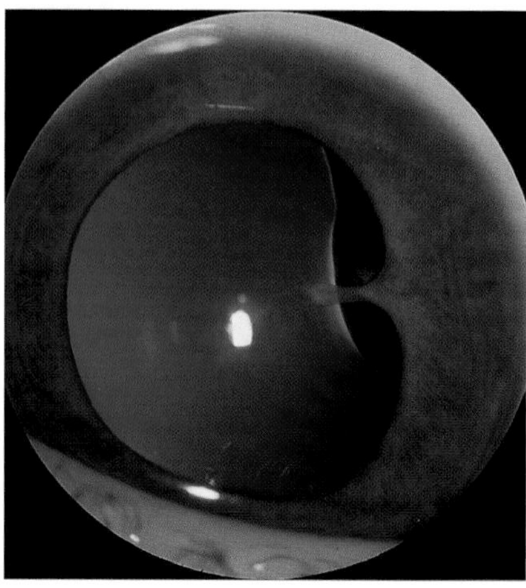

Figure 5.15. Coloboma of the lens with remnant of the pupillary membrane. The patient had an ipsilateral capillary hemangioma of the upper eyelid and orbit.

cornea guttata, posterior embryotoxon, diffuse iris atrophy in a slightly microphthalmic eye (Fig. 5.14), aniridia, and remnants of the pupillary membrane.

Glaucoma is a known complication of anterior segment dysgenesis. One patient developed bilateral aphakic glaucoma shortly after surgery and another patient with anterior polar cataract developed glaucoma without having undergone cataract surgery (Parks MM, personal communication). Patients with anterior polar cataracts should be monitored carefully for the presence of glaucoma, especially following lens extraction.

COLOBOMA OF THE LENS

True colobomas of the lens are extremely rare. More frequently, irregularities in lens contour may occur with typical chorioretinal colobomas that involve the ciliary body and hence the zonules that attach to the inferior pole of the lens; this leads to flattening of the rounded inferior edge of the lens equator.[10,55] In diseases such as Marfan syndrome and simple ectopia lentis, subluxation of the lens may be associated with zonular defects and irregularities of the edge of the lens that have been erroneously referred to as colobomas. Kihara and co-workers[62] reported a patient with partially absorbed, disc-shaped cataract and a coloboma of the lens.

The constellation of coloboma of the lens, hypoplastic ciliary processes, breaks of the pars plicata, and retinal detachment has been described in a number of patients.[56,115] This syndrome is presumed to result from a localized or segmental, sometimes bilateral, malformation of the lens–zonule–ciliary body complex. Some of these patients have elevated intraocular pressure that resolves following retinal reattachment.

This author has examined a single patient with what appeared to be a true coloboma of the lens. The defect was superotemporal and was associated with an anterior adherent leukoma (Fig. 5.15). It is possible that an iridohyaloid vessel that failed to regress interfered with the normal zonular development in that sector and resulted in a lens coloboma.

DUPLICATION OF THE LENS

This is an extremely rare malformation. Lyford and Roy[75] reported a case associated with unilateral arhinencepahly and uveal coloboma with subsequent cataract formation in one of the lenticular structures. Hemady and co-workers[49] described a patient with a large globe, an hourglass cornea, and duplication of the lens (Fig. 5.16). The etiology of this most unusual malformation is unknown.

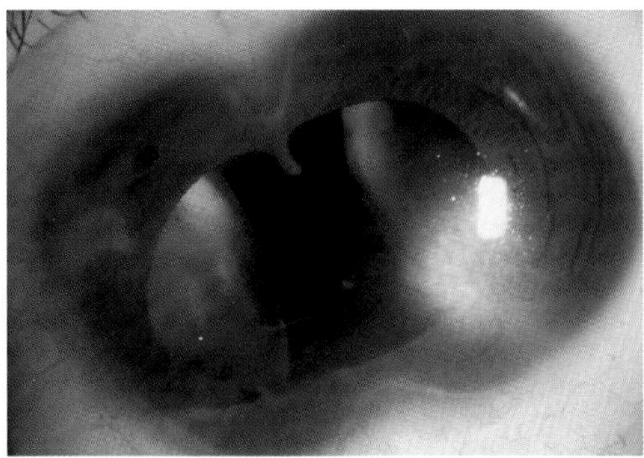

Figure 5.16. Duplication of the lens. (Courtesy of Dr. Ramzi Hemady. Reproduced with permission from Hemady et al.[49])

REFERENCES

1. Akazawa K, Yamane S, Shiota H, Naito E. A case of retinoblastoma associated with Rieger's anomaly and 13q deletion. *Jpn J Ophthalmol* 1981;25:321–325.

1a. Akarsu AN, Turacli ME, Aktan SG, et al. A second locus (GLC3B) for primary congenital glaucoma (buphthalmos) maps to the 1p36 region. *Hum Mol Genet* 1996;5:1199–1203.

2. Alkemade P. *Dysgenesis Mesodermalis of the Iris and Cornea.* Amsterdam, The Netherlands: Royal Van Gorcum, 1969.

3. Alward W, Murray J. Axenfeld-Rieger syndrome. In *Molecular Genetics of Ocular Diseases.* New York: Wiley-Liss, 1995:31–50.

4. Anyane-Yeboa K, Mackay C, Taterka P, et al. Cleft lip and palate corneal opacities and profound psychomotor retardation: A newly recognized syndrome? *Cleft Palate J* 1983; 20:246.

5. Appelmans M, Michiels J, Forez J. Malformations symmetriques du segment anterieur de l'oeil (syndrome de Peters). *Bull Soc Belge Ophtalmol* 1950;94:283–289.

6. Axenfeld T. Embryotoxon corneae posterius. *Ber Deutsch Ophthalmol Ges* 1920;42:301–302.

7. Bahn C, Falls H, Varley G, et al. Classification of corneal endothelial disorders based on neural crest origin. *Ophthalmology* 1984;91: 558–563.

8. Baqueiro A, Hein P Jr. Familial congenital leukoma. Case report and review of the literature. *Am J Ophthalmol* 1960;50:810.

9. Bateman J, Maumenee I, Sparkes R. Peters' anomaly associated with partial deletion of the long arm of chromosome 11. *Am J Ophthalmol* 1984;97:11–15.

10. Bavbek T, Ogut M, Kazokoglu H. Congenital lens coloboma and associated pathologies. *Doc Ophthalmol* 1993;83:312–322.

11. Beauchamp G. Anterior segment dysgenesis keratolenticular adhesion and aniridia. *J Pediatr Ophthalmol Strabismus* 1979;17:55.

11a. Berry V, Ionides AC, Moore TA, et al. A locus for autosomal dominant anterior polar cataract on chromosome 17p. *Hum Mol Genet* 1996; 5:415–419.

12. Boel M, Timmermans J, Emmery L, Dralands G, Fryns J, Van den Berghe H. Primary mesodermal dysgenesis of the cornea (Peters' anomaly) in two brothers. *Hum Genet* 1979;51:237–240.

13. Brodsky M, Cunniff C. Ocular abnormalities in the Alagille syndrome (arteriohepatic syndrome). *Ophthalmology* 1993;100:1767–1774.

14. Brown G, Shields J, Ogelsby R. Anterior polar cataracts associated with bilateral retinoblastoma. *Am J Ophthalmol* 1979;87:276–277.

15. Burian H, Rice M, Allen L. External visibility of the region of Schlemm's canal. *Arch Ophthalmol* 1957;57:651–658.

16. Cabral de Almeida J, Reis D, Llerena J Jr, Neto J, Lopes Pontes R, Middleton S, et al. Short stature brachydactyly and Peters' anomaly (Peters-plus syndrome): Confirmation of autosomal recessive inheritance. *J Med Genet* 1991;28:277–279.

17. Chen J, Mackey D, Fuller H, Serravalle S, Olsson J, Denton M. X-linked megalocornea: Close linkage to DXS87 and DXS94. *Hum Genet* 1989;83:292–294.

18. Chisholm I, Chudley A. Autosomal dominant iridogoniodysgenesis with associated somatic anomalies: Four-generation family with Rieger's syndrome. *Br J Ophthalmol* 1983;67: 529–534.

19. Cibis G, Waeltermann J, Harris D. Peters' anomaly with ring 21 chromosomal abnormality. *Am J Ophthalmol* 1985;100:733–734.

20. Cook C, Sulik K. Keratolenticular dysgenesis (Peters' anomaly) as a result of acute embryonic insult during gastrulation. *J Pediatr Ophthalmol Strabismus* 1988;25:60.

21. Cross H, Jorgenson R, Levin L, et al. The Rieger syndrome: An autosomal dominant disorder with ocular dental and systemic abnormalities. *Perspect Ophthalmol* 1979;3:3.

22. Crowford R. Iris dysgenesis with other anomalies. *Br J Ophthalmol* 1967;51:438–440.

23. David R, MacBaeth L, Jenkins T. Aniridia associated with microcornea and subluxated lenses. *Br J Ophthalmol* 1978;62:118–121.
24. De Hauwere R, Leroy J. Adrienssens K, Van Heule R. Iris dysplasia orbital hypertelorism and psychomotor retardation: A dominantly inherited developmental syndrome. *J Pediatr* 1973;82:679–681.
25. DeRespinis P, Wagner R. Peters' anomaly in a father and son. *Am J Ophthalmol* 1987;104:545–546.
26. Dohlman C. Familial congenital cornea guttata in association with anterior polar cataracts. *Acta Ophthalmol* 1951;29:445–471.
27. Elliott J, Feman S, O'Day D, et al. Hereditary sclerocornea. *Arch Ophthalmol* 1985;103: 767–679.
28. Eriksson A, Lehmann W, Forsius H. Congenital cornea plana in Finland. *Clin Genet* 1973;4:301–310.
29. Feingold M, Shiere F, Fogels H, Donaldson D. Rieger's syndrome. *Pediatrics* 1969;44: 564–569.
30. Felix C. Congenitale familiaere cornea plana. *Klin Monatsbl Augenheilkd* 1925;74:710–716.
31. Fishman A, Ackerman J, Kanarek I, et al. Cornea plana: A case report. *Ann Ophthalmol* 1982;14:47–48.
32. Forsius H. Studien ueber Cornea plana congenita bei 19 Kranken in 9 Familien. *Acta Ophthalmol* 1961;39:203–221.
33. François J, Neetens A. Microcornee associee a une hydrophthalmie et à d'autres anomalies hereditaires. *Acta Genet Med Gemelloe* 1955;4:217.
34. Friedman M, Wright E. Hereditary microcornea and cataracts in 5 generations. *Am J Ophthalmol* 1952;35:1017.
35. Frydman M, Weinstock A, Cohen H, Savir H, Varsano I. Autosomal recessive Peters' anomaly typical facial appearance failure to thrive hydrocephalus and other anomalies: Further delineation of the Krause-Kivlin syndrome. *Am J Med Genet* 1991;40:34–40.
36. Fryns J, Van Den Bergh H. Rieger syndrome and interstitial 4q26 deletion. *Genet Counsel* 1992;3:153–154.
37. Ferguson J, Hicks E. Rieger's anomaly and glaucoma associated with partial trisomy 16q. Case report. *Arch Ophthalmol* 1987;105:323.
38. Glaser T, Walton D, Maas R. Genomic structure, evolutionary conservation and aniridia mutations in the human PAX6 gene. *Nature Genet* 1992;2:232–239.
39. Godde-Jolly D, Bonnin M. Opacitees corneennes centrales congenitales par anomalie de developpement embryologique due segment anterieur de l'oeil (syndrome de Peters). *Bull Soc Ophtalmol Fr* 1966;66:917–922.
40. Gollamudi SR, Traboulsi EI, Chamon W, Stark WJ, Maumenee IH. Visual outcome after surgery for Peters' anomaly. *Ophthalmic Genet* 1994;15:31–35.
41. Green J, Johnson G. Congenital cataract with microcornea and Peters' anomaly as expressions of one autosomal dominant gene. *Ophthalmic Paediatr Genet* 1986;7:187–194.
42. Gregor Z, Hitchings R. Rieger's anomaly: A 42-year follow-up. *Br J Ophthalmol* 1980;64: 56–58.
43. Hanson I, Fletcher J, Jordan T, Brown A, Taylor D, Adams R, et al. Mutations at the PAX6 locus are found in heterogeneous anterior segment malformations including Peters' anomaly. *Nature Genet* 1994;6:168–173.
44. Tang HK, Chao LY, Saunders GF. Functional analysis of paired box missense mutations in the PAX6 gene. *Hum Mol Genet* 1997;6: 381–386.
45. Harman N. Hereditary anterior polar cataract and microphthalmia. *Traus Ophthalmol Soc UK* 1909;31:139–140.
46. Gunderson CA, Stone R, Pfeiffer R, Freedman S. Corneal coloboma aphokia and retinal neovascularization with anterior segment dysgenesis (Peters' anomaly). *Ophthalmologica,* 1996;210:361–366.
47. Harris R, Brownstein S, Little J. Peters' anomaly with congenital aphakia. *Can J Ophthalmol* 1980;15:91–94.
48. Heinemann M, Breg R, Cotlier E. Rieger's syndrome with pericentric inversion of chromosome 6. *Br J Ophthalmol* 1979;63:40–44.
49. Hemady R, Blum S, Sylvia B. Duplication of the lens, hourglass cornea, and cornea plana. *Arch Ophthalmol* 1993;111:303.
50. Henkind P, Marinoff G, Manas A, Freidman A. Bilateral corneal dermoids. *Am J Ophthalmol* 1973;76;972–977.
50a. Héon E, Sheth BP, Kalenak JW, Sunden SL, Streb LM, Taylor CM, Alward WL, Sheffield VC, Stone EM. Linkage of autosomal dominant iris hypoplasia to the region of the Rieger syndrome locus (4q25). *Hum Mol Genet* 1995;4:1435–1439.
51. Herve J, Warnet J, Jeaneau-Bellego E, Portnoi M, Taillemitte J, Herve F. Monosomie partielle du bras court d'un chromosome 10 associée à un syndrome de Rieger et à un

deficit immunitaire partiel type Di George. *Ann Pediatr* 1984;31:77–80.

52. Hol F, Hamel B, Geurds M, Hansmann I, Nabben F, Daniels O, et al. Localization of Alagille syndrome to 20p11.2-p12 by linkage analysis of a three generation family. *Hum Genet* 1995;95:687–690.
53. Holmark J, Jensen D. Anterior chamber cleavage syndrome. A typical case of Peters' anomaly with primary aphakia. *Acta Ophthalmol* 1972;50:877–886.
54. Holmstrom G, Reardon W, Baraitser M, Elston J, Taylor D. Heterogeneity in dominant anterior segment malformations. *Br J Ophthalmol* 1991;75:591–597.
55. Huismans H. Zur Atiologie des Linsenkoloboms. *Klin Monatsbl Augenheilkd* 1978;172: 884–887.
56. Ijima Y, Wagai K. Matsuura Y, Ueda M, Miyazaki I. Retinal detachment with breaks in the pars plicata of the ciliary body. *Am J Ophthalmol* 1989;108:349–355.

56a. Ionides AC, Berry V, Mackay DS, et al. A locus for autosomal dominant posterior polar cataract on chromosome 1p. *Hum Mol Genet* 1997;6:47–51.

57. Jaafar M, Robb R. Congenital anterior polar cataract. A review of 63 cases. *Ophthalmology* 1984;91:249–254.
58. Johnston M, Noden D, Hazelton R, Coulombre JL, Coulombre AJ. Origins of avian ocular and periocular tissues. *Exp Eye Res* 1979;29:27–43.
59. Jorgenson R, Levin L, Cross H, Yoder F, Kelly T. The Rieger syndrome. *Am J Med Genet* 1978;2:307–318.
60. Judisch G, Phelps C, Hanson J. Rieger's syndrome—A case report with a 15-year follow-up. *Arch Ophthalmol* 1979;97:2120–2122.

60a. Junemann A, Gusek GC, Naumann GO. Optical sector iridectomy: An alternative to perforating keratoplasty in Peters' anomaly. *Klin Monatsbl Augenheilkd* 1996;209:117–124.

61. Kanai A, Wood T, Polack F, Kaufman HE. The fine structure of sclerocornea. *Invest Ophthalmol* 1971;10:687–694.
62. Kihara Y, Shimomura Y, Omoto T, Fukuda M. Unilateral disc-shaped cataract with coloboma of the lens. *Jpn J Ophthalmol* 1988; 32:31–34.
63. Kivlin J, Fineman R, Crandall AS, Olson RJ. Peters' anomaly as a consequence of genetic and nongenetic syndromes. *Arch Ophthalmol* 1986;104:61–64.
64. Kleinmann R, Kazarian E, Raptopoulos V, Braverman LE. Primary empty sella and Rieger's anomaly of the anterior segment of the eye: A familial syndrome. *N Engl J Med* 1981;304:90–93.
65. Koster R, van Balen A. Congenital corneal opacity (Peters' anomaly) combined with buphthalmos and aniridia. *Ophthalmic Paediatr Genet* 1985;6:247–255.
66. Kraft S, Judisch G, Grayson D. Megalocornea: A clinical and echographic study of an autosomal dominant pedigree. *J Pediatr Ophthalmol Strabismus* 1984;21:190–193.

66a. Krantz ID, Piccoli DA, Spinner NB. Alagille syndrome. *J Med Genet* 1997; 34:152–157.

67. Krause U, Koivistom M, Rantakallio P. A case of Peters' anomaly with spontaneous corneal perforation. *J Pediatr Ophthalmol* 1969;6: 145–149.
68. Kupfer C, Kuwabara T, Stark W. The histopathology of Peters' anomaly. *Am J Ophthalmol* 1975;80:653–660.
69. Larsen V, Eriksson A. Cornea plana. *Acta Ophthalmol* 1949;27:275–286.
70. Legius E, de Die-Smulders C, Verbaak F, Habex H, Decorte R, Marynen P, et al. Genetic heterogeneity in Rieger eye malformation. *J Med Genet* 1994;31:340–341.
71. Lewis R. Mapping the gene for X-linked cataracts and microcornea with facial, dental and skeletal features to Xp22: An appraisal of the Nance-Horan syndrome. *Trans Am Ophthalmol Soc* 1989;87:658–728.
72. Lewis R, Nussbaum R, Stambolian D. Mapping X-linked ophthalmic diseases. IV. Provisional assignment of the locus for X-linked congenital cataracts and microcornea (the Nance-Horan syndrome) to Xp22.2-p22.3. *Ophthalmology* 1990;97:110–120.
73. Li H, Yang J, Jacobson RD, Pasco D, Sundin O. PAX6 is first expressed in a region of ectoderm anterior to the early neural plate: Implication for stepwise determination of the lens. *Dev Biol* 1994;162:181–194.

73a. Li L, Krantz ID, Deng Y, et al. Alagille syndrome is caused by mutations in human Jagged1, which encodes a ligand for Notch1. *Nature Genet* 1997;16:243–251.

74. Lubin J. Oculocutaneous albinism associated with corneal mesodermal dysgenesis. *Am J Ophthalmol* 1981;91:347–350.
75. Lyford J, Roy F. Arhinencephaly unilateralis, uveal coloboma, and lens reduplication. *Am J Ophthalmol* 1977;77:315–318.
76. Mackey D, Buttery R, Wise G, Denton M. Description of X-linked megalocornea with

identification of the gene locus. *Arch Ophthalmol* 1991;109:829–833.
77. Manschot W. Primary congenital aphakia. *Arch Ophthalmol* 1963;69:71–77.
78. Mattos J, Contreras F, O'Donnell F Jr. Ring dermoid syndrome: A new syndrome of autosomal-dominantly inherited bilateral annual limbal dermoids with corneal and conjunctival extension. *Arch Ophthalmol* 1980;98:1059–1061.
79. Mayer U, Bialasiewicz A. Ocular findings in a 4 p− deletion syndrome (Wolf-Hirschhorn). *Ophthalmic Paediatr Genet* 1989;10:62–72.
80. Mears A, Mirzayans F, Gould D, Pearce W, Walter M. Autosomal dominant iridogoniodysgenesis anomaly maps to 6p25. *Am J Hum Genet* 1996;59:1321–1327.
81. Miller M, Epstein R, Sugar J, et al. Anterior segment anomalies associated with the fetal alcohol syndrome. *J Pediatr Ophthalmol Strabismus* 1984;21:8–18.
82. Motegi T, Nakamura K, Terakawa T, Oohira A, Minoda K, Kishi K, et al. Deletion of a single chromosome band 4q26 in a malformed girl: Exclusion of Rieger syndrome associated gene(s) from the 4q26 segment. *J Med Genet* 1988;25:628–633.
83. Murray J, Bennett S, Kwitek A, Small K, Schinzel A, Alward W, et al. Linkage of Rieger syndrome to the region of the epidermal growth factor gene on chromosome 4. *Nature Genet* 1992;2:46–49.
84. Nakanishi I, Brown S. The histopathology and ultrastructure of congenital central corneal opacity (Peters' anomaly). *Am J Ophthalmol* 1971;72:801–812.
85. Neuhauser G, Kaveggia E, France T, Opitz JM. Syndrome of mental retardation seizures, hypotonic cerebral palsy and megalocornea, recessively inherited. *Z Kinderheilkd* 1975; 120:1–18.
85a. Nischall KK, Hingorani M, Bentley CR. Ocular ultrasound in Alagille syndrome: A new sign. *Ophthalmology* 1977;104:79–85.
85b. Oda T, Elkahloun AG, Pike BL, et al. Mutations in the human Jagged1 gene are responsible for Alagille syndrome. *Nature Genet* 1997;16:235–242.
86. Pearce W, Kerr C. Inherited variation in Rieger's malformation. *Br J Ophthalmol* 1965;49: 530–537.
87. Peters A. Ueber angeborene Defektbildung der Descemetschen Membran (Anatomische Untersuchung eines Falles von angeborener Hornhauttrubung ringformiger vorderer Synechie und Fehlen der Descemetschen Membran im Hornhautzentrum). *Klin Monatsbl Augenheilkd* 1906;44:27, 105–119.
88. Phillips J, Del Bono E, Haines J, Pralea A, Cohen J, Greff L, et al. A second locus for Rieger syndrome maps to chromosome 13q14. *Am J Hum Genet* 1996;59:613–619.
89. Polack F, Graue E. Scanning electron microscopy of congenital corneal leukomas (Peters' anomaly). *Am J Ophthalmol* 1979;88:169–178.
90. Polomeno R, Cummings C. Autosomal dominant cataracts and microcornea. *Can J Ophthalmol* 1979;14:227–229.
91. Pouliquen Y, Graf B, Saraux H, Bisson J, Frouin M-A. Etude histologique et ultrastructurale dans deux cas de syndrome de Peters. *Arch Ophtalmol Rev Gen Ophtalmol* 1971;31:695–708.
92. Puklin J, Riely C, Simon R, Cotlier E. Anterior segment and retinal pigmentary abnormalities in arteriohepatic dysplasia. *Ophthalmology* 1981;88:337–347.
93. Rand E, Spinner N, Piccoli D, Whitington P, Taub R. Molecular analysis of 24 Alagille syndrome families identifies a single submicroscopic deletion and further localizes the Alagille region within 20p12. *Am J Hum Genet* 1995;57:1068–1073.
94. Rieger H. Beitrage zur Kenntnis seltener Missbildungen der Iris: ueber Hypoplasie des Irisvorderblattes mit Verlagerung und Entrundung der Pupille. *Albrecht von Graefes Arch Klin Exp Ophthalmol* 1935;133:602.
95. Rieger H. Erbfrangen in der Augenheilkunde. *Albrecht von Graefes Arch Klin Exp Ophthalmol* 1941;143:277–299.
96. Saal H, Arunstein R, Weinbaum P, Poole A. Autosomal recessive Robinow-like syndrome with anterior chamber cleavage anomalies. *Am J Med Genet* 1988;30:709–718.
97. Sadeghi-Nejad A, Senior B. Autosomal dominant transmission of isolated growth hormone deficiency in iris-dental dysplasia (Rieger's syndrome). *J Pediatr* 1974;85:644–648.
97a. Sarfarazi M, Akarsu AN, Hossain A, et al. Assignment of a locus (GLC3A) for primary congenital glaucoma (buphthalmos) to 2p21 and evidence for genetic heterogeneity. *Genomics* 1995;30:171–177.
98. Schanzlin D, Goldberg D, Brown S. Hallerman-Streiff syndrome associated with sclerocornea aniridia and a chromosomal abnormality. *Am J Ophthalmol* 1980;90:411–415.

99. Scheie H, Yanoff M. Peter's anomaly and total posterior coloboma of the retinal pigment epithelium. *Arch Ophthalmol* 1972; 87:525–530.
100. Semina E, Reiter R, Leysens N, Alward W, Small K, Datson N, et al. Cloning and characterization of a novel bicoid-related homeobox transcription factor gene, RIEG, involved in Rieger syndrome. *Nature Genet* 1996; 14:392–399.
101. Shields M. Axenfeld-Rieger syndrome: A theory of mechanism and distinctions from the iridocorneal endothelial syndrome. *Trans Am phthalmol Soc* 1983;81:736–784.
102. Shields M, Buckley E, Klintworth G, Thresher R. Axenfeld-Rieger syndrome. A spectrum of developmental disorders. *Surv Ophthalmol* 1985;29:387–409.
103. Skuta G, Sugar J, Ericson E. Corneal endothelial cell measurement in megalocornea. *Arch Ophthalmol* 1983;101:51–53.
104. Spallone A. Retinal detachment in Axenfeld-Rieger syndrome. *Br J Ophthalmol* 1989; 73:559–562.
105. Stathacopoulos R, Bateman J, Sparkes R, Hepler R. The Rieger syndrome and a chromosome 13 deletion. *J Pediatr Ophthalmol Strabismus* 1987;24:198–203.
105a. Stoilov I, Akarsu AN, Sarfarozi M. Identification of three different truncating mutations in cytochrome P4501B1 (CYP1B1) as the principal cause of primary congenital gloucoma (buphthalmos) in families linked to the GLC3A locus on chromosome 2p21. *Hum Mol Genet* 1997;6:641–647.
106. Stone D, Kenyon K, Green W, Ryan S. Congenital central corneal leukoma (Peters' anomaly). *Am J Ophthalmol* 1976;81: 173–193.
107. Tabbara K, Khouri F, Der Kaloustian V. Rieger's syndrome with chromosomal anomaly. *Can J Ophthalmol* 1973;8:488–491.
108. Tabuchi A, Matsuura M, Hirokawa M. Three siblings with Peters' anomaly. *Ophthalmic Paediatr Genet* 1985;5:205–212.
109. Tahvanainen E, Forsius H, Karila E, Ranta S, Eerola M, Weissenbach J, et al. Cornea plana congenita gene assigned to the long arm of chromosome 12 by linkage analysis. *Genomics* 1995;26:290–293.
110. Toppare M, Kitapci F, Dilmen U, Kaya I, Senses D. Periumbilical skin length measurements in the newborn. *Clin Genet* 1995; 47:207–209.
111. Townsend W. Congenital corneal leukomas 1 Central defect in Descemet's membrane. *Am J Ophthalmol* 1974;77:80.
112. Traboulsi E, Lustbader J, Lemp M. Keratoconus in Alagille syndrome. *Am J Ophthalmol* 1989;108:332–333.
113. Traboulsi E, Maumenee I. Peters' anomaly and associated congenital malformations. *Arch Ophthalmol* 1992;110:1739–1742.
114. Traboulsi E, Weinberg R. Familial congenital cornea guttata with anterior polar cataracts. *Am J Ophthalmol* 1989;108:123–125.
115. Uemura A, Uto M. Bilateral retinal detachment with large breaks of pars plicata associated with coloboma lentis and ocular hypertension. *Jpn J Ophthalmol* 1992;36:97–102.
116. Van Schooneveld M, Delleman J, Beemer F, Bleeker-Wagemakers E. Peters'-plus: A new syndrome. *Ophthalmic Paediatr Genet* 1984; 4:141–146.
117. Vaux C, Sheffield L, Keith C. Voullaire L. Evidence that Rieger syndrome maps to 4q25 or 4q27. *J Med Genet* 1992;29:256–258.
118. Verloes A, Dodinval P. Rieger anomaly and uveal coloboma with associated anomalies. Third observation of a rare oculo-palato-osseous syndrome—The Abruzzo-Erikson syndrome. *Ophthalmic Paediatr Genet* 1990; 11:41–47.
119. Vermeij-Keers C. Primary congenital aphakia and the rubella syndrome. *Teratology* 1975; 11:257–266.
120. Von Noorden G, Baller R. The chamber angle in split-pupil. *Arch Ophthalmol* 1963;70: 598–602.
121. Walsh F, Wageman M. A pedigree of hereditary cataract illustrating sex limited type. *Bull Johns Hopkins Hosp* 1939;61:125.
122. Walter M, Mirzayans F, Mears A, Hickey K, Pearce W. Autosomal dominant iridogoniodysgenesis and Axenfeld-Rieger syndrome and genetically distinct. *Ophthalmology* 1996;103:1907–1915.
123. Walther C, Gruss P. PAX6, a murine paired-box gene expressed in the developing CNS. *Development* 1991;113:1435–1449.
124. Waring G, Rodrigues M. Ultrastructure and successful keratoplasty of sclerocornea in Mieten's syndrome. *Am J Ophthalmol* 1980; 90:469–475.
125. Waring G, Rodrigues M, Laibson P. Anterior chamber cleavage syndrome: A step-ladder classification. *Surv Ophthalmol* 1976;20: 3–27.
126. Weiland H, Vermeij-Keers C, Salimans M, Fleuren G, Verwey R. Parvovirus B19 associ-

ated with fetal abnormality. *Lancet* 1987; 1:682–683.

127. Wells K, Pulido J, Judisch G, Ossoinig K, Fisher T, LaBrecque D. Ophthalmic features of Alagille syndrome (arteriohepatic syndrome). *J Pediatr Ophthalmol Strabismus* 1993;30:130–135.
128. Wilcox L Jr, Bercovitch L, Howard R. Ophthalmic features of chromosome deletion 4p− (Wolf-Hirschhorn syndrome). *Am J Ophthalmol* 1978;86:834–839.
129. Wilson M. Congenital iris ectropion and new classification for anterior segment dysgenesis. *J Pediatr Ophthalmol Strabismus* 1990;27: 48–55.
130. Wolter J, Hall R, Mason G. Unilateral primary congenital aphakia. *Am J Ophthalmol* 1964; 58:1011–1016.
131. Wood W, Green W, Marr W. Megalocornea: A clinicopathologic clinical case report. *Md State Med J* 1974;23:57–60.

6

Aniridia

ELIAS I. TRABOULSI
DANPING ZHU
IRENE H. MAUMENEE

Aniridia (absence of the iris), or "irideremia" in earlier literature, was first described by Baratta in 1819[1a] and the first pedigree was published by Gutbier in 1834.[32] The delayed appearance of glaucoma as one of the major complications of aniridia was recognized as early as 1888 by Hirschberg[39] and 1898 by Foster.[16] The association of aniridia and nephroblastoma (Wilms' tumor) was first reported in 1953 by Brusa and Torricelli.[5] This association is commonly referred to as Miller syndrome because of the 1964 report by Miller and coworkers[57] of six cases of aniridia among 440 cases of patients with Wilms' tumor. In 1968, Fraumeni and Glass[19] drew attention to the syndrome of aniridia, Wilms' tumor, mental retardation, and ambiguous genitalia. This syndrome was attributed to contiguous gene defects on 11p13 by Riccardi et al.[70] in 1978. Mannens and co-workers[54] mapped familial aniridia to 11p13 in 1989. The human aniridia gene was finally cloned by Ton et al.[82] and by Glaser and co-workers,[27] and proved to be a member of a class of developmental genes called PAX genes because of their similarity to the Drosophila gene paired. Mutations in the PAX6 or aniridia gene have since been identified in numerous patients and families with the disease.

DEFINITION, MORPHOLOGY, AND HISTOPATHOLOGY

Aniridia is a misnomer applied to a bilateral malformation of the eye in which the most prominent abnormality is near-total absence of the iris (Fig. 6.1). A stump of tissue is invariably present at the base of the iris and gonioscopy may be required for its adequate visualization.[17] The diagnosis of aniridia is more difficult to make in patients who have a substantial amount of remaining iris tissue (Fig. 6.2). Several families have been described in which some members have clinical aniridia and others have atypical iris defects ranging from radial clefts or atypical colobomas to more extensive absence of iris tissue (Fig. 6.3).[12,40,83] The most characteristic clinical morphological feature of the iris in aniridia is a focal or total circumferential absence of the pupillary rim and iris sphincter muscle together with absence of central iris tissue (Fig. 6.2). Residual iris tissue appears normal in some patients, or has focal areas of

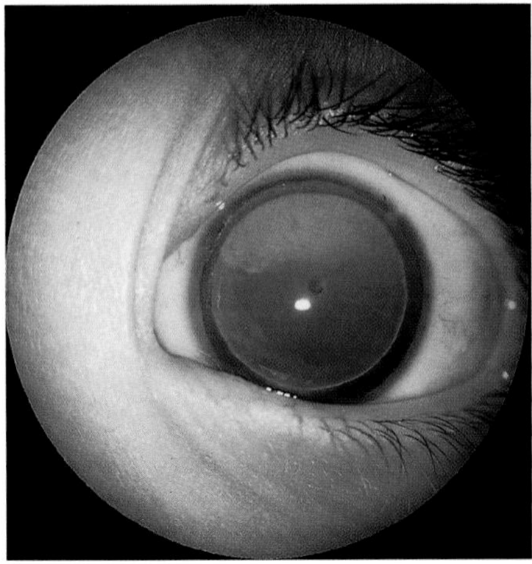

Figure 6.1. Aniridia with small anterior polar lens opacity.

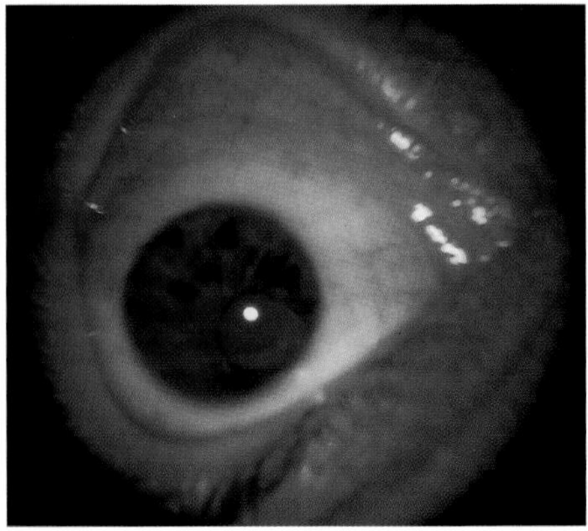

Figure 6.3. Atypical colobomata and iris defects in a patient with aniridia. Her daughter had a classic aniridia phenotype.

absence of the stroma and or iris pigment epithelium, with pseudopolycoria in others (Fig. 6.3).

In a report of a large family with relatively well-preserved visual function, Elsas and coworkers[12] classified aniridia into four genetic types. In an autosomal dominant type I there is near-total absence of iris tissue with foveal hypoplasia, optic nerve hypoplasia, nystagmus, corneal pannus, subluxation of the lens, and secondary glaucoma. In type II, such as the family they reported, also inherited in an autosomal dominant fashion, iris defects are the prominent ocular findings but occur in a wide range of severity; visual function is preserved with a lower incidence of cataracts and glaucoma; most patients with this type of aniridia

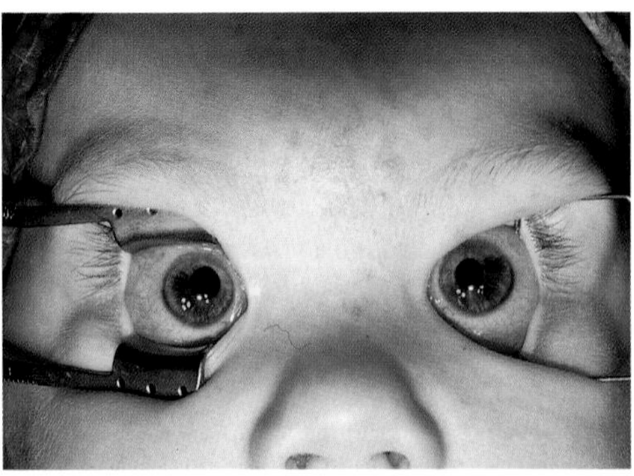

Figure 6.2. Baby with atypical iris defects and congenital large pupil. The pupillary sphincter is absent. Diagnosis: aniridia.

do not have nystagmus. In type III, aniridia occurs with cerebellar ataxia and mental retardation; this very rare condition is inherited in an autosomal recessive fashion and is known as the Gillespie syndrome (*vide infra*).[22] Type IV aniridia in their classification scheme refers to the Wilms' tumor-aniridia-genitourinary abnormalities-retardation (WAGR) or Miller syndrome that results from a deletion of a contiguous set of genes in band 13 of the short arm of chromosome 11.[85] Aniridia can also occur in association with malformations of the globe such as Peters' anomaly or congenital anterior staphyloma,[46] or with microcornea and subluxed lenses.[10] Aniridia may be a feature of multisystem malformation syndromes and chromosomal abnormalities such as a ring chromosome 6,[51] the syndrome of multiple ocular malformations and mental retardation described by Walker and Dyson[87] and Hamming et al.,[34] the syndrome of aniridia, other ocular malformations, dysmorphic features and mental retardation described by Edwards et al.[11] and the syndrome of aniridia and absence of the patella.[58] Finally, unilateral aniridia may be present in malformed eyes. It may be accompanied by anterior segment dysgenesis, congenital glaucoma, megalophthalmos, microphthalmos, aphakia, and malformations of the retina.

Margo[55] reported the histopathologic findings in the anterior segment of several eyes from patients with aniridia. There was iris and ciliary body hypoplasia, anomalous development and incomplete cleavage of the anterior chamber angle, and attenuation of Bowman's membrane. According to Margo,[55] acquired, as opposed to congenital, ocular abnormalities in these eyes included corneal pannus, peripheral anterior synechiae, and lenticular degeneration. Margo[55] observed that the two patients who had anomalous development of the anterior chamber angle had a microscopic deletion of chromosome 11p.

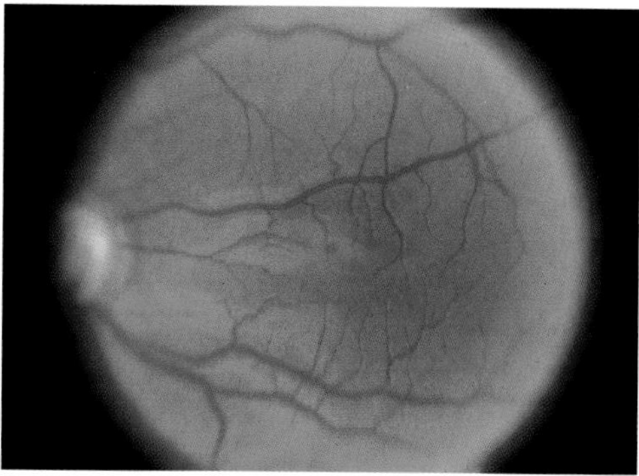

Figure 6.4. Foveal hypoplasia in a patient with aniridia.

EPIDEMIOLOGY

In a study conducted across the state of Michigan, Shaw et al.[75] found 118 cases of aniridia in a population of 7.6 million. They calculated an estimated incidence of 1 in 56,000 live births. One-third of cases were sporadic and the rest were familial. In the first report of aniridia and interstitial delection of 11p from Europe, Warburg et al.[90] cited the prevalance of aniridia in Denmark to be 1 in 100,000

CLINICAL FINDINGS

Two-thirds to three-fourths of cases are familial. Males are as frequently affected as females. Babies with aniridia are often referred to an ophthalmologist because of fixed and dilated pupils or because of nystagmus. Poor vision, cataracts, and a diagnosis of Rieger anomaly or of keratitis may be the presenting signs or symptoms in older patients. Photophobia may be present but is not a constant finding. In the family reported by Shaw et al.,[75] photophobia was not a prominent symptom; 7 of 40 examined patients had ectopia lentis.

Congenital poor visual function in aniridia is due to macular, foveal, and optic nerve hypoplasia (Fig. 6.4).[49,73] Acquired causes of visual loss include cataract, glaucoma, keratopathy, and anisometropic or strabismic amblyopia.[73]

Ocular abnormalities associated with aniridia include persistent pupillary membrane,[35] congenital cataracts (Figs. 6.5, 6.6),[6] ectopia lentis (Fig. 6.7), developmental glaucoma, corneal pannus, and progressive keratopathy (Figs. 6.8, 6.9),[6,53,64,65] persistence of the retina over pars plana, and foveal hypoplasia. Traboulsi et al.[83] reported the occurrence of a pit of the optic nerve head and of a morning glory disc anomaly in a girl with familial aniridia whose mother had atypical iris defects and cataracts (Fig. 6.3). Weiss and co-workers[91] performed specular microscopic studies in nine patients with aniridia and demonstrated normal morphology and number of endothelial cells.

In most families with aniridia, visual acuity is less than 20/60 in all patients and less than 20/200 in over 60%, glaucoma develops in 70%, and cataracts are present in about 85% of cases. Nystagmus is not a universal finding and occurs in 85%–92% of cases. Dislocated lenses were detected in 35% of patients in one series[75] and

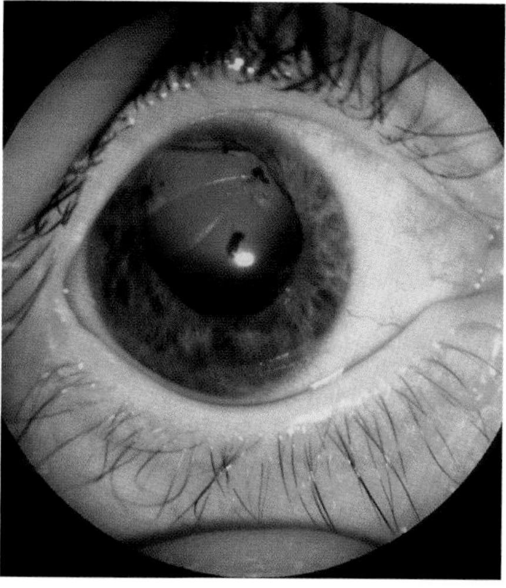

Figure 6.5. Cortical spoke cataract in a patient with aniridia.

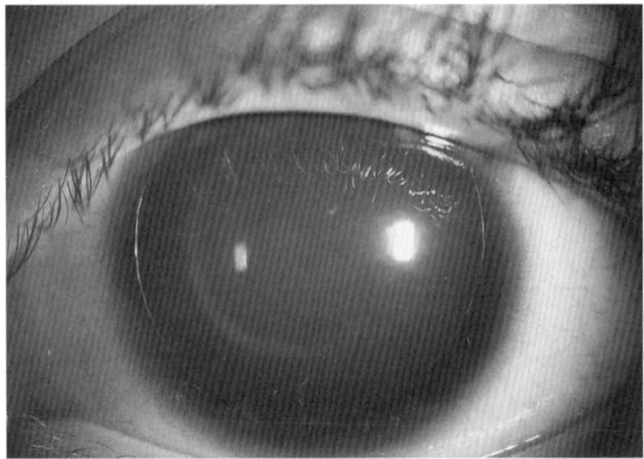

Figure 6.6. Lamellar cataract in a patient with aniridia.

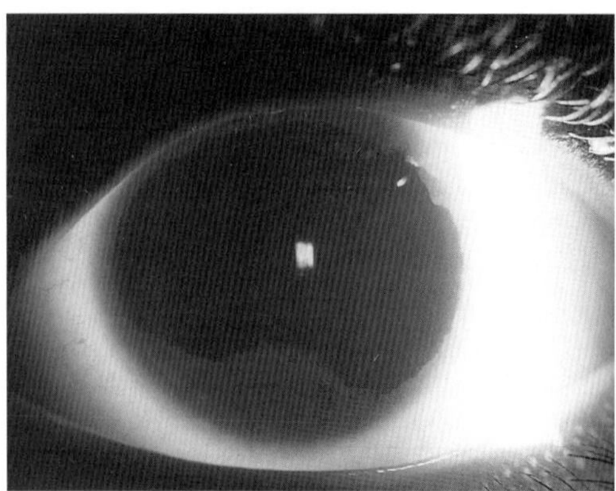

Figure 6.8. Early keratopathy in a child with familial aniridia.

in 18% of cases in another.[30] Eventual blindness from uncontrolled glaucoma and/or progressive corneal opacification is the outcome in many patients. In some families such as the ones reported by Elsas and co-workers[12] and Hittner et al.,[40] visual function is surprisingly well preserved. Of 38 members of a large Pennsylvania Irish pedigree, 56% of 32 whose vision could be accurately tested had 20/30 vision or better. Acuity was less than 20/200 in only one eye of four patients and both eyes of one patient. The reduced vision was due to amblyopia, corneal edema after cataract surgery, or age-related macular degeneration. Vision was not reduced to less than 20/70 because of aniridia in any patient. Nystagmus was not present in any patient. Only 18% of patients had cataracts and 13% had glaucoma. Both cataracts and glaucoma increased in prevalence with age.

The types of cataracts in aniridia vary from classical anterior polar (Fig. 6.1) or pyramidal, to lamellar rings (Fig. 6.6), nuclear opacities, and cortical spokes (Fig. 6.5). In many patients with cataracts, visual acuity is relatively good and compatible with what one would expect from foveal hypoplasia, despite the presence of apparently extensive lenticular opacities. This may be due to the presence of sectors of clear lens space through which the aniridic patient can see. Lens extraction is best deferred in these patients because of the low potential for visual improvement and the possible increased risk of glaucoma associated with cataract surgery in an eye with anterior segment dysgenesis.

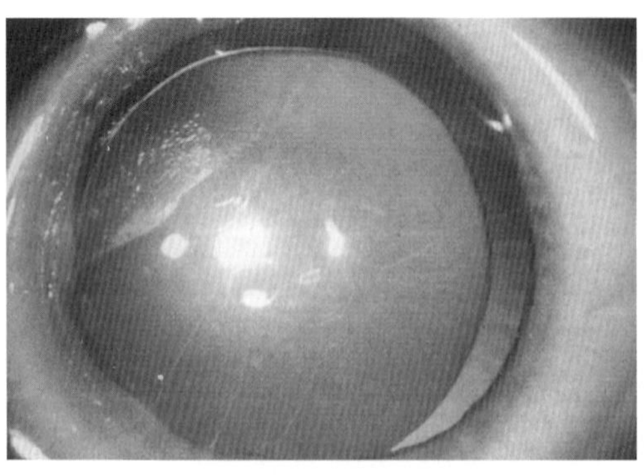

Figure 6.7. Lens subluxation in a patient with aniridia.

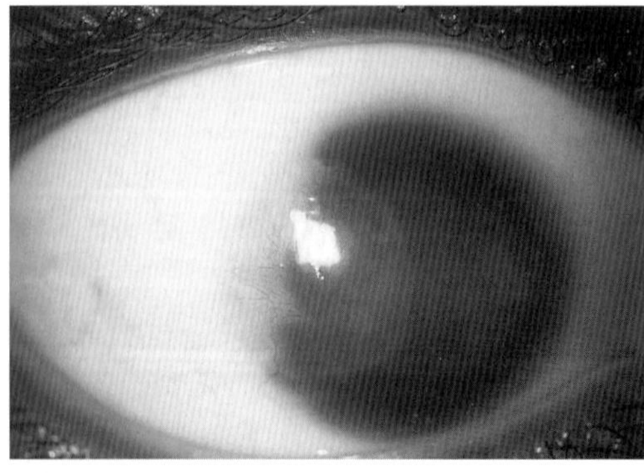

Figure 6.9. Advanced keratopathy in an adult with familial aniridia.

Grant and Walton[29] attributed the development of glaucoma in aniridia to progressive closure of the anterior chamber angle by the residual iris stump. In a group of 25 patients with aniridia but no glaucoma, gonioscopy revealed no attachment of the iris stroma to the trabecular meshwork and no ectropion of the edge of the iris stump. In contradistinction, in 31 patients with aniridia and glaucoma, there were varied forms and stages of adhesions between the iris stump and angle structures. The extent of adhesions seemed to progress with increasing age and there was a correlation between the extent of the adhesions and the severity of the glaucoma. In a small proportion of patients with aniridia, however, the iris stump did not adhere to the angle, but there was a thin layer of amorphous tissue covering the angle.

In a study of 19 patients with aniridia, Mackman and co-workers[53] found that a progressive corneal dystrophy develops in almost all patients after the age of 2.5 years. The superficial corneal opacification and pannus start in the 6 and 12 o'clock positions and go on to involve the whole circumference of the cornea. The corneal dystrophic changes progress from the periphery to the center. Corneal erosions result in secondary scarring in some patients. Kivlin et al.[45] were the first investigators to report a family with autosomal dominant keratitis. Pearce and co-workers[65] reported another family with dominant keratitis and foveal hypoplasia, and suggested that this disease may represent a variant of aniridia. Indeed, linkage analysis mapped the disease in that family to 11p13 and mutation analysis showed a mutation in the PAX6/aniridia gene exon 11 splice-acceptor site.[59] Nishida and co-workers[64] attributed the corneal pathology in aniridia to a total absence of the limbal girdles of Vogt and corneal epithelial limbal stem cells. Using biomicroscopy and impression cytology in eight patients with aniridia, these authors showed that the conjunctival epithelium extended over the limbus and onto the opaque and vascularized peripheral cornea. Koroma et al.[45a] showed that Pax6 is expressed strongly in adult surface epithelia of the cornea and conjunctiva. In these cells the gene may regulate structural or secretory specializations and might play a role in the maintenance and proliferation of corneal stem cells.[45a]

GENETICS

Mendelian Inheritance

Familial aniridia is clearly dominantly inherited. The Gillespie syndrome is autosomal recessive, and most cases of WAGR and 11p13 deletion are sporadic. In a large pedigree reported by Grove et al.,[30] with 77 affected individuals in 5 generations, there was complete penetrance of the gene. No parents with normal eyes gave birth to an affected child, and there were no cases of unilateral aniridia.

11p − Syndrome (WAGR Syndrome, Miller Syndrome)

The association of aniridia and an abnormality of 11p was first reported by Ladda and co-workers[48] in 1974 in a 19-month-old boy with a rearrangement between chromosomes 8 and 11. Although the initial interpretation was that of an interstitial deletion of 8p, further analysis revealed a net loss of chromosomal material from 11p. Godde-Salz and Behmke[28] reported another case of aniridia, mental retardation, and an unbalanced translocation of chromosomes 8q and 11p. A causal relationship of del (11p13) to the WAGR complex was first suggested by Riccardi and co-workers.[70] Hittner and co-workers[41] reported a patient with a deletion of 11p that was inherited from an unaffected mother with a balanced rearrangement of chromosome 11. Riccardi et al.[68] presented monozygotic twins with a deletion of 11-13 who were concordant for aniridia but discordant for Wilms' tumor, suggesting that 11p13 deletion is permissive, but not sufficient, for Wilms' tumor. Hotta and co-workers[43] studied eight cases of aniridia with high-resolution G-banding and found two with an interstitial deletion of 11p. One of the two patients developed Wilms' tumor.

The gene for red blood cell catalase was mapped to 11p13 and a dosage effect was demonstrated for individuals with triplication or deletion of that chromosomal region. Ferrell and Riccardi[15] studied 12 individuals with aniridia, Wilms' tumor, or both and without a microscopically detectable deletion of 11p13. All patients had normal levels of catalase, demonstrating that catalase levels are not helpful in detecting submicroscopic 11p13 deletions in patients with aniridia or Wilms' tumor. Riccardi and co-workers[69] reported two patients with aniridia and Wilms' tumor and a normal karyotype. One of the two patients had very little loss of iris tissue and was labeled as having iris dysplasia by the authors; she also had corneal opacification and vascularization. Narahara and co-workers[61] studied two patients with the 11p− syndrome using high-resolution chromosome banding and assayed for levels of catalase. They determined that the WAGR complex and the catalase gene map to 11p1305-p1306 and that catalase was more distally placed. Simola and co-workers[77] reported a three-generation family with aniridia and translocation t(4;11)(q22;p13) but without Wilms' tumor. These authors suggested that the loci for aniridia and Wilms' tumor susceptibility were separate and that the WAGR complex is caused by a mutation of more than one gene located at 11p13. Pettenati et al.[66] described a father and daughter with isolated aniridia and a balanced translocation t(5;11)(q13.1;p13). Other reports of a single break at 11p13 resulting in apparently isolated aniridia include those of Niikawa et al.[63] and Moore et al.[60] Turleau and co-workers[85] reported their observations on three patients with the del 11p/aniridia complex and reviewed 37 cases from the literature. These authors made the following observations: (*1*) there were twice as many affected males as females; (*2*) the chromosomal rearrangements were extremely variable ranging from familial insertions to translocations and interstitial deletions; (*3*) aniridia appeared to be the only constant clinical feature of the complex associated with a deletion of 11p13, although the same authors[84] later reported a patient with a deletion of 11p13 and Wilms' tumor, genitourinary (GU) abnormalities, and retardation but no aniridia; (*4*) tumors appeared to develop in about one-third of cases with 11p−; (*5*) genital abnormalities were present in the majority of male patients and included cryptorchidism, hypospadias, and abnormalities of internal organs; (*6*) mental retardation was a constant feature of the complex but was variable in severity; (*7*) growth retardation was present in 9 of 14 reliable observations; and (*8*) additional malformations were rare and included renal abnormalities, tetralogy of Fallot, microcephaly, and polydactyly.

Cotlier et al.[8] reported monozygotic twins with aniridia and cataracts, one of whom developed Wilms' tumor. In a study of four patients with WAGR and deletions of 11p13, Glaser and co-workers[25] demonstrated close physical linkage between the gene for the β subunit of follicle-stimulating hormone (FSHB) and the WAGR locus and suggested that the position of the aniridia gene is immediately proximal to FSHB on 11p.

In addition to aniridia, GU malformations resulting in ambiguous genitalia in male patients, mental retardation, and Wilms' tumor, patients with 11p13 deletion syndrome have rather characteristic facial dysmorphic features with a long narrow face, high nasal root, ptosis, small palpebral fissures, and low-set poorly lobulated ears.[20] Jotterand and co-workers[44] reported three cases of 11p13 deletion syndrome which included a patient who was mosaic for the deletion and who had markedly asymmetric ocular abnormalities with iridocorneal adhesions in one eye and localized absence of the lens zonules in the other eye.

Mapping Studies and Linkage Analysis

Mannens and co-workers[54] were the first investigators to map familial aniridia to 11p13 by demonstrating linkage between the disease locus, catalase, and D11S151 in a large Dutch family. They excluded linkage with markers on 2p25, a region that was proposed to be the site for the aniridia region by Ferrell and co-workers[14] in their linkage study of the family reported by Hittner and co-workers.[40] More recent linkage studies of the same family by this last group of investigators showed that the gene for aniridia in that family indeed maps to 11p13.[52]

PAX6—The Aniridia Gene

Using positional cloning and DNA samples from patients with aniridia and deletions involving the 11p13 aniridia locus (AN2), Ton and co-workers[82] cloned a cDNA that they presumed to be complementary to AN2. The gene contained two phylogenetically conserved DNA binding motifs, a homeobox, and a paired box, characteristic of the PAX family of developmental genes (Fig. 6.10) (see also Chapter 1 by Sundin for a discussion of developmental genes).[31,38,80] This gene was found to be the human homologus of the murine Pax6 gene which, when mutated, results in the small eye (Sey) phenotype. Homozygous Sey/Sey mice are anophthalmic, lack nasal structures, and die shortly after birth.[37] Hemizygous Sey/+ mice are microphthalmic and have a range of anterior segment abnormalities ranging from colobomas to iris hypoplasia and lenticulo-iridocorneal adhesions.[36,37] A neuropathological study of Small eye mice showed that there was a delay of premigratory neurons and an impairment of axonal growth and differentiation. This eventually results in a broad spectrum of neuronal migration disorders of the neocortical roof.[72] The murine Pax6 gene is mapped to a region of chromosome 2 in the mouse, which is syntenic to the aniridia locus on chromosome 11 in humans, giving further support that Sey is the murine homolog of the aniridia gene.[24,86]

PAX6 is expressed in the fetal eye, forebrain, cerebellum, and olfactory bulbs.[82,88] In the developing eye Sey is expressed first in the optic sulcus and subsequently in the eye vesicle, in the lens, in the differentiating retina and finally in the cornea. Glaser and co-workers[27] described the complete genomic structure of the human PAX6 gene and discovered mutations in familial and sporadic cases. Using mutation analysis of the PAX6 gene, other investigators identified numerous mutations in patients with aniridia. Most mutations result in premature termination of translation and truncated proteins. This haploinsufficiency leads to the aniridia phenotype. There remains, however, a significant proportion (up to 50%) of patients with aniridia in whom PAX6 mutations cannot be detected using mutation analysis and direct sequencing of the gene and some of its regulatory elements. Linkage analysis has not provided evidence for more than one genetic locus for aniridia. All familial cases investigated to date have mapped to 11p13. Fantes and co-workers[13] reported two families with aniridia and cytogenetic rearrangements that involved 11p13 where the aniridia gene was intact. Breakpoints in both families were at least 85 kb distant to the 3′ end of PAX6. These authors proposed that a position effect resulting from an inappropriate chromatin environment has led to the mutant phenotype, despite a physically intact PAX6 gene.

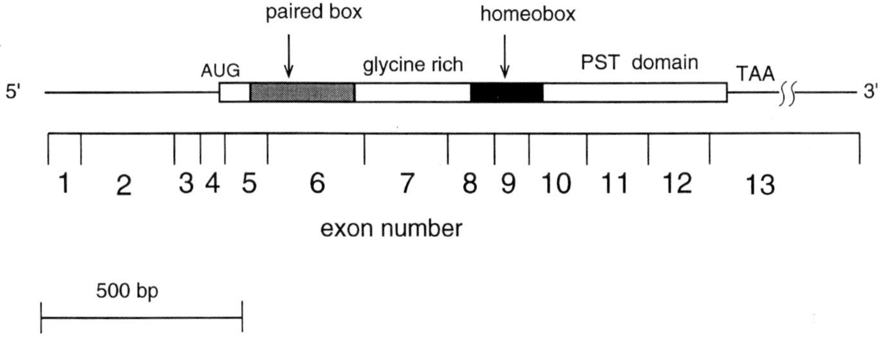

Figure 6.10. Genomic structure of the PAX6 gene.

At the laboratory of the Johns Hopkins Center for Hereditary Eye Diseases, PAX6 exons were amplified from genomic DNA using oligonucleotide primers flanking intron–exon junctions as described by Glaser et al.[27] Mutations were detected by single-strand conformational polymorphism (SSCP), heteroduplex analysis, or reverse transcription of total RNA from lymphoblastoid cells and direct sequencing of the cDNA.

Four new mutations in the paired-box domain resulted in a premature stop codon, a frame shift due to insertion or deletion, or a splice error. Mutations were not found in a pedigree with an atypical phenotype with 20/20 visual acuity and partial aniridia. In this family there was positive linkage of a CA repeat marker in intron 8 to the disease phenotype with a lod score of 2.52 at $\theta = 0$ in 19 known meioses with 14 affected individuals. A PAX6 mutation could not be found in a patient who carries a chromosome 11p15p13-q13 inv ins and 20/20 vision. The disease in this last patient is possibly due to a position effect despite having an intact PAX6 gene.

Some PAX6 mutations give rise to panocular effects with signs that are less severe or different from classic aniridia. For example, a missense mutation (R26G) caused a heterogeneous syndrome of anterior segment malformations including iris hypoplasia and Peters' anomaly.[36] A nonsense mutation in codon S353 produces a truncated protein in the PST domain and is associated with normal irides, cataracts, and late onset of cone dystrophy.[23] These two truncated PST domains have partial transcriptional activity, possibly accounting for the milder phenotype.[23] An exon 11 splice-acceptor mutation caused the autosomal dominant keratitis (APK) in one family.[59] Yanagisawa and colleagues[94] reported a missense mutation at nucleotide 799. This C to T transition was associated with a phenotype dominated by foveal hypoplasia and, according to the authors, no iris defects.

Axton and co-workers[1] were able to detect PAX6 mutations in 90% of patients with aniridia uncomplicated by associated anomalies. They used three mutation detection techniques: (*1*) protein truncation test; (*2*) SSCP; and (*3*) chemical cleavage of mismatch. They concluded that SSCP analysis of individually amplified exons, with which nine of ten mutations were seen, was the most useful detection method for PAX6.[1]

EYELESS

The *Drosophila melanogaster* gene eyeless (ey) is the homologue of PAX6 in humans and Pax6 in the mouse. Eyeless flies have partial or total absence of their compound eyes. Hypomorphic (weak) alleles lead to the reduction or absence of the compound eyes but do not affect the ocelli or simple eyes. Null alleles are not available now but presumably affect all eyes and are lethal when homozygous. The proteins encoded by ey, Sey, and AN2 share 94% sequence identity in the paired domain and 90% identity in the homeodomain. Furthermore, there are similarities in the flanking sequences and some of the splice sites in the paired box and in the homeobox are conserved between the fly and mammalian genes, indicating that the genes are orthologous.[33] Evidence that ey is the master control gene for eye morphogenesis came from the experiments of Halder and co-workers,[33] who induced the formation of ectopic eye structures in other parts of the body of *D. melanogaster* through targeted expression of the ey complementary DNA. These investigators were able to induce the growth of ectopic eye structures on the wings, the legs, and the antennae. The eyes appeared normal and consisted of groups of fully differentiated omatidia with a complete set of photoreceptor cells.

OTHER OCULAR MALFORMATIONS RESULTING FROM PAX6 MUTATIONS

Hanson and co-workers[36] described a child with Peters' anomaly (central corneal leukoma, absence of the underlying portion of Descemet's membrane and a variable extent of lenticulo-irido-corneal adhesions) and deletion of one copy of the PAX6 gene. The patient did not have other systemic malformations but had a slight developmental delay. The same authors also reported affected members of a family with dominantly inherited anterior segment malformations and an R26G mutation in one copy of the PAX6 gene. This family was comprised of a mother and daughter with iris hypoplasia and posterior embryotoxon, a son with Peters' anomaly, and another son with iris hypoplasia. Hanson and co-workers[36] also examined mice with the Small eye phenotype and observed that a proportion of Sey/+ mice with nonsense mutations in the Pax6 gene have anterior segment malformations resembling Peters' anomaly. There are two reports of patients with an aniridia phenotype in one eye and a Peters' phenotype in the other eye.[3,79]

ANIRIDIA × ANIRIDIA MATINGS

Grove et al.[30] reported two such matings in a large family. One couple had no children. A second couple had a total of six children. One girl with aniridia lived to 11 months and died of central nervous system problems; three boys died at less than 24 hours of age; there was also one spontaneous abortion at 3 months of gestation and one near-term intrauterine fetal death. Elsas and co-workers[12] also reported one mating between aniridics; the couple had four living children: three had aniridia and one was normal; there was a stillborn child with unknown phenotype. Other cases are those reported by Hodgson and Saunders,[42] who described the necropsy findings in a stillborn girl whose mother and father had aniridia. There were two previous miscarriages at 10 weeks of gestation. The fetus had absence of the palpebral fissures and eyes. The nasal bones were completely absent and the nasal cavity was small. Both parietal bones had elliptical defects at their posterior medial aspects and overlapped the occipital bone. The adrenals were absent. The skeletal, urogenital, alimentary, cardiovascular, and respiratory systems appeared normal. The thyroid and thymus were normal. The brain was macerated. Glaser et al.[23] reported a family where two mutations of the PAX6 gene segregated independently, causing either aniridia or a syndrome of cataracts and late-onset corneal dystrophy. A compound heterozygote for the mutations at codons 103 and 353 had severe craniofacial and central nervous system defects and no eyes. This study demonstrates a dosage effect of the PAX6 gene and its critical role in the development of eye and brain structures.

MALFORMATION SYNDROMES WITH ANIRIDIA

Ring Chromosome 6

Levin and co-workers[51] reported an infant with anterior segment dysgenesis, glaucoma, unilateral aniridia, hydrocephalus, and a ring chromosome 6. His karyotype was XY, r(6) (p24-q26). The breakpoint appeared to be at the 6q22 region with loss of material from 6p and 6q. This patient does not have classic aniridia but does have an absence of iris tissue in one eye from anterior segment dysgenesis.

Aniridia and Inversion of Chromosome 9

A single family with autosomal dominant aniridia and pericentric inversion of chromosome 9 has been reported by Gabriel et al.[21] The association is presumed to be fortuitous because chromosome 9 is known for its high susceptibility for structural arrangements and the absence of evidence for a locus for aniridia on chromosome 9 to date.

Aniridia, Ptosis, and Systemic Malformations

Hamming et al.[34] described a woman and her two children with aniridia, ptosis, and several systemic abnormalities including obesity and mental retardation in the children and alopecia, cardiac abnormalities and frequent abortions in the mother. No chromosomal studies were performed. This family may have the same syndrome described by Walker and Dyson.[87]

Aniridia, Microcornea, and Spontaneous Absorption of the Lens

Yamamoto and co-workers[93] described a three-generation family with aniridia, microcornea, and spontaneously reabsorbed cataract.[93] Corneal diameter was 10 mm in five of six eyes and 7 mm in one; iris hypoplasia was severe in some and mild in others, and membranous remnants of spontaneously reabsorbed cataracts were present in four of six eyes while aphakia was present in one and a cataract in the last eye.

Aniridia with Ptosis, Microcornea, and Glaucoma

One family with this constellation of clinical findings was described by Cohen and Nelson.[7] Two additional families of ptosis and aniridia are those reported by Shields and Reed[76] and by Bergamini et al.[2] The South African Ndebele family described by David et al.[10] also had dislocated lenses.

Gillespie Syndrome

Gillespie[22] reported a brother and sister with an autosomal recessive syndrome of aniridia, mental retardation, and ataxia. The parents were healthy and nonconsanguineous. The 22-year-old sister had normal eye movements and no nystagmus. Her irides were reduced to a stump with festooned edges and there were no cataracts. The discs were small and there were no macular reflexes. She was dysarthric and mentally retarded. The deep tendon reflexes were normal and there was past-pointing on the finger-to-nose test. The karyotype was normal. Her 19-year-old brother had similar ocular and neurologic abnormalities. Gillespie likened this syndrome to that described by Marinesco et al.[56] and by Sjögren and Larsson,[78] except that his patients had aniridia instead of cataracts in the reports by the latter two authors. Additional reports of patients with the Gillespie syndrome include those of Sarsfield[71] of one male patient, Lechtenberg and Ferreti[50] of an 18-month-old girl, and Crawfurd et al.[9] of a brother-sister pair and the son of the affected woman. François and co-workers[18] described two sisters. Wittig and co-workers[92] reported two Brazilian brothers from a sibship of three with partial aniridia, cerebellar ataxia, and moderate mental retardation. The karyotype was normal. There was cerebellar hypoplasia in both patients and the younger sibling had pulmonic stenosis. The authors attributed the syndrome to a recessive gene. Nevin and Lim[62] reported a girl with Gillespie syndrome who had an enlarged basal cistern with prominent folia of the cerebellum and a dilated fourth ventricle. Nelson et al.[61a] described two unrelated patients with this syndrome. One patient, whose parents were consanguineous, had cerebral and cerebellar atrophy with white matter changes, suggesting that patients with Gillespie syndrome have more extensive central nervous system involvement than previously described. Glaser and co-workers[26] studied the PAX6 gene for mutations in several patients with the Gillespie syndrome and failed to find mutations, suggesting that another developmental gene was possibly responsible for this condition.

Aniridia and Absence of the Patella

Mirkinson and Mirkinson[58] reported a family where a boy, his father, and his maternal grandmother had aniridia and hypoplastic or absent patellae. No other families with this combination of malformation have been reported since.

DIFFERENTIAL DIAGNOSIS

There is no difficulty in diagnosing aniridia in the patient with near-total absence of the iris, nystagmus, and foveal hypoplasia. Some patients with significant amounts of remaining iris tissue may be misdiagnosed as having the Rieger anomaly. Also, adults with essential iris atrophy (Chandler syndrome) must be differentiated. It is rare that ectopia lentis et pupillae and traumatic or iatrogenic iridectomies may mimic aniridia.

TREATMENT

Diagnostic Studies

It is essential to make an early accurate diagnosis in order to anticipate the development of Wilms' tumor in nonfamilial cases. These patients should have analysis of their chromosomes looking for a deletion of 11p13. Breslow and Beckwith[4] reported an incidence of aniridia of 8.2 of 1000 cases in 200 patients with Wilms' tumor registered with the National Wilms' Tumor study. Fraumeni and Glass[19] reported that Wilms' tumor developed in 7 of 28 patients with aniridia. One of the seven patients had familial aniridia and the rest were sporadic cases. Pilling[67] found Wilms' tumor in 7 of 20 patients with sporadic aniridia but in none of 6 patients with familial aniridia. The average age at diagnosis of the tumor was 22 months in Pilling's series and 1.8 years in Fraumeni and Glass's series. When Wilms' tumor is not associated with aniridia it is diagnosed at an average age of 3.6 years.

Finding an intragenic mutation in PAX6 reduces the risk of developing Wilms' tumor to almost zero, as it is assumed that the contiguous Wilms' tumor gene on 11p13 is normal. PAX6 gene analysis is performed on a research basis in a number of laboratories. A list of PAX6 mutations can be retrieved at the following internet page: http://www.hgu.mrc.ac.uk/Softdata/PAX6.

All patients with sporadic aniridia should have intravenous pyelograms, renal ultrasonograms, or MRI studies to rule out Wilms' tumor beginning by age 1 year. The imaging studies are repeated every 3–6 months until the age of 4 years. Ultrasonographic examinations of the kidneys may alternate with pyelograms. These studies are not necessary in familial cases of aniridia as these are presumably due to intragenic mutations of the PAX6 gene.

Family members should be examined for the presence of mild degrees of iris hypoplasia, or for aniridia with good visual function, although it is more likely that the disease is either consistently severe or consistently mild within an individual pedigree.

Cataracts

Cataracts are extracted if they produce significant decrease in visual acuity in addition to the visual loss inherent to the aniridia proper. Some patients have anterior polar or other types of congenital cataracts, whereas others develop cataracts later in life. Ectopia lentis is a less common finding but should be looked for if a lens extraction is contemplated.

Keratopathy

Corneal opacification and decompensation may result from repeated glaucoma surgery but is more commonly due to superficial opacification, vascularization, or pannus formation. Penetrating keratoplasty has been performed with a variable degree of success in some patients.[47] More recently, Tan and co-workers[81] have reported successful treatment of the keratopathy of aniridia using limbal transplantation. These authors performed limbal allograft transplantation in 18 patients with a number of superficial corneal problems, including 4 with aniridia. Visual acuity improved markedly in three patients and modestly in one patient. This is a logical modality of treatment in view of the defective limbal stem cells in patients with aniridia.

Strabismus

Strabismus adds a cosmetic handicap to the visual impairment in patients with aniridia. Strabismus surgery may be performed at the discretion of the physician and family.

Glaucoma

Glaucoma is the main cause of acquired visual loss in aniridia. Patients should be screened for its presence at regular intervals. Glaucoma develops in 50%–75% of cases in late childhood or early adulthood. However, it may be present in the first year of life. In the family reported by Elsas et al.,[12] glaucoma was present in 13% of cases. The low incidence of ocular complications in this last family was presumed to be due to mild expression of the aniridia gene. Aniridic glaucoma may be due to trabeculodysgenesis but has been observed to follow occlusion of the filtering angle by the iris stump.[89] Goniotomy has been advocated in the past as the procedure of choice for aniridic glaucoma,[74] but medical therapy should be tried first in older individuals with aniridic glaucoma. Walton[89] recommends and performs prophylactic goniotomies in patients with aniridia in the hope of preventing the progressive occlusion of anterior chamber angle structures by the iris stump. He reported good prophylaxis of glaucoma in patients treated in this fashion, but the follow-up period in his group of patients was limited. In patients in whom goniotomy and/or trabeculotomy have been unsuccessful, filtering surgery may be required. Trabeculectomy with antimetabolites or valve implants may be used. Cyclodestructive procedures including cyclocryotherapy, cyclodiathermy, or transcleral diode laser applications are often required to control intraocular pressure.

Grant and Walton[29] reported that medical treatment in the form of miotics, epinephrine, or carbonic anhydrase inhibitors could be helpful for a prolonged period. Goniosurgery was performed in 15 cases but did not cure the glaucoma; in nine eyes, goniosurgery improved the responsiveness to medical treatment. Filtering procedures were performed on nine eyes of seven patients but were unsuccessful. Cyclodialysis was also unsuccessful and cyclocryotherapy was helpful in one eye but resulted in phthisis bulbi in another. Grant and Walton[29] had suggested the performance of prophylactic goniotomies in patients of aniridia to prevent the formation of progressive iridotrabecular adhesions and glaucoma. Nine such goniotomies were performed over 7 years. None of those patients developed glaucoma, but the authors acknowledge that follow-up was limited. Grant and Walton recommend prophylactic surgery only in those patients whose angles show progressive changes that, in their opinion, lead to glaucoma. One-third of the angle circumference is operated first, followed by another third. In 1986, Walton[89] reported his experience in the use of goniosurgery in the prevention and treatment of aniridic glaucoma. Fifty-one prophylactic operations were performed on 28 eyes of 16 patients with a follow-up period ranging from 1 to 11 years (average 2 years). The average age at surgery was 4 years. Two patients had elevation of intraocular pressure 3 and 7 years after surgery. The remaining eyes maintained normal pressures, including 12 eyes followed for 6 or more years. In a second group of patients with aniridic glaucoma, 18 operations are performed on 14 eyes with only two procedures resulting in control of intraocular pressure. These goniotomies were done after failure of medical treatment. All patients required additional surgical interventions after the failure of goniotomy to reduce intraocular pressure. Walton[89] considered all eyes with aniridia and without glaucoma to be candidates for prophylactic goniotomy. He did not require the observation of progressive angle closure by peripheral iris tissue to initiate surgical management.

Other Considerations

Dark glasses or tinted contact lenses may be helpful in patients with significant light sensitivity.

REFERENCES

1. Axton R, Hanson I, Danes S, et al. The incidence of PAX6 mutation in patients with simple aniridia: An evaluation of mutation detection in 12 cases. *J Med Genet* 1997;34:279–286.

1a. Baratta G. Observazioni pratiche sulle principali malattie degli orchi Milano, 1818, Tomo 2, p. 349, as cited by Jungken C: Ueber den angebornen mangel der iris. *J Chir Augen-Heilkd (Berlin)* 1821;2:677.

2. Bergamini I, Ferraris F, Inghirami L. Su di una singalara sindrome neuro-oftalmology congenita e familiare (potosi palpebrali aniridia cateratta nistagma subatrofia ottica). *Riv Ofo-Neuro-Oftal* 1966;41:81–104.

3. Beauchamp G. Anterior segment dysgenesis keratolenticular adhesion and aniridia. *J Pediatr Ophthalmol Strabismus* 1978;17:55–58.

4. Breslow N, Beckwith J. Epidemiological features of Wilms' tumor: Results of the National Wilms' Tumor Study. *J Natl Cancer Inst* 1982;68:429–436.

5. Brusa P, Torricelli C. Nefroblastoma di Wilms' ed affezioni renali congenite nella casistica dell'IIPAI di Milano. *Minerv Pediatr (Torino)* 1953;5:457–463.

6. Callahan A. Aniridia with ectopia lentis and secondary glaucoma. *Am J Ophthalmol* 1949;32:28.

7. Cohen S, Nelson L. Aniridia with congenital ptosis and glaucoma: A family study. *Ann Ophthalmol* 1988;20:53–57.

8. Cotlier E, Rose M, Moel S. Aniridia, cataracts and Wilms' tumor in monozygous twins. *Am J Ophthalmol* 1978;86:129–132.

9. Crawfurd M, Harcourt R, Shaw P. Nonprogressive cerebellar ataxia, aplasia of pupillary zone of iris and mental subnormality (Gillespie's syndrome) affecting 3 members of a non-consanguinous family in 2 generations. *J Med Genet* 1979;16:373–378.
10. David R, MacBeath L, Jenkins T. Aniridia associated with microcornea and subluxed lenses. *Br J Ophthalmol* 1978;62:118–121.
11. Edwards, J, Lampert R, Hammer M, et al. Ocular defects and dysmorphic features in three generations. *J Clin Dysmorphol* 1984;2:8.
12. Elsas F, Maumenee I, Kenyon K, Yoder F. Familial aniridia was preserved ocular function. *Am J Ophthalmol* 1977;83:718–724.
13. Fantes J, Redeker B, Breen M, Boyle S, Brown, J, Fletcher J, et al. Aniridia-associated cytogenetic rearrangements suggest that a position effect may cause the mutant phenotype. *Hum Mol Genet* 1995;4:415–422.
14. Ferrell R, Chakravarti A, Hittner H, Riccardi V. Autosomal dominant aniridia: Probable linkage to the acid phosphatase-1 locus on chromosome 2. *Proc Natl Acad Sci USA* 1980;77:1580–1582.
15. Ferrell R, Riccardi V. Catalase levels in patients with aniridia and/or Wilms' tumor: Utility and limitations. *Cytogenet Cell Genet* 1981;31:120–123.
16. Foster M. Congenital irideremia. *Arch Ophthalmol* 1898;25:593.
17. François J. La gonioscopie. *Prog Ophtalmol* 1955;4:19–129.
18. François J, Lentini F, De Rouck F. Gillespie's syndrome (incomplete aniridia cerebellar ataxia and oligophrenia). *Ophthalmic Paediatr Genet* 1984;4:29–32.
19. Fraumeni J Jr, Glass A. Wilms' tumor and congenital aniridia. *JAMA* 1968;206:825–828.
20. Fryns J, Beirinckx J, DeSutter E, Derluyn, J, François J, Van den Berghe H. Aniridia-Wilms' tumor association and 11p interstitial deletion. *Eur J Pediatr* 1981;136:91–92.
21. Gabriel K, Savir H, Shabtai F. Chromosome 9 pericentric inversion in familial aniridia. *Metab Ophthalmol* 1978;2:213–214.
22. Gillespie F. Aniridia cerebellar ataxia and oligophrenia in siblings. *Arch Ophthalmol* 1965;73:338–341.
23. Glaser T, Jepeal L, Edwards J, Young R, Favor J, Maas R. PAX6 gene dosage effect in a family with congenital cataracts aniridia anophthalmia and central nervous system defects. *Nature Genet* 1994;7:463–469.
24. Glaser T, Lane J, Housman D. A mouse model of the aniridia-Wilms' tumor deletion syndrome. *Science* 1990;250:823–827.
25. Glaser T, Lewis W, Bruns G, Watkins P, Rogler C, Shows T, et al. The β-subunit of follicle-stimulating hormone is deleted in patients with aniridia and Wilms' tumor allowing a further definition of the WAGR locus. *Nature* 1986;321(6073):882–887.
26. Glaser T, Ton C, Mueller R, Petzlerler M, Oliver C, Nevin N, et al. Absence of PAX6 gene mutations in Gillespie syndrome (partial aniridia cerebellar-ataxia and mental-retardation). *Genomics* 1994;19:145–148.
27. Glaser T, Walton D, Maas R. Genomic structure evolutionary conservation and aniridia mutations in the human PAX6 gene. *Nature Genet* 1992;2:232–239.
28. Godde-Salz E, Behmke H. Aniridia mental retardation and an unbalanced reciprocal translocation of chromosomes 8 and 11 with an interstitial deletion of 11p. *Eur J Pediatr* 1981;136:93–96.
29. Grant W, Walton D. Progressive changes in the angle in congenital aniridia with development of glaucoma. *Am J Ophthalmol* 1974;78:842–847.
30. Grove J, Shaw M, Bourque G. A family study of aniridia. *Arch Ophthalmol* 1961;65:81–94.
31. Gruss P, Walther C. Pax in development. *Cell* 1992;69:719–722.
32. Gutbier S. Iridermia seu defectu iridis congenito. *Dissert Inaug Wirceb def Gothae* 1834;14.
33. Halder G, Callaerts P, Gehring W. Induction of ectopic eyes by targeted expression of the eyeless gene in *Drosophila*. *Science* 1995;267(5205):1788–1792.
34. Hamming N, Miller M, Rabb M. Unusual variant of familial aniridia. *J Pediatr Ophthalmol Strabismus* 1986;23:195.
35. Hamming N, Wilensky J. Persistent pupillary membrane associated with aniridia. *Am J Ophthalmol* 1978;86:118–120.
36. Hanson I, Fletcher J, Jordan T, Brown A, Taylor D, Adams R, et al. Mutations at the PAX6 locus are found in heterogeneous anterior segment malformations including Peters' anomaly. *Nature Genet* 1994;6:168–173.
37. Hill R, Favor J, Hogan B, Ton C, Saunders G, Hanson I, et al. Mouse small eye results from mutations in a paired-like homeobox-containing gene. *Nature* 1991;354:522–525.
38. Hill R, Hanson I. Molecular genetics of the Pax gene family. *Curr Opin Cell Biol* 1992;4:967–972.

39. Hirschberg J. Angeborener Irismangel mit spaterer Linsen-Verschiebung wie Trubung und Drucksteigerung. *Centralblatt Prakt Augenheilkd* 1888;12:13.
40. Hittner H, Riccardi V, Ferrell R, Borda R, Justice J. Variable expressivity of autosomal dominant aniridia by clinical electrophysiologic and angiographic criteria. *Am J Ophthalmol* 1980;89:531–539.
41. Hittner H, Riccardi V, Francke U. Aniridia caused by a heritable chromosome 11 deletion. *Trans Am Acad Ophthalmol* 1979;86:1173–1183.
42. Hodgson S, Saunders K. A probable case of the homozygous condition of the aniridia gene. *J Med Genet* 1980;17:478–480.
43. Hotta Y, Fujiki K, Ishida N, Kato K, Nakajima A, Takamatsu H. High resolution G-banding analysis in anirida. *Ophthalmic Paediatr Genet* 1987;8:145–150.
44. Jotterand V, Boisjoly H, Harnois C, Bigonesse P, Laframboise R, Gagne R, et al. 11p13 deletion Wilms' tumor and anitidia: Unusual genetic non-ocular and ocular features in three cases. *Br J Ophthalmol* 1990;74:568–570.
45. Kivlin J, Apple D, Olson R, Manthey R. Dominantly inherited keratitis. *Arch Ophthalmol* 1986;104:1621–1623.
45a. Koroma BM, Yang JM, Sundin OH. The Pax-6 homeobox gene is expressed throughout the corneal and conjunctival epithelia. *Invest Ophthalmol Vis Sci* 1997;38:108–120.
46. Koster R, van Balen A. Congenital corneal opacity (Peters' anomaly) combined with buphthalmos and aniridia. *Ophthalmic Paediatr Genex* 1985;6:1.
47. Kremer I, Rajpal RK, Rapuano CJ, Cohen EJ, Laibson PR. Results of penetrating keratoplasty in aniridia. *Am J Ophthalmol* 1993;115(3):317–320.
48. Ladda R, Atkins L, Littlefield J. Computer-assisted analysis of chromosomal abnormalities: detection of a deletion in aniridia/Wilms' tumor syndrome. *Science* 1974;185:784.
49. Layman P, Anderson D, Flynn J. Frequent occurrence of hypoplastic optic disks in patients with aniridia. *Am J Ophthalmol* 1974;77:513–516.
50. Lechtenberg R, Ferreti C. Ataxia with aniridia of Gillespie: A case report. *Neurology* 1981;31:95–97.
51. Levin H, Ritch R, Barathur R, Teekhasaenee C, Margolis S. Aniridia congenital glaucoma and hydrocephalus in a male infant with ring chromosome 6. *Am J Med Genet* 1986;25:281–287.
52. Lyons LA, Martha A, Mintz-Hittner HA, Saunders GF, Ferrell RE. Resolution of the two loci for autosomal dominant aniridia, AN1 and AN2, to a single locus on chromosome 11p13. *Genomics* 1992;13(4):925–930.
53. Mackman G, Brightbill F, Optiz J. Corneal changes in aniridia. *Am J Ophthalmol* 1979;87:497–502.
54. Mannens M, Bleeker-Wagemakers E, Bliek J, Hoovers J, Mandjes I, van Tol S, et al. Autosomal dominant aniridia linked to the chromosome 11p13 markers catalase and D11S151 in a large Dutch family. *Cytogenet Cell Genet* 1989;52:32–36.
55. Margo C. Congenital aniridia: A histopathologic study of the anterior segment in children. *J Pediatr Ophthalmol Strabismismus* 1983;20:192–198.
56. Marinesco G, Draganesco G, Vasilus O. Nouvelle maladie familiale caracterisee par une cataracte congenitale et un arret du developpement somato-neuro-psychique. *Encephale* 1931;26:97–102.
57. Miller R, Fraumeni J Jr, Manning M. Association of Wilms' tumor with aniridia hemihypertrophy and other congenital malformations. *N Engl J Med* 1964;270:922.
58. Mirkinson A, Mirkinson N. A familial syndrome of aniridia and absence of the patella. *Birth Defects Orig Art Ser* 1975;XI (5):129–131.
59. Mirzayans F, Pearce W, MacDonald I, Walter M. Mutation of the PAX6 gene in patients with autosomal dominant keratitis. *Am J Hum Genet* 1995;57:539–548.
60. Moore J, Hyman S, Antonarakis S, Mules E, Thomas G. Familial isolated aniridia associated with a translocation involving chromosomes 11 and 22 [t(1122)(p13q122)]. *Hum Genet* 1986;72:297–302.
61. Narahara K, Kikkawa K, Kimira S, Kimoto H, Ogata M, Kasai R, et al. Regional mapping of catalase and Wilms' tumor-aniridia genitourinary abnormalities and mental retardation triad loci to the chromosome segment 11p1305-p1306. *Hum Genet* 1984; 66:181–185.
61a. Nelson J, Flaherty M, Grattan-Smith P. Gillespie syndrome: A report of two further cases. *Am J Med Genet* 1997;71:134–138.
62. Nevin N, Lim J. Syndrome of partial aniridia cerebellar ataxia and mental retardation—

Gillespie syndrome. *Am J Med Genet* 1990;35:468.

63. Niikawa N, Fukushima Y, Tanigushi N, Iizuka S, Kajii T. Chromosome abnormalities involving 11p13 and low erythrocyte catalase activity. *Hum Genet* 1982;60:373–375.
64. Nishida K, Kinoshita S, Ohashi Y, Kuwayama Y, Yamamoto S. Ocular surface abnormalities in aniridia. *Am J Ophthalmol* 1995;120(3):368–375.
65. Pearce W, Mielke B, Hassard D, Climenhaga H, Climenhaga D, Hodges E. Autosomal dominant keratitis: A possible aniridia variant. *Can J Ophthalmol* 1995;30:131–137.
66. Pettenati M, Weaver R, Burton B. translocation t(511)(q131p13) associated with familial isolated aniridia. *Am J Med Genet* 1989;34:230–232.
67. Pilling G. Wilms' tumor in seven children with congenital aniridia. J Pediatr Surg 1975;10:87.
68. Riccardi V, Hittner H, Francke U, Yunis J, Ledbetter D, Borges W. The aniridia-Wilms' tumor association: The critical role of chromosome band 11p13. *Cancer Genet Cytogenet* 1980;2:131–137.
69. Riccardi V, Hittner H, Strong L, Fernbach D, Lebo R, Ferrell R. Wilms' tumor with aniridia/iris dysplasia and apparently normal chromosomes. *J Pediatr* 1982;100:574–577.
70. Riccardi V, Sujansky E, Smith A, Francke U. Chromosomal imbalance in the aniridia-Wilms' tumor association: 11p interstitial deletion. *Pediatrics* 1978;61:604–610.
71. Sarsfield J. The syndrome of congenital cerebellar ataxia aniridia and mental retardation. *Dev Med Child Neurol* 1971;13:508–511.
72. Schmahl W, Knoedlseder M, Favor J, Davidson D. Defects of neuronal migration and the pathogenesis of cortical malformations are associated with Small eye (Sey) in the mouse a point mutation at the Pax-6 locus. *Acta Neuropathol* 1993;86:126–135.
73. Shaffer R, Cohen J. Visual reduction in aniridia. *J Pediatr Ophthalmol* 1975;12:220–222.
74. Shaffer R, Walton DJ. *Congenital and Pediatric Glaucomas*. St. Louis: C. V. Mosby, 1970.
75. Shaw M, Falls H, Neel J. Congenital aniridia. *Am J Hum Genet* 1960;12:389–415.
76. Shields M, Reed J. Aniridia and congenital ptosis. *Ann Ophthalmol* 1975;7:203–211.
77. Simola K, Knuutila S, Kaitila I, Pirkola A, Pohja P. Familial aniridia and translocation t(411)(q22p13) without Wilms' tumor. *Hum Genet* 1983;63:158–161.
78. Sjögren T, Larsson T. Oligophrenia in combination with congenital ichthyosis and spastic disorders: A clinical and genetic study. *Acta Psychiatr Neurol Scand* 1957;32(suppl 113):1–112.
79. Stone D, Kenyon K, Green W, Ryan S. Congenital central corneal leukoma (Peters' anomaly). *Am J Ophthalmol* 1976;81:173–193.
80. Strachan T, Read A. PAX genes. *Curr Opin Genet Dev* 1994;4:427–438.
81. Tan DT, Ficker LA, Buckley RJ. Limbal transplantation. *Ophthalmology* 1996;103:29–36.
82. Ton C, Hirvonen H, Miwa H, Well M, Monaghan P, Jordan T, et al. Positional cloning and characterization of a paired box- and homeobox-containing gene from the aniridia region. *Cell* 1991;67:1059–1074.
83. Traboulsi E, Jurdi-Nuwayhid F, Torbey N, Frangieh G. Aniridia atypical iris defects optic pit and the morning glory disc anomaly in a family. *Ophthalmic Paediatr Genet* 1986;7:131–135.
84. Turleau C, de Grouchy J, Nihoul-Fekete C, Dufier J, Chavin-Colin F, Junien C. Del 11p13/nephroblastoma without aniridia. *Hum Genet* 1984;67:455–456.
85. Turleau C, de Grouchy J, Tournade M-F, Gagnadoux M-F, Junien C. Del 11p/aniridia complex. Report of three patients and review of 37 observations from the literature. *Clin Genet* 1984;26:356–362.
86. Van der Meer-de Jong R, Dickinson M, Woychik R, Stubbs L, Hetherington C, Hogan B. Location of the gene involving the small eye mutation on mouse chromosome 2 suggests homology with human aniridia (AN2). *Genomics* 1990;7:270–275.
87. Walker F, Dyson C. Dominantly inherited aniridia associated with mental retardation and other eye anomalies. *Birth Defects Orig Art Ser* 1974;10:147.
88. Walter C, Gruss P. Pax-6, a murine paired box gene, is expressed in the developing CNS. *Development* 1991;113:1435–1449.
89. Walton D. Aniridic glaucoma: The results of gonio-surgery to prevent and treat this problem. *Trans Am Ophthalmol Soc* 1986; 84:59.
90. Warburg M, Mikkelsen M, Andersen S, Geertinger P, Larsen H, Vestermark S, et al. Aniridia and interstitial deletion of the short arm of chromosome 11. *Metab Pediatr Ophthalmol* 1980;4:97–102.
91. Weiss J, Demartini D, Brown R, Forster R.

Specular microscopy in aniridia. *Cornea* 1987;6:27–31.

92. Wittig E, Moreira C, Freire-Maia N, Vianna-Morgante A. Partial aniridia cerebellar ataxia and mental deficiency (Gillespie syndrome) in two brothers. *Am J Med Genet* 1988; 30:703–708.
93. Yamamoto Y, Hayasaka S, Setogawa T. Family wtih aniridia, microcornea and spontaneously reabsorbed cataract. *Arch Ophthalmol* 1988;106:502–504.
94. Yanagisawa H, Okuyama T, Yamada M. PAX6 missense mutation in isolated foveal hypoplasia. *Nature Genet* 1996;13(2):141–142.

7

Congenital Anomalies of the Optic Nerve Head

MARYAM AROICHANE
ELIAS I. TRABOULSI

There is a wide variation in the normal morphology of the optic nerve head. The ophthalmoscopic appearance of the optic disc depends on the size of the scleral canal, the orientation of the optic nerve as it exits from the globe, the location of the edge of the retinal pigment epithelial and other retinal layers as they approach the circumference of the optic nerve head, the error of refraction, the size of the optic cup, and the variability of the branching pattern of the retinal vasculature and their exit from the papilla. It is important to differentiate between variations of the normal appearance of the nerve head and malformations that may be associated with reduced vision or with significant brain or other systemic defects. Table 7.1 categorizes optic nerve anomalies as they are listed in this chapter.

ABNORMALITIES OF SIZE OF THE OPTIC DISC

Aplasia of the Optic Nerve

Congenital aplasia of the optic nerve was first described in 1854 by von Graefe[276] in a 10-year-old boy with a blind esotropic eye and absent optic nerve and retinal vessels. This anomaly is characterized by absence of the optic disc, optic nerve, retinal ganglion cells, and retinal vessels. Aplasia of the optic nerve is very rare and can occur in otherwise healthy patients,[26,161a,170] although early deaths have been reported.[16,100,124,251,295] Viral infection[100] and/or environmental factors such as acetone exposure[125] may be implicated in this congenital anomaly. Family history is not consistent with Mendelian inheritance. Incidence is equal in males and females.

Eyes with optic nerve aplasia have no light perception. Therefore, direct pupillary reaction is absent and there is a relative pupillary afferent defect on the affected side. Stimulation of the normal eye results in a consensual response in the eye with optic nerve aplasia and a normal direct pupillary reaction in the normal eye. In the case described by Howard et al.,[125] esotropia was present but no nystagmus was observed. Corneal sensation is usually normal.

Ocular abnormalities associated with optic nerve aplasia include microphthalmia, enophthalmos, ptosis, smaller corneal diameter, and absent Descemet's membrane and endothelium. The iridocorneal angle may be underdeveloped with an embryonic configuration[295] and

Table 7.1. Optic Nerve Anomalies

Abnormalities of size of the optic nerve head	Congenital pigmentation of the optic disc
Aplasia of the optic nerve	Bergmeister papilla
Hypoplasia of the optic nerve	Myelinated nerve fibers
Megalopapilla	Congenital vascular anomalies
Cavitary malformations of the optic nerve head	Peripapillary vascular loops
Optic disc coloboma	Cilioretinal arteries
Morning glory disc anomaly	Optociliary veins
Peripapillary staphyloma	Disc drusen
Optic pit	
Congenital tilted disc	

iridocorneal adhesions. The iris may have patchy areas of hypoplasia or coloboma or may resemble aniridia.[100] The lens may be cataractous. There may be persistence and hyperplasia of the primary vitreous. Posterior segment abnormalities include avascular retina, hyperplasia, hypoplasia or normal pigmentation of the retinal pigment epithelium (RPE), and retinal detachment.[125]

Visual evoked potentials show increased signals in the ipsilateral occipital cortex suggesting increased decussation of the temporal retinal nerve fibers of the normal contralateral eye. The electroretinogram (ERG) may be flat, but if it is present, the a and b waves are diminished.[26,161a] The intravenous fluorescein angiogram shows no retinal vessels.[26,125,161a] There is no detectable shadow of the optic nerve on ultrasonography, and the electrooculogram (EOG) is abnormal.[125]

The optic foramen is small on the side of the aplasia.[161a] Computerized tomography shows a smaller orbit and globe on the affected side. Magnetic resonance imaging can document absence of the optic nerve, and a chiasm and lateral geniculate body that are smaller than normal.[170] In two reports, chromosomal studies were normal.[100,251]

Histopathologic studies of this condition have shown microphthalmia, a scleral type of organization of collagen in the cornea, and absence of Descemet's membrane and corneal endothelium. Embryonic iridocorneal angle, anterior synechiae, patchy iris hypoplasia, persistent hyperplastic primary vitreous (PHPV), retinal dysplasia and rosette formation, and an abnormal or deficient RPE[16,100,124,287,295] have all been described in association with aplasia of the optic nerve. Chorioretinal colobomas and staphylomas may also be present. Macular differentiation is poor.[251] Remnants of the dural sheath may be present and attach to the posterior aspect of the globe.

Associated anomalies of the visual pathways in the central nervous system (CNS) include smaller or absent chiasm[170,251,295] and smaller optic tract and lateral geniculate body. Other CNS malformations such as anencephaly, hydranencephaly,[251] lissencephaly, arhinencephaly, encephalocele, and partial agenesis of the medulla, pons, and cerebellum have also been reported. Osteogenesis imperfecta and cleft lip and palate have also been described.[100] There is one report of a blind infant with mitochondrial disease and optic nerve aplasia.[31]

Optic nerve aplasia is a congenital, nonhereditary condition of unknown etiology. Chromosomal studies have been normal. Scheie and Adler[235] hypothesized that the fetal fissure failed to form and close, causing mesenchyme to be misdirected and failure of normal retinal and optic disc vascularization. However, as pointed out by Weiter et al.,[287] the presence of the dural sheath, which is derived from mesoderm, suggests that ventral invagination of the optic vesicle causes nerve fiber misdirection and secondary atrophy. Yanoff and colleagues[295] hypothesized that primary failure of ganglion cells to develop and send out axons results in lack of induction of mesodermal ingrowth. Hotchkiss and Green[124] suggested that failure of mesodermal induction was secondary to a neuronal defect in the ganglion cell layer.

An animal model for optic nerve aplasia and hypoplasia has been described. Ocular retardation (*or*) is a recessive gene mutation in the mouse that causes microphthalmia, cataracts, progressive degeneration of the retina, and aplasia of the optic nerve.[215] In the homozygous stage, this fully penetrant mutation causes degeneration of cells of the optic cup and failure of the embryonic fissure to close early in the development of the eye. These phenomena seem to occur before the arrest of retinal and optic nerve development with secondary disappearance of retinal vessels and cataract formation.

The esotropia can be operated as in the case of Howard et al.,[125] commented on by Kearns, who recommended a high plus lens in front of the affected eye to improve the cosmetic appearance of the microphthalmic eye. Neuroimaging studies should be performed to document other associated CNS malformations.

Hypoplasia of the Optic Nerve

Optic nerve hypoplasia (ONH) is a nonprogressive, segmental or diffuse, congenital abnormality of one or both optic nerves characterized by a decreased number of axons in the involved nerve that otherwise has normal glial and supportive mesodermal tissue.[124,184]

Optic nerve hypoplasia should be suspected in patients with long-standing nonprogressive visual impairment of unclear etiology and in patients with midfacial abnormalities. Males are affected as frequently as females and bilateral occurrence is more common than unilateral disease.[2,23,243,281] Patients with unilateral or asymmetric ONH may present with strabismus. Those with bilateral severe disease are usually examined because of poor vision and nystagmus. Visual acuity may be normal in the presence of visual field defects and mild disease.

Ophthalmoscopically, the nerve head is reduced in size because of the decreased number of axons (Figs. 7.1, 7.2). There may or may not be a surrounding hypopigmented halo, a so-called "double-ring sign." The double-ring sign indicates that a small optic nerve is present in a wider scleral canal.[124,184] The degree of optic nerve hypoplasia is extremely variable and tends to be more severe in bilateral cases. Mild ONH is difficult to diagnose because of problems in measuring optic nerve head diameter. The variability in appearance of the optic nerve head in different racial groups, and the accompanying myopia or hyperopia add to the measurement difficulties. In cases where a mild degree of hypoplasia is suspected, fundus photographs allow objective measurements of optic nerve diameter and calculation of diameter to retinal arterial vessel diameter ratio or to other retinal landmaks such as the distance from the center of the disc to the fovea.[10,297] The retinal vessels can be of normal caliber but are frequently tortuous. The macula may be normal or there may be blunted macular and foveal reflexes, reflecting the decrease in number of nerve fibers.[184]

Hypoplasia can also involve the optic disc in a segmental manner, often superiorly. Segmental optic nerve hypoplasia has been reported in children of insulin-dependent diabetic mothers

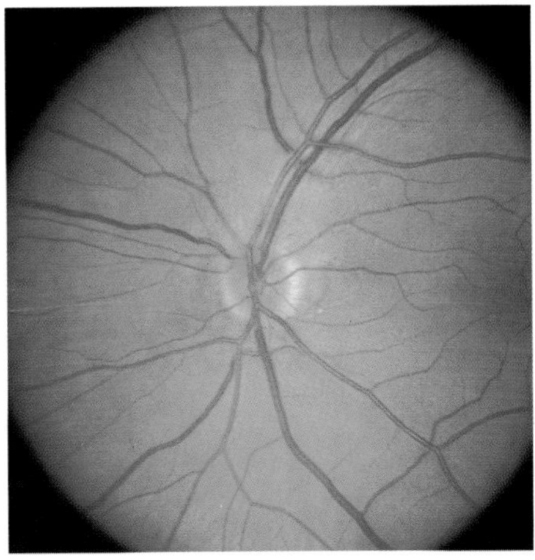

Figure 7.1. Optic nerve hypoplasia. Patient also has adult-onset glaucoma.

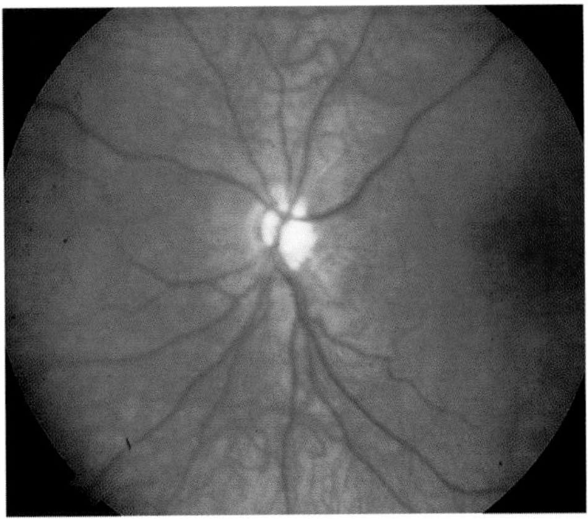

Figure 7.2. Eight-year-old girl with optic nerve hypoplasia. Vision is with no light perception. There was a trace direct pupillary reaction. (Courtesy of Dr. Scott Brodie.)

in the absence of other systemic abnormalities.[141,201,202] A distinct form of ONH is the homonymous hemioptic hypoplasia described by Hoyt and colleagues[131] in patients with unilateral congenital retrochiasmatic lesions involving the optic pathways resulting in nasal and temporal segmental hypoplasia in the eye contralateral to the lesion. The ipsilateral optic disc may or may not be normal.[193] The mechanism involved in homonymous hemioptic hypoplasia is presumed to be a transsynaptic degeneration of the optic tract that is secondary to lesions of the occipital cortex.[128,193]

Visual acuity in ONH is variable and can be normal or markedly decreased depending on preservation of the papillomacular bundle.[37] Treatment of any associated amblyopia can result in improvement of vision.[294]

A variety of visual field defects may be present in patients with optic nerve hypoplasia and depend on the severity and location of nerve fiber loss. Bitemporal visual field defects and generalized constriction are most commonly seen in severe hypoplasia,[2] whereas inferior altitudinal field defects that spare fixation predominate in segmental hypoplasia.[201] Bitemporal field defects may indicate the presence of midline defects in the central nervous system.[77,224]

Optic nerve hypoplasia should be differentiated from the crowded disc in high hypermetropia, hence refraction should always be performed. There seems to be an associated increase in incidence of axial myopia,[8,288] as well as other refractive errors including astigmatism.[298] Also, hypoplastic discs have been incorrectly diagnosed as atrophic because of the surrounding pallor; the disc itself, however, is pink in color but is smaller than normal.

Cibis and Fitzgerald[57] performed electroretinographic studies on patients with ONH and found abnormalities in 35% of cases. These findings suggested transsynaptic degeneration beyond the ganglion cell layer. The EOG is usually normal. When normal, the ERG helps distinguish ONH from Leber congenital amaurosis.[90] Visual evoked responses are usually reduced in amplitude and correlate with the degree of visual acuity loss.[169,247] Color vision has not been systematically assessed in patients with ONH.

On histopathologic sections the ganglion cells and optic nerve fibers are reduced in number, but the outer retinal layers are normal. The double ring sign appears to be due to an overgrowth of retinal pigment epithelial cells toward the center of the optic disc.[124,184] The ocular and systemic conditions associated with ONH include aniridia, albinism, colobomatous microphthalmia, Aicardi syndrome, Potter syndrome, Klippel-Trenaunay syndrome, facio-auriculo-vertebral sequence, Duane syndrome, Meckel syndrome, 13q– syndrome, trisomy 18, and nevus sebaceous of Jadassohn.

Of most interest and significance is the association of ONH with midline brain abnormalities. Optic nerve hypoplasia is present in 25% of patients with absence of the septum pellucidum,[72] and 27% of patients with ONH have partial or complete absence of the septum pellucidum.[2] Septo-optic dysplasia, or De Morsier syndrome, is characterized by variable degrees of ONH and absence of the septum pellucidum or corpus callosum, mental retardation, spasticity, and impairment of taste and smell. Patients with septo-optic dysplasia also have problems learning tasks that require spatial orientation. Pituitary dysfunction and endocrinologic abnormalities may result from hypothalamic maldevelopment.[169,182,291] Growth hormone deficiency is the most common endocrinologic abnormality in patients with septo-optic dysplasia. Growth hormone deficiency and growth retardation usually become evident in the third or fourth year of life.[65,151] Hypothyroidism, diabetes insipidus, and hyperprolactinemia may also be present.[9,126,169] Pituitary dysfunction in patients with septo-optic dysplasia may lead to prolonged neonatal hyperbilirubinemia, hypotonia or infantile hypoglycemia without hyperinsulinemia. Cells of the supraoptic and paraventricular nuclei were found to be abnormally small and few in number in a patient with severe bilateral ONH and pituitary dysfunction.[199] Other associations include hydranencephaly, arhinencephaly, aniridia, cyclopia, orbital encephalomeningocele, hypotelorism,[7] and holoprosencephaly.[85]

Magnetic resonance imaging (MRI) has allowed better visualization of the hypoplastic optic nerve and its associated CNS abnormalities. The thinning and attenuation of the prechiasmatic intracranial optic nerve(s) are well delineated.[41] In bilateral cases, the chiasm is smaller than normal. MRI abnormalities in patients with ONH fall into one of the following categories: (*1*) isolated ONH, (*2*) absence of the septum pellucidum, (*3*) posterior pituitary ectopia, (*4*) cerebral hemispheric migration anomalies (schizencephaly, cortical heterotopia), and (*5*) perinatal hemispheric injury (periventricular leukomalacia, encephalomalacia).[41]

MRI can be used to acquire prognostic information concerning neurodevelopment and growth hormone deficiency. Brodsky et al.[41] showed that patients with posterior pituitary ectopia (MRI group 3) were at highest risk for pituitary hormone deficiency. The presence of anomalies in categories 4 and 5 correlated well with the presence of neurodevelopmental defects. Interestingly, these authors[41] have found that isolated absence of the septum pellucidum can be associated with normal neurodevelopmental and endocrinologic function.

Failure of differentiation of the retinal ganglion cell layer between the 12 and 17 mm stages of retinal development has been proposed to explain ONH.[184] This suggests selective involvement of ganglion cells as other cells from the inner neuroblastic retinal layer are normal. This theory does not account for the associated brain anomalies. Another theory suggests that inadequate target organs, e.g., CNS structures, prevent the development of ascending optic nerve fibers.[5,77] Finally, excessive death (apoptosis) of ganglion cells following their exuberant development may be a plausible pathogenetic mechanism in optic nerve hypoplasia.[206] Possible etiologic factors for the development of ONH include maternal diabetes mellitus[189,201] postmaturity, and young maternal age.[72,169] Gestational intake of anticonvulsants, quinine, lysergic acid, diethylamide, and phencyclidine has also been associated with ONH. Nearly half of the patients with fetal alcohol syndrome have ONH[154,257] and 12.5% of mothers of children with ONH admit to alcohol abuse during pregnancy.[2] Cytomegalovirus infection during pregnancy has been implicated in abnormal optic nerve development in four patients.[121]

Autosomal dominant inheritance of ONH has been reported in five members of one family[111] and in at least one mother–daughter pair. Other genetics anomalities associated with ONH include interstitial duplication of chromosome 7(q22-q34),[255] and ring chromosome 21 mosaicism (syndrome of lens dislocation associated with ONH and systemic anomalies).[172]

Patients with bilateral ONH should undergo neuroradiologic evaluaton for associated pituitary or other midline brain defects. MRI may show abnormalities of the septum pellucidum, posterior pituitary ectopia, dilated ventricles, encephalocele, porencephaly, holoprosencephaly, or encephalomalacia.[83,166] On the other hand, an apparently normal septum pellucidum on computed tomography does not invalidate a clinical diagnosis of septo-optic dysplasia.[292]

Patients with unilateral ONH and strabismus should undergo a trial of occlusion therapy for any superimposed anisometropic amblyopia.[97,294] Optic nerve hypoplasia is compatible with good visual acuity if the maculopapillary bundle is spared.[25] Whether children with bilateral ONH should undergo routine endocrinologic evaluation early in life and periodically thereafter remains a controversial subject. The workup should certainly be performed in the presence of suggestive symptomatology or if there is growth retardation. Endocrinologic abnormalities are treated as needed. The prediatrician should be an active participant in the management of patients with ONH.

Megalopapilla

Megalopapilla was described by Kraupa and others[28,89,148] as an abnormally large optic disc with no anatomical defects. This condition is usually bilateral with a large cup-to-disc ratio that mimics low-tension glaucoma (Fig. 7.3). The optic cup is round or larger horizontally than vertically. The neuroretinal rim appears pale and megalopapilla may mimic optic atrophy.[50] This has been attributed to the spreading out of axons over a larger rim area. This condition can be unilateral or bilateral, the former being more frequent.[176]

Visual acuity is usually normal or mildly decreased from anisometropic or strabismic amblyopia. Visual field tracings may demonstrate

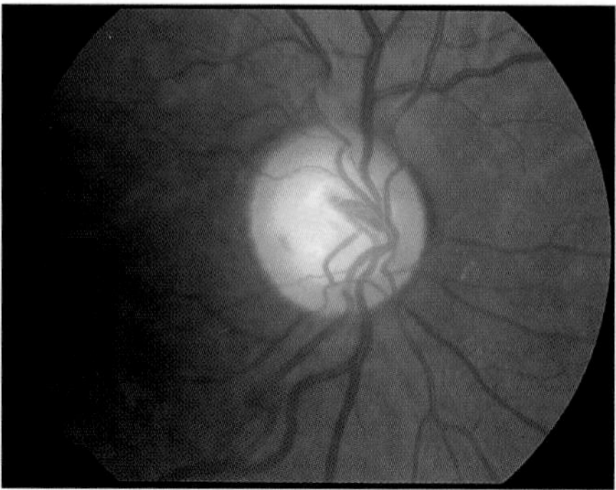

Figure 7.3. Megalopapilla. The cup-to-disc ratio is large. The rim is healthy.

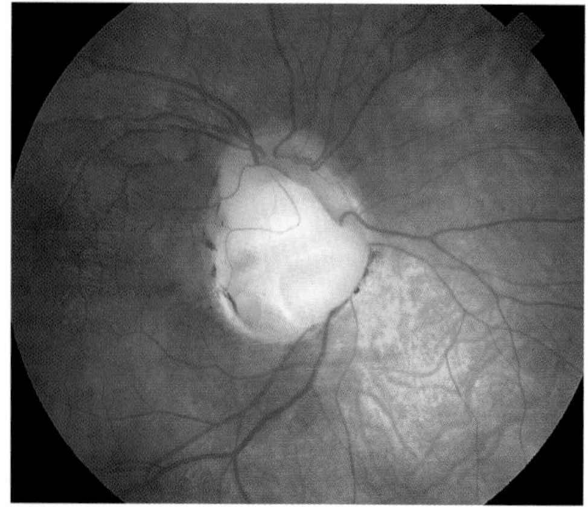

Figure 7.4. Typical coloboma of the optic nerve head that results from faulty closure of the fetal fissure.

an enlarged blind spot or peripheral constriction. The report of megalopapilla in a child with basal encephalocele[106] suggests that optic axonal migration is modified early in embryogenesis. Neuroimaging is recommended if midfacial anomalies such as hypertelorism, cleft palate, cleft lip, and depressed nasal bridge are present.[37] This condition has been described with mandibulofacial dysostosis of the Franceschetti–Zwhalen type[164] and with retinochoroidal coloboma.[62]

CAVITARY MALFORMATIONS OF THE OPTIC NERVE HEAD

Optic Disc Coloboma

This anomaly results from incomplete closure of the embryonic fissure and takes a spectrum of forms ranging from notches to holes and large defects of one or more anatomical structures along the fetal fissure line.[197a] When the optic disc is involved, a large excavated white area devoid of neuroretinal tissue replaces part of the optic disc and may extend inferiorly (Fig. 7.4). Optic disc coloboma can be unilateral or bilateral. Autosomal dominant inheritance has been described,[231] but the abnormality also occurs sporadically. Optic disc coloboma can be isolated or may be associated with multiple systemic abnormalities such as the CHARGE association,[56,198,214,225] Walker-Warburg syndrome,[283,284] Goltz focal dermal hypoplasia,[108,282] Goldenhar syndrome,[18,157] Aicardi syndrome,[52,127] linear nevus sebaceous syndrome,[168] Rubinstein-Taybi syndrome,[221] basal encephalocele,[153,256] arachnoid cyst,[219] or intraorbital cyst with ocular motility restriction.[289] Optic disc coloboma has been described with deletion of the long arm of chromosome 7[210] as well as with Edward syndrome (trisomy 18).[274] Weaver and colleagues[285] reported two cases of renal disease in association with optic disc coloboma.

The optic disc coloboma is usually decentered inferiorly reflecting the inferotemporal location of the embryonic fissure. The superior neuroretinal rim is generally spared. There usually is enlargement of the excavated papillary area, with the deepest part located inferiorly, a glistening white surface, and retinal vessels entering and existing from the borders of the defect.[3,43,132,136,213,240] Other colobomatous defects along the choroidal fissure can be present in the adjacent retina and choroid. Visual acuity may be normal or markedly decreased and is difficult to predict from the appearance of the optic disc. Strabismus may be present.[218,249]

Optic disc colobomas can be complicated by macular holes[22] and serous macular detachment[158] that can reattach spontaneously or may require treatment. Several modalities have been employed for the treatment of serous retinal detachment in optic disc coloboma including bed rest, steroids, vitrectomy, scleral buckling procedures, gas-fluid exchange and photocoagulation.[234] Congenital optic disc anomalies associated with nonrhegmatogenous retinal detachment include pits, morning glory disc anomaly, peripapillary staphyloma, and typical uveal coloboma involving the optic disc.[47] The source of the subretinal fluid is unknown. Savell and Cook[231] failed to demonstrate that the cerebrospinal fluid (CSF) was the source for subretinal fluid by radioisotope cisternography.

The colobomatous area is devoid of retina, choroid, and sclera. The defect is lined by fibrous tissue and may contain well-formed hypoplastic or gliotic retina.[47] The lamina cribrosa is located more posteriorly or is absent.[58,290] The presence of intrascleral smooth muscle strands oriented in a concentric fashion around the distal optic nerve on histopathological examination may be responsible for optic disc contractility in rare cases of optic disc coloboma.[87,290]

Sensory serous macular detachment may rarely occur, sometimes with spontaneous reattachments.[27] The cause of retinal detachment in optic disc coloboma is unknown. Mechanisms involved in the retinal detachment may be related to communication of the subretinal space with the CSF or with the vitreous cavity or to leakage from the peripapillary capillaries.

Visual field defects associated with optic disc coloboma include generalized constriction,[3,43] altitudinal defects,[3,213] cecocentral scotomas,[136,218] enlargement of the blind spot,[136] arcuate scotomas, and ring scotomas.[213,231]

Distinguishing a typical optic disc coloboma from the morning glory disc anomaly can be difficult in some cases but is important to establish because the morning glory disc anomaly is sporadic, whereas optic disc coloboma can be inherited and patients have to be offered genetic counseling.[268]

Morning Glory Disc Anomaly

The morning glory disc anomaly (MGDA) is characterized by an enlarged, excavated, and funnel-shaped optic disc with a central white glial tuft and a raised annulus of pigmentary chorioretinal changes at its edge.[115,250] The descriptive term "morning disc anomaly" was coined by Kindler[142] in 1970 because of the resemblance to the morning glory flower.

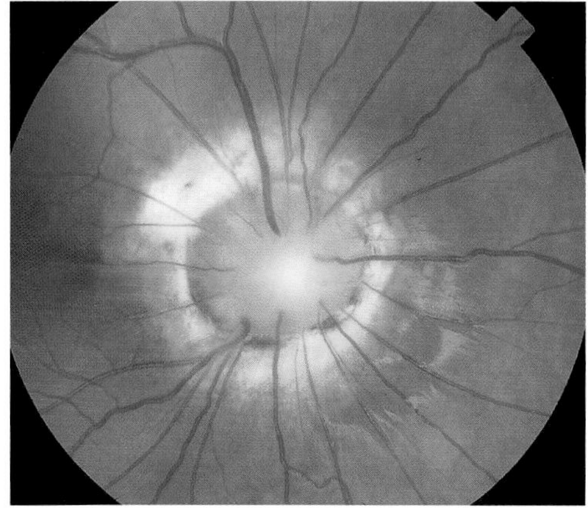

Figure 7.5. "Morning glory" anomaly of the optic nerve head.

The appearance of the optic nerve head is variable and various degrees of dysplasia may be present. The optic disc configuration depends on the size of the posterior scleral opening, which is usually ectatic, the amount surrounding chorioretinal pigmentation, the vascular pattern, and the amount of gliosis and remnants of the hyaloid system at the center of the disc (Figs. 7.5, 7.6).[204,271] The macula is usually dragged nasally to the edge of the disc and the yellow macular xanthophyll pigment is frequently noticeable at that location. The

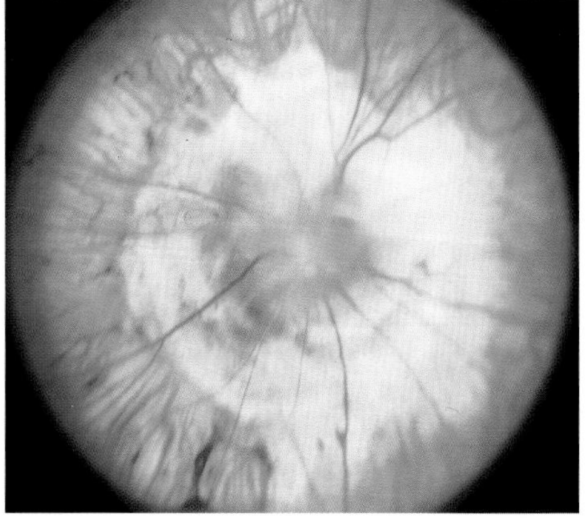

Figure 7.6. Large "morning glory" anomaly of the optic nerve head. There is a tuft of glial tissue in the center of the disc. The vessels exist in a radial fashion from the nerve head. The peripapillary scleral opening is very large.

retinal arterioles and venules emerge in a radial pattern from the enlarged scleral canal and may be bridged by vascular arcades close to the optic nerve head. Other straight arterioarterial bridging vessels can be seen more peripherally.

The majority of cases of MGDA are unilateral with equal involvement of the left and right eyes. Bilaterality of this condition can occur.[21,204] Males and females are affected equally. One-half of patients with MGDA present with strabismus. The abnormality is otherwise discovered during routine examination of older children. The MGDA is almost never familial.[39,268]

A large optic nerve head with excessive glial tissue may lead to a white pupillary reflex or leukocoria, hence MGDA is on the differential list of retinoblastoma and a white pupillary reflex. Patients may present with a total retinal detachment that occurs in up to 30% of cases.[55,114,116] The detachment is usually nonrhegmatogenous (except for one case report,[61] where the hole was in the optic disc defect) and its exact etiology is unknown. Communication between the subarachnoid and subretinal spaces with seepage of cerebrospinal fluid under the retina has been postulated to be the cause of retinal detachment in MGDA.[133,275] Spontaneous retinal reattachment has been reported.[112]

Contractile movements can be seen in a MGDA. Pollock[204] suggested that this contractility was due to variation in subretinal fluid volume. The presence of heterotopic smooth muscle fibers in colobomas may be a mechanism contributing to this singular phenomenon of contractility.[209] Amaurosis fugax can occur in association with retinal vein dilatation.[109,237]

Visual impairment is variable but generally substantial; visual acuity ranges from 20/30 to poor light perception. Poor vision results from retinal and optic nerve dysplasia but may also be partly due to strabismic or anisometropic amblyopia.

Associated ocular anomalies in the affected eye include strabismus, remnants of the pupillary membrane, cataract, aniridia, persistence of the hyaloid system,[53] ciliary body cyst, vitreous cyst, retinal detachment, foveal dysplasia, epiretinal membranes, and microphthalmos.[271] Retinal vascular tortuosity, optic pits, microphthalmos, anterior segment dysgenesis, Duane retraction syndrome, and remnants of the pupillary membrane have been reported in the fellow eye.[271] There may be an accompanying pulsating peripapillary staphyloma.[277]

The association of the morning glory disc anomaly with basal encephaloceles of the transsphenoidal or transethmoidal type is well known. Hypopituitarism can also be associated with the encephaloceles and affects growth hormones and antidiuretic hormone production.[21,134,181] Pituitary dwarfism has also been reported in patients with MGDA.[81] Transsphenoidal encephaloceles are part of a more complex malformation that includes midfacial anomalies such as hypertelorism, depressed nasal bridge, and cleft lip and/or palate.[106] The osseous defect in the anterior skull base allows the herniation of hypothalamopituitary structures. Agenesis of the corpus callosum and an absent chiasm are other intracranial anomalies that have been reported with MGDA. Congenital renal abnormalities can also occur and have been observed by one of the authors (E.I.T.) in a boy with preauricular tags, patent ductus arteriosus, and unilateral renal agenesis.[269]

The funnel-shaped junction of the optic nerve with the posterior aspect of the globe as well as the posterior sclerochoroidal defects and the exacavation of the optic disc are apparent on computed tomography.[163,271] The neuroimaging studies also uncover associated brain malformations such as encephaloceles and agenesis of the corpus callosum.[186] Fluorescein angiography detects the abnormal arteriovenous communications.[42,271] If peripapillary contractions are present, they may be demonstrable with B-scan ultrasonography.

The MGDA probably results from failure of the posterior sclera and the lamina cribrosa of the optic nerve head to form. This leads to herniation of intraocular contents through the defect and formation of the conical deformity.[167] This process interferes with regression of the hyaloid vasculature and remnants of the hyaloid system are frequently observed in the center of the malformed papilla. It is possible that this process also interferes with closure of the most posterior aspect of the optic fetal fissure leading to a typical colobomatous component to the MGDA. In some cases it is difficult to distinguish between an optic nerve coloboma resulting from failure of closure of the fetal fissure and a MGDA. Optic pit, MGDA, and peripapillary contractile staphyloma may constitute a spectrum of malformations with the same etiology.[260,269,271,293] In peripapillary contractile staphyloma, myofibroblastic differentiation of some of the mesenchymal tissue at the disc edge is presumed to lead to contractions that have been observed clinically and recorded by ultrasonography.

Some cases of MGDA are probably misdiagnosed as typical uveal colobomas at the optic disc. Slusher and co-workers[244] reported a large kindred where cavitary optic disc anomalies ranging from optic pits to large anomalous discs and typical colobomas were inherited in an autosomal dominant fashion. The great majority of cases with MGDA and optic pits, however, are isolated and the recurrence risk in siblings is negligible.

Visual prognosis is very poor in patients who present with profound visual loss in the affected eye. Careful refraction and treatment of associated strabismic or anisometropic amblyopia may result in some recuperation of vision in rare instances.[271] Cryotherapy at the nerve head, scleral buckling, vitrectomy, and retinal tamponade with gas or fluid have been tried for treatment of the retinal detachment that occurs in about 30% of cases. Poor visual outcome usually follows despite retinal reattachment in some cases.[167,275]

Peripapillary Staphyloma

In this malformation, the scleral ectasia that surrounds the optic disc is deeper than in the morning glory anomaly. The disc lies in the bottom of the excavation and has a normal retinal vascular pattern despite the molding of vessels over the ectatic sclera (Fig. 7.7). The disc may show a varying degree of pallor. In contrast to the morning glory anomaly, peripapillary staphyloma does not have the central glial tuft. The walls and margins of the staphyloma may display atrophic pigmentary changes in the RPE and choroid. This rare condition is usually unilateral. Several reports documented the contractility of peripapillary staphylomas.[53,144,145,293] Seybold and Rosen[237] described

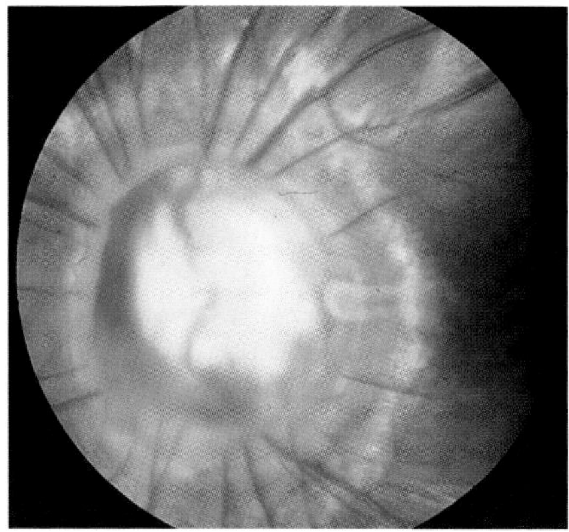

Figure 7.7. Peripapillary staphyloma. Macular xanthophyll is seen in a fold on the temporal edge of the staphyloma. A posterior scleral defect was evident on ultrasonography and on computed tomography. (Courtesy of Dr. Mohamad S. Jaafar.)

a patient with atypical peripapillary staphyloma who presented with transient visual obscurations.

Visual acuity is usually decreased although cases with nearly normal vision have been described.[51] Refractive states include emmetropia or myopia.[47] Theories proposed to explain the mechanism by which peripapillary staphylomas contract include (*1*) pressure balance and muscular contractions,[293] (*2*) association with respiratory cycle and pressure on the neck veins,[144,260] (*3*) histopathological reports of smooth muscle in peripapillary staphyloma and MGDA suggesting a common embryogenic pathogenesis for these two congenital anomalies,[204] (*4*) presence of an atavistic retractor bulbi muscle,[293] and (*5*) autonomic cholinergic mechanism comparable to iris sphincter as hypothesized by Kral and Svarc[145] to explain the staphyloma contraction in response to light stimulation.

The relatively normal appearing optic disc and retinal vessels in peripapillary staphyloma suggest that development of these structures is completed before occurrence of the staphyloma. Pollock[204] postulated that clinical features of peripapillary staphylomas are most consistent with decreased peripapillary structural support with resulting herniation of unsupported tissues through the staphyloma. Clinical differentiation of peripapillary staphyloma from morning glory syndrome can be difficult.

The ophthalmoscopic findings that help distinguish the two include the deep cup-shaped excavation, relatively normal optic disc, and absent glial tuft in peripapillary staphyloma versus the tapering funnel-shaped excavation, absence of normal disc structure, and central glial tuft in MGDA.

Optic Pit

A pit of the optic nerve head is an oval, round, triangular, or even slitlike excavation of variable color, depth, and location in the disc substance. Pits may be single or multiple and the optic nerve head may be normal or increased in size.[45,46] Optic pits could be considered part of a continuum of cavitary malformations of the optic nerve head which includes the morning glory disc anomaly.[271]

Optic pits affect males and females equally. About 10%–15% are bilateral.[47] The diagnosis is made by ophthalmoscopy and may be helped by intravenous fluorescein angiography. Pits vary from one-tenth of a disc diameter (0.15 mm) to one-half or more disc diameter in size (Figs. 7.8, 7.9). They may be white, gray, greenish, or even black and are most often located in the inferotemporal aspects of the disc touching, or distant from, the disc margin. Up to three optic pits have been reported in one disc. They are often associated with cilioretinal arteries.[47,266] Pulsations of the glial tissue have been reported in optic pits.[93] At least two families with dominant inheritance of optic pits[12,247a] and another with cavitary malformations of the optic nerve head have been reported.[244] Ocular anomalies associated with optic disc pit are microphthalmos with cyst[239] and aniridia and morning glory disc anomaly.[269]

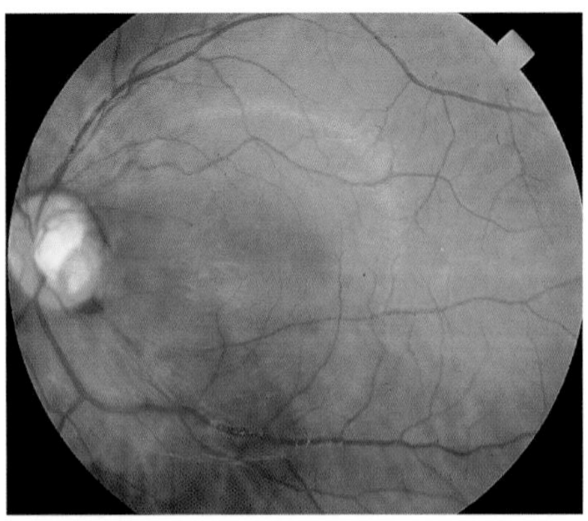

Figure 7.8. Inferotemporal optic pit with demarcated serous macular detachment.

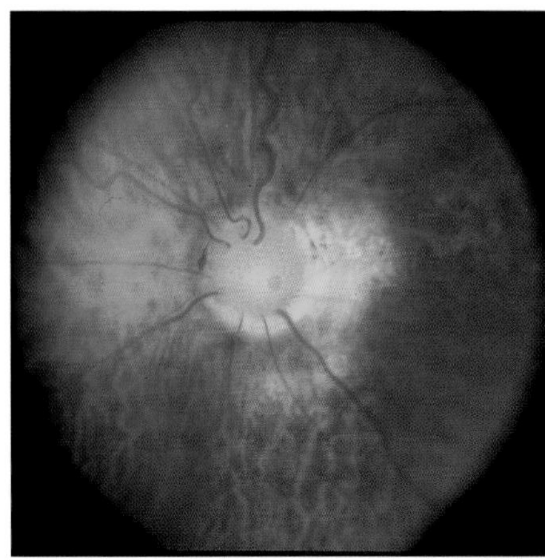

Figure 7.9. Optic pit occupies the entire nerve head. Patient was misdiagnosed with glaucoma. (Courtesy of Dr. Irene H. Maumenee.)

Visual acuity is normal unless there is associated serous retinal detachment. Visual field defects include paracentral arcuate scotoma attached to an enlarged blind spot,[45,146] nasal steps, arcuate scotomas, paracentral scotomas, cecocentral scotomas, and generalized field constriction.[7,228]

Serous detachment of the retina in the macular area occurs in more than one-third of patients usually in the third and fourth decades of life and is the major cause of visual loss that complicates this congenital malformation that may otherwise go unnoticed (Fig. 7.8).[30,146,222,258,259] The etiology of the serous detachment is still debated. Irvine et al.[133] reported the case of a young boy with MGDA who underwent an optic nerve sheath fenestration where a communication between the vitreous, the optic disc, and the subarachnoid space was demonstrated. Lincoff and associates[159] suggested that the macular lesion starts as an area of schisis in the inner retinal layers, which communicates with the pit, then an outer layer macular hole develops, and the outer retinal layer detachment progresses around the macular hole, leading to a serous macular detachment. Bonnett[30] proposed a mechanism of tractional retinal detachment combined with a rhegmatogenous component in the roof of the optic pit as an explanation for serous macular detachment. Akiba and colleagues[4] suggested that vitreous anomalies associated with optic disc pits (anomalous Cloquet canal and posterior vitreous detachment) cause traction on the optic pit and may exacerbate serous macular detachment. Spontaneous reattachments of the serous detachment can occur.[45,245] Possible sources of the subretinal fluid include the vitreous cavity, subarachnoid space, blood vessels at the base of the pit, and peridural orbital space.[7,30,47,158] Another rare complication is the development of subretinal neovascularization at the disc margin.[32]

Ultrasonography can demonstrate the presence of coexistent anomalies such as microphthalmos with cyst. The intravenous fluorescein angiogram studies show that only pits with serous macular detachment will have late staining, whereas pits without serous macular detachment remain hypofluorescent throughout the angiogram.[103]

On histopathology, there is herniation of abnormal retina and glial tissue through a defect in the lamina cribosa, which is usually surrounded by a connective tissue capsule in contact with the meninges.

Gass[99] believes that optic pits are due to anomalous development of the primordial optic nerve papilla and failure of complete resolution of the peripapillary neuroectodermal folds that are part of the normal development of the optic nerve head. Other authors have, probably erroneously, attributed the development of pits to failure of closure of the ocular fetal fissure in the region of the nerve head. Although pits and typical chorioretinal colobomata have been reported to coexist, a common etiology for both is highly unlikely. On the other hand, pits have been described in fellow eyes of patients with MGDA; one author (E.I.T.) believes that both cavitary anomalies share a common embryologic etiology.[269] The temporal location of many optic pits does not correspond to the inferonasal position of the embryonic fissure.[37]

A significant proportion of eyes with optic pits go on to develop serous macular detachment with loss of visual acuity. In a study of the natural history of optic pits with serous detachment of the macula, Sobol and coworkers[245] showed that 12% of patients had eventual visual acuity of 20/200 or less. There is no effective therapy for the visual complications from optic pits. Bed rest, bilateral patches, laser photocoagulation (Fig. 7.10), and systemic corticosteroids have all been tried. Vitrectomy with gas-fluid exchange has been tried with limited success in reattaching the retina and improving vision.[66,160] Laser photocoagulation[6,266] has been tried in the treatment of both macular detachment and peripapillary neovascularization in this condition.[6,135,180]

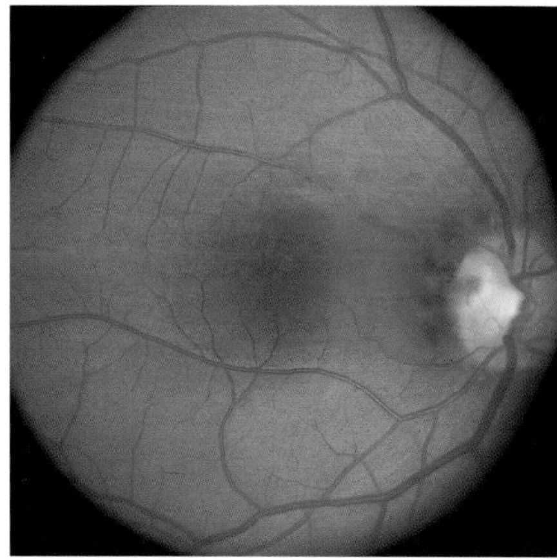

Figure 7.10. Temporal optic pit with laser marks at the edge of the disc. The laser was used to seal presumed leakage of fluid through the pit and under the retina that produced serous macular detachment.

Congenital Tilted Disc

Several synonyms for congenital tilted disc have been employed in the literature including Fuchs coloboma, inferior conus, inversion or dysversion of the optic disc, nasal fundus ectasia, congenital crescent, and congenital conus. They all describe situs inversus of the optic disc with inferior nasal thinning of the choroid and retinal pigment epithelium associated with myopic astigmatism. The descriptive term "tilted disc" takes its origin from the observation that the vertical axis of the oval disc is directed at an oblique angle with the upper and temporal portion of the optic disc being anterior to the

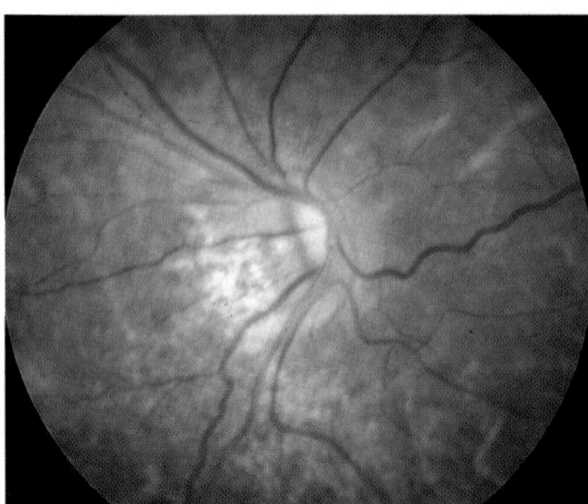

Figure 7.11. Tilted disc. Blood vessels exit from the nerve head, course nasally first, and then turn to go to the temporal part of the fundus.

lower nasal aspect and sometimes creating confusion with papilledema. The retinal vessels arise from the superotemporal region rather than from the nasal aspect of the optic disc, hence the term *situs inversus* (Fig. 7.11). This condition is usually nonhereditary except for a pedigree with dominant inheritance associated with lacquer cracks.[33]

There is posterior ectasia of the inferonasal retina and choroid with myopic astigmatism, the plus axis being parallel to the ectatic region.[296] The etiology of this malformation is unknown but the location suggests some type of colobomatous defect.[7] The longer horizontal diameter gives the ovoid aspect of the disc. Hypopigmentation of the RPE and choroid in the inferonasal region leads to the D-shaped inferonasal crescent, which remains unchanged throughout life.[102] The vessels sweep nasally from the nerve head before reaching the temporal area. Visual acuity may be reduced. A portion of the optic disc may be elevated, leading to a mistaken diagnosis of papilledema. Choroidal neovascularization has been described in association with tilted disc syndrome.[205]

Some patients have a bitemporal hemianopia that does not respect the midline. Hypotheses to explain this field defect include (*1*) a refractive scotoma from myopic astigmatism of the inferonasal conus, (*2*) distortion of photoreceptors, which accounts for the residual field defect once refractive errors are corrected, and (*3*) decreased number of axons entering the defective inferonasal disc.[73] This superotemporal depression of the island of vision usually affects midsize isopters, sparing larger and smaller ones. The margins of the defect may be sloping. Perimetry with a −4.00D lens eliminates the visual field depression, confirming the refractive nature of the defect. In some cases, the field defect persists even with a −4.00D lens, due to an abnormal inferonasal retina.[179,212] Threshold perimetry of patients with tilted disc has revealed a more homogeneous field loss.[36] The tilted disc syndrome has been described in patients with true bitemporal hemianopia harboring a congenital suprasellar brain tumor.[139,196,263]

The optic nerve enters the globe in an oblique fashion. The circular retinal opening does not match the scleral canal, which is contracted on one side. This discrepancy between the retinal and scleral openings leads to the D-shaped appearance of the tilted disc. Fewer than normal retinal nerve fibers enter the defective side of the disc leading to a visual field defect.[73] Giuffré[102] hypothesized that atrophy of the ganglion cells occurs after an anomalous closure of the embryonic fissure. This theory would explain the inferonasal quadrant hypoplasia and the upward shift of vessels.[102]

The localized ectasia of the fundus can be visualized with B-scan ultrasonography. The A-scan can show an increased dural diameter of the optic nerve as a result of the oblique optic nerve entry into the globe.[241] Alterations in electrofunctional testing include decreased scotopic and photopic ERGs, pathological EOGs, and abnormal latencies of visual evoked potentials (VEPs) that might be related to decreased retinal sensitivity.[105] The reported ERG abnormality could be attributed to the association of tilted discs with X-linked recessive congenital stationary night blindness.[118,203]

Craniofacial anomalies such as hypertelorism and Crouzon and Apert syndromes have been described in association with tilted discs.[171] Ehler-Danlos type III,[86] hemifacial atrophy and congenital horizontal gaze palsy,[217] and familial dextrocardia and exotropia[84] are other conditions reported with tilted discs.

Any patient with tilted discs and a superior bitemporal hemianopia that respects the vertical midline needs to undergo neuroimaging studies to rule out a suprasellar tumor. Optical correction of the refractive error and penalization treatment of amblyopia improve visual acuity.

Congenital Optic Disc Pigmentation

Congenital optic disc pigmentation is a descriptive term for melanin deposition anterior to, or within, the lamina cribrosa leading to a grayish discoloration of the optic disc (Fig. 7.12). This extremely rare condition was reported in a child with interstitial deletion of chromosome 17[40] and in Aicardi syndrome.[262]

Four types of pigmentation have been described: (*1*) occasional pigment flecks on the optic disc or in the lamina cribrosa, (*2*) dense plaques on or contiguous to the disc, (*3*) stripes of pigment on the disc, and (*4*) slate gray coloration of the disc.[176] The first three types described by Reese[209] and by Mann[165] are probably developmental in origin. Theories that have been proposed to explain congenital optic disc pigmentation include the incorporation of pigment-bearing tissues in the lamina cribrosa, extension of the RPE into the disc margins, and metaplasia of pigmented cells within the optic disc.[63] Brodsky et al.[40] describe congenital optic disc pigmentation as discrete, irregular, and granular in appearance. The slate gray color of the entire disc was described by Beauvieux[19] in 1926 and by Halbertsma[113] in 1937. Beauvieux[19] presented three female infants with poor vision and absent or near absent pupillary reactions. The patients had some systemic abnormalities (one patient with athetosis) and ocular abnormalities (epicanthi, myopia, posterior polar cataract, nystagmus). Vision improved as the gray appearance of the disc disappeared. Beauvieux[19] suggested that delayed myelination was responsible for the transient discoloration of the disc in these infants. Transient grayish appearance of the optic disc can also be seen in normal neonates and in albinotic patients and often disappears during the first years of life. This discoloration is nonspecific in normal neonates unless it is accompanied by clinical signs of delayed visual maturation or albinism.[38,40]

Bergmeister Papilla

Bergmeister papilla is a benign anomaly that describes an optic nerve head with veillike remnants of the primary vitreous in its center or covering it (Fig. 7.13). The glial tissue may extend along a vessel. This small blue-white or gray prepapillary fibrous glial tuft on an optic disc with an absent or small cup does not involve retinal vessels and may be part of a more widespread hyaloid vascular abnormality.[7] Vascular loops seen in conjunction with this anomaly can project into the vitreous cavity from the optic disc and pulsate with heartbeat.[69] Occlusion of this prepapillary vascular loop in adults

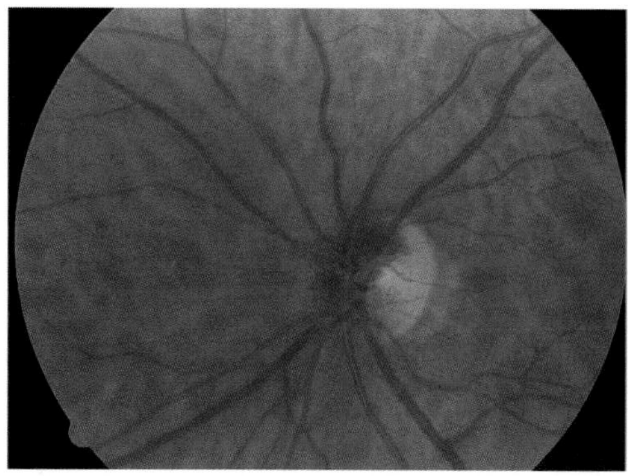

Figure 7.12. Presumed congenital melanosis of the optic nerve head in a 60-year-old man. The pigmentation did not change over 4 years of follow-up.

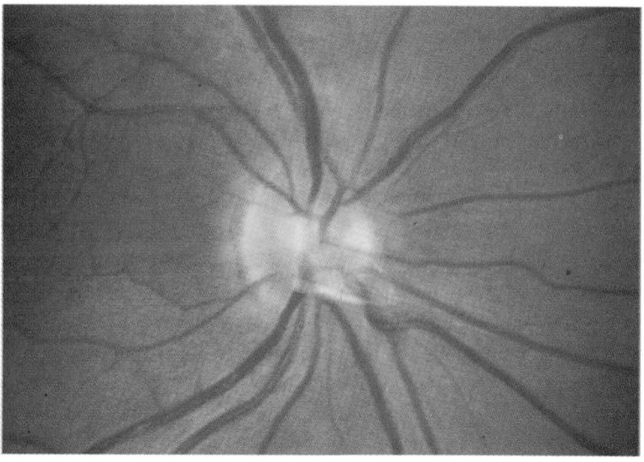

Figure 7.13. Bergmeister papilla. There is a small veil of glial tissue on the superior aspect of the nerve head.

can involve retinal arterioles[44] and cause visual loss.

Rhodes[211] suggested that Bergmeister papilla is the result of a focal glial proliferation, perhaps from traction between the vitreal surface and the disc, progressively dislocating Bergmeister papilla from the disc and forming a glial sheath.

Agatston[3a] classified remnants of the primary vitreous and included De Beck's[68] initial observations. He divided the primary vitreal remnants into 12 parts: (*1*) shreds of tissue on the optic nerve, (*2*) a membrane on the disc, (*3*) cystic remnants on the disc, (*4*) massive connective tissue on the disc, (*5*) a rudimentary strand attached to the disc, (*6*) a strand on the disc and posterior capsule of the lens, (*7*) a strand that extends from the disc to the lens, (*8*) a similar strand containing a patent blood vessel, (*9*) a strand attached to the lens alone, (*10*) a posterior capsular cataract, (*11*) striae on the posterior capsule, and (*12*) a persistent canal without vascular remnant.[176]

Bergmeister papilla has been described with bilateral renal agenesis in Potter syndrome,[48] with retinochoroidal[104] or optic disc colobomas,[64] and in trisomy 18 (Edward syndrome).[200]

Myelinated Nerve Fibers

Retinal nerve fibers do not normally have myelin. Intraocular myelination occurs in 0.3%–0.98% of ophthalmic patients[75] and is considered to be ectopic myelinization.[254] Males are affected twice as frequently as females and unilateral cases (80%)[74] predominate. A commonly used synonym is medullation of the retinal nerve fibers.

In the fifth month of gestation, myelination starts in the lateral geniculate ganglion and proceeds centrifugally toward the chiasm and optic nerves, in the reverse direction of the optic nerve fiber growth. The chiasm is myelinated around the sixth month of gestation. Normally, myelin production stops at the lamina cribrosa. Myelin is produced by oligodendroglial cells that are usually absent from the retina but that are present in the CNS. The presence of myelinated retinal nerve fibers suggests heterotopic oligodendrocytes or glial cells within the retinal nerve fiber layer,[252] or a congenital defect in the lamina cribrosa. Autopsy studies have failed to demonstrate an abnormal lamina cribrosa.[82,252,254]

Nerve fibers are usually normal in function and structure. The myelination is in contact with the optic disc in 81% of cases.[254] Myelin follows the pattern of retinal nerve fibers taking an arcuate, fan or flamelike shape (Fig. 7.14). The myelinated fibers are usually located near the upper and lower poles of optic disc, often adjacent to the disc. In some instances, the myelinated fibers appear as feathery patches in the retinal periphery. Because the fibers are in a superficial location, they obscure retinal vessels.

The majority of patients have normal visual acuity. A subgroup of patients with unilateral myelinated retinal nerve fibers will have anisometropia with severe myopia, amblyopia, and strabismus.[122,173,253] High myopia and amblyopia can be treated effectively with a good visual outcome even if macular involvement is present,[261] although some patients will not respond to amblyopia therapy.[78] The axial length is increased in eyes with myelinated fibers.[174,253] Merritt[173] reported a relative afferent pupillary defect (RAPD) and amblyopia in association with myelinated fibers. Amblyopia by itself can cause a mild RAPD. In another series, none of six patients with myelinated fibers had a RAPD, but four had an abnormal photostress test.[78] Field defects associated with myelinated nerve fibers are related to the size and extent of the congenital anomaly. The field defect is usually smaller than the size of myelination.[254] Intravenous fluorescein angiogram shows hypo-

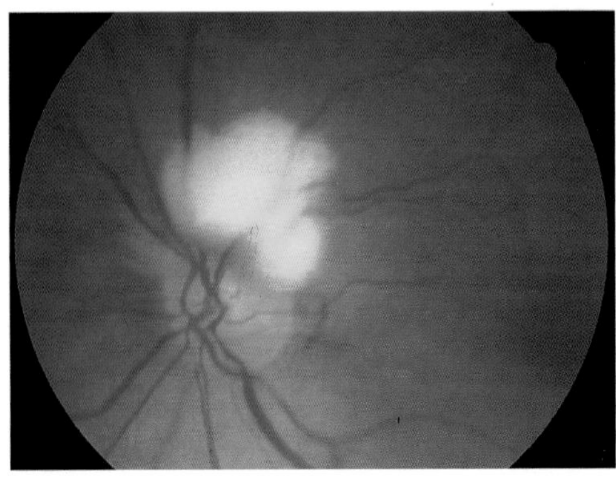

Figure 7.14. Tuft of myelinated nerve fibers along the superior nerve bundle.

fluorescence from the masking effect of the myelinated nerve fibers and early patchy filling of the choroid.[78] Patients may have reduced amplitudes of VEP.[120]

Myelinated fibers remain stable during life or can undergo optic atrophy from different causes such as syphilis,[278] a pituitary tumor,[110,226] glaucoma,[96] central retinal artery occlusion,[14] branch retinal artery occlusion,[264] optic neuritis in multiple sclerosis,[238] anterior ischemic optic neuropathy (AION),[233] and trauma.[150] An extraordinary appearance of myelinated fibers in adult life.[1,11] suggests remyelination by oligodendrocytes that migrated from surrounding intact glia or differentiation of spongioblasts into oligodendrocytes. Baber and colleagues[13] reported progression of myelinated nerve fibers in a child.

Patients with myelinated fibers are usually normal although some cases have been reported in association with craniofacial dysostoses[88] and in the Gorlin-Goltz (autosomal dominant multiple basal cell nevi carcinoma syndrome with variable expressivity).[71] Traboulsi et al.[270] reported a new syndrome of extensive myelinated nerve fibers associated with a severe vitreoretinopathy, retinal dystrophy, and skeletal malformations in the form of ectrodactyly. Other associations of myelinated fibers include congential cataracts, persistence of the hyaloid system, uveal coloboma, epilepsy, dolichocephaly, and neurofibromatosis type I.[143]

Visual acuity may improve in some patients who undergo amblyopia therapy. The visual prognosis in patients with macular involvement is guarded.[120]

CONGENITAL VASCULAR ANOMALIES

Prepapillary Vascular Loops

Liebreich[156] was the first to describe prepapillary vascular loops. Liebreich,[156] Little,[161] and Walker[279] thought that the loops represented an incompletely regressed hyaloid system. Goldstein and Wexler[107] studied prepapillary loops histopathologically and found them to be branches of the central retinal artery. These preretinal arterial loops originate from a main branch of the central retinal artery on the optic disc. The loop may be single and may have a corkscrew appearance.[69] They may be either arterial or venous and are independent from the embryonic hyaloid artery as suggested by Hirschberg.[119] Eighty-three percent to 95% of prepapillary loops are arterial.[24,44] Cilioretinal arteries are often associated with prepapillary vascular loops.[44,157a]

Arterial loops may project into the vitreous cavity several millimeters but do not reach the posterior aspect of the lens.[47] Nine percent to 17% of cases are bilateral.[69] Oxilia[197] reported that 70% of the preretinal arterial loops are located inferiorly on the disc.

Visual acuity is usually normal unless events such as vitreous hemorrhage, branch retinal artery occlusion,[157a] hyphema, and amaurosis fugax occur. Kinking or twisting of the loop with subsequent thrombosis is a possible mechanism for occlusion of the loop. Intravenous fluorescein angiogram demonstrates normal choroidal filling.[69]

Cilioretinal Arteries

These arteries arise from the ciliary circulation around the margin of the optic disc or from an optic pit. Usually of no significance, cilioretinal arteries become important in retinal vascular occlusive disease. They can be selectively occluded with infarction of the retinal area they supply, or this area will be selectively spared in cases of central retinal artery occlusion. Justice and Lehman found that 90% of cilioretinal arteries are temporal and 5% are nasal with the remainder located superiorly and inferiorly.[137] In the latter study, cilioretinal arteries were detected by intravenous fluorescein angiogram in up to 50% of normal individuals.[137] Optic disc drusen have been reported in association with cilioretinal arteries.[80] Barroso et al.[15] reported four cilioretinal arteries associated with a dysplastic disc.

Optociliary Veins

Optociliary veins can be congenital with abnormal arrangement of the veins[35,79,147] or may be acquired. They may be ectatic or tortuous with sheathed vessels and secondary gliosis.[286] Laminar flow on fluorescein angiography confirms the venous filling of these vessels.[76] The blood in optociliary veins is derived from the central retinal vein and flows back via peripapillary choroidal channels. Connection between retinal veins and choroidal veins to vortex veins can be single or multiple.[95]

Chronic obstruction of the central retinal vein will cause capillaries to become enlarged and blood is shunted to the choroid. The optociliary shunt may resolve after surgical relief of increased intracranial pressure. These optociliary shunts have been reported in association with optic nerve glioma,[129] chronic papilledema,[76] and craniopharyngiomas.[286] They also occur in sphenoorbital meningioma in conjunction with disc pallor and visual loss (triad of optociliary shunt, disc astrophy, and visual loss).[95] One hypothesis for the development of optociliary shunt is that constriction of the central retinal vein by any form of compression in the retrobulbar space creates a bypass of the blood flow.

Histopathological examination of optociliary shunts by Salzmann[229] and Elschnig[79] showed that compression of the central retinal vein by an optic nerve tumor favors the development of shunts. A gradual obstruction will produce disc swelling, and optic nerve fiber atrophy occurs with time exposing the optociliary shunt.

Disc Drusen

Drusen or hyaline bodies were first described by Liebreich[155] in 1868. This anomaly may be transmitted as an irregular dominant trait,[130,162,242] with males and females equally affected, and whites more often than others.[34] In 75% of cases, drusen are bilateral.[162] About 10%–15% of patients have unilateral drusen with a normal contralateral optic nerve head.[187,220] Drusen are rare in early childhood and are usually identified in or after the second decade of life.[123] Their incidence increases in adulthood and ranges between 3.4 and 20 per 1000.[162]

Visual acuity is usually normal unless there are other ophthalmologic abnormalities.[130,187,220] Patients with optic disc drusen and progressive visual loss may harbor intracranial masses such as pituitary tumors,[188,248] meningiomas,[20,115a,177,194,223] craniopharyngiomas,[149] ophthalmic artery aneurysms,[67] cerebral abscesses,[92] and other space-occupying lesions.[54,187,220] The · prevalence of ametropia is the same as in the general population.[187,220]

Papilledema secondary to increased intracranial pressure must be ruled out in patients with elevated optic nerve heads. In such cases, neuroimaging studies and appropriate referrals are crucial in the management of the patient. If indeed, pseudopapilledema is due to the presence of optic disc drusen, then neuroimaging is not necessary unless there is a decreased visual acuity that cannot be explained on the basis of the ophthalmologic evaluation. The distinction between optic disc drusen and papilledema might be difficult in some cases. Ultrasonography is very helpful in distinguishing between these two entities: the optic disc will highly reflect ultrasound in patients with drusen, whereas increased subarchnoid fluid around the optic nerve and a positive 30° test may be demonstrated in patients with elevated intracranial pressure and papilledema.

The optic disc with drusen is not hyperemic and the surface vessels are not obscured (Figs. 7.15, 7.16). The physiologic cup is absent and the papilla appears smaller than normal.[185] Anomalous branching of vessels, increased tortuosity, and vascular loops[80] have all been described with optic disc drusen. A higher frequency of cilioretinal arteries in patients with disc drusen suggests some vascular anomaly or

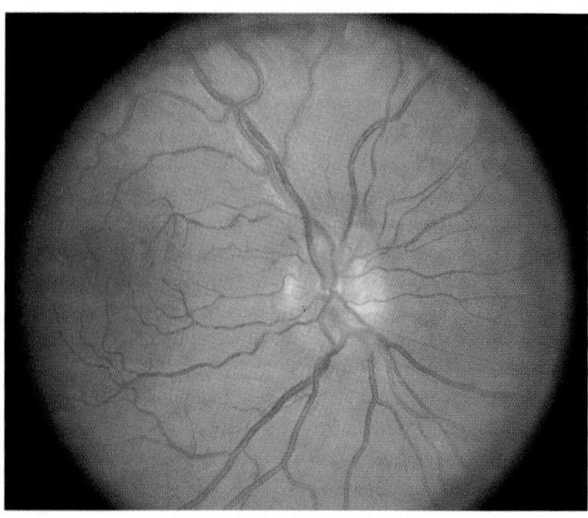

Figure 7.15. Buried drusen of the optic nerve. (Courtesy of Dr. John Gillis.)

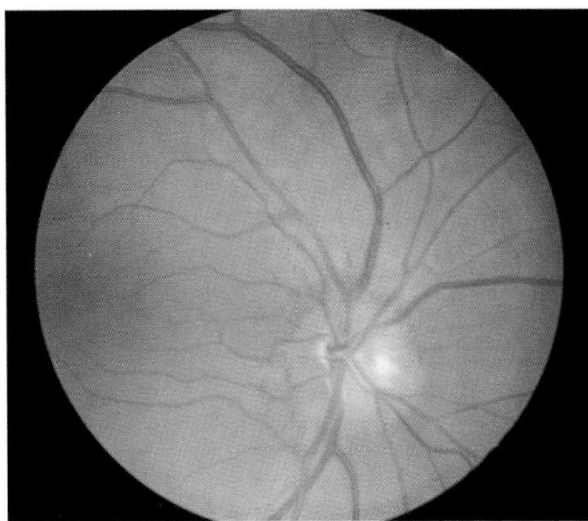

Figure 7.16. Buried drusen of the optic nerve head. Some of the colloid bodies are visible on the surface of the disc.

local circulatory disturbances.[70,117] The elevation is confined to the disc and does not extend to the peripapillary area. The disc borders may have a moth-eaten appearance. Spontaneous venous pulsations can be seen in the presence of optic disc drusen (only 20% of the normal population have spontaneous venous pulsations) but are consistently absent in papilledema. Furthermore, the nerve fiber layer adjacent to the disc in papilledema is swollen, obscuring retinal vessels.

Illuminating the peripapillary area with a vertical slit of light either with the direct ophthalmoscope or with a 90-D lens may make some buried drusen visible, appearing as brilliant yellow concretions.

Hemorrhages may be associated with optic disc drusen. They may be small on the surface of the disc, large, with or without extension into the vitreous cavity, or deep in the peripapillary area.[230] Visual symptoms in optic disc drusen are related to hemorrhages originating from associated neovascularization, compression of nerve fibers, or from vascular complications. Patients with optic disc drusen without systemic vascular abnormalities are predisposed to complications such as anterior ischemic optic neuropathy,[59,101,129,138] central retinal artery occlusion,[190,208,273] and central retinal vein occlusion.[265] Objective signs of an optic neuropathy such as relative afferent pupillary defect and acquired dyschromatopsia may be present.[17,175]

Visual field defects involve the lower nasal fields most frequently[223] but may be sectorial or arcuate. There may be enlargement of the blind spot[123] or concentric constriction of the entire visual field, reflecting a slowly progressive neuropathy.[91,152] Buried drusen cause field defects less frequently than superficial ones.[175]

Red-free filter fundus photographs[178] can demonstrate the particular autofluorescence property of optic disc drusen.[140] Drusen stain in late stages of fluorescein angiography.[229a] Ultrasonography[29,191] (Fig. 7.17) and computed tomography, but not magnetic resonance imaging,[175,185] are very useful in detecting drusen, especially if they are calcified.

Several reports have described the association of retinitis pigmentosa with optic disc drusen.[98,183,192,195,207,216,280] Pseudoxanthoma elasticum is another disease in which optic disc drusen may be seen.[60] They also occur in Alagille syndrome.

Histopathologic studies of drusen have shown deposits of hyaline material inside and outside the cells of the capillaries as well as alterations in the vessel walls of the disc.[94] Other histologic features include concentric laminations and calcifications, and negative staining for amyloid.[94] Different hypotheses have been proposed to explain the development of optic disc drusen including the presence of vascular anomalies,[227] a small optic nerve,[185] and a disorder of axoplasmic transport.[246] Seitz and Kersting[236] suggested that op-

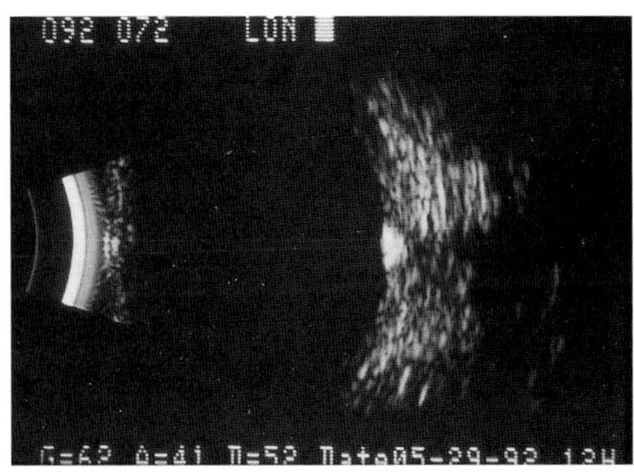

Figure 7.17. Ultrasonogram of the globe (B-scan) reveals highly reflective shadow of the drusen in the nerve head area.

tic disc drusen are derived from axoplasmic degeneration; their theory is supported by the findings of Tso,[272] who studied optic disc drusen ultrastructurally, and suggested that the drusen derive from abnormal intracellular calcified mitochondria that are extruded from the axon. The ongoing calcification process persists even after extracellular expulsion of the material.

Optic disc drusen are considered a progressive optic neuropathy, producing nerve fiber damage and visual field defects. Visual acuity is preserved unless another ocular or neurologic process is present. If the decrease in vision cannot be explained, an intracranial process needs to be ruled out. Careful follow-up and treatment of associated ocular conditions are important. In cases of bleeding from a neovascular membrane with optic disc drusen, photocoagulation can be performed.

REFERENCES

1. Aaby AA, Kushner BJ. Acquired and progressive myelinated nerve fibers. *Arch Ophthalmol* 1985;103:542–544.
2. Acers TE. Optic nerve hypoplasia: Septo-optic-pituitary dysplasia syndrome. *Trans Am Ophthalmol Soc* 1981;79:425–457.
3. Adler FH. Bilateral partial colobomata of the optic nerve. *Am J Ophthalmol* 1937;20:777–778.

3a. Agatston SA. Congenital cyst of the optic nerve. *Am J Ophthalmol* 1944;27:278–279.

4. Akiba J, Kakehashi A, Hikichi T, Trempe C. Vitreous findings in cases of optic nerve pits and serous macular detachment. *Am J Ophthalmol* 1993;116:38–41.
5. Andersen SR, Bro-Rasmussen F, Tygstrup I. Anencephaly related to ocular development and malformation. *Am J Ophthalmol* 1967; 64(suppl):559–566.
6. Annesley W, Brown G, Bolling J, et al. Treatment of retinal detachment with congenital optic pit by Krypton laser photocoagulation. *Graefes Arch Clin Exp Ophthalmol* 1987; 225:311–314.
7. Apple DJ, Rabb MF, Walsh PM. Congenital anomalies of the optic disc. *Surv Ophthalmol* 1982;27:3–41.
8. Aroichane M, Barsoum-Homsy M, Roy MS, et al. Computerized image analysis of optic nerve hypoplasia. *Invest Ophthalmol Vis Sci* 1992;33(suppl):1225.
9. Arslanian SA, Rofus WE, Foley TP, Becker DJ. Hormonal, metabolic, and neuroradiologic abnormalities associated with septo-optic dysplasia. *Acta Endocrinol* 1984;139: 249–254.
10. Awan KJ. Ganglionic neuroretinal aplasia and hypoplasia: Aplasia and hypoplasia of the optic nerve. *Ann Ophthalmol* 1976;8(10):1193–1202.
11. Baarsma GS. Acquired medullated nerve fibres. *Br J Ophthalmol* 1980;64:651–652.
12. Babel J, Farpour H. L'origine génétique des fossettes colobomateuses du nerf optique. *J Genet Hum* 1967;16:187–198.
13. Baber HA, Logani S, Kozlov KL, Arnold AC, Bateman B. Progression of retinal nerve fiber myelination in childhood. *Am J Ophthalmol* 1994;118:515–517.
14. Bachman R. Schwund markhaltiger nervenfasern in der netzhaut nach embolie der artere centralis retinae. *Albrecht von Graefes Arch Ophthalmol* 1922;107:10.
15. Barroso LH, Ragge NK, Hoyt WF. Multiple cilioretinal arteries and dysplasia of the optic disc. *J Clin Neuro-Ophthalmol* 1991; 11:278–279.
16. Barry DR. Aplasia of the optic nerves. *Int Ophthalmol* 1985;7:235–242.
17. Barry WE, Tredici TJ. Drusen of the optic disc with visual field defects and Marcus Gunn phenomenon (aeromedical consultation service case report). *Aerospace Med* 1972; 43:203–206.
18. Baum JL, Feingold M. Ocular aspects of Goldenhar's syndrome. *Am J Ophthalmol* 1973;75:250–257.
19. Beauvieux J. La pseudo-atrophie optique des nouveau-nés (dysgénésie myélinique des voies optiques). *Ann Oculist* 1926;163: 881–921.
20. Ben Zur PH, Lieberman TW. Drusen of the optic nerves and meningioma: A case report. *Mt Sinai Med J* 1972;39:188–196.
21. Beyer WB, Quencer RM, Osher RH. Morning glory syndrome: A functional analysis including fluorescein angiography, ultrasonography, and computerized tomography. *Ophthalmology* 1982;89:1362–1364.
22. Biedner B, Klemperer I, Dagan M, Yassur Y. Optic disc coloboma associated with macular hole and retinal detachment. *Ann Ophthalmol* 1993;25:350–352.

23. Billson FA. Clinical significance of optic nerve hypoplasia. *Trans Ophthalmol Soc NZ* 1973; 25:179–180.
24. Bisland T. Vascular loops in the vitreous. *Arch Ophthalmol* 1953;49:514.
25. Bjork A, Laurell CG, Laurell U. Bilateral optic nerve hypoplasia with normal visual acuity. *Am J Ophthalmol* 1978;86(4):524–529.
26. Blanco R, Salvador F, Galan A, Gil-Gibernau JJ. Aplasia of the optic nerve: Report of three cases. *J Pediatr Ophthalmol Strabismus* 1992; 29:228–231.
27. Bochow TW, Olk RJ, Knupp JA, Smith ME. Spontaneous reattachment of a total retinal detachment in an infant with microphthalmos and an optic nerve coloboma. *Am J Ophthalmol* 1991;112:347–348.
28. Bock R. Une nouvelle anomalie congénitale: La mégalopapille. *Confin Neurol* 1943;9: 407–408.
29. Boldt HC, Byrne SF, DiBernardo C. Echographic evaluation of optic disc drusen. *J Clin Neuro-Ophthalmol* 119;11:85–91.
30. Bonnet M. Serous macular detachment associated with optic nerve pits. *Graefe's Arch Clin Exp Ophthalmol* 1991;229:526–532.
31. Boor R, Rochels R, Walther B, Reitter B. Aplasia of the retinal vessels combined with optic nerve hypoplasia, neonatal epileptic seizures, and lactic acidosis due to mitochondrial complex I deficiency. *Eur J Pediatr* 1992; 151:519–521.
32. Borodic GE, Gragoudas ES, Edward WO, et al. Peripapillary subretinal neovascularization and serous macular detachment: Association with congenital optic nerve pits. *Arch Ophthalmol* 1984;102:229–231.
33. Bottoni FG, Eggink CA, Cruysberg JRM, Verbeek AM. Dominant inherited tilted disc syndrome and lacquer cracks. *Eye* 1990; 4:504–509.
34. Boyce SW, Platia EV, Green WR. Drusen of the optic nerve head. *Ann Ophthalmol* 1978;10:695–704.
35. Braune. Ein Beitrag zur Kenntnis optikociliorer gefässe. *Klin Monatsbl Augenheilkd* 1905;43:579–588.
36. Brazitikos PD, Safran AB, Simona F, Zulauf M. Threshold perimetry in tilted disc syndrome. *Arch Ophthalmol* 1990;108:1698–1700.
37. Brodsky MC. Congenital optic disk anomalies. *Surv Ophthalmol* 1994;39:89–112.
38. Brodsky MC. Congenital optic nerve abnormalities. In *Pediatric Ophthalmology and Strabismus,* K.W. Wright, ed. St. Louis: C. V. Mosby, 1995:785–797.
39. Brodsky MC. Morning glory disc anomaly or optic disc coloboma? (Letter) *Arch Ophthalmol* 1994;112:153.
40. Brodsky MC, Buckley EG, McConkie-Rosell A. The case of the gray optic disc. *Surv Ophthalmol* 1989;33:367–372.
41. Brodsky MC, Glasier CM, Pollock SC, et al. Optic nerve hypoplasia: Identification by magnetic resonance imaging. *Arch Ophthalmol* 1990;108:562–567.
42. Brodsky MC, Wilson RS. Retinal arteriovenous communications in the morning glory disc anomaly (letter). *Arch Opththalmol* 1995;113:410–411.
43. Brown GC. Optic nerve hypoplasia and colobomatous defects. *J Pediatr Ophthalmol* 1982;19:90–93.
44. Brown GC, Magargal L, Augsburger JJ, Shields JA. Preretinal arterial loops and retinal arterial occlusion. *Am J Ophthalmol* 1979; 87:646–651.
45. Brown GC, Shields JA, Goldberg RE. Congenital pits of the optic nerve head. II. Clinical studies in humans. *Ophthalmology* 1980; 87:51–65.
46. Brown GC, Shields JA, Patty E, et al. Congenital pits of the optic nerve head. I. Experimental studies in Collie dogs. *Arch Ophthalmol* 1979;97:1341–1344.
47. Brown G, Tasman W. *Congenital Anomalies of the Optic Disc.* New York: Grune & Stratton, 1983.
48. Brownstein S, Kirkham TH, Kalousek DG. Bilateral renal agenesis with multiple congenital ocular anomalies. *Am J Ophthalmol* 1976;82:770–774.
49. Buys Y, Enzenauer R, Crawford JS. Myelinated nerve fibers and refractory amblyopia: A case report. *Ann Ophthalmol* 1993;25:353–355.
50. Bynke H, Holmdahl G. Megalopapilla: A differential diagnosis in suspected optic atrophy. *Neuro-Ophthalmology* 1981;2:53–57.
51. Caldwell JBH, Sears ML, Gilman M. Bilateral peripapillary staphyloma with normal vision. *Am J Ophthalmol* 1971;71:423–425.
52. Carney SH, Brodsky MC, Good WV, et al. Aicardi syndrome: More than meets the eye. *Surv Ophthalmol* 1993;37:419–424.
53. Cennamo G, Sammartino A, Fioretti F. Morning glory syndrome with contractile

peripapillary staphyloma. *Br J Ophthalmol* 1983;67:346–348.

54. Chambers JW, Walsh FB. Hyaline bodies in the optic discs: Report of ten cases exemplifying importance in neurologic diagnosis. *Brain* 1951;74:95–108.
55. Chang S, Haik BG, Ellsworth RM, et al. Treatment of total retinal detachment in morning glory syndrome. *Am J Ophthalmol* 1984;97:596–600.
56. Chestler RJ, France TD. Ocular findings in the CHARGE syndrome: Six case reports and a review. *Ophthalmology* 1988;95:1613–1619.
57. Cibis GW, Fitzgerald KM. Optic nerve hypoplasia in association with brain anomalies and abnormal ERG. *Doc Ophthalmol* 1994; 86:11–22.
58. Coats G. The pathology of coloboma at the nerve entrance. *R London Ophthalmol Hosp Rep* 1908;17:178–224.
59. Cohen DN. Drusen of the optic disc and the development of field defects. *Arch Ophthalmol* 1971;85:224–226.
60. Coleman K, Ross MH, McCabe M, Coleman R, Mooney D. Disk drusen and angioid streaks in pseudoxanthoma elasticum. *Am J Ophthalmol* 1991;112:166–170.
61. Coll GE, Chang S, Flynn TE, Brown GC. Communication between the subretinal space and the vitreous cavity in the morning glory syndrome. *Graefes Arch Clin Exp Ophthalmol* 1995;233:441–443.
62. Collier M, Adias L. Les anomalies congénitales des dimensions papillaires. *Clin Ophthalmol* 1960;2:1–23.
63. Collins TE. Metaplasia of the tissues of the eyeball. *Trans Ophthalmol Soc UK* 1927; 47:124–155.
64. Connolly WES, Polomeno RC. Optic disc colobomas. *Can J Ophthalmol* 1983;18:299–301.
65. Costin G, Murphree AL. Hypothalamic-pituitary function in children with optic nerve hypoplasia. *Am J Dis Child* 1985;139(3): 249–254.
66. Cox MS, Witherspoon CD, Morris RE, Flynn HW. Evolving techniques in the treatment of macular detachment caused by optic nerve pits. *Ophthalmology* 1988;95:889–896.
67. Cunningham RD, Sewell JJ. Aneurysm of the ophthalmic artery with drusen of the optic nerve head. *Am J Ophthalmol* 1971;72: 743–745.
68. De Beck D. Persistent remains of fetal hyaloid artery. *Monogr Am Ophthalmol* 1890;3:1–78.
69. Degenhart W, Brown GC, Augsburger JJ, Magargal L. Prepapillary vascular loops: A clinical and fluorescein angiographic study. *Ophthalmology* 1981;88:1126–1131.
70. Dejean C, Leplat G, Hervouet F. *L'embryologie de l'oeil et sa tératologie.* Paris: Masson, 1958.
71. DeJong P, Bistervels B, Cosgrove J, DeGrip G, Leys A, Goffin M. Medullated nerve fibers. A sign of multiple basal cell nevi (Gorlin's syndrome). *Arch Ophthalmol* 1985; 103:1833–1836.
72. de Morsier G. Etudes sur les dysraphies crânio-encéphaliques. III. Agénésie du septum lucidum avec malformation du tractus optique. La dysplasie septo-optique. *Schweiz Arch Neurol Psychiatr* 1956;77:267–292.
73. Dorrell D. The tilted disc. *Br J Ophthalmol* 1978;62:16–20.
74. Duke-Elder S, Scott GI. Neuro-ophthalmology. In *System of Ophthalmology,* S. Duke-Elder, ed. St. Louis: C.V. Mosby, 1971: 273.
75. Duke-Elder S. Normal and abnormal development. Congenital deformities. In *System of Ophthalmology,* vol. 3, part 2. St. Louis: C. V. Mosby, 1963:661.
76. Eggers HM, Sanders MD. Acquired optociliary shunt veins in papilloedema. *Br J Ophthalmol* 1980;64:267–271.
77. Ellenberger C, Runyan TE. Holoprosencephaly with hypoplasia of the optic nerves, dwarfism, and agenesis of the septum pellucidum. *Am J Ophthalmol* 1970;70:960–967.
78. Ellis GS, Frey T, Gouterman RZ. Myelinated nerve fibers, axial myopia, and refractory amblyopia: An organic disease. *J Pediatr Ophthalmol Strabismus* 1987;24:111–119.
79. Elschnig A. Ueber opticociliare Gefässe. *Klin Monatsbl Augenheilkd* 1898;36:93–96.
80. Erkkila H. The central vascular pattern of the eyeground in children with drusen of the optic disc. *Graefes Arch Klin Exp Ophthalmol* 1976;199:1–10.
81. Eustis HS, Sanders MR, Zimmerman T. Morning glory syndrome in children: Association with endocrine and central nervous system anomalies. *Arch Ophthalmol* 1994;112: 204–207.
82. Eversbusch O. Eine neue form von missbildung der papilla nervi optici ver bundeen mit ausgendhnter ver breitung markhaltiger sehn-

nervenfasern und congenitaler hochgradiger kurzsichtigkeit. *Klin Monatsbl Augenheilkd* 1885;23:1–24.
83. Fielder AR, Levene MI, Trounce JQ, Tanner MS. Optic nerve hypoplasia in infancy. *J Roy Soc Med* 1986;79:25–29.
84. Fishman JE, Spaier AH, Cohen MM. Familial dextrocardia, divergent strabismus, and situs inversus of the optic disc. *Am J Med Sci* 1976;271:225–231.
85. Fitz CR. Holoprosencephaly and septo-optic dysplasia. *Pediatr Neuroradiol* 1994;4:263–281.
86. Forman AR. Situs inversus of the disc in the Ehler-Danlos syndrome, type III. *Ophthalmology* 1979;86:844–846.
87. Foster JA, Lam S. Contractile optic disc coloboma. *Arch Ophthalmol* 1991;109;472–473.
88. Franceschetti A. Fibres à myéline de la rétine et dyscranie. *Bull Soc Ophthalmol Fr* 1938; 51:573–577.
89. Franceschetti A, Bock RH. Megalopapilla: A new congenital anomaly. *Am J Ophthalmol* 1950;33:227–235.
90. François J, De Rouck A. Electroretinographical study of the hypoplasia of the optic nerve. *Ophthalmologica* 1976;172:308–330.
91. François J, Verriest G. Les druses de la papille. *Ophthalmologica* 1958;136:289–325.
92. François P. Les verrucosités hyalines de la papille. *Ann Oculist* 1949;182:249–278.
93. Friberg TR, McLellan TG. Vitreous pulsations, relative hypotony, and retrobulbar cyst associated with a congenital optic pit. *Am J Ophthalmol* 1992;116:767–769.
94. Friedman DH, Henkind P, Gartner S. Drusen of the optic disc: A Histopathological study. *Trans Ophthalmol Soc UK* 1975;95:4–9.
95. Frisen L, Hoyt WF, Tengroth BM. Optociliary veins, disc pallor and visual loss. *Acta Ophthalmol* 1973;51:241–249.
96. Fuchs A. *Diseases of the Fundus Oculi.* London: Lewis, 1951:14.
97. Gardner HB, Irvine AR. Optic nerve hypoplasia with good visual acuity. *Arch Ophthalmol* 1972;88:255–258.
98. Gartner S. Drusen of the optic disk in retinitis pigmentosa. *Am J Ophthalmol* 1987; 103:845.
99. Gass JDM. Serous detachment of the macula secondary to congenital pit of the optic nerve head. *Am J Ophthalmol* 1969;67:821–841.
100. Ginsberg J, Bove KE, Cuesta MG. Aplasia of the optic nerve with aniridia. *Ann Ophthalmol* 1980;12:433–439.
101. Gittinger JW, Lessell S, Bondar RL. Ischemic optic neuropathy associated with optic disc drusen. *J Clin Neuro-Ophthalmol* 1984;4: 79–84.
102. Giuffré G. Hypothèse sur la pathogénie du syndrome de dysversion papillaire. *J Fr Ophthalmol* 1985;8:565–572.
103. Giuffré G. Optic pit syndrome. *Doc Ophthalmol* 1986;64:187–199.
104. Giuffré G. Remnants of Bergmeister's papilla and retinochoroidal colobomas. *Ann Ophthalmol* 1987;19:316–318.
105. Giuffré G, Anastasi M. Electrofunctional features of the tilted disc syndrome. *Doc Ophthalmol* 1986;62:223–230.
106. Goldhammer Y, Smith JL. Optic nerve anomalies in basal encephalocele. *Arch Ophthalmol* 1975;93:115–118.
107. Goldstein I, Wexler D. The preretinal artery. An anatomic study. *Arch Ophthalmol* 1929; 1:324.
108. Gorlin RJ, Pindborg JJ, Cohen MM. *Syndromes of the Head and Neck,* 2nd ed. New York: McGraw-Hill, 1976:310–314.
109. Graether JM. Transient amaurosis in one eye with simultaneous dilatation of retinal veins. *Arch Ophthalmol* 1963;70:342–345.
110. Gupta A, Khandalavala B, Bansal RK, Jain IS, Grewal SPS. Atrophy of myelinated nerve fibers in pituitary adenoma. *J Clin Neuro-Ophthalmol* 1990;10:100–102.
111. Hackenbruch Y, Meerhoff E, Besio R, Cardoso H. Familial bilateral optic nerve hypoplasia. *Am J Ophthalmol* 1975;79:314–320.
112. Haik BG, Greenstein SH, Smith ME, Abramson DH, Ellsworth RM. Retinal detachment in the morning glory disc anomaly. *Ophthalmogy* 1984;91:1638–1647.
113. Halbertsma KTA. Pseudo-atrophy of the optic nerve in infant two months old. *Ned Tiidschr Geneeskd* 1937;81:1230–1236.
114. Hamada S, Ellsworth RM. Congenital retinal detachment and the optic disk anomaly. *Am J Ophthalmol* 1971;71:460–464.
115. Handman M. Erbliche, vermutlich angeborene zentrale gliose Entartung des Sehnerven mit besonderer Beteiligung der Zentralgefasse. *Klin Monatsbl Augenheilkd* 1929;83:145.
115a. Harms H. Fall von drusenpapillen. *Klin Monatsbl Augenheilkd* 1960;136:122.
116. Harris MJ, De Bustros S, Michels RG, et al. Treatment of combined traction-rhegmatogenous retinal detachment in the morning glory syndrome. *Retina* 1984;4:249–252.

117. Hayreh SS. The optic disc. In *Aspects of Neuro-Ophthalmology,* S. I. Davidson, ed. London: Butterworths, 1974:45–85.
118. Heckenlively JR, Martin DA, Rosenbaum AL. Loss of electroretinographic oscillatory potentials, optic atrophy, and dysplasia in congenital stationary night blindness. *Am J Ophthalmol* 1983;96:526–534.
119. Hirschberg J. Ein Fall von prapapillarer Gefasschlinge der netzhautschlagader. *Z Prakt Augenheilkd* 1885;9:205–206.
120. Hittner HM, Antoszyk JH. Unilateral peripapillary myelinated nerve fibers with myopia and/or amblyopia. *Arch Ophthalmol* 1987; 105:943–948.
121. Hittner HM, Desmond MM, Montgomery JR. Optic nerve manifestations of cytomegalovirus infection. *Am J Ophthalmol* 1976;81: 661–665.
122. Holland PM, Anderson B. Myelinated nerve fibers and severe myopia. *Am J Ophthalmol* 1976;81:597–599.
123. Hoover DL, Robb RM, Petersen RA. Optic disc drusen in children. *J Pediatr Ophthalmol Strabismus* 1988;25:191–195.
124. Hotchkiss ML, Green WR. Optic nerve aplasia and hypoplasia. *J Pediatr Ophthalmol Strabismus* 1979;16:225–240.
125. Howard MA, Thompson JT, Howard RO. Aplasia of the optic nerve. *Trans Am Ophthalmol Soc* 1993;91:267–281.
126. Hoyt CS, Billson FA. Optic nerve hypoplasia: Changing perspectives. *Aust N Z J Ophthalmol* 1986;14:325–331.
127. Hoyt CS, Billson F, Ouvrier R, et al. Ocular features of Aicardi's syndrome. *Arch Ophthalmol* 1978;96:291–295.
128. Hoyt WF. Congenital occipital hemianopia. *Neuro-Ophthalmol Jpn* 1985;2:252–259.
129. Hoyt WF, Beeston D. *The Ocular Fundus in Neurologic Disease.* St. Louis: C. V. Mosby, 1966.
130. Hoyt WF, Pont ME. Pseudopapilledema: Anomalous elevation of optic disk. Pitfalls in diagnosis and management. *JAMA* 1962; 181:191–196.
131. Hoyt WF, Rios-Montenegro EN, Behrens MM, Eckelhoff RJ. Homonymous hemioptic hypoplasia: Funduscopic features in standard and red-free illumination in three patients with congenital hemiplegia. *Br J Ophthalmol* 1972;56:537–545.
132. Hugues HL. A case of bilateral coloboma of the optic disc. *Br J Ophthalmol* 1947;31: 689–692.
133. Irvine AR, Crawford JB, Sullivan JH. The pathogenesis of retinal detachment with morning glory and optic pit. *Retina* 1986; 6:146–150.
134. Itakura T, Miyamoto K, Uematsu Y, Hayashi S, Komai N. Bilateral morning glory syndrome associated with sphenoid encephalocele. Case report. *J Neurosurg* 1992;77:949–951.
135. Jack MK. Central serous retinopathy with optic pit treated with photocoagulation. *Am J Ophthalmol* 1969;67:519–521.
136. Jennings JE. Coloboma of the optic nerve. *Am J Ophthalmol* 1924;7:788.
137. Justice J, Lehman RP. Cilioretinal arteries: A study based on review of stereo fundus photographs and fluorescein angiographic findings. *Arch Ophthalmol* 1976;94:1355–1358.
138. Karel I, Otradovec J, Peleska M. Fluorescein angiography in circulatory disturbances in drusen of the optic disc. *Ophthalmologica* 1972;164:449–462.
139. Keane JR. Suprasellar tumors and incidental optic disc anomalies: Diagnostic problem in two patients with hemianopic temporal scotomas. *Arch Ophthalmol* 1977;95: 2180–2183.
140. Kelley JS. Autofluorescence of drusen of the optic nerve head. *Arch Ophthalmol* 1974; 92:263–264.
141. Kim RY, Hoyt WF, Lessell S, Narahara MH. Superior segmental optic hypoplasia: A sign of maternal diabetes. *Arch Ophthalmol* 1989;107:1312–1315.
142. Kindler P. Morning glory syndrome: Unusual congenital optic disk anomaly. *Am J Ophthalmol* 1970;69:376–384.
143. Kiso K. Beitrage zur kenntnis von der vererbung der markhaltigen sehnervenfasern der netzhaut. *Graefes Arch Clin Exp Ophthalmol* 1928;120:154–174.
144. Konstas P, Katikos G, Vatakas LC. Contractile peripapillary staphyloma. *Ophthalmologica* 1971;172:379–381.
145. Kral K, Svarc D. Contractile peripapillary staphyloma. *Am J Ophthalmol* 1971;71:1090–1092.
146. Kranenburg EW. Crater-like holes in the optic disc and central serous retinopathy. *Arch Ophthalmol* 1960;64:912–924.
147. Kraupa E. Die anastomosen an papillen-und netzhautvenen. *Arch Augenheilkd* 1915;78: 182–207.
148. Kraupa E. Beitrage zur morphologie des augenhintergrundes: III. *Klin Monatsbl Augenheilkd* 1921;67:15–26.

149. Kurus E. Zur Definition der drusenpapille. *Ber Dtsch Ophthalmol Ges* 1955;59:46–47.
150. Kushner BJ. Optic nerve decompression. *Arch Ophthalmol* 1979;97:1459–1461.
151. Lambert SR, Hoyt CS, Narahara MH. Optic nerve hypoplasia. *Surv Ophthalmol* 1987; 32:1–9.
152. Lansche RK, Rucker CW. Progression of defects in visual fields produced by hyaline bodies in optic disks. *Arch Ophthalmol* 1957;58:115–121.
153. Lewin ML, Shuster MM. Transpalatal correction of basilar meningocele with cleft palate. *Arch Surg* 1965;90:687–693.
154. Lewis DD, Woods SE. Fetal alcohol syndrome. *Am Fam Phys* 1994;50:1035–1036.
155. Liebreich R. In discussion of Iwanoff A. Ueber neuritis optica. *Klin Monatsbl Augenheilkd* 1868;6:426–427.
156. Liebreich R. Demonstration of diseases of the eye. Pesistent hyaloid artery and vein. *Trans Pathol Soc London* 1871;22:222.
157. Limaye SR. Coloboma of the iris and choroid and retinal detachment in oculoauricular dysplasia (Goldenhar syndrome). *Eye Ear Nose Throat Monthly* 1972;51:28–31.
157a. Limaye SR, Tang RA, Pilkerton AR. Cilioretinal circulation and branch arterial occlusion associated with preretinal arterial loops. *Am J Ophthalmol* 1980;89:834–839.
158. Lin CCL, Tso MOM, Vygantas CM. Coloboma of optic nerve associated with serous maculopathy, A clinicopathologic correlative study. *Arch Ophthalmol* 1984;102:1651–1654.
159. Lincoff H, Lopez R, Kreissig I, et al. Retinoschisis associated with optic nerve pits. *Arch Ophthalmol* 1988;106:61–67.
160. Lincoff H, Yannuzzi L, Singerman L, Kreissig I, Fisher Y. Improvement in visual function after displacement of the retinal elevations emanating from optic pits. *Arch Ophthalmol* 1993;111:1071–1079.
161. Little WS. A case of persistent hyaloid artery. *Trans Am Ophthalmol Soc* 1881;5: 211–213.
161a. Little LE, Whitmore PV, Wells TW. Aplasia of the optic nerve. *J Pediatr Ophthalmol* 1976;13:84–88.
162. Lorentzen SE. Drusen of the optic disk, an irregularly dominant hereditary affection. *Acta Ophthalmol* 1961;39:626–643.
163. Mafee MF, Jampol LM, Langer BG, Tso MOM. Computed tomography of the optic nerve colobomas, morning glory anomaly, and colobomatous cyst. *Radiol Clin N Am* 1987;25:693–699.
164. Malbran JL, Roveda JM. Megalopapilla. *Arch Oftal B Aires* 1951;26:331–335.
165. Mann I. *Developmental Abnormalities of the Eye,* 2nd ed. Philadelphia: Lippincott, 1957.
166. Manelfe C, Rochiccioli P. CT of septo-optic dysplasia. *Am J Roentgenol* 1979;133:1157–1160.
167. Manschot WA. Morning glory syndrome: A histopathological study. *Br J Ophthalmol* 1990;74:56–58.
168. Marden PM, Venters HD. A new neurocutaneous syndrome. *Am J Dis Child* 1966; 112:79–81.
169. Margalith D, Jan JE, McCormick AQ, et al. Clinical spectrum of optic nerve hypoplasia: review of 51 patients. *Dev Med Child Neurol* 1984;26(3):311–322.
170. Margo CE, Hamed LM, Fang E, Dawson WW. Optic nerve aplasia. *Arch Ophthalmol* 1992;110:1610–1613.
171. Margolis S, Siegel IM. The tilted disc syndrome in craniofacial diseases. In *Neuro-Ophthalmology Focus 1980,* J. L. Smith, ed. New York: Masson, 1979:97–116.
172. Meire FM, Fryns JP. Lens dislocation and optic nerve hypoplasia in ring chromosome 21 mosaicism. *Ann Genet* 1994;37:150–152.
173. Merritt JC. Myelinated nerve fibers associated with afferent pupillary defect and amblyopia. *J Pediatr Ophthalmol* 1977;14:139–140.
174. Mets M, Price RL. Contact lenses in the management of myopic anisometropic amblyopia. *Am J Ophthalmol* 1981;91:484–489.
175. Miller NR. Optic disc drusen. *Medical Retina,* vol. 2. St. Louis: C. V. Mosby, 1989:807–823.
176. Miller NR. Anomalies of the optic disc. *Walsh and Hoyt's Clinical Neuro-Ophthalmology,* vol. I, 4th ed. Baltimore: Williams & Wilkins, 1982:343–373.
177. Miller NR, Fine SL. The ocular fundus in neuro-ophthalmologic diagnosis. In *Sights and Sounds in Ophthalmology,* vol. 3. St. Louis: Mosby-Year Book, 1977.
178. Miller NR, George TW. Monochromatic (red-free) photography and ophthalmoscopy of the peripapillary retinal nerve fiber layer. *Neuro-Ophthalmology Focus 1980,* J. L. Smith, ed. New York: Masson, 1979:43–51.
179. Mimura O, Shiraki K. Shimo-Oku M. Fundus controlled perimetry in the tilted disc syndrome. *Jpn J Ophthalmol* 1980;24:105–111.
180. Montenegro M, Bonnet M. Fossettes colobomateuses de la papille: Revue clinique et

thérapeutique de 21 cas. *J Fr Ophthalmol* 1989;12:411–419.

181. Morioka M, Marubayashi T, Masumitsu T, Miura M, Ushio Y. Basal encephaloceles with morning glory syndrome, and progressive hormonal and visual disturbances: Case report and review of the literature. *Brain Dev* 1995;17:196–201.
182. Morishima A, Aranoff GS. Syndrome of septo optic-pituitary dysplasia: The clinical spectrum. *Brain Dev* 1986;8:233–239.
183. Morton AS, Parsons JH. Hyaline bodies at the optic disc. *Trans Ophthalmol Soc UK* 1903;23:135–153.
184. Mosier MA, Lieberman MF, Green WR, Knox DL. Hypoplasia of the optic nerve. *Arch Ophthalmol* 1978;96:1437–1442.
185. Mullie MA, Sanders MD. Computed tomographic diagnosis of buried drusen of the optic nerve head. *Can J Ophthalmol* 1985;20: 114–117.
186. Murphy BL, Griffin JF. Optic nerve coloboma (morning glory syndrome): CT findings. *Radiology* 1994;191:59–61.
187. Mustonen E. Pseudopapilloedema with and without verified optic disc drusen: A clinical analysis: I. *Acta Ophthalmol* (Copenh) 1983;61:1037–1056.
188. Mustonen E. Optic disc drusen and tumours of the chiasmal region. *Acta Ophthalmol* 1977;55:191–200.
189. Nelson M, Lessel S, Sadun AA. Optic nerve hypoplasia and maternal diabetes mellitus. *Arch Neurol* 1986;43:20–25.
190. Newman NJ, Lessell S, Brandt, EM. Bilateral central retinal artery occlusions, disk drusen, and migraine. *Am J Ophthalmol* 1989;107: 236–240.
191. Noel LP, Clarke WN, MacInnis BJ. Detection of drusen of the optic disc in children by B-scan ultrasonography. *Can J Ophthalmol* 1983;18:266–268.
192. Novack RL, Foos RY. Drusen of the optic disk in retinitis pigmentosa. *Am J Ophthalmol* 1987;103:44–47.
193. Novakovic P, Taylor DSI, Hoyt WF. Localizing patterns of optic nerve hypoplasia—Retina to occipital lobes. *Br J Ophthalmol* 1988;72:176–182.
194. Okun E. Chronic papilledema simulating hyaline bodies of the optic disc. *Am J Ophthalmol* 1962;53:922–927.
195. Oliver GH. Hyaline bodies at the optic disc in a case of retinitis pigmentosa. *Ophthalmoscope* 1913;11:716–718.
196. Osher RH, Schatz NJ. A sinister association of the congenital tilted disc syndrome with chiasmal compression. In *Neuro-Ophthalmology Focus 1980,* J. L. Smith, ed. New York: Masson, 1979:117–123.
197. Oxilia E. Anomalie vascolari della retina: Ansa Arteriosa prepapillare. *Ann Ottalmol Clin Ocul* 1946;73:408–427.

197a. Pagon RA. Ocular coloboma. *Surv Ophthalmol* 1981;25:223–236.

198. Pagon RA, Graham JM, Zonana J, Yong SL. Coloboma, congenital heart disease, and choanal atresia with multiple anomalies: CHARGE association. *J Pediatr* 1981;99: 223–227.
199. Patel H, Tze WJ, Crichton JU, et al. Optic nerve hypoplasia with hypopituitarism. Septo-optic dysplasia with hypopituitarism. *Am J Dis Child* 1975;129:175–180.
200. Pe'er J, Braun JT. Ocular pathology in trisomy 18 (Edwards' syndrome). *Ophthalmologica* 1986;192:176–178.
201. Petersen RA, Walton DS. Optic nerve hypoplasia with good visual acuity and visual field defects: A study of children of diabetic mothers. *Arch Ophthalmol* 1977;95:254–258.
202. Petersen RA, Holmes LB. Optic nerve hypoplasia in infants of diabetic mothers. *Arch Ophthalmol* 1986;104:1587.
203. Pinckers A, Lion F, Notting JGA. X-chromosomal recessive night blindness and tilted disc anomaly. *Ophthalmologica* 1978;176:160–163.
204. Pollock S. The morning disc anomaly: Contractile movement, classification, and embryogenesis. *Doc Ophthalmol* 1987;656:439–460.
205. Prost M, De Laey JJ. Choroidal neovascularization in tilted dics syndrome. *Int Ophthalmol* 1988;12:131–135.
206. Provis JM, van Driel D, Billson FA, Russell P. Human fetal optic nerve: Overproduction and elimination of retinal axons during development. *J Comp Neurol* 1985;238(1): 92–100.
207. Puck A, Tso MOM, Fishman GA. Drusen of the optic nerve associated with retinitis pigmentosa. *Arch Ophthalmol* 1985;103:231–234.
208. Purcell JJ, Goldberg RE. Hyaline bodies of the optic papilla and bilateral acute vascular occlusions. *Ann Ophthalmol* 1974;6:1069–1076.
209. Reese AB. Pigmentation of the optic nerve. *Arch Ophthalmol* 1933;9:560.

210. Reynolds JD, Golden WL, Zhang Y, Hiles DA. Ocular abnormalities in terminal deletion of the long arm of chromosome seven. *J Pediatr Ophthalmol Strabismus* 1984;21:28–32.
211. Rhodes RH. Development of the human optic disc: Light microscopy. *Am J Anat* 1978; 153:601–616.
212. Riise D. The nasal fundus ectasia. *Acta Ophthalmol (Suppl)* 1975;126:103–108.
213. Rintoul RJ. Colobomatous cupping of the optic disc. *Br J Ophthalmol* 1971;55:396–399.
214. Risse JF, Guillaume JB, Boissonot M, Bonneau D. Un syndrome polymalformatif inhabituel: Association CHARGE à un morning glory syndrome unilatéral. *Ophthalmologie* 1989;3:196–198.
215. Robb RM, Silver J, Sullivan RT. Ocular retardation *(or)* in the mouse. *Invest Ophthalmol Vis Sci* 1978;17:468–473.
216. Robertson DM. Hamartomas of the optic disc with retinitis pigmentosa. *Am J Ophthalmol* 1972;74:526–531.
217. Rothkoff L, Biedner B. Congenital horizontal gaze paralysis, facial hemiatrophy, and situs inversus of the optic disc: A case report. *Acta Ophthalmol* 1979;57:1091–1095.
218. Rosenbaum J. Coloboma of the optic nerve with remains of the hyaloid artery. *Br J Ophthalmol* 1929;13:407–408.
219. Rosenberg LF, Burde RM. Progressive visual loss caused by an arachnoid brain cyst in a patient with an optic nerve coloboma. *Am J Ophthalmol* 1988;106:322–325.
220. Rosenberg MA, Savino, PJ, Glaser JS. A clinical analysis of pseudopapilledema: I. Population, laterality, acuity, refractive error, ophthalmoscopic characteristics, and coincident disease. *Arch Ophthalmol* 1979;97:65–70.
221. Roy FH, Summitt RL, Hiatt RL, et al. Ocular manifestations of the Rubinstein-Taybi syndrome: Case report and review of the literature. *Arch Ophthalmol* 1968;79:272–278.
222. Rubenstein K, Ali M. Complications of optic disc pits. *Trans Ophthalmol Soc UK* 1978; 98:195–200.
223. Rucker CW. Defects in visual fields produced by hyaline bodies in optic disks. *Arch Ophthalmol* 1944;32:56–59.
224. Rush JA, Bajandas FJ. Septo-optic dysplasia (De Morsier syndrome). *Am J Ophthalmol* 1978;86:202–205.
225. Russell-Eggit IM, Blake KD, Taylor DSI, Wyse RKH. The eye in the CHARGE association. *Br J Ophthalmol* 1990;74:421–426.
226. Sachsalber A. Schwund markhaltiger nervenfasern in der netzhaut bei intzündlicher atrophie des sehnerven infolge eines tumor cerebri. *Z Augenheilkd* 1905;13:739–750.
227. Sacks JG, O'Grady RB, Chormokos E, Leestma J. The pathogenesis of optic nerve drusen: A hypothesis. *Arch Ophthalmol* 1977; 95:425–428.
228. Sadun AA. Optic disc pits and associated serous macular detachment. *Medical Retina*, vol. 2. St. Louis: C. V. Mosby, 1989:799–805.
229. Salzmann M. Zur Anatomie der angeborenen Sichel nach innen-unten. *Graefes Arch Ophthalmol* 1893;39:131–150.
229a. Sanders MD, Ffytche TJ. Fluorescein angiography in the diagnosis of drusen of the disc. *Trans Ophthalmol Soc UK* 1967;87:457–468.
230. Saunders MD, Gay AJ, Newman M. Hemorrhagic complications of drusen of the optic disc. *Am J Ophthalmol* 1971;71:204–217.
231. Savell J, Cook JR. Optic nerve colobomas of autosomal-dominant heredity. *Arch Ophthalmol* 1976;94:395–400.
232. Savino PJ, Glaser JS, Rosenberg MA. A clinical analysis of pseudopapilledema: II. Visual field defects. *Arch Ophthalmol* 1979;97: 71–75.
233. Schachat AP, Miller NR. Atrohy of myelinated retinal nerve fibers after acute optic neuropathy. *Am J Ophthalmol* 1981;92:854–856.
234. Schatz H, McDonald HR. Treatment of sensory retinal detachment associated with optic nerve pit or coloboma. *Ophthalmology* 1988; 95:178–186.
235. Scheie HG, Adler FH. Aplasia of the optic nerve. *Arch Ophthalmol* 1941;26:61–70.
236. Seitz R, Kersting G. Die drusen der sehnervenpapille und des pigmentepithels. *Klin Monatsbl Augenheilkd* 1962;140:75–88.
237. Seybold ME, Rosen PN. Peripapillary staphyloma and amaurosis fugax. *Ann Ophthalmol* 1977;9:139–141.
238. Sharpe JA, Sanders MD. Atrophy of myelinated nerve fibres in the retina in optic neuritis. *Br J Ophthalmol* 1975;59:229–232.
239. Sherman J, Bass SJ, Ajax G, Noble KG, Nath S. Optic pit, microphathalmos and orbital cyst. *Ophthalmic Pediatr Genet* 1988;9:131–133.
240. Shipman JS. Coloboma of the optic nerve associated with posterior lenticonus. *Arch Ophthalmol* 1934;11:503–512.
241. Singh J. Echographic features of tilted optic disk. *Ann Ophthalmol* 1985;17:382–384.
242. Singleton EM, Kinsbourne M, Anderson WB. Familial pseudopapilledema. *South Med J* 1973;66:796–802.

243. Sharf B, Hoyt CS. Optic nerve hypoplasia in children. Association with anomalies of the endocrine and CNS. *Arch Ophthalmol* 1984;102:62–67.
244. Slusher MM, Weaver RG, Greven CM, et al. The spectrum of cavitary optic disc anomalies in a family. *Ophthalmology* 1989;96:342–347.
245. Sobol WM, Blodi CF, Folk JC, et al. Long-term visual outcome in patients with optic nerve pit and serous retinal detachment of the macula. *Ophthalmology* 1990;97:1539–1542.
246. Spencer WH. Drusen of the optic disc and aberrant axoplasmic transport. *Ophthalmology* 1978;85:21–38.
247. Sprague JB, Wilson WB. Electrophysiologic findings in bilateral optic nerve hypoplasia. *Arch Ophthalmol* 1981;99:1028–1029.
247a. Stefkost, Campochiarol, Wang P, Li Y, Zhu D, Traboulsi EI. Dominant inheritance of optic pits. *Am J Ophthalmol* 1997;124:112–113.
248. Steifel JW, Smith JL. Hyaline bodies (drusen) of the optic nerve and intracranial tumor. *Arch Ophthalmol* 1961;65:814–816.
249. Steinberg T. Coloboma of the optic nerve. *Am J Ophthalmol* 1943;26:846–849.
250. Steinkuller PG. The morning glory disc anomaly. Case report and literature review. *J Pediatr Ophthalmol Strabismus* 1980;17:81–87.
251. Storm RL, PeBenito R. Bilateral optic nerve aplasia associated with hydranencephaly. *Ann Ophthalmol* 1984;16:988–992.
252. Straatsma BR, Foos RY, Heckenlively JR, Christensen RE. Myelinated retinal nerve fibers: Clinicopathologic study and clinical correlations. *Excerpta Med* 1978;32:36.
253. Straatsma BR, Heckenlively JR, Foos RY, Shahinian JK. Myelinated retinal nerve fibers associated with ipsilateral myopia, amblyopia and strabismus. *Am J Ophthalmol* 1979;88:506–510.
254. Straatsma BR, Foos RY, Heckenlively JR, Taylor GN. Myelinated retinal nerve fibers. *Am J Ophthalmol* 1981;91:25–38.
255. Stratton RF, DuPont BR, Mattern VL, et al. Interstitial duplication of 7(q22-q34). *Am J Med Genet* 1993;47:380–382.
256. Streletz LJ, Schatz NJ. Transsphenoidal encephalocele associated with hypopituitary dwarfism. In *Neuro-Ophthalmology Symposium,* vol. 7, J. L. Smith and J. Glaser, eds. C. V. Mosby, 1973;78–86.
257. Stromland K. Ocular abnormalities in the fetal alcohol syndrome. *Acta Ophthalmol (Suppl)* 1985;171:1–50.
258. Sugar HS. Congenital pits of the optic disc with acquired macular pathology. *Am J Ophthalmol* 1962;53:307–311.
259. Sugar HS. Congenital pits of the optic discs and their equivalents (congenital colobomas and coloboma-like excavations) associated with submacular fluid. *Am J Ophthalmol* 1967;63:298–307.
260. Sugar HS, Beckman H. Peripapillary staphyloma with respiratory pulsation. *Am J Ophthalmol* 1969;68:895–897.
261. Summers CG, Romig L, Lavoie JD. Unexpected good results after therapy for anisometropic amblyopia associated with unilateral peripapillary myelinated nerve fibers. *J Pediatr Ophthalmol Strabismus* 1991;28:134–136.
262. Taylor D. Congenital tumors of the anterior visual pathways. *Br J Ophthalmol* 1982;66:455–463.
263. Taylor D, Eustace P. Optic disc anomalies in congenital chiasmal tumors. Paper presented at the 3rd International Neuro-Ophthalmology Congress, Valbella, Switzerland, March 16–20, 1980.
264. Teich SA. Disappearance of myelinated retinal nerve fibers after a branch retinal artery occlusion. *Am J Ophthalmol* 1987;103:835–837.
265. Ten Doesschate MJL, Manshot WA. Optic disc drusen and central retinal vein occlusion. *Doc Ophthalmol* 1985;59:27–31.
266. Theodossiadis G. Treatment of retinal detachment with congenital optic pit by krypton laser photocoagulation. *Graefes Arch Clin Exp Ophthalmol* 1988;226:299.
267. Theodossiadis GP, Kollia AK. Cilioretinal arteries in conjunction with a pit of the optic disc. *Ophthalmologica* 1992;204:115–121.
268. Traboulsi EI. Morning glory disc anomaly or optic disc coloboma? (Letter) *Arch Ophthalmol* 1994;112(2):153.
269. Traboulsi EI, Jurdi-Nuwayhid F, Torbey NS, et al. Aniridia, atypical iris defects, optic pit and the morning glory disc anomaly in a family. *Ophthalmic Pediatr Genet* 1986;7:131–135.
270. Traboulsi EI, Lim JI, Pyeritz R, Goldberg HK, Haller JA. A new syndrome of myelinated nerve fibers, vitreoretinopathy, and skeletal malformations. *Arch Ophthalmol* 1993;111:1543–1545.
271. Traboulsi EI, O'Neill JR. The spectrum in the morphology of the so-called "morning glory disc anomaly." *J Pediatr Ophthalmol Strabismus* 1988;25:93–98.

272. Tso MOM. Pathology and pathogenesis of drusen of the optic nerve head. *Ophthalmology* 1981;88:1066–1080.
273. Uehara M, Inomata H, Yamana Y, Taniguchi Y, Tsuji K. Optic disk drusen with central retinal artery occlusion. *Jpn J Ophthalmol* 1982;26:10–17.
274. Velzeboer CMJ, Van der Harten JJ, Koole FD. Ocular pathology in trisomy 18: A histopathological report of three cases. *Ophthalmic Pediatr Genet* 1989;10:263–269.
275. von Fricken MA, Dhungel R. Retinal detachment in the morning glory syndrome: Pathogenesis and management. *Retina* 1984;4:97–99.
276. von Graefe A. Ganzliches fehlen der netzhautgefasse. *Graefes Arch Ophthalmol* 1854;1:403–404.
277. Vuori ML. Morning glory disc anomaly with pulsating peripapillary staphyloma: A case history. *Acta Ophthalmol* 1987;65:602–606.
278. Wagenmann A. Schwund markhaltiger nervenfasern in der retina in folgre von genuiner sehnerveatrophiebei tabes dorsalis. *Graefes Arch Ophthalmol* 1894;40:250–258.
279. Walker CH. Thrombosis of the inferior temporal branch of the arteria centralis retinae in an eye with a persistent hyaloid artery and vein caused by exposure to direct sunlight. *Trans Ophthalmol Soc UK* 1903;23:279–281.
280. Walker CH. Diseases of the retina and optic nerve: A case of hyaline bodies at the disc. *Trans Ophthalmol Soc UK* 1915;35:366–370.
281. Walton DS, Robb RM. Optic nerve hypoplasia, A report of 20 cases. *Arch Ophthalmol* 1970;4:572–578.
282. Warburg M. Focal dermal hypoplasia: Ocular and general manifestations with a survey of the literature. *Acta Ophthalmol* (Copenh) 1970;48:525–536.
283. Warburg M. Update of sporadic microphthalmos and coloboma. *Ophthalmic Pediatr Genet* 1992;13:111–122.
284. Warburg M. The heterogeneity of microphthalmia in the mentally retarded. *Birth Defects Orig Art Ser* 1971;VII:136–154.
285. Weaver RG, Cashwell LF, Lorentz W, Whiteman D, Geisinger KR, Ball M. Optic nerve coloboma associated with renal disease. *Am J Med Gen* 1988;29:597–605.
286. Weiter JJ. Retinociliary vein associated with a craniopharyngioma. *Ann Ophthalmol* 1979;13:751–754.
287. Weiter JJ, McLean IW, Zimmerman LE. Aplasia of the optic nerve and disc. *Am J Ophthalmol* 1977;83:569–576.
288. Weiss AH, Ross EA. Axial myopia in eyes with optic nerve hypoplasia. *Graefes Arch Clin Exp Ophthalmol* 1992;230:372–377.
289. Wiggins RE, von Noorden GK, Boniuk M. Optic nerve coloboma with cyst: A case report and review. *J Pediatr Ophthalmol Strabismus* 1991;28:274–277.
290. Willis R, Zimmerman LE, O'Grady R, et al. Heterotropic adipose tissue and smooth muscle in the optic disc, association with isolated colobomas. *Arch Ophthalmol* 1972;88:139–146.
291. Wilson PW, Easly RB, Bolander FF, et al. Evidence for a hypothalamic defect in septo-optic dysplasia. *Arch Intern Med* 1978;138:1276–1277.
292. Wilson DM, Enzmann DR, Hintz RL, Rosenfeld G. Computed tomographic findings in septo-optic dysplasia: Discordance between clinical and radiological findings. *Neuroradiology* 1984;26:279–283.
293. Wise JB, Maclean AL, Gass JDM. Contractile peripapillary staphyloma. *Arch Ophthalmol* 1966;75:626–630.
294. Yang LL, Lambert SR. Reappraisal of occlusion therapy for severe structural abnormalities of the optic disc and macula. *J Pediatr Ophthalmol Strabismus* 1995;32:37–41.
295. Yanoff M, Rorke LB, Allman MI. Bilateral optic system aplasia with relatively normal eyes. *Arch Ophthalmol* 1978;96:97–101.
296. Young SE, Walsh FB, Knox DL. The tilted disk syndrome. *Am J Ophthalmol* 1976;82:16–23.
297. Zeki SM, Dutton GN. Reappraisal of the ratio of disc to macula/disc diameter in optic nerve hypoplasia. *Br J Ophthalmol* 1991;75:538–541.
298. Zeki SM. Optic nerve hypoplasia and astigmatism: A new association. *Br J Ophthalmol* 1990;74:297–299.

8

Congenital Abnormalities of the Retinal Pigment Epithelium

ARTURO SANTOS
MICHAEL HUMAYUN
ELIAS I. TRABOULSI

After the optic vesicle has formed and invaginated to become the optic cup, and during the fifth week of gestation, the outer wall of the optic cup is composed of a mitotically active pseudostratified columnar epithelium. With the expansion of the cup, the outer cells arrange themselves in a monolayer and take on a cuboidal appearance. The apical surfaces of these future retinal pigment epithelial (RPE) cells are reflected into short projections against the future photoreceptor outer segments. The RPE cells are the site of earliest melanin production in the body. Melanization of the RPE begins in the posterior pole of the developing eye, proceeds anteriorly, and is completed by the end of the sixth week of gestation. The RPE cells produce a basement membrane which becomes the inner portion of Bruch's membrane.[42]

The RPE is one of the most reactive human tissues. It can undergo hyperplasia, hypertrophy, migration, metaplasia, and atrophy. Examples of all these morphologic changes are encountered in congenital abnormalities that affect this layer of tissue.[19] Congenital abnormalities of the retinal pigment epithelium may be divided into focal, diffuse, and mixed categories. In focal lesions, such as congenital hypertrophy of the retinal pigment epithelium (CHRPE), only a circumscribed group of cells are morphologically different from the rest of the RPE. In some metabolic diseases, such as albinism, however, all RPE cells are abnormal. In other conditions, yet, such as familial adenomatous polyposis, there are focal lesions in addition to a diffuse RPE involvement. A clinicopathologic classification of these abnormalities is given in Table 8.1.

FOCAL ABNORMALITIES

Congenital Hypertrophy of the Retinal Pigment Epithelium

Patches of congenital hypertrophy of the retinal pigment epithelium are present at birth and have no malignant potential.[10] CHRPE was first described by Reese and Jones in nine patients

Parts of this chapter also appear in *The Retinal Pigment Epithelium*, edited by Michael F. Marmor and Thomas J. Wolfensberger. New York: Oxford University Press, 1998.

Table 8.1. Classification of Congenital Abnormalities of the Retinal Pigment Epithelium

Focal Abnormalities
Congenital hypertrophy of the retinal pigment epithelium
Congenital grouped pigmentation of the retinal pigment epithelium
Solitary albinotic spot of the retinal pigment epithelium
Congenital grouped albinotic spots of the retinal pigment epithelium
Diffuse Abnormalities
Albinism
Albinoidism
Diffuse and Focal Abnormalities
Familial adenomatous polyposis

as *benign melanoma of the RPE.*[52] The hypertrophic nature of the pigment epithelial cells in these lesions was demonstrated by Kurz and Zimmerman[34] and by Buettner.[6] The term *congenital hypertrophy of the retinal pigment epithelium* was introduced by Buettner and has become widely accepted.[6] Gass classified focal congenital anomalies of the retinal pigment epithelium and proposed to call CHRPE *solitary melanotic nevi of the retinal pigment epithelium.*[19] Although some of the fundus lesions in intestinal polyposis are histologically similar to CHRPE, we reserve the term *CHRPE* for the solitary, non-polyposis-related, lesion. We chose the term POFL-FAP, or simply POFL (*pigmented ocular fundus lesion of familial adenomatous polyposis*) to describe any of the pleomorphic morphologic or histopathologic types of pigmented ocular lesion in patients with polyposis (*vide infra*).

Symptoms

Patients are generally asymptomatic and CHRPE lesions are incidental findings on routine ophthalmoscopy. In a case-control study of pigmented fundus lesions in polyposis, Traboulsi and associates found that an isolated patch of CHRPE of any size was present in about one-third of normal individuals.[63] Only 2% or less of individuals have bilateral patches of CHRPE.[36,49]

Ophthalmoscopy

Typically, CHRPE appears as an isolated, dark gray to black, flat or minimally elevated, round lesion located at the level of the RPE. The lesion has well-demarcated, smooth, or scalloped margins.[6,18,49] The dark lesion is almost always surrounded by a white halo that is internal to a darker rim, producing a double outline (Fig. 8.1). In some cases, punched-out areas of depigmentation develop in the center of the lesion and coalesce in a cauliflower-like fashion. CHRPE varies from 100 μm to 5 mm in diameter. Rare large lesions may involve up to one-quarter of the fundus.[19] CHRPE is typically located in the retinal periphery but may surround part of the optic nerve head. There is no apparent predilection for any particular fundus quadrant.[6] Uncommon clinical findings include pigmented areas adjacent to the anterior border of the lesion and the presence or the appearance of linear streaks near or across the CHRPE.[9] The retina and retinal vessels overlying the CHRPE appear normal. There may be occasional focal intraretinal pigmentation near the margin of the lesion.[6] Enlargement of the depigmented areas inside these lesions has been well described (Figs. 8.1 and 8.2).[6,9,19] Concentric enlargement of the whole lesion has also been observed.[5,9,19,44] Chamot and associates reported the clinical characteristics of CHRPE in 35 patients followed for 1, and up to 14 years with serial fundus photographs.[9] Progressive enlargement of the depigmented area inside the lesions was observed in 83% of patients, and concentric enlargement was documented in 74%. This progression is very slow and may be detected only after careful examination of serial fundus photographs. Norris and Cleasby reported a patient in whom a CHRPE lesion doubled in surface area over a period of 13 years.[44] Slight widening of the margins of CHRPE lesions was documented by Boldrey and Schwartz in two patients who were followed for more than 7 years.[5]

Ancillary Diagnostic Tests

Patients with CHRPE may have visual field defects that correspond to the location and size of the fundus abnormality. In younger patients the scotoma tends to be relative, whereas in

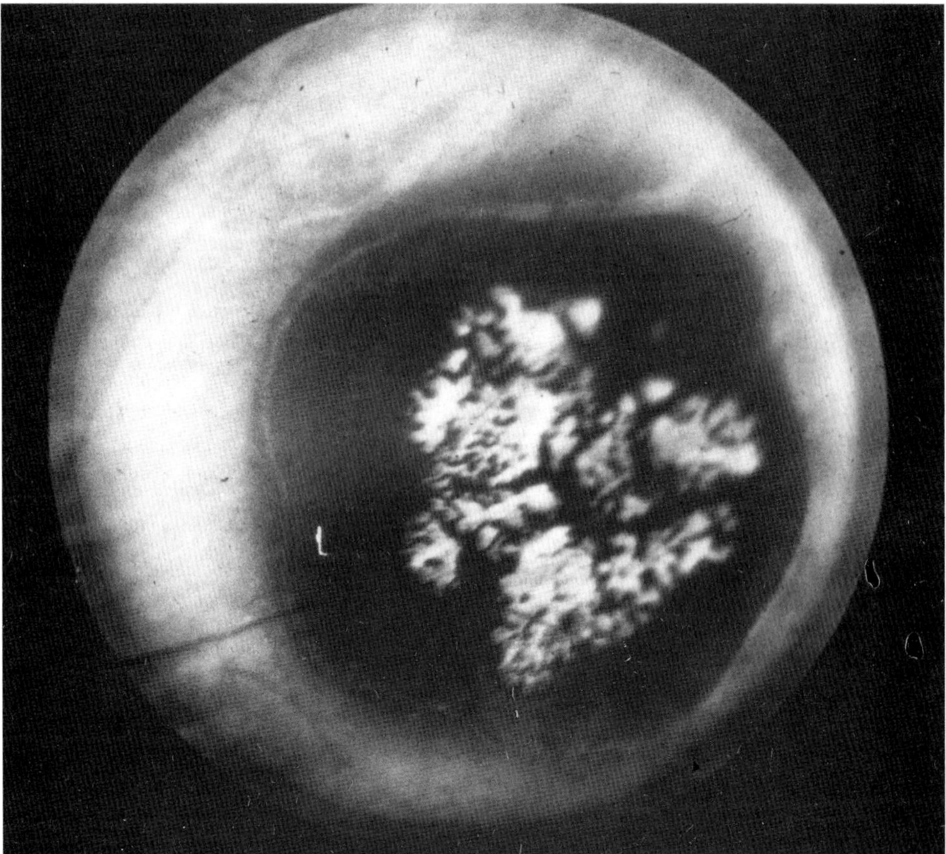

Figure 8.1. Congenital hypertrophy of the retinal pigment epithelium (CHRPE). A large, isolated, dark flat round lesion with well-demarcated smooth margins, surrounded by a white halo. There are multiple areas of depigmentation in the center of the lesion.

older patients it is absolute.[6] The scotomas are generally asymptomatic. Electroretinographic and electrooculographic responses are normal.[6] On angiography CHRPE lesions totally block the normal background choroidal fluorescence. The normal choriocapillaris flush can be observed through the central depigmented areas. Choroidal fluorescence has also been observed through the hypopigmented halo that surrounds some of the lesions. The retina and the retinal vasculature that overly patches of CHRPE, as well as the RPE and choroid in these areas, usually exhibit a normal fluorescein angiographic pattern.[6] However, in five cases Cleary and co-workers described vascular nonperfusion with obliteration of the retinal capillary bed, retinal capillary leakage, and presumed neovascularization.[8]

Associated Findings

Solitary patches of congenital hypertrophy of the retinal pigment epithelium are not associated with systemic diseases such as familial adenomatous polyposis.[2,6,49] However, patches of CHRPE have been observed in a newborn with multiple abnormalities of the spinal cord, thorax, and skull; these findings were thought to be consistent with a diagnosis of spondylothoracic dysplasia.[10] Champion and Daicker reported a 6-year-old girl with microcephaly, epilepsy, spastic tetraparesis, persistent left upper vein, dysplastic fingernails and toenails, and congenital glaucoma; a diagnosis of Donohue syndrome was considered.[10] Kurz and Zimmerman reported a 19-year-old woman with syringomyelia, a history of poliomyelitis, spinal fusion for

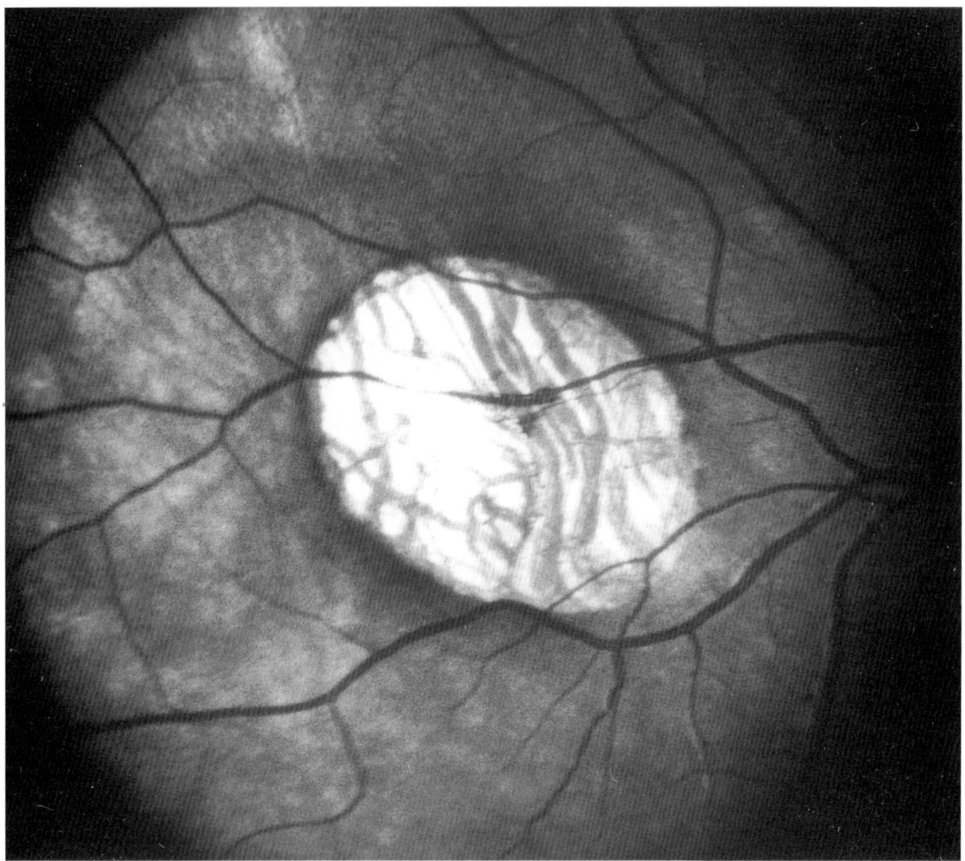

Figure 8.2. Completely depigmented patch of congenital hypertrophy of the retinal pigment epithelium (CHRPE).

scoliosis, several scattered cutaneous nevi, and "cafe-au-lait" spots.[34] A possible association of CHRPE with neurofibromatosis has also been suggested.[59] Patients with isolated CHRPE are not at greater risk of developing intestinal cancer.[60]

Histopathology

The lesions of CHRPE consist of a single layer of hypertrophied (tall), maximally pigmented retinal pigment epithelial cells (Fig. 8.3).[6,10,19,70] Segmental hyperplasia and focal atrophy of the RPE cells have also been observed in these lesions.[70] In a morphometric analysis of a CHRPE lesion performed by Lloyd and coworkers the density of the RPE cells that constituted the lesion was found to be 1.7 times greater than the density of adjacent normal peripheral RPE cells.[37] The hypertrophic RPE cells contain an increased number of large, round pigment granules instead of the football-shaped melanin granules of normal RPE (Fig. 8.4).[6,34] Initially, these granules were thought to be lipofuscin,[6] however, several authors have excluded the presence of lipofuscin in CHRPE lesions using fluorescence microscopy and identified these granules as enlarged melanin granules.[10,37,70] Retinal photoreceptors that overly CHRPE are variably degenerated.[6,34,37,70] Bruch's membrane is thickened as a result of thickening of the basement membrane of the hypertrophied RPE cells. The choriocapillaris and choroid underneath the lesion are normal.[6] The inner retinal layers and retinal vasculature are unremarkable. The hypopigmented halo that surrounds some of the lesions consists of less-pigmented hypertrophied RPE cells. In

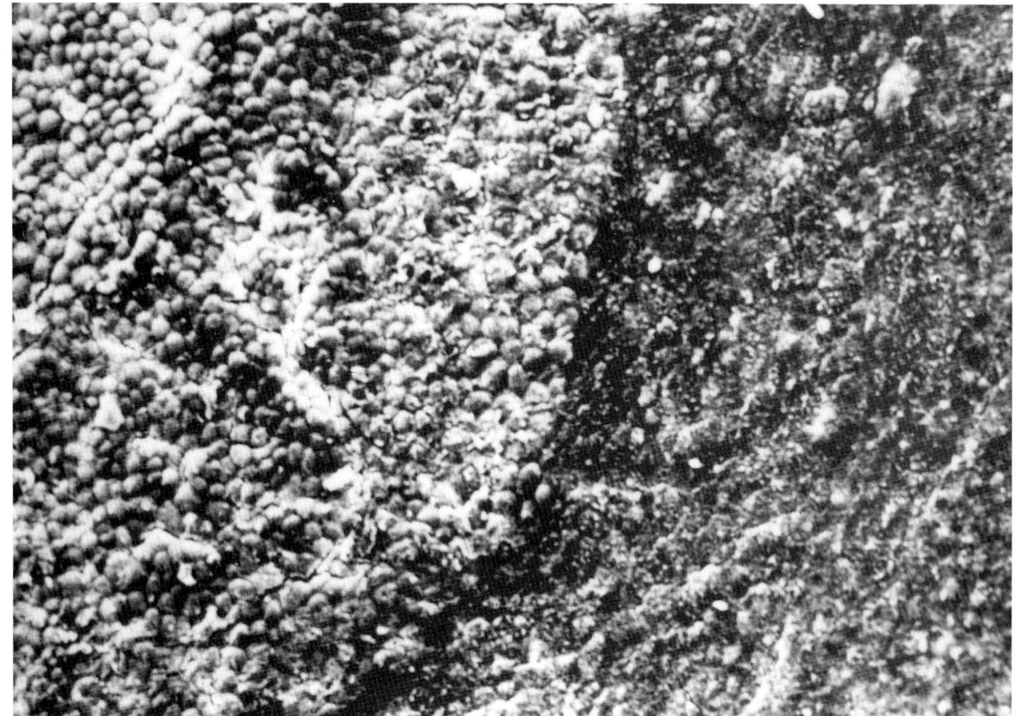

Figure 8.3. Abrupt transition is shown between the congenital hypertrophy of the retinal pigment epithelium (CHRPE) (left) and adjacent normal retinal pigment epithelium (RPE) at the lesion's smoothly curved temporal margin. Compared with the cobblestoned surface of the lesion, the adjacent RPE is relatively flat. (Scanning electron microscopy; original magnification ×160.) (Reprinted by permission from Lloyd et al., ref. 37.)

the central depigmented areas, both hypertrophied RPE cells and retinal photoreceptors are absent and are replaced by glial cells.[6]

Pathogenesis

The congenital nature of CHRPE was confirmed by Champion and Daicker.[10] These authors reported a term neonate with multiple congenital anomalies, including CHRPE, who died shortly after birth. Based on the absence of lipofuscin pigment in CHRPE, it has been hypothesized that the abnormal RPE cells comprising the lesion lack the capacity to phagocytose and digest photoreceptor outer segments, leading to degeneration of rods and cones and to visual field defects.[37] The pathogenic mechanisms for the enlargement of some lesions and for the development of pigmented areas and linear streaks adjacent to or overlying lesions remain unknown. Some histopathologic features, such as hypertrophy, segmental hyperplasia, and focal atrophy of the RPE cells found in CHRPE, may help explain the slow growth of some of these lesions.[10] In view of the benign clinical course of CHRPE, such changes in pigmentation and increases in size of the lesion should not be considered signs of malignant degeneration.[9]

Differential Diagnosis

The ophthalmoscopic characteristics of CHRPE, and the occasional use of fluorescein angiography and ultrasonography aid in differentiating this lesion from other pigmented retinal, RPE, and choroidal lesions.[49,60] The differential diagnosis includes choroidal melanoma, choroidal nevus, melanocytoma, hyperplasia of the RPE, pigmented ocular fundus lesions (POFLs) associated with familial adenomatous polyposis (FAP), congenital grouped pigmenta-

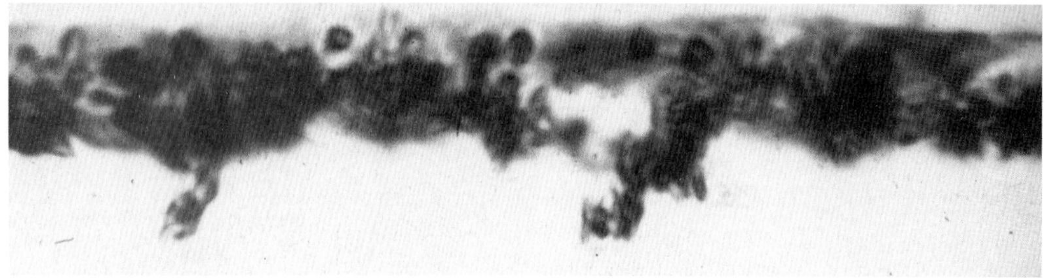

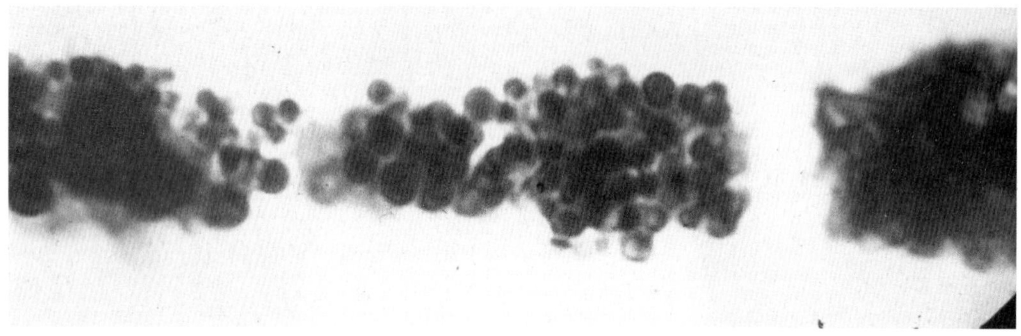

Figure 8.4. Pigment granules within congenital hypertrophy of the retinal pigment epithelium (CHRPE) lesions are more spheroidal (**bottom**) and more variable in size than in normal pigment epithelium (**top**) (×900. Armed Forces Institute of Pathology Neg. 61-3087). (Reprinted by permission from Kurz and Zimmerman, ref. 34.)

tion of the retinal pigment epithelium, sunburst lesions of sickle cell disease, hemorrhage beneath the RPE, old chorioretinitis, "pavingstone" degeneration, and enclosed bays of the ora serrata. In contradistinction to choroidal melanoma, CHRPE lesions are flat and have well-demarcated margins and characteristic depigmented changes.[6,37,49,60] Choroidal melanomas have tapering boundaries, may hyperfluoresce on angiography, and may show low internal reflectivity on ultrasonography.[59] The POFLs associated with intestinal polyposis are pleomorphic and have different ophthalmoscopic characteristics from solitary CHRPE; they are multiple and bilateral.

Congenital Grouped Pigmentation of the Retinal Pigment Epithelium

Congenital grouped pigmentation of the retinal pigment epithelium, a condition characterized by multiple, well-circumscribed, flat lesions that are arranged in clusters, giving the appearance of animal footprints, was initially recognized by Mauthner.[40] The term *grouped pigmentation of the fundus* was first used by Hoeg to describe lesions that resembled animal tracks.[26] Egerer reviewed all cases reported before 1976.[16] Eighty-four percent of lesions were unilateral; 59% involved a single quadrant of the fundus; and none were inherited. Two familial instances have been described.[14,51] De Jong and Delleman described a father and son with grouped pigmentation of the RPE, suggesting autosomal dominant inheritance with variable expressivity.[14] Renardel de Lavalette and associates reported on a mother and daughter, also suggesting dominant inheritance.[51] Of patients examined in a general ophthalmic practice, 0.12% have grouped pigmentation of the RPE.[13] The entity has also been called *melanosis retinae, bear or animal tracks, nevoid pig-*

mentation of the fundus, familial grouped pigmentation of the retinal pigment epithelium,[13] *grouped pigmentation of the retina,*[39] and *congenital grouped pigmentation of the retina.*[3]

Symptoms

Congenital grouped pigmentation of the retinal pigment epithelium is asymptomatic and is detected during routine examinations of the eye.[71]

Ophthalmoscopy

Grouped pigmentation of the RPE consists of multiple, small, variable sized, well-circumscribed, uniformly pigmented, flat lesions that vary from 0.1 to 0.5 disc diameter (DD) and are arranged in clusters in one or more sectors of the fundus.[3,34,39,58] The smaller spots are usually located at the apex of each cluster and closer to the posterior pole; this leads to the appearance suggestive of animal footprints or bear tracks (Fig. 8.5).[26,40,47,58]

Ancillary Diagnostic Tests

Visual field, color vision, and dark adaptation tests are normal.[14,71] Similarly, electroretinography, electrooculography, and visually evoked cortical potentials, have been found to be normal in patients with grouped pigmentation of the RPE.[14,71] Fluorescein angiography shows blocked choroidal fluorescence by the RPE lesions in the early arteriovenous phase. The boundaries of larger lesions may hyperfluoresce. No leakage of dye is observed during any phase of the angiogram. The choroid, retinal pigment epithelium, and retinal vasculature are not involved and show a normal fluorescein angiographic pattern.[71]

Associated Findings

Congenital grouped pigmentation of the RPE occasionally occurs in association with other anomalies of the eye such as convergent strabismus,[26] macular coloboma,[38] Rieger anomaly,[14]

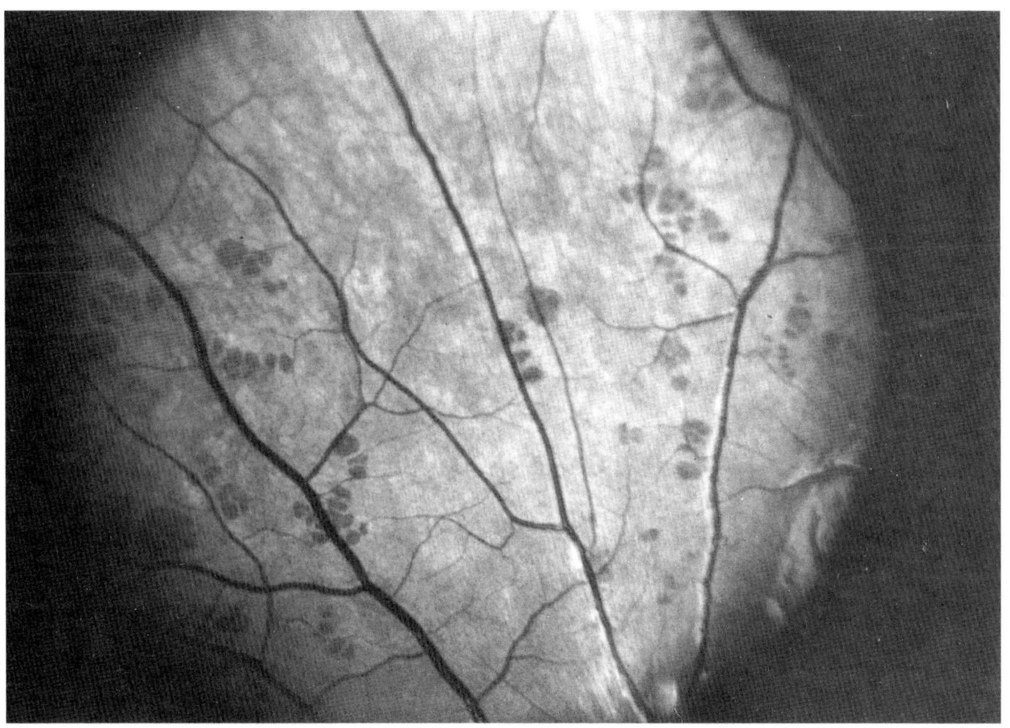

Figure 8.5. Grouped pigmentation of the retinal pigment epithelium. Multiple small, uniformly pigmented, flat lesions are arranged in clusters, producing so-called animal footprints or bear tracks.

and retinoblastoma.[50] No association has been reported with extraocular abnormalities. Patients with grouped pigmentation of the RPE are not at a greater risk of developing intestinal cancer.[60]

Histopathology

The histopathologic features of grouped pigmentation of the RPE were mentioned in the French literature in 1904 and in the Italian literature in 1938.[12,47] In a light microscopic study by Shields and Tso, the pigmented lesions were formed of focal areas of increased concentration of pigment granules in otherwise normal RPE cells.[58] Pigment granules were large and football-shaped. The overlying photoreceptors were normal. Regillo and associates described the histopathologic and ultrastructural features of grouped pigmentation of the RPE in one eye of a 2-year-old child with retinoblastoma.[50] There was an abrupt transition between hyperpigmented and surrounding normal RPE. The height of RPE cells in the pigmented lesions did not differ significantly from that of uninvolved cells. The pigment granules, however, were 1.6 times larger in greatest dimension in the involved cells compared to normal cells. Melanosomes were larger in the hyperpigmented cells but retained their normal football shape. The basement membrane of the RPE under the lesion and in uninvolved areas was not thickened.

Pathogenesis

This benign condition of unknown etiology is congenital and nonprogressive.[60] The presumed normal function of the RPE cells may explain the normal electrophysiological responses and visual fields usually reported in patients with grouped pigmentation of the RPE.

Differential Diagnosis

The differential diagnosis of grouped pigmentation of the RPE includes sector retinitis pigmentosa, inflammatory conditions such as rubella retinopathy, pigment proliferation secondary to trauma or hemorrhage,[60] congenital hypertrophy of the retinal pigment epithelium, and pigmented ocular fundus lesions associated with familial adenomatous polyposis.

Solitary Albinotic Spot of the Retinal Pigment Epithelium

This condition was described by Schlernitzauer and Green in 1971 as *peripheral retinal albinotic spots*.[55] The lesions were noted during the routine processing of two autopsy eyes. Later, Gass noted an identical lesion during gross examination of a fresh autopsy eye of an adult patient and labeled this *congenital amelanotic freckle of the RPE*.[18] These lesions were documented in 6 of 842 individuals examined during a mass screening of members of a small Maryland community.[55]

Clinical Features

Cases of solitary albinotic spot of the RPE are discovered during routine ophthalmic examinations and are asymptomatic. The lesions are focal, round, sharply circumscribed white spots, one-fourth to one disc diameter in size, usually located in the midperiphery of the fundus (Fig. 8.6). Underlying large choroidal vessels are usually visible within the lesions.[19]

Histopathology

On microscopic examination, there is an abrupt transition between the lesion and the normal surrounding RPE. The retinal pigment epithelial cells that form the lesion are slightly flatter than those in adjacent areas. These cells have virtually no pigment granules. The pigment granules observed at the borders of the lesion are football-shaped. The underlying Bruch's membrane, choriocapillaris, and choroid are normal. The overlying photoreceptors and internal retinal layers are also normal (Fig. 8.7).[55]

Pathogenesis

This lesion is thought to be congenital. The absence of all pigment in the RPE cells suggests

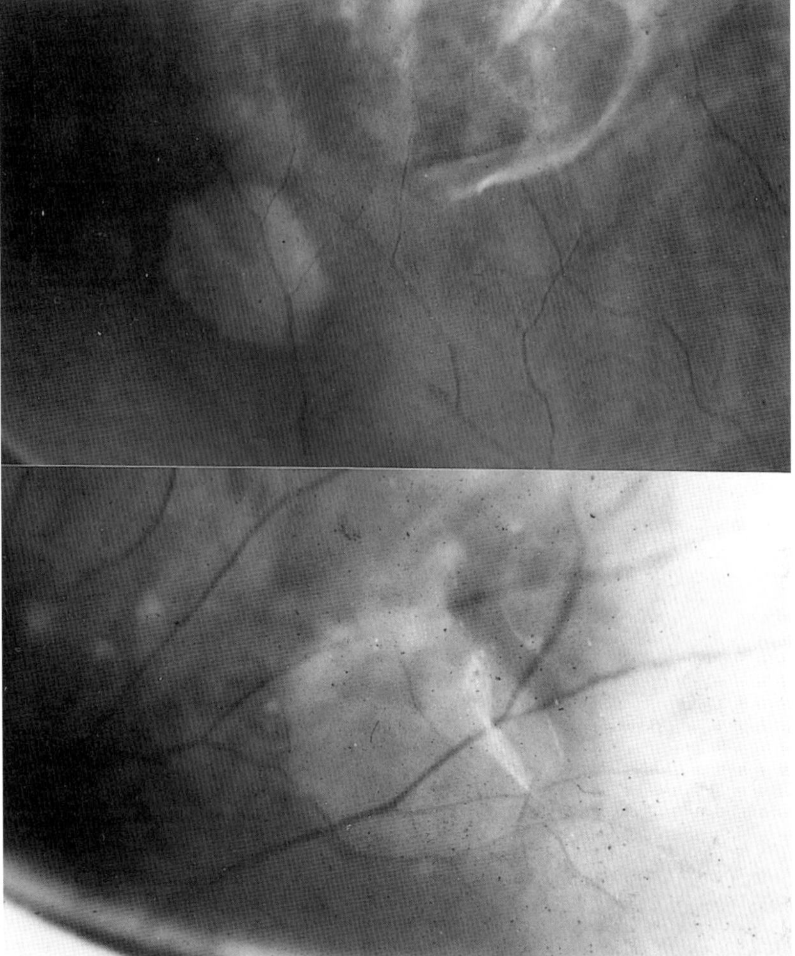

Figure 8.6. Gross photographs of a peripheral albinotic spot noted in one autopsy eye of a 59-year-old man. (Reprinted by permission from Schlernitzauer and Green, ref. 55.)

that the lesion contains no melanin or white pigment from birth.[19]

Differential Diagnosis

The differential diagnosis of this condition includes a completely depigmented CHRPE and nonpigmented choroidal nevi.[19]

Congenital Grouped Albinotic Spots of the Retinal Pigment Epithelium

This is a very rare abnormality of the RPE. To date, only nine cases have been reported.[17,19] Because of the ophthalmoscopic appearance it is also known as *polar bear tracks.*[19]

Symptoms

This condition may be observed in one or both eyes of typically asymptomatic healthy children or adults.

Ophthalmoscopy

Gass described the grouped albinotic spots of the RPE as sharply circumscribed placoid, chalky white lesions of the same size, shape,

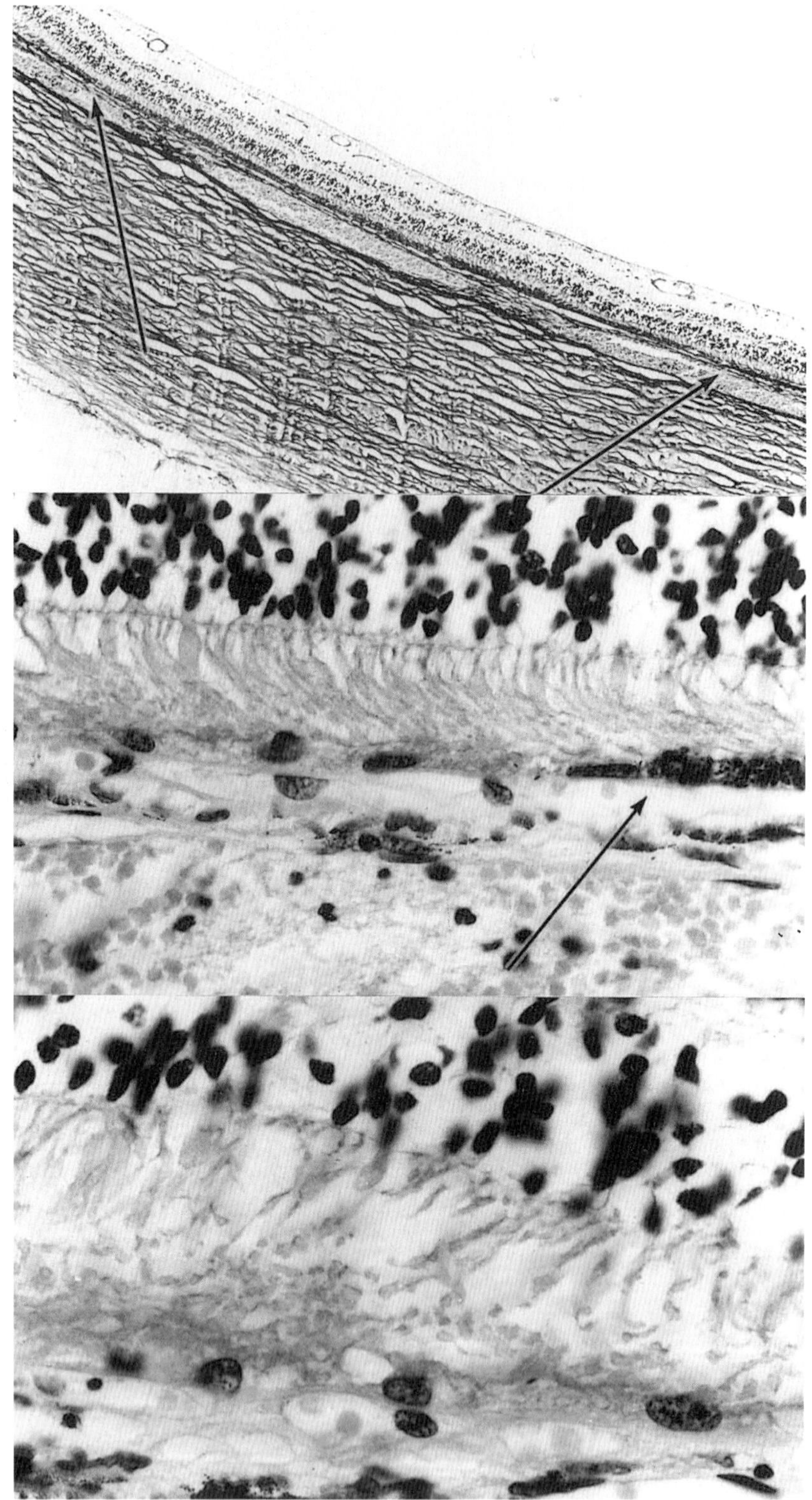

Figure 8.7.

and distribution of congenital grouped pigmentation of the RPE.[19] The spots appear to be slightly elevated and to lie at the level of the RPE. They may be uniformly thick or may have a dimpled appearance. There is focal narrowing of the major retinal vessels as they course over some of the larger lesions. Choroidal vessels may be visible beneath some lesions. Melanotic or partially melanotic spots may accompany albinotic ones. The lesions may be widely scattered in both eyes, or centered in one quadrant or less of the fundus. In some patients, small albinotic spots are present in the macular area.[17,19]

Ancillary Diagnostic Tests

The electroretinographic and electroculographic recordings are normal in patients with this condition.[17,19] Dark adaptation is also normal.[19] Fluorescein angiography slows early hyperfluorescence corresponding to most of the albinotic spots. There is no leakage of dye or staining of the lesions.[19]

Associated Findings

Gass reported the case of an 11-year-old girl with bilateral widespread albinotic spots, who at the age of 14 years, had severe visual loss from subretinal neovascularization in one eye.[19]

Histopathology

To date, there is no histopathologic information about these lesions.

Figure 8.7. Photographs of the retinal pigment abnormality. (**Top**) Overall view showing the extent of the lesion (arrows indicate the borders) (periodic acid–Schiff, ×45). (**Middle**) Higher power view of the border of the lesion, showing the abrupt transition from normal-appearing retinal pigment epithelial cells to the abnormal cells (arrow) (hematoxylin & eosin, ×575). (**Bottom**) View of the center of a lesion showing the somewhat flattened retinal pigment epithelial cells that lack pigment and that rest on a normal-appearing Bruch's membrane and choriocapillaris (hematoxylin & eosin, ×800). (Reprinted by permission from Schlernitzauer and Green, ref. 55.)

Pathogenesis

The biomicroscopic and angiographic findings locate these lesions at the level of the RPE.[19] Based on this clinical appearance, Gass postulated that polar bear tracks could consist of hypertrophied RPE cells packed with white pigment.[19] Because choroidal neovascularization is uncommon in children, it is possible that this complication reported in a 14-year-old patient with this condition occurred at the site of one of the lesions.[19]

Differential Diagnosis

The ophthalmoscopic appearance and the fluorescein angiographic findings in grouped albinotic spots of RPE are similar to those of nonfamilial stationary night blindesss of Kandori. In this disorder, the retinal flecks are described as "dirty yellow" in color, and they do not affect the peripapillary or macular areas. In addition, mild changes are found in the dark adaptation test.[29] All eight patients reported by Gass denied nyctalopia, and in two of them the dark adaptation test was normal.[19]

DIFFUSE ABNORMALITIES

Familial Adenomatous Polyposis

Familial adenomatous polyposis (FAP) is an autosomal dominant condition characterized by the development of hundreds of adenomatous colonic polyps and the inevitable progression to colon cancer if a colectomy is not performed (Fig. 8.8).[22] When FAP is associated with extracolonic manifestations, such as benign soft tissue and bony tumors, jaw lesions, and desmoid tumors, the condition is termed Gardner syndrome.[20,21] Patients with FAP are also at higher risk for developing extracolonic cancers of the thyroid, adrenal glands, and liver.[33] The association of pigmented ocular fundus lesions (POFLs) with Gardner syndrome and the clinical significance of these lesions in identifying patients at risk of developing polyps was first described by Blair and Trempe.[2] The lesions were first labeled *congenital hypertrophy of the retinal pigment epi-*

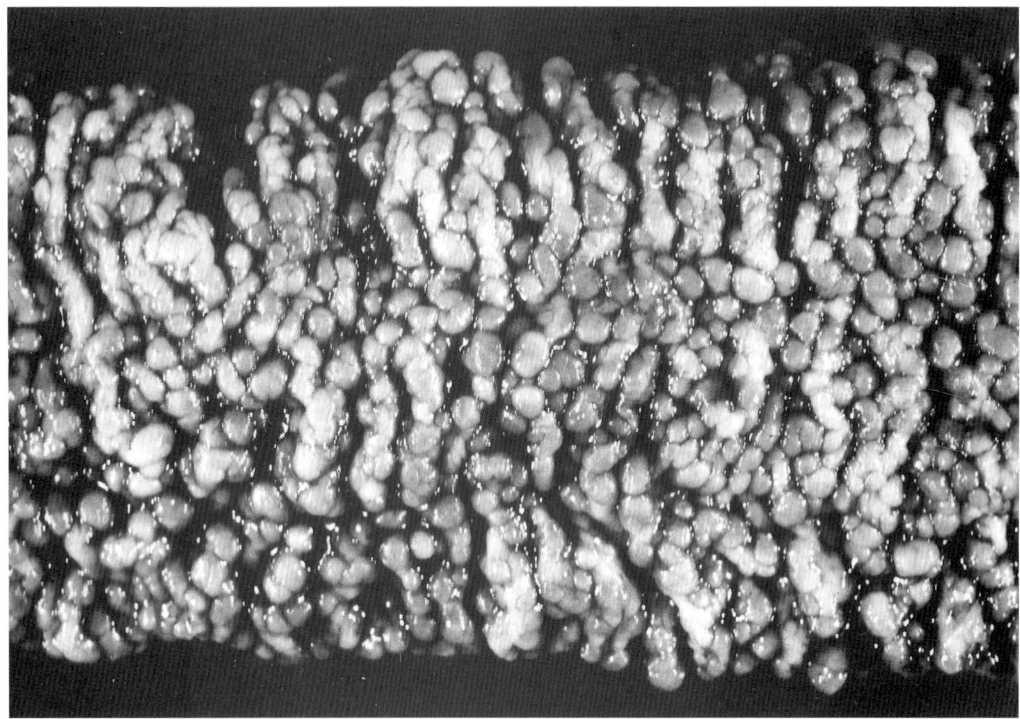

Figure 8.8. Colectomy specimen from a patient with familial adenomatous polyposis (FAP). Hundreds of adenomatous colonic polyps are present on the mucosal aspect of colon.

thelium (CHRPE) because of their similarity to isolated CHRPE. Histopathologic and clinical studies have, however, allowed the differentiation of CHRPE from the polymorphic POFLs of FAP. The use of multiple POFLs as specific and reliable markers of FAP with extracolonic manifestations has been demonstrated in a number of studies.[36,63,65] Traboulsi and associates have shown that the presence of four or more POFLs predicts a carrier status of the FAP gene in family members at risk of the disease.[63,64]

Symptoms

Although multiple POFLs are usually present in patients with FAP, they do not cause symptoms unless the macula is involved, in which case visual acuity may be reduced.[63]

Ophthalmoscopy

These lesions are multiple and bilateral. The vast majority are less than 0.5 DD in size. Various morphologic forms can be observed in combination in the same subject. The most common type of lesion is small, flat, round, and hyperpigmented. This type of POFL occurs predominately in the equator and fundus midperiphery. Larger lesions, usually ovoid to round in shape, are present close to the posterior pole and vary in color from light grayish-brown to black. Other POFLs are tear-shaped, coffee bean-shaped, pencil-shaped, or irregular. The larger lesions exhibit variable degrees of hypopigmentation and lacunae formation. Some have a hypopigmented halo or a hypopigmented tail (Fig. 8.9). Most of the lesions ap-

Figure 8.9. Various types of pigmented ocular fundus lesions (POFLs) in familial adenomatous polyposis. (**A**) Midperiphery of retina with three small pigmented lesions (arrowheads). (**B**) An oval, dark lesion with a hypopigmented tail. (**C**) A round lesion with mild pigmentary disturbance at the edges. Two satellite lesions are present (arrows). (**D**) An oval lesion in a blond fundus. (**E**) A large, lightly pigmented lesion and one smaller pen-shaped lesion. (**F**) A lesion with two areas of hypopigmentation (°) and a hypopigmented halo.

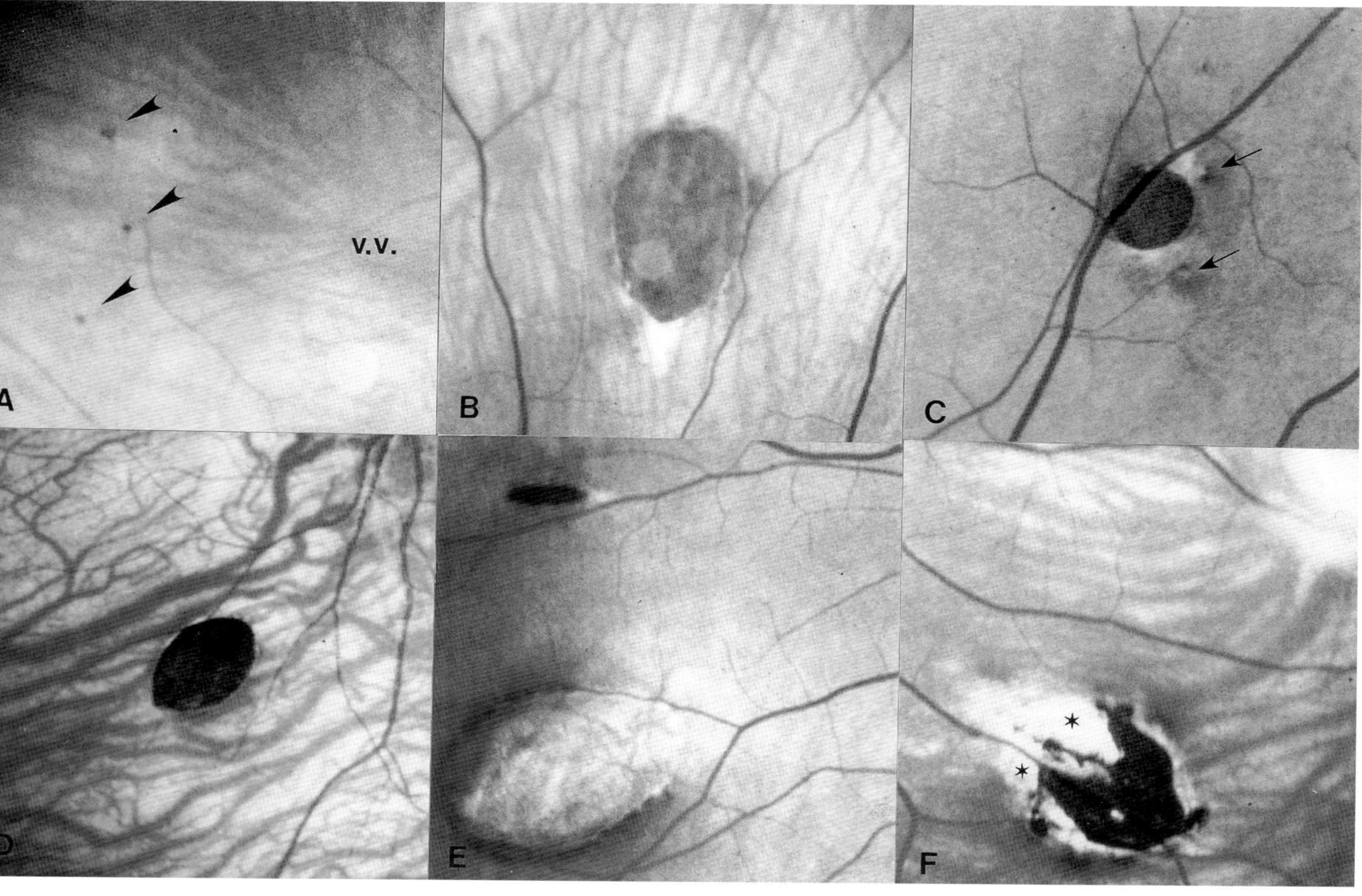

Figure 8.9.

pear flat with binocular biomicroscopy; others, however, are minimally elevated.[54] Schmidt and associates described hyperpigmentation of the RPE underlying retinal vessels and longitudinally oriented RPE changes that followed the course of retinal vessels.[56] The number of POFLs is variable among families but appears to be consistent within a kindred.[53] Some of the lesions are difficult to identify by indirect ophthalmoscopy. Three-mirror contact lens examination has been recommended.

Ancillary Diagnostic Test

Visual field scotomas corresponding to large lesions have been reported.[54] Electroretinographic and electrooculographic studies in patients with Gardner syndrome reveal no abnormalities.[54,62] On fluorescein angiography, the hyperpigmented RPE totally blocks background choroidal fluorescence. A normal choriocapillaris flush is observed through the hypopigmented or depigmented lacunae present in some lesions.[54] Retinal vascular changes such as capillary nonperfusion, microaneurysm formation, and chorioretinal anastomoses are occasionally present in association with CHRPE.[11]

From a systemic perspective, examination of the colon for polyps should be performed annually, commencing at 10 years of age, in patients at risk for the disease.[27] Determination of disease status in children is done by ocular examination, panoramic X-rays of the mandible to detect opaque jaw lesions,[45] testing of the APC (adenomatous polyposis coli) gene is used to detect mutations, or a combination of the above.

Syndromes with POFLs

Gardner syndrome refers to FAP with extracolonic manifestations such as POFLs, benign soft tissue and bony tumors, jaw lesions, and desmoid tumors. Orbital osteomas have been reported in a few patients with Gardner syndrome,[28,69] and epidermal cysts of the eyelid skin may occur in these patients.[21]

Turcot syndrome is a variant of FAP in which patients develop brain tumors. Patients with Turcot syndrome may also have multiple POFLs [Traboulsi, personal observation].[43]

Sheriff and Hegab reported three siblings with microcephaly and retinal/RPE abnormalities that included some lesions described as similar to those of FAP. Two had focal areas of chorioretinal atrophy, and one had a whitish round lesion in front of retinal vessels. None of these three patients had stigmata of intestinal polyposis.[57]

Histopathology

The focal hyperpigmented lesions of FAP are present on a background of diffuse involvement of the RPE.[30,66] RPE cells outside focal lesions are slightly enlarged and contain large round melanin granules. These large round granules are different from the football-shaped melanin granules of normal RPE. Melanin and lipofuscin granules are also present in the hypertrophied RPE cells of patients with Gardner syndrome.[66] There is a thickening of Bruch's membrane under the focal lesions (Figs. 8.10, 8.11, and 8.12). Traboulsi and associates classified POFLs-FAP into four histopathological categories: *(1)* lesions formed of a single layer of hypertrophic RPE cells, *(2)* lesions consisting of a small mound of two to three cell layers of RPE located between the inner collagenous layer of Bruch's membrane and thickened RPE basement membrane, *(3)* thicker lesions composed of seven to eight cell layers of hyperplastic RPE cells, and *(4)* hyperplastic, darkly pigmented lesions that occupy the full thickness of the retina (Fig. 8.13).[66] These authors also proposed that POFLs are best classified as adenomas of the RPE.

Molecular Genetics of FAP

Herrera and associates reported a patient with Gardner syndrome and a deletion involving the long arm of chromosome 5.[25] Following this report, the gene for FAP, designated as APC, was mapped to chromosome 5q21-q22[4,15,35,41] and was later cloned,[24,31] allowing mutation analysis of patients with this condition. Several reports describe the correlation between the type of mutation and the clinical phenotype of FAP.[7,23,32,48,61] Mutations in exons 1–8 of the

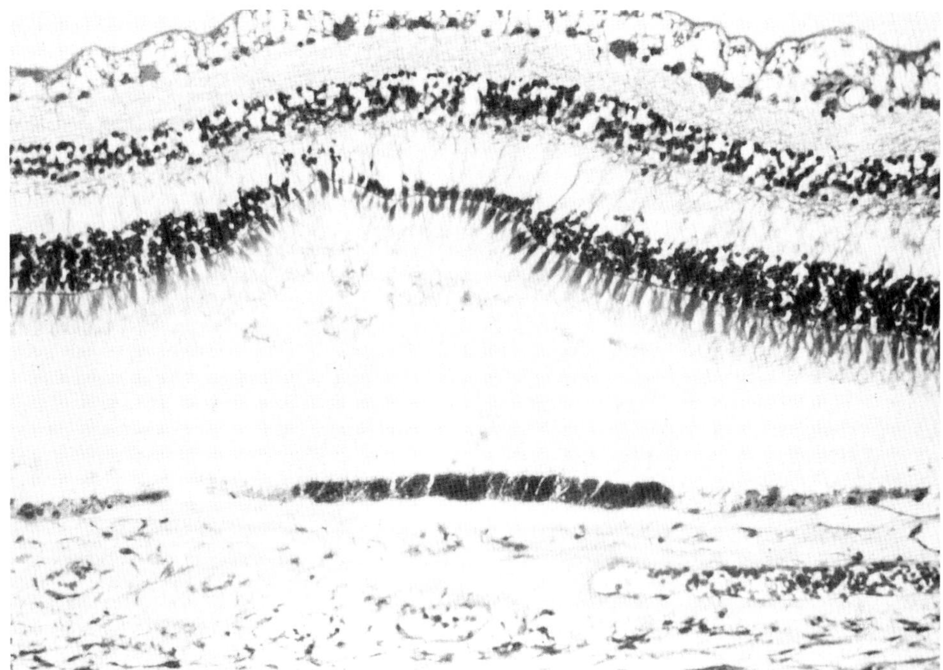

Figure 8.10. A 0.3 mm posterior pole lesion consists of tall, darkly pigmented retinal pigment epithelial cells. There is partial loss of outer and inner photoreceptors and of the outer nuclear layer (hematoxylin & eosin, ×175). (Reproduced by permission from Traboulsi et al., ref. 66.)

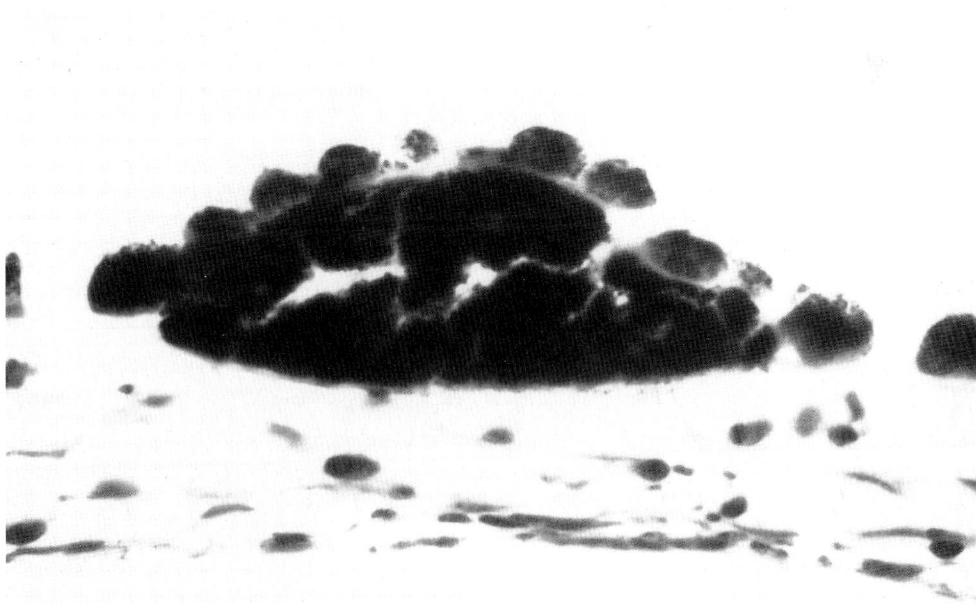

Figure 8.11. This lesion measured 0.15 mm in diameter and was located 6.5 mm posterior to the temporal ora serrata. This mound-shaped lesion consists of an aggregate of large, densely pigmented cells containing spherical pigment granules located between Bruch's membrane and the basement membrane of the overlying hypertrophic retinal pigment epithelium (periodic acid–Schiff, ×725). (Reproduced by permission from Traboulsi et al., ref. 66.)

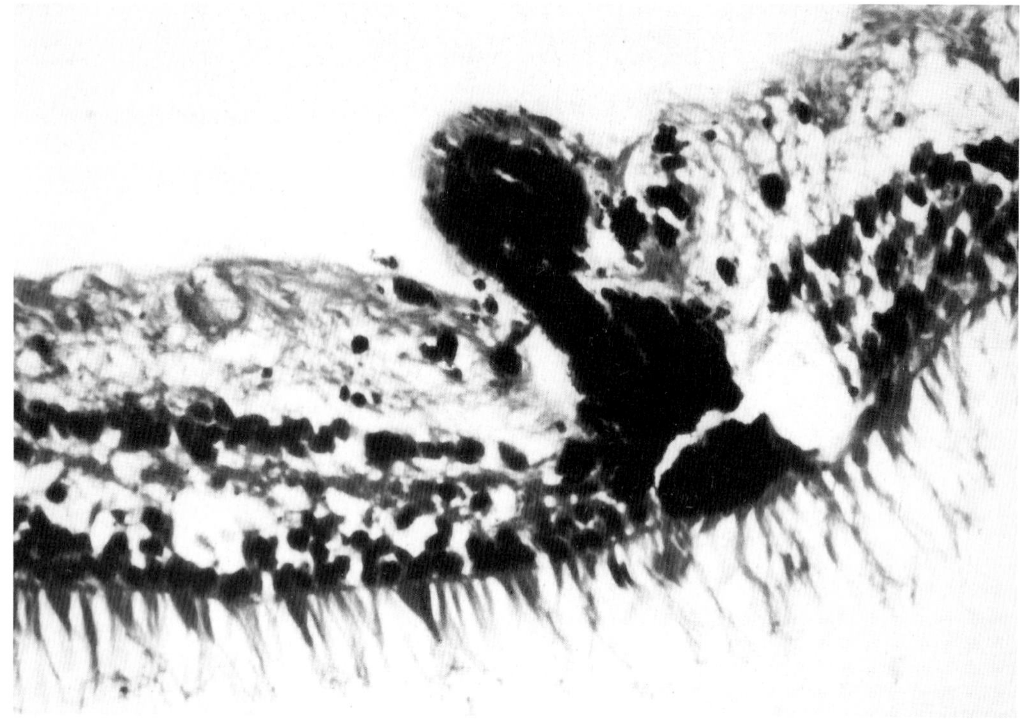

Figure 8.12. A 0.5 mm area of full-thickness intraretinal involvement by pigmented cells located 4 mm posterior to the inferonasal ora serrata (hematoxylin & eosin, ×480). (Reproduced by permission from Traboulsi et al., ref. 66.)

APC gene are associated with a POFL-negative phenotype,[46,67,68] while those in exons 10–15 are generally associated with a POFL-positive phenotype.[46,67,68]

Pathogenesis of Ocular Abnormalities in FAP

POFLs are congenital and have been observed in a premature neonate.[1] These lesions presumably do not increase in number or in size with age. Based on the histopathologic findings of diffuse and focal RPE abnormalities, Traboulsi et al.[66] and Kasner and associates[30] have suggested a generalized effect of the FAP gene on the RPE. The visual field scotomas corresponding to the location of some of the focal lesions are explained by the overlying photoreceptor atrophy. The electroretinogram and the electrooculogram measure mass responses of the photoreceptors and RPE; the normal values recorded in patients with Gardner syndrome indicate the absence of a detectable functional diffuse abnormality. Further studies on the role of the protein product of the APC gene in the RPE are needed to determine the pathology of the diffuse and focal abnormalities.

POFLs as a Clinical Marker for FAP

The presence of four or more POFLs is a reliable presymptomatic, highly specific (>90%), and relatively sensitive (70%–80%) clinical marker for FAP. This biologic marker is especially helpful in families where multiple affected individuals have numerous POFLs because of the intrafamilial consistency of expression of the ocular trait. The absence of the ocular trait, however, does not rule out the disease in any family.

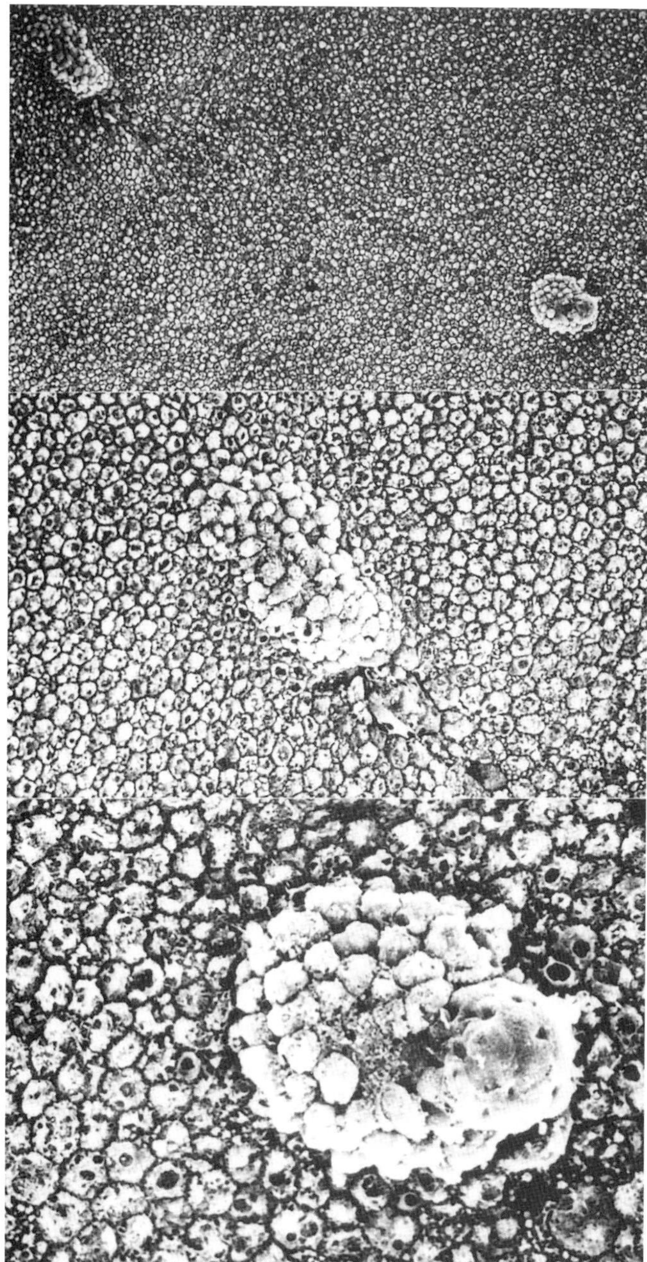

Figure 8.13. (**Top**) Scanning electron microscopic appearance of two discrete lesions composed of a cluster of enlarged retinal pigment epithelium surrounded by normal-appearing 10.0 μm hexagonal retinal pigment epithelial cells. One lesion has a posterior trail of enlarged retinal pigment epithelial cells (×100). (**Middle**) The first lesion is 140.0 μm in diameter, elevated, and consists of large 15.0–17.0 μm cells that appear multilayered. A linear trail of large 20.0–50 μm retinal pigment epithelial cells extends posteriorly for about 100 μm (×250). The second lesion is 100.0 μm in diameter and is similar to the first, except for a posterior trail of only one cell (×500). (Reproduced by permission from Traboulsi et al., ref. 66.)

Differential Diagnosis

The differential diagnosis of POFLs-FAP includes solitary CHRPE, choroidal nevus or melanoma, melanocytoma, hyperplasia of the RPE, congenital grouped pigmentation of the retinal pigment epithelium, sunburst lesions of sickle cell disease, hemorrhage beneath the RPE, old chorioretinitis, paving-stone degeneration, and enclosed oral bays. Patients with Peutz–Jeghers syndrome and hereditary nonpolyposis colorectal cancer also have colonic polyps but no POFLs.[64]

REFERENCES

1. Aiello LP, Traboulsi EI. Pigmented fundus lesions in a preterm infant with familial adenomatous polyposis. *Arch. Ophthalmol* 1993;111: 302–303.
2. Blair NP, Trempe CL. Hypertrophy of the retinal pigment epithelium associated with Gardner's syndrome. *Am J Ophthalmol* 1980;90: 661–667.
3. Blake EM. Congenital grouped pigmentation of the retina. *Trans Am Ophthalmol Soc* 1926; 24:223–233.
4. Bodmer WF, Bailey CS, Bodmer J et al. Localization of the gene for familial adenomatous polyposis on chromosome 5. *Nature* 1987;328: 614–616.
5. Boldrey EE, Schwartz A. Enlargement of congenital hypertrophy of the retinal pigment epithelium. *Am J Ophthalmol* 1982;94:64–66.
6. Buettner H. Congenital hypertrophy of the retinal pigment epithelium. *Am J Ophthalmol* 1975;79:177–189.
7. Caspari R, Friedl W, Boker T et al. Familial adenomatous polyposis: mutation at codon 1309 and early onset of colon cancer. *Lancet* 1994; 343:629–632.
8. Cleary PE, Gregor Z, Bird AC. Retinal vascular changes in congenital hypertrophy of the retinal pigment epithelium. *Br J Ophthalmol* 1976; 60:499–503.
9. Chamot L, Zografos L, Klainguti G. Fundus changes associated with congenital hypertrophy of the retinal pigment epithelium. *Am J Ophthalmol* 1993;115:154–161.
10. Champion R, Daicker BC. Congenital hypertrophy of the retinal pigment epithelium: Light microscopic and ultrastructural findings in young children. *Retina* 1989;9:44–48.
11. Cohen SY, Quentel G, Guiberteau B, Coscas GJ. Retinal vascular changes in congenital hypertrophy of the retinal pigment epithelium. *Ophthalmology* 1993;100:471–474.
12. Ciotola G. Melanosi delta retina. *Ann Ottalmol Clin Ocul* 1938;66:543–552.
13. de Jong PTVM, Delleman JW. Familial grouped pigmentation of the retinal pigment epithelium *Br J Ophthalmol* 1988;72:439–441.
14. de Jong PTVM, Delleman JW, Witmer JP, Zeilstra C. Riegers' anomaly with retinal pigmentations. *Ophthalmologica* 1979;178:107–108.
15. Dunlop MG, Wyllie AH, Steel CM et al. Linked DNA markers for presymptomatic diagnosis of familial adenomatous polyposis. *Lancet* 1991; 337:313–316.
16. Egerer I. Die gruppierte (oder navoide) Pigmentation des Augenhintergrundes. *Klin Monatsbl Augenheilkd* 1976;168:672–677.
17. Fuhrmann C, Bopp S, Laqua H. Congenital grouped albinotic spots: a rare anomaly of the retinal pigment epithelium. *Ger J Ophthalmol* 1992;1:103–104.
18. Gass JDM. *Stereoscopic Atlas of Macular Diseases Diagnostic and Treatment.* 3rd ed. St. Louis: C.V. Mosby, 1987, pp. 606–624.
19. Gass JDM. Focal congenital anomalies of the retinal pigment epithelium. Eye 1989;3:1–18.
20. Gardner EJ. A genetic and clinical study of intestinal polyposis, A predisposing factor for carcinoma of the colon and rectum. *Am J Hum Genet* 1951;3:167–176.
21. Gardner EJ, Richards RC. Multiple cutaneous and subcutaneous lesions occurring simultaneously with hereditary polyposis and osteomatosis. *Am J Hum Genet* 1953;5:139.
22. Gebert HF, Jagelman DG, McGannon E. Familial polyposis coli. *Am Fam Physician* 1986;33:127–137.
23. Giardiello FM, Krush AJ, Petersen GM et al. Phenotypic variability of familial adenomatous polyposis in 11 unrelated families with identical APC gene mutation. *Gastroenterology* 1994; 106:1542–1547.
24. Groden J, Thliveris A, Samowitz W et al. Mutational analysis of patients with adenomatous polyposis: Identical inactivating mutations in unrelated individuals. *Am J Hum Genet* 1993:52: 263–272.
25. Herrera L, Kakati S, Gibas L et al. Gardner syndrome in a man with interstitial deletion of 5q. *Am J Med Genet* 1986;25:473–476.
26. Hoeg N. Die gruppierte Pigmentation des Augengrundes. *Klin Monastsbl Augenheilkd* 1911;49:49–77.

27. Jagelman DG. Familial polyposis coli and hereditary cancer of the colon. *Curr Ther Gastroenterol Liver Dis* 1986;2:228–233.
28. Jones EL, Cornell WP. Gardner's syndrome. Review of the literature and report on a family. *Arch Surg* 1966;92:287–300.
29. Kandori F, Setogawa T, Tamai A. Electroretinographical studies on "flek retina with congenital nonprogressive nightblindness." *Yonago Acta Med* 1966;10:98–108.
30. Kasner L, Traboulsi EI, De la Cruz Z, Green WR. A histopathologic study of the pigmented fundus lesions in familial adenomatous polyposis. *Retina* 1992;12:35–42.
31. Kinzler KW, et al. Identification of FAP locus genes from chromosome 5q21. *Science* 1991; 253:661–665.
32. Koorey DJ, McCaughan GW, Trent RS, Gallagher ND. Exon eight APC mutation account for a disproportionate number of familial adenomatous polyposis families. *Hum Mutat* 1994; 3:12–18.
33. Krush AJ, Traboulsi EI, Offerhaus JA et al. Hepatoblastoma, pigmented ocular fundus lesions, and jaw lesions in Gardner syndrome. *Am J Med Genet* 1988;29:323–332.
34. Kurz GH, Zimmerman LE. Vagaries of the retinal pigment epithelium. *Int Ophthalmol Clin* 1962;2:441–464.
35. Leppert M, Dobbs M, Scambler P et al. The gene for familial polyposis coli maps to the long arm of chromosome 5. *Science* 1987;238:1411–1413.
36. Lewis RA, Crowder WE, Eierman LA et al. The Gardner syndrome. Significance of ocular features. *Ophthalmology* 1984;91:916–925.
37. Lloyd WC III, Eagle RC Jr, Shields JA et al. Congenital hypertrophy of the retinal pigment epithelium electron microscopic and morphometric observations. *Ophthalmology* 1990;97: 1052–1560.
38. McGregor IS. Macular coloboma with bilateral grouped pigmentation of the retina. *Br J Ophthalmol* 1945;39:132–136.
39. Mann WA Jr. Grouped pigmentation of the retina. *Arch Ophthalmol* 1932;8:66–71.
40. Mauthner L. *Lehrbuch der Ophthalmoscopie.* Vienna: Tendler, 1868, p. 388.
41. Meera Khan P, Tops CM, Broek M et al. Close linkage of a highly polymorphic marker (D5S37) to familial adenomatous polyposis (FAP) and confirmation of FAP localization on chromosome 5q21-q22. *Hum Genet* 1988;79:183–185.
42. Mund M, Rodriquez M, Fine B. Light and electron microscopic observations on the pigmented layers of the developing human eye. *Am J Ophthalmol* 1972;73:167–182.
43. Munden PM, Sobol WM, Weingeist TA. Ocular findings in Turcot syndrome (glioma-polyposis). *Ophthalmology* 1991;98:111–114.
44. Norris JL, Cleasby GW. An unusual case of congenital hypertrophy of the retinal pigment epithelium. *Arch Ophthalmol* 1976;94:1910–1911.
45. Offerhaus GJ, Levin LS, Giardello FM et al. Occult radiopaque jaw lesions in familial adenomatous polyposis coli and hereditary nonpolyposis colorectal cancer. *Gastroenterology* 1987;93:490–497.
46. Olshwang S, Tiret A, Laurent-Puig P et al. Restriction of ocular fundus lesions to a specific subgroup of APC mutations in adenomatous polyposis coli patients. *Cell* 1993;75:959–968.
47. Parsons JH. Some anomalies of pigmentation. In *Dixième Congres International d'Ophthalmologie.* Lausanne: G. Bridel, 1905, p. 152.
48. Paul P, Letteboer T, Gerlbert L et al. Identical APC exon 15 mutations result in a variable phenotype in familial adenomatous polyposis. *Hum Mol Genet* 1993;2:925–931.
49. Purcell JJ Jr, Shields JA. Hypertrophy with pigmentation of the retinal pigment epithelium. *Arch Ophthalmol* 1975;93:1122–1126.
50. Regillo CD, Eagle RC Jr, Shields JA et al. Histopathologic findings in congenital grouped pigmentation of the retina. *Ophthalmology* 1993; 100:400–405.
51. Renardel de Lavalette VW, Cruysberg JRM, Deutman AF. Familial congenital grouped pigmentation of the retina. *Am J Ophthalmol* 1991;112:406–409.
52. Reese AB, Jones IS. Benign melanomas of the retinal pigment epithelium. *Am J Ophthalmol* 1956;42:207–212.
53. Romania A, Zakov N, McGannon E et al. Congenital hypertrophy of the retinal pigment epithelium in familial adenomatous polyposis. *Ophthalmology* 1989;96:879–884.
54. Santos A. Morales L, Hernandez-Quintela E et al. Congenital hypertrophy of the retinal pigment epithelium associated with familial adenomatous polyposis. *Retina* 1994;14:6–9.
55. Schlernitzauer DA, Green WR. Peripheral retinal albinotic spots. *Am J Ophthalmol* 1971; 72:729–732.
56. Schmidt D, Lung CE, Wolff G. Changes in the retinal pigment epithelium close to retinal vessels in familial adenomatous polyposis. *Graefes Arch Clin Exp Ophthalmol* 1994;232:96–102.
57. Sheriff SMM, Hegab S. A syndrome of multiple fundal anomalies in siblings with microcephaly

without mental retardation. *Ophthalmic Surg* 1988;19:353–355.

58. Shields JA, Tso MOM. Congenital grouped pigmentation of the retina. *Arch Ophthalmol* 1975;93:1153–1155.
59. Shields JA. Tumors and related lesions of the pigment epithelium. In *Diagnosis and Management of Intraocular Tumors.* St. Louis: C.V. Mosby, 1983, pp. 389–400.
60. Shields JA, Shields CL, Pankajkumar G et al. Lack of association among typical congenital hypertrophy of the retinal pigment epithelium, adenomatous polyposis, and Gardner's syndrome. *Ophthalmology* 1992;99:1709–1713.
61. Spirio L, Olschwang S, Groden J et al. Alleles of the APC gene: An attenuated form of familial polyposis. *Cell* 1993;75:951–957.
62. Stein EA, Brady KD. Ophthalmologic and electrooculographic findings in Gardner's syndrome. *Am J Ophthalmol* 1988;106:326–331.
63. Traboulsi EI, Krush AJ, Gardner EJ et al. Prevalence and importance of pigmented ocular fundus lesions in Gardner's syndrome. *N Engl J Med* 1987;316:661–667.
64. Traboulsi EI, Maumenee IH, Krush AJ et al. Pigmented ocular fundus lesions in the inherited gastrointestinal polyposis syndromes and in hereditary nonpolyposis colon cancer. *Ophthalmology* 1988;95:964–969.
65. Traboulsi EI, Maumenee IH, Krush AJ et al. Congenital hypertrophy of the retinal pigment epithelium predicts colorectal polyposis in Gardner's syndrome. *Arch Ophthalmol* 1990; 108:525–526.
66. Traboulsi EI, Murphy SF, De la Cruz ZC et al. A clinicopathologic study of the eyes in familial adenomatous polyposis with extracolonic manifestations (Gardner's syndrome). *Am J Ophthalmol* 1990;110:550–561.
67. Traboulsi EI, Apostolides J, Giardiello FM et al. Pigmented ocular fundus lesions and APC mutations in familial adenomatous polyposis. *Ophthalmic Genet* 1996;17:167–174.
68. Wallis YL, MacDonald F, Hulter M et al. Genotype-phenotype correlation between position of constitutional APC gene mutation and CHRPE expression in familial adenomatous polyposis. *Hum Genet* 1994;94:543–548.
69. Whitson WE, Orcutt JC, Walkinshaw MD. Orbital osteoma in Gardner's syndrome. *Am J Ophthalmol* 1986;101:236–241.
70. Wirz K, Lee WR, Coaker T. Progressive changes in congenital hypertrophy of the retinal pigment epithelium. An electron microscopic study. *Graefes Arch Clin Exp Ophthalmol* 1982; 219:214–221.
71. Yoshida T, Adachi-Usami E, Kimura T. Three cases of grouped pigment of the retina. *Ophthalmologica* 1995;209:101–105.

9

Inheritance of Refractive Errors

ARLENE V. DRACK

The refractive status of a given human eye depends upon the refractive powers of the cornea and lens, the axial length, the refractive index of the aqueous and vitreous, and the age of the person in question. Except in patients who have certain types of intraocular surgery e.g. silicone oil to repair retinal detachments, the effect of the aqueous and vitreous on the refractive status may be considered constant, each of these two components having a refractive index of 1.33620. The major determinants of refraction are therefore the cornea, the lens, and the axial length. The size, shape, and power of these components at birth are determined largely by inheritance, although mitigating factors in the intrauterine environment, and the configuration of the eyelids and bony orbits may also play a role. At birth 75% of normal infants are hyperopic.[8] The mean refraction during the first year of life is +1.25 diopters (D) with the majority of children having less than 3–4D of hyperopia.[4,19,25] Hyperopia may increase until about age 7 years or may steadily decrease. Fifteen to 30% of infants and children have astigmatism of 1.00 diopter or more.[12] This moderate hyperopia is easily compensated for by the large accommodative amplitude of youth. Children can accommodate at least 14D up to age 10 years; this drops to about 10D at age 20, and down to 4.5D by age 40 years, at which point symptoms of presbyopia usually begin.

The moderate hyperopia of infancy is generally produced by a very short axial eye length (AEL). The average AEL at birth is 17 mm; this rapidly increases to 20 mm by the end of the first year,[15] with continued rapid growth to age 2 years, then a slow increase to the adult norm of approximately 24 mm. The short infant AEL is partly offset by a very steep cornea averaging 51D at birth that flatterns to 44D by about 6 weeks of age.[15] The infant's cornea has a diameter of 10 mm versus the adult size of 12 mm. The power of the crystalline lens averages 34D at birth and decreases to 28D by 6 months of age.[15] These rapid relatively large changes in the refractive components over the first few months of life explain the need for frequent refraction and change of spectacles or contact lenses in infants who have undergone cataract extraction. Emmetropization, the process of the refractive components of the eye changing to complement each other to produce emmetropia as the eye grows, generally proceeds by the cornea increasing in diameter and getting flatter as the axial length gets longer and the lens flattens. If these factors cancel each other out properly, emmetropia is reached at about 9–12 years with no refractive change in normal eyes after age 13 years.[26]

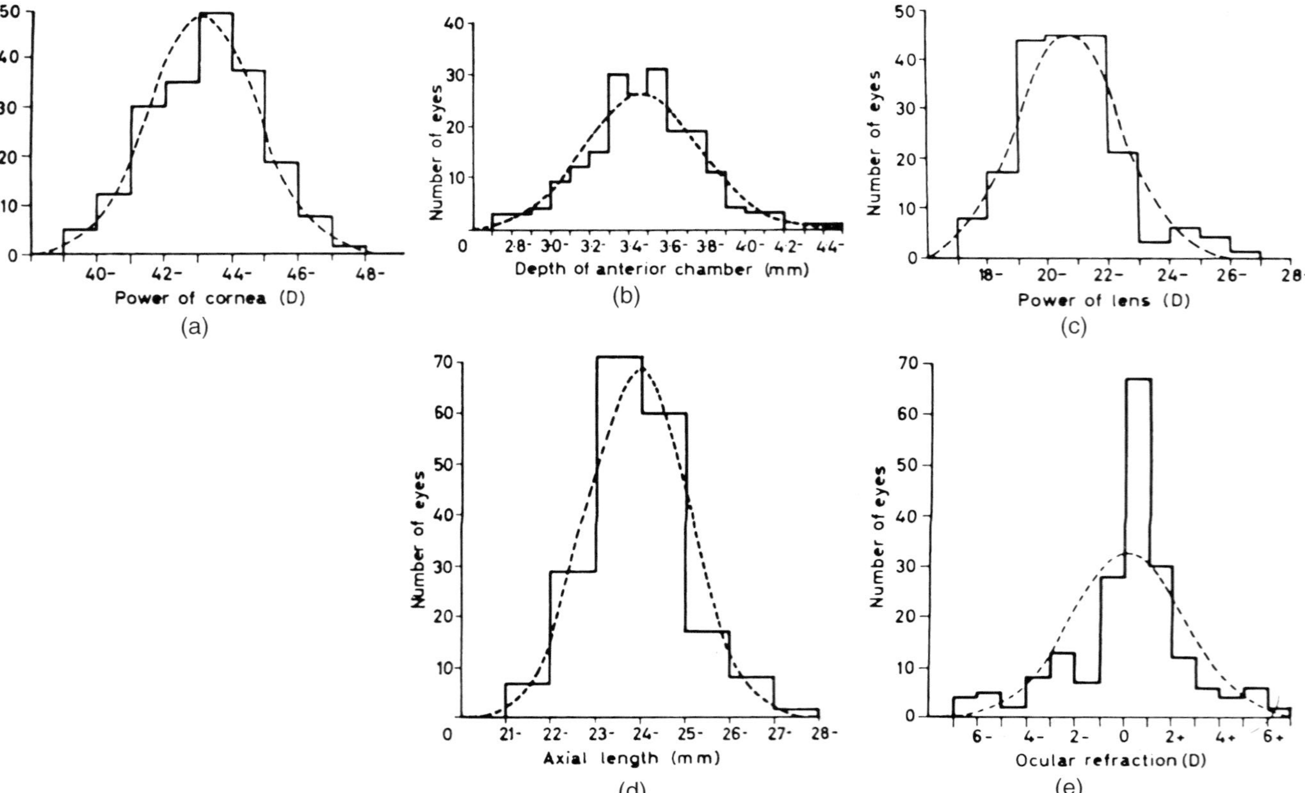

Figure 9.1. Cures of distribution of refraction and its components in the population (194 eyes). *a:* Distribution of corneal power in diopters (D). *b:* Distribution of anterior chamber depth in millimeters. *c:* Distribution of crystalline lens power in diopters. *d:* Distribution of axial eye length in millimeters. *e:* Distribution of refraction in diopters. (From Sorsby.[27])

Not surprisingly, this complex process frequently does not end in emmetropia. Refractive errors are the result of one or more components of refraction falling outside of the normal range, or of the combination of several high-normal or low-normal components that together result in ametropia. Refractive errors are by far the most common ocular disorders, with myopia alone causing symptoms of decreased vision in 25% of the U.S. population.[9] Presbyopia affects almost everyone eventually. Although not all refractive errors are inherited in a simple Mendelian fashion, genetic factors certainly play a key role in most cases.

The distribution of refractive errors in the population follows a bell-shaped curve with an excess around emmetropia as seen in Fig. 9.1e. The separate refractive components of the eye—i.e., the power of the cornea, lens, anterior chamber depth, and axial length—also follow roughly bell-shaped distributions for the population (see Fig. 9.1a–d). Axial length may actually have a bimodal distribution with a second peak of increased AEL causing high myopia (Fig. 9.2). Emmetropia is the result of a cornea and lens that correlate with axial length to form a clear image on the retina. Moderate ametropia represents a mild failure of correlation of the components—in general, all components are within normal limits but are borderline high or low enough to give ametropia when combined. High refractive errors are generally the result of one or more components (usually axial length) being outside the normal range. Refractions from +4.00D to −6.00D are usually the result of *correlation ametropia,* and those above this range are due to *component ametropia.* These two categories of refractive errors may have different etiologies and genetic components.

Like height, pigmentation, and other characteristics, the size and shape of the eyeball (i.e., the refraction) are inherited. However, as the foregoing discussion indicates, the genetics of refraction depend on inheritance of genes that determine at least three different structures (cornea, lens, AEL) as well as a postulated correlation or "emmetropization factor." Environmental or other factors such as the shape of lids and orbits and vascular supply may also

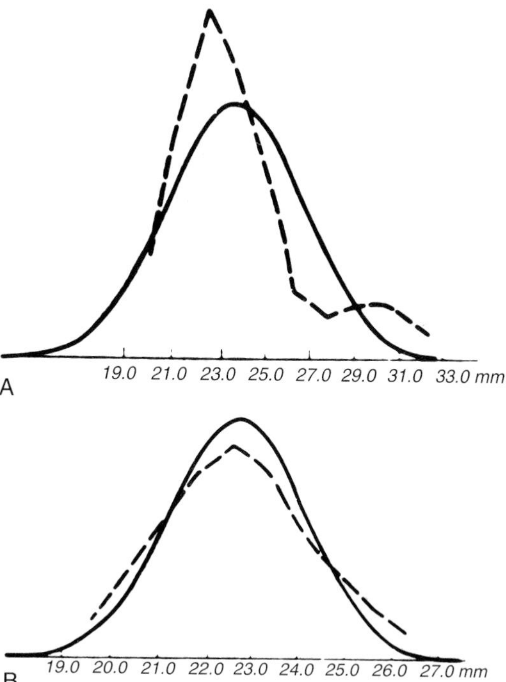

Figure 9.2. Distribution curves of axial eye length (AEL). *A:* Calculated AEL in millimeters for all eyes. Dotted line is distribution curve—note second peak at higher axial lengths. Solid line is binomial curve. *B:* Calculated AEL for the same sample excluding all eyes with refraction greater than −6D. Note that now the distribution curve (dotted line) is a normal distribution similar to the binomial curve (solid line). Tron thus suggested that myopia of more than −6D represents a deviation from the normal distribution of axial length and is therefore not physiologic. (From Tron EJ. The optical elements of the refractive power of the eye. In F. Ridley and A. Sorsby, eds. *Modern Trends in Ophthalmology.* London: Buttersworth and Co., 1940:245. Reprinted in Curtin.[9])

be involved. In this chapter we examine the existing data from the literature to develop a general scheme of inheritance of refractive errors. This data takes the form of pedigree analysis of emmetropia versus various refractive errors, population studies evaluating differences between ethnic groups and genetic/geographic isolates, and twin studies. Also useful are linkage analysis and gene mutation analysis of individuals or families with specific refractive errors, study of specific ocular and systemic syndromes that include refractive errors, and consideration of refractive errors in the context of associated environmental influences.

PEDIGREE ANALYSIS

Emmetropia

A study of families having either a parent or offspring with an unusual refraction correlated all of the components of refraction as well as refraction itself in 21 families. A high correlation was found between parents and children for all factors except axial length.[27] In another study of 28 unselected "normal" families, there was no correlation of refractive components between parents, however, there were fairly high parent/offspring and midparent/offspring (i.e., the average of the two parents' refractions compared to each child's refraction) correlation coefficients. Highest correlation was for lens power (0.580 midparent/offspring) and corneal power (0.401). Lowest correlation was for AEL (0.076).[27]

Hyperopia

There are many pedigrees reported in which hyperopia is transmitted in an autosomal recessive or autosomal dominant fashion. Pedigrees have been reported for Mendelian transmission of low, intermediate, and high hyperopia. Often various degrees are present within the same pedigree. It is, of course, important to take into account the age of the patients at the time of the study since hyperopia decreases with age. The relative frequency of the different modes of inheritance as well as the contribution of the different components of refraction are not known.

Hyperopia with squint, or accommodative esotropia (ET), has also been reported to be transmitted in a Mendelian fashion in some families. This will be considered separately.

Myopia

Many published pedigrees demonstrate autosomal dominant or autosomal recessive inheritance of myopia. In some pedigrees the degree of myopia is quite similar among family members; in others it differs widely.[27] Again, age of family members at time of examination would be important to know in this regard since myopia generally increases during puberty and early adulthood. High, or pathologic, myopia with early onset of lacquer cracks and macular changes has most often been reported to be recessive, however, as X-linked pedigree has been described recently.[16] In this report, some family members had nystagmus. No electroretinograms were performed so this pedigree cannot be differentiated from congenital stationary night blindness (CSNB) without further workup. CSNB will be discussed in the Refractive Errors with Associated Features section of this chapter. Another X-linked myopia family has been reported in which myopia, astigmatism, optic nerve hypoplasia, deuteranopia, and decreased best corrected vision was found.[17] This may represent a distinct syndrome.

A cross-sectional volunteer sample of 716 school children in the first, third, and sixth grades done in Orinda, California, found that of children with two myopic parents, 12.2% were myopic.[31] Of the children with one myopic parent, 8.2% were myopic, and of children with no myopic parents, only 2.7% were myopic. In children not myopic at the start of the study, 11% of those with two myopic parents became myopic over the 3-year study period. Only 5% of those with one myopic parent and 1.9% of those with no myopic parents became myopic over the same time period. In addition, children with a family history of myopia had, on average, less hyperopia, deeper anterior chambers, and longer vitreous chambers even before they became myopic. All of this implies a strong role for genetics in the initial shape and subsequent growth of the eye in myopia. However, using time spent at work as an additional predictive factor significantly improved the predictive value.[31]

Although these data are unique and important, they have several shortcomings. Parental refractive error was determined by a questionnaire, and the sample was overwhelmingly Caucasian. As will be seen in subsequent sections, myopia in Asians tends to be associated with a different ocular configuration than Caucasians, and prevalence among Caucasians, Asians, and blacks differs widely enough to postulate different mechanisms and patterns, making these study results ungeneralizable.

Of 1319 parents enrolled in the Framingham Offspring Eye Study, 1585 offspring had eye examinations over a 3-year period to examine correlation of myopic refraction between siblings.[30] There was a high correlation of myopic refractive error between siblings, but this association decreased with increasing age difference between siblings. This seems to suggest an environmental effect that siblings closer in age would be more likely to have in common.

In a study on Eskimos from Greenland it was found that the individual components of refraction were highly heritable, but overall refraction was not. Lens power was the only factor not measured in this study and thus it appears that changes in lens size or shape caused the discordance in refraction.[2]

Astigmatism

Sorsby[27] considers high astigmatism an abortive form of keratoconus. There are published pedigrees of both autosomal dominant and autosomal recessive inheritance. Sorsby[27] notes that in many patients with classic keratoconus in one eye, there is a high degree of astigmatism in the other and that in some pedigrees certain members have keratoconus whereas others have simple astigmatism. Few other studies are available.

Anisometropia

Significant anisometropia is most often the result of differences in axial length between the two eyes.[27] This is usually sporadic but at least two pedigrees have been published that demonstrate Mendelian inheritance; in one, twin sisters had anisometropia and one twin had a daughter with similar anisometropia. In the other, 3 of 11 siblings of nonconsanguineous parents had high anisomyopia.[27] In other monozygotic twins, mirror-image anisomyopia has been reported. In rare cases anisometropia is caused by a global congenital defect of one eye such as Peters' anomaly, persistent hyperplastic primary vitreous (PHPV), or unilateral caratact with microphthalmia. These are usually sporadic conditions when unilateral.

POPULATION STUDIES

People with ancestors from the same geographic region generally share many of the same genes, and thus have physical features in common. With the advent of rapid transportation and immigration/emigration, these genetic types are no longer clustered as tightly as previously, but certain genetic traits can be traced back to an ancestral region or group of people. Although some inherited or genetic conditions, such as schizophrenia and Down syndrome, occur equally in all populations, others, such as sickle cell disease in Africans, juvenile X-linked retinoschisis in Finns, Tay-Sachs disease in Ashkenazi Jews, and Avellino corneal dystrophy in Italians, are highly overrepresented in certain groups. In some cases, this is because the heterozygous state confers an advantage. For example, sickle cell disease carriers (heterozygotes) are more resistant than normals to malaria, which was endemic in certain geographic regions. Thus, sickle cell hemoglobinopathy is not restricted to people of a certain skin color or race, but to people with ancestors in this geographic region. In other cases a founder effect explains the prevalence. If a carrier of an X-linked or autosomal dominant disorder happens to be one of a few settlers of a small community and produced many offspring, that community will be relatively enriched with that particular mutation. Dominant disorders such as North Carolina macular dystrophy and Nougaret congenital stationary night blindness are in this group. Similarly, if a small group of people become geographically or socially isolated and thus have consanguineous matings as was true of the Ashkenazi Jewish settlers in the Pale,[13] recessive disorders become more prevalent in that community.

Refractive errors fall into the category of disorders that vary greatly from population to population. Because people from the same geographic region share similar genes, this is an argument for the strong genetic role in the development of refractive errors. On the other hand, people in the same geographic region also share the same diet, climate, and living conditions by and large. As we shall see, population studies of refractive errors have also demonstrated the important role of these nongenetic factors.

The best studied refractive error across various populations and ethnic groups is myopia. In the 1920s Sorsby set out to investigate whether Jews in London had a higher prevalence of myopia than the general population. An article written by other authors of the era proposed this to be the case and suggested that Jewish immigrants were less fit for English society because of it; Goodman[13] feels Sorsby's study may have been an attempt to counteract this. In fact, after careful study, Sorsby did find an increased prevalence of myopia among Jewish boys who spent long hours studying. He did not state that this was the cause. However, this set into motion several elegant studies of myopia in different populations and among family members as well as the role of near work in its development.

Populations may be assigned to a "racial group" based on anthropomorphic features (skin color, hair type, etc.), polymorphic gene frequencies (such as blood groups that roughly divide people into three major categories), and rare or special characteristics or genetic subtypes that occur in only one ethnic group. However, individuals cannot readily be assigned to a "race" in the scientific sense. Thus, all studies of refractive error are flawed by judgments of group assignment. In addition, since the refractive state changes with age, many studies are not comparable due to different groups studied, or combinations of ages within the group. Finally, in children and young adults, accommodation plays an important role in the measurement of refractive error. Since a 10-year-old child has 14D of accommodation, if cycloplegia were not used, or were incomplete, a false "myopia" of up to −14.00D might be recorded. Some studies did not use cycloplegia, and others do not state whether or not it was used. By the same token, any study that does not use adequate cycloplegia of its subjects will grossly underestimate hyperopia in any pediatric population. In spite of these many shortcomings, a few very clear trends are present in studies of refractive error in populations: Jewish people tend to have a higher prevalence of myopia than the non-Jewish population of the same area. Sorsby's[27] study in Britain found 33.5% of Jewish children 10–14 years of age to be myopic. He found the prevalence of myopia to be one-third lower in non-Jewish children. The male to female ratio was 2 : 1 for Jews. Asians, particularly Chinese and Japanese, have a much higher prevalence of myopia than Caucasians or blacks with average frequencies of 50%, 26%, and 12.5%, respectively.[9] Unlike Caucasian myopic eyes that tend to have deep anterior chambers, Asian eyes with myopia usually have shallow anterior chambers. Finally, females have significantly higher rates of pathologic or high myopia than males, with a ratio of 4.2% : 1% in Denmark and 1% : 0.4% in the United States.[9]

These data support the strong role that genetics and inheritance play in refractive errors as presumably people in these various racial, ethnic, or gender groups share common genes. However, several other interesting factors must be considered.

A recent study of myopia in young Jewish adults showed a striking prevalence of high myopia in young Jewish men who are Orthodox and studied the Talmud, a book with tiny print, many hours a day.[33] The next highest prevalence was in males who studied at the Yeshiva, but fewer hours a day. The lowest prevalence of myopia found was in girls who, in this traditional society, studied far less. These data confirm the higher prevalence of myopia in Jewish males that Sorsby found. They are at odds with the sex distribution data from other populations where there was equal distribution of low myopia among males and females, and a female predominance for high myopia. These data are in agreement with the many studies that have demonstrated a correlation between myopia and the number of years spent in school, number of reading hours per day, certain occupations, and higher reading test scores.[9]

Rosner and Belkin[24] found that in U.S. males years of schooling and intelligence level weigh equally in association with myopia by regression analysis. Teasdale et al.[28] found the same for 18-year-old Danish males and further noted no correlation between amount of myopia and degree of intelligence or years of schooling (i.e., higher myopia did not correlate with higher intelligence, only presence of *any* myopia). The Framingham Offspring Eye Study Group found that among males both age and years of education were related to myopia, whereas among females age was, but years of education was not.[30] Thus, in evaluating population data, the nature–nurture debate is still very much alive and shared activities as well as shared genes may play a role.

The higher rates of myopia in Asians are indisputable, but the rates have increased over time in Japan, corresponding to increasing industrialization. The prevalence is also highest in university students, who do a lot of close work, with 81% of this group exhibiting myopia.[9]

Eskimos had almost no myopia (<1%) when a study was first done in 1950.[6] Lifestyle was mostly rural and many areas did not use electric lights. Myopia rose to 30%–36% or higher over the succeeding years in which diet changed, school became prevalent, and electric lighting became available.[9] The genetic background of the people did not change. The myopia was found in young Eskimos but not adults.

There is also an association between myopia and early menarche in women.[9] Thus, estrogen levels or other hormonal factors may be involved, rather than a specific gene on the X chromosome.

Twin Studies

Dizygotic or fraternal twins are the result of two eggs fertilized by two sperm in which both happen to implant and grow in the uterus at the same time. Monozygotic or identical twins are the result of one fertilized egg that subsequently divides into two separate embryos. Thus, dizygotic twins do not share more genetic material than any other two siblings. Monozygotic twins have identical genes and thus, if refraction is genetically determined in the main, should have identical refractions.

Jablonski (cited by Sorsby[27]), in 1922, undertook the first study of refractive errors in 28 pairs of monozygotic twins and used 23 pairs of dizygotic twins as controls.[27] He found a startling concordance of myopia, hyperopia, emmetropia, or astigmatism between monozygotic twins. This was not the case in dizygotic twins.

The most important study of refraction in twins was done by Sorsby.[27] He studied 78 pairs of monozygotic twins, 40 pairs of same sex dizygotic twins, and 48 pairs of unselected control pairs with regard to all of the individual components of refraction, as well as refractive error. For the monozygotic twins, concordance was very high for all components as well as total refractions: 70.6% for refraction, 66.7% for anterior chamber (A/C) depth, 70.5% for lens thickness, and 83.3% for axial length. There was little difference in concordance whether the twins were emmetropic, myopic or hyperopic. In the other two groups there was only minimal concordance for refraction or its components, and even when there was concordance for refraction, the components did not correlate.

In reviewing several studies of refraction in monozygotic twins, Curtin[9] noted that up to 2.00D of difference in refraction may be present between identical twins, but two separate studies found that 90% of twins' refractions did not differ by more than 1.00D. Sorsby and Meyer-Schwickerath (cited by Sorsby[27]) noted that the greatest concordance between monozygotic twins occurred in those with refractions closest to emmetropia.[27] Several studies have reported monozygotic twin pairs in which one twin was emmetropic and the other a moderate (up to −5.50D) myope. We have also seen such twin pairs, but in our experience many such twin pairs were born prematurely and the more myopic twin was the smaller twin with worse retinopathy of prematurity, usually treated with cryotherapy or laser (personal data).

Importantly, studies of monozygotic twins reared apart found no difference in the amount of myopia between twins who did a lot of near work and those who did not.[9] However, the difference between the refractions of emmetropic twins was 0.14D+/−0.02D, whereas the difference between myopic twins' refraction averaged 3.08D ± 0.53D, a 20× increase in variability. This suggests an environmental effect on an inherited predisposition. Minkovitz et al.[21] found a much higher correlation of axial length, refractive error, and intraocular lens (IOL) calculation between monozygotic than dizygotic twin pairs, although even between monozygotic twins there was an average 1D difference between IOL powers for the right eye. Corneal topography, however, was not more similar between monozygotic than dizygotic twins.

REFRACTIVE ERRORS WITH ASSOCIATED FEATURES

Many studies have failed to find a correlation between height and/or weight and refractive error in otherwise normal subjects. However, Teikari[29] did find that male myopes were on average taller than male nonmyopes in his population, although no such differences were found for females. A correlation between higher IQ (intelligence quotient) and myopia, and increased level of education has been documented repeatedly as mentioned previously, though which is cause and which is effect remain unknown.

Many genetic syndromes and congenital birth defects as well as progressive systemic disorders have a high refractive error as an associated feature. A partial list is given in Table 9.1, but the full list is too extensive for this chapter. Suffice it to say that a refractive error significantly outside the norm for a patient's age should raise a red flag and other systemic associations should be sought.

Refractive errors are often associated with other ocular disorders (Table 9.2). High hyperopia predisposes to central retinal vein occlusion and angle closure glaucoma. High myopia predisposes to retinal detachment, cataract, and open-angle glaucoma. In rare cases, a refractive error may be protective; myopia lessens the risk of proliferative and nonproliferative diabetic retinopathy in some patients.[5] Anisometropia may be associated with syndromes involving asymmetric facies such as linear sebaceous nevus syndrome and hemimicrosomia or may be secondary to early onset glaucoma, asymmetric retinopathy of prematurity, or anterior segment anomalies of only one eye. In ectopia lentis and keratoconus among other bilateral disorders, progression is often asymmetric and may lead to anisometropia. This can cause dense amblyopia if not detected and treated early in life.

Peripapillary myelinated nerve fibers are associated with high myopia in the affected eye in some patients causing marked anisometropia. This induces both organic and anisometropic

Table 9.1. Systemic Conditions Associated with Refractive Errors

Hyperopia	Myopia	Astigmatism	Anisometropia
WAGR*	Down syndrome	Craniosynostosis/Crouzon syndrome	Linear nevus sebaceous
Albinism	Sticker syndrome	Down syndrome (keratoconus)	Hemifacial microsomia
Senior-Loken syndrome	Spondyloepiphyseal dysplasia congenita	Ehlers-Danlos syndrome (keratoconus)	Sturge-Weber syndrome
	Fabry disease	Bardet-Biedl syndrome (keratoconus)	
	Ehlers-Danlos syndrome	Albinism	
	Marfan syndrome		
	Postaxial polydactyly and progressive myopia		
	Homocystinuria		

*Wilms' tumor, aniridia, growth retardation.

Table 9.2. Ocular Conditions Associated with Refractive Errors

Hyperopia	***Astigmatism***
Accommodative esotropia	Congenital ptosis
Leber's congenital amaurosis	Coloboma
Ocular albinism	Keratoconus
Myopia	Forceps injury
Retinitis pigmentosa	Eyelid hemangioma
Congenital stationary night blindness	***Anisometropia***
Achromatopsia	Myelinated nerve fibers
Microcornea	Congenital/juvenile glaucoma
Coloboma	Retinopathy of prematurity
Choroideremia	Amblyopia
Gyrate atrophy	Hemangioma of eyelid
Fundus flavimaculatus	
Progressive bifocal chorioretinal atrophy	
Myelinated nerve fibers (often unilateral)	
Wagner syndrome	
FEVR*	
Retinopathy of prematurity	
Vitreous hemorrhage in early childhood	

*Familial exudative vitreoretinopathy.

amblyopia, and best corrected vision of only 20/200 is often the best outcome possible even with contact lens therapy and amblyopia (patching) therapy.[10,18] There is no evidence for inheritance; most cases are sporadic.

Isolated ptosis as well as hemangioma of the upper eyelid have been associated with high myopia. The etiology may be the same as for deprivation or "lid suture" myopia in kittens and monkeys.[23] Ptosis may be inherited as a dominant; hemangioma is usually sporadic. Vitreous hemorrhage can also induce axial myopia in young children's eyes. Retinopathy of prematurity is associated with myopia and this type of myopia is caused largely by increases in lens thickness and only minimally by increased axial length.[14] The effect is likely environmental not genetic.

Ptosis, or brow or orbit abnormalities as seen in the various craniosynostosis syndromes can produce astigmatism. Surgery to correct ptosis may not change the cylinder and can actually increase it. Astigmatism may also be seen in conditions with a primary malformation of the cornea such as limbal or corneal dermoids, or iris colobomas. Craniosynostosis is often autosomal dominant; iris coloboma may be as well. Dermoids may be part of Goldenhar syndrome and are usually sporadic.

Waardenburg published two pedigrees of autosomal dominant inheritance of accommodative esotropia (ET), but penetrance was incomplete.[27] Some members had esophoria, others hyperopia only, and others the full accommodative ET, making polygenic inheritance likely.

We have studied two families with esotropia and hyperopia looking for correlation of refractive components.[32] In both families, refractive components of children were similar to those of parents with the exception of axial length. In one family (Fig. 9.3), the only child without esotropia was also the only myope, with an increased axial length compared to his siblings. Hyperopia correlated with ET, but ET did not resolve with full hyperopic correction. Thus, we agree with Sorsby[27] that hyperopia is probably a precipitating factor for esotropia in these fami-

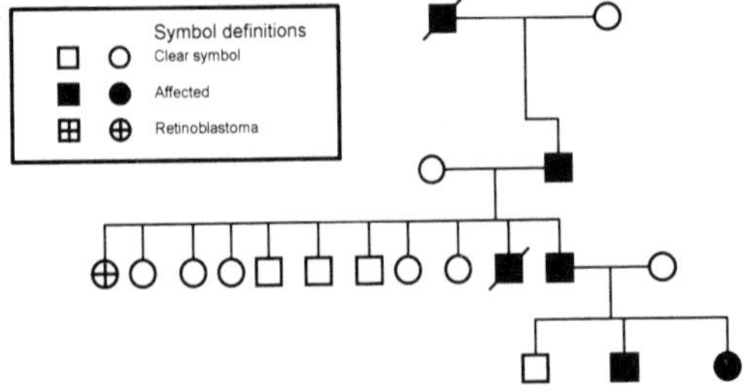

Figure 9.3. Autosomal dominant esotropia from pedigree 1.

lies, but that it may be inherited separately from another esotropia factor. In our second family (Fig. 9.4), there was probable pseudodominant inheritance. Only the mother in generation II has hyperopia and manifest esotropia. The father has esophoria and decreased stereopsis. One of the offspring in generation III has high hyperopia but no esotropia. Hyperopes in this family had short axial lengths. Thus, although hyperopia may be inherited in a Mendelian fashion, and may be most commonly caused by inheriting a short axial length, the factors that lead to esotropia do not appear to be inextricably linked, even in families where both hyperopia and esotropia occur. In addition, esophoria may have an additive genetic effect when combined with genetic factors for hyperopia and/or esotropia as seen in Waardenburg's pedigree from 1932, and our second family from 1995.

MOLECULAR GENETICS OF REFRACTIVE ERRORS

High myopia with retinal detachments associated with early onset arthropathy and characteristic radiologic findings constitute the Stickler syndrome. This autosomal dominant disorder is caused by mutations in the COL2A1 gene in about 50% of families.[1,11] This type of collagen is found in abundance in joints and vitreous, thus the myopia is caused by a vitreoretinopathy. Even in Stickler pedigrees, the amount of myopia may be variable; we have a large family with one patient and five of eight siblings affected. One child, however, has only unilateral high myopia. Thus even in cases of known genetic mutation there may be mitigating features. The role of mutations in this gene in isolated myopia is not known. Few molecular genetic studies of isolated myopia have been done. In one study when 214 patients with myopia < -6.00D and 124 patients with myopia of -6.25D to -30D were compared to normal controls regarding Rh and acid phosphatase status, a p value of <0.05 was found for low myopes for Rh status on chromosome 1 and for high myopes for acid phosphatase on chromosome 2. Although these data are difficult to interpret especially given the large mix-

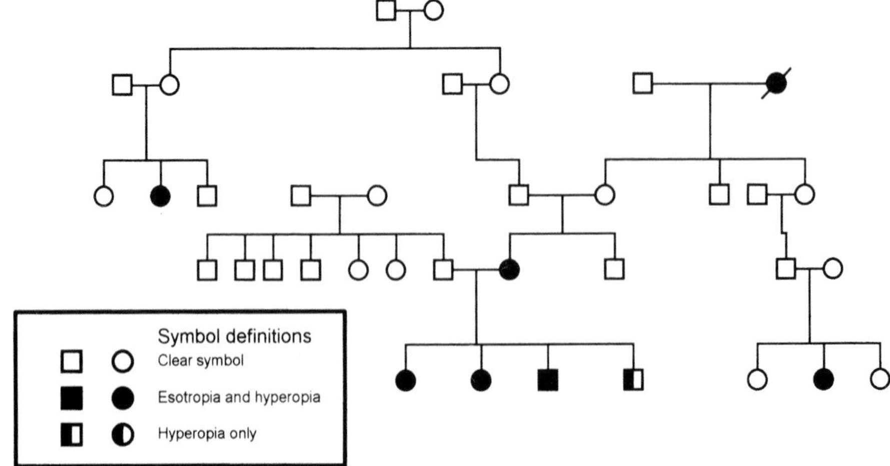

Figure 9.4. Autosomal dominant hyperopia with possible pseudodominant esotropia from pedigree 2.

ture of unrelated patients with different types of myopia in the groups, and the soft nature of these markers, they represent an attempt to use molecular genetic techniques to develop candidate loci for myopia.[22] Segregation analysis was used to explore whether a major gene, dominant or recessive, is likely to be responsible for refraction. One hundred eighty-five families of Japanese decent and 192 families of European decent all living in Hawaii were studied.[3] Parent-parent, sibling-sibling, and midparent/offspring correlations for refraction were similar to those of Sorsby discussed previously. Correlation of refraction between siblings and between midparent/offspring was again high. However, segregation analysis was not suggestive of either Mendelian dominant or recessive inheritance in either ethnic group. When myopes were separated from the general population and analyzed separately, again no Mendelian inheritance was suggested. Polygenic inheritance was also not strongly supported in either the general population or myopes. The authors therefore suggest refraction is largely determined by nongenetic factors. Although these data are very interesting, this conclusion does not agree with clinical experience in many, many cases, nor with copious twin studies.

CONCLUSIONS

Identical twin studies showing up to 90% correlation of refraction between monozygotic twins leave little doubt that the principal components of refraction are inherited. The fact that correlation is not 100%, and that the correlation weakens with ametropia, particularly high myopia, proves that refraction is not completely genetically programmed, at least not by a single gene. Other intrauterine, polygenic, or environmental influences certainly play a role. Refractive errors of all types can be inherited in a simple Mendelian fashion in some families. Even in such families, however, the degree of ametropia may vary widely among affected individuals.

In most people the refractive state is a complex trait. A genetic substrate is inherited and other factors act upon it. Much work is needed to elucidate the genes responsible for normal ocular component development, and the ways they change postnatally. Clues may come from genetic defects elucidated in disorders which feature refractive errors, such as Stickler syndrome. Currently, if a high refractive error is present, an associated syndrome should be sought. If the refractive error appears to be isolated, signs of other ocular disorders should be sought. A careful family history may reveal the inheritance pattern of isolated refractive errors for a given family. If none is apparent, patients must be informed that while simple Mendelian frequencies cannot be given, cases of X-linked, autosomal recessive, and autosomal dominant transmission have been reported for almost every type of refractive error and cannot be ruled out for a single individual. Myopes in particular tend to have myopic children, and hyperopes, especially those with esophorias, may impart increased risk of ET to their offspring. The relationship between astigmatism and keratoconus is not well known, but given the pedigrees available it seems prudent to discourage eye rubbing in families with high astigmatism since this has been linked with keratoconus development. In all eye conditions, early recognition and treatment in childhood help make normal vision possible and early examination may prevent amblyopia in those with a family history of refractive errors.

REFERENCES

1. Ahmad NN, Ala-Kokko L, Knowlton RG, et al. Stop codon in the procollagen II gene (COL2A1) in a family with Stickler syndrome. *Proc Natl Acad Sci USA* 1991;88:6624–6627.
2. Alsbirk PH. Specular change in anterior chamber depth, a refractive component of high heritability. *Doc Ophthalmol* 1980;28:53.
3. Ashton GC. Segregation analysis of ocular refraction and myopia. *Hum Hered* 1985;35: 232–239.
4. Atkinson J, Braddick OJ, Durden K, et al. Screening for refractive error in 6–9-month-old infants by photorefraction. *Br J Ophthalmol* 1984;68:105–112.
5. Baker RS, Rand LT, Krolewski AS, et al. Influence of HLADR phenotype and myopia on the risk of nonproliferative and proliferative diabe-

tic retinopathy. *Am J Ophthalmol* 1986;102(6): 693–700.

6. Bind E. Carrying optometric services to the Eskimos of the Eastern Arctic. *Am J Optom Arch Acad Optom* 1950;47:24.
7. Brown EVL. Net average yearly change in refraction of atropinized eyes from birth to beyond middle age. *Arch Ophthalmol* 1938;19: 719–734.
8. Cook RC, Glasscock RE. Refractive and ocular findings in the newborn. *Am J Ophthalmol* 1951;34:1407–1412.
9. Curtin BJ. *The Myopias: Basic Science and Clinical Management.* New York: Harper & Row, 1985.
10. Ellis GS, Frey T, Gouterman RZ. Myelinated nerve fibers axial myopia, and refractory amblyopia: An organic disease. *J Pediatr Ophthalmol Strabismus* 1987;24(3):111–119.
11. Francomano CA, Liberfarb RM, Hirose T, et al. The Stickler syndrome: Evidence for close linkage to the structural gene for type II collagen. *Genomics* 1987;1:293–296.
12. Fulton AB, Dobson V, Salem D, et al. Cycloplegic refractions in infants and young children. *Am J Ophthalmol* 1980;90:239–247.
13. Goodman RM. *Genetic Disorders of the Jewish People.* Baltimore: Johns Hopkins University Press, 1979.
14. Gordon RA, Donzis PB. Myopia associated with retinopathy of prematurity. *Ophthalmology* 1986;93(12):1593–1598.
15. Gordon RA, Donzis PB. Refractive development of the human eye. *Arch Ophthalmol* 1986;103:785–789.
16. Gregg FM, Feinberg EB: X-linked pathologic myopia. *Ann Ophthalmol* 1992;24(8):310–312.
17. Haim M, Fledelius HC, Skarsholm. X-linked myopia in a Danish family. *Acta Ophthalmol* 1988;66(4):450–456.
18. Hittner HM, Antoszyk JH: Unilateral peripapillary myelinated nerve fibers with myopia and/or amblyopia. *Arch Ophthalmol* 1987;105(7): 943–948.
19. Ingram RM. Refraction of 1 year old children after atropine refraction. *Br J Ophthalmol* 1979;63:343–347.
20. Katz M. *The Human Eye as an Optical System in Clinical Ophthalmology,* vol. 33, T. Duane, ed. Edward Jaeger, assoc. ed. Philadelphia: Harper & Row, 1985:10, 51.
21. Minkovitz JB, Essary LR, Walker RS, et al. Comparative corneal topography and refractive parameters in MZ and DZ twins. *Invest Ophthalmol Vis Sci* (Suppl) 1993;34:Abstract #2531.
22. Olmedo MV, Munoz JI, Rodriquez-Cid A, et al. Two different genetic markers for high and low myopia. *Eur J Ophthalmol* 1995;2(4):196–199.
23. Raviola E, Wiesel TN. An animal model of myopia. *N Engl J Med* 1985;312(25):1615.
24. Rosner M, Belkin M. Intelligence, education and myopia in males. *Arch Ophthalmol* 1987; 105(11):1508–1511.
25. Slataper FJ. Age norms of refraction and vision. *Arch Ophthalmol* 1950;43:466–481.
26. Sorsby A, Benjamin B, Sheridan M. Refraction and its components during the growth of the eye from the age of 3 years. In *Medical Research Council (Great Britain) Special Report Series No. 301.* London: Medical Research Council, 1961:1–67.
27. Sorsby A. *Ophthalmic Genetics,* 2nd ed. London: Butterworths, 1970.
28. Teasdale TW, Fuchs J, Goldschmidt E. Degree of myopia in relation to intelligence and education level. *Lancet* 1988;2(8624):1351–1354.
29. Teikari JM. Myopia and stature. *Acta Ophthalmol* 1987;65(6):673–676.
30. Framingham Offspring Eye Study Group. Familial aggregation and prevalence of myopia in the Framingham Offspring Eye Study. *Arch Ophthalmol* 1996;114:326–332.
31. Zadnik K, Satariano WA, Mutti DO, et al. The effect of parental history of myopia on children's eye size. *JAMA* 1994;271(17):1323–1327.
32. Zummo A, Drack A. Autosomal dominant congenital esotropia. Posters presented at Association for Research in Vision and Ophthalmology and American Association for Pediatric Ophthalmology and Strabismus Annual Meetings, 1995.
33. Zylbermann R, Landau D, Berson D. The influence of study habits on myopia in Jewish teenagers. *J Pediatr Ophthalmol Strabismus* 1993;30:319–322.

II.

Hereditary Disorders of the Anterior Segment of the Eye

10

Congenital Glaucoma

DAVID S. WALTON

Children may be born with glaucoma caused by primary, often hereditary defects in the aqueous filtration system, or they may develop this disease as a consequence of other ocular abnormalities or genetic syndromes (Table 10.1). If clinical findings such as buphthalmos or breaks in Descemet's membrane are present, an early onset of glaucoma is suggested and the term *congenital glaucoma* is commonly used, even when the disease is recognized later in the first year of life or thereafter. The use of other terms such as *infantile glaucoma, late-recognized infantile glaucoma,* and *juvenile glaucoma* often relates to the time of recognition of the clinical problem, and they are less descriptive of the underlying pathologic defect.

The most common type of infantile glaucoma is primary congenital open-angle glaucoma (PCOAG). The medical literature on this disease became abundant following its recognition as a subtype of glaucoma in the nineteenth century and includes an excellent review by DeLuise and Anderson.[3]

CLINICAL MANIFESTATIONS

Congenital glaucoma may not be easily recognized at birth if it is associated with only mild ocular anterior segment abnormalities and minimal symptomatology. Symptoms and signs are highly variable, but there is typically abnormal light sensitivity, squinting of the eyelids, and epiphora with exposure to even normal levels of light. In contrast, some children may be completely asymptomatic, especially during the first few months of life. Symptoms generally worsen slowly, but a remittent course is not unusual.

Infants are often initially referred for evaluation of corneal haze or opacification (Fig. 10.1). The corneal defects are secondary to the unsuspected elevated intraocular pressure. Progressive enlargement of the cornea and anterior segment occurs and is typically associated with stromal opacification and horizontal breaks in Descemet's membrane (Haab striae). Abnormal deepening of the anterior chamber is a constant finding. With progression of untreated congenital glaucoma, there is increasing myopia with eventual extreme enlargement of the globe, and in some patients permanent corneal scarring and dislocation of the lens. There is temporal cupping of the optic disk early in the first year of life and advanced circumferential cupping in patients with persistent elevation of intraocular pressure.

The severity of PCOAG is estimated in terms of the magnitude of the anterior segment devel-

Table 10.1. Classification of Primary and Secondary Childhood Glaucoma

I. Primary glaucomas
  A. Congenital open-angle glaucoma
    1. Congenital
    2. Infantile
    3. Late recognized
  B. Autosomal dominant juvenile glaucoma
  C. Primary angle-closure glaucoma
  D. Glaucoma associated with systemic abnormalities
    1. Sturge–Weber syndrome
    2. Neurofibromatosis (NF-1)
    3. Stickler syndrome
    4. Oculocerebrorenal (Lowe) syndrome
    5. Rieger syndrome
    6. Hepatocerebrorenal syndrome
    7. Marfan syndrome
    8. Rubinstein–Taybi syndrome
    9. Infantile glaucoma associated with mental retardation and paralysis
    10. Oculodentodigital dysplasia
    11. Open-angle glaucoma associated with microcornea and absence of frontal sinuses
    12. Mucopolysaccharidosis
    13. Trisomy 13
    14. Cutis marmorata telangiectasia congenita
    15. Warburg syndrome
    16. Kniest syndrome (skeletal dysplasia)
    17. Michel syndrome
    18. Nonprogressive hemiatrophy
  E. Glaucoma associated with ocular abnormalities
    1. Congenital glaucoma with iris and pupillary abnormalities
    2. Aniridia
      a. Congenital glaucoma
      b. Acquired glaucoma
    3. Congenital ocular melanosis
    4. Sclerocornea
    5. Iridotrabecular dysgenesis
    6. Peters' anomaly
    7. Iridotrabecular dysgenesis and ectropion uveae
    8. Posterior polymorphous dystrophy
    9. Idiopathic or familial elevated episcleral venous pressure
    10. Anterior corneal staphyloma
    11. Congenital microcoria with myopia
    12. Congenital hereditary endothelial dystrophy
    13. Congenital hereditary iris stromal hypoplasia
II. Secondary glaucomas
  A. Traumatic glaucoma
    1. Acute glaucoma
      a. Angle concussion
      b. Hyphema
      c. Ghost cell glaucoma
    2. Late-onset glaucoma with angle recession
    3. Arteriovenous fistula
  B. Glaucoma secondary to intraocular neoplasm
    1. Retinoblastoma
    2. Juvenile xanthogranuloma
    3. Leukemia
    4. Melanoma
    5. Melanocytoma
    6. Iris rhabdomyosarcoma
  C. Glaucoma secondary to uveitis
    1. Open-angle glaucoma
    2. Angle-blockage glaucoma
      a. Synechial angle closure
      b. Iris bombé with pupillary block
  D. Lens-induced glaucoma
    1. Subluxation-dislocation and pupillary block
      a. Marfan syndrome
      b. Homocystinuria
    2. Spherophakia and pupillary block
    3. Chronic open-angle glaucoma associated with angle defects
  E. Glaucoma secondary to surgery for congenital cataract
    1. Lens material blockage of the trabecular meshwork (acute or subacute)
    2. Pupillary block
    3. Chronic open-angle glaucoma associated with angle defects
  F. Steroid-induced glaucoma
  G. Glaucoma secondary to rubeosis
    1. Retinoblastoma
    2. Coats disease
    3. Medulloepithelioma
    4. Familial exudative vitreoretinopathy
  H. Secondary angle-closure glaucoma
    1. Retinopathy of prematurity
    2. Microphthalmos
    3. Nanophthalmos
    4. Retinoblastoma
    5. Persistent hyperplastic primary vitreous
    6. Congenital pupillary iris–lens membrane
  I. Glaucoma associated with increased venous pressure
    1. Carotid or dural-venous fistula
    2. Orbital disease
  J. Glaucoma secondary to maternal rubella
  K. Glaucoma secondary to intraocular infection
    1. Acute recurrent toxoplasmosis
    2. Acute herpetic iritis
  L. Malignant glaucoma

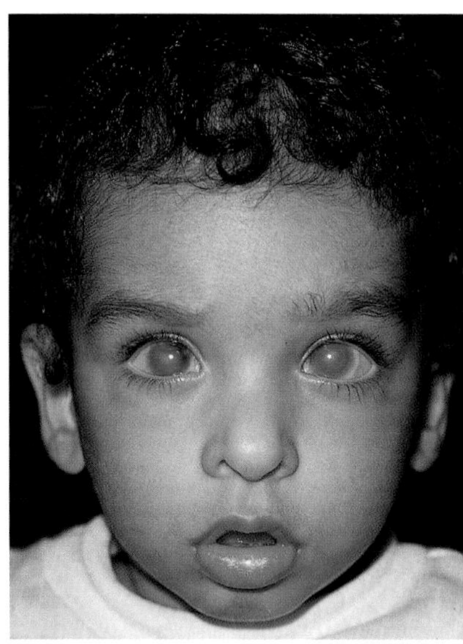

Figure 10.1. Patient with bilateral congenital glaucoma, buphthalmos, and corneal opacification.

opmental defects and of the functional abnormalities caused by the elevated intraocular pressure. Infants with severe primary anatomic defects are often recognized in the newborn period. Other patients, in contrast, may not have their glaucoma recognized for years, even into the second decade of life, and may have only moderate visual loss secondary to the disease process. The extremely variable manifestations of this disease cannot be overemphasized. When PCOAG is severe, cloudy and enlarged corneas are present in the newborn child and there is bilateral ocular involvement. The anterior chambers are deep, and gonioscopy reveals little evidence of filtration angle structures. The iris appears to insert anteriorly into the peripheral cornea. In some patients careful inspection will reveal evidence of a narrowed trabecular meshwork. No scleral spur or ciliary body band is evident. There are no abnormal iris processes or exaggeration of Schwalbe's line. The irides are often abnormal in patients with severe PCOAG. The iris leaf appears straight and does not have the normal convexity over the lens. The stroma is thin and lacks the normal development of crypts. Fine, radial blood vessels are often present in the iris, but none are visualized in the angle except at the iris root, where they are often seen to knuckle posteriorly. An almost constant finding in eyes with severe PCOAG is enlargement of the pupil, which can be so large as to mimic aniridia in one or both eyes. Such abnormal pupils react normally to light. A narrow ectropion of the iris frill is typically present and is often the most easily recognized pupillary–iris defect through the cloudy cornea.

Most children with PCOAG, however, have mild or only moderate anterior segment abnormalities. The cornea is moderately enlarged with diffuse epithelial edema. Localized corneal opacification at the level of Descemet's membrane and into the posterior stroma is generally associated with a break in Descemet's membrane. The iris and pupils are normal. There are no characteristic gonioscopic findings. Schwalbe's line is unremarkable and the trabecular meshwork appears normal. The scleral spur is often not definable in several circumferential meridians. the ciliary body band is abnormally translucent, suggesting thickening or increased opacification. In some patients, the ciliary body band may be narrowed but there is no anterior insertion of the iris. Gonioscopic abnormalities are nearly always bilateral, even in patients with unilateral glaucoma. The elevated intraocular pressure in patients with PCOAG is also capable of spontaneous normalization. Such patients present with corneal enlargement, breaks in Descemet's membrane, angle defects, optic nerve abnormalities, and a normal intraocular pressure.

The assessment of intraocular pressure in infants and children is often challenging, producing variable results when measurements are performed in suboptimal conditions. Readings are falsely high in uncooperative children or are lower than their actual levels in children examined under general anesthesia. Several pieces of information should be obtained in patients with suspected PCOAG: reliable intraocular pressure (IOP) measurements, careful assessment of the primary ocular defects by biomicroscopy and gonioscopy, and evaluation for secondary abnormalities such as high errors of refraction and amblyopia.

DIFFERENTIAL DIAGNOSIS OF PRIMARY CONGENITAL OPEN-ANGLE GLAUCOMA

Young infants with cloudy corneas are appropriately evaluated for glaucoma. Older children with large cup-to-disc ratio also become glaucoma suspects. Rarely is a child discovered to have glaucoma associated with symptoms of progressive myopia or decreasing hyperopia. When an elevated eye pressure is documented and glaucoma confirmed by optic nerve head appearance and visual field defects in older children, familiarity with the causes of glaucoma in childhood helps the clinician identify potential underlying or associated conditions (Table 10.1).

Often, and because of uncertain and nonreliable IOP measurements, children without glaucoma but with cloudy corneas continue to be assessed for glaucoma. This consideration for the potential damage from untreated glaucoma is appropriate, but it is more important to consider other conditions that cause cloudy corneas in children without glaucoma (Table 10.2).

Table 10.2. Causes of Pediatric Cloudy Corneas

Glaucomas
Birth trauma
Metabolic disease
Niemann–Pick disease
Mucopolysaccharidosis
Mucolipidosis
Generalized gangliosidosis
Cystinosis
Hypovitaminosis A
Corneal disease
Posterior polymorphous dystrophy
Peters' anomaly
Anterior staphyloma
Keratitis
Neurotrophic keratitis
Hereditary endothelial dystrophy
Sclerocornea

EPIDEMIOLOGY OF CONGENITAL PRIMARY OPEN-ANGLE GLAUCOMA

Primary congenital open-angle glaucoma is rare, with a reported incidence of 1 : 10,000 patients seen for ophthalmologic care.[12] In the Middle East, PCOAG is much more common than in Western societies, with an estimated incidence of 1 : 2500 births.[10] Most cases are sporadic, without a family history of the disease. Approximately 75% of patients have bilateral glaucoma.[3] Patients diagnosed in the newborn period typically have bilateral and more severe disease, whereas patients recognized later in life more frequently have unilateral milder glaucoma. In the United States and Europe the disease has been found more frequently in males but has been reported more frequently in Japanese girls.[3,17]

GENETICS

There is a consensus that primary congenital chronic open-angle glaucoma is inherited. There is also evidence of genetic heterogeneity given the occurrence of the disease in diverse clinical settings with, and without, associated systemic disease (Table 10.1). Nongenetic primary congenital glaucoma, for example, occurs in congenital rubella or in association with Sturge–Weber syndrome.

The mode of inheritance of primary congenital open-angle glaucoma remains uncertain in many cases. Analysis of families has suggested recessive, dominant, multifactorial, and polygenic inheritance.[4,7,7a,14] Review of 344 families with at least one member with congenital glaucoma revealed 36 families with at least one other affected first-degree relative.[5] Twenty-four families had affected siblings; 11 families, affected parents; and 1 family, affected sibling and parent.[5] Analysis of these families suggested genetic heterogeneity and polygenic inheritance. In a review of 67 Arab patients cared for in Jerusalem, a family history of an affected sibling was given in 9 of 67 (13%) patients with no involvement of parents or grandparents.[6] Consanguinity was present in approximately one-half of the families, suggesting autosomal recessive inheritance. In another review of 64 families, 9 (14%) had more than one affected member, including 3 parents, 4 siblings, and 2 monozygotic twins.[14] An equal occurrence in parents and siblings and absence in distant relatives suggested multifactorial inheritance. The occurrence of both bilateral and unilateral PCOAG in sets of twins has been repeatedly described.[15] Human leukocyte antigen (HLA) histocompatibility studies have revealed inconsistent results when patients with primary congenital glaucoma were compared to unrelated controls.[9,11] Steroid testing of parents of children affected with primary congenital glaucoma and matched controls suggested that the genetic carrier state for infantile glaucoma is not related to open-angle adult glaucoma.[17]

Congenital glaucoma has been reported in association with numerous chromosomal abnormalities. Defects have included trisomy 13, 14, 18, and 21 and monosomy 10p−, 13q−, 18q−, 45X, 46XX, 46YY, as well as numerous occurrences of balanced translocation.[2,8,16]

After excluding two candidate regions on chromosomes 6p and 11,[1,1a] Sarfarazi and coworkers[15a] mapped one gene (GLC3A) for autosomal recessive primary congenital glaucoma to 2p21 in 11 of 17 Turkish families. The same investigators later identified the location of another gene (GLC3B) at 1p36, and presented evidence for at least one more genetic locus for primary congenital glaucoma.[1b] The human cytochrome P4501B1 gene (*CYP1B1*) had been mapped to the 2p21 region and was analyzed by Stoilov and co-workers[16a] for mutations in patients with GLC3A. Homozygous frameshift mutations resulting in null alleles were found in five families and the gene was expressed in the trabecular meshwork.[16a]

Reports of large series often give little information about individual patients included under the broad classification of congenital glaucoma. When reviewing descriptions of patients and families with primary congenital open-angle glaucoma, or when classifying one's own patients, it is important to carefully evaluate the anterior segment findings associated with the glaucoma. This permits the recognition of such entities as iris hypoplasia and glaucoma with angle dysgenesis and associated iris defects, both of which are most often inherited in an autosomal dominant fashion.

Severe primary congenital glaucoma of the newborn should probably not be grouped with the less severe glaucoma recognized later in infancy. The occurence of both types in siblings, however, suggests that these disorders are variable expressions of a common genetic defect (Walton, personal observation).

The recurrence risk in siblings may be as high as 25%, especially if parents are consanguineous. The recurrence risk in offspring is probably low unless the glaucoma is a manifestation of an autosomal dominant anterior segment dysgenic syndrome.

TREATMENT OF PRIMARY CONGENITAL OPEN-ANGLE GLAUCOMA

Treatment should be initiated promptly after the diagnosis is established. Medical treatment will often decrease the intraocular pressure but will rarely control it satisfactorily. Surgery is hence indicated to effect permanent reduction of the intraocular pressure.

Medical treatment consists of agents that decrease the rate of aqueous humor formation. Acetazolamide given by mouth (15 mg/kg/day) is the most effective initial therapy. Dorzolamide, a topical carbonic anhydrase inhibitor, also deserves consideration; one drop is given two to three times per day. Topical beta blockers also suppress aqueous formation and may be of help; they are given in addition to the topical or systemic carbonic anhydrase inhibitor.

Goniosurgery, filtration surgery, and implant surgery are the three options for the management of congenital glaucoma. In goniosurgery (goniotomy, trabeculotomy), the abnormal trabeculum is incised to enhance the passage of fluid into the filtering channels. For many patients with congenital glaucoma this can be a very effective operation. Children with more severe defects of the filtration channels often do not respond to goniosurgery, and filtration procedures may be required to bypass the malfunctioning system, creating a new egress passage for the aqueous humor. The results of this type of surgery may be disappointing due to the failure of the new passage to remain patent. When the filtration angle defect is seen on gonioscopy to be mild to moderate, with a visible ciliary body band, angle survery is effective in 75% of cases. Repeat surgery in an unoperated area may be necessary to achieve an adequate lowering of the eye pressure. In case of failure of classic filtration surgery, implants (Molteno, Ahmed, others) may be used to drain the aqueous fluid from the eye by way of a silicone tube to an episcleral reservoir.

Treatment of congenital glaucoma is difficult, specialized, and sometimes disappointing. With persistent careful monitoring, however, the outcome of therapy can be viewed with guarded optimism. Attention to occlusion therapy and correction of optical defects are important to prevent amblyopia. Genetic counseling is essential and should rely on the individual family structure and general available statistics.

REFERENCES

1. Akarsu AN, Turacli ME, Houssain A, Barsoum-Homsy M, Chevrette L, Aktan G, Sarfarazi M. Genetic linkage study of primary congenital glaucoma (abstract). *Invest Ophthalmol Vis Sci* 1995;36:abstract #2577.

1a. Akarsu AN, Turacli ME, Aktan SG, Hossain A, Barsoum-Homsy M, Chevrette L, Sayli BS, Sarfarazi M. Exclusion of primary congenital glaucoma (buphthalmos) from two candidate regions of chromosome arm 6p and chromosome 11. *Am J Med Genet* 1996;61:290–292.

1b. Akarsu AN, Turacli ME, Aktan SG, Barsoum-Homsy M, Chevrette L, Sayli BS, Sarfarazi M. A second locus (GLC3B) for primary congenital glaucoma (buphthalmos) maps to the 1p36 region. *Hum Mol Genet* 1996;5:1199–1203.

2. Boughton WL, Rosenbaum KN, Beauchamp GR. Congenital glaucoma and other ocular abnormalities associated with pericentric inversion of chromosome 11. *Arch Ophthalmol* 1983;101:594–597.

3. DeLuise VP, Anderson DR. Primary infantile glaucoma (congenital glaucoma). *Surv Ophthalmol* 1983;28:1–19.

4. Demenais F, Bonaiti C, Briard ML, Feingold J, Frezal J. Congenital glaucoma. Genetic models. *Hum Genet* 1979;46:305–317.

5. Demenais F, Elston RC, Bonaiti C, Briard ML, Kaplan EB, Namboodini KK. Segregation analysis of congenital glaucoma: Approach by 2 different models. *Am J Hum Genet* 1981; 33:300–306.

6. Elder MJ. Congenital glaucoma in the West Bank and Gaza Strip. *Br J Ophthalmol* 1993; 77:413–416.

7. Gencik A, Gencikova A, Gerince A. Genetic heterogeneity of congenital glaucoma. *Clin Genet* 1980;17:241.

7a. Gencik A. Epidemiology and genetics of primary congenital galucoma in Slovakia. Description of a form of primary glaucoma in gypsies with autosomal recessive inheritance and complete penetrance. *Dev Ophthalmol* 1989;16: 76–115.

8. Gustavson AU, Berggren L, Svedberg B, Tornquist P. Congenital glaucoma resulting from a chromosomal translocation. *Acta Ophthalmol* 1992;70:285–288.

9. Hvidberg A, Kessing V, Svejgaard D. HLA histocompatibility antigens in primary congenital glaucoma. *Glaucoma* 1979;1:134–136.

10. Jaafar MS. Care of infantile glaucoma patients. In *Ophthalmology Annual*, R. D. Reinecke, ed. New York; Raven Press, 1988:15.

11. Kumar R, Ararwal H, Murthy H, Vaidya C, Sood NA. Histocompatibility antigens in Indian patients with congenital glaucoma. *Glaucoma* 1991;13:171–173.

12. Lehrfeld L, Reber J. Glaucoma at the Wells Hospital (1925–1935). *Arch Ophthalmol* 1937; 18:712–738.

13. Leighton DA, Phillips CI. Infantile glaucoma: Steroid testing in parents of affected children. *Br J Ophthalmol* 1970;54:27–30.

14. Merin S, Morin D. Heredity of congenital glaucoma. *Br J Ophthalmol* 1972;56:414–417.

15. Rasmussen DH, Ellis PP. Congenital glaucoma in identical twins. *Arch Ophthalmol* 1970;84: 827–830.

15a. Sarfarazi M, Akarsu AN, Hossain A, Turacli E, Aktan SG, Barsoum-Homsy M, Chevrette L, Sayli BS. Assignment of a locus (GLC3A) for primary congenital glaucoma (buphthalmos) to 2p21 and evidence for genetic heterogeneity. *Genomics* 1995;30:171–177.

16. Stambolian D, Quin G, Emanuel BS, Zackai E. Congenital glaucoma associated with chromosomal abnormality. *Am J Ophthalmol* 1988;106:625–627.

16a. Stoilov I, Akarsu AN, Sarfarazi M. Identification of three different truncating mutations in cytochrome P4501B1 (*CYP1B1*) as the principal cause of primary congenital glaucoma (buphthalmos) in families linked to the GLC3A locus on chromosome 2p21. *Hum Mol Genet* 1997;6:641–647.

11

Genetics of Open-Angle Glaucoma

JANEY L. WIGGS

The primary open-angle glaucomas are those forms of the disorder that are not associated with other anatomical abnormalities of the eye or with other physiologic phenomena of the eye, nor do they result from ocular manifestations of systemic disease. Primary open-angle glaucoma can be divided into two main subtypes according to age of onset: juvenile open-angle glaucoma (JOAG), which generally develops before the age of 40, and adult-onset open-angle glaucoma (usually abbreviated COAG, or POAG), which generally develops after the age of 40. Genetic factors have been determined to be at least partly responsible for these disorders, suggesting that specific gene defects may play a role in the development of the disease.

Despite many decades of research, little is known about the precise molecular defects and abnormal biochemical pathways that result in glaucoma. This is especially true for the primary glaucomas, which are not characterized by any recognizable anatomical defect. An obstruction to the outflow of aqueous humor through the trabecular meshwork is probably a major cause of the increase in intraocular pressure in open-angle glaucoma, but the processes that lead to this obstruction have not been identified.[32] Enzymes, structural proteins, and proteins involved in the embryogenesis and development of the eye may be important to the normal physiology of the trabecular meshwork, and defects in the genes coding for these proteins might play a role in the genetic predisposition to the disease.

Identifying a gene for even a rare type of glaucoma would have a dramatic impact on the diagnosis and treatment of this condition, and it would provide valuable new insights into the pathophysiology of glaucoma in general. The demonstration that the function of a particular enzyme or structural protein is impaired in patients affected with glaucoma may lead to the development of new drug therapy that could more effectively treat the disease. The description of specific DNA mutations could form the basis of diagnostic tests that would be useful in the identification of individuals at risk for glaucoma so that early detection and treatment could be accomplished. Because the destructive process created by the disease is usually painless and very gradually progressive, it often goes unnoticed by the patient until it has reached an advanced and irreversible stage. If left untreated, the disease results in absolute irreversible blindness. The availability of a test that could identify individuals at risk for glaucoma at the earliest premorbid stages of the disease, combined with effective treatment based on the specific defect causing the disorder, would greatly improve the prognosis of this condition.

JUVENILE OPEN-ANGLE GLAUCOMA

Juvenile glaucoma has been defined as a form of primary open-angle glaucoma that develops during the first two decades of life. The age of onset is variable but is typically between the ages of 3 and 20 years. Primary juvenile glaucoma has been previously classified as *true juvenile glaucoma, neglected infantile (congenital) glaucoma, presenile glaucoma,* and *angle-closure glaucoma.* The discussion in this chapter refers to the form of juvenile glaucoma previously classified as "true juvenile glaucoma." The disease process is characterized by a severe high-pressure glaucoma that can result in significant damage to the optic nerve, leaving affected individuals with little useful vision early in life. There are no known associated systemic findings.

Characteristic clinical features often include a high incidence of myopia. Affected eyes do not show signs of buphthalmos. The cornea does not demonstrate breaks in Descemet's membrane. Gonioscopy typically shows a normal appearance to the angle structures. Generally there is no evidence of increased pigment deposition in the angle or other findings consistent with the pigment dispersion syndrome. Some patients with juvenile open-angle glaucoma may have an increased number of iris processes, some of which have an anterior insertion crossing the scleral spur and posterior trabecular meshwork (Fig. 11.1). This is not a consistently identified finding, however, and these patients do not have any of the other findings associated with Axenfeld–Rieger anomaly, including posterior embryotoxon.[36] Nor do they appear to have a Barkan membrane covering the angle, as is typical of patients affected by congenital glaucoma. One histopathologic study suggested that a thick compact tissue on the anterior chamber side of Schlemm's canal was present in ten cases of juvenile glaucoma. In these ten patients, the mechanism of glaucoma was postulated to be a developmental immaturity of the trabecular meshwork.[29] Other specific anatomical abnormalities have not been identified in patients with juvenile glaucoma.

Patients affected by juvenile open-angle glaucoma develop a severe high-pressure glaucoma that usually requires surgical treatment for adequate control. Patients have been treated effectively by goniotomy and trabeculectomy, although the reports of the surgical outcomes are largely anecdotal. Comparative studies designed to determine the efficacy of various surgical procedures for the treatment

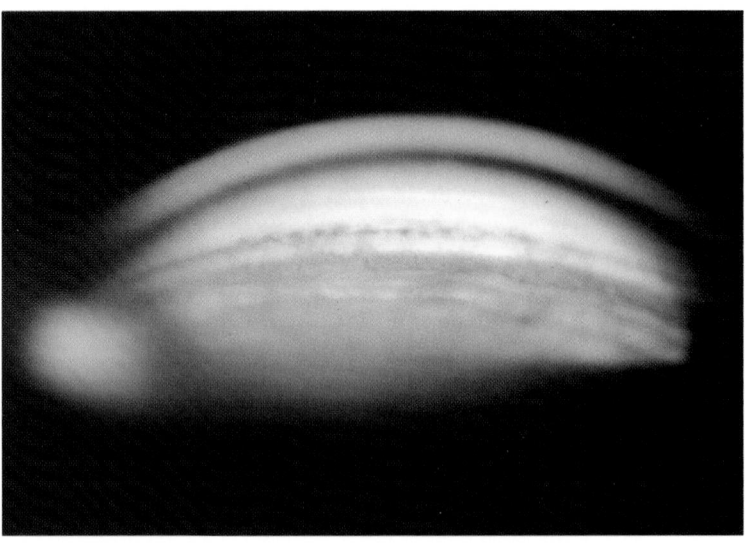

Figure 11.1. Gonioscopy of angle structures in juvenile glaucoma. Goniophotography was performed using the Humphrey–Zeiss 40 SLP slit-lamp camera.

of juvenile glaucoma have not appeared in the recent literature.

A number of pedigrees affected with juvenile open-angle glaucoma demonstrating an autosomal dominant mode of inheritance have been reported (Fig. 11.2).[1,6,8,16,17,23,27,28,35] Familial hypoplasia of the iris and unusually darkly pigmented irides (Ian of Blackberry Eyes) have also been reported associated with the glaucoma in pedigrees affected with autosomal dominant juvenile glaucoma.[33] In the pedigrees studied, the penetrance appears to approach 100% after age 20, although formal studies of penetrance have not been performed.

In a single pedigree affected with autosomal dominant juvenile glaucoma without any associated anterior segment dysgenesis, Sheffield et al., using short tandem-repeat genetic markers for genetic linkage analysis, demonstrated that a gene responsible for this condition is located within a 30 cM region on the long arm of chromosome 1 (1q21-q31).[27] This result has subsequently been confirmed by several similar studies.[16,23,35]

The chromosomal region that contains the putative gene was initially narrowed down to less than an 8 cM interval on chromosome 1.[23,27,35] Stone and co-workers investigated five candidate genes in a 3 cM region containing the gene and found three different mutations in the TIGR (trabecular meshwork-induced glucocorticoid response protein) gene in five of eight families with juvenile open-angle glaucoma, in one family with adult-onset glaucoma, and in about 3% of unselected patients with adult-onset glaucoma.[28a] The TIGR protein is expressed in trabecular meshwork and ciliary body and is postulated to cause an elevation in intraocular pressure by obstructing the outflow passages.

The extent that phenotypic heterogeneity may exist among a genetically homogeneous collection of individuals affected by glaucoma remains unknown. Substantial variability in the phenotypic expression of a single gene defect has been observed in other ocular disorders, including retinitis pigmentosa,[5] juvenile macular degeneration,[19] and aniridia.[12] To investigate the phenotypic heterogeneity of juvenile glaucoma, we have compared the clinical features identified as genetically linked to the 1q21-q31 locus of affected individuals from five affected pedigrees. The average age of diagnosis was 18.5 years (range 5–30 years), and the average initial intraocular pressure was 38.5 mm Hg (range 30–53 mm Hg). Of affected individuals, 87% were myopic and 83% required surgical treatment for glaucoma. There were no uni-

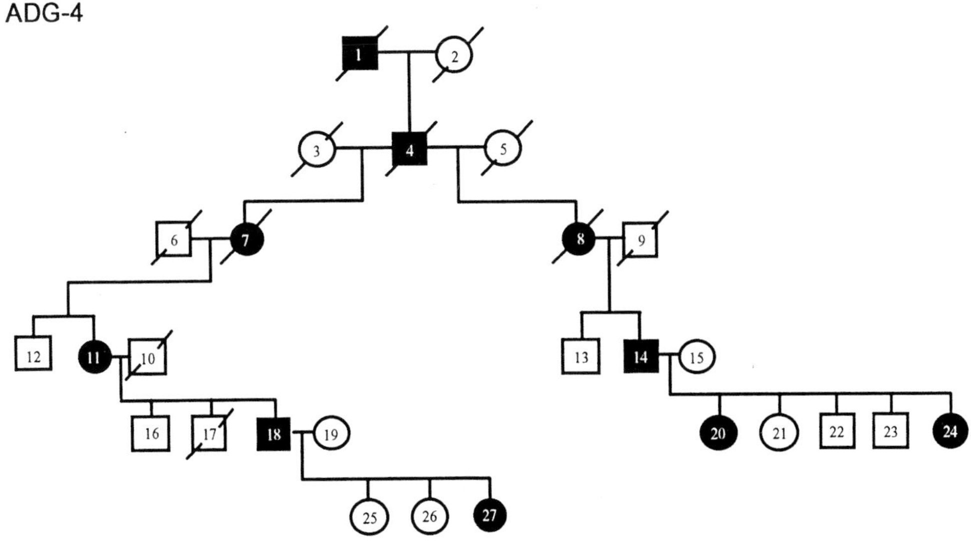

Figure 11.2. Juvenile glaucoma pedigree. Affected individuals are shown as solid circles (females) or squares (males). Deceased individuals are indicated with slashes.

formly associated systemic or ocular abnormalities.[36]

The identification of one locus containing a gene responsible for juvenile glaucoma allows the investigation of the role of that gene in other forms of glaucoma. Like juvenile glaucoma, pigmentary glaucoma affects young individuals. Thus, several investigators have speculated that pigmentary glaucoma may be related to primary open-angle glaucoma and may be a form of primary juvenile glaucoma.[4] To investigate the role of the juvenile glaucoma gene in the pigment dispersion syndrome, three pedigrees affected by the pigment dispersion syndrome and pigmentary glaucoma were identified and analyzed for genetic linkage to markers located in the chromosome 1q21-q31 region. The results of these experiments indicate that the gene responsible for the pigment dispersion syndrome is not located in this region of the human genome and that the pigment dispersion syndrome is genetically distinct from the form of juvenile glaucoma caused by the gene mapped to chromosome 1q21-q31. Recently, one locus containing a gene responsible for the pigment dispersion syndrome and pigmentary glaucoma has been mapped to 7q35-36.[4a]

Among our collection of juvenile glaucoma pedigrees genetically linked to the 1q21-q31 region, we have observed one individual who may be a nonpenetrant carrier of the disease gene. This result, together with other reports of possible reduced penetrance in juvenile glaucoma pedigrees,[18] suggests that the phenotypic expression of the glaucoma-predisposing gene may be variable. This notion is supported by the variation in severity of the disease in a pair of monozygotic twins.[36] It is possible that other genes or environmental factors may contribute to the full expression of the juvenile glaucoma gene located in the 1q21-q31 region. However, confirmation of the phenotype–genotype relationship can be accomplished only after the gene is sequenced and specific mutations are identified in affected individuals.

Two pedigrees affected by juvenile glaucoma that do not demonstrate positive linkage to genetic markers located in the 1q21-q31 region have been identified.[36] When the clinical features of these two pedigrees were compared to those that are genetically linked to 1q21-q31, two differences were noted. First, affected individuals from one of the unlinked pedigrees have early onset of the disease, associated with severe optic nerve deterioration before the age of 10. However, the affected individuals have intraocular pressures in the 25- to 30-mmHg range, rather than the very high intraocular pressures that characterize the pedigrees linked to the 1q21-q31 region.

The clinical features of the other pedigree not demonstrating linkage to the 1q21-q31 region are similar to the five linked pedigrees except that this pedigree is of African-American descent. The observation that two families affected by juvenile glaucoma are not linked to the 1q21-q31 region suggests that other gene(s) located elsewhere in the human genome are responsible for the disease process in these families. This result indicates that juvenile glaucoma may be a genetically heterogeneous disorder.

The pathogenesis of juvenile glaucoma is unknown. Because highly elevated intraocular pressure is a strikingly consistent feature of pedigrees linked to 1q21-q31, it is possible that there is defective outflow function of the trabecular meshwork in affected patients. An immediate result of the characterization of the gene product may be the identification of specific proteins in the trabecular meshwork that could be altered to create novel and possibly more effective methods to lower intraocular pressure.

ADULT-ONSET PRIMARY OPEN-ANGLE GLAUCOMA

Primary open-angle glaucoma of adult onset (POAG) is the most prevalent form of glaucoma, affecting 7 to 8 million Americans. This disease typically affects individuals after the fifth decade and results in the characteristic optic neuropathy common to all forms of glaucoma. Compelling data indicate that susceptibility to POAG is inherited; in fact, the prevalence of POAG in first-degree relatives of affected patients has been documented to be as high as 7 to 10 times that of the general population.[2,9,13,22] It is likely that the incidence of

POAG in family members of affected patients is even higher, given the older age at diagnosis and the lack of patient awareness of the disease. Patients affected by POAG are more likely to develop an increase in intraocular pressure in response to dexamethasone eye drops, and this trait has been shown to be inherited.[26] Several twin studies have suggested a high concordance of glaucoma between monozygotic twins, consistent with a significant genetic predisposition to the disease.[10,30] The higher prevalence of POAG among black Americans compared with white Americans may reflect an underlying genetic difference in susceptibility to this disorder.[31] POAG has been weakly associated with inheritance of various genetic markers, including the Duffy blood group on chromosome 1 and the inability to taste phenylthiocarbamide.[3]

Recently, loci possibly responsible for some cases of POAG have been identified on human chromosomes 3q21-24[3a] and 2cen-q13.[3b] These results are consistent with the hypothesis that a significant proportion of POAG is inherited. However, because of the complex inheritance pattern of POAG, it is likely that additional genes will be found to be associated with it.

The variability in the age of onset of the disease, the apparent incomplete penetrance of the condition in some pedigrees, and the prevalence of the disease all suggest that more than one gene may be responsible for this disorder. Patients affected by POAG also vary with respect to the relationship between increased intraocular pressure and deterioration of the optic nerve. These observations are consistent with the conclusion that POAG is not inherited as a simple single-gene disorder but as a complicated "complex trait."

Complex inherited disorders are commonly found in the human population. The genetic analysis of common conditions does not follow the Mendelian inheritance patterns of single-gene disorders. For example, a trait may be present in every generation of an affected pedigree, suggesting autosomal dominant inheritance, but less than 50% of individuals at risk for the disease actually express the disease phenotype. This pattern of inheritance is consistent with an autosomal dominant model but with incomplete penetrance of the disease trait. However, a similar pattern of inheritance can be created by an autosomal recessive trait, if a high incidence of heterozygous carriers are present in the studied population. Because the mode of inheritance (i.e., autosomal dominant versus autosomal recessive) cannot be precisely defined by the apparent segregation of the disease trait, the inheritance pattern in this example would be consistent with that of a complex trait.

Common traits have complicated patterns of inheritance for several different reasons. These disorders are phenotypic traits frequently found in the human population. This fact alone suggests that mutations in more than one gene may be responsible for a common phenotype. If mutations in different genes can independently cause a certain disease, then two individuals belonging to the same family can have the same disease phenotype but have developed the disease according to independent mechanisms that are the result of mutations in two different and unrelated genes. The genetic term that describes this phenomena is "phenocopy" and it simply means that mutations in more than one gene can result in the same phenotypic trait. The observed laws of Mendelian genetics hold only for inherited traits that are the result of mutations in single genes. When more than one gene is responsible for a certain trait, the observed frequency and transmission of that trait does not follow the segregation laws that Mendel observed for simple dominant and recessive traits.

Another factor to consider when analyzing the segregation of disease traits that follow a complex pattern is the possibility of incomplete penetrance or incomplete expression of a predisposing mutation. Penetrance is a parameter that measures the expression of a genetic mutation, or the extent that mutations in a gene result in the appearance of a specific trait. Mathematically penetrance is defined by the ratio of "disease, or expressed trait" to "genetic mutation." A trait inherited with high penetrance is found in almost every individual with a mutation in the gene responsible for that trait. Traits with low values of penetrance are found in only a fraction of the individuals who carry mutations in the gene responsible for the trait. Because every individual carrying a mutation does not reliably develop the disease trait, a reduction in penetrance can mask the actual segregation pattern of the responsible gene.

Several different mechanisms may lead to a reduction in penetrance of some inherited traits. One hypothesis invokes the role of influential environmental factors. Environmental factors can modulate the expression of a particular genetic mutation that may otherwise lie dormant. It is theoretically possible that a combination of genetic and environmental factors may be necessary for the full expression of the disease. Because the full development of the disease trait would be dependent on environmental factors as well as inherited factors, the expression of the disease trait would be variable among individuals carrying a predisposing mutation. The segregation of the predisposing mutation would follow a Mendelian pattern; however, because of the additional requirement for the contributing environmental factor, the expression of the disease trait in an affected pedigree would not necessarily follow the expected pattern for a Mendelian trait.

The full expression of a disease phenotype caused by a specific mutation in one responsible gene may also be influenced by mutations in other genes. Secondary genes responsible for the modulation of the expression of a specific genetic mutation may be referred to as "modifier genes." Modifier genes may be inherited completely independently from the gene directly responsible for the disease trait. Not every individual who inherits the mutation responsible for the disease trait will also inherit a form of the modifier gene that is required for full expression of the disease. Hence, the analysis of the segregation of the disease trait in an affected pedigree will not appear to follow the rules of simple Mendelian genetics.

Modifier genes may also lead to a reduction in expression of a mutation that otherwise could cause the full disease phenotype. This effect can also lead to a complicated or non-Mendelian pattern of inheritance. For example, a disease may be caused by mutations in a gene that is typically inherited as an autosomal dominant trait. However, if mutations in a second gene can alter the expression of the disease gene, an individual inheriting mutated forms of both genes may not develop the disease. The genetic analysis of a pedigree affected by mutations in the disease gene and the modifier gene is not likely to be consistent with an autosomal dominant or an autosomal recessive pattern.

The origins of the genetic complexity of POAG are likely to stem from the diversity of ocular tissues and cell types potentially involved in the disease process. Many studies have suggested that defects in the trabecular outflow pathways are responsible for the elevation of intraocular pressure that is associated with a majority of cases of POAG.[24] However, the cell type and biochemical processes that are altered in the disease have not yet been identified. It is possible that mutations in a number of genes encoding for different proteins can alter the normal function of the ocular outflow pathways. Many patients with elevated intraocular pressure do not develop the characteristic degeneration of the optic nerve that is the ultimate cause of blindness in these individuals.[31] Indeed, elevation of intraocular pressure is an important risk factor for the disease but does not by itself define the disease process. Individuals who do develop degeneration of the optic nerve may have sustained additional gene defects that render the retinal ganglion cell and optic nerve more susceptible to damage. The complex inheritance of POAG is likely to be, at least in part, due to the diversity of affected tissue type and function leading to phenocopy, and possibly to multigenic requirements for full expression of the disease phenotype.

Conversely, individuals with the full POAG phenotype, including optic nerve damage, may have inherited mutations that increase their vulnerability to the attack of certain environmental factors that potentially contribute to the disease process. For example, certain toxic substances, such as free radicals, may cause significant damage to the trabecular meshwork. It is possible that some individuals affected by POAG have inherited a predisposing mutation that only becomes manifest if the critical component of the trabecular meshwork receives sufficient exposure to such toxic substances. Although the predisposing mutation would follow a Mendelian inheritance pattern, the disease process would be variable among individuals at risk because of the unpredictable contribution of toxin exposure.

A challenging aspect of the genetic analysis of complex traits is the identification of genes that may be responsible for these common disorders. In examining the segregation of a disease trait that exhibits complex inheritance, one must sort out which individuals are affected because of mutations in separate genes and then wonder if the unaffected individuals are only unaffected because they have not been in the "correct" predisposing environment. Finally, the possibility of secondary or modifier genes must always be included in the analysis, especially when the penetrance of the disease trait appears low.

In general, the genetic analysis of complex traits is simpler if the pedigrees selected for the investigation are as clinically homogeneous as possible. The use of strict criteria for the definition of affected status will select for the most clinically homogeneous population, which has the greatest chance of being the most genetically homogeneous population. When possible a quantitative trait should be selected as the defining feature of the affected individuals, and any subjective component of the clinical diagnosis should be deemphasized.

The size and structure of pedigrees used for the analysis are also important to consider. In general, pedigrees composed of multiply affected generations with large subships of affected individuals provide the most genetic information. However, large pedigrees are also more likely to be plagued by an increased incidence of phenocopy, especially with phenotypic traits commonly found among the studied population.

Methods to map genes responsible for homogeneous single-gene disorders have been well defined. Recently, these methods such as traditional two-point lod score analysis have also met some success with several complex traits, such as hypertension[15] and Alzheimer disease.[21] However, the problems of reduced penetrance and genetic heterogeneity often make this approach impossible for common disorders. New statistical methods have been developed and applied to the identification of disease-susceptibility loci for complex traits. These methods include robust sibpair studies,[7,14] affected pedigree member studies[21,34] and two-trait locus linkage studies (i.e., the disease is caused by two or more genes at separate loci).[11,20,25] The important feature of these methods is they do not assume a specific model or mode of inheritance for the analyses. As stated earlier, many pedigrees affected by a complex trait demonstrate a segregation pattern that can be consistent with several models of inheritance. To perform simple two-point linkage analyses, a particular model (i.e., autosomal dominant or autosomal recessive), must be assumed. If an incorrect assumption is made, the entire analysis is erroneous and can lead to inaccurate conclusions. The ability to use statistical methods that do not require assumption of a specific model has led the way for mapping studies designed to identify genes responsible for complex traits.

Once the gene(s) responsible for POAG is mapped and characterized, it will remain a difficult task to determine the genetic risk of the disease based on the known predisposing mutations. Because multiple genes and mutations are likely to be independently responsible for the common POAG phenotype, the identification of the specific disease-causing mutation in any one individual will require screening many segments of DNA for potential defects. If mutations in ten different genes can all cause adult-onset glaucoma, then, using current technology, it will be a tedious and expensive procedure to screen all the patients at risk for the disease for mutations in all ten genes. Population studies of mutation frequency will aid this effort by identifying the more commonly responsible mutations. If a patient does not have a common mutation, then a decision regarding further testing for rarer mutations will have to be made, and ultimately the cost/benefit ratio of this decision process will have to be evaluated. Certainly for a disease such as glaucoma, where preventive therapy is available, the benefit of identifying a smaller number of rarer mutations in a fraction of the population may be worth the expense.

Assessing the risk that a person carrying a predisposing mutation will develop the disease can be difficult for a complex disorder. The development of the disease may depend on environmental as well as genetic factors, and the relative impact of contributing factors may be difficult to establish. Ultimately, the prognosis based on mutation detection will depend on further investigations into the extent that other factors may contribute to the disease process. Ideally, the penetrance values should be correlated with specific mutations, as it is possible that penetrance will vary with individual mutations. Specifically, depending on the biological process interrupted by a particular mutation, the role of environmental factors or contributing factors from other genes may vary. Correlation studies between specific genetic mutations (or genotypes) and the ultimate phenotype should define penetrances of individual mutations and will identify the mutations that are more or less susceptible to various other influences, such as environmental factors. It is possible that a mutation in one gene responsible for POAG will be very dependent on certain environmental factors for full expression, whereas another mutation will be quite insensitive to these same environmental conditions. Accurate risk assessment for the patient will be dependent on studies performed to define these features of individual mutations in the various genes that may increase the susceptibility to the disease.

Primary open-angle glaucoma is one of the leading causes of blindness worldwide. Because of its prevalence, and because of the significant morbidity caused by the disease, the genetic factors responsible for POAG will be very important to identify and characterize. In recent years human genetics has had a tremendous impact on the theory of medicine, and in years to come will likely have a similar impact on the diagnosis and treatment of inherited conditions. Human traits commonly found in the population, such as POAG, will be among the most important to understand, diagnose, and treat. Yet these common disorders are also the most challenging to study. The redundancy of responsible genes and mutations, the variable expression of predisposing mutations, and the interplay between environmental factors and modifying genes all contribute to make the genetic analysis of common disorders complex indeed. The identification of genes responsible for this and other common human disorders, and the stepwise delineation of factors contributing to the development of the disease phenotype will greatly enhance our understanding of human genetics and human biology and will provide the critical knowledge that will ultimately reduce the morbidity and mortality caused by these conditions.

REFERENCES

1. Allen TD, Ackerman WG. Hereditary glaucoma in a pedigree of three generations. *Arch Ophthalmol* 1942;27:139–157.
2. Becker B, Kolker AE, Roth FD. Glaucoma family study. *Am J Ophthalmol* 1960;50:557.
3. Becker B, Morton WR. Phenylthiourea taste testing and glaucoma. *Arch Ophthalmol* 1964;72:323–327.

3a. Wirtz MK, Samples JR, Kramer PL, Rust K, Topinka JR, Yount J, Koler RD, et al. Mapping a gene for adult-onset primary open-angle glaucoma to chromosome 3q. *Am J Hum Genet* 1997;60:296–304.

3b. Sarfarazi M, Akarsu AN, Hossain A, Turacli ME, Aktan SG, Barsoum-Homsy M, Chevrette L, et al. Assignment of a locus (GLA3A) for primary congenital glaucoma (buphthalmos) to 2p21 and evidence for genetic heterogeneity. *Genomics* 1995;30:171–177.

4. Becker B, Podos SM. Krukenberg's spindles and primary open-angle glaucoma. *Arch Ophthalmol* 1966;76:635.

4a. Andersen J, Pralea AM, DelBono E, Haines JL, Gorin M, Schuman JS, Mattox CG, Wiggs JL. A gene responsible for the pigment dispersion syndrome maps to chromosome 7q35-36. *Arch Ophthalmol* 1997;115:384–388.

5. Berson EL, Rosner B, Sandberg MA, Dryja TP. Ocular findings in patients with autosomal dominant retinitis pigmentosa and a rhodopsin gene defect (Pro-23-His). *Arch Ophthalmol* 1991;109:92–101.
6. Courtney RH, Hill E. Hereditary juvenile glaucoma simplex. *JAMA* 1931;97:1602–1609.
7. Dawson DV, Kaplan EB, Elston RC. Extensions to sib-pair linkage tests applicable to disorders characterized by delayed onset. *Genet Epidemiol* 1990;7:453.
8. Dorozynski A. Privacy rules blindside French glaucoma effort [news]. *Science* 1991;252:369–370.
9. Drance SM, Schulzer M, Thomas B, Douglas GR. Multivariate analysis in glaucoma: Use of discriminant analysis in predicting glaucomatous visual field damage. *Arch Ophthalmol* 1981;99:1019–1022.
10. Goldschmidt E. The heredity of glaucoma. *Acta Ophthalmol (Copenh)* 1973;120:27.
11. Haines JL, St. George-Hyslop PH, Rimmler JB, Yamaoka L, Kazantsev A, Tanzi RE, Gusella JF, Roses AD, Pericak-Vance MA. Inheritance of multiple loci in familial Alzheimer's disease. In *Alzheimer's Disease: Advances in Clinical and Basic Research.* B. Corain, K. Iqbal, M.

Nicolini, B. Winblad, H. Wisniewski, and P. Zatta, eds. Chichester, England: Wiley, 1992, pp. 221–226.

12. Hanson IM, Fletcher JM, Jordon T et al. Mutations at the PAX6 locus are found in heterogeneous anterior segment malformations including Peters' anomaly. *Nature Genet* 1994;6: 168–173.
13. Hart WM Jr, Yablonski M, Kass MA et al. Multivariate analysis of the risk of glaucomatous visual field loss. *Arch Ophthalmol* 1979; 97:1455.
14. Haseman JK, Elston RC. The investigation of linkage between a quantitative trait and a marker locus. *Behav Genet* 1972;2:3–19.
15. Jeunemaitre X, Soubrier F, Kotelevtsev YV, et al. Molecular basis of human hypertension: Role of angiotensinogen. *Cell* 1992;71:169.
16. Johnson AT, Drak AV, Kwitek AE et al. Clinical features and linkage analysis of a family with autosomal dominant juvenile glaucoma. *Ophthalmology* 1993;100:524–529.
17. Martin JP, Zorab EC. Familial glaucoma in nine generation of South Hampshire family. *Br J Ophthalmol* 1974;58:536–542.
18. Morissette J, Cote G, Anctil JL et al. A common gene for juvenile and adult-onset primary open-angle glaucoma confined on chromosome 1q. *Am J Hum Genet* 1995;56:1431–1442.
19. Nichols BE, Sheffield VC, Vandenburgh K et al. Butterfly-shaped pigment dystrophy of the fovea caused by a point mutation in codon 167 of the RDS gene. *Nature Genet* 1993;3:202–7.
20. Ott J. *analysis of Human Genetic Linkage (Revised Edition)*. Baltimore: The John Hopkins University Press, 1991.
21. Pericak-Vance MA, Bebout JL, Gaskell PC Jr., Yamaoka LH, Hung W-Y, Alberts MJ, Wlaker AP, Barlett RJ, Haynes CA, Welsh KA, Earl NL, Heyman A, Clark CM, Roses AD. Linkage studies in familial Alzheimer disease: Evidence for chromosome linkage. *Am J Hum Genet* 1991;48:1034.
22. Perkins ES. Family studies in glaucoma. *Br J Ophthalmol* 1974;58:529.
23. Richards JE, Lichter PR, Boehnke M et al. Mapping of a gene for autosomal dominant juvenile-onset open-angle glaucoma to chromosome 1q. *Am J Hum Genet* 1994;54:5462–5470.
24. Rohen JW. Why is intraocular pressure elevated in chronic simple glaucoma? Anatomical considerations. *Ophthalmology* 1983;90:758.
25. Schork NJ, Boehnke M, Terwillinger JD, Ott J. Two-trait-locus linkage analysis: A powerful strategy for mapping complex genetic traits. *Am J Hum Genet* 1993;53:1127–1138.
26. Schwartz JR, Reuling FH, Feinleib M et al. Twin heritability study of the effect of corticosteroids on intraocular pressure. *J Med Genet* 1972;9:137.
27. Sheffield VC, Stone EM, Alward WL et al. Genetic linkage of familial open angle glaucoma to chromosome 1q21-q31. *Nature Genet* 1993;4:47.
28. Stokes WH. Hereditary primary glaucoma. *Arch Ophthalmol* 1940;24:885–909.

28a. Stone EM, Fingert JH, Alward WLM, Nguyen TD, Polansky JR, Sunden SLF, Nishimura D, Clark AF, Nystuen A, Nichols BE, Mackey DA, Ritch R, Kalenak JW, Craven ER, Sheffield VC. Identification of a gene that causes primary open angle glaucoma. *Science* 1997; 275:668–670.

29. Tawara A, Inomata H. Developmental immaturity of the trabecular meshwork in juvenile glaucoma. *Am J Ophthalmol* 1984;98:82–97.
30. Teikari JM. Genetic factors in open-angle (simple and capsular) glacoma: A population-based twin study. *Acta Ophthalmol (Copenh)* 1987; 65:715.
31. Tielsch JM, Sommer A, Katz J, Royall RM, Quigley HA, Javitt J. Racial variation in the prevalence of primary open-angle glaucoma: The Baltimore Eye Survey. *JAMA* 1991; 266:369.
32. Tripathi RC. Pathologic anatomy of the outflow pathways of aqueous humor in chronic simple glaucoma. *Exp Eye Rres* 1977; 25(suppl):403.
33. Weatherill JR, Hart CT. Familial hypoplasia of the iris stroma associated with glaucoma. *Br J Ophthalmol* 1969;53:433–438.
34. Weeks DE, Lange K. The affected-pedigree member method of linkage analysis. *Am J Hum Genet* 1988;42:315.
35. Wiggs JL, Haines JL, Paglinauan C et al. Genetic linkage of autosomal dominant juvenile glaucoma to 1q21-q31 in three affected pedigrees. *Genomics* 1994;21:299–303.
36. Wiggs JL, Del Bono EA, Schuman JS et al. Clinical features of five pedigrees genetically linked to the juvenile glaucoma locus on chromosome 1q21-q31. *Ophthalmology* 1995;102: 1782–1789.

12

Cataracts

J. BRONWYN BATEMAN

The lens of the eye is normally transparent as a result of the tertiary structure of the proteins. Any opacity is termed a cataract regardless of the cause, and the resulting level of visual impairment depends on the location within the lens as well as the density and size; some cataracts do not impair vision. In adults, interference with or blurring of vision is the major effect of a cataract; in infants and children, a cataract has more significant implications. In an infant or young child, a cataract may interfere with the development of the central nervous system pathways responsible for vision and cause amblyopia.

EMBRYOGENESIS OF THE EYE

The optic vesicle develops as an evagination of the neuroectodermal layer from the forebrain; invagination of the anterior surface forms the "optic cup." The overlying surface ectoderm increases in thickness and forms a central pit; progressive infolding forms the single cell layered wall of the primary lens vesicle. By the 8–9 mm stage, the posterior cells of the lens vesicle elongate and fill the cavity. This primary or embryonal nucleus forms the acellular capsule. The lens continues to grow throughout life by proliferation and subsequent elongation of equatorial epithelial fibers below the capsule. As these secondary lens fibers extend, the junctions form "sutures."

CLASSIFICATION

Pediatric cataracts should be classified by etiology. Most are either genetic in origin or related to an intrauterine infection. Despite careful evaluation, some may remain unclassifiable. Important characteristics include the size, density and position of the opacity, the age of onset and rate of progression, and laterality. In general, larger and/or denser opacities usually reduce vision more than smaller and/or less dense ones; cataracts in the posterior portion of the lens are more visually significant than those in the anterior region. Pediatric cataracts with an onset early in life may seriously impair the development of central vision. The gestational age at the time of cataract formation will determine the region of the lens affected. Unilateral opacities are less likely to be genetic in origin. Children with cataracts frequently have other anomalies present. Several studies indicate that many will have some associated abnormality of ocular structure and/or other nonocular organ systems.

GENETIC BASES

Isolated Cataracts

The great majority of isolated inherited congenital cataracts occur in an *autosomal dominant* pattern. Penetrance is usually high and morphology varies considerably from one family to the next. Morphology may vary among family members.[105,117,118,135,151,211,217] Although symmetry is common,[67,105,135,151,211] unilaterality and reduced penetrance has been documented[23,156]; interocular phenotypic variability has been reported.[183] Autosomal dominant congenital cataracts, depending on the size, density, and location, may not cause significant visual impairment. Well-documented pedigrees include, but are not limited to, total, anterior[41,86,176] and posterior polar,[121,204] coralliform or stellate,[89] fetal and cortical,[34] nuclear,[105,117,135] and zonular cataracts (Figs. 12.1–12.3).[67,74,87,151] The nomenclature remains vague.

In addition to phenotypic heterogeneity, genetic heterogeneity has been confirmed by the combination of linkage analyses and, in one family, identification of the gene defect. A congenital cataract gene represented the first localization of a disease to an autosome; the Coppock cataract, a zonular pulverulent (dustlike) opacity, was closely linked to the Duffy blood group locus on chromosome 1 in 1963.[163] Additional mappings have confirmed genetic heterogeneity (Table 12.1).[114] Chromosomal rearrangements associated with isolated congenital cataracts have implicated other locations.[130,160]

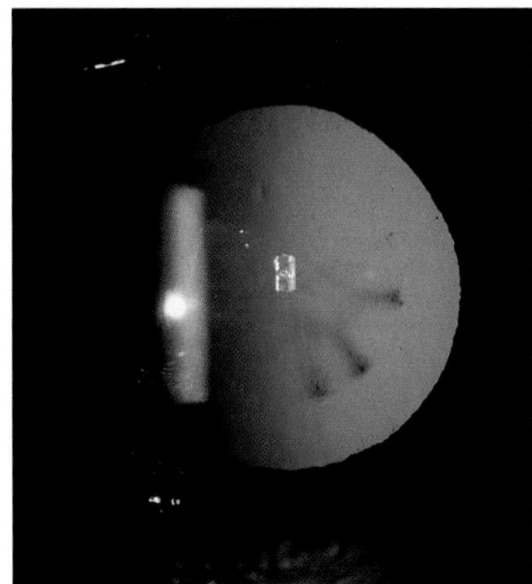

Figure 12.2. Star-shaped cataract in a patient from a family with other members who have embryonal opacities. The disease is inherited in an autosomal dominant pattern.

Cortical cataracts are associated with age and are sometimes termed "senile" cataract[81,94,109]; female gender,[81,109] education,[81,109] nonwhite race,[81,109] diabetes,[109] and exposure to sunlight[81,200] are risk factors. Based on segregation, sibling correlational, and commingling analyses, age-related cataracts are related to a major gene effect.[76]

X-linked cataracts are uncommon but well documented. Affected males exhibit dense con-

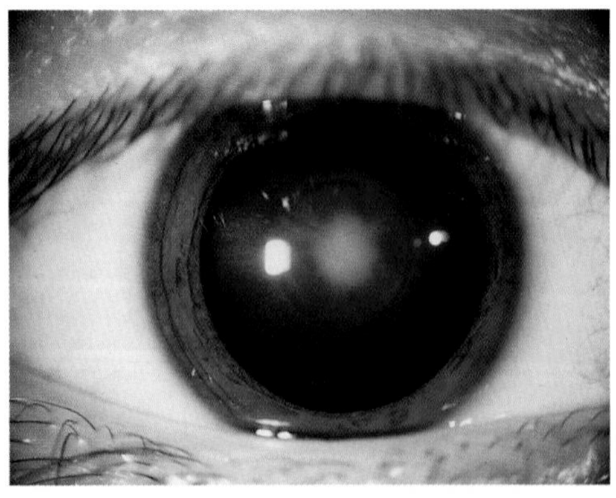

Figure 12.1. Autosomal dominant embryonal nuclear cataract.

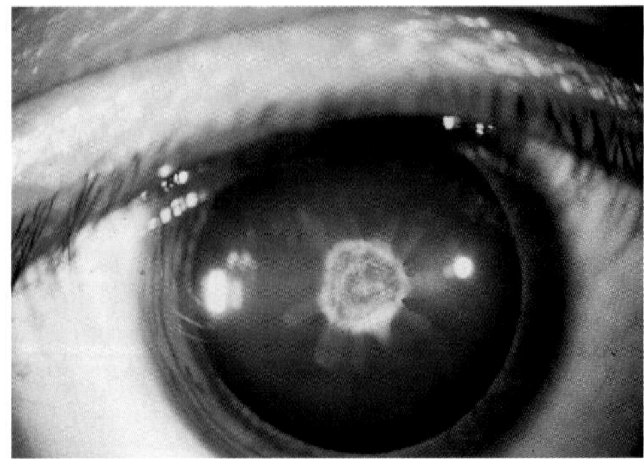

Figure 12.3. Autosomal dominant posterior subcapsular cataract.

Table 12.1. Mapping of Autosomal Dominant Cataracts

Type	Chromosomal Location	Gene Defect	Reference
Central, zonular	1p36	unknown	46
Coppock (zonular pulverulent)	1q21-q25	unknown	163, 85
Coppock-like	1q21-q25	unknown	34
Coppock-like	2q33-35	activation of γE-crystalline pseudogene	113, 20, 45
Zonular, central, stellate, anterior polar	16q21	unknown	45
Posterior polar	16q22.1	unknown	121, 166
Anterior polar	17p	unknown	15
Zonular	17q11-12	unknown	142
Coppock-like	17q24	unknown	11
Cerulean	22q	unknown	98

genital cataracts, microcornea, and low-set ears. Female carriers have variable sutural cataracts that do not affect visual acuity and normal to slightly small corneal diameters (Fig. 12.4). Dental abnormalities have been described in both heterozygous and hemizygous individuals. The gene has been mapped to the p21.1-p22.3 region of the X chromosome[110,194] but is not yet cloned.

Autosomal recessively inherited congenital cataracts are much less common. Reported pedigrees usually occur in endogamous societies.[52,131,144,188] Some previously reported cases may represent undetected galactokinase deficiency and enzymatic disorder recently described.

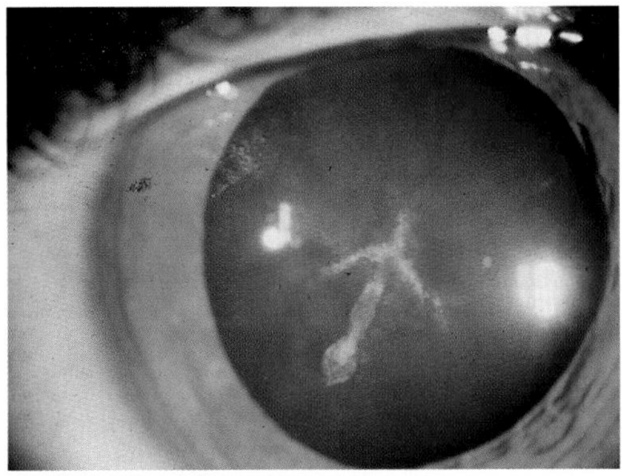

Figure 12.4. Sutural opacity in a obligate carrier for X-linked congenital cataracts. (Courtesy of Dr. Irene H. Maumenee.)

Hereditary Cataracts Associated with Ocular Abnormalities

Cataracts may be associated with isolated ocular anomalies that are inherited. Norrie disease, an X-linked recessive disorder, consists of microphthalmia, retinal dysplasia, and cataracts; mental retardation and deafness also may be present. Aniridia, both in the isolated autosomal dominant and sporadic form, is frequently associated with cataracts. Colobomatous microphthalmos may be accompanied by cataract; although an X-linked variety exists, autosomal dominant and other forms of the disease such as the form that occurs with chromosomal rearrangements are common. Cataracts and microphthalmia without coloboma may occur by X-linked recessive or autosomal dominant inheritance. Microcornea associated with cataracts may be inherited in an autosomal dominant manner. In conjunction with microcornea,[56,70,128,150,175] the asymmetry may be more evident.[175,183]

Hereditary Cataracts Associated with Systemic Abnormalities

Metabolic Disease

Galactosemia (galactose-1-phosphate uridyl transferase deficiency) is a recessively inherited generalized disorder associated with acquired cataract formation (Fig. 12.5*F*). The cataract results from accumulation of the osmotically active sugar dulcitol (galactitol), a product of

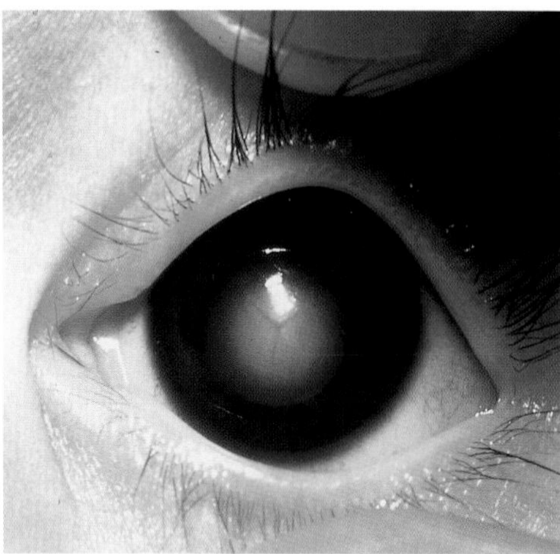

Figure 12.5. Cataract due to untreated galactosemia. (Courtesy of Dr. Sherwin J. Isenberg.)

aldose reductase activity on galactose. The lens opacity may occur as early as the first few weeks of life and may be arrested and possibly reversed if galactose is removed from the diet. The disease is usually severe and leads to death if untreated. Diagnosis is made by enzymatic analysis of erythrocytes.

Galactokinase deficiency, a recessively inherited enzymatic disorder first identified by Gitzlemann in 1965,[67a] is characterized by galactosuria and cataract formation as early as 27 days of age (Fig. 12.6). No other systemic manifestations of the disorder have been reported, and mental development is normal. Regression of cataracts may occur after dietary control. Diagnosis is made by enzymatic analysis of erythrocytes. The carrier state has been estimated to be as high as 1%, and the incidence of the homozygote state has been estimated to be between 1/46,000 births and 1/100,000 births. The gene has been cloned and mapped to chromosome 17q24; mutations in individuals with cataracts have been identified.[195] Cataracts have been noted in adult heterozygotes.[193]

Glucose-6-phosphate dehydrogenase deficiency, an X-linked recessive disorder, has been reported to be associated with cataracts.[129,141]

Fabry disease, inherited in an X-linked recessive pattern, results from defective activity of alpha-galactosidase (ceramide trihexosidase). Ocular abnormalities of the corneal epithelium, lens, and venous system are evident in both female carriers and affected males (Fig. 12.7). Lens opacities may take one of two forms: A spokelike cataract present beneath the posterior lens capsule is unique and usually requires slit-lamp biomicroscopy for detection; this form is present in 37% of hemizygotes and 14% of heterozygotes.[186] The second type of lens opacity is an anterior subcapsular deposit, typically inferior and wedge-shaped, with the base toward the equator of the lens. This type has been noted in 35% of hemizygotes but not in heterozygotes.[186] Visual acuity is rarely impaired by the cataracts.

Mannosidosis, an autosomal recessive disorder of mannosidase deficiency, is characterized by progressive mental deterioration and skele-

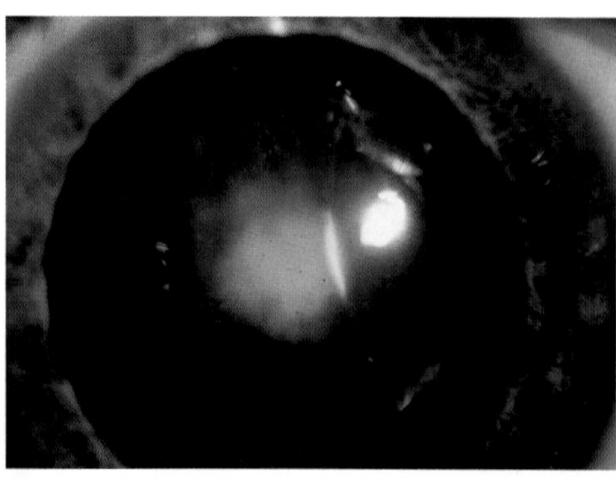

Figure 12.6. Cataract due to galactokinase deficiency. (Courtesy of Dr. Irene H. Maumenee.)

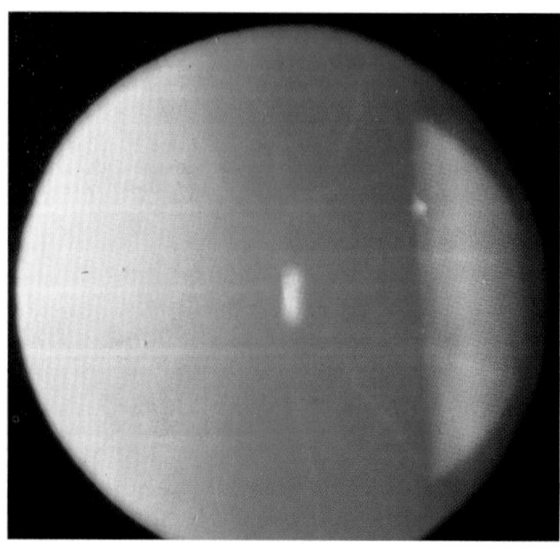

Figure 12.7. Fabry disease cataract.

tal abnormalities; affected children develop coarse features. On ocular examination characteristic spokelike cataracts emanating from a central point in the posterior cortex may be observed.[10] The spokes differ from those found in Fabry disease by their increased width and symmetry; the level within the lens has not been reported. Definitive diagnosis is made by enzymatic assay of fibroblasts and/or leukocytes.

Refsum syndrome is an autosomal recessive disorder characterized by progressive peripheral neuropathy, cerebellar ataxia, and atypical retinitis pigmentosa. Cataracts have been noted in 80% of the patients and frequently develop in the late teens or twenties. Congenital cataracts have been reported in this disorder.[32]

Wilson disease (hepatolenticular degeneration) may be associated with "sunflower cataracts" (chalcosis lentis), a copper deposition in the lens (Fig. 12.8).[25] The distinctive appearance of the cataract is that of a greenish central disc in the anterior capsule with circumferential radiating linear opacities. The cataract usually does not impair vision.

Renal Disease

Oculo-cerebro-renal or Lowe syndrome is inherited in an X-linked recessive manner and characterized by mental retardation, renal abnormalities (Fanconi-type aminoaciduria) and ocular manifestations. The defective gene is a phosphatidylinositol 4,5-biphosphate 5-phosphatase, a Golgi complex protein similar to platelet 5-phosphatase.[13,139,199,236] Congenital cataracts of the nuclear, polar, or complete type are a consistent feature; glaucoma frequently develops. Up to 100% of female heterozygotes exhibit cortical and/or central opacities that do not impair vision (Fig. 12.9).[31,39,65]

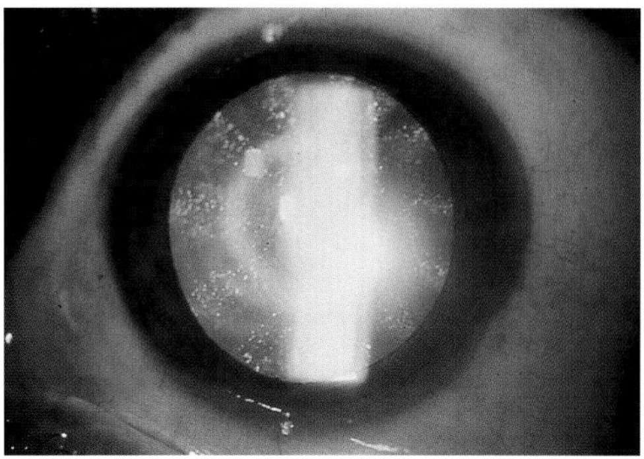

Figure 12.9. Obligate carrier of Lowe syndrome. (Courtesy of Dr. Otis Paul.)

Alport syndrome,[4a] is characterized by a progressive glomerulopathy and sensorineural deafness. Affected males typically develop renal disease in their teens; females, later in life. The hearing loss is acquired. Reported lenticular changes include anterior lenticonus (conical protrusion of anterior central lens) (Fig. 12.10) and posterior subcapsular cataracts; additional ocular changes include retinal pigment epitheliopathy; less commonly, arcus juvenilis has been reported. Ocular abnormalities occur in approximately 30% of cases and primarily in males.[86a]

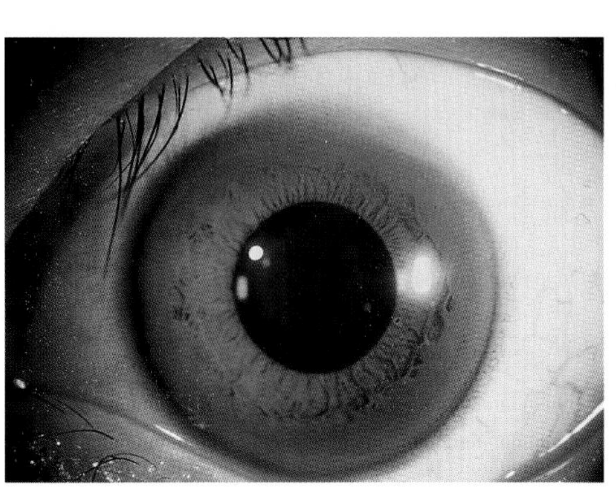

Figure 12.8. Sunflower cataract caused by Wilson disease.

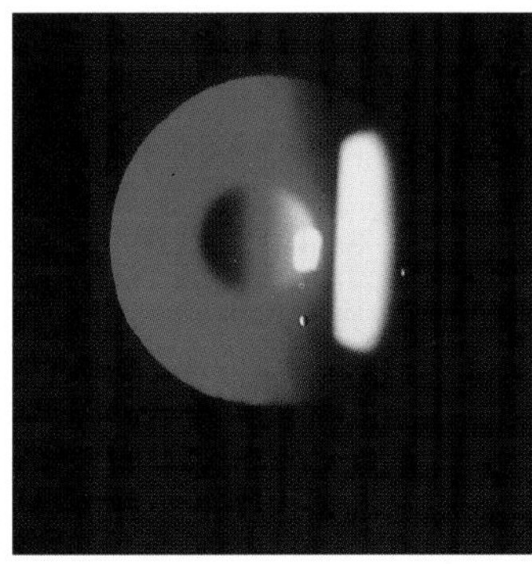

Figure 12.10. Anterior lenticonus in patient with Alport syndrome.

The mode of inheritance has long been debated. There are at least three forms of the disease: X-linked recessive, autosomal recessive, and autosomal dominant. The X-linked recessive is due to mutations in the α5 (type IV) collagen chain,[162] and the autosomal recessive is caused by mutations of the α3(IV) and α4(IV) collagen genes.[77,96,107,126] The autosomal dominant form, benign familial hematuria, is caused by a mutation of α4(IV).[107a] Alport syndrome may be associated with diffuse esophageal leimyomatosis, a proliferation of smooth muscle tumors; disruption of both the α5(IV) and α6(IV) collagen genes, which are closely mapped, has been implicated.[77,237]

Immunohistologic studies of type IV collagen in anterior lens capsules from affected males support absence of the α3, α2, and the α5 chains.[29]

Musculoskeletal Disease

Chondrodysplasia punctata, a bone dysplasia characterized by punctate epiphyseal and extraepiphyseal calcification, exhibits all single-gene forms of inheritance: autosomal recessive, autosomal dominant, and both X-linked dominant and recessive. Cutaneous abnormalities may occur in any of the forms but is most prominent in the X-linked dominant form, with a whorled pattern of thick white adherent scales on a background of erythemous skin[43]; there is palmar and plantar hyperkeratosis. The milder autosomal dominant variety, sometimes termed Conradi-Hunermann, is characterized by asymmetrical dwarfing, joint contractures, and a flat face with a depressed bridge of the nose; cataracts have been found in 18% of this group.[119,191] The recessive or rhizomelic form of the disease is associated with symmetric dwarfism and is usually lethal in infancy or childhood; congenital cataracts occur in 72% of these cases.[192] The rhizomelic type is a peroxisomal disorder.[80] The more recently described are X-linked dominant and recessive forms, both of which are associated with congenital cataracts.[36,73,146b] The X-linked recessive has been mapped to the short arm.[214,312] Prenatal diagnosis is feasible by ultrasonography.[154]

Myotonic dystrophy is inherited in an autosomal dominant fashion and is characterized by muscle weakness and wasting; the facial muscles, sternomastoids, and distal limb muscles are most affected. Myotonia is a prominent and insidious symptom. Other prominent features include dysfunction of smooth muscle, particularly of the gastrointestinal tract and heart; sudden death in adults is not uncommon. Widespread endocrine disturbances including testicular atrophy and glucose intolerance are common; despite reduced spermatogenesis, males may be fertile. The disease may be particularly severe in neonates and children, if the mother is the transmitting parent. The features include severe hypotonia and facial diplegia; respiratory distress and feeding difficulties are common. Affected infants do not exhibit myotonia. Mental retardation is a prominent feature of childhood myotonic dystrophy. Mitochondrial DNA does not appear to influence the congenital onset type.[152]

The disease is associated with multiple ocular changes including ptosis, enophthalmos, ocular myotonia (extraocular muscle pareses), xerophthalmia, cataracts, hypotony, and pigmentary abnormalities of the macula. The cataracts are the most common manifestation[12] and may take any of three forms: a characteristic iridescent crystalline dust, unique to myotonic dystrophy (Fig. 12.11); the less specific small, white "snowball-like" opacities (Fig. 12.12); or typical aging changes (Fig. 12.13). The cataracts, rarely evident before age 10 years, may be noted in adolescence, sometimes as the

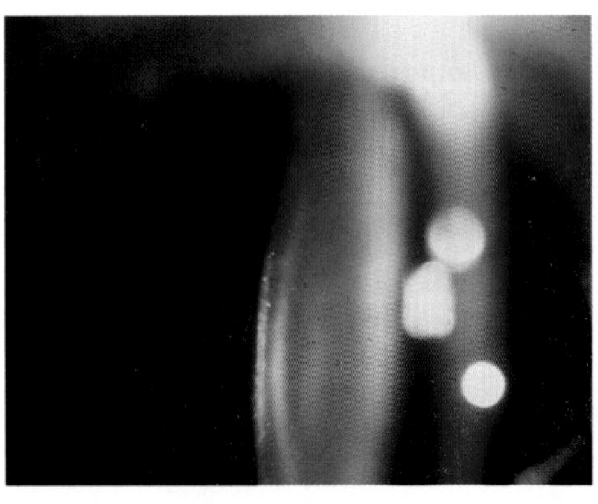

Figure 12.11. Green and blue Christmas tree cataracts in anterior lens of patient with myotonic dystrophy. (Courtesy of Dr. John R. Heckenlively.)

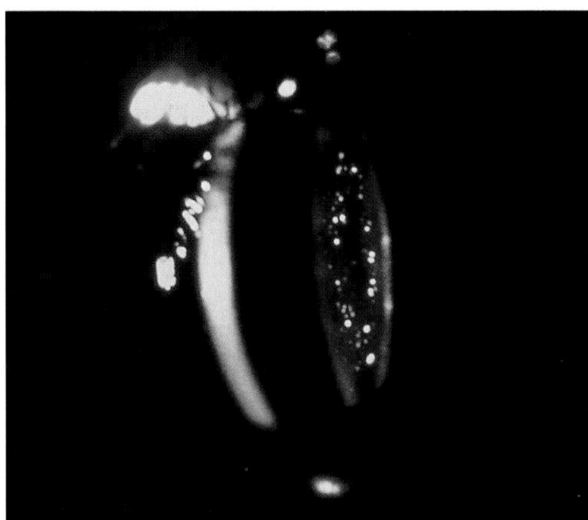

Figure 12.12. Snowball-like cataracts in a patient with myotonic dystrophy. (Courtesy of Dr. Hilel Lewis.)

initial sign of the disease.[12,159] Uncommonly, the disease may be ascertained by cataract screening.[91]

The genetic basis of the disease is a (CTG)n trinucleotide repeat expansion in the 3′-untranslated region of a protein kinase-encoding gene, DMPK, which is on the long arm of chromosome 19.[115] The unstable repeat impairs posttranscriptional processing of transcripts.[88,100] The mutation rate is believed to be low, and a common Eurasian origin of the myotonic dystrophy mutation has been postulated.[230] The penetrance is high by adulthood.

Albright hereditary osteodystrophy (AHO) is a skeletal dysplasia characterized by short stature, obesity, and mental retardation. Additional findings include brachymetacarpy, subcutaneous calcifications, tetanic symptoms, cataracts, and intracranial calcification. There are two forms of the disorder: pseudohypoparathyroidism (PH) and pseudo-pseudohypoparathyroidism (PPH), which are associated with hypocalcemic and normocalcemic states, respectively. The disease is caused by resistance to parathyroid and other hormones. Both forms of AHO may occur in the same pedigree, and cataract formation occurs in both. Autosomal dominant inheritance seems most likely; the phenotype may be dependent on the gender of the parent transmitting the mutation. The defective gene is Gs alpha, the alpha subunit of the G protein, which couples hormone receptors to stimulation of adenylate cyclase.[112,184]

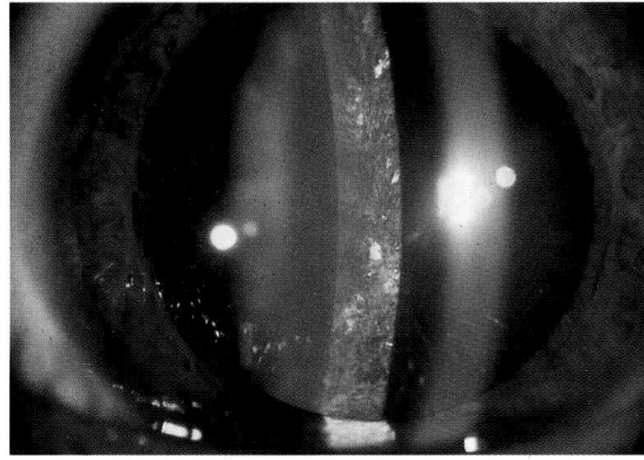

Figure 12.13. Water clefts in lens of a 20-year-old patient with myotonic dystrophy.

Stickler syndrome is associated with normal to tall stature, joint laxity with arthritis, cleft palate, and sensorineural deafness (up to 80% of patients).[67d] Ocular abnormalities are common and include moderate to severe myopia and retinal detachment. Cataracts may be evident in the teenage years. The disease is inherited in an autosomal dominant pattern. Three genes, type II collagen[1,53] and two type XI collagens ($\alpha 1$ and $\alpha 2$)[167,210] have been identified as causing the syndrome if mutated. Snead and associates[190] have proposed that clinical differences may be related to the genetic defect.

Robert syndrome, consisting of tetraphocomelia, cleft lip and palate, and prominence of the phallus, may be associated with ocular hypertelorism and congenital cataracts. The malformations are similar to those found in thalidomide-exposed fetuses and infants. The inheritance pattern is autosomal recessive.[72,79,104,170]

Connective Tissue Disease

All syndromes associated with dislocation of the lens may be associated with cataract formation.

Central Nervous System Disorders

The *Marinesco-Sjögren syndrome,* a central nervous system (CNS) disorder, is characterized by progressive cerebellar ataxia, abnormal hair, congenital cataracts, and mental retardation. Strabismus may also be evident in this

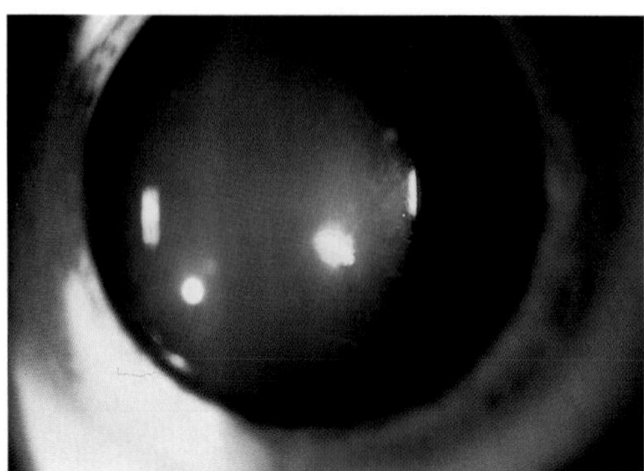

Figure 12.14. Posterior subcapsular cataract in a patient with neurofibromatosis. (From Dr. Muriel Kaiser-Kupfer.)

disorder. Inheritance pattern is autosomal recessive.

Sjögren syndrome is a recessively inherited CNS disorder that manifests with congenital cataracts and mental retardation.

Meckel syndrome is an autosomal recessive disorder with multisystem abnormalities similar to those of trisomy 13. The ocular abnormalities include anophthalmos/microphthalmos, partial aniridia, congenital cataract, retinal dysplasia, and optic nerve abnormalities.[55,124]

Neurofibromatosis type 2 is a less common form of neurofibromatosis and is characterized by bilateral acoustic neuromas; other features include other tumors, including paraspinal neurofibromas, meningiomas, and, less frequently, spinal astrocytomas and schwannomas. Ophthalmologic features include posterior subcapsular cataracts,[19,157] which can be diagnostic (Fig. 12.14), and retinal hamartomas.[19,157] Optic nerve gliomas are not a feature. The gene product, termed *schwannomin* or *merlin,* is a member of a superfamily thought to link cytoskeletal elements to cell membranes and a tumor suppressor gene.[16,171,173]

Dermatologic Disorders

Cockayne syndrome, a recessively inherited disorder, is characterized by dwarfism with prognathism, mental retardation, deafness, thickening of the skull bones, photosensitivity, retinal degeneration, optic atrophy, and cataracts. Cataracts were reported to occur at birth in one of Cockayne's original patients. Patients with this disorder have a normal infancy. Cells from affected individuals are abnormally sensitive to ultraviolet radiation and are defective in the repair of transcriptionally active genes. The defective gene has been cloned and encodes a transcriptional regulator.[78]

Rothmund-Thomson syndrome is an autosomal recessive condition characterized by atrophic telangiectatic dermatosis, cataracts, short stature, hypogonadism, absent or sparse hair, and defective dentition.[201] There is no gender predilection and most reported cases have been in Caucasians. The skin changes develop between 3–6 months of age. Loss of body hair usually occurs within the first year of life and remains absent or sparse throughout life. Cataracts are reported in 75% of patients and typically develop rapidly between the ages of 18 months and 7 years (Fig. 12.15).[92] The cataracts are usually bilateral and require surgical removal. Additional ocular abnormalities include microcornea and band keratopathy of the cornea.

Incontinentia pigmenti or Block-Sulzberger syndrome, a generalized ectodermal dysplasia inherited in an X-linked dominant pattern, is usually evident at birth but may be noted as late as 2 years of age. Initially the lesions may take the form of bullous eruptions, which develop into characteristic pigmented streaks and flecks. Additional changes include delayed appearance or hypoplasia of dentition and skeletal abnormalities. The most prominent ocular anomaly is a retinal detachment that may be

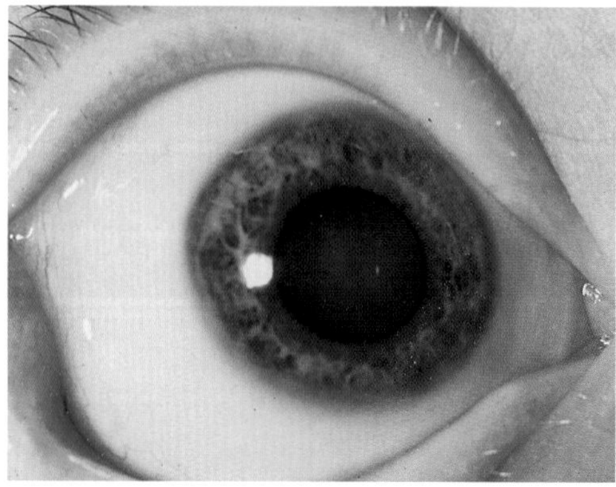

Figure 12.15. Cataract in a boy with Rothmund–Thomson syndrome. (From the late Dr. David Friendly.)

misdiagnosed as retinoblastoma if congenital. Isolated cataracts have been reported. The gene has been mapped to Xp28.[36a]

Ichthyosis is characterized by scaling and drying of skin; rare cases of presumed congenital cataracts have been reported. Congenital coronary opacities have been reported in a patient with ichthyosis vulgaris, which is inherited in an autosomal dominant pattern. Congenital cataracts have also been associated with ichthyosiform erythroderma, the congenital form of the disease, which is inherited in an autosomal recessive pattern.

Craniofacial Malformations

Hallermann-Streiff syndrome or François syndrome consists of dyscephaly, beaked nose, mandibular hypoplasia, cutaneous atrophy, and proportionate short stature. Ocular abnormalities are common and include hypotrichosis, blue sclera, variable microphthalmia, and congenital cataracts. Spontaneous resorption of the cataractous lens has been reported.[190a] Although pedigrees demonstrating a dominant mode of inheritance have been described, the majority of cases are sporadic.

Rubinstein-Taybi syndrome is characterized by broad thumbs and great toes, a characteristic facies, and mental retardation. Ocular abnormalities are common and include antimongoloid lid fissures and highly arched brows. Other ocular abnormalities, including congenital cataracts, coloboma, dacryostenosis, and glaucoma, are less frequently present.[22]

Smith-Lemli-Opitz syndrome is characterized by microcephaly, ptosis, upturned nares, micrognathia, hypotonia, polydactyly and syndactyly of the toes, hypospadias and cryptorchidism, mental retardation, and pyloric stenosis. Infantile cataracts have been noted.[35a] Inheritance is autosomal recessive.

Marshall syndrome includes saddle nose, infantile and juvenile cataracts, high myopia, and sensorineural deafness. Stature is normal. Inheritance is autosomal dominant with complete penetrance. It has been suggested that Marshall syndrome may be synonymous with Stickler syndrome.[13a]

The *cerebro-oculo-facial-skeletal syndrome* (COFS): COFS, first described in 1974,[146a] is a degenerative disorder characterized by hypotonia, microcephaly, microphthalmia, cataracts, blepharophimosis, micrognathia, camptodactly, flexion contractures, and rocker-bottom feet. Death is common during the first few years of life. Cataracts may be infantile. The inheritance pattern is believed to be autosomal recessive.

Disordes Rarely Associated with Cataracts

Cataracts have rarely been associated with Ellis-Van Creveld syndrome (chondroectodermal dysplasia), Prader-Willi syndrome, Bardet-Biedl syndrome, phenylketonuria, Swartz-Jampel syndrome, oxycephaly, cerebro-hepatorenal syndrome (Zellweger), and Noonan syndrome.

CHROMOSOMAL ABNORMALITIES

Trisomy 13 (Patau Syndrome)

Trisomy 13 was initially described by Patau and colleagues[143] in 1960. Although the major diagnostic criteria include microphthalmia, cleft lip/palate, and polydactyly, nearly every organ system may be involved. Most infants have normal birthweights and are hypotonic; about half have a cleft lip/palate. Many have a characteristic face with sloping forehead and bulbous nose. Life-threatening abnormalities include cardiovascular and central nervous system malformations; perinatal death is common and 97% die by age 6 months.[67c] Additional anomalies include polycystic renal cortices, biseptate uterus in females, undescended testes and abnormal insertion of phallus in males, hyperconvex nails, muscle and skeletal abnormalities, capillary cutaneous defects, and cutaneous scalp defects. The central nervous system is markedly affected, with defects including absence of rhinencephalon, union of ventricles and thalami, defects of corpus callosum, falx cerebri, and commissures, and arhinencephaly with absence of olfactory nerves and lobes; microcephaly is common.

Ophthalmologic abnormalities are common in trisomy 13 and include colobomatous microphthalmia, cyclopia, cataracts, corneal opacities, glaucoma, persistent hyperplastic primary vitreous, intraocular cartilage, and retinal dysplasia.[4,68,83]

Trisomy 8

Trisomy of chromosome 8 only occurs in a mosaic form in live births. Many organ systems may be involved in the disorder. The facial features are characteristic with a prominent forehead, broad-based nose, everted upper lip, high-arched and/or cleft palate, stretched lingual frenulum, micrognathia, and large, dysplastic ears with a prominent antihelix. The neck is short and broad; the trunk of the body tends to be long and thin. Skeletal anomalies include structural and numerical vertebral abnormalities, spina bifida, scoliosis, pectus carinatum, absent patellae, and hip abnormalities. Renal and ureteral anomalies and cardiac defects are common. Ophthalmologic features include hypertelorism, downward slanting of the palpebral fissures, strabismus, blepharoptosis, blepharophimosis, corneal opacities, cataracts, heterochromia of the irides, and colobomatous microphthalmia.[7,24,54,133,148,164,165,172,213]

Trisomy 18 (Edwards Syndrome)

Trisomy 18, initially identified in 1960,[44] causes serious birth defects including a low birthweight; microcephaly; a characteristic facies with fawnlike ears, micrognathia, high arched palate, a narrow bifrontal diameter, and prominent occiput; hypertonicity; poor muscle development; hand flexion with overlapping of second and fifth fingers; and limited hip abduction. Rocker-bottom feet, webbing of toes, and dorsiflexion of a short great toe are common. Renal anomalies including horseshoe kidney and collecting duct malformations, cardiac malformations, pyloric stenosis, eventration of the diaphragm, and Meckel's diverticulum may occur. Apneic spells and failure to thrive are serious complications. The majority (95%) die before 1 year of age.[170a]

The most common ophthalmologic anomalies include epicanthus, hypertelorism, and hypoplastic supraorbital ridges. Corneal opacities, congenital glaucoma, cataract, microcornea, retinal depigmentation, colobomatous microphthalmia, and cyclopia occur less frequently.[83,145,180]

Trisomy 21 (Down Syndrome)

The most common trisomy among live births is chromosome 21 or Down syndrome, deriving its eponym from Langdon Down, who first described the clinical features in 1866.[42] Systemic findings include hypotonia; brachycephaly; a large protruding tongue; small nose with a low, small bridge; small, poorly defined ears; short, thick neck; stubby hands with a single palmar crease; clinodactyly of the fifth digit with hypoplasia of middigital phalanges; short, stubby feet with a wide gap between first and second toes; and cardiac malformations. Affected individuals have a higher incidence of leukemia. Males are usually sterile; females, on occasion, are fertile.[161]

The ocular features include epicanthus, upward slanting of the palpebral fissures, myopia, strabismus, nystagmus, blepharitis, ectropion of the eyelids, keratoconus, Bushfield spots of the irides, infantile glaucoma, congenital or acquired cataracts, and an increased number of retinal vessels crossing the disc margin.[26,28,66,185,203]

Trisomy 22

Trisomy 22 causes severe growth and development retardation, craniofacial anomalies including microcephaly, arhinencephaly, depressed nasal bridge with a flat nose, preauricular skin tags; dysplastic ears and high arched or cleft palate, and micrognathia; other features include cardiac, pulmonary, and gastrointestinal malformations. Individuals with partial or mosaic trisomy 22 have been well described; trisomy 22 in a live birth is rare. Ophthalmologic manifestations include epicanthus, hypertelorism, upward or downward slanting of the palpebral fissures, blepharoptosis, strabismus, synophrys, cataract, dislocated lenses, optic nerve hypoplasia, colobomatous microphthalmia, and persistent hyperplastic primary vitreous.[8,177,189,212,216]

Monosomy 21

Complete or partial deletion of chromosome 21 causes prenatal growth retardation and craniofacial features including microcephaly, prominent nose, downturned corners of the mouth, micrognathia, and cleft lip and/or palate. Death results from recurrent respiratory infections and gastrointestinal illness. Ophthalmologic manifestations include epicanthus, downward slanting of the palpebral fissures, Peters' anomaly of the anterior segment, cataracts, and microphthalmia.[58,146,169,225]

Deletion 2q

Partial monosomy of the long arm of chromosome 2 is characterized by relatively nonspecific findings including microcephaly, thin nasal bridge and a short upturned nose, low-set and/or dysplastic ears, micrognathia, and cleft or arched palate; additional features include cardiac and lung malformations, cystic gonads, and digital anomalies. The ophthalmic manifestations include downslanting of the palpebral fissures, epicanthus, narrow palpebral fissures, thick eyebrows and lashes, blepharoptosis and blepharophimosis, corneal opacities, cataracts, optic nerve hypoplasia, nystagmus, and colobomatous microphthalmia.[57,61,127,158,232]

Deletion 3q

Partial monosomy of the long arm of chromosome 3 is extremely rare. Features include microcephaly, growth retardation, an unusual facial appearance with cleft lip/palate, cardiac malformations, and clubfeet. Ophthalmologic features include narrow palpebral fissures, epicanthus, blepharoptosis, strabismus, cataract, and colobomatous microphthalmia.[5,6,64,209]

Deletion 4p (Wolf-Hirschhorn Syndrome)

The physical findings in partial deletion of the short arm of chromosome 4 include microcephaly, seizures, prominent glabella, midline scalp defects, preauricular dimple, cleft lip/palate or high arched palate, deformed nose, hemangiomas, hydrocephalus, and undescended testes and hypospadias in males.[227] Colobomatous microphthalmia is common as is hypertelorism, epicanthus, and downward slanting of the palpebral fissures and strabismus; blepharoptosis, corneal opacities (Peters' anomaly), the anterior segment abnormalities of Rieger anomaly, and cataracts may occur.[99,122,218]

Deletion 5p (Cri-du-chat Syndrome)

The syndrome due to the partial deletion of the short arm of chromosome 5 was described originally by Lejeune and his colleagues.[106] Affected individuals have a low birthweight and are hypotonic; the neonatal growth rate is slow. The catlike cry is most noticeable in infancy and attributable to an abnormality in structure of the larynx. Findings include microcephaly with a round face, micrognathia, low-set ears, and cardiac malformations.

Ophthalmologic features include an upward- or downward slanting of the palpebral fissures, hypo- or hypertelorism, epicanthus, blepharoptosis, myopia, reduced tear production, strabismus with or without reduced abduction, cataracts, glaucoma, tortuous retinal vessels, foveal hypoplasia, optic atrophy, and colobomatous microphthalmia.[59,83,103,111,179,228]

Deletion 13q

Partial monosomy for chromosome 13 caused by either deletion of part of the long arm or ring 13 results in similar phenotypes including microcephaly and trigonocephaly; facial features include a prominent bridge of the nose; small chin; large, low-set, malformed ears; and facial asymmetry. Other features include absent or hypoplastic thumbs, cardiac and renal malformations, anal atresia, and features of Noonan syndrome; males may have hypospadias and undescended testes. Ophthalmologic findings include hypertelorism, upward- or downward slanting and/or narrow palpebral fissures, epicanthus, strabismus, blepharoptosis, cataract, retinoblastoma, Rieger syndrome, and colobomatous microphthalmia.[3,102,120,136,137,140,168,196,202,215,223]

Deletion 18p

The physical findings associated with the deletion (total or partial) of the short arm of chromosome 18 are broad. In the mildest form, affected individuals have microcephaly, mild mental retardation, short stature, webbed neck, and immunoglobulin abnormalities.[69] In the most severe form, median facial dysplasia with cebocephaly and/or incomplete morphogenesis of the brain may occur with digital anomalies such as short fingers, high-set thumb(s), and syndactyly. Cardiac, renal, and gastrointestinal malformations are uncommon but may be evident. The ophthalmologic features consistently include hypertelorism, epicanthus, blepharoptosis, and strabismus. Cataracts, retinal dysplasia, colobomatous microphthalmia, and synophthalmia/cyclopia have been reported.[59,83,103,111,179]

Deletion 18q

Partial deletion of the long arm of chromosome 18 produces a syndrome marked by mental and growth retardation with hypotonia. The facies are striking with microcephaly, midface hypoplasia, a carplike mouth with downward slanting margins, and a prominent antihelix and/or antitragus of the ears with a narrow or atretic canal and hearing loss. Cardiac and genitourinary malformations are common. The fingers taper markedly with a high frequency of whorl patterns and simian creases may be evident. Toes may have abnormal placement with the third toe placed above the second and fourth. Dimples may be evident on knuckles, knees, elbows, and shoulders. Ophthalmologic abnormalities include epicanthus, hypertelorism, downward slanting of the palpebral fissures, nystagmus, strabismus, corneal abnormalities, cataracts, blue sclerae, dysplastic or atrophic optic nerve heads, and colobomatous microphthalmia.[35,38,49,111,134,178,205,224]

Duplication 2p

Partial trisomy of the short arm of chromosome 2 is characterized by craniofacial features including microcephaly, a prominent forehead and/or glabella, short nose with a broad bridge and prominent tip, high-arched palate, micrognathia, pointed chin, and low-set and dysplastic ears; cardiac and/or genitourinary malformations, and skeletal and/or digital anomalies may be present. Ophthalmologic features include hypertelorism, epicanthus, strabismus, narrow palpebral fissures, blepharoptosis and blepharophimosis, nasolacrimal duct obstruction, cataract, retinal detachment and dysplasia, tortuosity of the retinal vessels, optic atrophy, persistent hyperplastic primary vitreous, and microphthalmia.[75,123,155,233]

Duplication 3q

Partial trisomy of the long arm of chromosome 3 is rare and characterized by acrocephaly, brachycephaly, hirsutism, facial features similar to de Lange syndrome, synophrys, long eyelashes, hypogenitalism in both males and females, and cardiac malformations. Ophthalmologic manifestations are common and include hypertelorism, epicanthus, upward- or downward slanting of the palpebral fissures, synophrys, strabismus, nasolacrimal duct obstruction, cataract, corneal opacities, congenital glaucoma, nystagmus, and colobomatous microphthalmia.[2,30,48,62,97,174,182,197,209,221,235]

Duplication 5p

Partial trisomy of the short arm of chromosome 5 is rare and the general features are relatively nonspecific; ophthalmic manifestations are common. Affected individuals have macrodolicho-scaphocaphaly, low-set ears, depressed nasal bridge, macroglossia, micrognathia, cardiac malformations, long fingers, club feet, and seizures. Ophthalmologic features include hypertelorism, upward slanting and/or narrowing of the palpebral fissures, epicanthus, strabismus, cataracts, nystagmus, and colobomatous microphthalmia.[27,95,108]

Duplication 9p

Trisomy of the short arm of chromosome 9 is characterized by relatively consistent facial features including a brachycephaly, bulbous nose, low-set and/or dysplastic ears, short philtrum, downturned corners of the mouth, cleft lip/palate, and a "worried appearance." Mental retardation and microcephaly occur in all cases. Delayed bone maturation, cardiac anomalies and skeletal anomalies such as brachydactyly, clinodactyly, and nail hypoplasia may be evident. Ophthalmologic features include hypertelorism, downward slanting of the palpebral fissures, entropion, strabismus, cataracts, optic atrophy, and enophthalmos.[125,164,198,206,222,231]

Duplication 10q

Duplication of the long arm of chromosome 10 is characterized by severe growth retardation. Craniofacial features include microcephaly, high forehead, midfacial hypoplasia with a broad nasal bridge, an upturned nose, microstomia, micrognathia, cleft lip/palate, and a short neck. Additional features include skeletal anomalies such as generalized laxity, scoliosis, and camptodactyly, and cardiac and renal malformations. Ophthalmologic manifestations include hypertelorism, epicanthus, downward slanting and/or narrow palpebral fissures, strabismus, enophthalmia, blepharoptosis and blepharophimosis, cataract, and microphthalmia.[14,50,60,93,101,153,234]

Duplication 15q

Duplication of long arm of chromosome 15 results in mental and postnatal growth retardation with microcephaly associated with craniofacial features including microdolichocephaly, prominent occiput, sloping forehead, large, low-set ears, prominent bulbous nose, long philtrum, and a midline crease in the upper lip, high-arched palate, and micrognathia. Ophthalmologic manifestations include downward slanting of the palpebral fissures, narrow palpebral fissures, epicanthus, strabismus, blepharoptosis, cataract, retinal detachment, and microphthalmia.[33,63,71,181,229]

Duplication of band 1 of the long arm of chromosome 15 causes severe mental retardation with the craniofacial features of an oval face with prominent supraorbital and zygomatic regions, full cheeks, a large nose, low-set ears, and a high-arched or cleft palate; microcephaly may be evident. Additional features include limb anomalies such as short, thick digits and rocker-bottom feet, cardiac malformations, and seizures. Signs and symptoms of the Prader-Willi syndrome may be evident. Ophthalmologic manifestations include deeply set eyes, strabismus, and microphthalmia.[82,147]

Triploidy

Triploidy causes multiple congenital anomalies and severe intrauterine growth retardation; the condition is lethal. Affected fetuses/infants have central nervous system malformations including hydrocephalus and hypoplasia of the cortex and/or cerebellum and anomalies of internal organs including the genitourinary, cardiac, intestinal, and endocrine systems. Hydatidiform mole may develop. Ophthalmologic features include hypertelorism, cataracts, glaucoma, and colobomatous microphthalmia.[17,68,187,208]

Turner Syndrome

Turner[207] described several females with sexual infantilism, webbed neck, and cubitus valgus, establishing as a clinical syndrome a previously described endocrinologic disorder. The absence of "sex chromatin" in most Turner syndrome patients was reported independently by three groups in 1954.[37,149,220] The first published 45,X karyotype was confirmed by many laboratories within the same year.[51] Approximately 80% of females with Turner syndrome have 45 chromosomes, a single X, and no "sex chromatin" (Barr bodies). The remaining 20% have other chromosomal variants. The unifying cytogenetic characteristic is the presence of a cell line that does not have two normal X chromosomes; it may lack the second X chromosome completely or have an abnormal second X chromosome (ring, fragment, deletion). Some patients are mosaic (45,X/46,XX) or have a long-arm isochromosome (46,X,i(Xq)) (an isochromosome is an abnormal chromosome with duplication of one arm forming two arms of equal length).

The typical findings in Turner syndrome are sexual infantilism, short stature, webbed neck, broad shield chest with widely spaced nipples, increased carrying angle, small uterus, and multiple pigmented nevi. Recurrent ear infections are common. The ovaries consist of fibrous streaks with few or no follicles, and failure to feminize may be the presenting problem in the older girl with few of the physical stigmata. Coarctation of the aorta is common and may account for early childhood death. Autoimmune diseases, particularly Hashimoto thyroiditis and diabetes, have been associated with the syndrome. Turner syndrome in some newborn infants is characterized by lymphedema of the hands and feet, which may persist into adulthood. Blepharoptosis and strabismus are the most common ocular abnormalities. Cataracts may occur, particularly in association with diabetes. Refractive errors, corneal scars, blue sclera, and a variety of other anomalies have been reported.[9] The incidence of color blindness in females with 45,X Turner syndrome equals that seen in normal males, since only one X chromosome is present.

NONHEREDITARY CATARACTS

Dysgeneses

The most common area of disturbance of the lens capsule formation are the anterior and posterior regions. Opacities of the posterior axial structures are often associated with incomplete dissolution of the embryonic hyaloid vascular system or the anterior capsule when elements of the embryonal vascular sheath which surround the lens may persist through fetal development. Persistent hyperplastic primary vitreous (PHPV) is believed to be caused by incomplete progression of the development of the eye with persistence of the hyaloid vascular system. The eye is microphthalmic and cataracts are present in most anterior forms of the disease. The posterior lens may have vascular infiltration and the hyaloid system may be patent.[67b] Anterior polar cataracts may be nongenetic and usually have minimal effect on vision. A Mittendorf dot is a discrete opacity that occurs just nasal to the visual axis at the level of the posterior capsule and is believed to be due to a remnant of the fibrovascular hyaloid tissue attached to or immediately posterior to the central posterior capsule. Posterior lenticonus is a central ectatic deformity of the posterior lens capsule and is usually associated with cataracts that may be progressive. Infantile cataracts may be secondary and occur as a result of retinoblastoma, inflammatory disease or retinopathy of prematurity.

Infectious Embryopathies

Transplacental infection of the eye may occur with all of the organisms that can infect the fetus including rubella, herpes simplex, herpes zoster, cytomegalovirus, and varicella. Cataracts, as well as glaucoma, microphthalmia, transient corneal clouding, retinopathy, and intraocular inflammation, occur as a result of intrauterine rubella infection. The cataracts may be unilateral or bilateral and live rubella virus has been recovered from several ocular tissues and from the lens aspirate as late as the teenage years.

REFERENCES

1. Ahmad NN, Ala-Kooko L, Knowlton RG, Jimenez SA, Weaver EF, Maguire JI, Tasman W, Prockop DJ. Stop codon in the procollagen II gene (COL2A1) in a family with the Stickler syndrome (arthro-ophthalmolpathy) *Proc Natl Acad Sci USA* 1991;88:6624–6627.
2. Allderdice PW, Browne N, Murphy DP. Chromosome 3 duplication q21→qter deletion p25→pter syndrome in children of carriers of a pericentric inversion inv(3)(p25q21). *Am J Hum Genet* 1975;27:699–718.
3. Allderdice PW, Davis JG, Miller OJ et al. The 13q- deletion syndrome. *Am J Hum Genet* 1969;21:499–512.
4. Allen JC, Venecia G, Opitz JM. Eye findings in the 13 trisomy syndrome. *Eur J Pediatr* 1977;124:179–183.

4a. Alport AC. Hereditary familial congenital hemorrhagic nephritis. *Br Med J* 1927; 1:504–506.

5. Alvarado M, Bocian M, Walker AP. Interstitial deletion of the long arm of chromosome 3: Case report, review, and definition of a phenotype. *Am J Med Genet* 1987;27:781–786.
6. Alvarez-Arratia MC, Rivera H, Moller M, Valdivia A, Vigueras A. De nove del(3)(q2800). *Ann Genet* 1984;27:109–111.

7. Anneren G, Frodis E, Jorulf H. Trisomy 8 syndrome. *Helv Paediatr Acta* 1981;36:465–472.
8. Antle CM, Pantzar JT, White VA. The ocular pathology of trisomy 22: Report of two cases and review. *J Pediatr Ophthalmol Strabismus* 1990;27:310–314.
9. Antonakou G, Levine R, Chrousos GP et al. Ocular findings in Turner syndrome. A prospective study. *Ophthalmology* 1984;91:926–928.
10. Arbisser AI, Murphree AL, Garcia CG, Howell RR. Ocular findings in mannosidosis. *Am J Ophthalmol* 1976;82:465–471.
11. Armitage MM, Kivlin JD, Ferrell RE. A progressive early onset cataract gene maps to human chromosome 17q24. *Nature Genet* 1995;9:37–40.
12. Ashizawa T, Kejtamancik JF, Kiw J, Perryman MB, Epstein HF, Koch DD. Diagnostic value of ophthalmologic findings in myotonic dystrophy: Comparison with risks calculated by haplotype analysis of closely linked restriction fragment length polymorphisms. *Am J Med Genet* 1992;42:55–60.
13. Attree O, Olivos IM, Okabe I, Bailey LC, Melson KL, Lewis RA, McInnes RR, Nussbaum, RL: The Lowe's oculocerebrorenal syndrome gene encodes a protein highly homologous to inositol polyphosphate-5-phosphatase. *Nature* 1992;358:239–242.
13a. Ayme S, Preus M. The Marshall and Stickler syndromes objective rejection of lumping. *J Med Genet* 1984;21:34–38.
14. Bass HN, Sparkes RS, Crandall F, Tannenbaum SM. Familial partial trisomy 10q(q23-qter) syndrome and paracentric inversion 3 (q13 q26) in the same patient. *Ann Genet* 1978;21:74–77.
15. Berry V, Ionides ACW, Moore AT, Plant C, Bhattacharya SS, Shiels A. A locus for autosomal dominant anterior polar cataract on chromosome 17p. *Hum Mol Genet* 1996;5;415–419.
16. Bianchi AB, Hara T, Ramesh V, Gao J, Klein-Szanto AJ, Morin F, Menon AG, Trofatter JA, Gusella JF, Seizinger BR et al. Mutations in transcript isoforms of the neurofibromatosis 2 gene in multiple human tumour types. *Nature Genet* 1994;6:185–192.
17. Blackburn W, Miller R, Peyton W, Superneau DW, Cooley NR Jr, Zellweger H, Wertelecki W. Comparative studies of infants with mosaic and complete triploidy: An analysis of 55 cases of birth defects. *Birth Defects Orig Art Ser.* New York: March of Dimes Birth Defects Foundation, 1982;18(3B):251–274.
18. Boucher CA, King SK, Carey N, Krahe R, Winchester CL, Rahman S, Creavin T, Meghji P, Bailey ME, Chartier FL et al. A novel homeodomain-encoding gene is associated with a large CpG island interrupted by the myotonic dystrophy unstable (CTG)n repeat. *Hum Mol Genet* 1995;4:1919–1925.
19. Bouzas EA, Freidlin V, Parry DM, Eldridge R, Kaiser-Kupfer MI. Lens opacities in neurofibromatosis 2: Further significant correlations. *Brit J Ophthalmol* 1993;77:354–357.
20. Brakenhoff RH, Henskens HAM, van Rossum MWPC, Lubsen NH, Schoenmakers JGG. Activation of the γE-crystallin pseudogene in the human hereditary Coppock-like cataract. *Hum Mol Genet* 1994;3:279–283.
21. Breg WR, Steele MW, Miller OJ, Warburton D, deCapoa A, Allderdice PW. The cri-du-chat syndrome in adolescents and adults: Clinical finding in 13 older patients with partial deletion of the short arm of chromosome No. 5(5p-). *J Pediatr* 1970;77:782–791.
22. Brei TJ, Burke MJ, Rubinstein JH. Glaucoma and findings simulating glaucoma in the Rubinstein-Taybi syndrome. *J Pediatr Ophthalmol Strabismus* 1995;32:248–252.
23. Buckers M. Erbleiden des auges. Handb d Erbkrankh 1938;5:125–128. As cited in Waardenburg PJ, Franceschetti A, Klein D. *Genetics and Ophthalmology,* Vol. 1. Oxford: Blackwell Scientific, 1961, p. 867.
24. Burd L, Kerbeshian J, Fisher W, Martsolf JT. A case of autism and mosaic of trisomy 8. *J Autism Dev Disord* 1985;15:351–352.
25. Cairns JE, Williams HP, Walshe JM. "Sunflower cataract" in Wilson's disease. *Br Med J* 1969;3:95–96.
26. Caputo AR, Wagner RS, Reynolds DR, Guo SQ, Goel AK. Down syndrome. Clinical review of ocular features. *Clin Pediatr* 1989;29:355–358.
27. Carnevale A, Hernandez M, Limon-Toledo I, Frias S, Castillo J, del Castillo V. A clinical syndrome associated with dup(5p). *Am J Med Genet* 1982;13:277–283.
28. Catalano RA. Down syndrome. *Surv Ophthalmol* 1990;34:385–398.
29. Cheong HI, Kashtan CE, Kin Y, Kleppel MM, Michael AF. Immunohistologic studies of type IV collagen in anterior lens capsules of patients with Alport syndrome. *Lab Invest* 1994;70:553–557.
30. Chrousos GA, O'Neill JF, Traboulsi EI, Rich-

mond A, Rosenbaum KN. Ocular findings in partial trisomy 3q. A case report and review of the literature. *Ophthalmic Paediatr Genet* 1988;9:127–130.

31. Cibis GW, Waeltermann JM, Whitcraft CT, Tripathi RC, Harris DJ. Lenticular opacities in carriers of Lowe's syndrome. *Ophthalmology* 1986;93:1041–1045.
32. Claridge KG, Gibberd FB, Sidey MC. Refsum disease. The presentation and ophthalmic aspects of Refsum disease in a series of 23 patients. *Eye* 1992;6:371–375.
33. Cohen MM, Ornoy A, Rosenmann A, Kohn G. An inherited translocation t(4;15) (p16;q22) leading to two cases of partial trisomy 15. *Ann Genet* 1975;18:99–103.
34. Conneally PM, Wilson AF, Merritt AD, Helveston EM, Palmer CG, Wang LY. Confirmation of genetic heterogeneity in autosomal dominant forms of congenital cataracts from linkage studies. *Cytogenet Cell Genet* 1978;22:295–297.
35. Corney MJ, Smith S. Early development of an infant with 18q- syndrome. *J Ment Defic Res* 1984;28(Pt 4):303–307.

35a. Cotlier E, Rice P. Cataracts in the Smith-Lemli-Opitz syndrome. *Am J Ophthalmol* 1971;72:955–959.

36. Curry CJR, Magenis E, Brown M. Inherited chondrodysplasia punctata due to a deletion of the terminal short arm of an X-chromosome. *N Engl J Med* 1984;311:1010–1015.

36a. Curtis AR, Lindsay S, Boye E, Clarke AJ, Landy SJ, Bhattacharya SS. A study of X chromosome activity in two incontinentia pigmenti families with probable linkage to Xq28. *Eur J Hum Genet* 1994;2:51–58.

37. Decourt L, De Silva Sasso W, Chiorboli E, Fernandes JM. Sobre o sexo genetico nas pacientes dom sindrome de Turner. *Rev Assoc Med Bras* 1954;1:203–206.
38. de Grouchy J, Royer P, Salmon C, Lamy M. Deletion partielle des bras longs du chromosome 18. *Pathol Biol* 1964;12:579–582.
39. Delleman JW, Bleeker-Wagemakers EM, van Veelen AW. Opacities of the lens indicating carrier status in the oculo-cerebro-renal (Lowe) syndrome. *J Pediatr Ophthalmol* 1977;14:202–212.
40. DiLiberti JH, McKean R, Webb MJ, Williams G. Trisomy 5p: Delineation of clinical features. *Birth Defects Orig Art Ser.* New York: March of Dimes Birth Defects Foundation, 1977;8(3C):185–194.
41. Dohlman CH. Familial congenital cornea guttata in association with anterior polar cataract. *Acta Ophthalmol* 1951;29:445–473.
42. Down JLH. Observations on an ethnic classification of idiots. *Clin Lect Rep Lond Hosp* 1866;3:259–262.
43. Edidin DV, Esterly NB, Bamzai AK, Fretzin DF. Chondrodysplasia punctata. Conradi-Hunermann syndrome. *Arch Dermatol* 1977; 113:1431–1434.
44. Edwards JH, Harnden DG, Cameron AH, Crosse VM, Wolff OH. A new trisomic syndrome. *Lancet* 1960;1:787–789.
45. Eiberg H, Marner E, Rosenberg T, Mohr J. Marner's cataract (CAM) assigned to chromosome 16: Linkage to haptoglobin. *Clin Genet* 1988;34:272–275.
46. Eiberg H, Lund AM, Warburg M, Rosenberg T. Assignment of congenital cataract Volkmann type (CCV) to chromosome 1p36. *Hum Genet* 1995;96:33–38.
47. Farrell JW, Morgan KS, Black S. Lensectomy in an infant with cri-du-chat syndrome and cataracts. *J Pediatr Ophthalmol Strabismus* 1988;25:131–134.
48. Fear C, Briggs A. Familial partial trisomy of the long arm of chromosome 3 (3q). *Arch Dis Child* 1979;54:135–138.
49. Felding I, Kirstoffersson U, Sjostrom H, Noren O. Contribution to the 18q- syndrome. A patient with del(18)(q22.3qter). *Clin Genet* 1987;31:206–210.
50. Forabosco A, Bernasconi S, Giovannelli G, Dutrillaux B. Trisomy of the distal third of the long arm of chromosome 10. Report of a new case due to a familial translocation t(10;18)(q24;p11). *Helv Paediatr Acta* 1975; 30:289–295.
51. Ford EC, Jones KW, Polani PE, de Almeida JC, Briggs JH. A sex-chromosome anomaly in a case of gonadal dysgenesis (Turner's syndrome). *Lancet* 1959;1:711–713.
52. Forsius H, Arentz-Grastvedt, Eriksson AW. Juvenile cataract with autosomal recessive inheritance. A study from the Aland Islands, Finland. *Acta Ophthalmol* 1992;70:26–32.
53. Francomano CA, Liberfarb RM, Hirose T, Maumenee IH, Streeten EA, Meyers DA, Pyeritz RE. The Stickler syndrome: Evidence for close linkage to the structural gene for type II collagen. *Genomics* 1987;1:293–296.
54. Frangoulis M, Taylor C. Corneal opacities—A diagnostic feature of the trisomy 8 mosaic syndrome. *Br J Ophthalmol* 1983;67: 619–622.

55. Fried K, Liban E, Lurie M, Friedman S, Reisner SH. Polycystic kidneys associated with malformations of the brain, polydactylyand other birth defects in new born sib. *J Med Genet* 1971;8:285–290.
56. Friedman MW, Wright ES. Hereditary microcornea and cataract in five generations. *Am J Ophthalmol* 1952;35:1017–1021.
57. Frydman M, Steinberger J, Shabtai F, Katznelson MBM, Varsano I. Interstitial deletion 2q14q21. *Am J Med Genet* 1989;34:476–479.
58. Fryns JP, D'hondt F, Goddeeris P, van den Berghe. Full monosomy 21: A clinically recognizable syndrome? *Hum Genet* 1977;37: 155–259.
59. Fryns JP, Kleczkowska A, Vinken L, Geutjens J, Smeets E, Van Den Berghe H. Acrocentric/18p translocation in two mentally retarded males. *Ann Genet* 1986;29:107–111.
60. Fryns JP, Logghe N, van Eygen M, van den Berghe H. New chromosomal syndromes: Partial trisomy of the distal portion of the long arm of chromosome number 10 (10q24->10qter): A clinical entity. *Acta Paediatr Belg* 1979b;32:141–143.
61. Fryns JP, van Bosstraeten B, Malbrain H, van den Berghe H. Interstitial deletion of the long arm of chromosome 2 in a polymalformed newborn—Karyotype: 46,XX,del(2)(q21;q24). *Hum Genet* 1977;39:233–238.
62. Fryns JP, van Eygen M, Logghe N, van den Berghe H. Partial trisomy for the long arm of chromosome 3 (3(q21->qter)+) in a newborn with minor physical stigmata. *Hum Genet* 1978;40:333–339.
63. Fujimoto A, Towner JW, Ebbin AJ, Kahlstrom EJ, Wilson MG. Inherited partial duplication of chromosome no. 15. *Am J Med Genet* 1974;11:287–291.
64. Fujita H, Meng, J, Kawamura M, Tozuka N, Ishii F, Tanaka N. Boy with a chromosome del (3)(q12q23) and blepharophimosis syndrome. *Am J Med Genet* 1992;44:434–436.
65. Gardner RJ, Brown N: Lowe's syndrome: Identification of carriers by lens examination. *J Med Genet* 1976;13:449–454.
66. Ginsberg J, Ballard ET, Buchino JJ, Kinkler AK. Further observations of ocular pathology in Down's syndrome. *J Pediatro Ophthalmol Strabismus* 1980;17:166–171.
67. Girardet M: Une novelle famille de cataracte poussiereuse centrale (cataracta centralis pulverulents). *Opthalmologica* 1943;105:24–36.
67a. Gitzlemann R. Deficiency of erythrocyte galactokinase in a patient with galactose diabetes. *Lancet* 1965;2:670–671.
67b. Goldberg M. The 54th Jackson Memorial Lecture. Persistent fetal vasculature (PFV): an integrated interpretation of signs and symptoms associated with persistent hyperplastic primary vitreous (PHPV). *Am J Ophthalmol* 1997;124:587–626.
67c. Goldstein H, Nielsen KG. Rates and survival of individuals with trisomy 13 and trisomy 18. *Clin Genet* 1988;34:366–372.
67d. Gorlin RJ, Cohen MM, Levin LS. *Syndromes of the Head and Neck*, 3rd Ed. New York: Oxford University Press, 1990, 1008 pp.
68. Gorlin RJ. Classical chromosome disorders. In *New Chromosomal Syndromes,* J. J. Yunis, ed. New York: Academic Press, 1977, pp. 59–117.
69. Gorlin RJ, Yunis J, Anderson VE. Short arm deletion of chromosome 18 in cebocephaly. *Am J Dis Child* 1968;115:473–476.
70. Green JS, Johnson GJ. Congenital cataract with microcornea and Peters' anomaly as expressions of one autosomal dominant gene. *Ophthalmic Paediatr Genet* 1986;7:187–194.
71. Gregoire MJ, Boue J, Junien C, Pernot C, Gilgenkrantz S, Zergollern L. Duplication 15q22qter and its phenotypic expression. *Hum Genet* 1981;59:429–433.
72. Grosse FR, Pandel C, Wiedemann H. The tetraphocomelia-cleft palate syndrome. *Humangenetik* 1975;28:353–356.
73. Happle R. X-linked dominant chondrodysplasia punctata: A review of literature and report of a case. *Hum Genet* 1979;53:65–73.
74. Harman NB. Congenital cataract. A pedigree of five generations. *Trans Ophthalmol Soc UK* 1909;29:101–108.
75. Heathcote JG, Sholdice J, Walton JC, Willis NR, Sergovich FR. Anterior segment mesenchymal dysgenesis associated with partial duplication of the short arm of chromosome 2. *Can J Ophthalmol* 1991;26:35–43.
76. Heiba IM, Elston RC, Klein BEK, Klein R. Evidence for a major gene for cortical cataract. *Invest Ophthalmol Vis Sci* 1995;36:227–235.
77. Heidet L, Dahan K, Zhou J et al. Deletions of both alpha 5(IV) and alpha 6(IV) collagen genes in Alport syndrome and in Alport syndrome associated with smooth muscle tumours. *Hum Mol Genet* 1995;4:99–108.
78. Henning KA, Li L, Iyer N, McDaniel LD, Reagan MS, Legerski R, Schultz RA, Stega-

nini M, Lehmann AR, Mayne LV et al. The Cockayne syndrome group. A gene encodes a WD repeat protein that interacts with CSB protein and a subunit of RNA polymerase II TFIIH. *Cell* 1995;82:555–564.

79. Herrmann J, Opitz JM. The SC phocomelia and the Roberts syndrome: Nogoloci aspects. *Eur J Pediatr* 1977;125:117–134.
80. Heymans HAS, Oorthuys JWE, Nelck G, Wanders RJA, Dingemans KP, Schutgens RBH. Peroxisomal abnormalities in rhizomelic chondrodysplasia punctata. *J Inherited Metab Dis* 1986;9(suppl 2):329–331.
81. Hiller R, Sperduto RD, Ederer F. Epidemiologic associations with nuclear, cortical, and posterior subcapular cataracts. *Am J Epidemiol* 1986;124:916–925.
82. Hood OJ, Rouse BM, Lockhart LH, Bodensteiner JB. Proximal duplications of chromosome 15: Clinical dilemmas. *Clin Genet* 1986:29:234–240.
83. Howard RO. Chromosomal abnormalities associated with cyclopia and synophthalmia. *Trans Am Ophthalmol Soc* 1977;75:505–538.
84. Howard RO. Ocular abnormalities in the cri-du-chat syndrome. *Am J Ophthalmol* 1972; 73:949–954.
85. Human Gene Mapping 5 (1979). Fifth international workshop on human gene mapping. *Birth Defects Orig Art Ser* 1979;15:10.
86. Jaafar MS, Robb RM. Congenital anterior polar cataract. A review of 63 cases. *Ophthalmology* 1984;91:249–254.
86a. Jacobs M, Jeffrey B, Kriss A, Taylor D, Sa G, Bakratt M. Ophthalmologic assessment of young patients with Alport syndrome. *Ophthalmology* 1992;99:1039–1044.
87. Jankiewicz H, Freeberg DD. A six-generation pedigree of congenital zonular cataract. *Am J Optom Arch Am Acad Optom* 1956;33: 555–557.
88. Jansen G, Bachner D, Coerwinkel M, Wormskamp N, Hameister H, Wieringa B. Structural organization and developmental expression pattern of the mouse WD-repeat gene DMR-N9 immediately upstream of the myotonic dystrophy locus. *Hum Mol Genet* 1995;4:843–852.
89. Jordan M. Stammbaumuntersuchungen bei Cataracta stellata coralliformis. *Klin Monatsbl Augenheilkd* 1955:126;469–475.
90. Kaye LD, Rathner AD, Beauchamp GR, Meyers SM, Estes ML. Ocular findings associated with neurofibromatosis type II. *Ophthalmology* 1992;99:1424–1429.
91. Kidd A, Turnpenny P, Kelly K, Clark C, Church W, Hutchinson C, Dean JC, Haites NE. Ascertainment of myotonic dystrophy through cataract by selective screening. *J Med Genet* 1995;32:519–523.
92. Kirkham TH, Werner EB. The ophthalmic manifestations of Rothmund's syndrome. *Can J Ophthalmol* 1975;10:1–4.
93. Klep-de Pater JM, Bijlsma JB, de France HF, Leschot NJ, Duijndam-van den Berge M, van Hemel JO. Partial trisomy 10q. *Hum Genet* 1979;46:29–40.
94. Klein BEK, Klein R, Linton KLP. Prevalence of age-related lens opacities in a population: The Beaver Dam Eye Study. *Ophthalmology* 1992;99:546–552.
95. Khodr GS, Cadena G, Le KL, Kagan-Hallet KS. Duplication (5p14->pter): Prenatal diagnosis and review of the literature. *Am J Med Genet* 1982;12:43–49.
96. Knebelmann B, Forestier L, Drouot L, et al. Spice-mediated insertion of an Alu sequence in the COL4A3 mRNA causing autosomal recessive Alport syndrome. *Hum Mol Genet* 1995;4:675–679.
97. Kondo I, Hirano T, Hamaguchi H, Ohta Y, Haibara S, Nakai H, Takita H. A case of trisomy 3q21->qter syndrome. *Hum Genet* 1979;46:141–147.
98. Kramer P, Yount J, Mitchell T, LaMorticella D, Carrero-Valenzuela R, Lovrien E, Maumenee I, Litt M. A second gene for cerulean cataracts maps to the β crystallin region on chromosome 22. *Genomics* 1996;35:539–542.
99. Kozma C, Hunt M, Meck J, Traboulsi E, Scribanu N. Familial Wolf-Hirschhorn syndrome associated with Rieger anomaly of the eye. *Ophthalmic Paediatr Genet* 1990;11:23–30.
100. Krahe R, Ashizawa T, Abbruzzese C, Roeder E, Carango P, Giancanelli M, Funanange VL, Siciliano MJ. Effect of myotonic dystrophy trinucleotide repeat expansion on DMPK transcription and processing. *Genomics* 1995; 28:1–14.
101. Kroyer S, Niebuhr E. Partial trisomy 10q occurring in a family with a reciprocal translocation t(10;18)(q25;q23). *Ann Genet* 1975; 18:50–55.
102. Kuchle HJ, Normann J, Lubbering I. Ein beitrag zum kongenitalen zystenauge. *Klin Monatsbl Augenheilkd* 1986;188:239–241.
103. Kuchle M, Kraus J, Rummelt C, Naumann GOH. Synophthalmia and holoprosencephaly in chromosome 18p deletion defect. *Arch Ophthalmol* 1991;109:136–137.

104. Latta RJ, Graham CB, Aase J, Scham SM, Smith DW. Larsen's syndrome: A skeletal dysplasia with multiple joint dislocations and unusual facies. *J Pediatr* 1971;78:291–298.
105. Lee JB, Benedict WL. Hereditary nuclear cataract. *Arch Ophthalmol* 1950;44:643–650.
106. Lejeune J, Lafourcade J, Berger R et al. Trois cas de deletion partielle du bras curt d'un chromosome 5. *CR Acad Sci (Paris)* 1963; 257:3098–3102.
107. Lemmink HH, Mochizuki T, van den Heuvel LP, Schroder CH, Barrientos A, Monnens LA, van Oost BA, Brunner HG, Reeders ST, Smeets HJ. Mutations in the type IV collagen alphe 3 (COL4A3) gene in autosomal recessive Alport syndrome. *Hum Mol Genet* 1994; 3:1269–1273.
107a. Lemmink HH, Nillesen WN, Mochizuki T, Schroder CH, Brunner HG, van Gost BA, Monnens LA, Smeets HJ. Benign familial hematuria due to mutation of the type IV collagen α4 gene. *J Clin Invest* 1996;98:1114–1118.
108. Leschot NJ, Lim KS. Complete trisomy 5p: De Novo translocation t(2;5)(q36;p11) with isochromosome 5p. *Hum Genet* 1979;46: 271–278.
109. Leske MC, Chylack LT, Wu S. The lens opacities case control study: Risk factors for cataract. *Arch Ophthalmol* 1991;109:24–51.
110. Lewis RA, Nussbaum RL, Stambolian D. Mapping X-linked ophthalmic diseases. IV. Provisional assignment of the locus for X-linked congenital cataracts and microcornea (the Nance-Horan syndrome) to Xp22.2-p22.3. *Ophthalmology* 1990;97:110–120.
111. Lurie IW, Lazjuk GI. Partial monosomies 18. *Humangenetik* 1972;15:203–222.
112. Luttikhuis ME, Wilson LC, Leonard JV, Trembath RC. Characterization of a de novo 43-bp deletion of the Gs alpha gene (GNAS1) in Albright hereditary osteodystrophy. *Genomics* 1994;21:455–457.
113. Lubsen NH, Renwick JH, Tsui L-C, Breitman ML. A locus for a human hereditary cataract is closely linked to the γ-crystallin gene family. *Proc Natl Acad Sci USA* 1987;84:489–492.
114. Lund AM, Eiberg H, Rosenberg T, Warburg M. Autosomal dominant congenital cataract; linkage relations; clinical and genetic heterogeneity. *Clin Genet* 1992;41:65–69.
115. Mahadevan MS, Baird S, Bailly JE, Shutler GG, Sabourin LA, Tsilfidis C, Neville CE, Barang M, Korneluk RG. Isolation of a novel G protein-coupled receptor (GPR4) localized to chromosome 19q13.3. *Genomics* 1995;30: 84–88.
116. Mansour AM, Traboulsi EI, Khawwam E, Dudin GE, Der Kaloustian VM. Eye findings in interstitial deletion of band q12 of chromosome 5. *Ophthalmic Paediatr Genet* 1984; 4:117–119.
117. Marner E. A family with eight generations of hereditary cataract. *Acta Ophthalmol* 1949; 27:537–551.
118. Marner E, Rosenberg T, Eiberg H. Autosomal dominant congenital cataract. Morphology and genetic mapping. *Acta Ophthalmol* 1989;67:151–158.
119. Massey JY, Roy FH. Ocular manifestations of Conradi disease. *Arch Ophthalmol* 1974;92: 524–526.
120. Martin NJ, Harvey PJ, Pearn JH. The ring chromosome 13 syndrome. *Hum Genet* 1982; 61:18–23.
121. Maumenee IH. Classification of hereditary cataracts in children by linkage analysis. *Trans Am Acad Ophthalmol Otolaryngol* 1979;86: 1554–1558.
122. Mayer UM, Bialasiewicz AA. Ocular findings in a 4p- deletion syndrome (Wolf-Hirschhorn). *Ophthalmic Paediatr Genet* 1989;10: 69–72.
123. Mayer U, Schwanitz G, Grosse KP, Etzold R. Trisomie partielle 2p par translocation familiale 2/6. *Ann Genet* 1978;23:172–176.
124. Mecke S, Passarge E. Encephalocele, polycystic kidneys and polydactyly as an autosomal recessive trait simulating certain other disorders: The Meckel syndrome. *Ann Genet* 1971;14:97–103.
125. Milot JA, Noel L-P, Lemieux N, Richer C-L. Ocular and cytogenetic findings in three new cases of trisomy 9p. *Metab Pediatr Syst Ophthalmol* 1987;10:89–94.
126. Mochizuki T, Lemmink HH, Mariyama M, Antignac C, Gubler MC, Pirson Y, Verellen-Dumoulin C, Chan B, Schroder CH, Smeets HJ et al. Identification of mutations in the alpha 3(IV) and alpha 4(IV) collagen genes in autosomal recessive Alport syndrome. *Nature Genet* 1994;8:77–81.
127. Moller M, Garcia-Cruz D, Rivera H, Sanchez-Corona J, Cantu JM. Pure monosomy and trisomy 2q24.2-q3105 due to an inv ins (7;2)(q21.2;q3105q24.2) segregating in four generations. *Hum Genet* 1984;68:77–86.
128. Mollica F, Li Volti S, Tomarchio S et al. Autosomal dominant cataract and microcornea associated with myopia in a Sicilian family. *Clin Genet* 1985;28:42–46.

129. Moro F, Gorgone G, Li Volti S, Cavallaro N, Faro S, Curreri R, Mollica F. Glucose-6-phosphate dehydrogenase deficiency and incidence of cataract in Silicy. *Ophthalmic Paediatr Genet* 1985;5:197–200.
130. Moross T, Vaithilingam SS, Styles S, Gardner HA. Autosomal dominant anterior polar cataracts associated with a familial 2 : 14 translocation. *J Med Genet* 1984;21:52–53.
131. Mostafa MSE, Temtamy S, El-Gammal MY, Abdel Sayed SI, Abdel-Salam M, El-Baroudy R. Genetic studies of congenital cataract. *Met Pediatr Ophthalmol* 1981;5:233–242.
132. Muroya K, Ogata T, Rappold G, Kink A, Nakahori Y, Fukushimi Y, Aizu I, Matsuo N. Refinement of the locus for X-linked recessive chondrodysplasia punctata. *Hum Genet* 1995; 95:577–580.
133. Nakamura Y, Nakamura H, Fukuda S, Hashimoto T, Maruyama M. Bilateral cystic nephroblastomas and multiple malformations with trisomy 8 mosaicism. *Hum Pathol* 1985; 16:754–756.
134. Nance WE, Higdon SH, Chown B, Engel E. Partial E-18 long-arm deletion. *Lancet* 1968; 1:303.
135. Nettleship E, Ogilvie FM. A peculiar form of hereditary congenital cataract. *Trans Ophthalmol Soc UK* 1906;26:191–206.
136. Nichols WW, Miller RC, Hoffman E et al. Interstitial deletion of chromosome 13 and associated congenital anomalies. *Hum Genet* 1979;52:169–173.
137. Niebuhr E. Partial trisomies and deletions of chromosome 13. In *New Chromosomal Syndromes,* J. J. Yunis, ed. New York: Academic Press, 1977, pp. 273–299.
138. Niebuhr E. The cri-du-chat syndrome. *Hum Genet* 1978;44:227–275.
139. Olivos-Glander IM, Janne PA, Nussbaum RL. The oculocerebrorenal syndrome gene product is a 105-kD protein localized to the Golgi complex. *Am J Hum Genet* 1995;57:817–823.
140. Onufer CN, Stephan MJ, Thuline HC, Char F. Chromosome 13 long arm interstitial deletion associated with features of Noonan phenotype. *Ann Genet* 1987;30:236–239.
141. Orzalesi N, Sorcinelli R, Guiso G. Increased incidence of cataracts in male subjects deficient in glucose-6-phosphate dehydrogenase. *Arch Ophthalmol* 1981;99:69–70.
142. Padma T, Ayyagari R, Murty JS, Basti S, Fletcher T, Rao GN, Kaiser-Kupfer M, Hejtmancik JF. Autosomal dominant zonular cataract with sutural opacities localized to chromosome 17q11-12. *Am J Hum Genet* 1995; 57:840–845.
143. Patau K, Smith DW, Therman E, Inhorn SL, Wagner HP. Multiple congenital anomaly caused by an extra autosome. *Lancet* 1960; 1:790–793.
144. Pearce WG, Mackay JA, Holmes TM, Morgan K, Fowlow SB, Shokeir MH, Lowry RB. Autosomal recessive juvenile cataract I Hutterites. *Ophthalmic Paediatr Genet* 1987;8: 119–124.
145. Pe'er J, Braun JT. Ocular pathology in trisomy 18 (Edward's syndrome). *Ophthalmologica* 1986;192:176–178.
146. Pellissier MC, Philip N, Voeleckel-Baeteman MA, Mattei MG, Mattei JF. Monosomy 21: A new case confirmed by in situ hybridization. *Hum Genet* 1987;75:95–96.
146a. Pena SD, Shokeir MHK. Autosomal recessive cerebro-oculo-facio-skeletal syndrome. *Clin Genet* 1974;5:285–293.
146b. Petit C, Melki J, Levilliers J, Serville F, Weissenbach J, Maroteaux P. An interstitial deletion in Xp22.3 in a family with X-linked recessive chondrodysplasia punctata and short stature. *Hum Genet* 1990;85:247–250.
147. Pettigrew AL, Gollin SM, Greenberg F, Riccardi VM, Ledbetter DH. Duplication of proximal 15q as a cause of Prader-Willi syndrome. *Am J Med Genet* 1987;28:791–802.
148. Pfeiffer RA. Trisomy 8. In *New Chromosomal Syndromes,* J. J. Yunis, ed. New York: Academic Press, 1977, pp. 197–217.
149. Polani PE, Hunter WF, Lennox B. Chromosomal sex in Turner's syndrome with coarctation of the aorta. *Lancet* 1954;2:120–121.
150. Polomeno RC, Cummings C. Autosomal dominant cataracts and microcornea. *Can J Ophthalmol* 1979;14:227–229.
151. Poos F. Ueber eine familiar aufgetretene besondere Schichtstarform: "Cataracta zonlaris pulverulents." *Klin Monatsbl Augenheilkd* 1926;76:502–507.
152. Poulton J, Harley HG, Dasmahapatra J, Brown GK, Potter CG, Sykes B. Mitochondrial DNA does not appear to influence the congenital onset type of mytonic dystrophy. *J Med Genet* 1995;32:732–735.
153. Prieur M, Forabosco A, Dutrillaux B, Laurent C, Bernasconi S, Lejeune J. La trisome 10q24→10qter. *Ann Genet* 1975;18:218–221.
154. Pryde PG, Bawle E, Brandt F, Romero R, Treadwell MC, Evans MI. Prenatal diagnosis

of nonrhizomelic chondrodysplasia punctata (Conradi-Hunermann syndrome). *Am J Med Genet* 1993;47:426–431.
155. Pueschel SM, Scola PS, Mendoza T. Partial trisomy 2p. *J Ment Defic Res* 1987;31: 293–298.
156. Rados A. Central pulverulent (discoid) cataract and its hereditary transmission. *Arch Ophthalmol* 1947;38:57–77.
157. Ragge NK, Baser ME, Klein J, Nechiporuk A, Sainz J, Pulst SM, Riccardi VM. Ocular abnormalities in neurofibromatosis 2. *Am J Ophthalmol* 1995;120:634–641.
158. Ramer JC, Ladda RL, Frankel CA, Beckford A. A review of phenotype-karyotype correlations in individuals with interstitial deletions of the long arm of chromosome 2. *Am J Med Genet* 1989;32:359–363.
159. Reardon W, MacMillan JC, Myring J, Harley HG, Rundle SA, Beck L, Harper PS, Shaw DJ. Cataract and myotonic dystrophy: The role of molecular diagnosis. *Br J Ophthalmol* 1993;77:579–583.
160. Reese PD, Tuck-Muller CM, Maumenee IH. Autosomal dominant congenital cataract associated with chromosomal translocation [t(3;4)(p26.2;p15)]. *Arch Ophthalmol* 1987; 105:1382–1384.
161. Reiss JA, Lovrien EW, Hecht F. A mother with Down's syndrome and her chromosomally normal infant. *Ann Genet* 1971;14: 225–227.
162. Renieri A, Bruttini M, Galli L, Zanelli P, Neri T, Rossetti S, Turco A, Heiskari N, Zhou J et al. X-linked Alport syndrome: An SSCP-based mutation survey over all 51 exons of the COL4A5 gene. *Am J Hum Genet* 1996; 58:1192–1204.
163. Renwick JH, Lawler SD. Probable linkage between a congenital cataract locus and the Duffy blood group locus. *Ann Hum Genet* 1963;27:67–84.
164. Rethore M-O, Aurias A, Couturier J, Dutrillaux B, Prieur M, Lejeune J. Chromosome 8: Trisome complete et trisomies segmentaires. *Ann Genet* 1977;20:5–11.
165. Riccardi VM. Trisomy 8: An international study of 70 patients. *Birth Defects Orig Art Ser.* New York: March of Dimes Birth Defects Foundation, 1977;13(3C):171–184.
166. Richard J, Maumenee IH, Rowe S, Lovrien EW. Congenital cataract possibly linked to haptoglobin. *Cytogenet Cell Genet* 1984; 37:570.
167. Richards A, Yates JRW, Williams R, Payne SJ, Pope FM, Scott JD, Snead MP. A family with Stickler syndrome type 2 has a mutation in the COL11A1 gene resulting in the substitution of glycine 97 by valine in α1(XI) collagen. *Hum Mol Genet* 1996;5:1339–1343.
168. Rivera H, Gonzalez-Flores SA, Rivas F, Sanchez-Corona J, Moller M, Cantu JM. Monosomy 13q32.3->qtr: Report of two cases. *J Med Genet* 1985a;22:142–145.
169. Rivera H, Rivas F, Plascencia L, Cantu JM. Pure monosomy 21pter-q21 in a girl born to a couple 46,XX,t(14;21)(p12;q22) and 46,XY,t(5;18)(q32;q22). *Ann Genet* 1983;26: 234–237.
170. Romke C, Froster-Iskenius U, Heyne K et al. Roberts syndrome and SC phocomelia. A single genetic entity. *Clin Genet* 1987;321: 170–177.
170a. Root S, Carey JC. Survival in trisomy 18. *Am J Med Genet* 1994;49:170–174.
171. Roulear GA, Merel P, Lutchman M, Sanson M, Zucman J, Marineau C, Hoang-Xuan K, Demczuk S, Desmaze C, Plougastel B et al. Alteration in a new gene encoding a putative membrane-organizing protein causes neurofibromatosis type 2. *Nature* 1993;363: 515–521.
172. Rutzler L, Briner J, Sauer F, Schnid W. Mosaik-trisomie-8. *Helv Paediatr Acta* 1974; 29:541–553.
173. Ruttledge MH, Sarrazin J, Rangaratnam S, Phelan CM, Twist E, Merel P, Delattre O, Thomas G, Nordenskjold M, Collins VP et al. Evidence for the complete inactivation of the NF2 gene in the majority of sporadic meningiomas. *Nature Genet* 1994;6:180–184.
174. Salazar D, Rosenfeld W, Verma RS, Jhaveri RC, Dosik H. Partial trisomy of chromosome (3q12→qter) owing to 3q/18p translocation. *Am J Dis Child* 1979;133:1006–1008.
175. Salmon JF, Wallis CE, Murray AND. Variable expressivity of autosomal dominant microcornea with cataract. *Arch Ophthalmol* 1988; 106:505–510.
176. Sander P. A family affected with keratoconus and anterior polar cataract. *Br J Ophthalmol* 1931;15:23–25.
177. Schinzel A. Incomplete trisomy 22. *Hum Genet* 1981;56:269–273.
178. Schinzel A, Hayashi K, Schmid W. Structural aberrations of chromosome 18. II. The 18q-syndrome. Report of three cases. *Humangenetik* 1975;26:123–132.

179. Schinzel A, Schmid W, Luscher U, Nater M, Brook C, Steinmann B. Structural aberrations of chromosome 18. I. The 18p-syndrome. *Archiv Genet* 1974;47:1–15.
180. Schlessel JS, Brown WT, Lysikiewicz A, Schiff R, Zaslav AL. Monozygotic twins with trisomy 18: A report of discordant phenotype. *J Med Genet* 1990;27:640–642.
181. Schnatterly P, Bono KL, Robinow M, Wyandt HE, Kardon N, Kelly TE. Distal 15q trisomy: Phenotypic comparison of nine cases in an extended family. *Am J Hum Genet* 1984; 36:444–451.
182. Schwanitz G, Schmid R-D, Grosse G, Grahn-Liebe E. Translocation familiale 3/22 mat avec trisomie partielle 3q. *J Genet Hum* 1977;25:141–150.
183. Scott MH, Hejtmancik JF, Wozencraft LA, Reuter LM, Parks MM, Kaiser-Kupfer MI. Autosomal dominant congenital cataract. Interocular phenotypic variability. *Ophthalmology* 1994;101:866–871.
184. Shapira H, Mouallem M, Shapiro MS, Weisman Y, Farfel Z. Pseudohypoparathyroidism type Ia: Two new heterozygous frameshift mutations in exons 5 and 10 of the Gs alpha gene. *Hum Genet* 1996;97:73–75.
185. Shapiro MB, France TD. The ocular features of Down's syndrome. *Am J Ophthalmol* 1985;99:659–663.
186. Sher NA, Letson RD, Desnick RJ. The ocular manifestations in Fabry's disease. *Arch Ophthalmol* 1979;97:671–676.
187. Sherard J, Bean C, Bove B et al. Long survival in a 69,XXY triploid male. *Am J Med Genet* 1986;25:307–312.
188. Shokeir MH, Lowry RB. Juvenile cataract in Hutterites. *Am J Med Genet* 1985;22: 495–500.
189. Shokeir MHK. Complete trisomy 22. *Clin Genet* 1978;14:139–146.
190. Snead MP, Payne SJ, Barton DE, Yates JR, al-Imara L, Pope FM, Scott JD. Stickler syndrome: Correlation between vitreoretinal phenotypes and linkage to COL 2A1. *Eye* 1994;8:609–614.
190a. Soriano JM, Funk J. Spontaneous bilateral lens resorption in a case of Hallermann-Streiff. *Klin Monatsbl Augenheilk* 1991;199: 195–198.
191. Spranger JW, Bidder U, Voelz C. Chondrodysplasi punctata (chondrodystropia calcificans) type Conradi-Hunermann. *Fortsch Geb Rontgenstr Nuklearmed* 1970;113:717–725.
192. Spranger JW, Bidder U, Voelz C. Chondrodysplasia punctata (chondrodystropia calcificans). II der Rhizomele typ. *Fortschr Geb Rontgenstr Nucklearmed* 1971;114:327.
193. Stambolian D, Scarpino-Myers V, Eagle RC Jr, Hodes B, Harris H. Cataracts in patients heterozygous for galactokinase. *Invest Ophthalmol Visual Sci* 1986;27:429–433.
194. Stambolian D, Lewis RA, Buetow I, Bond A, Nussbaum R. Nance-Horan syndrome: Localization within the region Xp21.1-Xp22.3 by linkage analysis. *Am J Hum Genet* 1990; 47:13–19.
195. Stambolian D, Ai Y, Sidjanin D, Newburn K, Sathe G, Rosenberg M, Bergsma DJ. Cloning of the galactokinase cDNA and identification of mutations in two families with cataracts. *Nature Genet* 1995;10:307–312.
196. Stathacopoulos RA, Bateman JB, Sparkes RS, Hepler RS. The Rieger syndrome and a chromosome 13 deletion. *J Pediatr Ophthalmol Strabismus* 1987;24:198–203.
197. Steinbach P, Adkins WN, Caspar H et al. The dup(3q) syndrome: Report of eight cases and review of the literature. *Am J Med Genet* 1981;10:159–177.
198. Subrt I, Blehova B, Pallova B. Trisomy 9p resulting from maternal 9/21 translocation. *Hum Genet* 1976;32:217–220.
199. Suchy SF, Olivos-Glander IM, Nussbaum RL. Lowe syndrome, A deficiency of phosphatidylinositol 4,5-bisphosphate 5-phosphatase in the Golgi apparatus. *Hum Mol Genet* 1995;4:2245–2250.
200. Taylor HR, West SK, Rosenthal FS et al. Effect of ultraviolet radiation on cataract formation. *N Engl J Med* 1988;319:1429–1433.
201. Taylor WB. Rothmund's syndrome-Thomson syndrome. *Arch Dermatol* 1957;75:236–244.
202. Telfer MA, Clark CE, Casey PA, Cowell HR, Stroud HH. Long arm deletion of chromosome 13 with exclusion of esterase D from 13q32-13qter. *Clin Genet* 1980;17:428–432.
203. Traboulsi EI, Levine E, Mets M, Parelhoff ES, O'Neill JF, Gaasterland DE. Infantile glaucoma in Down's syndrome (trisomy 21). *Am J Ophthalmol* 1988;105:389–394.
204. Tulloh CG. Heredity of posterior polar cataract with report of a pedigree. *Br J Ophthalmol* 1955;39:374–379.
205. Turleau C, Chavin-Colin F, Narbouton R, Asensi D, de Grouchy J. Trisomy 18q-. Trisomy mapping of chromosome 18 revisited. *Clin Genet* 1980a;18:20–26.
206. Turleau C, de Grouchy J, Roubin M, Chavin-Colin F, Cachin O. Trisomie 9p pure

47,XX,+del(9)(q11) chez le pere. *Ann Genet* 1975b;18:125–129.

207. Turner HH. A syndrome of infantilism, congenital webbed neck and cuitus valgus. *Endocrinology* 1938;23:566–574.
208. Uchida I, Freeman VCP. Triploidy and chromosomes. *Am J Obstet Gynecol* 1985; 151:65–69.
209. van Essen AJ, Kok K, van den Berg A, de Jong B, Stellink F. Partial 3q duplication syndrome and assignment of D385 to 3q25-3q28. *Hum Genet* 1991;87:151–154.
210. Vikkula M, Mariman EC, Lui VC, Zhidkova NI, Tiller GE, Goldring MB, van Beersum SE, de Waal Malefijt MC, van den Hoogen FH, Rogers HH et al. Autosomal dominant and recessive osteochondrodysplasias associated with the COL11A2 locus. *Cell* 1995; 80:431–437.
211. Vogt A. Weitere ergebnisse der Spaltlampenmikroskopie des vorderen Bulbusabschnittes *Archiv Ophthalmol* 1921;107:196–240.
212. Voiculescu I, Back E, Duncan AMV, Schwaibold H, Schempp W. Trisomy 22 in a newborn with multiple malformations. *Hum Genet* 1987;76:298–301.
213. Walravens PA, Greensher A, Sparks JW, Wesenberg RL. Trisomy 8 mosaicism. *Am J Dis Child* 1974;128:564–566.
214. Wang I, Franco B, Ferrero GB, Chinault AC, Weissenbach J, Chumakov I, Le Paslier D, Levilliers J, Klink A, Rappold GA et al. High-density physical mapping of a 3-Mb region in Xp22.3 and refined localization of the gene for X-linked recessive chondodysplasia punctata (CDPX1) *Genomics* 1995;26:229–238.
215. Weiss A, Margo CE. Bilateral microphthalmos with cyst and 13q deletion syndrome. Case report. *Arch Ophthalmol* 1987;105:29.
216. Wertelecki W, Breg WR, Graham JM, Iinuma K, Puck SM, Sergovich FR. Trisomy 22 mosaicism syndrome and Ullrich-Turner stigmata. *Am J Med Genet* 1986;23:739–749.
217. Wibail R, Meunier A: Cataractes congénitales hérditaires du noyau embryonnaire. *Bull Soc Belge Ophtalmol* 1950;95:339–345.
218. Wilcox LM, Bercovitch L, Howard RO. Ophthalmic features of chromosome deletion 4p-(Wolf-Hirchhorn syndrome). *Am J Ophthalmol* 1978;86:834–839.
219. Wilkins LE, Brown JA, Nance WE, Wolf B. Clinical heterogeneity in 80 home-reared children with cri-du-chat syndrome. *J Pediatr* 1983;102:528–533.
220. Wilkins L, Grumbach MM, van Wyk JJ. Chromsomal sex in "ovarian agenesis." *J Clin Endocrinol* 1954;14:1270–1271.
221. Wilson GN, Dasouki M, Barr M. Further delineation of the dup(3q) syndrome. *Am J Med Genet* 1985;22:117–123.
222. Wilson GN, Raj A, Baker D. The phenotypic and cytogenetic spectrum of partial trisomy 9. *Am J Med Genet* 1985;20:277–282.
223. Wilson L, Hodes BL, Martin AO, Elias S, Ogata E, Simpson JL. Cytogenetic analysis of a case of "13q-syndrome." *J Pediatr Ophthalmol Strabismus* 1980;17:63–67.
224. Wilson MG, Towner JW, Forsman I, Siris E. Syndromes associated with the deletion of the long arm of chromosome 18[del(18q)]. *Am J Med Genet* 1979;3:155–174.
225. Wisniewski K, Dambska M, Jenkins EC, Sklower S, Brown WT. Monosomy 21 syndrome: Further delineation including clinical, neuropathological, cytogenetic and biochemical studies. *Clin Genet* 1983;23:102–110.
226. Wohrle D, Kennerknecht I, Wolf M, Enders H, Schwemmle S, Steinbach P. Heterogeneity of DM kinase repeat expansion in different fetal tissues and further expansion during cell proliferation in vitro: Evidence for a causal involvement of methyl-directed DNA mismatch repair in triplet repeat stability. *Hum Mol Genet* 1995;4:1147–1153.
227. Wolf U, Reinwein H, Porsch R, Schroter R, Baitsch H. Defizienz an den hurzen Armen eines Chromosoms Nr. 4. *Humangenetik* 1965;1:397–413.
228. Wulfsberg EA, Sparks RS, Klisak IJ, Teng A. Trisomy 18 phenotype in a patient with an isopseudodicentric 18 chromosome. *J Med Genet* 1984;21:151–153.
229. Wyandt HE, Magenis RE, Hecht F. Abnormal chromosomes 14 and 15 in abortions, syndromes, and malignancy. In *New Chromosomal Syndromes,* J. J. Yunis, ed. New York: Academic Press, 1977:301–338.
230. Yamagata H, Miki T, Nakagawa M, Johnson K, Deka R, Ogihara T. Association of CTG repeats and the 1-kb Alu insertion/deletion polymorphism at the myotonin protein kinase gene in the Japanese population suggests a common Eurasian origin of the myotonic dystrophy mutation. *Hum Genet* 1996;97: 145–147.
231. Young RS, Reed T, Hodes ME, Palmer CG. The dermatoglyphic and clinical features of the 9p trisomy and partial 9p monosomy syndromes. *Hum Genet* 1982;62:31–39.

232. Young RS, Shapiro SD, Hansen KL, Hine LK, Rainosek DE, Guerra FA. Deletion 2q: Two new cases with karyotypes 46,XY, del(2)(q31q33) and 46,XX,del(2)(q36). *J Med Genet* 1983;20:199–202.
233. Yunis E, Gonzalez J, Zuniga R, Torres de Caballero OM, Mondragon A. Direct duplication 2p14->2p23. *Hum Genet* 1979;48: 241–244.
234. Yunis JJ, Lewandowski RC Jr. Partial duplication 10q and duplication 10p syndromes. In *New Chromosomal Syndromes*, J. J. Yunis, ed. New York: Academic Press, 1977.
235. Yunis E, Quintero L, Castaneda A, Ramirez E, Leibovici M. Partial trisomy 3q. *Hum Genet* 1979;48:315–320.
236. Zhang X, Jefferson AB, Auethavekiat V, Majerus PW. The protein deficient in Lowe syndrome is a phosphatidylinositol-4,5-bisphosphate 5-phosphatase. *Proc Natl Acad Sci USA* 1995;92:4853–4856.
237. Zhou J, Mochizuki T, Smeets H, Antignac C, Laurila P, de Paepe A, Tryggvason K, Reeders ST. Deletion of the paired alpha 5(IV) and alpha 6(IV) collagen genes in inherited smooth muscle tumors. *Science* 1993;261: 1167–1169.

13

Corneal Dystrophies

SHU WUN CHANG
SUHAS TULI
DIMITRI T. AZAR

Corneal dystrophies are hereditary disorders that affect the central part of both corneas and are not associated with inflammation. They are generally inherited in an autosomal dominant fashion with variable expressivity.

Although the genetic basis of all dystrophies has not been fully elucidated, more dystrophies are being linked to mutations in specific genes. With recombinant DNA technology it has become possible to study the molecular basis of individual genes and their expression.

Lattice, granular, and Avellino dystrophies have been mapped to the same region on chromosome 5q.[90] The mapping has been further refined to a genetic distance of 2 cM on the same chromosome for lattice type I dystrophy,[122] and the gene has been identified as coding for kerato-epithelin.[238a] Type 2 lattice corneal dystrophy is clinically more similar to lattice corneal dystrophy type 1 (LCDI) than to granular dystrophy. Yet type 2 lattice corneal dystrophy was mapped to chromosome 9,[71] and LCD I and granular dystrophy map to chromosome 5q. Another interesting fact is that patients may show evidence of lattice type 1 dystrophy in the primary graft, and granular dystrophy in the regraft specimens.[90] This illustrates that some other factor, probably also genetic, is capable of modulating phenotypic expression of the primary disease-causing mutation. Existing classifications of corneal dystrophies have been based on the layer of the cornea that is affected. However, involvement of more than one layer can occur simultaneously. For example, Reis–Bückler dystrophy, which was also mapped to chromosome 5q,[315] not only affects Bowman's layer but has been found to be associated with granular deposits in the stroma[233] and with lattice type 1 dystrophy.[203] Thus, a classification based on the genetic localization of corneal dystrophies may emerge with further gene mapping and identification. Also with time there is a possibility that some conditions not conventionally considered to be dystrophies might be reclassified as such. For example, polymorphic amyloid degeneration has been reported in three siblings, indicating that it may be hereditary.[340]

The use of a gene-based classification will improve the understanding of the pathogenesis of these disorders. It may be possible to modulate the course of these diseases based on knowledge of their biochemical defects. At present, however, the current classification scheme based on the involvement of different layers of the cornea allows ophthalmologists to allocate corneal dystrophies to distinct phenotypic categories, whether or not these categories are genetically related (Table 13.1).

Table 13.1. Classification: Based on the Affected Layer of the Cornea

Epithelium	Meesman's dystrophy
Epithelial basement membrane	Map/dot/fingerprint dystrophy
Bowman's membrane	Reis–Bücklers dystrophy Anterior membrane dystrophy of Grayson–Wilbrandt Honeycomb dystrophy of Thiel and Behnke Subepithelial mucinous corneal dystrophy
Stroma	Granular dystrophy Granular-lattice dystrophy Lattice dystrophy Macular dystrophy Gelatinous droplike dystrophy Fleck dystrophy Central crystalline dystrophy of Schnyder Marginal crystalline dystrophy of Bietti Central cloudy dystrophy of François Parenchymatous dystrophy of Pillat Posterior amorphous dystrophy
Pre-Descemet's dystrophy	Typical pre-Descemet's dystrophy Associated with ichthyosis Polymorphic stromal dystrophy Cornea farinata
Endothelial dystrophies	Fuchs' endothelial dystrophy Congenital hereditary endothelial dystrophy Posterior polymorphous dystrophy

DYSTROPHIES OF THE EPITHELIUM, EPITHELIAL BASEMENT MEMBRANE, AND BOWMAN'S LAYER

Juvenile Hereditary Epithelial Dystrophy (Meesman Dystrophy)

First described clinically by Pameijer in 1935[254] and histopathologically by Meesman and Wilke in 1939,[219] this rare autosomal dominant dystrophy[324] has incomplete penetrance (as low as 60%) and variable expressivity.[185,219,220,254,318,324] A recessive form has also been reported that was described by Stocker and Holt, who found 20 affected individuals in a group of 200 descendants of Moravian settlers.[324]

Clinical Features

Patients range in age from 7 months to 70 years. The disease process begins early in life. There is bilateral, symmetric, and diffuse corneal involvement, especially in the interpalpebral zone. Clusters of tiny round cysts in the epithelium appear as discrete white spots on focal illumination and as refractile, clear, cyst-like structures on retroillumination (Fig. 13.1*A* and *B*).[318] Positive staining with fluorescein can be seen due to rupture of superficial cysts. Some of the cysts near the limbus may occur in whorls or wedge-shaped clusters.[219] Refractile lines may be formed by coalescence of cysts. Patients remain asymptomatic until the fourth or fifth decades of life when photophobia, redness, and pain occur because of recurrent erosions due to rupture of cysts. Later, subepithelial gray opacities appear. There may be blurring of vision,[324] but visual acuity remains good in most cases. Visual disturbances are due to irregularity of the corneal surface and to mild opacification. The central corneal thickness and corneal sensations are reduced, particularly in younger patients.

Differential Diagnosis

The epithelial cysts of this disease may be confused with the epitheliopathy that develops in contact lens wearers, toxicity from local anesthetics, vernal conjunctivitis, meibomitis, or dry

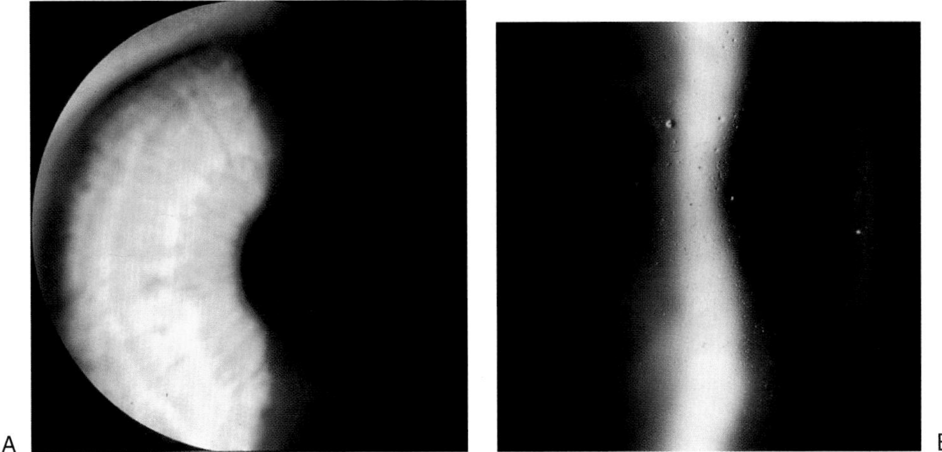

Figure 13.1 A, B. Meesman's dystrophy. **B.** Note the diffuse uniform microcystic changes involving superficial and deep epithelial layer. (**B.** Courtesy of Dr. William Power.)

eyes. These conditions are nonfamilial, however. Map dot, fingerprint dystrophy is not characterized by the uniform and diffuse distribution of the cysts of Meesman dystrophy.

Histopathology

The primary pathology in Meesmann dystrophy lies in the basal epithelium, which shows accumulation of an abnormal intracytoplasmic substance described as a "peculiar" fibrillogranular material that causes cell death. This material reacts with periodic acid and Schiff's reagent and stains with Hale's colloidal iron.[339] Cysts are actually areas of cellular degeneration and contain PAS-positive (periodic acid–Schiff) material. There is thickening of the basement membrane[44,86,185] and increase in glycogen content of the basal epithelial cells. The increased glycogen content is believed to represent increased cell turnover.[60,185]

Electron Microscopy

The epithelium shows degenerative changes including intense vacuolation.[241] Cysts have a corrugated wall consistent with acantholysis. An electron-dense fibrillogranular "peculiar" substance is found in the cytoplasm of affected cells.[44,86,185] Some believe that the abnormal material is derived from tonofilaments and is in close relation to the desmosomes.[339] Others have found electron-dense bodies similar to lysosomes in the epithelial cells.[241] The basement membrane is thickened and appears to have two zones. The thicker zone is rich in collagen fibrils mimicking abnormal anchoring fibrils. Frequent intercalated fibroblasts are seen in the thinner zone, which is poor in fibrils and may represent a repair phenomenon.[339] Bowman's layer and the superficial stroma are unaffected.

Treatment

Because the symptoms are minimal, treatment is rarely required. It includes symptomatic management of recurrent erosions with hypertonic saline, therapeutic contact lenses, or epithelial debridement. Debridement of the epithelium is usually followed by reappearance of symptoms. Superficial keratectomy is curative but is rarely warranted.[60] In recent years phototherapeutic keratectomy (PTK) with the excimer laser has emerged as an alternative treatment of recalcitrant recurrent erosions. With PTK the epithelial defect sites are ablated to a depth of 3–4 μm with reportedly promising results[70,83,93,136,148,246,248,264,276,314] Lamellar and penetrating keratoplasty are rarely indicated.[44,324] Although the dystrophy is known to recur in grafts, the disease may be less severe after recurrence.

Epithelial Basement Membrane Dystrophy

The underlying pathology in all anterior corneal dystrophies is localized to the abnormal epithelial–basement membrane adhesion complex and manifests clinically as recurrent erosions. The primary alteration in the epithelial–basement membrane adhesion complex could be either due to a dystrophic epithelium, epithelial basement membrane, or Bowman's membrane, in combination with or without production of abnormal substances.

Clinical Features

Also known as fingerprint/map/dot dystrophy, Cogan microcystic dystrophy, fingerprint dystrophy, anterior basement membrane dystrophy, and dystrophic recurrent erosion, this is probably the anterior corneal dystrophy most frequently encountered in clinical practice.[60,61,166,343,373] It is bilateral, with no definite hereditary pattern. Autosomal dominant forms have been reported.[34,96,188] Changes similar to fingerprint/map/dot dystrophy are seen in about 76% of the normal population above the age of 50 years.[362] There is an overlap between the epithelial changes that occur in normal individuals following trauma and genetically determined dystrophies. This may reflect the limited ways that the anterior cornea can respond to a variety of insults. The name fingerprint/map/dot dystrophy very aptly describes the clinical appearance of the disorder and represents the historical sequence of recognition of its individual clinical components. Cogan first described microcystic dystrophy of the cornea in five unrelated women who had bilateral grayish-white spherical lesions of varying sizes. Histopathology revealed cysts and an abnormal basement membrane. Maplike dystrophy was described by Guerry in 1965,[126] who had earlier reported fingerprint lines.[125]

Cogan dystrophy affects predominantly white women above 30 years of age. However, it can occur as early as 4–8 years of age in familial cases. In nonfamilial cases, recurrent erosions occur for a few years, with spontaneous improvement and no significant residual visual acuity loss (Fig. 13-2*A–F*).[348] Maps are geographic circumscribed gray lesions best seen with broad oblique illumination and are the most common and earliest clinical manifestation of fingerprint/map/dot dystrophy. They appear in varying shapes and sizes and do not stain with fluorescein. They are better appreciated on retroillumination and a dilated pupil and have a well-defined border at one end, and blend with the surrounding clear cornea at the other end (Fig. 13.2). Dots are cysts or fine blebs seen as gray-white intraepithelial opacities in close proximity to the maplike patches. Best visualized on retroillumination, dots vary in size. The superficial microcysts may stain positively with fluorescein, whereas deeper ones do not indicate unruptured microcysts. Fingerprint lines are the least frequently encountered of the three lesions. They are branching refractile lines with club-shaped terminations[188] and are best seen on retroillumination. They predominate in the central and midperipheral cornea surrounding the maps, and fluorescein may highlight them. Leashes of long, thick fingerprint lines are called "mare's tails." Combinations of maps and dots are encountered most frequently, followed by maps alone. It is rare that fingerprints are present along with maps and dots, whereas dots alone are never seen. visual acuity is minimally affected. Visual loss occurs due to irregular astigmatism.

Histopathology and Pathogenesis

The basic pathology in fingerprint/map/dot dystrophy is the synthesis of abnormal basement membrane and is responsible for the whole spectrum of clinical manifestations. Erosions are due to absence of hemidesmosomal connections of the epithelial cells in areas with abnormal basement membrane. Maps are formed by multilaminar basement membrane[32] and extension of projections of abnormal basement membrane into the epithelium. Dots are pseudocysts filled with cytoplasmic and nuclear debris, and lipid. Cysts form in areas with intraepithelial extensions of aberrant basement membrane. Epithelial cells beneath the aberrant basement membrane become vacuolated and liquefied. The wall of the pseudocyst has a corrugated appearance on electron microscopy due to the villous processes of the surrounding

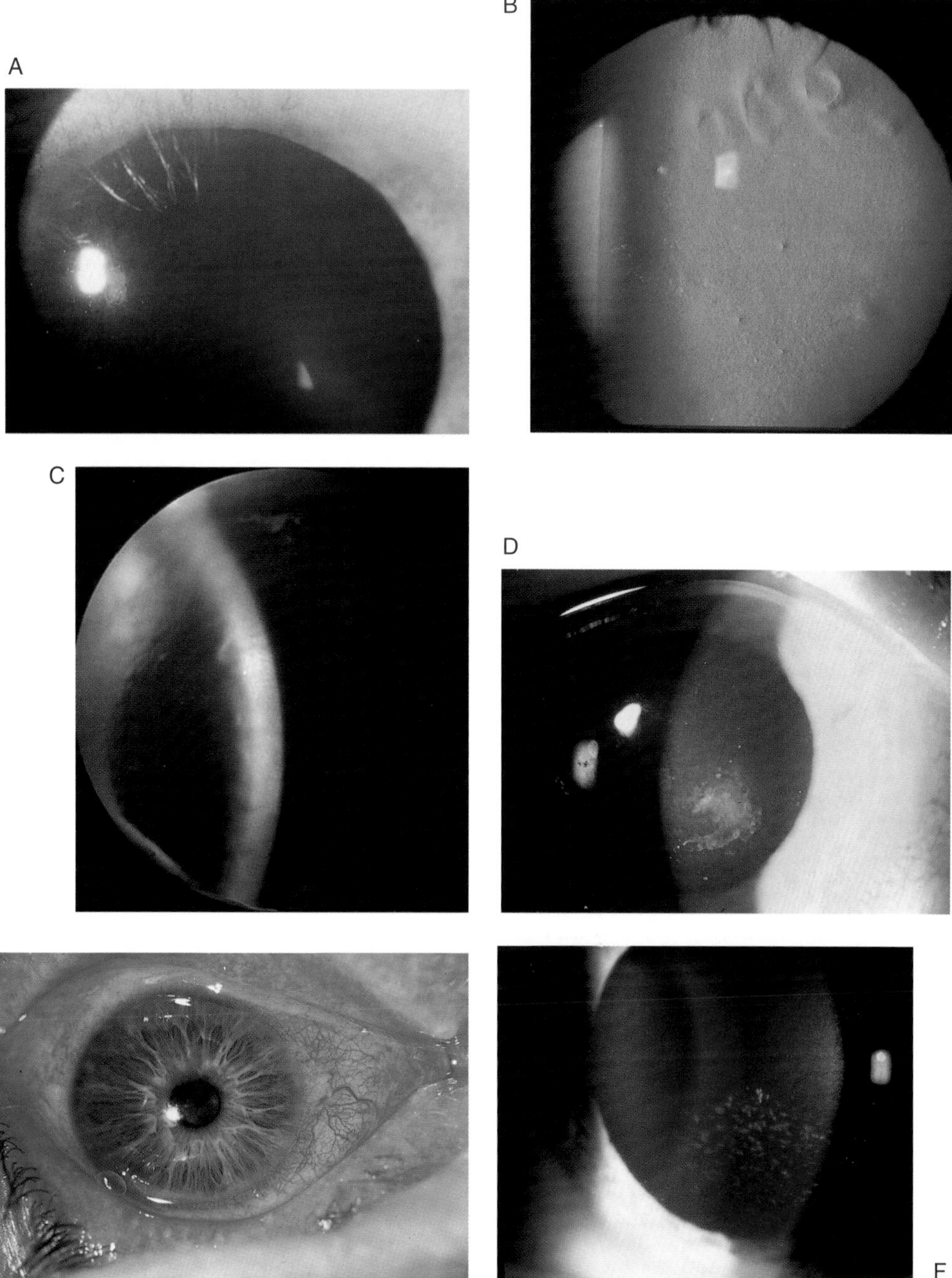

Figure 13.2. **A, B.** Clinical appearance of a 35-year-old female with map/dot/fingerprint dystrophy by direct illumination (**A**) and by retroillumination (**B**). **C, D.** Recurrent erosion syndrome. Loose epithelium (**C**) and epithelial defects (**D**) may recur frequently in patients with map/dot/fingerprint dystrophy. **E.** Therapeutic soft contact lens used to allow reformation of the epithelial adhesion structures. **F.** A 35-year-old man with epithelial basement membrane dystrophy and persistent recurrent corneal erosion and 20/40 visual acuity after anterior stromal puncture. (A, B, and F reproduced with permission from: Phototherapeutic Keratectomy, Azar DT, Steinert RF, and Stark WJ, eds. Igaku Shoin, Tokyo Japan.)

epithelial cells that project into the pseudocyst. Rupture of these cysts causes recurrent erosions. Linear projections of fibrillogranular material into the epithelium with thickening of the basement membrane is responsible for fingerprints.

Differential Diagnosis

Fingerprint lines are also seen in Fuchs dystrophy and a variety of other conditions.[33,38] Traumatic erosions show similar features, but the changes are localized to the traumatized area.[40] Blebs are bubblelike structures seen on retroillumination and are uniform in size and shape. Cases with blebs only were earlier designated *bleblike dystrophy.* Nets are refractile lines or rows of blebs. Neither blebs nor nets are associated with recurrent erosions.[35,36]

Treatment

In the early stages, treatment consists of symptomatic management of recurrent erosions with hypertonic saline and double patching, and a thin, loosely fitting, high water content soft contact lens. Epithelial debridement has been reported to be successful in severe cases.[247] In

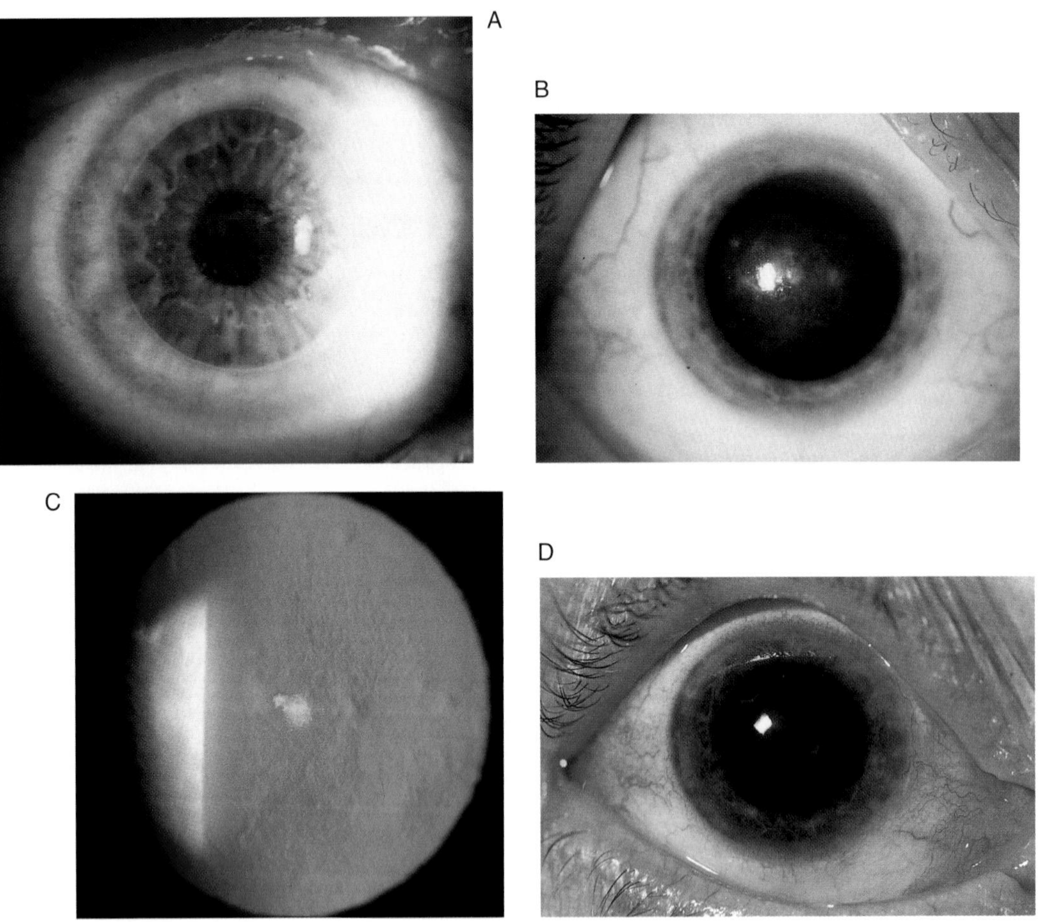

Figure 13.3. **A.** Clinical appearance of cornea of 26-year-old woman with recurrent Reis–Bücklers dystrophy in a graft presenting with 20/40 vision. **B, C.** A 57-year-old man with Reis–Bückler's dystrophy resulting in 20–80 vision who underwent phototherapeutic keratectomy (PTK). Preoperative appearance, by direct illumination and by retroillumination, respectively. **D.** Postoperative appearance of the eye at 1 month postoperatively. Visual acquity improved 20/50. **E.** At 6 months postoperatively. Visual acuity regressed to 20–70. **F, G.** Appearance of cornea, by direct illumination and retroillumination, respectively, at 20 months postoperatively with similar visual acuity. **H.** Honeycomb dystrophy. (A–G: reproduced with permission from: Phototherapeutic Keratectomy, Azar DT, Steinert RF, and Stark WJ, eds. Igaku Shoin, Tokyo Japan.)

recalcitrant cases superficial keratectomy and a soft contact lens relieve symptoms.[48] Anterior stromal puncture with a 23- to 25-gauge needle to a 0.1 mm depth induces new basement membrane formation and a fibrocytic reaction and may help decrease recurrences.[159] There are several reports of treatment of recalcitrant recurrent erosions with excimer laser phototherapeutic keratectomy with success rates ranging from 74% to 100%.[70,83,93,136,148,246,248,264,276,314] If visual symptoms are due to epithelial irregularity, they can be treated with a hard contact lens, which also decreases the severity of basement membrane changes.

Reis–Bücklers Dystrophy

This condition was first reported by Reis in 1917 as a superficial corneal annular dystrophy with geographic opacities.[22,278] A later description was given in more detail by Bücklers in another family. The mode of inheritance is autosomal dominant with variable expressivity. Two other dystrophies, Thiel–Behnke and Grayson–Wilbrandt, which were earlier thought to be distinct entities, are now considered to be variants of Reis–Bücklers dystrophy.

Clinical Features

Reis–Bücklers dystrophy manifests in the first decade of life with recurrent episodes of ocular irritation, photophobia, and watering. These attacks are due to recurrent erosions, which decrease in frequency with time as Bowman's layer is progressively replaced with scar tissue.[151,278] Attacks typically occur four to five times a year and stabilize after the third decade of life, around which time visual acuity is reduced. The diffuse opacification and irregular surface contribute to the decrease in visual acuity (Fig. 13.3*A*–*H*).

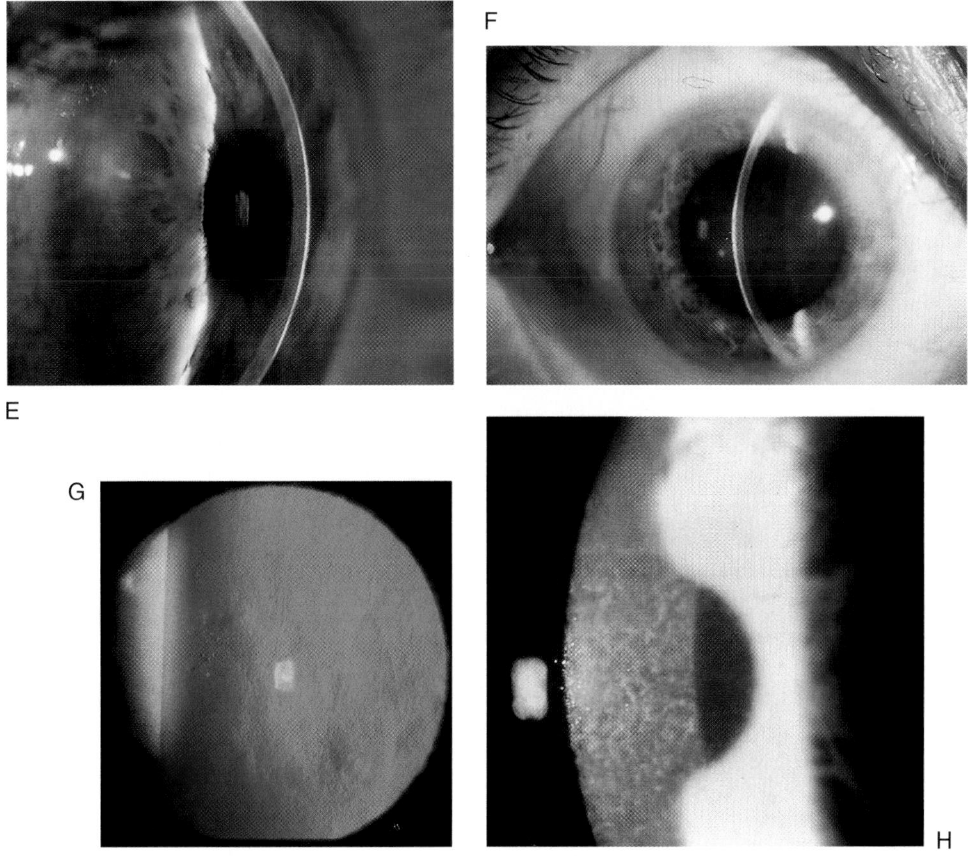

Figure 13.3. Continued.

Lesions are located centrally and in the midperipheral cornea, giving an annular or ring-shaped appearance. The peripheral cornea is spared and the intervening areas are essentially normal, although a diffuse haze that extends to the limbus can be seen by retroillumination. There is gradual fine reticular opacification of the anterior cornea in the early stages. Superficial gray-white opacities develop at the level of Bowman's layer. These opacities are linear, geographic, honeycombed, or ringlike and cause progressive corneal clouding[151,256,278] and are best seen with broad oblique illumination. Corneal sensations are decreased[129,160,372] and prominent corneal nerves[151] may be seen.

Etiology

The structural alterations in Reis–Bücklers dystrophy could be either due to *(1)* anomalous fibrous tissue production by anterior stromal keratocytes causing destruction of Bowman's layer, *(2)* abnormal basal epithelium causing activation of anterior stromal keratocytes, which leads to scar formation and secondary destruction of Bowman's layer, or *(3)* primary dystrophy of Bowman's layer causing secondary alterations in the epithelium and stroma. Immunolocalization of laminin and bullous pemphigoid antigen favors an epithelial defect as the primary cause for this dystrophy.[196] Basement membrane collagens have been localized in the anterior stroma, further implicating an epithelium problem[56] in the pathogenesis of this dystrophy.

Histopathology

Light Microscopy. Bowman's layer is replaced with a fibrocellular material and projects into the epithelium.[123,129,143,151,155,160,259,281,372,377] The basal epithelial layers degenerate and the basement membrane breaks down and is absent in places. The posterior epithelial layer has a sawtooth configuration. In places where Bowman's layer is intact, this material accumulates between the epithelium and Bowman's layer. The posterior stroma, Descemet's membrane, and endothelium are unaffected.

Electron Microscopy. Ultrastructurally, the fibrocellular layer consists of large collagen fibrils (diameter 250–400 Å) with a regular periodicity interspersed with short curly filaments with a diameter of 100 Å. There is disorganization of the epithelial–basement membrane adhesion structures with loss of hemidesmosomes.[5] The basal epithelium shows degenerative changes. There is cytoplasmic vacuolization, mitochondrial swelling, and clumping of nuclear chromatin. Occasionally the epithelial basement membrane of the bulbar conjunctiva may show reduplication.[377]

Linkage Studies

The clinical features of Reis–Bücklers dystrophy resemble granular dystrophy, and there has been a lot of debate whether they are different entities or part of a wide spectrum of manifestations of the same disease.[35,179,233,302,356] Granular corneal dystrophy has been linked to chromosome 5q.[82,122] Kompf et al. were able to show some evidence of linkage of Reis–Bücklers dystrophy on chromosome 6.[179] More recent studies, however, have localized the gene to 5q![315]

Treatment

Management of this disorder includes treatment of recurrent erosions in the early stages. Recurrent erosions can be treated conventionally with hypertonic saline, double patching of the eye, or soft contact lenses. Debridement can be done in cases with recalcitrant erosions. Phototherapeutic keratectomy with the excimer laser has been shown to be very successful[54,128,136,189,217,253,277,296,314] for the treatment of Reis–Bücklers dystrophy. PTK is performed to a depth ranging from 18 to 100 μm following epithelial debridement or ablation. Superficial keratectomy and keratoplasty[129,151,281,376] are warranted when visual acuity is significantly reduced or if the symptoms are debilitating. Recurrences may occur after keratectomy or keratoplasty.[50,250,377]

Anterior Membrane Dystrophy of Grayson-Wilbrandt

Grayson and Wilbrandt[118] described a corneal dystrophy similar to Reis–Bücklers dystrophy in two generations of one family. The onset of this disease occurs at 10–11 years of age, which is slightly later than in Reis–Bücklers dystrophy. Recurrent erosions are infrequent and visual acuity is variably affected. Slit-lamp examination reveals gray-white moundlike opacities at the level of Bowman's layer projecting into the epithelium. The intervening areas are clear and the peripheral cornea is spared. The corneal sensation is normal. Histopathologic examination reveals PAS-positive material at the level of the basement membrane. There are interruptions of Bowman's layer. In one patient,[87] ultrastructural examination revealed accumulation of fibrocellular material above an intact Bowman's membrane with thickening of the basement membrane. Thus, Grayson–Wilbrandt dystrophy is a variant of Reis–Bücklers dystrophy and the differentiating features are its later onset and the fact that the corneal sensations are normal and visual acuity is not severely reduced. Grayson–Wilbrandt dystrophy has also been described in members of a Japanese family who developed bilateral ring-shaped corneal opacities in adolescence.[184]

Honeycomb Dystrophy of Thiel and Behnke

Another variant of Reis–Bücklers dystrophy, honeycomb dystrophy of Thiel and Behnke is a bilateral autosomal dominant disorder with onset in early childhood.[335] Patients suffer from progressive recurrent erosions that cease later in life and are followed by a decrease in visual acuity. A honeycomblike subepithelial opacification develops in the central cornea with sparing of the peripheral cornea. The corneal surface remains smooth and corneal sensations are normal.

Histopathologically, a fibrillogranular material is deposited under the epithelium with projections into the overlying cells. The epithelial basement membrane is thickened, split, or duplicated. These findings were seen in a patient with a family history of Reis–Bücklers dystrophy.[378] Reis–Bücklers dystrophy differs from this disease in that Bowman's layer is primarily affected in the former. However, in light of the family history of Reis–Bücklers dystrophy in some patients with Thiel–Behnke disease, honeycomb dystrophy is best considered a variant of the former. Wittebol-Post et al. reexamined the family reported to have the corneal dystrophy of Waardenburg and Jonkers, and their biomicroscopical and histopathological examination revealed findings similar to those of honeycomb dystrophy.[347,370]

Subepithelial Mucinous Corneal Dystrophy

Feder et al.[84] described a dystrophy in a family where patients ranged in age from 45 to 78 years. Recurrent erosions started in early childhood with progressively decreasing visual acuity. The visual acuity varied from 20/25 to 20/400. On slit-lamp examination the cornea showed a diffuse, bilateral, homogeneous subepithelial haze, most dense centrally and fading toward the limbus. There were irregularly shaped, dense, gray-white, subepithelial patches in the central and paracentral parts of the cornea. Some of these patches were elevated and distorted the anterior corneal contour. The epithelium was intact and the cornea was of normal thickness.

Light microscopic examination revealed degeneration of the epithelium without evidence of pseudocysts. A homogeneous eosinophilic layer was present anterior to Bowman's layer. There was thinning of the overlying epithelium, and the deposits were elevated above the level of the basement membrane. The material showed a positive PAS reaction and stained with Masson trichome and Alcian blue. It did not stain positively for hyalin, and Congo red staining was negative. Electron microscopy revealed irregular deposits of a fine fibrillar material consistent with proteoglycan, which is the main component of connective tissue mucins. The epithelial adhesion structures were absent in places where the basement membrane was disrupted. Immunohistochemical staining was positive for chondroitin 4-sulfate and dermatan sulfate. The dystrophy is similar to the Grayson–Wilbrandt variant of Reis–Bücklers corneal dystrophy clinically but differs from it histochemically. Corneas of patients with Grayson–Wilbrandt disease do not stain with Alcian blue or Masson trichrome.

Treatment includes management of recurrent erosions in the early stages. Penetrating keratoplasty and superficial keratectomy can be performed if vision is reduced. Because the disease is superficial, PTK with the excimer laser has potential for its treatment.

STROMAL DYSTROPHIES

Granular Dystrophy

Clinical Features

Granular dystrophy is also called Groenouw I or breadcrumb dystrophy. The mode of inheritance is autosomal dominant[4,9,229,308] with 100% penetrance. Lesions develop in the first or second decades of life. They are bilateral, symmetric, sharply demarcated grayish-white opacities of variable size and shape, or radial lines in the superficial stroma with intervening clear areas. The overlying epithelium is intact. Visual acuity is minimally affected in this early stage. Photophobia may occur due to scattering of light by the opacities. The opacities slowly progress, coalesce, and involve the deeper stroma. Some have a Christmas tree appearance; others are round with clear or solid centers, snowflake-like or appear like sponge imprints. Snowflakes are homogeneous opacities with sharp irregular margins. They are opaque on focal illumination and partially translucent on retroillumination. Opacities are variable in extent but never reach the limbus. Corneal sensations are intact. Intrafamilial similarities and interfamilial differences in clinical features have been reported.[232]

Several variants of granular dystrophy are recognized. In type I, or the progressive corneal dystrophy of Waardenburg and Jonkers,[347] the onset is in the first decade of life. The opacities are snowflake-like, forming a diffuse superficial stromal haze. The haze is best visualized on broad oblique illumination, Retroillumination reveals fine granularity and indirect illumination shows a myriad of fine punctate opacities (Figs. 13.4*A*, *B*, *E*, and *F*). Some patients experience recurrent erosions. Visual acuity may be severely affected by the fourth decade of life due to stromal opacification. The staining characteristics of this dystrophy, however, are similar to those of granular dystrophy. Some authors have considered this dystrophy a variant of Reis–Bücklers dystrophy.[370]

In type II granular dystrophy, opacities appear in the second decade. It is less severe and slower in progression[92] than type I. Opacities have a breadcrumb-like appearance, and patients do not usually suffer from recurrent erosions (Fig. 13.4*C* and *D*).

Rodrigues et al. described a dystrophy with onset in infancy. The deposits are superficial and cause painful recurrent erosions that require early surgical intervention. There are numerous deposits in the region of Bowman's layer and Bowman's layer is destroyed. The presence of classic granular dystrophy in parents or siblings may indicate that they are expressions of the same genotype.[127,291]

Although identical biomicroscopically, granular dystrophy patients show a normal immunoglobulin pattern on electrophoresis in contrast to patients with paraproteinemic crystalline keratopathy.[230]

Pathology

The stroma contains hyaline eosinophilic deposits that stain intensely with Masson trichrome, weakly with periodic acid–Schiff (PAS) stain, and negatively with Verhoeff stain. Congo red may stain the peripheral portions of the deposits.[110,146] The epithelial basement membrane and Bowman's membrane may be thin or absent in places.[207]

Ultrastructurally, electron-dense rodlike deposits (100–500 μm wide) are seen subepithelially, in between the stromal lamellae and intracytoplasmically in keratocytes.[127,186,371] the deposits are either filamentous, homogeneous, or have a moth-eaten pattern.[319,348,371] Tubular microfibrils can be seen surrounding these lesions. The deposits have positive Congo red staining, but they do not have the spatial orientation of amyloid.[289] Histochemically they contain tyrosine, tryptophan, and sulfur-containing amino acids.[110] Moller et al. demonstrated the presence of kappa and lambda light chains of immunoglobulin G.[231] The exact source of these deposits is unknown and it is speculated that either the keratocytes or the epithelium, or both, are responsible for their production.[200] In keratocyte-related dystrophies, recurrences

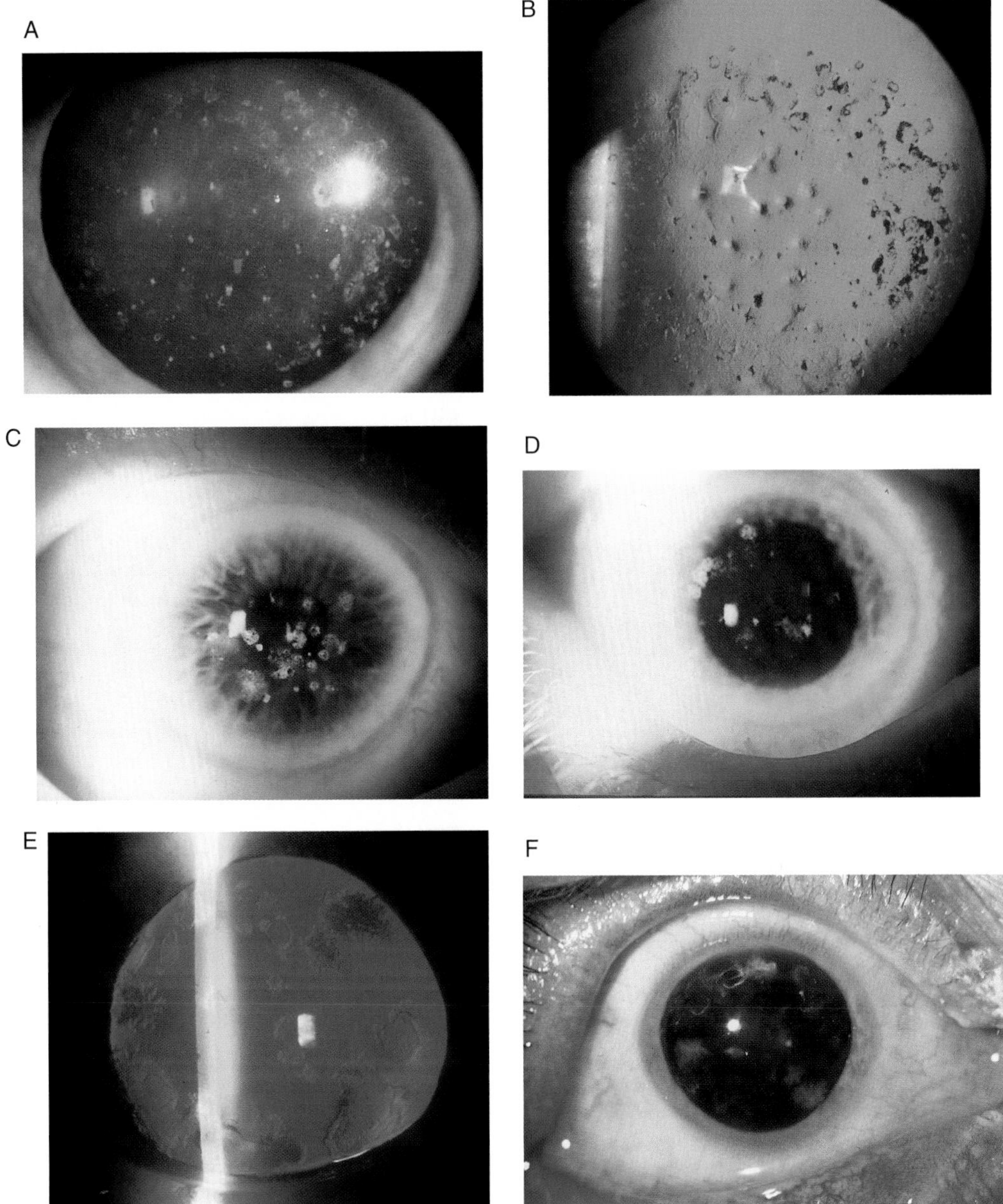

Figure 13.4. Clinical appearance of a patient with type I granular dystrophy by direct diffuse illumination (**A**) and by retroillumination (**B**). **C.** Clinical appearance of a patient with type II granular dystrophy showing breadcrumb-like appearance of hyaline deposits. **D.** Postoperative appearance 1 month after phototherapeutic keratectomy. Visual acuity of 20/20 was achieved despite residual deposits of hyaline material in the visual axis. **E, F.** Snowflake hyaline deposits of type I granular dystrophy. (A, B, and F reproduced with permission from: Phototherapeutic Keratectomy, Azar DT, Steinert RF, and Stark WJ, eds. Igaku Shoin, Tokyo Japan.)

after penetrating keratoplasty are expected to occur peripherally within the deeper donor tissue. The time taken to recur centrally would be expected to vary proportionally with the graft size, and the recurrences are expected sooner in lamellar grafts. These findings are observed in recurrent macular dystrophy but not in recurrent granular dystrophy, lending support to the epithelial etiology of granular dystrophy.

Degenerative changes are apparent in keratocytes with cytoplasmic vacuolization and dilatation of endoplasmic reticulum.[319] In recurrent cases of granular dystrophy, electron-dense deposits are seen in the epithelium. These deposits are crystalline granules that are either rod-shaped or trapezoid-shaped. The smaller granules are surrounded by 15 nm particles, whereas the larger granules are membrane bound.[150,369]

Linkage Studies

Granular dystrophy has been linked to chromosome 5q.[82] Linkage analysis for three clinically distinct stromal corneal dystrophies—lattice, granular, and Avellino (Fig. 13.5*A* and *B*)—revealed that the chromosomal location is the same on chromosome 5q for all three dystrophies. The gene causing each of the three dystrophies was located within a 10 cM region on chromosome 5,[326] and was found to code for a structural protein named kerato-epithelin.[238a]

Treatment

Patients are asymptomatic in the early stages. Intervening clear areas between the opacities allow unobstructed vision. As the disease progresses, visual acuity is reduced and superficial keratectomy may be beneficial.[228] In the superficial variant treatment with the excimer laser, PTK may be an attractive alternative to lamellar keratectomy (Fig. 13.4*D*). The goal of PTK is to remove the anterior corneal opacity and smooth out the anterior refractive surface. PTK is performed after removal of the epithelium either mechanically or by ablation with the excimer laser. If the epithelial surface is rough a smoothing agent or modulator fluid is used to create a more regular surface that is then treated. Variable success rates ranging from 66% to 100% have been reported.[51] Penetrating keratoplasty is required in the more advanced cases. Recurrences after keratectomy have been reported as early as one year[330,341] and are more frequent in the superficial variant. It is believed that in this disease homozygous patients present earlier, have a more severe form, and have earlier recurrences following surgical intervention.[73,308] Recurrences are seen as a diffuse haze in the peripheral graft or as granular lesions in the stroma (Fig. 13.6*A* and *B*). The diffuse haze occurs due to growth of fibrous tissue between the epithelium and Bowman's layer and it can be stripped by superficial keratectomy.

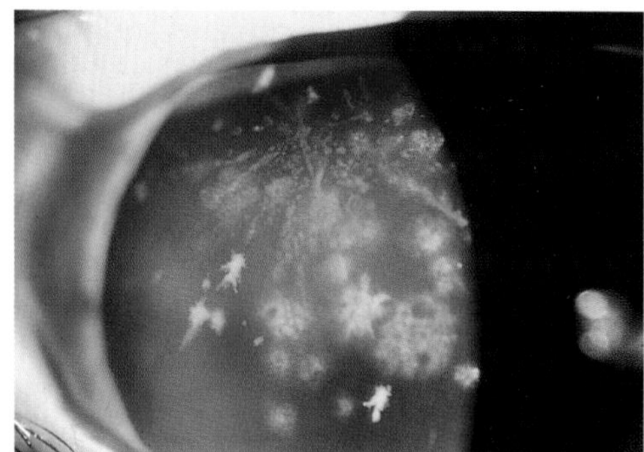

A

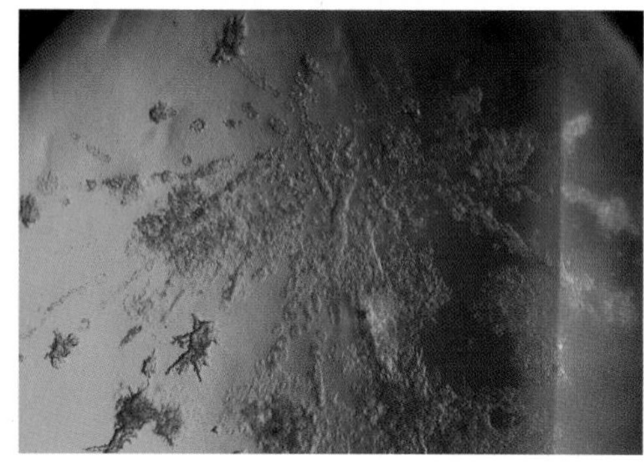

B

Figure 13.5. Avellino dystrophy by direct illumination (**A**) and retroillumination (**B**).

Avellino Corneal Dystrophy

This dystrophy was first described by Folberg et al. in 1988[89] who reported three families with histologic features of both granular and lattice dystrophies (Fig. 13.5). Because all of these

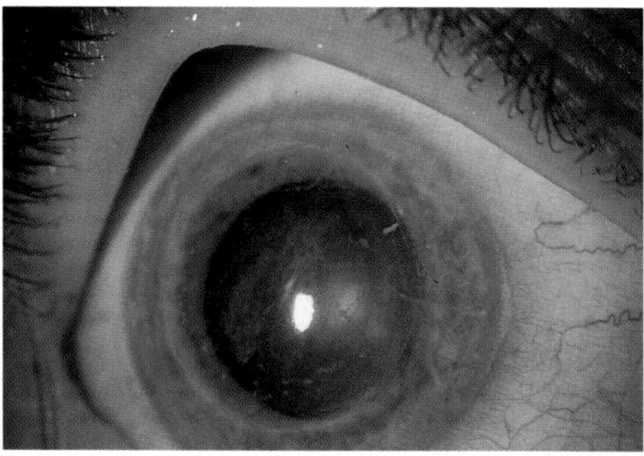

A

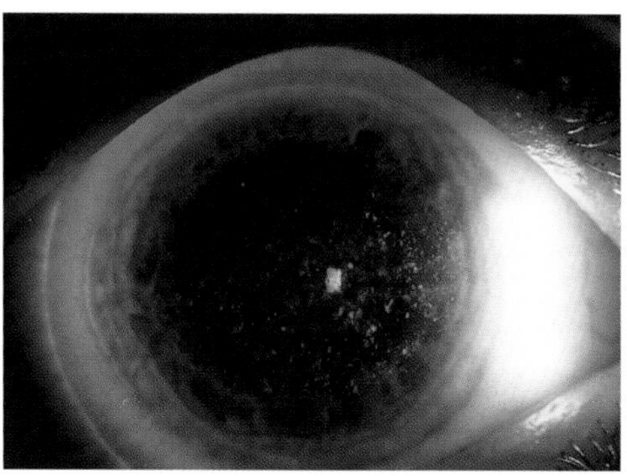

B

Figure 13.6. **A, B.** Recurrent granular dystrophy in a 56-year-old woman. **A.** Clinical appearance of recurrent granular dystrophy showing superficial mild diffuse opacification resulting in 20/7 visual acquity. **B.** Unoperated contralateral eye showing typical granular dystrophy and 20/100 visual acuity. Note the difference in clinical appearance between the two eyes. (Reproduced with permission from: Phototherapeutic Keratectomy, Azar DT, Steinert RF, and Stark WJ, eds. Igaku Shoin, Tokyo Japan.)

patients traced their origins to Avellino, Italy, it was later named Avellino corneal dystrophy by Holland and colleagues.[144] Earlier, reports had appeared in the literature that suggested that there may be a close relationship between lattice type 1 and granular dystrophy.[110,380] Amyloid deposits had been seen in patients with clinically typical granular dystrophy, and conversely, granular deposits had been detected in corneal buttons with otherwise typical lattice type 1 dystrophy.

Clinical Features

It is inherited as a simple autosomal dominant trait with very high penetrance (greater than 90%) and moderately variable expressivity. Both males and females are equally affected. The dystrophy usually appears in the first or second decade of life. A lot of interfamilial and intrafamilial differences are seen among patients. Three clinical signs characterize Avellino corneal dystrophy: *(1)* anterior stromal discrete, gray-white granular deposits, *(2)* mid- to posterior stromal lattice lesions and *(3)* anterior stromal haze.

The earliest clinical evidence of this condition is discrete granular deposits predominantly in the anterior third of the corneal stroma. Granules reach their mature size early and remain nearly stationary in size. They often coalesce to form linear opacities, especially in the inferior cornea. Lattice changes start later in life and increase proportionally as the patient ages. Initially they are found in the mid- and deep stroma and later involve the entire stroma. The lattice rods are thicker than those in lattice corneal dystrophy type 1 (LCD 1). The lattice component of Avellino dystrophy bears a resemblance to lattice corneal dystrophy type IIIA.[323] The last clinical sign to emerge is diffuse, ground-glass stromal haze located between the granular deposits.

Visual acuity is minimally affected, and depends on the predominant location of the deposits, which may be either central or peripheral. Patients complain of glare and decreased night vision. Recurrent erosions occur in the third and fourth decades of life, and the granular deposits that are superficial enough seem to be the cause of these erosions.[298] Recurrent erosions are more common in patients with Avellino corneal dystrophy than in patients with typical granular dystrophy, in whom they are unusual.

Pathology

Granular deposits are seen that demonstrate both a hyaline appearance by haematoxylin–eosin staining and bright-red staining with Masson's trichrome. Coexisting are numerous fusiform stromal deposits of amyloid that stain with Congo red and demonstrate birefringence and dichroism with the cross-polarization that is typical of lattice dystrophy.[90,144,307] The superficial granular deposits are ultrastructurally homogeneous and electron dense. Microfilaments suggestive of amyloid can be seen in some of these deposits.

Linkage Studies

Stone et al.[326] performed linkage analysis for three clinically distinct stromal corneal dystrophies—lattice, granular, and Avellino. They found that the chromosomal location is the same on chromosome 5q for all three dystrophies. Their initial strategy was to examine chromosomal loci that have been associated with amyloid deposits reported previously. At least 14 genes are known whose products are involved in amyloid deposits. Stone et al.[326] performed this analysis on one family with Avellino dystrophy. However, there was no linkage detected near the candidate regions. Thus Avellino dystrophy did not appear to be allelic with any of the previously characterized human amyloidosis.

Later Stone et al.[326] employed highly polymorphic markers distributed across the autosomal genome. They first found linkage of Avellino dystrophy to chromosome 5q in one family (linkage to marker Il-9) in the standard genome

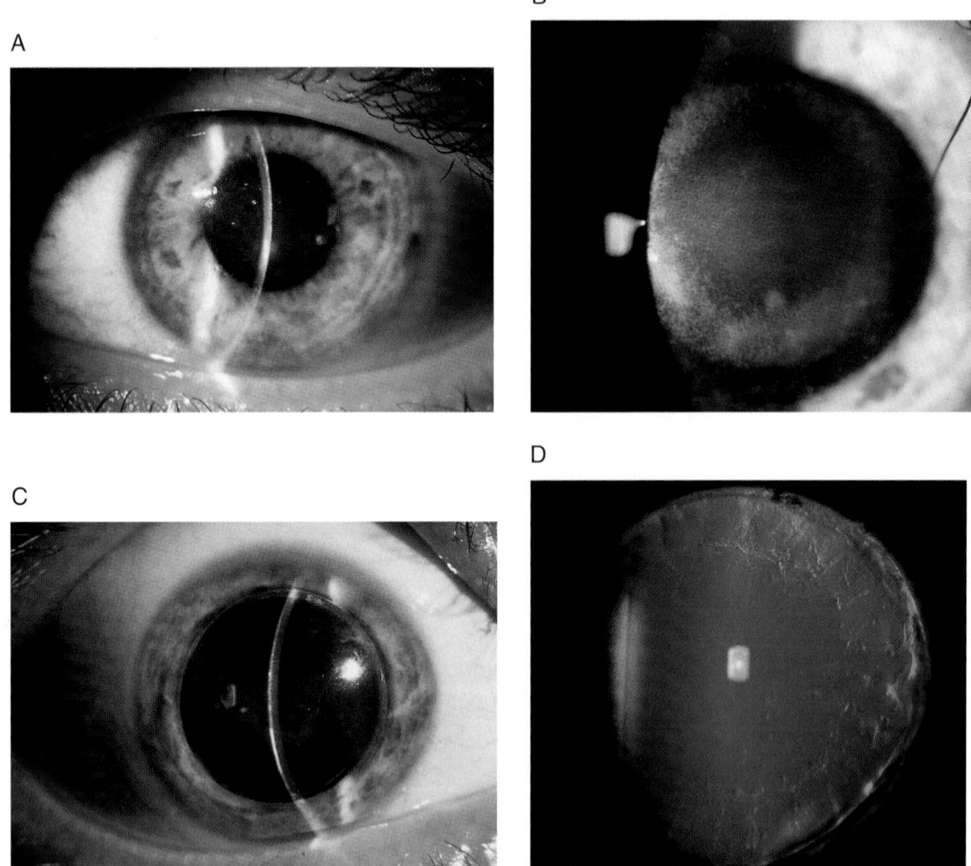

Figure 13.7. Clinical appearance of corneas of five brothers with lattice dystrophy who underwent phototherapeutic keratectomy (PTK). **A.** Member number one. Preoperative appearances of cornea by slit-beam illumination showing diffuse stromal haze. **B.** Clearing of the central corneal haze can be seen by broad illumination 3 months following PTK. **C, D.** Member number two. Pre-PTK and 6 months post-PTK, respectively. **E, F.** Member number three. Pre-PTK and at 3 months post-PTK, respectively. **G.** Member number four. At 5 months postoperatively. **H, I.** Member number five. At 5 and 14 months post-PTK, respectively. (Reproduced with permission from: Phototherapeutic Keratectomy, Azar DT, Steinert RF, and Stark WJ, eds. Igaku Shoin, Tokyo Japan.)

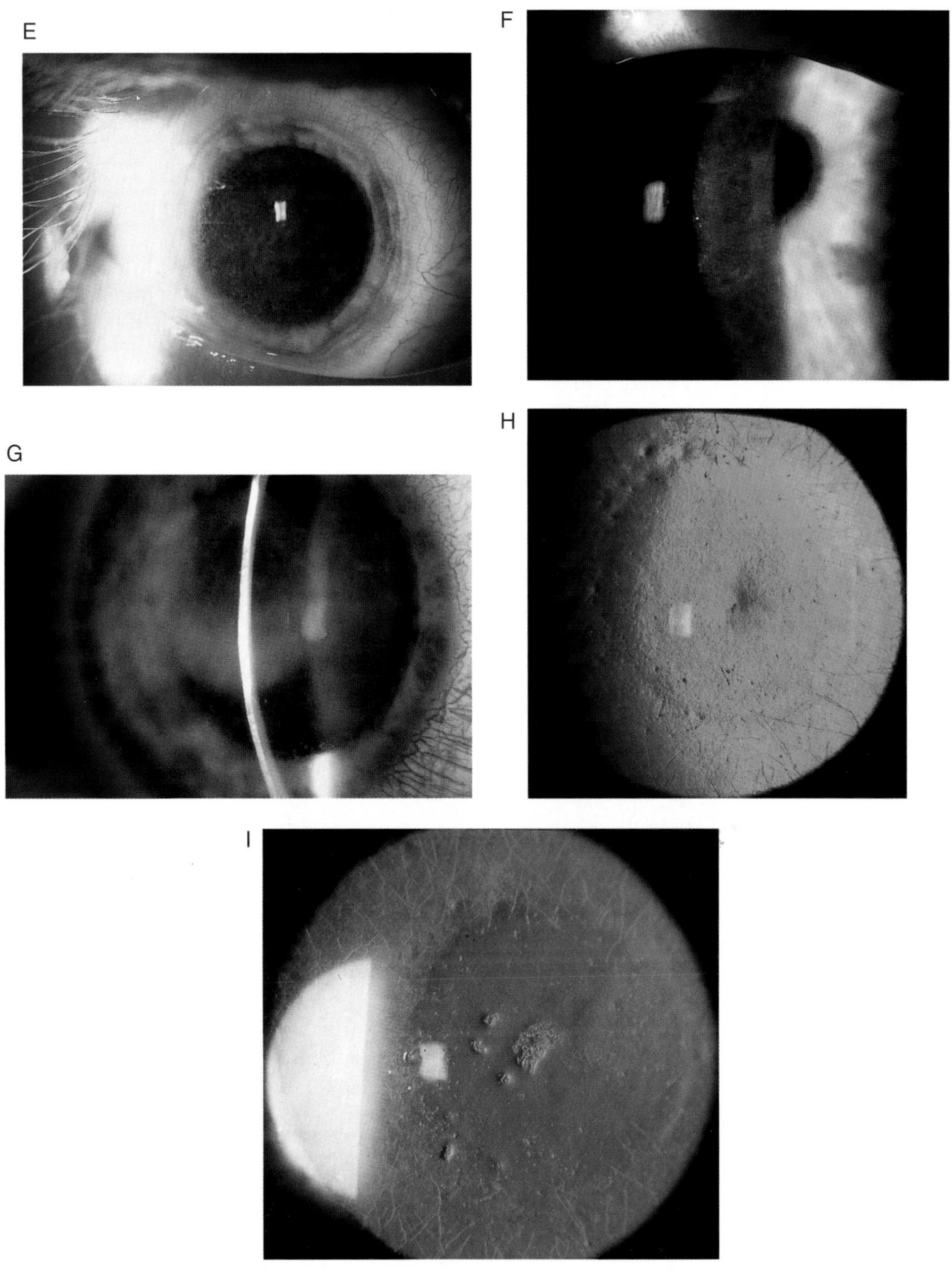

Figure 13.7. Continued.

screening test, following which they tested the remaining families of Avellino, lattice, and granular dystrophies for evidence of linkage at the same locus. They found significant linkage to 5q markers independently for each of the three corneal dystrophies. The gene causing each of the three dystrophies was located within a 10 cM region on chromosome 5. Recently, Gregory et al.[122] with linkage analysis studies on chromosome 5q bounded the region to a genetic distance of 2 cM for LCD1, thus refining linkage further. The three dystrophies are allelic conditions that result from mutations in the same gene on 5q that codes for kerato-epithelin.[238a]

Treatment

Treatment is conservative and includes hypertonic saline and bandage contact lenses for recurrent erosions. PTK with the excimer laser has been used to treat corneal erosions and to clear the central cornea of granular and lattice deposits.[53] Treatment for decreased visual acuity includes penetrating keratoplasty and is generally required late in the course of the disease. Recurrences have been reported following keratoplasty as late as 9 years after the graft.[144] The pattern of recurrence seems to follow the natural history of the disease with granular lesions being the first to appear.

Lattice Dystrophy

Also named Biber–Haab–Dimer dystrophy, lattice corneal dystrophy was first described by Biber in the 1890s. The mode of inheritance is autosomal dominant. As is expected of autosomal dominant diseases, it has variable penetrance and expressivity. It has been suggested

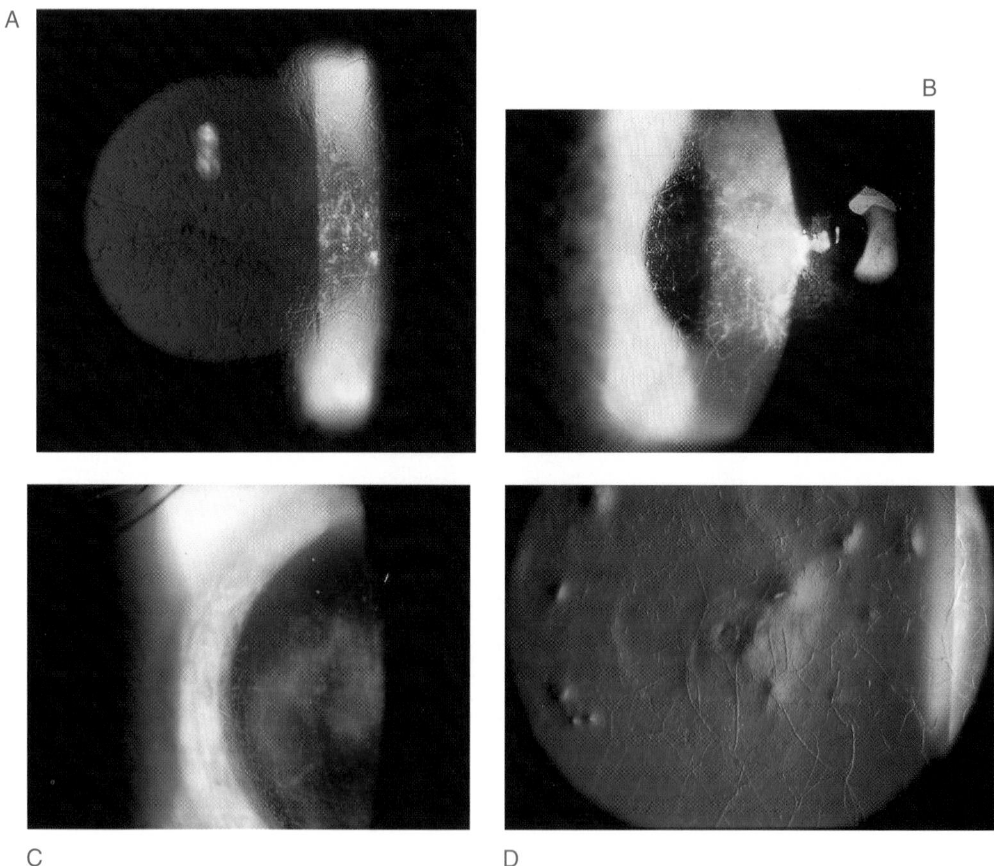

Figure 13.8. A, B, C. A 45-year-old man with a history of progressive lattice dystrophy. Appearance of cornea showing progression of dystrophy over 12 years resulting in 20/1000 visual acuity and a 2+ mean haze score. **D.** High magnification illustrating the lattice lines by retroillumination. (A–C reproduced with permission from: Phototherapeutic Keratectomy, Azar DT, Steinert RF, and Stark WJ, eds. Igaku Shoin, Tokyo Japan.)

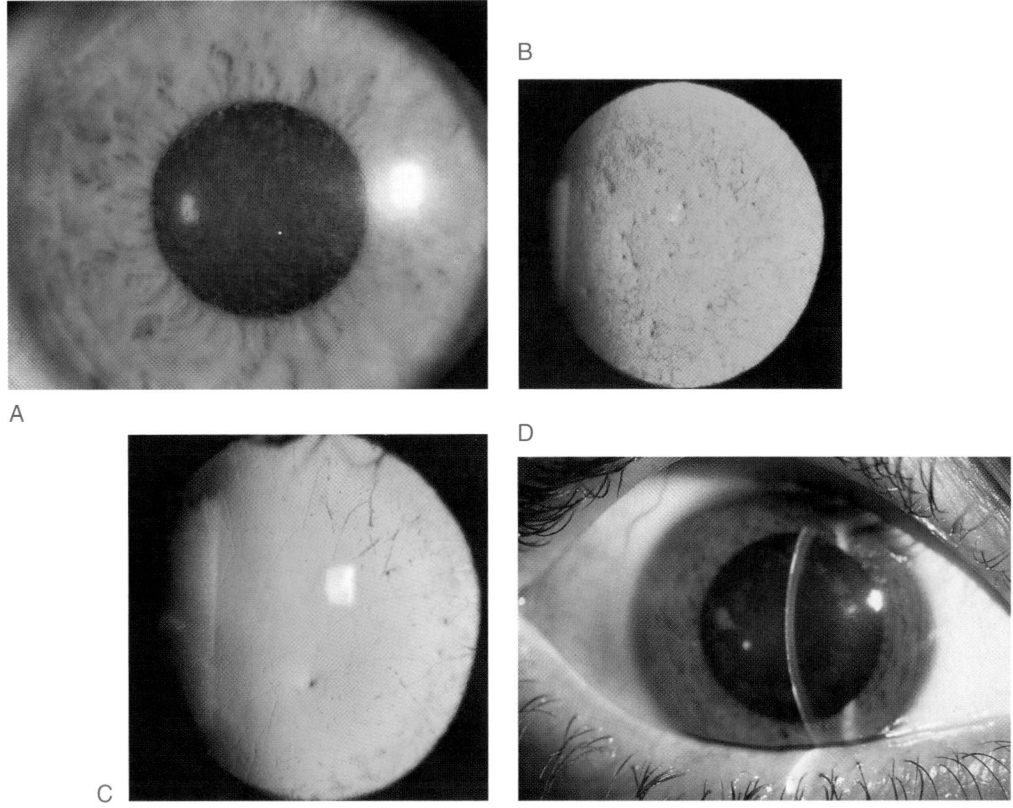

Figure 13.9. A 27-year-old woman with lattice dystrophy presenting with 20/200 vision who underwent phototherapeutic keratectomy (PTK). **A, B.** Pre-PTK appearance of the lesion by direct illumination and retroillumination, respectively. Note the confluence of lattice lines leading to generalized light scattering. **C.** Retroillumination of the eye at 1 month post-PTK, showing reduction of the lattice line intensity, with visual acuity of 20/80. **D.** A slit-lamp photograph of the eye at 18 months with similar visual acuity. (A, B, and F reproduced with permission from: Phototherapeutic Keratectomy, Azar DT, Steinert RF, and Stark WJ, eds. Igaku Shoin, Tokyo Japan.)

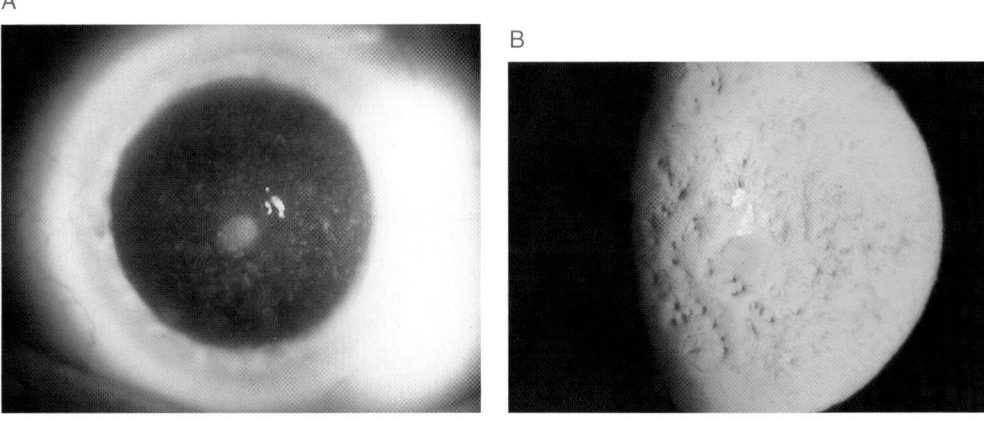

Figure 13.10. A 34-year-old man with lattice dystrophy resulting in 20/80 vision. **A, B.** Clinical appearance by direct illumination and retroillumination, respectively. Lattice lines are more difficult to observe in this patient. (Reproduced with permission from: Phototherapeutic Keratectomy, Azar DT, Steinert RF, and Stark WJ, eds. Igaku Shoin, Tokyo Japan.)

that lattice dystrophy type III may be autosomal recessive. The disease can be detected in only a few members of the affected family. Other members may show only recurrent erosions with minimal stromal opacification (Fig. 13.7*A*–*I*).[69] It is bilaterally symmetrical, although unilateral cases have been reported.[221,272,280] In unilateral cases it is later in onset with a less severe clinical course.

Clinical Features

It appears in the first decade of life. Rarely does it occur in the fourth decade or later.[69,274] In the early stages it appears as irregular lines and dots in the anterior axial stroma or as a diffuse haze in the center. The faint central haze in the center becomes more dense with time, and it is this central disc-shaped opacity that eventually causes reduced visual acuity and may obscure the underlying lattice pattern (Fig. 13.8*A*–*D*). The dots and lines increase in size and number with progression of time to become comma-shaped specks, thick ropy cords, and small nodules (Figs. 13.7 and 13.8*A*–*D*). On direct illumination it appears as gray opacities with irregular margins, and on retroillumination as refractile rods with a clear core and double contour. The lines extend to the periphery, and go deeper in the stroma and toward the epithelium (Fig. 13.8*D*). Small dots and opacities are usually present between the lines, and the intervening stroma is clear. As the opacities coalesce, a diffuse haze appears involving the anterior and midstroma (Figs. 13.9*A*–*D* and 13.10*A* and *B*). At this stage the lattice dystrophy may be difficult to distinguish from granular and macular dystrophies, but careful examination usually reveals the typical branching lattice lines. The lattice filaments range from fine lines to coarse bands with nodular dilatations. The lattice lines branch dichotomously near their central terminations and overlap one another at various stromal levels to create a lattice pattern. In advanced cases the lattice lines fluoresce under cobalt-blue slit-lamp illumination. Pseudofilaments may form due to the linear configuration of dots. Minute gray opacities in the superficial stroma may resemble granular or macular dystrophy in the early stages, but their refractile quality in lattice distinguishes them from other stromal dystrophies.

Epithelial erosions occur later in life and are the cause for irregular astigmatism and decreased visual acuity. They remain a serious problem till the third or fourth decade of life, after which they diminish in frequency. Involvement of the subepithelial area and Bowman's layer is the cause for recurrent erosions. The corneal sensations decrease with concomitant symptomatic improvement. Vascularization occurs rarely. Even in the late stages lattice lines and refractile opacities are visible that distinguish it from macular and granular dystrophy.

An association between vestibulocochleopathy and lattice corneal dystrophy has been reported in a case of nonfamilial amyloidosis.[344] Coexistence of progressive external ophthalmoplegia and corneal lattice dystrophy was seen in a family pedigree of 33 patients.[260]

Lattice dystrophy should be differentiated from polymorphic amyloid degeneration (parenchymatous dystrophy of Pillat),[204] which has stromal amyloid deposits seen in patients above 40 years of age. It is nonprogressive in nature and no hereditary pattern has been reported. Lattice lines can be produced by HEMA (hydroxyethylmethacrylate) contact lenses, they disappear on removal of the contact lens, however.

OTHER LATTICE DYSTROPHIES

Lattice Type II Corneal Dystrophy

Originally described by Meretoja[223–225] in 1969, this systemic amyloidosis is inherited as an autosomal dominant disorder. Also known as familial amyloid polyneuropathy type IV, the corneal changes appear in the third to fourth decade of life. Systemic involvement of the skin, peripheral nerves, and cranial nerves occurs later. It is less severe than lattice type I, with fewer dots and lattice lines that are radial, thicker, and extend to the limbus. Erosions are less frequent and vision is unaffected till the seventh decade of life. Recently seven cases of lattice type II dystrophy were described in Japan.[17]

Lattice Type III Corneal Dystrophy

Reported in two families in Japan[137,138] type III manifests as thick translucent lattice lines and diffuse subepithelial opacities. It is autosomal dominant, onset occurs after age 40, and vision is not affected until 70 years of age. Corneal erosions are not seen.[137,323] A variant of this dystrophy (lattice type IIIA) has a similar clinical appearance. However, the occurrence of recurrent erosions and its occurrence in whites differentiates it from lattice type III. Unilateral occurrence of type III lattice dystrophy has been reported in two cases and was confirmed electron microscopically by the presence of typical amyloid fibrils.[7,309]

Pathology

The epithelial layer of lattice dystrophies is irregular. Descemet's membrane and the endothelium are unaffected. Involvement of the epithelial or Bowman's layer can be confirmed by polarization microscopy. The deposits in lattice dystrophy are made up of amyloid, which has been confirmed by immunofluorescence,[30] Congo red, PAS, and Masson's trichrome staining. The deposits exhibit dichroism and manifest green birefringence.[100,140,315] Dichroism is demonstrated by alternate red and green color when viewed through a rotating polarizing filter; and green birefringence is demonstrated by an intermittent yellowish-green against a black background when the lesion is viewed through two rotating polarizing filters. The deposits show a greenish-yellow fluorescence on staining with thioflavine T. Crystal violet staining shows metachromasia. The amyloid protein is probably related to transthyretrin.[154,210] In type II lattice corneal dystrophy, amyloid deposits replace corneal nerves. Amyloid is also deposited systemically. Meretoja syndrome can be diagnosed retrospectively from corneal buttons based on the fact that monoclonal antibody to gelsolin faintly labels some deposits in lattice dystrophy type I as opposed to almost all the deposits in type II.[170,293]

Ultrastructurally the epithelium is of variable thickness. There is degeneration of the basal epithelium. The basement membrane is thickened and continuous without normal hemidesmosomes.[88,382] Bowman's membrane and superficial stroma contain amyloid structures, collagen fibrils, and fibroblasts. Bowman's layer may be thin, thick, or absent. The stroma contains large irregular deposits that distort the normal configuration of the corneal lamellae. They contain highly aligned short, delicate, nonbranching electron-dense fibrils with diameters of 80–100 Å.[102,218] There is a decrease in the number of keratocytes with evidence of degeneration.[100,140,154,177] Amyloid disrupts Bowman's layer and the epithelial basement membrane and is the cause for recurrent erosions.[88] Amyloid is a complex of chondroitin, sulfuric acid, and protein, and is found extracellularly. The amyloid seen in lattice dystrophy is distinct from amyloid in systemic amyloidosis or in primary or secondary amyloid degeneration of the cornea. There is no relationship to the corneal nerves.[223] Both lattice dystrophy type I and type III contain protein AA and protein AP.[137,138] Lattice dystrophy type II contains protein AA in some cases and protein AP in others.[137,323] Fluorescent staining for immune deposits like kappa chains, lambda chains, IgG, IgM, and IgA are negative,[235,363] which are seen in primary or secondary systemic amyloidosis. The deposition of amyloid occurs either due to release of lysosomal enzymes by abnormal keratocytes[101,103] or by abnormal keratocyte synthesis.[178,266] It is believed that sequestration of glycoprotein in the corneal stroma from plasma membranes of epithelial cells may stimulate amyloid deposition. Elastotic degeneration within amyloid deposits has been reported.[258] Antibodies to c-reactive protein in the epithelium of lattice dystrophy has been reported, although the significance is uncertain.[287]

Linkage Studies

Linkage analysis revealed that the location of the mutation was on chromosome 5q for lattice corneal dystrophy type 1.[326] Gregory et al.,[122] with linkage analysis studies on chromosome 5q, bounded the region to a genetic distance of 2 cM, thus refining linkage further for LCD1. Munier et al.[238a] found mutations in the gene on 5q coding for kerato-epithelin.

Lattice corneal dystrophy type II has been

shown to be caused by specific mutation in the gelsolin gene on chromosome 9q.[71] The amyloid protein found in patients with familial amyloidosis (FAF) has been found to be an internal degradation fragment of gelsolin with substitution of asparagine for aspartic acid at position 15, which is due to a guanine-to-adenine transversion. This mutation cosegregates with the disease phenotype and can be used as a diagnostic assay, including prenatal evaluation.[130] Until now, the diagnosis of FAF was based on clinical examination, and reliable results could be given between 20 and 30 years of age.

Treatment

Managing lattice dystrophy in the early stages includes treatment of recurrent erosions. PTK with the excimer laser is emerging as an attractive alternative to treat superficial corneal opacities and surface irregularities. The goal is to obviate more invasive procedures such as lamellar and penetrating keratoplasty. PTK has been reported to be very successful for the treatment of lattice dystrophy.[51] Penetrating keratoplasty is indicated when there is a decrease in visual acuity or, rarely, when the recurrent erosions become incapacitating. It is generally required in the third or fourth decade of life. Recurrence of lattice dystrophy in the graft is seen as early as 3 years postoperatively. Recurrences are more frequent in lattice dystrophy than in granular and macular dystrophies and are seen as dotlike filamentous subepithelial opacities or as a diffuse stromal haze (Fig. 13.11*A* and *B*).[222]

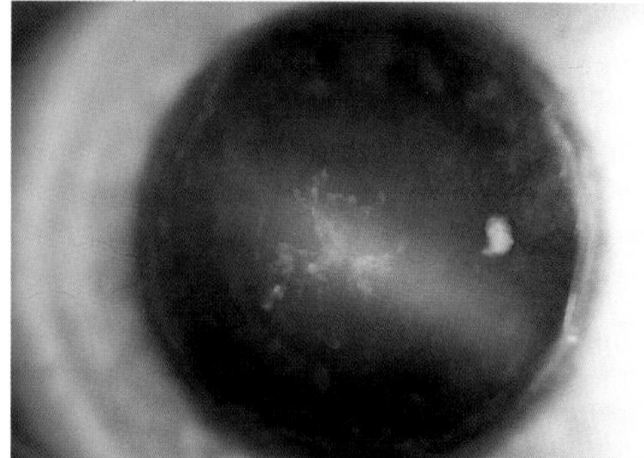

A

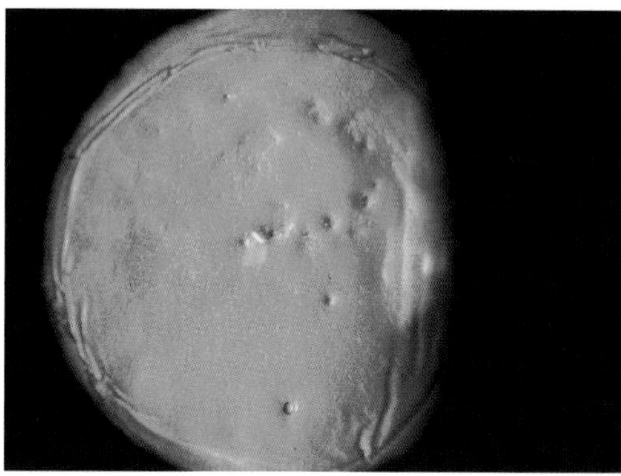

B

Figure 13.11. Clinical appearance of a 48-year-old man with recurrent lattice dystrophy in a graft by direct illumination (**A**) and by retroillumination (**B**). The recurrence is superficial, diffuse, and punctate rather than having a lattice configuration. (Reproduced with permission from: Phototherapeutic Keratectomy, Azar DT, Steinert RF, and Stark WJ, eds. Igaku Shoin, Tokyo Japan.)

Macular Dystrophy

Clinical Findings

Macular dystrophy is transmitted as an autosomal recessive trait. It is the least common of the three classic stromal dystrophies, but it is the most severe. The corneal changes usually are first noted between 3 and 9 years of age, when a diffuse clouding is seen in the central superficial stroma (Fig. 13.12). Unlike granular dystrophy, the macular opacities have indistinct

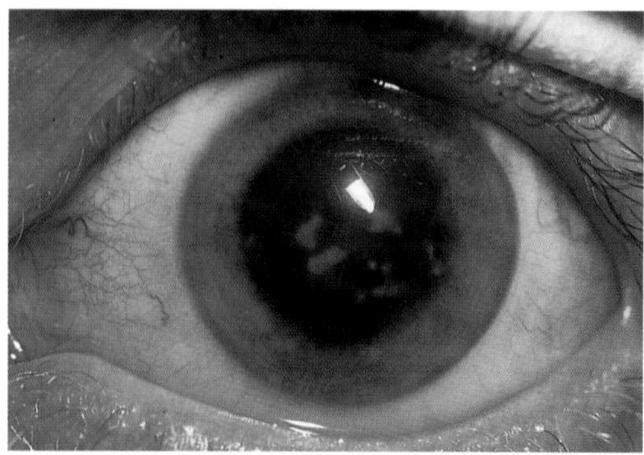

Figure 13.12. A 32-year-old woman with macular dystrophy resulting in 20/50 visual acuity. (Reproduced with permission from: Phototherapeutic Keratectomy, Azar DT, Steinert RF, and Stark WJ, eds. Igaku Shoin, Tokyo Japan.)

edges, the intervening stroma is not clear, and the clouding extends peripherally and into the deeper stroma as the disease progresses.

As the condition progresses, the cornea becomes increasingly cloudy. By the teens the opacification involves the entire thickness of the cornea and may extend out to the limbus. Within this sea of haziness are gray-white, denser opacities with ill-defined borders. These denser, macular opacities can protrude anteriorly, resulting in irregularity of the epithelial surface, or posteriorly, causing irregularity, grayness, and guttate appearance of Descemet's membrane. This may result in progressive loss of vision, irritation, and photophobia. These opacities can enlarge with time and coalesce. Corneal thinning confirmed by central pachometry has been documented.[74,80] In most cases vision is severely impaired by age 20 or 30. Recurrent erosions are seen, but they are less frequent than in lattice dystrophy. Heterozygous carriers do not manifest corneal abnormalities.

Biochemical studies have shown decreased activity of α-galactosidase in keratocytes from macular corneal dystrophy,[42] and previous evidence that the primary defect is in the synthetic pathway of the keratan sulfate proteoglycans.[42,135,175,242] The pathogenesis of macular dystrophy was thought to result from incomplete glycosaminoglacan sulfation.[242] This view was supported by the fact that monoclonal antibodies demonstrated the absence of sulfated keratan sulfate in the cornea and serum of patients with macular dystrophy (type 1).[173] However, a new subtype of macular dystrophy has been immunohistochemically identified in 1988, in which keratan sulfate is present in the cornea and serum (type 2).[78,379] Type 1 is most prevalent in Europe and North America. It is characterized by the absence of antigenic keratan sulfate in the cornea as well as in the serum; and it may represent a more widespread systemic disorder of keratan sulfate metabolism.[77] Type 2 may be more prevalent in Japan, based on a limited study by Santo et al.[305] A complete understanding of the cause of clinical and histopathologic differences between Japanese and Western distribution awaits future molecular biologic and genetic elucidation.

Histopathology

In macular dystrophy the cornea synthesizes chondroitin/dermatan sulfate proteoglycans that are larger than normal and oversulfated.[242] Histologically, macular dystrophy is characterized by the accumulation of glycosaminoglycans[97,152] (acid mucopolysaccharide) between the stromal lamellae, underneath the epithelium, within stromal keratocytes, and within the endothelial cells.[97,100,109,152,317,334] The glycosaminoglycans stain intensely with alcian blue and colloidal iron, minimally with PAS, and not at all with Masson's trichrome. Bifringence is decreased. Proteoglycan-specific cuprolinic blue staining has revealed that these proteoglycans accumulate and aggregate in both type 1 and type 2 macular dystrophy corneas. Degeneration of the basal epithelial cells and focal epithelial thinning is seen over the accumulated material.[334] Bowman's layer is thinned or absent in some areas.

Corneal stroma produces an X-ray diffraction pattern, the high-angle component that relates to the arrangement of atoms and groups of atoms into molecules and of collagen molecules into fibrils. Using synchrotron X-ray diffraction, Quantock et al. found that the interfibrillar spacing of collagen fibrils was significantly lower in type 1 macular dystrophy as compared to that of normal adult human corneas.[270] The authors suggested that this close-packing of collagen fibrils seemed to be responsible for the reduced thickness of the central cornea in macular dystrophy.[270]

Electron microscopy shows accumulation of mucopolysaccharide within stromal keratocytes.[109,176,195,236,317] The keratocytes are distended by numerous intracytoplasmic vacuoles, which appear to be the dilated cisternae of the rough endoplasmic reticulum. Some of these vacuoles are clear, but many contain fibrillar or granular material, and occasionally membranous lamellar material. The endothelium contains similar material. The posterior, nonbanded portion of Descemet's membrane is infiltrated by vesicular and granular material deposited by the abnormal endothelium. Quantock et al.[271] found abnormally large collagen fibrils that existed in localized regions, frequently adjacent to the vacuoles, and abnormal progeoglycans in an atypical variant of macular corneal dystrophy.

The accumulated material varies; its staining by different antikeratan sulfate antibodies differs between patients.[78,379] In some patients normal keratan sulfate is also absent from the serum and cartilage.[337,379] The keratocytes produce only glycoprotein precursors of keratan sulfate in culture.[134,135,174] The corneal deposits may contain an antigen associated with intermediate-type filament.[332] With the acridine orange technique, compensatory generalized hyperactivity of the lysosomal enzyme system has been demonstrated.[99]

As would be typical of an autosomal recessively inherited condition, macular dystrophy presumably results from deficiency of a hydrolytic enzyme (sulfotransferase) and may thus be considered a localized form of mucopolysaccharidosis.[175] The corneal pathology of macular corneal dystrophy, however, differs from that of the systemic mucopolysaccharidoses in several aspects. In the systemic mucopolysaccharidoses, the abnormal material accumulates in lysosomal vacuoles, whereas in macular dystrophy it accumulates in endoplasmic reticulum. In the systemic mucopolysaccharidoses, epithelial involvement is prominent, and Descemet's membrane usually is not affected.

Treatment

Good results are obtained from penetrating keratoplasty for macular dystrophy. Recurrences can be seen in both lamellar and penetrating grafts, but they usually are delayed for many years.[172,285] Host keratocytes invade the graft and produce abnormal glycosaminoglycan. The periphery of the graft is most affected, particularly the superficial and deep layers. Surprisingly, the endothelium and Descemet's membrane also are affected.

Fleck Dystrophy (François–Neetens)

Fleck dystrophy also has been called *speckled dystrophy* or *mouchetée dystrophy*. It is a rare dystrophy that is transmitted as an autosomal dominant trait.[8,14,25,62,117,255,269,329] The cornea in fleck dystrophy is characterized by numerous, tiny, small opacities scattered throughout the entire corneal stroma. The lesions are semiopaque, flattened opacities that may be oval, round, comma-shaped, granular, or stellate. The condition usually is detectable very early in life and in some patients is congenital. It is stationary with no loss of visual acuity and is usually noted during a routine examination. Some degree of photophobia may be present.[8,14] The lesions appear during the first decade of life and usually are bilateral, although they can be asymmetric or unilateral. Small opacities are present in all layers of the corneal stroma except Bowman's layer, and they involve the peripheral as well as the central stroma. Many have a doughnut-like appearance with a relatively clear center. These small opacities are well demarcated, and the intervening stroma is clear. They are best demonstrated by retroillumination. Corneal sensation is normal in most cases, but in some families sensation is decreased.[25]

Fleck dystrophy has been noted in association with a variety of disorders such as keratoconus (Fig. 13.13*A* and *B*),[25] limbal dermoids, central cloudy dystrophy, angioid streaks, papillitis, and punctate cortical lens opacities.[25,62,98,115,329] It is unclear whether the relationship is more than coincidental.

Histopathology

Histopathologic studies reveal abnormal, distended keratocytes throughout the stroma. Bowman's layer, epithelium, Descemet's membrane, and endothelium are normal. The keratocytes stain with oil red 0 and Sudan black B, indicating the presence of lipid, and alcian blue and colloidal iron, indicating the presence of mucopolysaccharide.[169,245] On electron microscopy the keratocytes are seen to contain varying numbers of membrane-limited intracytoplasmic vacuoles containing a fibrillogranular material.[245,321] Some of these vacuoles also contain membranous inclusions or pleomorphic, electron-dense deposits. The vacuoles appear to arise from the Golgi apparatus and therefore would be lysosomal vacuoles. Because of this, fleck dystrophy seems to be a storage disorder of glycosaminoglycans and complex lipids that is limited to the cornea.

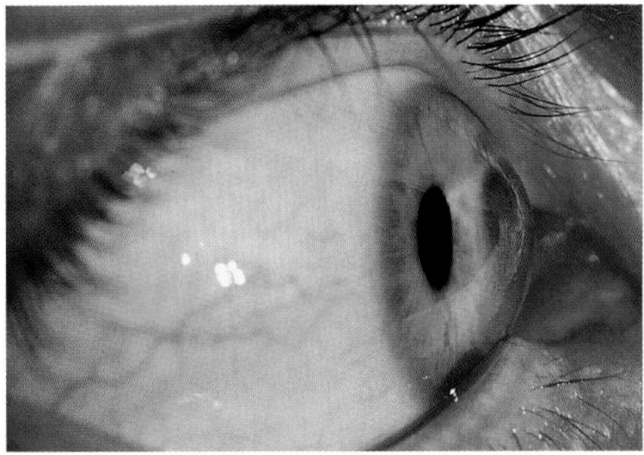

A

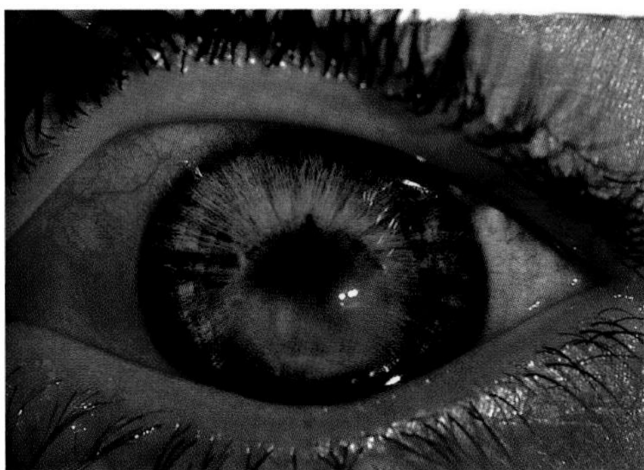

B

Figure 13.13. **A.** Keratoconus. **B.** Hydrops in a patient with keratoconus. Fleck dystrophy and Fuchs endothelial dystrophy have been associated with keratoconus.

Schnyder Crystalline Dystrophy

Central crystalline dystrophy is an autosomal dominant dystrophy characterized clinically by bilateral central corneal opacities that are sometimes associated with premature corneal arcus and limbal girdle of Vogt.[37,72,124] Xanthelasmas can also be seen in some cases. It occurs in early life and may be seen as early as 2 months of age.[72] Congenital cases are seen sporadically. Visual acuity usually is not affected, but occasionally it is moderately reduced. The main feature of the dystrophy is the presence of bilateral, axial, ring-shaped, or disciform opacities.[37,81,124,158,199,346] The opacities usually appear to consist of fine, polychromatic, needle-shaped crystals, but in some cases a disciform opacity is present without evident crystals.[72,211,358] Schnyder dystrophy is probably a dynamic clinicopathologic spectrum of disease, and the distribution of the corneal opacities could be subdivided into five morphologic types (Fig. 13.14*A–F*) type A: disk-shaped amorphous opacity without distinct crystals (Fig. 13.14A), type B: disk-shaped opacity composed of innumerable small, bright crystals in the form of needles and small iridescent plates with indistinct borders; type C: disk-shaped opacity composed of crystals, without a clear center, and with a garland-like outline (Fig. 13.14*B*); type D: ring-shaped amorphous opacity, with local crystal accumulation and with a clear center (Fig. 13.14*C*); and type E: ring-shaped opacity, composed of crystals and with a clear center (Fig. 13.14*D*). On rare occasions, clouding extends to the arcus,[348] but usually a clear cornea persists between the central opacification and the surrounding arcus (Fig. 13.14*C*).[20] The yellow-white opacity primarily involves Bowman's layer and anterior stroma but may extend into the deeper layers. The epithelium is normal and the intervening stroma usually is clear, but punctate white opacities can be scattered in the stroma (Fig. 13.14*E*), or the stroma can develop a milky opalescence.[81,158] Corneal sensation is normal and this is a feature that distinguishes Schnyder dystrophy from lipid neurotropic deposits (Fig. 13.14*F*). The opacities progress slowly and usually stabilize in later life. Progression is more frequent in patients with diffuse opacities (types A and D) than in those with crystalline deposits.[194]

The severity of dyslipidemia, which may[37,41,108,364] or may not[114,290,292,361] be associated with Schnyder dystrophy, usually does not correlate with the extent of opacification or the progression of the disease.[194] A significant number of patients have hyperlipidemia, but the type and severity of the hyperlipidemia vary.[81,158] Some individuals within a single family may have only crystalline dystrophy, others may have hyperlipidemia and crystalline dystrophy, and others have only hyperlipidemia. Chondrodystrophy and genu valgum also are associated with Schnyder dystrophy in some families.[37,81,106,158]

Histopathology

The main histopathologic feature of Schnyder dystrophy is the presence of phospholipid, cho-

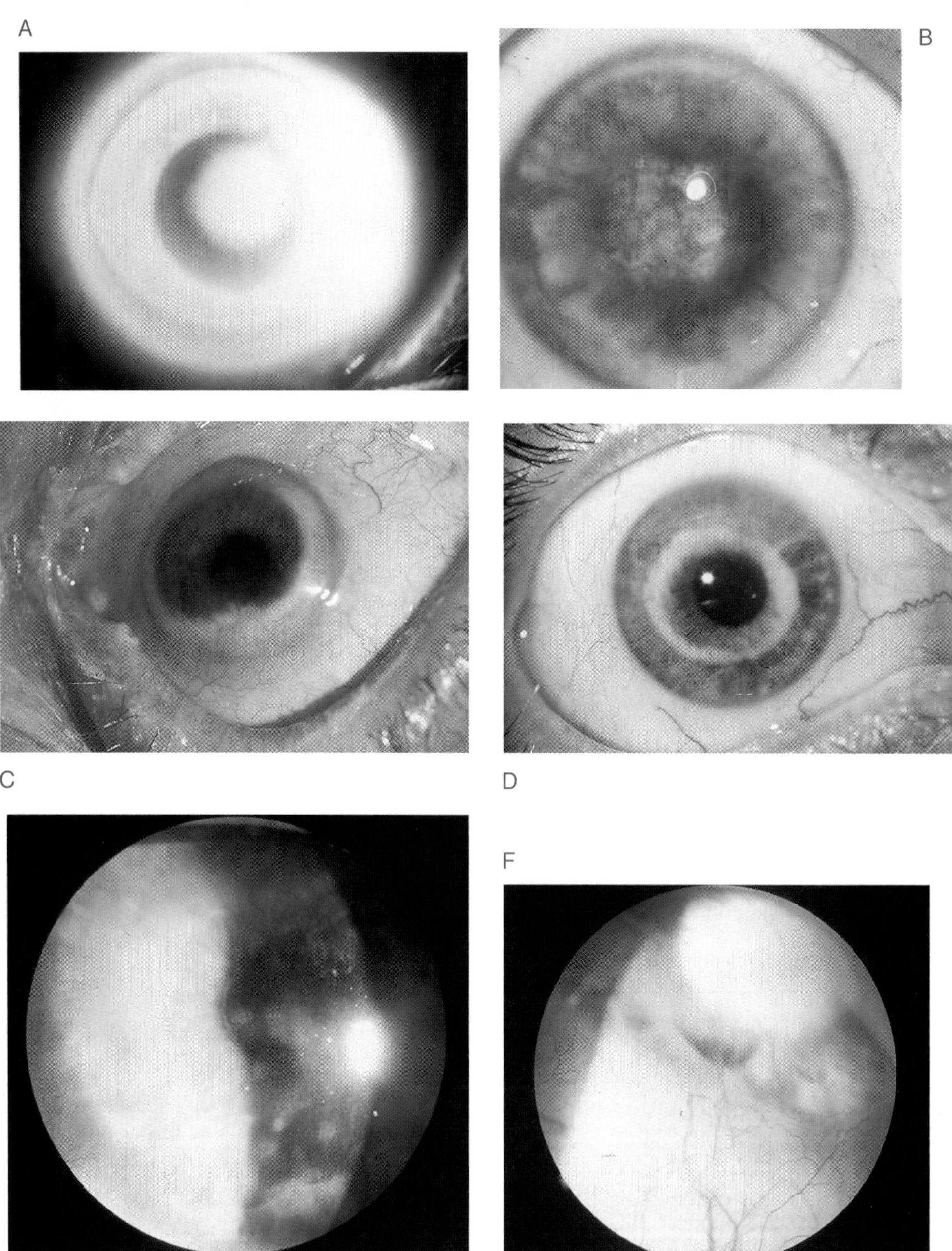

Figure 13.14. A. Clinical appearance of a patient with type A schnyder central crystalline dystrophy. **B.** Disk-shaped crystalline deposits in type C Schnyder dystrophy. **C.** Ring-shaped amorphous opacity of type D Schnyder dystrophy. **D.** Type E Schnyder dystrophy showing a ring-shaped opacity composed of crystals with a clear central area. This is similar to the corneal lipid deposits of Bietti dystrophy. **E.** Scattered early lipid deposits. **F.** Neurotrophic lipid deposition having a similar appearance of type A Schnyder dystrophy. Decreased corneal sensation and the presence of peripheral feeder vessel(s) diffentiate the former from the latter.

lesterol crystals, noncrystalline cholesterol, cholesterol esters, and neutral fats in the stroma.[158,290,346,361] The clinically apparent crystals correspond to cholesterol accumulations, both within keratocytes and extracellulary. Occasionally similar deposits have been noted in basal epithelial cells.[114] The deposits are most numerous in the anterior stroma, but they can extend posteriorly to Descemet's membrane.[104] Destruction of Bowman's layer and superficial stroma with disorganization of collagen have often been observed.

The pathogenesis of Schnyder dystrophy is unclear but is thought to involve a primary disorder of corneal lipid metabolism,[20,37,108] the severity of which may be altered by systemic hyperlipidemia. Burns et al.[43] administered radiolabeled cholesterol intravenously to a patient with crystalline dystrophy 2 weeks before keratoplasty. The radioactivity in the cornea was higher than that in the blood, suggesting active deposition of cholesterol in the cornea.

Phospholipid and unesterified cholesterol are important constituents of cell membranes. The increase of these lipids in Schnyder dystrophy suggests the possibility of a primary disorder of corneal metabolism, resulting in the accumulation of abnormal and subsequently unstable cell membranes. The primary abnormality could involve excess production or diminished breakdown of phospholipids, unesterified cholesterol, or other constituent of cell membranes. This concept can be supported by the findings that keratocytes and their membranes are abnormal in Schnyder dystrophy[37,41] and the characteristic membrane-bound vacuoles appearing to bud from degenerating keratocytes.[41] Both the vacuoles and keratocytes were noted to have similar trilamellar membranes.[211] Such budding could represent breakdown of unstable cell membranes in part composed of excess phospholipid and unesterified cholesterol. Mirshahi et al.[227] showed a much lower secretion of plasminogen activators by corneal fibroblasts from Schnyder dystrophy than that secreted by normal corneal fibroblasts. Because plasminogen activators are involved in extracellular matrix remodeling, the deficiency may be responsible for diminished breakdown of cell membranes in corneal dystrophy.

Treatment

In most cases of crystalline dystrophy the corneal disease requires no treatment. Serum lipid profiles should be obtained, although the severity of a systemic lipid abnormality does not necessarily correlate with the severity of the corneal disease. Elevated serum lipid levels and concomitant cardiovascular disease are associated features in some patients.[37] Efforts directed at visual improvement through such means as reduction of cholesterol intake have proven beneficial in only one case report.[333] Penetrating or lamellar keratoplasty can be performed for visual rehabilitation, but the dystrophy can recur.[37,108] Recurrence of crystalline deposits occurs sooner and in larger amounts in lamellar grafts than in full-thickness grafts.[72] Postoperative changes in the posterior layers of the cornea in Schnyder crystalline dystrophy may contribute to the comparatively poorer surgical outcomes obtained with lamellar grafts as compared to full-thickness grafts.[104]

Marginal Crystalline Dystrophy of Bietti

Bietti dystrophy is a form of Schnyder dystrophy associated with crystalline retinopathy. In 1937, Bietti first described crystalline fundus dystrophy with crystalline changes in the marginal cornea in three patients.[23] In the majority of patients with Bietti dystrophy[18,21,133,365] the first symptoms are noticed during the third decade of life and take the form of visual loss and decreased night vision. The corneal deposits are numerous, very small, yellowish-white, and are concentrated in the superficial layers of the cornea near the limbus. They are morphologically similar to type E Schnyder dystrophy. These punctate deposits can be found in the upper and lower areas or for 360°. Marginal crystalline dystrophy was described in two brothers who had crystalline material in the superficial stroma of the paralimbal cornea; their vision was not affected.[18] Both brothers also had fundus albipunctatus. The corneal dystrophy seems unchanged at a follow-up of 16–20 years, whereas the retinal crystals diminish with time.[133,360] Because this dystrophy shows familial clustering, an autosomal recessive mode of inheritance is assumed to be involved.[360] The reports published to date cover several ethnic groups. A recently described autosomal dominant inheritance pattern and the fact that many patients without corneal crystals remain asymptomatic[208,282,355] suggest that Bietti dystrophy may be two different diseases with different patterns of inheritance.

The clinical picture of a marginal corneal dystrophy and crystalline retinopathy provides little latitude with regard to the differential diagnosis, as few conditions show refractile bodies in both cornea and retina. The crystals of cystinosis are found throughout the entire cornea, not solely at the limbus, and appear in the choroid and retinal pigment epithelium but not the neuroretina.[304]

Histopathology

A metabolic storage disease has been suggested as a cause of crystalline corneal–retinal dystrophy.[360,365] Cholesterol, cholesterol esters, complex lipid inclusions, and immunoproteins[171] have been reported in corneal fibroblasts and circulating lymphocytes in the limbal reaction.[360,365]

Central Cloudy Dystrophy of François

Central cloudy dystrophy is transmitted as an autosomal dominant trait, with early onset and no progression with age.[31,327] It is characterized by axial clouding of the cornea, densest posteriorly and fading anteriorly and peripherally. The cloud is broken into segments by an interlacing network of clear lines, creating a mosaic pattern (Fig. 13.15). Sometimes the opacification extends to, or in rare cases involves, Bowman's layer; in this location the opacities are smaller and less numerous. Vision is not affected, and there are no other symptoms, so the diagnosis often is not made until late in life.

Most likely this condition is the same as posterior mosaic shagreen. It has been noted in association with fleck dystrophy,[65] fleck dystrophy and pseudoxanthoma elasticum,[66] and pre-Descemet dystrophy.[62]

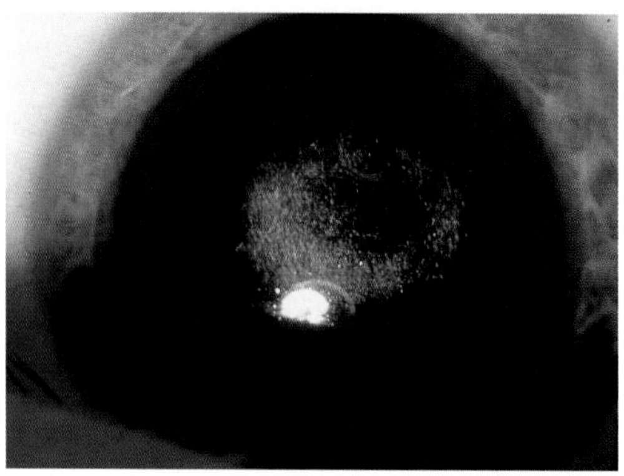

Figure 13.15. Central cloudy dystrophy of François. (Courtesy of Dr. William Power.)

Parenchymatous Dystrophy of Pillat

Parenchymatous dystrophy of the cornea is rare; only a few cases have been reported.[262,328] Thomsitt and Bron[336] called it *polymorphic stromal dystrophy*. Most likely this is a degenerative change and is the same as polymorphic amyloid degeneration.[204] Deep stromal opacities are seen, which are gray-white on focal illumination and clear on retroillumination. The deposits are punctate and filamentous and can be central, peripheral, or annular in distribution. The punctate opacities are polymorphic fleck-like, stellate, linear, or guttate. The filaments are identical to those seen in lattice dystrophy; they can have beading, striations, or dichotomous branching. The deposits usually are noted in patients in the sixth decade, and progression has not been demonstrated. Vision and corneal sensation are not affected. Although the condition has been noted in two siblings, no heritability has been demonstrated.

Posterior Amorphous Dystrophy

Clinical Manifestations

Posterior amorphous dystrophy, an autosomal dystrophy, has been described in only five families.[52,76,104,149,301] Changes have been noted as early as 16 weeks of age and thus may be present at birth. Progression has not been documented, and visual acuity is only mildly affected and is rarely worse than 20/40. Gray, amorphous sheetlike opacities can involve any portion of the stroma but are most prominent posteriorly. The sheetlike opacities may be irregular and broken with clear intervening stroma. They can affect the central or peripheral portions of the cornea or both. Descemet's membrane may show posterior bowing and distortion of the endothelial mosaic. Central corneal thinning, flattened keratometry, and hyperopia may be present. Various iris and angle abnormalities have been noted, including a prominent Schwalbe ring with numerous fine iris processes, pupillary remnants, corectopia, iridocorneal adhesions, and anterior stromal tags. It is important to differentiate this type of dystrophy from interstitial keratitis, since both can show posterior corneal opacification. However, no vascularization or inflammation is seen in posterior amorphous dystrophy. In view of the early onset, lack of progression, and association with iris abnormalities, this condition may be a dysgenesis rather than a dystrophy.[52]

Histopathology

Johnson et al.[149] described the keratoplasty specimen from a 5-year-old child, which demonstrated fracturing of the posterior stromal collagen lamellae, a thin Descemet's membrane, and focal attenuation of endothelial cells. Ultrastructural studies showed disorganization of the posterior stromal collagen.

Gelatinous Droplike Dystrophy (Primary Familial Amyloidosis of the Cornea)

Clinical Manifestation

Gelatinous droplike dystrophy is a rare familial disorder of the cornea, which is much more common in Japan.[6,111,239,240,273,354] It accounted for the greatest number of specimens in one Japanese study.[305] Early investigators in the United States termed the condition *primary familial amyloidosis of the cornea.*[167,322] A similar condition was described in the European literature in 1930.[192] The pattern of inheritance is unclear but is most likely autosomal recessive.[167]

The disorder usually appears in the first decade with photophobia, lacrimation, and decreased visual acuity. Early in the dystrophy the deposits are fairly flat and can resemble band-shaped keratopathy.[156] Examination shows bilateral, central, raised, multinodular, subepithelial mounds of amyloid. These are white on direct illumination and transparent on retroillumination but can become yellow and milky with time. Flat subepithelial opacities can be seen surrounding the mounds. The opacities increase in number and depth with age. In the late stages the cornea can have a diffuse, mulberry-like appearance. Vascularization, if present, is usually minimal. Anterior and posterior cortical lens changes may be associated.[167]

Histopathology

The amyloid nature of these deposits has been demonstrated histologically and ultrastructurally.[6,167,206,239,322] Bowman's layer usually is absent, and amyloid is deposited in the basal epithelial cells, and fusiform deposits similar to lattice dystrophy occur in the deeper stroma. A flat, more uniform layer of a similar material may surround the nodular masses. Amyloid can also deposit in the deep stroma.[305] In an unusual case, large amyloid deposits was found to a depth of two-thirds of the cornea, which contained needlelike cholesterol crystals.[305] Small spheroidal deposits showing positive reaction to Verhoeff iron hematoxylin were demonstrated at the periphery of the cornea in some cases. The type of corneal amyloid deposits containing protein AP but not protein AA or immunoglobulins may be different from that found in lattice dystrophy.[234]

The specimens obtained from the perilimbal conjunctiva showed amyloid deposits in the stroma.[305] This may support the idea that the epithelial cells, more precisely the limbal cells, are involved in the synthesis of amyloid fibrils and might have a role in the recurrence process. This also would explain the success observed when lamellar keratoplasty is combined with keratoepithelioplasty around the limbal area after a 360° peritomy.[303] However, the finding of stromal deposits suggests that keratocytes may participate in some way in the pathogenesis of this disease. Gelatinous droplike dystrophy and lattice dystrophy might be two facets of the same basic disorder, with the former representing the epithelial expression and the latter the stromal expression.[354]

Treatment

Treatment may include either superficial keratectomy or keratoplasty. Recurrence is seen after penetrating keratoplasty.[111,192,305] In fact, in one series, recurrences in a graft accounted for more than half the patients undergoing penetrating keratoplasty.[305]

PRE-DESCEMET DYSTROPHIES

Pre-Descemet dystrophy has several very rare subgroups. The vision is usually not affected and the patients usually do not feel discomfort. A clear pattern of heredity is not always obvious. A variety of fine posterior stromal opacities have been described in patients in the fourth decade or older (Fig. 13.16). Many of these may represent degenerative diseases rather than dystrophies.[348] However, some of these conditions have been reported in a number of family members, over two to four generations.[63,64,66,85,119] Typical comea farinata and pre-Descemet dystrophy had been reported affecting different members in one family.

Cornea Farinata

Cornea farinata is sometimes classified with pre-Descemet dystrophies, but it is more often considered an age-related degeneration. It consists of tiny, punctate, gray opacities in the deep stroma immediately anterior to Descemet's membrane. Sometimes larger and more polymorphous types of comma-shaped, circular, linear, filiform, and dotlike opacities are located in the pre-Descemet area. The opacities may be distributed axially or annularly. Visual acuity is usually not affected.

Grayson–Wilbrandt Dystrophy

Grayson and Wilbrandt[119] described primary pre-Descemet dystrophies that consisted of mixtures of six types of tiny, deep, stromal opacities: (*1*) dendritic or stellate, (*2*) boomerang, (*3*) circular or dot, (*4*) comma, (*5*) linear, and (*6*) filiform. The opacities resemble those in

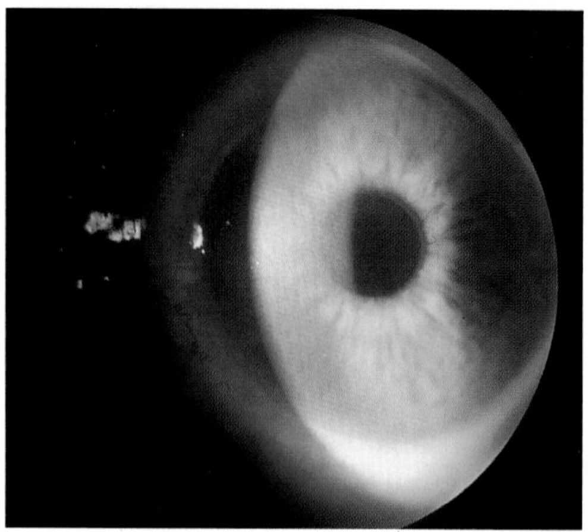

Figure 13.16. Pre-Descemet's dystrophy.

cornea farinata, but they are larger and more polymorphous. The deposits could be axial, peripheral, or diffuse. The type and location of the opacities were variable and affected by patient's age and presence or absence of coexisting ocular or systemic disease.

The pathologic condition of pre-Descemet dystrophy was limited to the keratocytes of the posterior stroma.[68,119] The keratocytes contained lipid-like material in their cytoplasmic vacuoles (secondary lysosomes). Ultrastructural study of these vacuoles revealed fibrillogranular and electron-dense lamellar inclusions, suggesting that the accumulated material most likely was lipofuscin, a degenerative "wear and tear" lipoprotein associated with aging. No extracellular deposition of a similar material was noted.

Punctiform and Polychromatic Pre-Descemet Dominant Dystrophy

A pedigree with more uniform, polychromatic deep stromal filaments in a diffuse pattern extending to the limbus[64] was described, affecting 46 family members from four generations, and the inheritance appeared to be autosomal dominant. No particular aggregations or annular patterns were appreciated, and Descemet's membrane and the endothelium were not clinically affected. No histopathologic specimens are available from this clinical variant.

Deep Filiform Dystrophy

Deep filiform dystrophy of Maeder and Danis[201] has been reported in association with keratoconus. The lesions consist of multiple filiform, gray opacities in the pre-Descemet area that affect the entire width of the cornea except for a perilimbal region. Yassa et al. reported a case with bilateral optically dense linear striae of variable lengths and a crisscross pattern forming a lacy network.[381] The opacities lie between the deep stromal lamellae immediately anterior to Descemet's membrane. Both corneas showed immunoglobulin deposited extracellularly in the posterior third of the stroma and intracellularly in the keratocytes of the posterior two-thirds. The collagen fibrils appeared to be both mechanically displaced and replaced by the accumulating material in the posterior third. Morphologically, the intracellular and extracellular material were similar. Ultrastructurally, the immunoglobulins were located within dilated cisternae of the rough endoplasmic reticulum in the keratocytes, indicating synthesis by the keratocytes rather than phagocytosis. Although the results of serum protein electrophoresis were within normal limits, the possibility of a dysproteinemia unable to be detected by currently available methods could not be excluded. Thus, in all cases diagnosed clinically as pre-Descemet dystrophy, one may consider examining the patient's serum for the possibility of dysproteinemia.

Similar opacities have been noted in association with other ocular or systemic abnormalities, and these have been called secondary pre-Descemet dystrophies, which also have been reported in patients with epithelial basement membrane dystrophy,[85] posterior polymorphous dystrophy,[85] ichthyosis (deep punctate dystrophy of Franceschetti and Maeder),[94,95] central cloudy corneal dystrophy,[66] pseudoxanthoma elasticum,[66] and in female carriers of sex-linked ichthyosis.[313]

ENDOTHELIAL DYSTROPHIES

The adult human corneal endothelial cells lack significant mitotic capability, and, as they undergo attrition, the surviving cells enlarge and spread to maintain an intact monolayer in order to remain functionally competent as a barrier and a pump in maintaining corneal deturgescence. Endothelial cell loss usually associates with aging and a variety of injuries, such as trauma, inflammation, drugs, and glaucoma. The earliest sign, corneal guttae, can progress to stromal edema, epithelial edema, and corneal scarring.[116] It is called *Fuchs dystrophy* when these changes are seen in the absence of contributory injury. Some such cases may be a result of unrecognized injury; many are related to normal aging or an accelerated aging of the endothelium; and some appear to be true dystrophies, with early onset and hereditary transmission.

Cornea Guttata

Vogt coined the term "guttae" to describe corneas containing multiple drop-like excrescences, or guttae, on their posterior surface (Fig. 13.17*A* and *B*). Cornea guttata is usually seen in middle-aged or older patients. Central corneal guttae without edema have been studied in several large series and have been noted in as many as 70% of patients over 40 years of age.[197] In addition to aging, they can be associated with corneal trauma and inflammation.[91,374,383]

Guttae are dewdrop-like, wart-like, or mushroom-like endothelial excrescences. They are abnormal basement membrane and fibrillar collagens elaborated by distressed or dystrophic endothelial cells. The endothelial cells over these excrescences become attenuated and eventually die prematurely. Brownish pigmentation, representing pigment phagocytosis by the endothelium, may often be seen at the level of the guttae, which appear as refractile circular excavations on the endothelial surface with direct illumination. They are black holes in the endothelial mosaic under specular microscope. Cornea guttata develops first in the central cornea and gradually spreads peripherally as the guttae become more numerous. Descemet's membrane can develop a beaten-metal appearance with time.

Guttae located in the periphery of the cornea

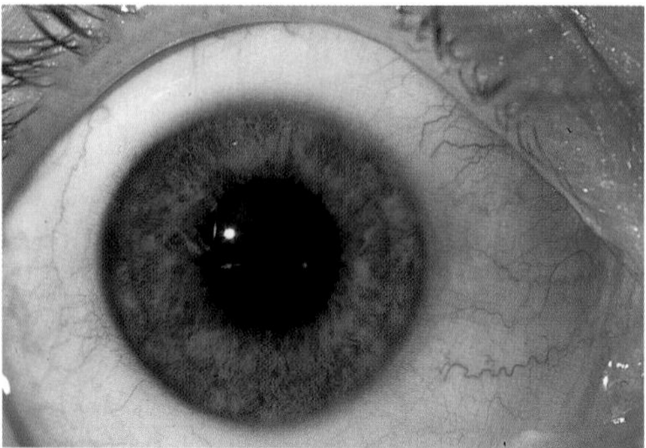

A

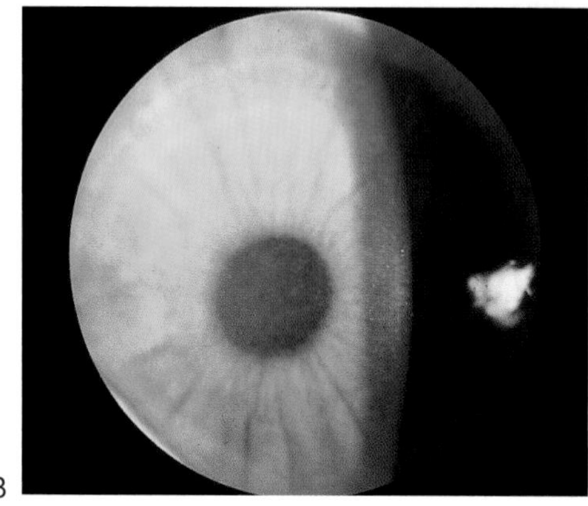

B

Figure 13.17. **A.** Asymptomatic cornea guttata. **B.** Guttae associated with epithelial granularity.

may be seen even in young individuals. These are called *Hassall–Henle bodies* and are of no clinical concern. When they become more numerous and central, this may foretell functional compromise of the endothelial cells to the extent that their barrier and pump functions become insufficient. In this event, stromal edema occurs, followed by epithelial edema and bullous keratopathy, and the condition is termed *Fuchs dystrophy* (Fig. 13.18*A–D*). However, mild to moderate cornea guttata can remain stationary for years without obligate dystrophic progression.

Secondary cornea guttata is usually associated with degenerative corneal disease, trauma, or inflammation. The corneal endothelial cells may be adversely affected by iritis, deep stromal inflammation or infection, and anterior segment surgery. In severe inflammation, the endothelial mosaic may be affected by the endothelial cell edema.[1,182,375] This condition resembles cornea guttata. On removal of the causative agent, these "pseudoguttae" subside,[182] whereas true corneal guttae are permanent. In some instances the endothelial change is not in guttate form, but rather the endothelium becomes increasingly diffusely opaque, giving the appearance of a grayish membrane.[1,57]

Fuchs Endothelial Dystrophy

Fuchs dystrophy is a bilateral condition that usually is noted in the fifth or sixth decade of life and is more common in women.[181] Autosomal dominant transmission has been demonstrated in some cases.[67,180,202,237,297] Some reports have suggested an association between Fuchs dystrophy and open-angle glaucoma,[47] but others have not found this relationship.[181,284] Pitts and Jay reported a significant association between Fuchs dystrophy and axial hypermetropia, shallow anterior chamber and angle-closure glaucoma[263] and propose a genetic linkage between the inheritance of an abnormal axial length and the inheritance of Fuchs dystrophy.

Recent reports in the literature document cases of coexistent bilateral Fuchs dystrophy and keratoconus (Fig. 13.13).[181,252] A retrospective review of 27 patients with Fuchs dystrophy reported a higher prevalence of cardiovascular disease than was present in age–sex-matched controls. The authors hypothesized that a common endothelial factor (i.e., vascular and corneal) may be responsible for the development of both diseases.[249] This rationale, however, is flawed in view of the different embryonic origins of the two endothelia.[3]

Pathophysiology

The fundamental defect in Fuchs dystrophy is the progressive deterioration of the endothelium. Early work by Burns et al. suggested that the initial defect in Fuchs dystrophy was a breakdown in the endothelial cell barrier function as manifested by an increased permeability to fluorescein.[45] However, using a more precise two-dimensional scanning fluorophotometer, Wilson et al.[366] and Wilson and Bourne[367] found no difference in the endothelial permeability between patients with advanced corneal guttae,

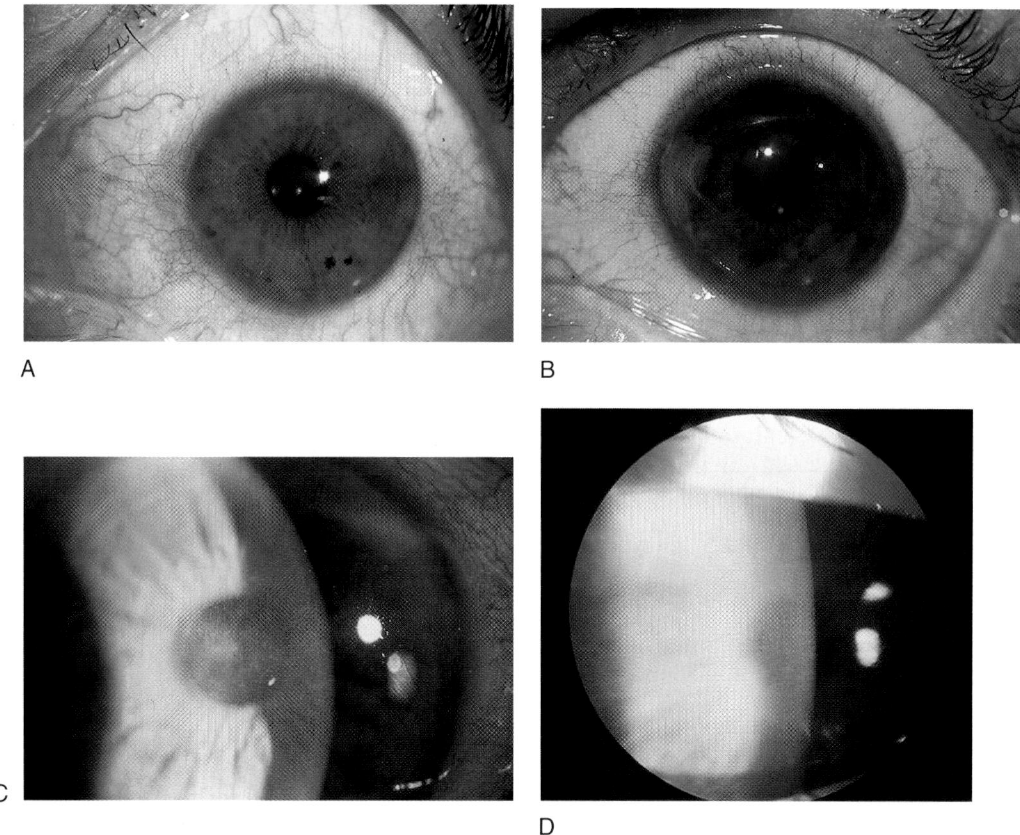

Figure 13.18. Fuchs endothelial dystrophy. **A.** Stage 1: Absent stromal edema. **B.** Stage 2: Localized stromal edema. **C.** Stage 2: Fluctuating vision and variable degrees of epithelial and stromal edema. **D.** Diffuse stromal and epithelial edema (stage 3).

mild corneal guttae, and normal age- and sex-matched controls. Moreover, the pump rate was found to be significantly decreased in patients with advanced guttae. These data suggest that an altered pump rate, not a leaky barrier, is the earliest defect seen in Fuchs dystrophy. Tuberville et al. found a significantly decreased cytochrome oxidase activity in the endothelial cells of patients with Fuchs dystrophy.[345] In individuals with moderated guttae, Geroski et al. suggest that the endothelium has an adaptive reserve pump capacity which is upregulated to maintain endothelial pump-leak rates when the endothelium is diseased.[113] Subsequent work has employed autoradiography, immunohistochemistry, lectin binding, and freeze-fracture with transmission electron microscopy to demonstrate that the Na-K ATPase pump site density is decreased in Fuchs dystrophy.[213,214,215,216,306]

Studies of Descemet's membrane in Fuchs dystrophy show that the basement membrane is altered not only morphologically but also biochemically. Scanning electron microscopy and energy-dispersive X-ray analysis demonstrate a 40%–50% decrease in the sulfur content and an increase in the calcium content in the guttate and nonguttate regions of Descemet's membrane.[286,306] Sodium dodecyl sulfate (SDS) polyacrylamide gel electrophoresis (PAGE) and two-dimensional mapping studies show that both normal corneas and Fuchs dystrophy corneas contain essentially the same stromal collagen types; however, a slight discrepancy is seen in the electrophoretic mobility of some of the collagen chains.[49] Fluorescein isothiocyanate conjugated (FITC) lectin studies demonstrate an increased deposition of normal sugars in Descemet's membrane [β-D-galactose (1-3)-D-*N*-acetylgalactosamine and terminal β-galactose] without the appearance of new or abnormal sugars.[49]

Biomicroscopic Appearance and Clinical Staging. On their own, guttae do not interfere with vision, but stromal edema does occur if endothelial cell function is sufficiently compromised. Stromal edema is more likely to occur with decreased endothelial cell density, yet the density may vary. The number of corneal guttae also does not correlate well, and stromal edema can occur in the absence of guttae.[1] With further impairment of endothelial function, epithelial edema develops. Epithelial edema can occur at different stages depending on the intraocular pressure. Elevations of intraocular pressure more readily cause epithelial edema in a cornea with compromised endothelium and stromal edema.

Stromal edema generally does not reduce the vision significantly until it becomes marked (approximately >0.65 mm), but it is usually not until epithelial edema develops that the patient becomes very symptomatic. Epithelial edema causes surface irregularity and haze and recurrent epithelial erosions. Decreased evaporation of the tears during sleep decreases their osmolarity, and in the early stage this leads to increased edema and decreased visual acuity on awakening, which clears as the day goes on. Vision can deteriorate similarly in humid atmospheric conditions. However, it becomes constantly impaired as corneal edema progresses.

Early epithelial edema appears as fine, clear cysts producing nodular elevations of the surface (bedewing) and can be difficult to diagnose. Indirect illumination reveals a slight clouding of the anterior cornea and sometimes microcysts. Sclerotic scatter (placing the slit beam at the limbus) is helpful in demonstrating the haze from epithelial edema. Topical fluorescein and cobalt blue lighting cause the microcysts to stand out by interrupting an otherwise smooth tear film. Fingerprint-like patterns and other linear opacities may be seen in the deep epithelium, probably caused by shifting of the overlying epithelium. Microcysts coalescence to form intraepithelial or subepithelial bullae. These markedly reduce vision and can rupture, causing photophobia, pain, and foreign-body sensation. Occasionally a ruptured bulla may become infected, creating an epithelial erosion. subepithelial fibrosis and vascularization can occur in more advanced cases, particularly with recurrent epithelial breakdown.

The clinical course of Fuchs dystrophy is divisible into four stages, usually spanning 20–30 years.[29,120] In *stage 1,* the patient is asymptomatic, but biomicroscopy reveals central corneal guttae, a variable amount of pigment on the posterior corneal surface, and a gray and thickened appearance of Descemet's membrane. This stage of Fuchs dystrophy is noted only retrospectively because it is identical to the appearance of central corneal guttae without edema. *Stage 2* is characterized by a painless decrease in vision and symptoms of glare, which are particularly severe on awakening. These symptoms are primarily due to varying degrees of epithelial and stromal edema. *Stage 3* is marked by the formation of epithelial and subepithelial bullae, which rupture, causing episodes of pain. In *stage 4,* the visual acuity may be reduced to hand motion, but the patient is free of painful attacks. The relief from pain coincides with the appearance of subepithelial scar tissue that lessens bullae formation but severely limits vision.

Histopathology. The main pathologic change in Fuchs dystrophy is in the endothelium.[142,145,147] Guttae are seen as nodular thickenings of Descemet's membrane. They are composed of collagen and most likely are abnormal products of the endothelial cells.[147]

The endothelium in Fuchs dystrophy is abnormal in a flat preparation, exhibiting displaced and crowded nuclei of various sizes and shapes. The few normal-appearing endothelial cell nuclei stain less intensely with hematoxylin than do the nuclei of the pleomorphic endothelial cells. In cross section, the cytoplasm of the endothelial cells is frequently thin or absent over areas of advanced guttae. The nuclei appear to be pushed into the areas between the prominent excrescences. The endothelial cell cytoplasm contains small to large vacuoles with occasional clumps of phagocytosed pigment. Sometimes the endothelium is too thin to be detected by light microscopy. Some of the endothelial cells take on morphologic features of fibroblasts and produce collagen.[142,147] Other cells show tonofilaments, surface microvilli, and desmosomes, similar to epithelial cells.[121] Normal-appearing cells are concentrated mainly at the corneal periphery, whereas fibroblast-like cells appear centrally.

Descemet's membrane becomes diffusely thickened because of deposition of collagenous basement membrane-like material on the posterior surface.[28,147,161,352] The warts are variable in appearance; they can be hemibroad-based fusiform protrusions. With hematoxylin and eosin, the staining intensity of these warts is identical to that of the anterior, fetal portion of Descemet's membrane. The anterior banded portion is relatively normal, whereas the posterior nonbanded layer is thinned or absent and is replaced by a posterior banded layer.[28,147] The thinness of the posterior nonbanded layer suggests that endothelial cell function becomes abnormal at an early age. The abnormal posterior collagenous layer of Fuchs dystrophy can be considered analogous to the deposition of excess collagen and basement membrane material found in other circumstances of the "endothelial distress syndrome."[349] Kenney et al. hypothesize that the changes seen in Descemet's membrane are due to the altered assembly of collagen molecules and that the fibrinolytic system may have a role in the pathogenesis of the disease.[161] Although no differences were found between the serum fibrinogen degradation products of patients with Fuchs dystrophy and controls, fibrinogen/fibrin was localized to the abnormal Descemet's membrane in Fuchs dystrophy corneas by immunofluorescence.[279] Oxatalan fibers, which normally are not present in posterior corneal tissue, have been localized around the guttae, but not in the central portion of the warts. These abnormal fibers may serve an anchoring and adhesive function by providing mechanical resistance to external forces.[79,107,275]

Epithelial edema appears first intracellularly in the basal cells. Later, interepithelial and subepithelial pockets of fluid are seen. Abnormalities of the basement membrane adhesion complexes develop because of repeated "liftoff" of the edematous epithelium. Although Bowman's layer usually remains intact, breaks may occasionally be found. Subepithelial deposition of collagen and basement membrane-like material can be noted.

Treatment

The medical management of Fuchs dystrophy is limited. Advanced corneal guttae in the absence of edema do not cause any significant vision loss or discomfort and thus require no treatment. Stage 2 disease with early epithelial edema may benefit from hyperosmotic drops and ointment; however, they have little effect on stromal edema.[29,120] Usually 5% NaCl drops are given four to eight times daily and 5% NaCl ointment at bedtime. Because of the increased severity of the symptoms in the morning, 5% NaCl eyedrops may be necessary every 15 minutes on awakening and less often as the day progresses. These drops may reduce epithelial edema and improve both comfort and vision. A hair dryer, held at arm's length and directed across the face, may help "dry out" the corneal surface and can be repeated two or three times a day. Incipient stromal and epithelial edema may sometimes be controlled temporarily by a reduction in the intraocular pressure (IOP), even if it is within normal limits.[29] Cycloplegic agents can relieve the discomfort associated with ciliary spasm. Topical corticosteroids appear to have little or no effect on the endothelial permeability or corneal thickness.

A loosely fit, high water content bandage contact lens is beneficial in alleviating discomfort resulting from bullae formation and rupture in stage 3 patients. It is particularly useful in making life more pleasant when corneal transplantation is not desired or recommended. Other alternatives for these patients include cautery of Bowman's layer or a conjunctival flap.

Penetrating keratoplasty is indicated once visual acuity is decreased to impair normal activities. The short-term results are quite good,[368] but long-term survival of these grafts is questionable. Some studies have found a relatively high incidence of graft failure.[251,325] Cataracts are often present, and combined keratoplasty and cataract extraction can be performed.[13,24,46,193] The relative value of separate versus combined procedures has not yet been determined. However, it is reasonable to state that even with flawless cataract surgery, a cornea with guttae is at increased risk for decompensation because of the preexisting endothelial disease. Most surgeons now perform combined procedures.[15] In the presence of a cataract, the indications for keratoplasty are not well defined. Some surgeons have recommended keratoplasty whenever the corneal thickness is greater than 0.60 mm,[226] whereas others suggest cataract extraction alone unless epithelial edema is present.[16] However, the use of a predetermined corneal thickness is not advocated as the corneal thickness can vary greatly in "clear" corneas.[2] Triple procedure is recommended for eyes with cataract *and* signs or symptoms or corneal edema.

Congenital Hereditary Endothelial Dystrophy

Initially described by Maumenee in 1960,[209] this congenital disorder of the endothelium is characterized clinically by diffuse, bilaterally symmetric corneal edema. Congenital hereditary endothelial dystrophy (CHED) can be inherited in both autosomal dominant and autosomal recessive forms. The recessive form is more common and more severe and relatively nonprogressive, whereas the dominant form is less severe and can be associated with deafness.[132,153,157,168,257,261,351] The recessive form is present at birth or develops in the neonatal period and is often associated with nystagmus. Patients with dominantly inherited disease have clear corneas early in life, but within a few years they develop slowly progressive opacification.[10,11,12,153] They do not develop nystagmus. In contrast to the recessive variety, progressive photophobia and tearing are the initial symptoms.

Astymtomatic relatives of patients with CHED can manifest corneal changes resembling those of posterior polymorphous dystrophy.[257] These individuals appear to have a higher risk of producing offspring with CHED.[191]

Clinical Manifestations

The essential feature of CHED is bilateral diffuse corneal edema, unrelated to commonly known etiologic factors, such as congenital glaucoma, intrauterine infections, or mucopolysaccharidosis. The clinical picture can vary from a mild haziness to a moderately severe, diffuse, homogeneous, gray-white, ground-glass appearance of the central cornea that extends to the periphery (Fig. 13.19). The corneal thickness is two to three times greater than normal, but corneal diameter is not enlarged. Macular or dot stromal opacities are sometimes present. Diffuse stromal cloudiness often prevents clinical evaluation of the endothelium and Descemet's membrane, but the latter can sometimes be seen as thickened and gray. Guttae are not present, there is no vascularization, and corneal sensation and intraocular pressure are normal. The corneal opacity may be stationary or show slow progression. Epithelial edema and bedewing can develop, but bullae and discomfort are rarely seen.

Histopathology

Congenital hereditary endothelial dystrophy appears to result from a degeneration of the endothelium, which may occur in utero or within the first year of life. Histologic study reveals nonspecific anterior and stromal changes consistent with long-standing secondary edema: basal epithelial cell swelling, base-

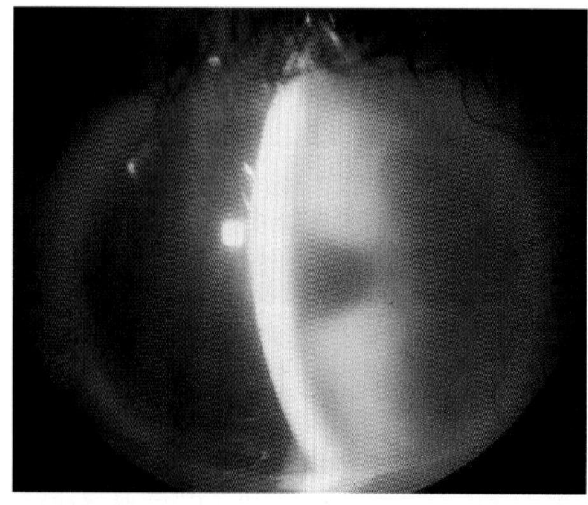

Figure 13.19. Congenital hereditary endothelial dystrophy.

ment membrane thickening and disruptions, and irregularities of Bowman's layer with pannus formation. However, in some patients ultrastructural examination discloses greatly enlarged stromal collagen fibrils sometimes measuring as much as 600 Å in diameter.

The anterior banded portion of Descemet's membrane is normal, indicating that the endothelium is functionally normal at least through the fifth month of gestation. However, sometime after the fifth month a defective endothelium secretes abnormal and excessive basement membrane, which accumulates as an aberrant, nonbanded posterior portion of Descemet's membrane.[12,157,162,163,165,294,320] The posterior layer consists of multilaminar basement membrane-like material with fine filaments and of collagen fibrils with a 550–1100 Å banded configuration. With the exception of the lack of guttae, these findings are similar to those in Fuchs dystrophy and thus represent another example of posterior collagen layer formation by either primarily or secondarily abnormal endothelium.[294,349,353] The rate at which the abnormal material is deposited is determined by the proportion of dystrophic endothelial cells. As more cells become abnormal, a disturbance in the synthetic activity leads to deposition of a totally abnormal posterior collagen layer. However, the presence of collagen type IV within the posterior collagen layer indicates a persisting "endothelial potential" of the degenerating cells.[312] In the majority of cases of CHED either simple degeneration or fibroblast-like transformation was observed.[55,164,165,168] It is postulated that in patients with a thin Descemet's membrane, complete endothelial loss occurred in utero such that only the fetal anterior portion of Descemet's membrane was secreted.[162] In contrast, thickened Descemet's membranes may be the product of dystrophic but persistent endothelium having secreted a hypertrophic posterior collagen layer. In one study the endothelial cells did not grow when placed in culture medium.[320] The frequent finding of enlarged stromal collagen fibrils suggest some primary developmental abnormality of both keratocytes and endothelium, perhaps qualifying this disorder as another example of mesenchymal dysgenesis.[164]

Linkage Studies[338]

Toma et al. have performed linkage analysis of 40 members of a 129-member, seven-generation family of CHED,[168,257] concluding that CHED is linked to chromosome 20. Multipoint analysis gave a maximum lod score between D20548 and D205471. This region lies within a region assigned to posterior polymorphous dystrophy.[136,338]

Treatment

Keratoplasty in such young children is considerably more difficult than in adults, but good results can be obtained in some cases.[63,66,348]

Posterior Polymorphous Dystrophy

Posterior polymorphous dystrophy (PPD) is an uncommon, but well-recognized, congenital disease affecting Descemet's membrane and endothelium. It is usually transmitted as a dominant trait, but recessive patterns of inheritance have been demonstrated in some pedigrees.[58,131,141] It is most often bilateral but can be asymmetric and, rarely, unilateral.[26] Some cases are clearly congenital, with cloudy corneas at birth. However, patients with PPD usually demonstrate normal vision and are asymptomatic, so the age of onset can be difficult to determine. Most cases are nonprogressive or very slowly progressive, but corneal edema develops in a small number of patients, necessitating a corneal graft in middle age.[121]

Clinical Manifestation

Posterior polymorphous dystrophy is characterized by deep corneal lesions of various shapes. It can be divided into three basic forms: vesicular, band, and diffuse. Nodular, grouped vesicular and blister-like lesions at the level of Descemet's membrane commonly occur.[316] Gray-white halos often surround the vesicular lesions (Fig. 13.20). The vesicles may be few or many, widely separated, clustered, or even confluent when they are termed geographic PPD by some investigators.[139,351] In band PPD, flat gray-white opacities, gray thickenings of Descemet's membrane, sinuous broad bands, or clear bands with

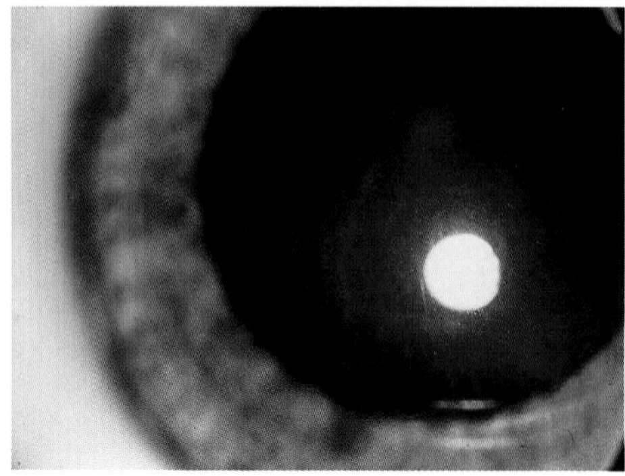

A

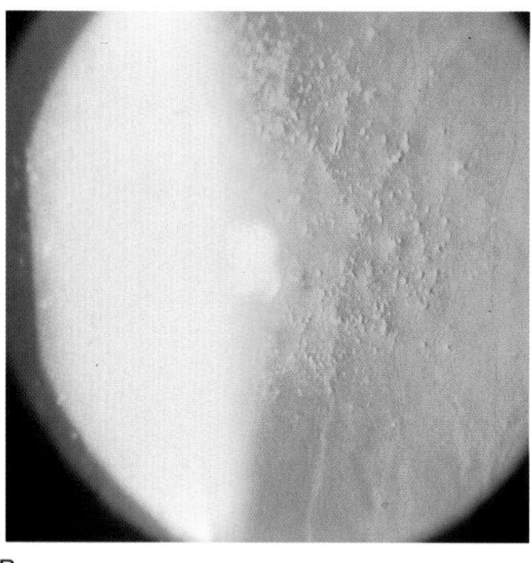

B

Figure 13.20. Posterior polymorphous dystrophy by direct illumination (**A**) and retroillumination (**B**).

white scalloped margins can be seen. The latter can be oriented vertically or horizontally and are often confused with Descemet's tears.[59] Diffuse PPD affects the entire posterior corneal surface or a large area of it and appears as a complicated swirled pattern of ridges and points in a Descemet's membrane of uneven thickness and translucency, often accompanied by full-thickness corneal edema. Both band and diffuse PPD, in addition to the signs mentioned above, show the classic PPD vesicles. The lesions stand out on retroillumination. Although careful biomicroscopy is usually adequate to establish the diagnosis,[59] specular microscopy may be helpful in differentiating posterior polymorphous dystrophy from other corneal endothelial disorders.[39,139] With specular microscopy the lesions are seen to contain abnormal pleomorphic cells, with indistinct borders and increased reflective highlights.[139,205] The endothelial cell density was considerably less than in normal age-matched individuals.[187]

Posterior polymorphous dystrophy can be associated with anterior segment dysgenesis, with prominent Schwalbe's ring, iridocorneal adhesions, abnormal iris processes, iris atrophy, corectopia, and ectropion uveae.[121] Intraocular pressure elevation occurs in approximately 15% of cases.[26,121,267,300] Band keratopathy,[121] calcium deposition in the deep stroma,[141] and anterior[112,359] and posterior keratoconus[121] have been reported.

Histopathology

Electron microscopic studies have revealed the main abnormality to be in the endothelial cell.[26,55,121,265,268,283,294,295,342] Three types of endothelial cell changes in posterior polymorphous dystrophy have been described: *(1)* degenerated endothelial cells, *(2)* fibroblast-like cells, and *(3)* epithelial-like cells. Islands of epithelial-like cells are found, which are larger than normal endothelial cells. These cells contain epithelial keratin and are connected by well-developed desmosomes. They can be multilayered and have extensive microvilli, intracytoplasmic filaments, and a decreased number of organelles. Although the epithelial-like endothelium was considered the pathologic hallmark of PPD, the most recent large study showed that this feature is present in less than two-thirds of cases.[212] When grown in culture, the abnormal endothelial cells maintain the abnormal characteristics observed in pathologic specimens.[288] However, the collagen synthetic capacity of the epithelium-like endothelium was similar to that of the normal epithelium and was much lower than that of normal native endothelium.[310] The abnormal endothelium can also extend across the trabecular meshwork and onto the iris.[183,295]

Pathologic examination of the specimens with the late manifestation of PPD showed a well-preserved anterior banded layer of Descemet's membrane, but the posterior portion may be thickened by abnormal multilaminar, basement membrane material. In a patient with early manifestation, however, the anterior banded zone of Descemet's membrane was thinned in the axial part of the cornea, contained defects in the paraxial part, and was absent at the periphery.[311] Corneal guttae and excavations of Descemet's membrane have been described.

The pathogenesis of PPD is unknown, but it has been suggested that there was an aberrant developmental differentiation of the endotheliogenic mesenchyme (neural crest),[19] possibly similar to the pathogenesis of the iridocorneal endothelial syndromes. The endothelial cells undergo transformation into epithelial-like cells, or that their embryonal precursors undergo abnormal differentiation. Ross et al. demonstrated the presence of cells staining positively for both endothelial antigen and cytokeratins supports the hypothesis that the cytokeratin-expressing epithelial-like cells found in corneas with posterior polymorphous dystrophy arise via a metaplastic process in which the phenotype of endothelial cells becomes progressively abnormal.[299] The angle and iris abnormalities may represent spread of these abnormal cells from the cornea, or they may be a broader reflection of the mesenchymal dysgenesis. Because the anterior banded portion of Descemet's membrane is normal in specimens with late manifestation, it is assumed that the abnormality develops late in gestation or shortly after birth. In a case with early manifestation, Sekundo et al.[311] suggested that failure to produce a continuous anterior banded zone of Descemet's membrane indicates an onset of the disease before the twelfth week of gestation. It appears that in PPD there is a mosaic of better preserved and dystrophic endothelial cells and that the presence or absence of the normal components of Descemet's membrane is determined by the proportion of dystrophic cells in the endothelial cell population.

Differential Diagnosis and Linkage Studies

Posterior polymorphous dystrophy and congenital hereditary endothelial dystrophy have been stated to be similar diseases. Both occur as part of the spectrum of a single entity based on observations that some ultrastructural features are similar.[55] Within one family some patients will only have a few vesicles and be diagnosed as having PPD, whereas others have severe stromal and epithelial edema that may be labeled CHED.[191] The largest family with autosomal dominant inheritance of CHED reported by Pearce et al.[257] and Kirkness et al.[168] had CHED linkage to a region of chromosome 20 assigned to PPD.[136,338] PPD can present as a cloudy cornea at birth and, therefore, must be differentiated from CHED and congenital hereditary stromal dystrophy (CHSD), as well as other conditions. Glaucoma, iridocorneal adhesions, and corneal edema can be present in both PPD and Chandler (iridocorneal endothelial) syndrome.

Treatment

In most cases no treatment is necessary, but occasionally keratoplasty is required when endothelial decompensation with stromal edema occurs. As with other corneal dystrophies, posterior polymorphous dystrophy may recur in the graft. In two cases histologic changes typical of PPD were observed in failed grafts 7 to 9 years after penetrating keratoplasty was performed for PPD.[27] The authors hypothesized that abnormal cells from the periphery of the host cornea repopulated the posterior graft surface, possibly after destruction of the donor endothelium. In rare instances corneal edema developing in adulthood has improved spontaneously.[58] If extensive angle and iris involvement is present, the resultant glaucoma can be very difficult to manage, and the prognosis for successful keratoplasty is very poor.

REFERENCES

1. Abbott RL et al. Specular microscopic and histologic observations in non-guttate corneal endothelial degeneration. *Ophthalmology* 1981;88:788.
2. Adamis AP, Filatov V, Tripathi BJ, Tripathi RC. Fuchs' endothelial dystrophy of the cornea. *Surv Ophthalmol* 1993;38:149–168.
3. Adamis AP, Molnar M, Tripathi BJ et al. Neuronal-specific enolase in human corneal endothelium and posterior keratocytes. *Exp Eye Res* 1985;41:665–668.

4. Akiya S, Brown S. Granular dystrophy of the cornea. *Arch Ophthalmol* 1970;84:179.
5. Akiya S, Brown SI. The ultrastructure of Reis–Bücklers dystrophy. *Am J Ophthalmol* 1971;72:549.
6. Akiya S, Ito I, Matsui M. Gelatinous drop-like dystrophy of the cornea. *Jpn J Clin Ophthalmol* 1972;56:815.
7. Akiya S, Nagaya K, Fukui A, Hamada T, Takahashi H, Furukawa H. Inherited corneal amyloidosis predominantly manifested in one eye. *Ophthalmologica* 1991;203(4):204–207.
8. Akova YA, Unlu N, Duman S. Fleck dystrophy of the cornea: A report of cases from three generations of a family. *Eur J Ophthalmol* 1994;4:123–125.
9. Andresen IL. Granular corneal dystrophy or Groenouw's diseases type 1. A challenge to Norwegian biochemists, genetists and ophthalmologists (Norwegian). *Tidsski Nor Laegeforen* 1995;115(3):355–356.
10. Antine BE. Congenital corneal dystrophy. *Am J Ophthalmol* 1970;70:656.
11. Antine BE. Congenital hereditary corneal dystrophy (CHCD). *South Med J* 1970;63: 946.
12. Antine BE. Histology of congenital hereditary corneal dystrophy. *Am J Ophthalmol* 1970; 69:964.
13. Aquavella JV, Shaw EL, Rao GN. Intraocular lens implantation combined with penetrating keratoplasty. *Ophthalmic Surg* 1977;8:113.
14. Aracena T. Hereditary fleck dystrophy of the cornea: Report of a family. *J Pediatr Ophthalmol* 1975;12:223.
15. Arentsen JJ, Laibson PR. Penetrating keratoplasty and cataract extraction: Combined vs nonsimultaneous surgery. *Arch Ophthalmol* 1978;96:75.
16. Arffa RC. Disorders of the endothelium. In *Grayson's Diseases of the Cornea,* 3rd ed. St. Louis: Mosby Year-Book, 1991.
17. Asaoka T, Amano S, Sunada Y, Sawa M. Lattice corneal dystrophy type II with familial amyloid polyneuropathy type IV. *Jpn J Ophthalmol* 1993;37:426–431.
18. Bagolini B, Ioli-Spada G. Bietti's tapetoretinal dygeneration with marginal corneal dystrophy. *Am J Ophthalmol* 1968;65:53–60.
19. Bahn CF, Galls HF, Varley GA. Classification of corneal endothelial disorders based on neural crest origin. *Ophthalmology* 1984; 91:558.
20. Barchiesi BJ, Eckel RH, Ellis PP. The cornea and disorders of lipid metabolism. *Surv Ophthalmol* 1991;36:1–22.
21. Bernauer W, Daicker B. Bietti's corneal-retinal dystrophy. *Retina* 1992;12:18–20.
22. Bücklers M. gber eine weitere familiare Hornhautdystrophie. *Klin Monatsbl Augenheilkd* 1949;114:386.
23. Bietti G. Ueber familiares Vorkommen von Retinitis punctata abcescens (verbunden mit Dystrophia marginalis cristallinea corneae). Glitzern des Glaskoerpers und anderen degenerativen Augenveaenderungen. *Klin Monatsbl Augenheilkd* 1937;99:737–756.
24. Binder PS. Intraocular lens power used in the triple procedure. *Ophthalmology* 1985;92: 1561.
25. Birndoft LA, Ginsberg SP. Hereditary fleck dystrophy associated with decreased corneal sensitivity. *Am J Ophthalmol* 1972;73:670.
26. Borchoff SA, Kuwabara T. Electron microscopy of posterior polymorphous degeneration. *Am J Ophthalmol* 1971;72:879.
27. Boruchoff SA, Weiner MJ, Albert DM. Recurrence of posterior polymorphous corneal dystrophy after penetrating keratoplasty. *Am J Ophthalmol* 1990;109:323.
28. Bourne WM, Johnson DH, Campbell RJ. The ultrastructure of Descemet's membrane. III. Fuchs' dystrophy. *Arch Ophthalmol* 1982; 100:1952–1955.
29. Bourne WM. Fuchs' corneal dystrophy. In *Current Ocular Therapy* 2nd ed. F. T. Fraunfelder, R. F. Hampton, eds. Philadelphia: W.B. Saunders, 1985, pp. 312–313.
30. Bowen RA, Hassard DTR, Wong VG et al. Lattice dystrophy of the cornea as a variety of amyloidosis. *Am J Ophthalmol* 1970;7: 822.
31. Bramsen T, Ehlers N, Baggesen KH. Central cloudy corneal dystrophy of François. *Acta Ophthalmol (Copenh)* 1976;54:221.
32. Broderick JD, Dark AJ, Pearce GW. Fingerprint dystrophy of the cornea. *Arch Ophthalmol* 1974;92:483.
33. Bron AJ, Brown NA. Some superficial corneal disorders. *Trans Ophthalmol Soc UK* 1971; 91:13.
34. Bron AJ, Buriless SEP. Inherited recurrent comeal erosion. *Trans Ophthalmol Soc UK* 1981;101:239.
35. Bron AJ, Tripathi RC. Anterior corneal mosaic: Further observations. *Br J Ophthalmol* 1969;53:760.
36. Bron AJ, Tripathi RC. Cystic disorders of the corneal epithelium. 1. Clinical aspects. *Br J Ophthalmol* 1969;53:760.
37. Bron AJ, Williams HP, Carruthers ME. Hereditary crystalline stromal dystrophy of

Schnyder: Clinical features of a family with hyperlipoproteinemia. *Br J Ophthalmol* 1973;56:383.

38. Bron AJ. Superficial fibrillary lines. A feature of the normal cornea. *Br J Ophthalmol* 1975; 59:133.
39. Brooks AMV, Grant G, Gillies WE. Differentiation of posterior polymorphous dystrophy from other posterior corneal opacities by specular microscopy. *Ophthalmology* 1989; 96:1639.
40. Brown NA, Bron AJ. Recurrent erosion of the cornea. *Br J Ophthalmol* 1976;60:84.
41. Brownstein S, Jackson WB, Onerheim RM. Schnyder's crystalline corneal dystrophy in association with hyperlipoproteinemia: histopathological and ultrastructural findings. *Can J Ophthalmol* 1991;26:273–279.
42. Bruner WE, Dejak TR, Grossniklaus HE, Stark WJ, Young E. Corneal alpha-galactosidase deficiency in macular corneal dystrophy. *Ophthalmic Paediatr Genet* 1985;5:179–183.
43. Burns RP, Connor W, Gipson I. Cholesterol turnover inhereditary crystalline corneal dystrophy of Schnyder. *Trans Am Ophthalmol Soc* 1978;76:184–196.
44. Burns RP. Meesmann's corneal dystrophy. *Trans Am Ophthalmol Soc* 1968;66:531.
45. Burns RR, Bourne WM, Brubaker RF. Endothelial function in patients with cornea guttata. *Invest Ophthalmol Vis Sci* 1981;20: 77–85.
46. Busin M et al. Combined penetrating keratoplasty, extracapsular cataract extraction, and posterior chamber intraocular lens implantation. *Ophthalmic Surg* 1987;18:272.
47. Buxton JN et al. Tonography in cornea guttata: A preliminary study. *Arch Ophthalmol* 1967;77:602.
48. Buxton JN, Fox ML. Superficial epithelial keratectomy in the treatment of epithelial basement membrane dystrophy. *Arch Ophthalmol* 1983;101:392.
49. Calandra A, Chwa M, Kenney MC. Characterization of stroma from Fuchs' endothelial dystrophy corneas. *Cornea* 1989;8:90–97.
50. Caldwell DR. Postoperative recurrence of Reis–Bücklers corneal dystrophy. *Am J Ophthalmol* 1978;85:567.
51. Campos M, Nielsen S, Szerenyi K, Garbus JJ et al. Clinical follow-up of phototherapeutic keratectomy for treatment of corneal opacities. *Am J Ophthalmol* 1993;115:433–440.
52. Carpel EF, Sigelman RJ, Doughman DJ. Posterior amorphous corneal dystrophy. *Am J Ophthalmol* 1977;83:629.
53. Cennamo G, Rosa N, Rosenwasser GOD, Sebastiani A. Phototherapeutic keratectomy in the treatment of Avellino dystrophy. *Ophthalmologica* 1994;208:198–200.
54. Chamon W, Azar DT, Stark WJ, Reed C, Enger C. Phototherapeutic keratectomy. *Ophthalmol Clin North Am* 1993;6:399–413.
55. Chan C, Green WR, Barraquer J, Barraquer SE, de la Cruz ZC. Similarities between posterior polymorphous and congenital hereditary endothelial dystrophies: A study of 14 buttons of 11 cases. *Cornea* 1982;1:155–172.
56. Chan CC, Cogan DG, Bucci FS, Barsley D, Crawford MA. Anterior corneal dystrophy with dyscollagenosis. (Reis-Bückler type?). *Cornea* 1993 Sept;12(5):451–460.
57. Chi HH, Teng CC, Katzin HM. Histopathology of primary endothelial-epithelial dystrophy of the cornea. *Am J Ophthalmol* 1958; 45:518.
58. Cibis GW et al. The clinical spectrum of posterior polymorphous dystrophy. *Arch Ophthalmol* 1977;95:1529.
59. Cibis GW, Tripathi RC. The differential diagnosis of Descemet's tears and posterior polymorphous dystrophy bands. *Ophthalmology* 1982;89:614.
60. Cogan DG et al. Microcystic dystrophy of the corneal epithelium. *Trans Am Ophthalmol Soc* 1964;62:213.
61. Cogan DG et al. Microcystic dystrophy of the cornea. *Arch Ophthalmol* 1974;92:470.
62. Collier M. Dystrophie nuageuse centrale et dystrophie ponctiforme prédescemédans une même famille. *Bull Soc Optalmol Fr* 1966; 66:57.
63. Collier M. Caracre heredo-familial de la dystrophie ponctiforme predescemetique. *Bull Soc Ophtalmol Fr* 1964;64:731.
64. Collier M. Dystrophie nuageuse centrale et dystrophie ponctiforme predescemetique. *Bull Soc Ophtalmol Fr* 1964;64:1034.
65. Collier MT. Dystrophie mouchete du parenchyme corneen avec dystrophie nuageuse centrale. *Bull Soc Ophtalmol Fr* 1964;64:608.
66. Collier MT. Elastorrhexie systee et dystrophies corneenees chez deux soerus. *Bull Soc Ophtalmol Fr* 1965;65:301.
67. Cross HE, Maumanee AE, Cantolino SJ. Inheritance of Fuchs' denodthelial dystrophy. *Arch Ophthalmol* 1971;85:268.
68. Curran RE, Kenyon KR, Green WR. Pre-Descemet's membrane corneal dystrophy. *Am J Ophthalmol* 1974;77:711.
69. Dark AJ, Thompson DS. Lattice dystrophy of

the cornea. A clinical and microscopic study. *Br J Ophthalmol* 1960;44:257.

70. Dausch D, Landesz M, Klein R, Schroder E. Phototherapeutic keratectomy in recurrent corneal erosion. *Refract Corneal Surg* 1993; 9:419–424.
71. de la Chapelle A et al. Gelsolin-derived familial amyloidosis caused by asparagine or tyrosine substitution for aspartic acid at residue 187. *Nature Genet* 1992;2:157–160.
72. Delleman JW, Winkelman JE. Degeneratio corneae cristallinea hereditaria: A clinical, genetical, and histological study. *Ophthalmologica* 1968;155:409–426.
73. Diaper CJ. Severe granular dystrophy: A pedigree with presumed homozygotes. *Eye* 1994; 8(pt 4):448–452.
74. Donnenfeld ED et al. Corneal thinning in macular corneal dystrophy. *Am J Ophthalmol* 1986;101:112.
75. Dreizen NB, Stulting RK, Cavanagh HD. Penetrating keratoplasty and cataract surgery in children. In *Ophthalmology Annual: Nineteen Eighty-Seven,* R. Reinecke, ed. Norwalk, CT: Appleton-Century Crofts, 1987.
76. Dunn SP, Krachmer JH, Ching SS. New findings in posterior amorphous dystrophy. *Arch Ophthalmol* 1984;102:236.
77. Edward D, Thonar EJ-MA, Srinivasan M et al. Macular corneal dystrophy of the cornea. A systemic disorder of keratan sulfate metabolism. *Ophthalmology* 1990;97:1194–1200.
78. Edward DP, Yue BYJT, Sugar J et al. Heterogeneity in macular corneal dystrophy. *Arch Ophthalmol* 1988;106:1579–1583.
79. Edwards JG. A study of the periodontium during orthodontic rotation of teeth. *Am J Orthodont* 1968;54:441–461.
80. Ehlen N, Bramsen T. Central thickness in corneal disorders. *Acta Ophthalmol* 1978; 56:412.
81. Ehlers N, Mathiessen M. Hereditary crystalline dystrophy of Schnyder. *Acta Ophthalmol (Copenh)* 1967;51:1.
82. Eiberg H, Moler HU, Berendt I, Mohr J. Assignment of granular corneal dystrophy Groenouw type 1 (CDGG1) to chromosome 5q. *Eur J Hum Genet* 1994;2(2):132–138.
83. Fagerholm P, Fitzsimmons TD, Orndahl M, Ohman L, Tengroth B. Phototherapeutic keratectomy: Long-term results in 166 eyes. *Refract Corneal Surg* 1993;9(2 suppl):76–81.
84. Feder RS, Jay M, Yue BYJT, Stock EL, O'Grady RB, Roth SI. Subepithelial micinous corneal dystrophy: Clinical and pathological correlations. *Arch Ophthalmol* 1993;111(8): 1106–1114.
85. Fernandez-Sasso D, Acosta JEP, Malbran E. Punctiform and polychromatic pre-Descemet's dominant corneal dystrophy. *Fr J Ophtalmol* 1979;63:336.
86. Fine BS et al. Meesman's epithelial dystrophy of the cornea. *Am J Ophthalmol* 1977;83:633.
87. Fogle JA, Green WR, Kenyon KR. Anterior corneal dystrophy. *Am J Ophthalmol* 1974; 77:529.
88. Fogle JA, Kenyon KR, Stark WJ, Green WR. Defective epithelial adhesion in anterior corneal dystrophies. *Am J Ophthalmol* 1975; 79:925–940.
89. Folberg R, Alfonso E, Croxatto JO et al. Clinically atypical granular corneal dystrophy with pathologic features of lattice-like amyloid deposits. A study of three families. *Ophthalmology* 1988;95:46–51.
90. Folberg R, Stone EM, Sheffield VC, Mathers WD. The relationship between granular, lattice type 1, and Avellino corneal dystrophies: A histopathologic study. *Arch Ophthalmol* 1994;112:1080–1085.
91. Forgacs J. Stries hyalines retrocorneennes postinflammatories en toiles araignees. *Ophthalmologica* 1963;145:301.
92. Forsius H et al. Granular corneal dystrophy with late manifestation, *Acta Ophthalmol (Copenh)* 1983;61:514.
93. Foster W, Grewe S, Atzler U, Lunecke C, Busse H. Phototherapeutic keratectomy in corneal diseases. *Refract Corneal Surg* 1993;9(2 suppl):85–90.
94. Franceschetti A, Maeder G. Dystrophie profonde de la cornee dans un cad d'ichthyose congenitale. *Bull Mem Soc Fr Ophtalmol* 1954;67:146.
95. Franceschetti A, Schlaeppi V. Degenerescence en bandelettes et dystophie predescemetique de la cornee dans un cas d'ichyhyose congenitale. *Dermatologica* 1957;115:217.
96. Franceschetti A. Hereditdre Rezidivierende Erosion der Homhaut. *Z. Agenheilkd* 1928; 66:309.
97. François J et al. Ultrastructural findings in macular dystrophy (Groenouw type II). *Ophthalmic Res* 175;7:80.
98. François J, Neetens A. Nouvelle dystrophie héhédofamiliale de parenchyme cornée (heérédo-dystrophie Mouchetée). *Bull Soc Belge Ophtalmol* 1957;114:641.
99. François J, Vicotria-Troncoso V, Maudgal PC, Victoria-Ihler A. Study of the lysosomes by

vital stains in normal keratocytes and in keratocytes from macular dystrophy of the cornea. *Invest Ophthalmol Vis Sci* 1976;15:559.

100. François J, Feh Jr J. Light microscopical and polarization optical study of lattice dystrophy of the cornea. *Ophthalmologica* 1972;164:1.
101. François J et al. Dégéné rescence marginale pellucide de la cornée. *Ophthalmologica* 1968;155:337.
102. François J, Hanssens M, Teuchy H. Ultrastructural changes in lattice dystrophy of the cornea. *Ophthalmic Res* 1975;7:321.
103. François J, Neetans A. Nouvelle dystrophie hérédofamiliare du parenchyme cornée. *Bull Soc Belge Ophtalmol* 1956;114:641.
104. Freddo RF, Polack FM, Leibowitz HM. Ultrastructural changes in the posterior layers of the cornea in Schnyder's corneal crystalline dystrophy. *Cornea* 1989;8:170–177.
105. Friend SH, Bernards R, Rogelj S, Weinberg RA, Rapaport JM, Albert DM, Dryja TP: A human DNA segment with properties of the gene that predisposes to retinoblastoma and osteosarcoma. *Nature* 1986;323:643–646.
106. Fry WE, Pickett WE. Crystalline dystrophy of the cornea. *Trans Am Ophthalmol Soc* 1950;48:220.
107. Fullmer HM, Lillie RD. The oxytalan fibre: A previously undescribed connective tissue fibre. *J Histochem Cytochem* 1958;6:425–430.
108. Garner A, Tripathi RC. Hereditary crystalline stromal dystrophy of Schnyder. II. Histopathology and ultrastructure. *Br J Ophthalmol* 1972;56:400–408.
109. Garner A. Histochemistry of corneal maculu dystrophy. *Invest Ophthalmol* 1969;9:473.
110. Garner A. Histochemistry of corneal granular dystrophy. *Br J Ophthalmol* 1969;53:799.
111. Gartry DS, Falcon MG, Cox RW. Primary gelatinous drop-like keratopathy. *Br J Ophthalmol* 1989;73:661.
112. Gasset AR, Zimmerman TJ. Posterior polymorphous dystrophy associated with keratoconus. *Am J Ophthalmol* 1974;78:525–527.
113. Geroski DH, Matsuda M, Yee RW et al. Pump function of the human corneal endothelium. *Ophthalmology* 1985;92:1–6.
114. Ghosh M, McCulloch C. Crystalline dystrophy of the cornea: A light and electron microscopic study. *Can J Ophthalmol* 1977;12:321.
115. Gellespie F, Covelli B. Fleck (Mouchetée) dystrophy of the cornea: Report of a family. *South Med J* 1963;56:1265.
116. Goer EL. Dystrophy of the corneal endothelium (cornea guttata), with a report of a histological examination. *Am J Ophthalmol* 1934;17:215.
117. Goldberg MF et al. Variable expression in flecked (speckled) dystrophy of the cornea. *Ann Ophthalmol* 1977;9:889.
118. Grayson M, Wilbrandt H. Dystrophy of the anterior limiting membrane of the cornea (Reis–Bücklers type). *Am J Ophthalmol* 1966;63:345.
119. Grayson M, Wilbrandt H. Pre-Descemet dystrophy. *Am J Ophthalmol* 1967;64:276.
120. Grayson M. *Diseases of the Cornea.* St. Louis: C.V. Mosby, 1991, pp. 417–424.
121. Grayson M. The nature of hereditary deep polymorphous dystrophy of the cornea: Its association with iris and anterior chamber dysgenesis. *Trans Am Ophthalmol Soc* 1974;72:516.
122. Gregory CY, Evans K, Bhattacharya SS. Genetic refinement of the chromosome 5q lattice corneal dystrophy type I locus to within a 2 cm interval. *J Med Genet* 1995;32:224–226.
123. Griffith DG, Fine BS. Light and electron microscopic observations in a superficial corneal dystrophy. *Am J Ophthalmol* 1967;63:1659.
124. Grop K. Clinical and histologic findings in crystalline corneal dystrophy. *Acta Ophthalmol (Copenh)* 1973;51(suppl 120):52.
125. Guerry D III. Fingerprint-like lines in the cornea. *Am J Ophthalmol* 1950;33:724.
126. Guerry DUP III. Observations on Cogan's microcystic dystrophy of the corneal epithelium. *Trans Am Ophthalmol Soc* 1965;63:320.
127. Haddad R, Font RL, Fine BS. Unusual superficial variant of granular dystrophy of the cornea. *Am J Ophthalmol* 1977;83:213.
128. Hahn TW, Sah WJ, Kim JH. Phototherapeutic keratectomy in nine eyes with superficial corneal diseases. *Refract Corneal Surg* 1994; 9(2 suppl)115–118.
129. Hall P. Reis-Bücklers dystrophy. *Arch Ophthalmol* 1974;91:170.
130. Haltia M, Levy E, Meretoja J, Madrid IV, Koivunen O, Frangione B. Gelsolin gene mutation-at codon 187-in familial amyloidosis. Finnish: DNA-diagnostic assay. *Am J Med Genet* 1992;42:357–359.
131. Hansen TE. Posterior polymorphous corneal dystrophy. *Acta Ophthalmol (Copenh)* 1983; 61:454.
132. Harboyan G et al. Congenital corneal hereditary dystrophy: Progressive sensorineural deafness in a family. *Arch Ophthalmol* 1971;85:27.
133. Harison RJ, Acheson RR, Dean-Hart JC.

Bietti's tapetoretinal degeneration with marginal corneal dystrophy (crystalline retinopathy): Case report. *Br J Ophthalmol* 1987; 71:220.
134. Hassell JR et al. Defective conversion of a glycoprotein precursor to keratan sulfate proteoglycan in macular corneal dystrophy. In *Extracellular Matrix*, S. Hawkes, J. L. Wang, eds. New York: Academic Press, 1982.
135. Hassell JR, Newsome DA, Krachmer JH, Rodrigues M. Macular corneal dystrophy: Failure to synthesize a mature keratan sulfate proteoglycan. *Proc Natl Acad Sci USA* 1980;77: 3705–3709.
136. Heon E, Mathers WD, Alward WLM, Weisenthal RW, Sunden SLF, Fishbaugh JA, Taylor CM, Krachmer JH, Sheffield VC, Stone EM. Linkage of posterior polymorphous dystrophy to 20q11. *Hum Mol Genet* 1995;4:485–488.
137. Hida T, Proia AD, Kigasawa K, et al. Clinical features of a new recognized type of lattice corneal dystrophy. *Am J Ophthalmol* 1987;104:241.
138. Hida T, Tsubota K, Kigasawa K, et al. Histopathologic and immunochemical features of lattice corneal dystrophy type III. *Am J Ophthalmol* 1987;104:249.
139. Hirst LW, Waring GO III. Clinical specular microscopy of posterior polymorphous endothelial dystrophy. *Am J Ophthalmol* 1983; 95:143.
140. Hogan M, Alvarado S. Ultrastructure of lattice dystrophy of the cornea: A case report. *Am J Ophthalmol* 1967;64:656.
141. Hogan MJ, Bietti G. Hereditary deep dystrophy of the cornea (polymorphous). *Am J Ophthalmol* 1968;65:777.
142. Hogan MJ, Wood I, Ne M. Fuchs' endothelial dystrophy of the cornea. *Am J Ophthalmol* 1974;78:363.
143. Hoizan M, Wood I. Reis-Bücklers corneal dystrophy. *Trans Ophthalmol Soc UK* 1971; 91:41.
144. Holland EJ, Daya SM, Stone EM, Folberg R, Dobler AA, Cameron D, Doughman DJ. Avellino corneal dystrophy: Clinical manifestations and natural history. *Ophthalmology* 1992;99:1564–1568.
145. Irvine AR. The role of the endothelium in bullous keratopathy. *Arch Ophthalmol* 1956;56: 338.
146. Iwamoto T et al. Ultrastructural variations in granular dystrophy of the cornea. *Graefes Arch Clin Exp Ophthalmol* 1975;194:1.
147. Iwamoto T, DeVoe AG. Electron microscopic studies on Fuchs' combined dystrophy. I. Posterior portion of the cornea. *Invest Ophthalmol* 1971;10:9.
148. John ME, Karr Van D, et al. Excimer laser phototherapeutic keratectomy for treatment of recurrent corneal erosion. *J. Cataract Refract Surg* 1994;20:179–180.
149. Johnson AT, Folberg R, Vrabec MP et al. The pathology of posterior amorphous corneal dystrophy. *Ophthalmology* 1990;97:104.
150. Johnson BL, Brown SI, Zaidman GW. A light and electron microscopic study of recurrent granular dystrophy of the cornea. *Am J Ophthalmol* 1981;92:49.
151. Jones ST, Stauffer LH. Reis-Bücklers corneal dystrophy. *Trans Am Acad Ophthalmol Otolaryngol* 1970;74:417.
152. Jones ST, Zimmerman LE. Histopathologic differentiation of granular, macular, and lattice dystrophies of the cornea. *Am J Ophthalmol* 1961;51:394.
153. Judisch GF, Maumenee IH. Clinical differentiation of recessive congenital hereditary endothelial dystrophy and dominant hereditary endothelial dystrophy. *Am J Ophthalmol* 1979;85:606.
154. Julien J. Familial amyloid neuropathies (review) (French). *Rev Neurol (Paris)* 1993; 149(10):517–523.
155. Kanai A, Kaufman HE, Polack FM. Electron microscopic study of Reis-Bücklers dystrophy. *Ann Ophthalmol* 1973;5:953.
156. Kanai A, Kaufman HE. Electron microscopic studies of primary band-shaped keratopathy and gelatinous drop-like corneal dystrophy in two brothers. *Ann Ophthalmol* 1982;14:535.
157. Kanai A. Further electron microscopic study of hereditary corneal edema. *Invest Ophthalmol* 1971;10:545.
158. Kaseras A, Price A. Central crystalline corneal dystrophy. *Br J Ophthalmol* 1970;54:659.
159. Katsev DA et al. Recurrent corneal erosion: Pathology of corneal puncture. *Cornea* 1991;10:418.
160. Kaufman HG and Clowe FW: Irregularities of Bowman's membrane. *Am J Ophthalmol* 1966;62:227.
161. Kenney MC, Labermeier U, Hinds D, Waring GO. Characterization of the Descemet's membrane isolated from Fuchs' endothelial dystrophy corneas. *Exp Eye Res* 1984;39: 267–277.
162. Kenyon KR, Maumenee AE. Further studies of congenital hereditary corneal dystrophy of the cornea. *Am J Ophthalmol* 1973;76:419.

163. Kenyon KR, Maumenee AE. The histological and ultrastructural pathology of congenital hereditary corneal dystrophy: A case report. *Invest Ophthalmol* 1968;7:475.
164. Kenyon KR. Mesenchymal dysgenesis in Peters' anomaly, sclerocornea and congenital endothelial dystrophy. *Exp Eye Res* 1975;21:125.
165. Keynon KR, Antine B. The pathogenesis of congenital hereditary endothelial dystrophy of the cornea. *Am J Ophthalmol* 1971;72:787.
166. King RG Jr, Geeraets R. Cogan-Guerry microcystic corneal epithelial dystrophy. *Med Coll Va Q* 1972;8:241.
167. Kirk HQ et al. Primary familial amyloidosis of the cornea. *Trans Am Acad Ophthalmol Otolaryngol* 1973;77:411.
168. Kirkness CM et al. Congenital hereditary corneal oedema of Maumenee: Its clinical features, management, and pathology. *Br J Ophthalmol* 1987;71:130.
169. Kiskaddon BM et al. Fleck dystrophy of the cornea: Case report. *Ann Ophthalmol* 1980; 12:700.
170. Kivela T, Tarkkanen A, McLean I, Ghiso J, Frangione B, Haltia M. Immunohistochemical analysis of lattice corneal dystrophies types I and II. *Br J Ophthalmol* 1993;77:799–804.
171. Klein M, Green WR. *Cit. Spencer Ophthalmic Pathology II: 1168.* Philadelphia: Saunders, 1984.
172. Klintworth GK et al. Recurrence of macular corneal dystrophy within grafts. *Am J Ophthalmol* 1983;95:60.
173. Klintworth GK, Meyer R, Dennis R, et al. Macular corneal dystrophy—Lack of keratan sulfate in serum and cornea. *Ophthalmic Paediatr Genet* 1986;7:139–143.
174. Klintworth GK, Smith CF. Abnormalities of proteoglycans and glycoproteins synthesized by corneal organ cultures derived from patients with macular corneal dystrophy. *Lab Invest* 1983;48:603.
175. Klintworth GK, Smith CF. Macular corneal dystrophy: Studies of sulfated glycosaminoglycans in corneal explant and confluent stromal cell cultures. *Am J Pathol* 1977;89:167.
176. Klintworth GK, Vogel FS. Macular corneal dystrophy: An inherited acid mucopolysaccharide storage disease of corneal fibroblasts. *Am J Pathol* 1964;45:565.
177. Klintworth GK. Lattice corneal dystrophy: An inherited variety of amyloidosis restricted to the cornea. *Am J Pathol* 1967;50:371.
178. Klintworth GK. Current concepts on the ultrastructural pathogenesis of macular and lattice corneal dystrophies. *Birth Defects Orig Art Ser* 1971;7:27.
179. Kompf J, Ritter H, Lisch W, Eidle EG, Bauer MP. Linkage analysis in granular corneal dystrophy (Groenouw I), Schnyder's crystalline corneal dystrophy, and Reis-Bücklers corneal dystrophy. *Graefes Arch Clin Exp Ophthalmol* 1989;227(6):538–540.
180. Krachmer JH et al. Inheritance of endothelial dystrophy of the cornea. *Ophthalmologica* 1980;181:301.
181. Krachmer JH, Purcell JJ, Young CW, Bucher KD. Corneal endothelial dystrophy. A study of 64 families. *Arch Ophthalmol* 1978;96: 2036–2039.
182. Krachmer JH, Schnitzer JI, Fratkin J. Cornea pseudoguttata: A clinical and histopathologic description of endothelial cell edema. *Arch Ophthalmol* 1981;99:1377.
183. Krachmer JH. Posterior polymorphous corneal dystrophy: a disease characterized by epithelial-like endothelial cells which influence management and prognosis. *Trans Am Ophthalmol Soc* 1985;83:413.
184. Kurome H, Noda S, Hayasaka S, Setogawa T. A Japanese family with Grayson-Wilbrandt variant of Reis-Bücklers corneal dystrophy. *Jpn J Ophthalmol* 1993;37:143–147.
185. Kuwabara R, Ciccarelli EC. Meesman's corneal dystrophy. *Arch Ophthalmol* 1964;71: 676.
186. Kuwabara Y, Akiya S, Obazawa H. Electron microscopic study of granular dystrophy, macular dystrophy, and gelatinous droplike dystrophy of the cornea. *Folia Ophthalmol Jpn* 1967;18:463.
187. Laganowski HC, Sherrard ES, Kerr Muir MG. The posterior corneal surface in posterior polymorphous dystrophy: A specular microscopical study. *Cornea* 1991;10:224–232.
188. Laibson PR, Krachmer JH. Familial occurrence of dot, map, and fingerprint dystrophy of the cornea. *Invest Ophthalmol* 1975;14: 397.
189. Lawless MA, Cohen PR, Rogers CM. Retreatment of undercorrected photorefractive keratectomy for myopia. *J Refract Corneal Surg* 1994;10(2 suppl):174–177.
190. Lee WH, Bookstein R, Hong F, Young LJ, Shew JY, Lee EY. Human retinoblastoma susceptibility gene: Cloning, identification, and sequence. *Science* 1987;235:1394–1399.
191. Levenson JE, Chandler JW, Kaufman HE. Affected asymptomatic relatives in congenital

hereditary endothelial dystrophy. *Am J Ophthalmol* 1973;76:967–971.

192. Lewkojewa EF. Uber einen Fall primärer Degenerationamyloidose der Kornea. *Klin Monatsbl Augenheilkd* 1930;85:117.
193. Linstrom RL, Harris WS, Doughman DJ. Combined penetrating keratoplasty, extracapsular cataract extraction, and posterior chamber intraocular lens implantation. *Am Intraocular Implant Soc J* 1981;7:130.
194. Lisch W et al. Schnyder's dystrophy: Progression and metabolism. *Ophthalmic Paediatr Genet* 1986;7:45.
195. Livni N, Abraham FA, Zauberman H. Groenouw's macular dystrophy: Histochemistry and ultrastructure of the cornea. *Doc Ophthalmol* 1974;37:327.
196. Lohse E, Stock EL, Jones JC et al: Reis-Bücklers corneal dystrophy: Immunofluorescent and electron microscope studies. *Cornea* 1989;8:200.
197. Lorenzetti DW et al. Central cornea guttata: incidence in the general population. *Am J Ophthalmol* 1967;64:1155.
198. Lubsen NH, Renwick JH, Tsui LC, Breitman ML, Schoenmakers JGG. A locus for a human hereditary cataract is closely linked to the y-crystallin gene family. *Proc Natl Acad Sci USA* 1987;84:489–492.
199. Luxenburg M. Hereditary crystalline dystrophy of the cornea. *Am J Ophthalmol* 1967;63:507.
200. Lyons CJ, McCartney AC, Kirkness CM, et al. Granular corneal dystrophy: Visual results and pattern of recurrence after lamellar or penetrating keratoplasty. *Ophthalmology* 1994;101:1812–1817.
201. Maeder G, Danis P. Surune nouvelle forme de dystrophie corneene (dystrophia filiformis profunda corneae) associe a un keratocone. *Ophthalmologica* 1947;114:246.
202. Magovern M et al. Inheritance of Fuchs' combined dystrophy. *Ophthalmology* 1979;86:1897.
203. Malbran ES, Meijide RF, Croxatto JO. Atypical corneal dystrophy with stromal amyloid deposits. *Cornea* 1988;7:210–213.
204. Mannis MJ et al. Polymorphic amyloid degeneration of the cornea. *Arch Ophthalmol* 1981;99:1217.
205. Mashima Y et al. Specular microscopy of posterior polymorphous endothelial dystrophy. *Ophthalmic Pediatr Genet* 1986;7:101.
206. Matsui M, Ito K, Akiua S. Histochemical and electron microscopic examinations on so-called gelatinous drop-like dystrophy of the cornea. *Folia Ophthalmol Jpn* 1972;23:466.
207. Matsuo N, Fujiwara H, Ofuchi Y. Electron and light microscopic observations in a case of Groenouw's corneal dystrophy and gelatinous droplike dystrophy of the cornea. *Folia Ophthalmol Jpn* 1967;18:436.
208. Mauldin WM, O'Connor PS. Crystalline retinopathy: Bietti's tapetoretinal degeneration without marginal corneal dystrophy. *Am J Ophthalmol* 1980;92:640–646.
209. Maumenee AE. Congenital hereditary corneal dystrophy. *Am J Ophthalmol* 1960;50:1114.
210. Maury CP, Teppo AM, Karinemi AL, Koeppen AH. Amyloid fibril protein in familial amyloidosis with cranial neuropathy and corneal lattice dystrophy (FAP type IV) is related to transthyretrin. *Am J Clin Pathol* 1988;89:359–364.
211. McCarthy M, Innis S, Dubord P, White V. Panstromal Schnyder corneal dystrophy. *Ophthalmology* 1994;101:895–901.
212. McCartney ACE, Kirkness CM. Comparison between posterior polymorphous dystrophy and congenital hereditary endothelial dystrophy of the cornea. *Eye* 1988;2:63–70.
213. McCartney MD, Robertson DP, Wood TO et al. ATPase pump site density in human dysfunctional corneal endothelium. *Invest Ophthalmol Vis Sci* 1987;28:1955–1962.
214. McCartney MD, Wood TO, McLaughlin BJ. Freeze-fracture label of functional and dysfunctional human corneal endothelium. *Curr Eye Res* 1987;6:589–597.
215. McCartney MD, Wood TO, McLaughlin BJ. Immunohistochemical localization of ATPase in human dysfunctional corneal endothelium. *Curr Eye Res* 1987;6:1479–1486.
216. McCartney MD, Wood TO, McLaughlin BJ. Moderate Fuchs' endothelial dystrophy ATPase pump site density. *Invest Ophthalmol Vis Sci* 1989;30:1560–1564.
217. McDonnell PJ, Seiler T. Phototherapeutic keratectomy with excimer laser for Reis-Bückler's corneal dystrophy. *Refract Corneal Surg* 1992;8:306–310.
218. McTigue JW, Fine BS. The stromal lesion in lattice dystrophy of the cornea. A light and electron microscopic study. *Invest Ophthalmology* 1964;3:355.
219. Meesman A, Wilke F. Klinische und Anatomische Untersuchungen Ueber eine Bisher Unbekannte, Dominant Vererbte Epitheldys-

trophie der Hornhaut. *Klin Monatsbl Augenheilkd* 1939;103:361.

220. Meesman A. Ueber eine Bisher Nicht Beschriebene Dominant Vererbte Dystrophia alis Corneae. *Ber Dtsch Ophthalmol Ges* 1938; 52:154.
221. Mehta RF. Unilateral lattice dystrophy of the cornea. *Br J Ophthalmol* 1980;64:53.
222. Meisler DM, Fine M. Recurrence of the clinical signs of lattice corneal dystrophy (type 1) in corneal transplants. *Am J Ophthalmol* 1984;97:210.
223. Meretoja J. Comparative histopathological and clinical findings in eyes with lattice corneal dystrophy of two types. *Ophthalmolgica* 1972;165:15.
224. Meretoja J. Familial systemic paraamyloidosis with lattice dystrophy of the cornea, progressive crania neuropathy, skin changes and various internal symptoms: A previously unrecognized heritable syndrome. *Ann Clin Res* 1969;1:314.
225. Meretoja J. Genetic aspects of familial amyloidosis with corneal lattice dystrophy and cranial neuropathy. *Clin Genet* 1973;4:173.
226. Miller CA, Krachmer JH. Endothelial dystrophies. In *The Cornea,* H. E. Kaufman et al., eds. New York: Churchill Linvingstone, 1988.
227. Mirshahi M, Mirshahi SS, Soria C, Lorans G, Soria J, Bureau J, Thomaidis A, Pouliquen Y. Secretion of plasminogen activators and their inhibitors in corneal fibroblasts. Modification of this secretion in Schnyder's lens corneal dystrophy. *CR Acad Sci III* 1990;311: 253–260.
228. Moller HU, Ehlers N. Early treatment of granular dystrophy (Groenouw type 1), *Acta Ophthalmol (Copenh)* 1985;63:597.
229. Moller HU, Ridgway AEA. Granular corneal dystrophy Groenouw type 1: A report of a probable homozygous patient. *Acta Ophthalmol (Copenh)* 1990;68:97–101.
230. Moller HU, Ehlers N, Bojsen-Moller M, Ridgway AE. Differential diagnosis between granular corneal dystrophy Groenouw type I and paraproteinemiccrystallinekeratopathy. *Acta Ophthalmol (Copenh)* 1993;71(4):552–555.
231. Moller HU, Bojsen-Moller M, Schroder HD, Nelson ME, Vegge T. Immunoglobulins in granular corneal dystrophy Groenouw type 1. *Acta Ophthalmol (Copenh)* 1993;71:548–551.
232. Moller HU. Interfamilial variability and intrafamilial similarities of granular corneal dystrophy Graenouw type I with respect to biomicroscopical appearance and symptomatology. *Acta Ophthalmol (Copenh)* 1989;67:669.
233. Moller HU. Granular corneal dystrophy Groenouw type 1 (GrC) and Reis-Bücklers corneal dystrophy (R-B): One entity? *Acta Ophthalmol (Copenh)* 1989;67:678–684.
234. Mondino BJ, Rabb MF, Sugar J, et al. Primary familial amyloidosis of the cornea. *Am J Ophthalmol* 1981;92:732.
235. Mondino BJ, Raj CVS, Skinner M et al. Protein AA and lattice corneal dystrophy. *Am J Ophthalmol* 1980;89:377.
236. Morgan G. Macular dystrophy of the cornea. *Br J Ophthalmol* 1966;50:57.
237. Mortelmans L. Forme familiale de la dystrophie corneene de Fuchs. *Ophthalmologica* 1952;123:88.
238. Moshegow CN, How WK, Wiffen SJ, Daya SM. Posterior amorphous corneal dystrophy. *Ophthalmology* 1996;103(3):474–478.

238a. Munier FL, Korvatska E, Djemai A, et al. Kerato-epithelin mutations in four 5q31-linked corneal dystrophies. *Nat Genet* 1997;15:247–251.

239. Nagataki S, Tanishima T, Sakomoto T. A case of primary gelatinous drop-like corneal dystrophy. *Jpn J Ophthalmol* 1972;16:107.
240. Nakaizumi K. A rare case of corneal dystrophy. *Nippon Ganka Gakkai Zasshi* 1914;18: 949.
241. Nakaniski I, Brown SI. Ultrastructure of epithelial dystrophy of Meesmann. *Arch Ophthalmol* 1975;93:259.
242. Nakazawa K, Hassell JR, Hascall VC, Lohmander S, Newsome DA, Krachmer J. Defective processing of keratan sulfate in macular corneal dystrophy. *J Biol Chem* 1984;259: 13751–13757.
243. Nathans J, Piantanida TP, Eddy RL, Shows TB, Hogness DS. Molecular genetics of inherited variation in human colour vision. *Science* 1986;232:203–210.
244. Nathans J, Thomas D, Hogness DS. Molecular genetics of human colour vision: The genes encoding blue, green, and red pigments. *Science* 1986;232:193–202.
245. Nicholson DH, Green WR, Cross HE. A clinical and histopathological study of François-Neetens speckled corneal dystrophy. *Am J Ophthalmol* 1977;83:554.
246. Niesen U, Thomann U, Schipper I. Phototherapeutic keratectomy (German). *Klin Monatsbl Augenheilkd* 1994;205(4):187–195.
247. Nirankari VS et al. An unusual case of epithe-

lial basement membrane dystrophy. *Am J Ophthalmol* 1989;107:552.

248. Ohman L, Fagerholm P, Tengroth B. Treatment of recurrent corneal erosions with the excimer laser. *Acta Ophthalmol (Copenh)* 1994;72:461–463.
249. Olsen T. Is there an association between Fuchs' endothelial dystrophy and cardiovascular disease? *Graefes Arch Clin Exp Ophthalmol* 1984;221:239–240.
250. Olson RJ, Kaufman HE. Recurrence of Reis-Bücklers corneal dystrophy in a graft. *Am J Ophthalmol* 1978;85:349.
251. Olson T, Ehlers N, Favini E. Long-term results of corneal grafting in Fuchs' endothelial dystrophy. *Acta Ophthalmol (Copenh)* 1984; 62:445.
252. Orlin SE, Raber IM, Eagle RC, Scheie HG. Keratoconus associated with corneal endothelial dystrophy. *Cornea* 1990;9:299–304.
253. Orndahl M, Fagerholm P, Fitzsimmons T, Tengroth B. Treatment of corneal dystrophies with excimer laser. *Acta Ophthalmol (Copenh)* 1994;72:235–240.
254. Pameijer JK. Ueber eine Fremdartige Familiere OberflEchliche HornhautverEnderung. *Klin Monatsbl Augenheilkd* 1935;95:516.
255. Patten JT et al. Fleck (Mouchetée) dystrophy of the cornea. *Ann Ophthalmol* 1976;8:25.
256. Paufique L, Bonnet M. La dystrophie cornéenne hérédito-familiale de Reis-Bücklers. *Ann Oculist* 1966;199:14.
257. Pearce WG, Tripathi RC, Morgan G. Congenital endothelial corneal dystrophy: Clinical, pathological and genetic study. *Br J Ophthalmol* 1969;53:477.
258. Pe'er J et al. Corneal elastosis within lattice dystrophy lesions: *Br J Ophthalmol* 1988; 72:183.
259. Perry HD, Fine BS, Caldwell CR. Reis-Bücklers' dystrophy. *Arch Ophthalmol* 1979;97: 664.
260. Petroutsos G, Kitsos G, Asproudis I, Melissamgos I, Psilas K. Association of progressive external ophthalmolplegia and lattice corneal dystrophy. *J Fr Ophtalmol* 1992;15(11): 592–595.
261. Pietruschka G. Ueber eine Familiare Endotheldystrophie der Hornhaut (in Kombination met Glaukom, Vitilgo, und Otoskklerose). *Klin Monatsbl Augenheilkd* 1960;136:794.
262. Pillat A. Zur frage der familiuaren Hornhautentartung: Unber eine einzigartige tiefe scholige und periphere gitterformige familire Hornhautdystrophie. *Klink Monatsbl Augenheilkd* 1939;104:571.
263. Pitts JF, Jay JL. The association of Fuchs's corneal endothelial dystrophy with axial hypermetropia, shallow anterior chamber, and angle closure glaucoma. *Br J Ophthalmol* 1990;74: 601–604.
264. Poirier C, Coulan P, Williamson W, Mortemousque B, Verin P. Results of therapeutic photokeratectomy using the Excimer laser. Apropos of 12 cases (review) (French). *J Fr Ophtalmol* 1994;17(4):262–270.
265. Polack FM et al. Scanning electron microscopy of posterior polymorphous corneal dystrophy. *Am J Ophthalmol* 1980;89:575.
266. Pouliquen Y et al. Itude en microscope Jlectronique d'une dystrophie grillagJe de Haab-Dimmer. *Arch Ophtalmol* (Paris) 1973; 33:485.
267. Pratt AW, Saheb ME, Leblanc R. Posterior polymorphous corneal dystrophy in juvenile glaucoma. *Can J Ophthalmol* 1976;11:180.
268. Presberg SE et al. Posterior polymorphous corneal dystrophy. *Cornea* 1985;4:239.
269. Purcell JJ Jr, Krachmer JH, Weingeist TA. Fleck corneal dystrophy. *Arch Ophthalmol* 1977;95:440.
270. Quantock AJ, Meek KM, Ridgway AEA, Bron AJ, Thonar EJMA. Macular corneal dystrophy: Reduction in both corneal thickness and collagen interfibrillar spacing. *Curr Eye Res* 1990;9:393–398.
271. Quantock AJ, Meek KM, Thonar EJMA, Assil KK. Synchrotron X-ray diffreaction in atypical macular dystrophy. *Eye* 1993;7:779–784.
272. Raab MF, Blodi F, Boniuk M. Unilateral lattice dystrophy of the cornea. *Trans Am Acad Ophthalmol Otolaryngol* 1974;78:440.
273. Ramsey MS, Fine BS. Localized corneal amyloidosis. *Am J Ophthalmol* 1972;75:560.
274. Ramsey RM. Familial corneal dystrophy lattice type. *Trans Am Ophthalmol Soc* 1957; 60:701.
275. Rannie I. Observations on the oxytalan fibre of the periodontal membrane. *Trans Eur Orthodont Soc.* 1963;39:127–136.
276. Rapuano CJ, Laibson PR. Excimer laser phototherapeutic keratectomy. *CLAO J* 1993;19: 235–240.
277. Rapuano CJ, Laibson PR. Excimer laser phototherapeutic keratectomy for anterior corneal pathology. *CLAO J* 1994;20:253–257.
278. Reis W. Familidre, Fleckige Homhautentartung. *Dtsch Med Wochenschr* 1917;43:575.
279. Reiss GR, Bourne WM. Fuchs' dystrophy and serum fibrinogen degradation products. *Am J Ophthalmol* 1985;100:615–616.
280. Reschmi CS, English FP. Unilateral lattice

dystrophy of the cornea: *Med J Aust* 1971; 1:966.

281. Rice NSC et al. Reis-Bücklers dystrophy, *Br J Ophthalmol* 1968;52:577.
282. Richards BW, Brodstein DE, Nussbaum JJ et al. Autosomal dominant crystalline dystrophy. *Ophthalmology* 1991;98:658–665.
283. Richardson WP, Hettinger ME. Endothelial and epithelial-like cell formations in a case of posterior polymorphous dystrophy. *Arch Ophthalmol* 1985;103:1520.
284. Roberts CW et al. Endothelial guttata and facility of aqueous outflow. *Cornea* 1984;3:5.
285. Robin AL et al. Recurrence of macular corneal dystrophy after lamellar keratoplasty. *Am J Ophthalmol* 1977;84:457.
286. Robinson MR, Streeten BW. Energy dispersive x-ray analysis of the cornea. Application to paraffin sections of normal and diseased corneas. *Arch Ophthalmol* 1984;102:1678–1682.
287. Rodrigues MM, Robey PG. C-reactive protein in human lattice corneal dystrophy. *Curr Eye Res* 1983;2:721.
288. Rodrigues MM et al. Posterior polymorphous dystrophy of the cornea: Cell culture studies. *Exp Eye Res* 1981;33:535.
289. Rodrigues MM et al. Microfibrillar protein and phospholipid in granular corneal dystrophy. *Arch Ophthalmol* 1983;101:802.
290. Rodrigues MM et al. Unesterified cholesterol in Schnyder's corneal crystalline dystrophy. *Am J Ophthalmol* 1987;104:147.
291. Rodrigues MM, Gaster RN, Pratt MV. Unusual superficial confluent form of granular corneal dystrophy. *Ophthalmology* 1983;90:1507.
292. Rodrigues MM, Kruth HS, Krachmer JH et al. Cholesterol localization in ultrathin frozen sections in Schnyder's corneal crystalline dystrophy. *Am J Ophthalmol* 1990;110:513–517.
293. Rodrigues MM, Rajgopalan S, Jones K, Nirankari V, Wisnewski J, Frangione B, Gorevic PD. Gelsolin immunoreactivity in corneal amyloid, wound healing and macular and granular dystrophies. *Am J Ophthalmol* 1993;115(5):644–652.
294. Rodrigues MM, Waring GO, Laibson PR, Weinreb S. Endothelial alterations in congenital corneal dystrophy. *Am J Ophthalmol* 1975;80:678.
295. Rodriques MM et al. Glaucoma due to endothelialization of the anterior chamber angle: A comparison of posterior polymorphous dystrophy of the cornea and Chandler's syndrome. *Arch Ophthalmol* 1980;98:832.
296. Rogers C, Cohen P, Lawless M. Phototherapeutic keratectomy for Reis-Bücklers corneal dystrophy. *Aust NZ J Ophthalmol* 1993;21:247–250.
297. Rosenblum P et al. Hereditary Fuchs' dystrophy. *Am J Ophthalmol* 1980;90:455.
298. Rosenwasser GOD, Sucheski BM, Rosa N, Pastena B, Sebastiani A, Sassani JW, Perry HD. Phenotypic variation in combined granular-lattice (Avellino) corneal dystrophy. *Arch Ophthalmol* 1993;111:1546–1552.
299. Ross JR, Foulks GN, Sanfilippo FP, Howell DN. Immunohistochemical analysis of the pathogenesis of posterior polymorphous dystrophy. *Arch Ophthalmol* 1995;113:340–345.
300. Rubenstein RA, Silverman JJ. Hereditary deep dystrophy of the cornea associated with glaucoma and ruptures in Descemet's membrane. *Arch Ophthalmol* 1968;79:123.
301. Roth SI, Mittelman D, Stock EL. Posterior amorphous corneal dystrophy. An ultrastructural study of a variant with histopathological features of an endothelial dystrophy. *Cornea* 1992;11:165–172.
302. Sajjadi SH, Javadi MA. Superficial juvenile granular dystrophy. *Ophthalmology* 1992; 99(1):95–102.
303. Sakuma A, Yokoyama T, Katou K, Kanai A. Lamellar kertoplasty combined with keratoepithelioplasty in four cases for recurrent gelatinous drop-like corneal dystrophy [in Japanese]. *Rinsho Ganka* 1991;45:527–530.
304. Sanderson PO, Kuwabara T, Stark WJ, Wong VG, Collins EM. Cystinosis. A clinical, histopathologic, and ultrastructural study. *Arch Ophthalmol* 1974;91:270–277.
305. Santo RM, Yamaguchi T, Kanai A, Okisaka S, Nakajima A. Clinical and histopathologic features of corneal dystrophies in Japan. *Ophthalmology* 1995;102:557–567.
306. Sasaki Y, Tuberville AW, Wood TO, McLaughlin BJ. Freeze fracture study of human corneal endothelial dysfunction. *Invest Ophthalmol Vis Sci* 1986;27:480–485.
307. Sassani J, Smith SG, Rabinowitz YS. Keratoconus and bilateral lattice-granular corneal dystrophies. *Cornea* 1992;11:343–350.
308. Schutz S. Hereditary corneal dystrophy. *Arch Ophthalmol* 1943;29:523.
309. Seitz B, Weidle E, Naumann GO. Unilateral typa III (Hida) lattice stromal corneal dystrophy (German). *Klin Monatsbl Augenheilkd* 1993;203(4):279–285.
310. Sekundo W, Lee WR, Aitken DA, Kirkness CM. Multirecurrence of corneal posterior

polymorphous dystrophy. An ultrastructural study. *Cornea* 1994;13:509–515.

311. Sekundo W, Lee WR, Kirkness CM, Aitken DA, Fleck B. An ultrastructural investigation of an early manifestation of the posterior polymorphous dystrophy of the cornea. *Ophthalmology* 1994;101:1422–1431.
312. Sekundo W, Marshall GE, Lee WR, Kirkness CM. Immuno-electron labelling of matrix components in congenital hereditary endothelial dystrophy. *Graefe's Arch Clin Exp Ophthalmol* 1994;232:337–346.
313. Sever RJ, Frost P, Weinstein G. Eye changes in icthyosis. *JAMA* 1968;206:2283.
314. Sher NA, Bowers RA, Zabel RW, Frantz JM et al. Clinical use of the 193-nm excimer laser in the treatment of corneal scars. *Arch Ophthalmol* 1991;109:491–499.
315. Small KW, Mullen L, Barletta J, Graham K, Glasgow B, Stern G, Yee R. Mapping of Reis-Bücklers corneal dystrophy to chromosome 5q. *Am J Ophthalmol* 1996;121:384–390.
316. Snell AC Jr, Irwin ES. Hereditary deep dystrophy of the cornea. *Am J Ophthalmol* 1958;45:636.
317. Snip RC, Kenyon DR, Green RD. Macular corneal dystrophy: ultrastructural pathology of the corneal endothelium and Descemet's membrane. *Invest Ophthalmol* 1973;12:88.
318. Snyder WB. Hereditary epithelial corneal dystrophy. *Am J Ophthalmol* 1963;55:56.
319. Somson E. Granular dystrophy of the cornea: an electron microscopic study. *Am J Ophthalmol* 1965;59:1001.
320. Stainer GA et al. Correlative microscopy and tissue culture of congenital hereditary endothelial dystrophy. *Am J Ophthalmol* 1982; 93:456.
321. Stankovic I, Stojanovic D. L'hérédodystrohie Mouchetée du parenchyme cornée. *Ann Oculist (Paris)* 1964;197:52.
322. Stock EI, Kielar RA. Primary familial amyloidosis of the cornea. *Am J Ophthalmol* 1976;82:266.
323. Stock EL, Feder RS, O'Grady RB, Sugar J, Roth SI. Lattice corneal dystrophy type 111A: Clinical and histopathologic correlations. *Arch Ophthalmol* 1991;109:354–358.
324. Stocker FW, Holt LB. Rare form of hereditary epithelial dystrophy. *Arch Ophthalmol* 1955;53:536.
324. Stocker FW, Holt LB. Rare form of hereditary epithelial dystrophy. *Arch Ophthalmol* 1955;53:536.
325. Stocker FW, Irish A. Fate of successful corneal graft in Fuchs' endothelial dystrophy. *Am J Ophthalmol* 1969;68:820.
326. Stone EM, Mathers WD, Rosenwasser GOD, Holland EJ, Folberg R, Krachmer JH, Nichols BE, Gorevic PD, Taylor CM, Streb LM, et al. Three autosomal dominant corneal dystrophies map to chromosome 5q. *Nature Genet* 1994;6:47–51.
327. Strachan IM. Central cloudy corneal dystrophy of François: Five cases in the same family. *Br J Ophthalmol* 1969;53:192.
328. Strachan IM. Pre-Descemetic corneal dystrophy. *Br J Ophthalmol* 1968;52:716.
329. Streeten BW, Falls HF. Hereditary fleck dystrophy of the cornea. *Am J Ophthalmol* 1961;51:275.
330. Stuart JC, Mund ML. Recurrent granular corneal dystrophy. *Am J Ophthalmol* 1975; 79:18.
331. Stulting RD et al. Penetrating keratoplasty in children. *Ophthalmology* 1984;91:1222.
332. Sundar-Raj N et al. Macular corneal dystrophy: Immunohistochemical characterization using monoclonal antibodies. *Invest Ophthalmol Vis Sci* 1987;28:1678.
333. Sysi R. Xanthoma corneae as hereditary dystrophy. *Br J Ophthalmol* 1950;34:369–374.
334. Teng CC.Macular dystrophy of the cornea: A histochemical and electron microscopic study. *Am J Ophthalmol* 1966;62:436.
335. Thiel HJ, Behnke H. Eine Bisher Unbekannte Subepitheliale Hereditaire Hornhautdystrophie. *Klin Monatsbl Augenheilkd* 1967;150: 862.
336. Thomsitt J, Bron AJ. Polymorphic stromal dystrophy. *Br J Ophthalmol* 1975;59:125.
337. Thonar EJ et al. Absence of normal keratan sulfate in the blood of patients with macular corneal dystrophy. *Am J Ophthalmol* 1986; 102:561.
338. Toma NMG, Ebenezer ND, Inglehearn CF, Plant C, Ficker LA, Bhattacharya SS. Linkage of congenital hereditary endothelial dystrophy to chromosome 20. *Hum Mol Genet* 1995;4: 2395–2398.
339. Tremblay M, Dube I. Meesman's corneal dystrophy: Ultrastructural features. *Can J Ophthalmol* 1982;17:24.
340. Trinkaus-Randall V, Tong M, Thomas P, Cornell-Bell A. Confocal imaging of the 64 subunits in the human cornea with aging. *Invest Ophthalmol Vis Sci* 1993;34:3103–3105.
341. Tripathi R, Garner A. Corneal granular dystrophy: A light and electron microscope study

of its recurrence in a graft. *Br J Ophthalmol* 1970;54:361.

342. Tripathi RC, Casey TA, Wise EG. Hereditary posterior polymorphous dystrophy: An ultrastructural and clinical report. *Trans Ophthalmol Soc UK* 1974;94:211.
343. Trobe JD, Laibson PR. Dystrophic changes in the anterior cornea. *Arch Ophthalmol* 1972;87:378.
344. Tsunoda I, Awano H, Kayama H, Tsukamoto T, Veno S, Fujiwara T, Watanabe M, Yamamoto T. Idiopathic AA amyloidosis manifested in autonomic neuropathy, vestibulocochleopathy and lattice corneal dystrophy. *J Neurol Neurosurg Psychiatry* 1994;57(5):635–637.
345. Tuberville AW, Wood TO, McLaughlin BJ. Cytochrome oxidase activity of Fuchs' endothelial dystrophy. *Curr Eye Res* 1986;5:939–947.
346. Van Went JM, Wibaut F. Een Zeldzane erfelijke hoornvliesaandoening. *Ned Tijdschr Geenskd* 1924;68:2996.
347. Waardenburg PJ, Jonkers GH. A specific type of dominant progressive dystrophy of the cornea, developing after birth. *Acta Ophthalmol Copenh*) 1961;39:919.
348. Waring GO III, Rodrigues MM, Laibson PR. Corneal dystrophies. I. Dystrophies of the epithelium, Bowman's layer and stroma. *Surv Ophthalmol* 1978;23:71–122.
349. Waring GO, Bourne WM, Edelhauser HF, Kenyon KR. The corneal endothelium. Normal and pathologic structure and function. *Ophthalmology* 1982;89:531.
350. Waring GO, Laibson PR. Keratoplasty in infants and children. *Trans Am Acad Ophthalmol Otolaryngol* 1977;83:283.
351. Waring GO, Rodrigues MM, Laibson PR. Corneal dystrophies. II. Endothelial dystrophies. *Surv Ophthalmol* 1978;23:147–168.
352. Waring GO. Posterior collagenous layer (PCL) of the cornea. *Arch Ophthalmol* 1982;100:122.
353. Waring GO. Ultrastructural classification of abnormal collagen tissue on the posterior cornea (posterior collagen layer). *Invest Ophthalmol Vis Sci* 1979;18(suppl):124.
354. Weber FL, Babel J. Gelatinous drop-like dystrophy. *Arch Ophthalmol* 1980;98:144.
355. Weber U, Owzarek J, Kluxen G, Bernsheimer H. Klinischer Verlauf bei Biettischer kristalliner tapetoretinaler Degeneration. *Klin Monatsbl Augenheilkd* 1983;259–261.
356. Weidle EG. Differentialdiagnose der Hornhautdystrophien vom Typ Groenouw 1, Reis-Bücklers and Thiel Behnke. *Fortscr Ophthalmol* 1989;86(4):265–271.
357. Weidle EG. Klinische and feingewebliche Abgrenzung der Reis-Bucklersschen Hornhautdystrophie. *Klin Monatsbl Augenheilk* 1989; 194(4):217–226.
358. Weiss JS. Schnyder crystalline dystrophy sine crystals. *Ophthalmology* 1996;103(3):465–473.
359. Weissman BA, Ehrlich M, Levenson JE, Pettit TH. Four cases of keratoconus and posterior polymorphous corneal dystrophy. *Optom Vis Sci* 1989;66:243–246.
360. Welch RB. Bietti's tapetoretinal degeneration with marginal corneal dystrophy: Crystalline retinopathy. *Trans Am Ophthalmol Soc* 1977;75:164–179.
361. Weller RO, Rodger FC. Crystalline stromal dystrophy: Histochemistry and ultrastructure of the cornea. *Br J Ophthalmol* 1986;64:46–52.
362. Werblin TP, Hirst LW, Stark WJ, Maumenee IH. Prevalence of map-dot-fingerprint change in the cornea. *Br J Ophthalmol* 1980;65:401.
363. Wheeler GE, Eiferman RA. Immunohistochemical identifications of the AA protein in lattice dystrophy. *Exp Eye Res* 1983;36:181.
364. Williams HP, Bron AJ, Tripathi RC, Garner A. Hereditary crystalline corneal dystrophy with an associated blood lipid disorder. *Trans Ophthalmol Soc UK* 1971;91:31–41.
365. Wilson DJ, Weleber RG, Klein ML, et al. Bietti's crystalline dystrophy: A clinicopathologic correlative study. *Arch Ophthalmol* 1989;107:213–221.
366. Wilson SE, Bourne WM, O'Brien PC et al. Endothelial function and aqueous humor flow rate in patients with Fuchs' dystrophy. *Am J Ophthalmol* 1988;106:270–278.
367. Wilson SE, Bourne WM. Fuchs' dystrophy. *cornea* 1988;7:2–18.
368. Wilson SE, Bourne WM. Effect of dexamethasone on corneal endothelial function in Fuchs' dystrophy. *Invest Ophthalmol Vis Sci* 1987;28(suppl):326.
369. Witschel H, Sundmacher R. Bilateral recurrence of granular dystrophy in the grafts. *Graefes Arch Clin Exp Ophthalmol* 1979; 209:179.
370. Wittebol-Post D, Van Schooneveld MJ, Pel V. The corneal dystrophy of Waardenburg and Jonkers. *Ophthalmic Paediatr Genet* 1989; 10(4):249–255.
371. Wittebol-Post D, van der Want JJ, van Bijster-

veld OP. Granular dystrophy of the cornea (Groenouw type 1): Is the keratocyte the primary source after all? *Ophthalmologica* 1987;195:169.

372. Wittehol-Post D, van Bijsterveld OP, Delleman JM. The honeycomb type of Reis-Bücklers dystrophy of the cornea: Biometrics and interpretation. *Ophthalmologica* 1987; 194:65.
373. Wolter JR, Fralick FB. Microcystic dystrophy of the corneal epithelium. *Arch Ophthalmol* 1966;75:380.
374. Wolter JR, Larson BF. Pathology of cornea guttata. *Am J Ophthalmol* 1959;48:161.
375. Wolter JR. Secondary cornea guttata in interstitial keratopathy. *Ophthalmologica* 1964; 148:289.
376. Wood TO et al. Treatment of Reis-Bücklers corneal dystrophy by removal of subepithelial fibrous tissue. *Am J Ophthalmol* 1978;85:360.
377. Yamaguchi T, Polack F, Valenti J: Reis-Bücklers corneal dystrophy. *Am J Ophthalmol* 1980;90:95.
378. Yamaguchi T, Polack FM, Rowsey JJ. Honeycombshaped corneal dystrophy: A variation of Reis-Bücklers dystrophy, *Cornea* 1982;I:71.
379. Yang CJ, SundarRaj N, Thonar EJ-MA, Klintworth GK. Immunohistochemical evidence of heterogeneity in macular corneal dystrophy. *Am J Ophthalmol* 1988;106:65–71.
380. Yanoff M et al. Lattice corneal dystrophy. *Arch Ophthalmol* 1977;95:651.
381. Yassa NH, Font RL, Fine BS, Koffler BH. Corneal immunoglobulin deposition in the posterior stroma. A case report including immunohistochemical and ultrastructural observations. *Arch Ophthalmol* 1987;105:99–103.
382. Zechner EM, Croxatto JO, Mabran ES. Superficial involvement in lattice corneal dystrophy. *Ophthalmologica* 1986;193(4):19309.
383. Zeporkes J. Glassy network in the anterior chamber: report of a case. *Arch Ophthalmol* 1933;10:517.

14

Keratoconus

YARON S. RABINOWITZ

Keratoconus is a clinical term used to describe a condition in which the cornea assumes a conical shape as a result of noninflammatory thinning of the stroma. This thinning induces irregular astigmatism, myopia, and corneal protrusion, resulting in mild to marked impairment of the quality of vision.[58] Keratoconus is a progressive disorder that ultimately affects both eyes, even though only one eye may initially show clinical signs of the disease. The disease classically has its onset at puberty and progresses until the third to fourth decade of life when it usually arrests. It may, however, commence later in life and progress or arrest at any age. Rarely is it found at birth. It is commonly an isolated condition despite multiple reports of its coexistence with other disorders.

The reported incidence of keratoconus varies from 50 to 230 per 100,000 (approximately 1/2000); the prevalence is 54.5 per 100,000.[21,27,48,53,58] The variability in the reported incidence reflects the subjective criteria often used to establish the diagnosis; subtle forms are often overlooked. Keratoconcus occurs in all ethnic groups with no male or female preponderance.

SYMPTOMS AND SIGNS

Symptoms are highly variable and depend in part on the stage of the progression of the disorder. In the early stages there may be no symptoms and the diagnosis may be made because of the ophthalmologist's inability to refract the patient to a clear 20/20, prompting keratometric studies. In advanced stages of the disease there is significant distortion and ultimately reduction of vision due to evolving ectasia or central scarring.

Clinical signs differ depending on the severity of the disease. Early in the disease process, the cornea may appear normal on slit-lamp biomicroscopy. There may be, however, slight distortion or steepening of the keratometer mires centrally or inferiorly. In such instances, it is helpful to dilate the pupil and to use retroillumination techniques and look for scissoring of the retinoscopic reflex or the "Charleaux" oil droplet sign in order to make a clinical diagnosis.[80] In mild or early cases where the cornea appears normal, but keratoconus is suspected, plotting the anterior topography of the central and paracentral cornea is extremely useful for confirming the diagnosis (see following paragraph on devices for detcting early keratoconus).[58] In moderate to advanced disease, there may be any one or combination of the following biomicroscopic signs: central or paracentral stromal thinning, most commonly in the inferior or inferotemporal cornea (Fig. 14.1); conical protrusion of the cornea; an iron line, partially or completely surrounding the cone, also known as a Fleischer ring; and Vogt striae or

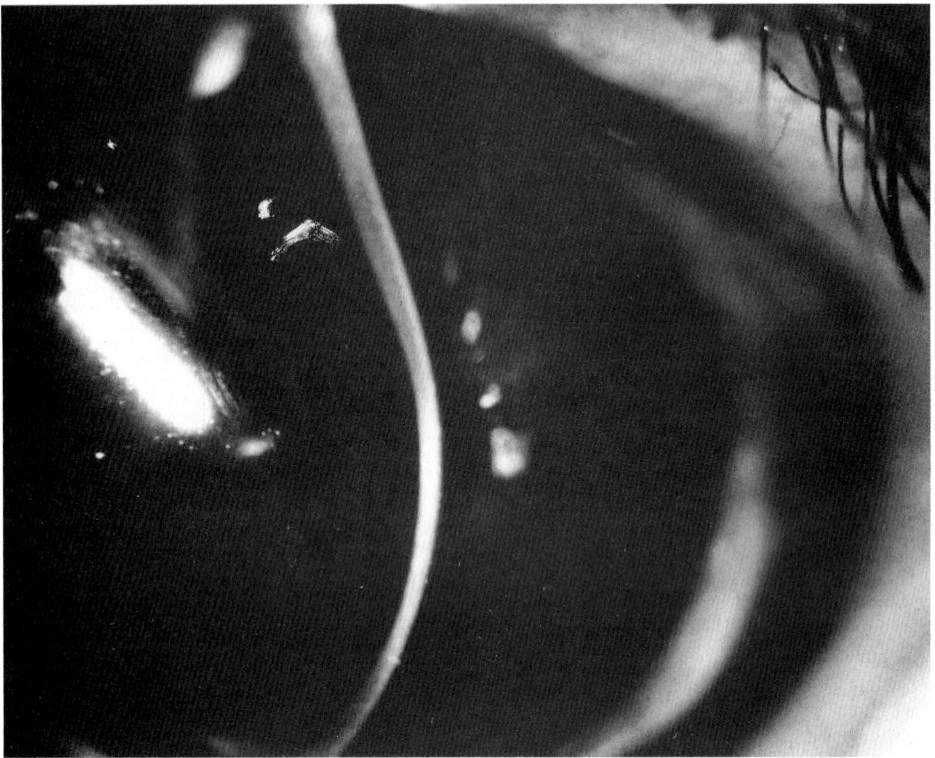

Figure 14.1. Paracentral inferior corneal thinning as seen on slit-lamp examination in a patient with keratoconus.

fine vertical lines in the deep stroma and Descemet's membrane that parallel the axis of the cone and disappear transiently on gentle digital pressure (Fig. 14.2). Other accompanying signs include epithelial nebulae, anterior stromal scars, enlarged corneal nerves, increased intensity of the corneal endothelial reflex, and the presence of subepithelial fibrillary lines.

Several devices are currently available for detecting the presence of early keratoconcus by mapping anterior corneal topography in the presence of a clinically normal cornea. These instruments include simple inexpensive ones such as a handheld keratoscope or Placido disk to expensive sophisticated devices such as computer-assisted videokeratoscopes. With the handheld keratoscope, such as the Klein keratoscope, early keratoconus is characterized by a downward deviation of the horizontal axis of the Placido disk reflections.[3,4] Amsler was the first to use such a device. In Amsler's[3,4] study of 600 patients, 22% had clinically obvious keratoconus in both eyes, 26% had clinical keratoconus in one eye and latent keratoconus in the other, and 52% had latent keratoconus bilaterally. Progression was highly variable and most often asymmetrical. The cone could remain stationary, progress rapidly over 3–5 years, and arrest or progress intermittently over an extended period of time. When Amsler reexamined 286 eyes 3–8 years after the diagnosis, only 20% of the entire group, but 66% of the latent cases, had progressed. Progression was most likely to occur in patients between 10 and 20 years of age, decreased slightly between 20 and 30 years, and was less likely to increase after age 30 years.[3,4] Munson's sign and Rizzuti's sign are useful adjunctive external signs associated with keratoconus.[65] Munson's sign refers to a V-shaped conformation of the lower lid produced by the ectatic cornea in, downgaze. Rizzuti's sign is a sharply focused beam of light near the nasal limbus, produced by lateral illumination of the cornea in patients

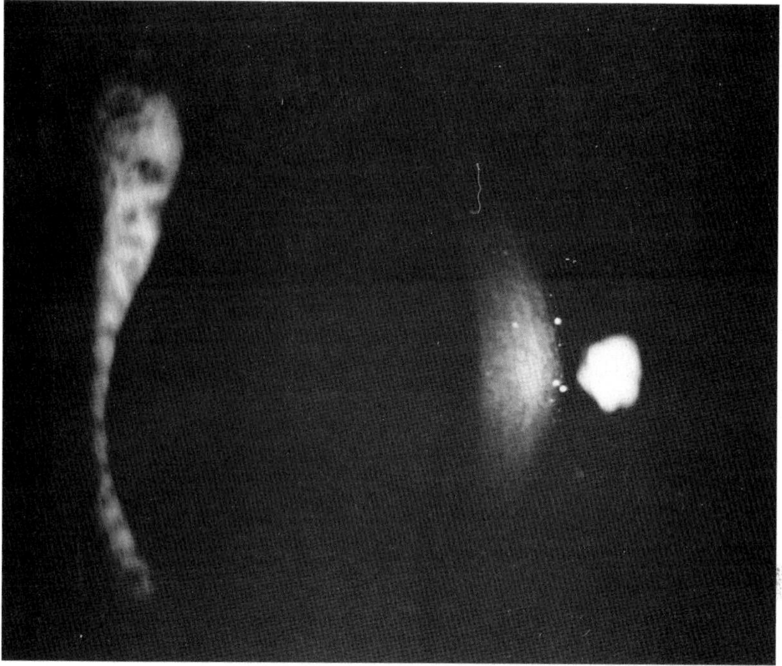

Figure 14.2. Vogt striae located at the level of Descemet's membrane noted on slit-lamp examination of the cornea.

with advanced keratoconus. Until recently, nine-ring photokeratoscopes such as the Corneascope (Keravision Co., Fremont, CA) were commonly used by cornea specialists and show compression of the mires inferiorly or inferotemporally in early keratoconcus (Fig. 14.3).[91] Computer-assisted videokeratoscopes such as the Topographic Modeling System (TMS-1, Computed Anatomy, New York, NY) measure the curvature of both central and paracentral corneal areas in one sitting. These devices, which have been described in detail, have been shown to be highly accurate and reproducible on spherical surfaces and in the central two-thirds of normal human corneas.[41,44,66,115] The 25-ring photokeratoscope mires can be superimposed on topographic maps for qualitative interpretation. Using this device, keratoconus appears as an area of increased surface power surrounded by concentric zones of decreasing surface power. Three features are common to keratoconus videokeratographs: (*1*) and area of increased surface power, (*2*) inferior-superior power asymmetry, and (*3*) skewed steep radial axes above and below the horizontal meridian that reflect the irregular astigmatism, which is the hallmark of keratoconus (Fig. 14.4).[81,82,116]

ACUTE HYDROPS

Patients with advanced disease may occasionally present with a sudden onset of visual loss accompanied by pain. On slit-lamp exam the conjunctiva may be injected and a diffuse stromal opacity is noted in the cornea. This condition is referred to as "hydrops" and is caused by breaks in Descemet's membrane with stromal imbibition of aqueous through these breaks. The edema may persist for weeks or months, usually diminishing gradually, with relief of pain and resolution of the redness and corneal edema ultimately being replaced by scarring (Fig. 14.5).

HISTOPATHOLOGY

Gross histopathological analysis of corneal buttons has revealed the presence of two types of

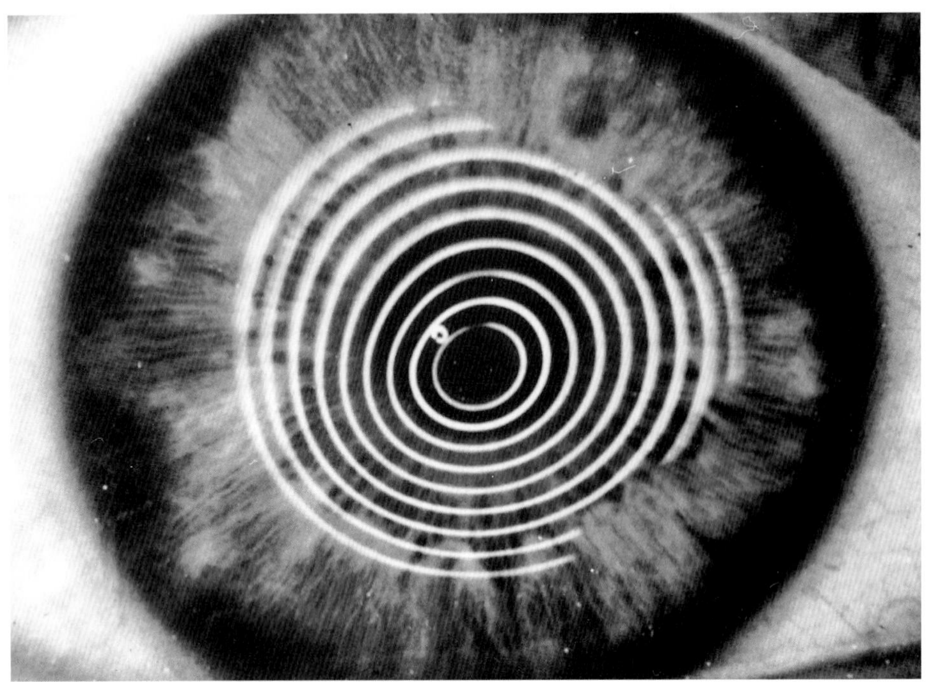

Figure 14.3. Egg-shaped mires or inferotemporal steepening detected with a Corneascope in a patient with early keratoconus.

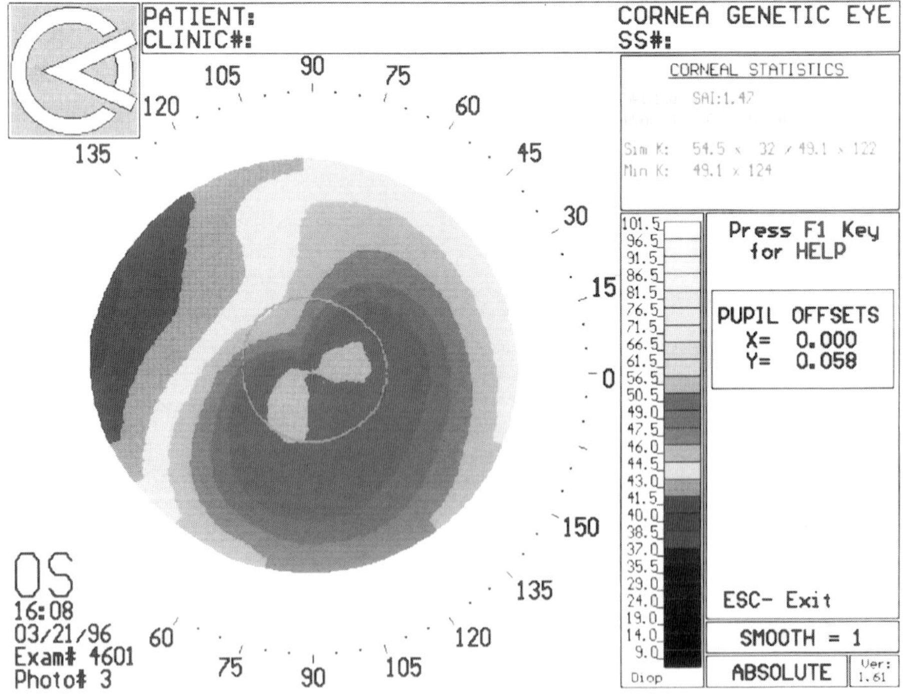

Figure 14.4. Keratoconus videokeratograph (TMS-1 videokeratoscope). Three characteristic features are localized steepening, inferior-superior dioptric asymmetry, and skewing of the steep radial axes above and below the horizontal meridian.

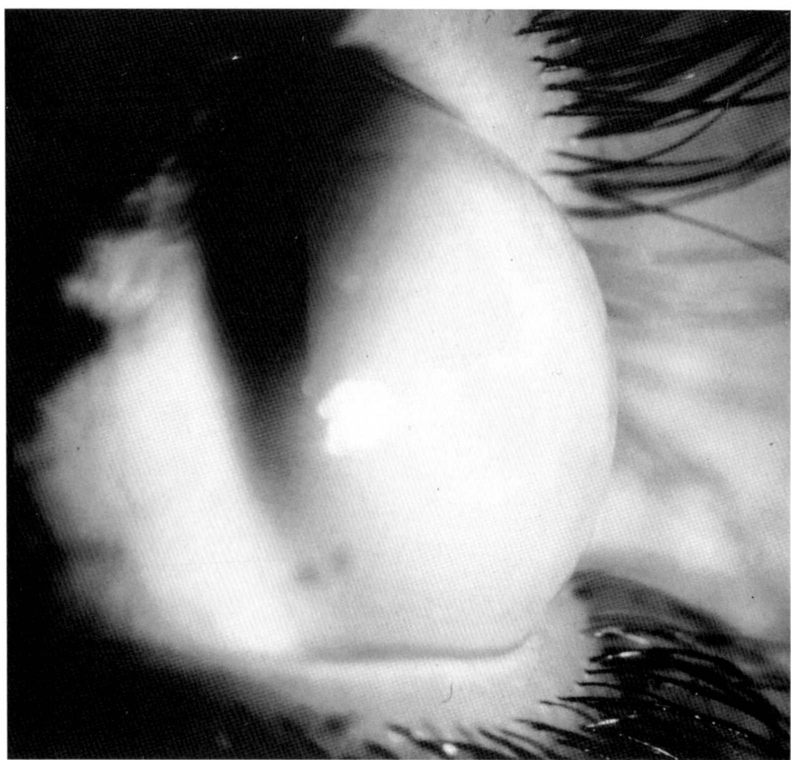

A

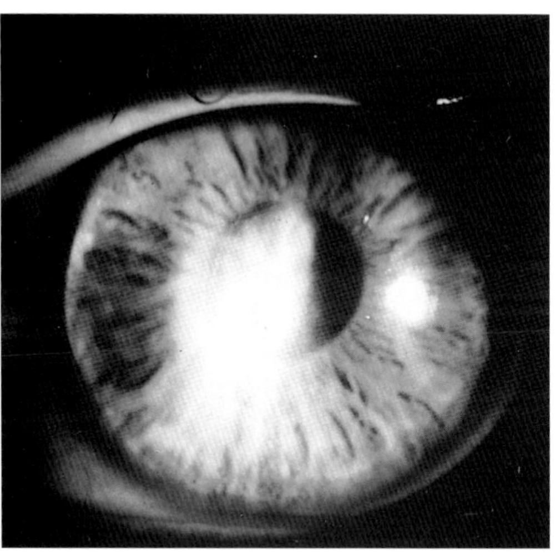

B

Figure 14.5. Acute hydrops. **A:** Stromal opacity as a result of corneal edema noted on initial presentation. **B:** Resolution of the hydrops with resultant corneal scarring in the same patient.

cones: nipple-type cones, located centrally, and oval- or sagging-type cones, located inferiorly or inferotemporally.[75] These types of cones can often also be distinguished biomicroscopically or using corneal topography.

Thinning of the corneal stroma, breaks in Bowman's membrane, and deposition of iron in the basal layers of the corneal epithelium comprise the classical histopathological triad of keratoconus (Fig. 14.6). Depending on the stage of the disease, every layer of the cornea may become involved in the pathological process. The epithelial basal cells may be degenerated and there may be breaks in Bowman's

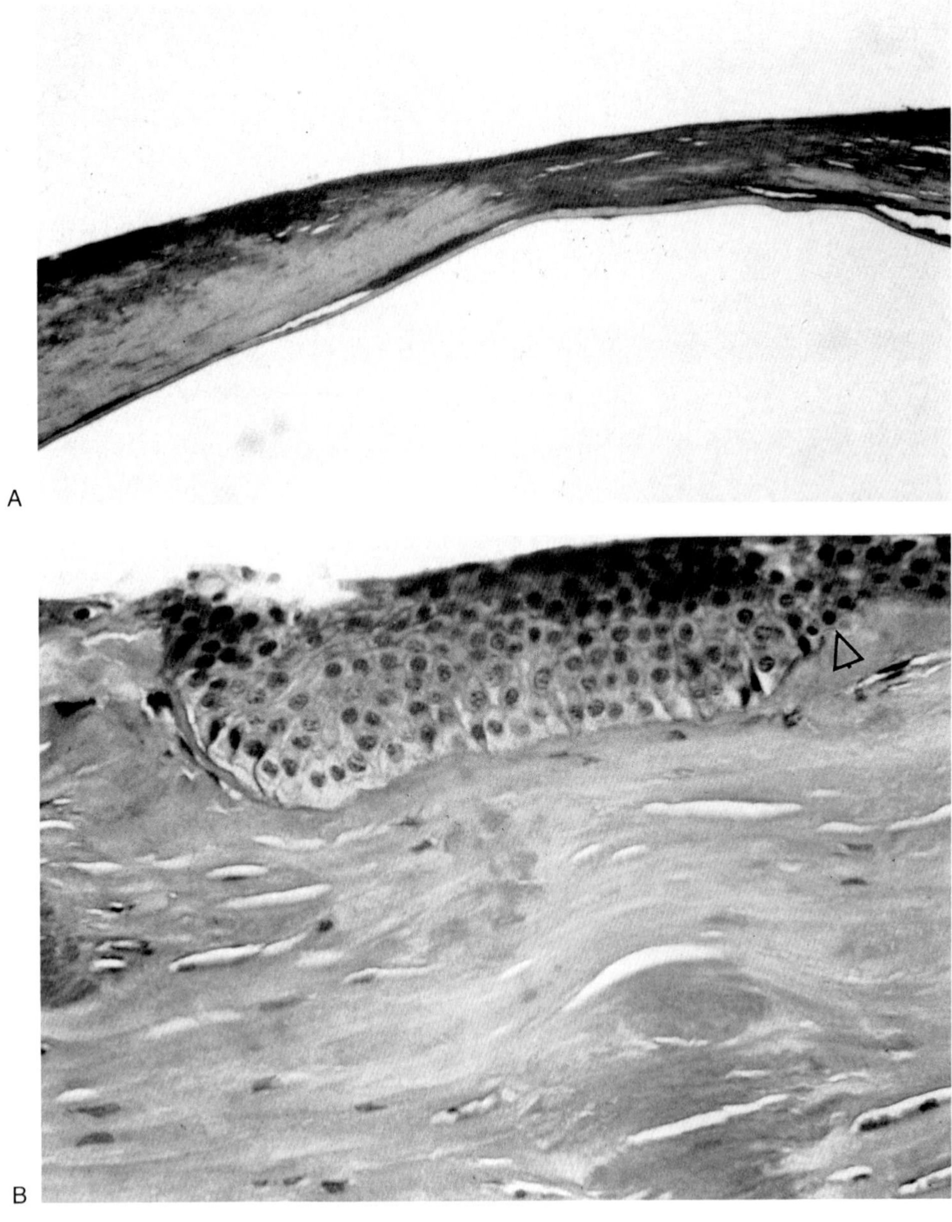

Figure 14.6. Classical histopathological features seen in keratoconus. **A:** Stromal thinning. **B:** Breaks in Bowman's membrane (arrowheads).

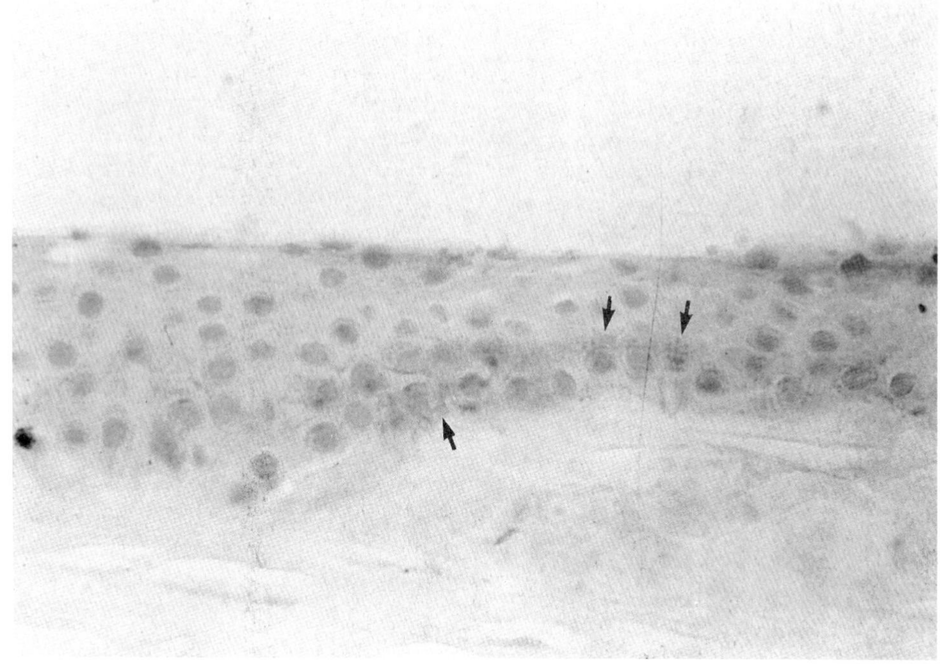

C

Figure 14.6. Continued. **C:** Deposition of iron in the basal epithelium (arrows).

membrane, accompanied by downgrowth of epithelial cells. On electron microscopy, particles may be seen within a thickened subepithelial basement membrane-like layer and between basal epithelial cells, and accumulation of ferritin particles within and between epithelial cells most prominently in the basal layer of the epithelium. There may be breaks of Bowman's layer that are filled by eruptions of underlying stromal collagen, periodic acid–Schiff-positive nodules, Z-shaped interruptions possibly due to separation of collagen bundles, and reticular scarring. There is compaction of the stroma with loss of normal arrangement of fibrils in the anterior stroma, and decrease in the number of collagen lamellae. There may be normal or degenerating fibroblasts in addition to keratocytes, and fine granular and microfibrillar material is present in association with keratocytes.[58] Descemet's membrane is rarely affected except for breaks that occur in association with acute hydrops. The endothelium is usually normal, except for reports of intracellular "dark structures," and pleomorphism and elongation of cells with their long axis toward the cone. Histopathological examination of corneal buttons in patients who have had acute hydrops reveals stromal edema. Descemet's membrane separates from the posterior surface and retracts into scrolls, ledges, or ridges. During the repair process, corneal endothelium extends over the anterior and posterior surfaces of the detached Descemet's membrane and denuded stroma. Endothelial integrity is usually reestablished 3–4 months after the acute event.[105]

ASSOCIATED DISORDERS

Keratoconus is most commonly an isolated condition, despite multiple single reports of its coexistence with other disorders (Table 14.1). More commonly recognized associations include Down syndrome, Leber's congenital amaurosis, and connective tissue disorders. Atopy, eye rubbing, and the wearing of hard contact lenses have also been associated with keratoconus. Six percent to 8% of cases reported to date have a positive family history of the disease or show evidence of familial transmission.[42,58]

Keratoconus is most commonly an isolated

Table 14.1. Conditions Associated with Keratoconus

Multisystem Disorders	
Alagille syndrome [89,108]	
Albers-Schonberg disease[32]	
Angelman syndrome[64]	
Apert syndrome[36]	
Autographism[50]	
Anetoderma[12]	
Bardet-Biedl syndrome[28,113]	
Down syndrome[19]	
Ehlers-Danlos syndrome[60]	
Goltz-Gorlin syndrome[118]	
Hyperornithemia[57]	
Ichthyosis[27]	
Kurz syndrome[119]	
Marfan syndrome[6]	
Mulvihill-Smith syndrome[87]	
Nail-patella syndrome[39]	
Neurocutaneous angiomatosis[30]	
Neurofibromatosis[113]	
Noonan syndrome[96]	
Osteogenesis imperfecta[8]	
Oculodentodigital syndrome[39]	
Pseudoxanthoma elasticum[113]	
Rieger syndrome[39]	
Rothmund syndrome[55]	
Tourette syndrome[24]	
Turner syndrome[70]	
Xeroderma pigmentosum	
Ocular Disorders	
Anetoderma and bilateral subcapsular cataracts[12]	
Aniridia[21]	
Ankyloblepharon[13]	
Bilateral macular coloboma[57]	
Blue sclerae[39]	
Congenital cataracts[57]	
Ectodermal and mesodermal anomalies[59]	
Floppy eyelid syndrome[68]	
Ocular Disorders—Continued	
Gyrate atrophy[57]	
Iridoschisis[22]	
Leber's congenital amaurosis[23]	
Macular coloboma and retinitis pigmentosa[31]	
Microcornea[57]	
Persistent pupillary membrane[57]	
Posterior lenticonus[14]	
Retinitis pigmentosa[27]	
Retinopathy of prematurity[100]	
Retrolental fibroplasia[63]	
Vernal conjunctivitis[38]	
Corneal Disorders	
Atopic keratoconjunctivitis[38]	
Axenfeld anomaly[104]	
Avellino corneal dystrophy[92]	
Chandler syndrome[35]	
Corneal amyloidosis[57]	
Deep filiform corneal dystrophy[57]	
Essential iris atrophy[10]	
Flecked corneal dystrophy[57]	
Fuchs corneal dystrophy[62]	
Iridocorneal dysgenesis[5]	
Lattice corneal dystrophy[47]	
Pellucid marginal degeneration[52]	
Posterior polymorphous dystrophy[20]	
Terrien's marginal degeneration[77]	
Other Disorders	
Congenital hip dysplasia[70]	
False chordae tendineae of left ventricle[57]	
Joint hypermobility[90]	
Mitral valve prolapse[97]	
Measles retinopathy[74]	
Ocular hypertension[9]	
Thalasselis syndrome[107]	

sporadic disorder with no associated systemic or ocular disease that are detectable by clinical evaluation. Of 300 consecutive patients with keratoconus screened for a genetic research study at the Cedars-Sinai Medical Center in Los Angeles, 2 (0.6%) had Down syndrome, 2 (0.6%) had neurofibromatosis, and 296 (99%) had no associated genetic disease. For the most part, the association of keratoconus with a systemic disease should be regarded as a chance event. For example, considering that the incidence of keratoconus is 1/2000 and the incidence of neurofibromatosis is 1/4000, there is a 1/8 million chance that these two disorders could occur together by chance alone (30 potential cases in the United States alone). Rare systemic associations with keratoconus are, however, particularly important if they occur as a result of a chromosomal abnormality, especially if the keratoconus and the chromosomal abnormality cosegregate within a given family. This might provide clues to the chromosomal location of the keratoconus gene(s). Cytogenetic studies should be performed in patients with mental retardation or other rare malformation syndromes associated with keratoconus. Patients with Down syndrome have been recognized to have a high incidence of keratoconus ranging from 0.5%–15%[19,99]; this is 10–300 times more common than the incidence of keratoconus is the general population. Similarly, a high incidence of keratoconus has been reported in patients with Leber's congenital amaurosis, affecting up to 30% of patients above above 15 years.[2] These two associations with keratoconus have been attributed to a higher incidence of eye rubbing in these disorders, resulting from an excess of blepharitis in Down syndrome and the oculodigital sign in Leber's amaurosis. A recent study of children in a school for the blind contradicts this commonly held theory and suggests that the association of Leber's with keratoconus is due to genetic factors rather than eye rubbing.[23]

Several reports suggest an association between keratoconus and connective tissue disorders such as osteogenesis imperfecta, subtypes of Ehlers-Danlos syndrome, and increased joint hypermobility.[8,51,67,90] The high incidence of joint hypermobility 22/44 (50%) as reported by Robertson,[90] is, however, disputed by two recent studies.[106,109] In the study by Tretter et al.,[109] 34 of 218 (15%) patients with keratoconus had joint hypermobility versus 10 of 183 (12%) normal age-matched controls; the difference between the two groups was not statistically significant. Other compelling evidence in support of a connective tissue abnormality in keratoconus does, however, exist and is based on two reports of an association between patients with advanced keratoconus and mitral valve prolapse.[7,97] Shariff et al.[97] reported that 58% of patients with advanced keratoconus who were scheduled to undergo cornea transplantation had mitral valve prolapse versus 7% of normal controls.

Many studies report a high association of eye rubbing in patients with keratoconus, but a cause-and-effect relationship is difficult to prove. A study at our institution found that patients with keratoconus patients rub their eyes significantly more often than normal controls: 174 of 218 (80%) keratoconus patients versus 106 of 183 (58%) normal age-matched controls ($p < 0.001$).[109] Contact lens wear is another form of mechanical trauma implicated in the pathogenesis of keratoconus.[34,45] Because patients may have worn contact lenses for mild myopic astigmatism before the diagnosis of keratoconus is made, it is extremely difficult to determine if the keratoconus or contact lens wear occurred first. It is possible, however, that mechanical trauma induced by eye rubbing and/or hard contact lens wear might act as an environmental factor enhancing the progression of keratoconus is genetically predisposed individuals.

Atopy is often cited as being highly associated with keratoconus. Review of the literature reveals conflicting data on the validity of this association.[86,114] We have not found a statistically significant difference between the prevalence of a history or symptoms of allergic disorders in patients with keratoconus and normal controls. At our institution, 96 of 218 (44%) keratoconus patients versus 66 of 183 (36%) normal age-matched controls ($p = 0.105$) had a history or symptoms of allergic disorders.[109]

ETIOLOGY AND PATHOGENESIS

Despite intensive biochemical investigation into the pathogenesis of this disorder, the underlying biochemical process and its etiology remain poorly understood. Corneal thinning appears to result from loss of structural components in the cornea. Theoretically, the cornea can become thinner because of fewer collagen lamellae, less collagen fibrils per lamella, closer packing of collagen fibrils, or various combinations of the above. These processes may result from defective formation of extracellular constituents of corneal tissue, a destruction of previously formed components, an increased distensibility of corneal tissue with sliding collagen fibers or collagen lamellae, or a combination of these mechanisms.[56]

Several biochemical and immunohistochemical studies of corneas with keratoconus suggest that the loss of corneal stroma after digestion by proteolytic enzymes could follow either increased levels of proteases and other catabolic enzymes[93] or decreased levels of proteinase inhibitors.[33] Studies of corneal alpha-1 proteinase inhibitor and alpha-2 macroglobulin (also a major proteinase inhibitor) confer further support to the hypothesis that the degradation process may be aberrant in keratoconus.[94] Both inhibitors can be demonstrated immunohistochemically in the epithelium, stroma, and endothelium of normal and pathologic human corneas. In contrast to normal corneas and corneas with other pathologic diseases, the staining intensity in the corneal epithelium of corneas with keratoconus corneas is markedly diminished. This decrease in alpha-2 macroglobulin in the cornea and stroma was confirmed by Western dot blot assays.[94] TIMP-1, another proteinase inhibitor that inhibits matrix metalloproteinase, was found not to be implicated in the increased levels of gelatinolytic activity in previous biochemical studies.[54,101]

Based on clinical observations and on our corneal topographic studies in families with keratoconus,it is our impression that keratoconus is the result of an as yet undetermined genetic abnormality. The heterogeneous nature of the disease suggests that different genetic subtypes exist. The high association of advanced keratoconus and mitral valve prolapse, and a recent study showing cosegregation of keratoconus with familial osteogenesis imperfecta, strongly point to an abnormality in connective tissue.[8,97] It is possible that environmental factors such as eye rubbing and/or rigid contact lens wear may cause progression of the disorder in genetically susceptible individuals. Despite the fact that the abnormality is unknown, genetic linkage analyses with DNA markers of large families with the inherited form of keratoconus have great potential for providing powerful pointers as to the underlying biochemical abnormality resulting in the noninflammatory corneal thinning.[18,101]

GENETICS

There is strong evidence in the literature to support a genetic basis for keratoconus. This includes eight reports of its occurrence in identical twins[25,58,73]; the bilateral nature of the disorder[61,81]; the high degree of nonsuperimposable topographic mirror image symmetry[116]; and multiple reports of its occurrence in family members in two and three generations.[29]

Of nine reported instances of keratoconus in monozygotic twins, all but one set of twins had keratoconus. In the one instance where keratoconus did not occur in the other twin, videokeratography was not performed. We have observed at least two sets of twins in whom one had clinical keratoconus while the other was affected using videokeratographic criteria only (Fig. 14.7); we have also examined two sets of dizygotic twins where one was affected and the other normal both clinically and using videokeratography. These observations represent the strongest evidence for a genetic basis of keratoconus, however, the fact that two twins often had differing degrees of the severity of the disorder suggests that environmental factors may play a role in the expression of the disease.

Several large series, including our own, have reported a positive family history in 6%–10% of patients.[43,109] The overwhelming majority of reports in the literature suggest an autosomal dominant mode of inheritance with variable expression and emphasis that subtle forms of the disorder such as keratoco-

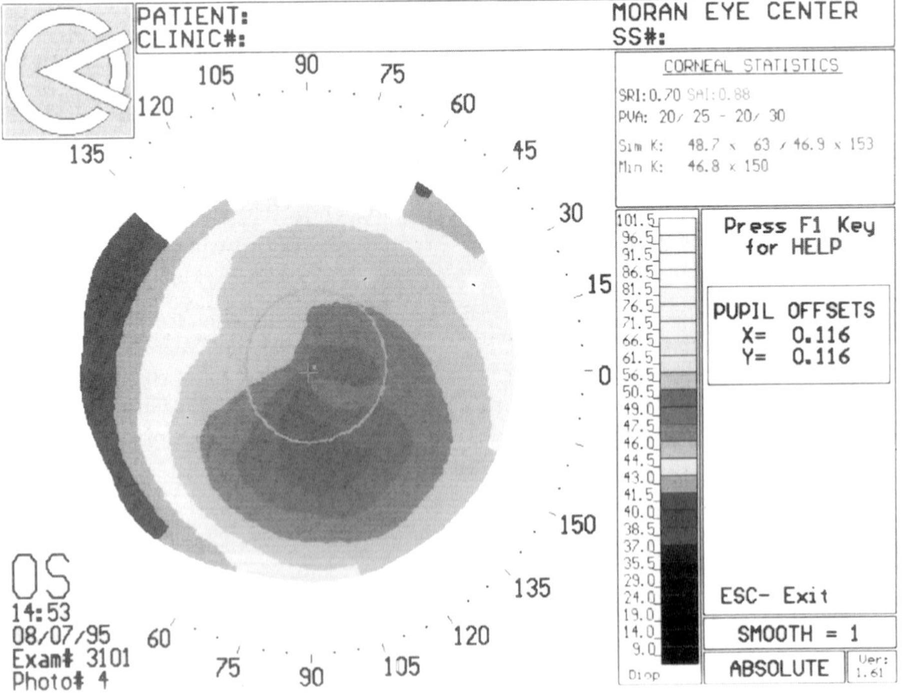

Figure 14.7. Videokeratography of forme fruste keratoconus in a clinically normal family member of a patient with familial keratoconus. The videokeratograph has similar but milder features to those noted in keratoconus.

nus fruste or mild irregular astigmatism need to be identified in order to resolve the mode of inheritance. At least 74 familial cases have been reported in the ophthalmic literature. These comprise the following: 21 cases cited by Falls and Allen,[26] including one of their own; 24 cases examined by Ihalainen[49] in a Finnish study; in 10 of 52 (19%) families examined by Hammerstien[43] keratoconus was detected in two or more relatives with a degree of penetrance estimated at approximately 20%; 7 pedigrees reported by Redmond,[88] who suggested that keratoconus fruste and high degrees of astigmatism represent incomplete expression of the keratoconus gene and should be taken into account in pedigree analysis; in all 5 families of patients with keratoconus reported by Rabinowitz et al.[84] the mode of inheritance was consistent with autosomal dominant transmission and variable expressivity (videokeratography was used to detect abortive forms of the disorder); and 7 families reported by Gonzalez and McDonnell,[40] who detected videokeratographic abnormalities in at least one parent of 7 sets of clinically normal parents of patients with keratoconus.

There are several reports favoring recessive inheritance.[29] In none of these reports, however, was there clear evidence that three generations were examined or that subtle forms of the disorder were sought to be included in the pedigree analysis.

To date there have been no well-designed genetic epidemiological studies in keratoconus and no reliable empiric risk estimates. Although most studies suggest a dominant mode of inheritance, formal segregation analyses need to be performed to accurately define hereditary patterns for the various subtypes of keratoconus. In order to do this, however, a very clear quantifiable and reproducible definition of "early" keratoconus in the absence of clinical signs is necessary. The introduction of computer-assisted videokeratoscopy into clinical practice provides an opportunity to do this. Research in this area provides a unique opportunity to determine true modes of inheritance and ultimately construct pedigrees for molecular genetic analysis in appropriate families with familial disease.[85]

DIFFERENTIAL DIAGNOSIS

It is important to distinguish keratoconus from other ectatic dystrophies and thinning disorders such as pellucid marginal degeneration, Terrien's marginal degeneration, and keratoglobus because the management and prognosis in these disorders differ markedly. The distinction can usually be made by careful slit-lamp evaluation and using corneal topography as an adjunct to differentiate these disorders in subtle cases.[81]

Pellucid marginal degeneration is characterized by a peripheral band of thinning of the inferior cornea from the 4 to 8 o'clock position. There is a 1–2 mm uninvolved area between the thinned zone and the limbus (Fig. 14.8). The corneal protrusion is most marked above the area of thinning and the central cornea is usually of normal corneal thickness. Like keratoconus, pellucid marginal degeneration is a progressive disorder that affects both eyes, sometimes in an asymmetric fashion. In moderate cases it can easily be differentiated from keratoconus by slit-lamp evaluation because of the classical location of the thinning. In early cases, the cornea may look relatively normal, and, in advanced cases, the disease may be very difficult to distinguish from keratoconus because thinning may progress to involve most, if not all, of the inferior cornea. In both early and advanced disease, videokeratography is very useful in making the distinction. The videokeratograph in pellucid marginal degeneration shows a classical butterfly-shaped appearance demonstrating large amounts of against-the-rule astigmatism as measured by simulated keratometry. Pellucid marginal degeneration can be differentiated from other peripheral thinning disorders such as Terrien's marginal degeneration in that the area of thinning is always epithelialized, clear, avascular, and without lipid deposition. Terrien's corneal degeneration affects a similar age group and also results in high astigmatism. However, it may affect both the superior and inferior corneas and is accompanied by lipid deposition and vascular invasion. Because of the large amounts of against-the-rule astigmatism, patients with pellucid marginal degeneration are much more difficult to fit with contact lenses

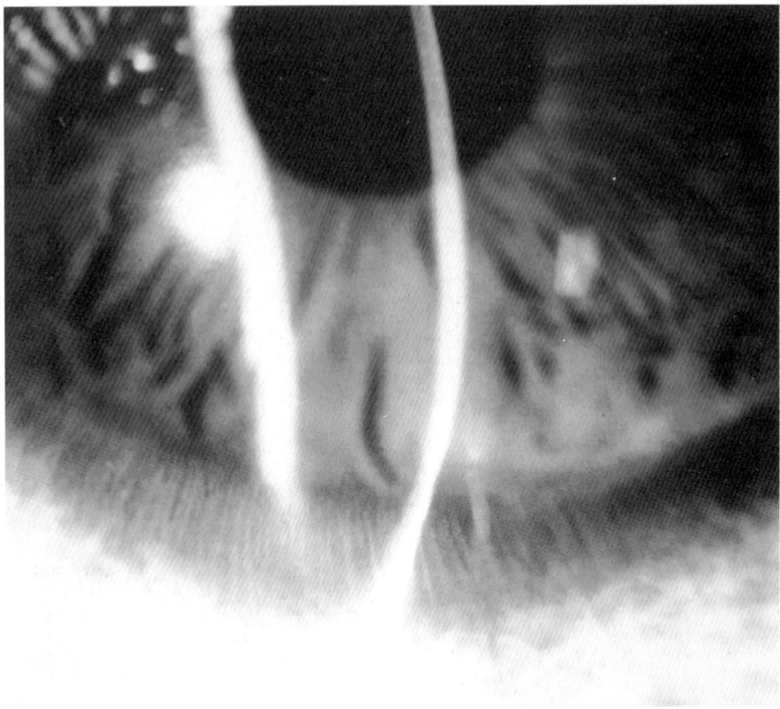

Figure 14.8. Slit-lamp photograph of a patient with pellucid marginal degeneration. Note the inferior thinning from the 4 to 8 o'clock position.

than patients with keratoconus, although aspheric or bispheric contact lenses should initially be attempted in early to moderate cases. In patients where contact lenses do not adequately correct vision or in patients who are contact lens intolerant, surgery may be considered. Patients with pellucid marginal degeneration are typically not good candidates for penetrating keratoplasty because the corneal thinning occurs so close to the limbus, increasing the chances of peripheral graft rejection, and because of the occurrence of very large postoperative astigmatism that might be extremely difficult to correct because of disparity in graft–host thickness. Crescentic lamellar keratoplasty is a useful initial surgical procedure in these patients. This procedure involves removing a crescentic inferior layer of ectatic tissue by lamellar dissection and replacing it with a thicker lamellar donor graft.[95] This will, in most instances, rid the patient of large amounts of against-the-rule astigmatism and in some instances make the patient contact lens tolerant, bypassing the need for a full-thickness procedure. In case of failure to tolerate contact lenses, a full-thickness, central-penetrating keratoplasty can be performed with a significantly reduced risk of graft rejection and postkeratoplasty astigmatism (Fig. 14.9).

Keratoglobus is a rare disorder in which the entire cornea is thinned most markedly near the corneal limbus as opposed to the localized thinning centrally or paracentrally noted in keratoconus.[17] The cornea may be thinned down to 20% of normal thickness and may assume a globular shape. In very advanced keratoconus, the entire cornea can also be thinned and assumes a globular shape, making it difficult to distinguish from keratoglobus. Invariably, however, and even in very advanced keratoconus, there will be a small area of uninvolved cornea superiorly. Keratoglobus is also bilateral but is usually present early in life and tends to be nonprogressive. Keratoglobus can be distinguished from megalocornea and congenital glaucoma by the normal corneal diameter and the reduced thickness in keratoglobus. Keratoglobus is an autosomal recessive disorder and is often associated with blue sclerae and other

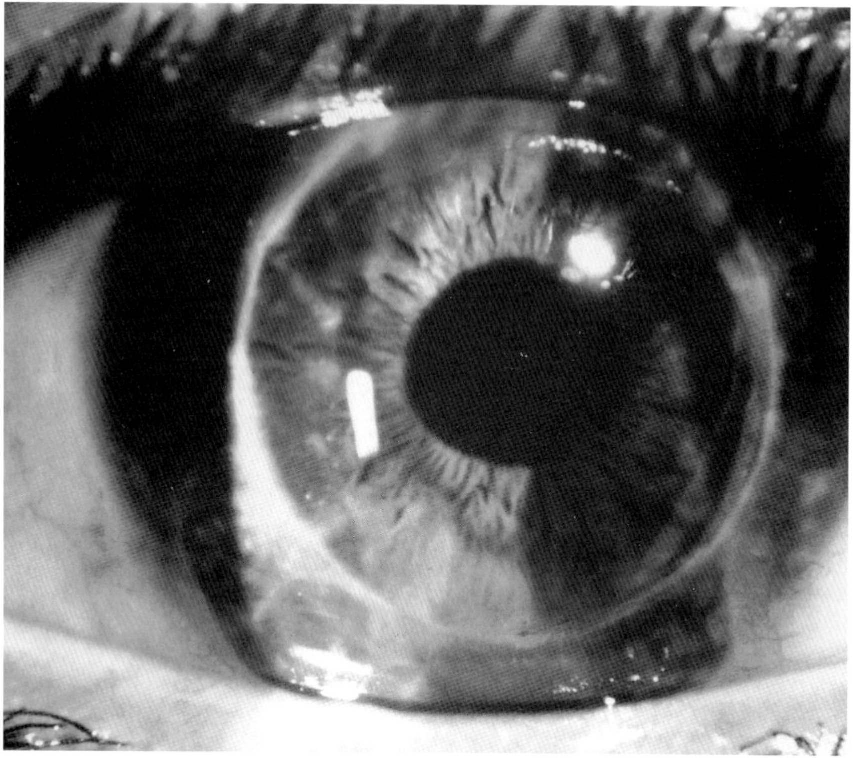

Figure 14.9. Postoperative slit-lamp photograph of a patient with pellucid marginal degeneration who has undergone a combined peripheral crescentic lamellar keratoplasty and central penetrating keratoplasty.

systemic features.[112] In contrast to keratoconus, the corneas in keratoglobus are prone to corneal rupture from even minimal trauma. As such, hard contact lenses are contraindicated and protective spectacles should be strongly encouraged. If the cornea is extremely thin a tectonic limbus to limbus lamellar keratoplasty should be considered to provide strength to the cornea and prevent it from rupturing. A superimposed full-thickness central keratoplasty might also be considered.

MANAGEMENT

The management of keratoconus varies depending on the state of progression of disease. Contact lenses are the mainstay of therapy in this disorder and are the treatment of choice in 90% of patients.[15,16,46] Patients with very early disease may be satisfied with glasses, but their vision is best corrected with contact lenses. The type of contact lens used also varies depending on the stage of the progression of the disease. Early on in the disease, soft lenses of toric design are adequate. As the disease progresses, more complex rigid gas-permeable lenses such as multicurve spherical-based lenses, aspheric lenses, and bispheric lenses are used. A hybrid lens that has a rigid central portion for obtaining best optics and a soft hydrophilic peripheral skirt is also popular. Contact lens fitting in keratoconus is complex, frustrating, and challenging, and has been embraced by few contact lens practitioners. The challenge is to keep the patient contact lens tolerant with good visual acuity in a cornea that may be changing in shape over time. Penetrating keratoplasty is the best and most successful option for patients who are not adequately visually rehabilitated by contact lenses. Because of the avascular and noninflammatory state of the cornea, this procedure is successful in 93%–96% of patients.[78,98] A patient with keratoconus has an approximately 10%–20% lifetime risk of needing a corneal transplant.[102,110] Indications for corneal transplantation in keratoconus include contact lens failure or intolerance, central scarring precluding good vision using contact lenses, and poor visual acuity despite tolerance of contact lenses. Corneas in keratoconus almost never perforate, and as such advanced thinning by itself is not an indication for surgery. Acute hydrops is also not an indication for penetrating keratoplasty, as in many instances the hydrops will resolve with scarring outside of the visual axis and flattening the cornea making the patients more contact lens tolerant. Patients with hydrops can be treated initially with cycloplegic agents, steroids, or nonsteroidal antiinflammatory agents, 5% sodium chloride solution, and, in rare instances, with bandage contact lenses.[103] Once the hydrops resolves, which can take up to 2–3 months, a determination as to surgical or contact lens management can be made. Patients who are candidates for penetrating keratoplasty should be counseled that in spite of the high success rate of surgery, there is still a 50% chance that they may need contact lenses, either because of residual myopia or postkeratoplasty astigmatism. To decrease the amount of myopia, several surgeons are performing keratoplasties with the donor and host trephines of equal size (usually 7.5 mm).[37] Although this does, in many instances, reduce the amount of myopia, patients who are axial myopes may still be left with large amounts of residual myopia.[111] There have been isolated reports of keratoconus reoccurring in the graft decades after surgery. These reports are extremly rare and it is not entirely clear whether this was from the disease recurring in the graft or from transplanted donor buttons with mild undetected disease.[1,69] Patients will, however, often ask about recurrence and these isolated reports should be mentioned within this context.

Acknowledgments: This work was supported in part by a grant from the National Institutes of Health (NEI 09052).

REFERENCES

1. Abelson MB, Collin HB, Gillete TE, Dohlman CH. Recurrent keratoconus after keratoplasty. *Am J Ophthalmol* 1980;90:672.
2. Alstrom CH, Olson O. Heredo-retinopathia congenitalis. Monohybride recessiva autosomalis. *Hereditas Genttiskt* 1957;43:1–177.
3. Amsler M. Le keratoconus fruste au javal. *Ophthalmologica* 1938;96:77–83.
4. Amsler M. Keratocone classique et keratocone fruste, arguments unitaries. *Ophthalmologica* 1946;111:96–101.
5. Archer DB, Sharma NK. Irido-corneal dysgenesis. *Trans Ophthalmol Soc UK* 1978;98(4): 510.
6. Austin MG, Schaefer RF. Marfan's syndrome with unusual blood vessel manifestations. *Arch Pathol* 1957;64:204–209.
7. Beardsley TL, Foulks GN. An association of keratoconus and mitral valve prolapse. *Ophthalmology* 1982;89:35–37.
8. Beckh U, Schonherr U, Naumann GO. Augenklinik mit Poliklinik, Universitat Erlangen-Nurnberg. Autosomal dominant keratoconus as the chief ocular symptom in Lobstein osteogenesis imperfecta tarda. *Klin Monatsbl Augenheilkd* 1995;206(4):268–272.
9. Bisaria KK. Bilateral keratoconus with ocular hypertension and the natural cure of one eye. *J All-India Ophthalmol Soc* 1967;15(5): 197–199.
10. Blair SD, Seabrooks D, Shields JW, Pillai S, Cavannagh H. Bilateral progressive essential iris atrophy and keratoconus with coincident features of posterior polymorphous dystrophy: A case report and proposed pathogenesis. *Cornea* 1992;11(3):255–261.
11. Blanksma LJ, Donders PC, Van Voorst Vader PC: Xeroderma pigmentosum and keratoconus. *Doc Ophthalmol* 1986;64(1)97–103.
12. Brenner S, Nemet P, Legum C. Jadassohn-type anectoderma in association with keratoconus and cataract. *Ophthalmologica* 1977;174: 181–184.
13. Brown IA. Ankyloblepharon associated with keratoconus. *Br J Ophthalmol* 1967;51(2): 138–139.
14. Buiuc S, Beschea G, Jaoblceastai L, Dimitriu G. A case of bilateral posterior lenticonus associated with keratoconus. *Rev Chir [Oftalmol]* 1978;22(4):229–300.
15. Buxton JN. Contact lenses in keratoconus. *Contact Intraocular Lens Med J* 1978;4:74.
16. Buxton JN, Keates RH, Hoefle FB. The contact lens correction of keratoconus. In *Contact Lenses. The CLAO Guide to Basic Service and Clinical Practice*, O.H. Diabezes, ed. Orlando FL: Grune & Stratton, 1984.
17. Cavara V. Keratoglobus and keratoconus. *Br J Ophthalmol* 1950;34:621.

18. Conneally PM, Rivas ML. Linkage analysis in man. *Adv Hum Genet* 1980;10:209–266.
19. Cullen JF, Butler HG. Mongolism (Down's syndrome) and keratoconus. *Br J Ophthalmol* 1963;47:321–330.
20. Driver PJ, Reed JW, Davis RM. Familial cases of keratoconus associated with posterior polymorphous dystrophy (letter). *Am J Ophthalmol* 1994;118:256–257.
21. Duke-Elder S, Leigh AG. *System of Ophthalmology. Diseases of the Outer Eye, vol. 8, part* 2. London: Henry Kimpton, 1965:964–976.
22. Eiferman RA, Law MW, Lane L. Iridoschisis and keratoconus. *Cornea* 1994;13:78–79.
23. Elder MJ. Leber congenital amaurosis and its association with keratoconus and keratoglobus. *J Pediatr Ophthalmol Strabismus* 1994;31: 38–40.
24. Enoch E, Itzahki A, Lakshminarayanan V, Comerford J, Lieberman M. Visual field defects detected in patients with Gilles de la Tourette syndrome: Preliminary report. *Int Ophthalmol* 1989;13(5):331–344.
25. Etzine S. Conical cornea in identical twins. *S Aftr Med J* 1954;28:154–155.
26. Falls HF, Allen W. Dominantly inherited keratoconus. Report of a family. *J Genet Hum* 1969;17:317.
27. Franceschetti A. Keratoconus. In *The Cornea. World Congress Cornea,* J.H. King, J.W. McTigue, eds. Washington, DC: Butterworths, 1965:152–168.
28. Francois J, Neetens A, Smets RM. Bardet-Biedl syndrome and keratoconus. *Bull Soc Belge Ophthalmol* 1982;203:117–121.
29. Francois J. Afflictions of the cornea. In *Heredity in Ophthalmology,* Vol. 8. J. Francois ed. St. Louis: C. V. Mosby, 1961:297–298.
30. Frasca G, Belmonte M. Neurocutaneous angiomatosis and keratoconus. A new syndrome entity? *Riv Oto-Neuro-Oftalmol* 1966;41(2): 119–130.
31. Freedman J, Gombos GM. Bilateral macular coloboma, keratoconus and retinitis pigmentosa. *Ann Ophthalmol* 1971;3:664–665.
32. Filip O, Golu T, Filip I, Scaueru N, Ciuchi V. Keratoconus in Albers-Schonberg disease (review) (Rumanian). *Oftalmologia* 1994;38: 247–251.
33. Fukuchi T, Yue B, Sugar J, Lam S. Lysosomal enzyme activities in conjunctival tissues of patients with keratoconus. *Arch Ophthalmol* 1994;112:1368–1372.
34. Gasset AR, Houde WI, Garcia-Bengochea H. Contact lens wear as an environmental risk factor for keratoconus. *Am J Ophthalmol* 1978;85:339–341.
35. Gasset AR, Worthen DM. Keratoconus and Chandler's syndrome. *Ann Ophthalmol* 1974;6(8):819–820.
36. Geerarts WJ. *Ocular syndromes,* 2nd ed. Philadelphia: Lea & Febiger, 1969:26.
37. Girard, LJ, Esnaola N, Rao R, Barnett L, Rand WJ. Use of grafts smaller than the opening for keratoconic myopia and astigmatism. *J Cataract Refract Surg* 1992;18(4):380–384.
38. Grayson M, Keates RH. *Manual of Diseases of the Cornea.* Boston: Little, Brown, 1969: 275–280.
39. Greenfield G, Romano A, Stein R, Goodman RM. Blue sclerae and keratoconus. Key features of a distant heritable disorder of connective tissue. *Clin Genet* 1973;4:8–16.
40. Gonzalez V, McDonnell PJ. Computer-assisted corneal topography of parents in keratoconus. *Arch Ophthalmol* 1992;110(10): 1413–1414.
41. Gormley DJ, Gersten M, Koplin RS, Lubkin V. Corneal modeling. *Cornea* 1988;7:30.
42. Hallerman W, Wilson EJ. Genetische betrachtungen uber den keratoconus. *Klin Monatsbl Augenheilkd* 1977;170:906–908.
43. Hammerstien W. Zur genetik des keratoconus. *Graefer Arch Klin Exp Ophthalmol* 1974; 190:293–308.
44. Hannush SB, Crawford SL, Waring GO III, Gemmill MC, Lynn MJ, Nizam A. Accuracy and precision of keratometry, photokeratoscopy, and corneal modeling on calibrated steel balls. *Arch Ophthalmol* 1989;107:1235–1239.
45. Harstien J. Keratoconus that developed in patients wearing corneal contact lenses. *Arch Ophthalmol* 1968;80:345–346.
46. Hartstien J. *Basics of Contact Lenses,* 3rd ed. San Francisco: American Academy of Ophthalmology, 1979.
47. Hoang-Xuan T, Elmaleh C, Dhermy P, Savoldelli M, D'Hermies F, Pouliquen Y. Association of a lattice dystrophy and keratoconus: Anatomo-clinical study apropos of a case. *Bull Soc Ophthalmol* 1989;89(1):35–38.
48. Hofstetter H. A keratoscopic survey of 13,395 eyes. *Am J Optom Acad Optom* 1959;36:3–11.
49. Ihalainen A. Clinical and epidemiological features of keratoconus: Genetic and external factors in the pathogenesis of the disease. *Acta Ophthalmol (Copenh)* 1986;178:5–64.
50. Iwaszkiewicz E. Keratoconus. II. Coexisting diseases and theories on its etiology and pathogenesis. *Klin Oczna* 1989;91(7–9):210–211.

51. Judisch F, Wariri M, Krachmer J. Ocular Ehlers-Danlos syndrome with normal lysyl hydrolase activity. *Arch Ophthalmol* 1976;94: 1489.
52. Kayazawa F, Nishimura K, Kodama Y, Tsuji T, Itoi M. Keratoconus with pellucid marginal corneal degeneration. *Arch Ophthalmol* 1984; 102(6):895–896.
53. Kennedy RH, Bourne WM, Dyer JA. A 48-year clinical and epidemiologic study of keratoconus. *Am J Ophthalmol* 1986;101:267–273.
54. Kenney MC, Chwa M, Opbroek AJ, et al. Increased gelatinolytic activity in keratoconus keratocyte cultures. A correlation to an altered matrix metalloproteinase-2/tissue inhibitor of metaloproteinase ratio. *Cornea* 1994;13: 108–113.
55. Kirkham TH, Werner EB. The ophthalmic manifestations of Rothmund's syndrome. *Can J Ophthalmol* 1975;10(1):1–14.
56. Klintworth GK, Damms T. Corneal dystrophies and keratoconus. Current opinion in ophthalmology. *Curr Sci* 1995;6:IV:44–56.
57. Klintworth GK. Degenerations, depositions and miscellaneous reactions of the ocular anterior segment. In *Pathobiology of Ocular Disease: A Dynamic Approach,* 2nd ed. A. Garner and G. K. Klintworth, eds. New York: Marcel Dekker, 1994:743–794.
58. Krachmer JH, Feder RS, Belin MW. Keratoconus and related noninflammatory corneal thinning disorders. *Surv Ophthalmol* 1984;28: 293–322.
59. Kremer I, Martini AM, Cohen EJ. Keratoconus associated with ectodermal and mesodermal anomalies (letter). *CLAO J* 1992;18(3):141.
60. Kuming BS, Joffe L. Ehlers-Danlos syndrome associated with keratoconus. *S Afr Med J* 1977;52:403–405.
61. Lee LR, Hirst LW, Readshaw G. Clinical detection of unilateral keratoconus. *Aust NZ J Ophthalmol* 1995;23(2):129–133.
62. Lipman RM, Rubenstein JB, Torczynski E. Keratoconus and Fuchs' corneal endothelial dystrophy in a patient and her family. *Arch Ophthalmol* 1990;108(7):993–994.
63. Lorfel RS, Sugar HS. Keratoconus associated with retrolental fibroplasia. *Ann Ophthalmol* 1976;8:449–450.
64. Lund AM. The Angelman syndrome. Does the phenotype depend on maternal inheritance? *Ugeskr Laeger* 1991;153(28):1993–1998.
65. Maguire LJ, Meyer RF. Ectatic Corneal Degenerations. In: *The Cornea* H. Kaufman, ed. Churchill Livingstone, New York: 1988: 485–510.
66. Maguire LJ, Wilson SE, Camp JJ, Verity S. Evaluating the reproducibility of topography systems on spherical surfaces. *Arch Ophthalmol* 1993;111:259–262.
67. Mckusick VA. *Heritable Diseases of Connective Tissue,* 4th ed. St. Louis: C. V. Mosby, 1972.
68. Negris R. Floppy eyelid syndrome associated with keratoconus. *J Am Optom Assoc* 1992;63(5):316–319.
69. Nirankari VS, Karesh J, Bastion F, et al. Recurrence of keratoconus in a donor cornea 22 years after successful keratoplasty. *Br J Ophthalmol* 1983;67:32.
70. Nucci P, Trabucchi G, Brancato R. Keratoconus and Turner's syndrome: A case report. *Optom Vis Sci* 1991;68(5):407–408.
71. Nucci P, Brancato R. Keratoconus and congenital hip dysplasia (letter). *Am J Ophthalmol* 1991;111(6):775–776.
72. Opbroek A, Kenney MC, Brown D. Characterization of a human corneal metalloproteinase inhibitor (TIMP-1). *Curr Eye Res* 1993; 12:877–883.
73. Parker J, Ko W, Pavlopoulos G, Wolfe PJ, Rabinowitz YS, Feldman ST. Videokeratography of keratoconus in monozygotic twins. *J Refract Surg* 1996;12:180–183.
74. Peduzzi MD, Torlai F, Delvecchio G. Bilateral pigmented retinopathy following measles: Long term follow up and possible association with keratoconus. *Eur J Ophthalmol* 1991; 1:148–150.
75. Perry HD, Buxton JN, Fine BS. Round and oval cones in keratoconus. *Ophthalmology* 1980;87:905–909.
76. Perlman JM, Zaidman GW. Bilateral keratoconus in Crouzon's syndrome. *Cornea* 1994; 13:80–81.
77. Pouliquen Y, Dhermy P, Renard G, Goichot-Bonnat L, Foster G, Savoldelli M. Maladie de Terrien, a propos de 6 observations. Etude ultrastructurale. *J Fr Ophthalmol* 1989; 12(8–9):503–520.
78. Price FW, Whitson WE, Marks RG. Graft survival in four common groups of patients undergoing penetrating keratoplasty. *Ophthalmology* 1991;98(3):322–328.
79. Rabinowitz YS, Nesburn AB, McDonnell PJ. Videokeratography of the fellow eye in unilateral keratoconus. *Ophthalmology* 1993;100:2: 181–186.
80. Rabinowitz YS, Klyce SD, Krachmer JH, Nordan L, Rowsey JJ, Sugar J, Wilson SE, Binder P, Damiano R, McDonald M, Neumann A, Seiler T, Thompson K, Wyzinski P. Videokera-

tography, keratoconus and refractive surgery. *Opin Refract Corneal Surg* 5:403–407.

81. Rabinowitz YS, Wilson SE, Klyce SD, eds. *Corneal Topography: Interpreting Videokeratography.* New York: Igaku Shoin Medical Publishers, 1993:63.
82. Rabinowitz YS, McDonnell PJ. Computer-assisted corneal topography in keratoconus. *Refract Corneal Surg* 1989;5,6:400–406.
83. Rabinowitz YS. Videokeratographic indices to aid in screening for keratoconus. *Refract Corneal Surg* 1975;11:5:371–379.
84. Rabinowitz YS, Garbus J, McDonnell PJ. Computer-assisted corneal topography in family members of keratoconus. *Arch Ophthalmol* 1990;108:365–371.
85. Rabinowitz YS, Maumenee IH, Lundergan MK, et al. Molecular genetic analysis in autosomal dominant keratoconus. *Cornea* 1992;11: 302–308.
86. Rahi A, Davies P, Ruben M, et al. Keratoconus and coexisting atopic disease. *Br J Ophthalmol* 1977;61:761–764.
87. Rau S, Duncker GI. Keratoconus in Mulvihill-Smith syndrome. *Klin Monatsbl Augenheilkd* 1994;205(1):44–46.
88. Redmond KB. The role of heredity in keratoconus. *Trans Ophthalmol Soc Aust* 1968;27: 52–54.
89. Ricci B, Lepore D, Iossa M, Santo A, Chiaretti A. Ocular anomalies in Alagille's syndrome [French]. Anomalies oculaires dans le syndrome d'Alagille, *J Fr Ophthalmol* 1991; 14(8–9):481–485.
90. Robertson I. Keratoconus and Ehlers Danlos syndrome. A new aspect of keratoconus. *Med J Aust* 1975;1:571–573.
91. Rowsey JJ, Reynolds AE, Brown R. Corneal topography. Corneascope. *Arch Ophthalmol* 1981;99:1093–1100.
92. Sassani JW, Smith SG, Rabinowitz YS. Keratoconus and bilateral lattice-granular corneal dystrophies. *Cornea* 1992;11(4):343–350.
93. Sawagamuchi S, Yue BYT, Sugar J, Giljoy JE. Lysosomal abnormalities in keratoconus. *Ophthalmology* 1989;107:1507–1510.
94. Sawagamuchi S, Twinning SS, Yue BY, et al. Alpha 2 macroglobulin levels in normal human and keratoconus corneas. *Invest Ophthalmol Vis Sci* 1994;35:4008–4014.
95. Schanzlin DJ, Samo EM, Robin JB. Crescentic lamellar keratoplasty in pellucid marginal degeneration. *Am J Ophthalmol* 1983;96:253.
96. Schwartz DE. Noonan's syndrome associated with ocular abnormalities. *Am J Ophthalmol* 1972;73:955–960.
97. Shariff KW, Casey TA, Colart J. Prevalence of mitral valve prolapse in keratoconus patients. *J R Soc Med* 1992;85(8)446–448.
98. Shariff KW, Casey TA. Penetrating keratoplasty for keratoconus: Complications and long term success. *Br J Ophthalmol* 1991; 75(3):142–146.
99. Shapiro MB, France T. The ocular features of Down's syndrome. *Am J Ophthalmol* 1985; 99:659.
100. Shammas HJ, McGaughey AS. Retinal disinsertion syndrome: Report of a case. *J Pediatr Ophthalmol Strabismus* 1979;16(5):284–286.
101. Shows TB, Sakaguchi AY, Naylor SL. Mapping the human genome, cloned genes, DNA polymorphisms, and inherited disease. *Adv Hum Genet* 1982;12:341–468.
102. Smiddy WE, Hamburg TR, Kracher GP, Stark WJ. Keratoconus. Contact lens or keratoplasty? *Ophthalmology* 1988;95:487–492.
103. Smolin G. Dystrophies and degenerations. In *The Cornea. Scientific Foundations and Clinical Practice.* G. Smolin and R. A. Thoft, eds. Boston: Little, Brown, 1987:449.
104. Stokes DW, Parrish CM. Axenfeld's anomaly associated with Down's syndrome. *Cornea* 1992;11(2)163–164.
105. Stone DL, Kenyon KR, Stark WJ. Ultrastructure of keratoconus with healed hydrops. *Am J Ophthalmol* 1976;82:450–458.
106. Street DA, Vinokur ET, Waring GO III, et al. Lack of association between keratoconus, mitral valve prolapse and joint hypermobility. *Ophthalmology* 1991;98:170–176.
107. Thalasselis A, Selim AA. Keratoconus-tetany-menopause: The new association. *Optom Vis Sci* 1991;68(5):357–363.
108. Traboulsi EI, Lustbader J, Lemp MA. Keratoconus in Alagille syndrome. *Am J Ophthalmol* 1989;108:332–333.
109. Tretter T, Rabinowitz YS, Yang H, et al. Aetiological factors in keratoconus. *Ophthalmology* (Supplement) 1995;102A:156.
110. Tuft SJ, Moodaley LC, Gregory WM, Davison CR, Buckley RJ. Prognostic factors of progression to keratoconus. *Ophthalmology* 1994; 101:3:439–447.
111. Tuft SJ, Fitzke FW, Buckley RJ. Myopia following penetrating keratoplasty for keratoconus. *Br J Ophthalmol* 1992;76(11):642–645.
112. Verrey F. Keratoglobe aigu. *Ophthalmologica* 1947;114:284.
113. Walsh FB, Hoyt WF. *Clinical Neuro-Ophthalmology,* 3rd ed. Baltimore: Williams & Wilkins, 1969:884–886.

114. Wachmeister L, Ingemannsson SO, Moller E. Atopy and HLA antigens in patients with keratoconus. *Acta Ophthalmol (Copenh)* 1982; 60:113.
115. Wilson SE, Verity SM, Conger DL. Accuracy and reproducibility of the corneal analysis system and topographic modeling system. *Cornea* 1992;11(1):28–35.
116. Wilson SE, Lin DTC, Klyce SD. The topography of keratoconus. *Cornea* 1991;10(1):2–8.
117. Wolter JR. Bilateral keratoconus in Crouzon's syndrome with unilateral acute hydrops. *J Pediatr Ophthalmol* 1977;14:141–143.
118. Zala L, Ettlin C, Krebs. Fokale dermale Hypoplasie mit Keratokonus. Osophaguspappillomen und Hidrokystomen. *Dermatologica* 1975;150:176–185.
119. Zolog N. [On congenital blindness (Kurz syndrome)] [French]. Observations sur la cecite congenitale (syndrome de Kurz). *Bull Mem Soc Fr Ophthalmol* 1969;82: 113–116.

III.

Retinal Dystrophies and Degeneration

15

Retinal Function Testing and Genetic Disease

JANET S. SUNNESS

A retinal evaluation is a critical step in understanding and diagnosing genetic disease. In addition to conditions that exclusively involve the retina, there are systemic disorders, such as storage diseases, in which determining whether or not the retina is involved will play an important part in diagnosis. As ophthalmologists, we are able to view the retina directly, and this often allows us to make diagnoses without additional functional testing. In a number of diseases, however, the clinical examination is inadequate for evaluating the patient's condition. Retinal function testing then becomes important in making the diagnosis and monitoring the progression of disease. It may be used to document and quantify a patient's symptoms, such as abnormalities in color vision or difficulty seeing at night. It may help in making a differential diagnosis of some retinal disorders, in distinguishing localized macular disorders from diffuse retinal disorders, and in distinguishing optic nerve disease from retinal disease. Genetic diseases may target the rod system or the cone system independently, and specific methods of psychophysical and electrophysiological testing can help to determine whether only one system is involved. As various therapies are proposed for these disorders, retinal function testing should help to determine whether they are beneficial in altering the natural course of a disease, and whether they have side effects affecting retinal function. An early alteration in a retinal function measure might serve as a surrogate outcome measure of the efficacy of an intervention, substituting for the years-long wait to determine if a disease has progressed clinically.

Beyond these advantages, specialized retinal function and electrophysiological testing may become more important in the future, as we gain a better understanding of the roles of the various genes in maintaining the structure and the function of the retina.[4] Visual psychophysicists[41] and electrophysiologists[18,31] can construct models of what part of the visual process would have to be affected to modify a given retinal function measure. As discussed below, they can design specific tests and analyses to examine such aspects as changes in rod phototransduction in retinitis pigmentosa, and whether rhodopsin or neural transmission changes are the cause of decreased dark adaptation in different forms of night blindness. Retinal function measures may provide insight into the roles of specific normal genes by providing better understanding of the pathological changes caused by mutations of that gene.

Table 15.1. Properties of Rods and Cones Important in Retinal Function Testing

Property	Rods	Cones
Maximum concentration in retina	15° from fovea	Foveal center
Predominant contribution to everyday vision	In dim light	In bright light
Rate of dark adaptation	Slow	Fast
Color vision	None	3 cone types for normal color vision
Maximal wavelength sensitivity	Blue-green (500 nm)	Green-yellow (560 nm)
Spatial resolving ability	Low	High (fine visual acuity)
Ability to detect flicker	Slow flicker only	Fast flicker

This chapter describes the specialized tests of retinal function—dark adaptation, electroretinography, electrooculography, and visual evoked potentials. Visual field testing is well understood by most ophthalmologists and researchers in visual function, so attention is focused on macular perimetry using a scanning laser ophthalmoscope, as it has been applied to genetic retinal disease. Color vision is discussed in Chapter 16 and is therefore not described here. Uses of these measures of visual function to diagnose and track the course of a disease are also described. In addition, some examples of the physiological and pathophysiological information we can learn from retinal function testing is discussed in the various sections. The examples given in this chapter are limited to studies of retinal degenerations and macular dystrophies; a broader treatment of the use of these tests in other disorders may be found in a number of fine articles and books.[5,8,9,14,17,20,32]

Many specialized visual function tests take advantage of the different properties of rods and cones to test selectively for one photoreceptor type. These properties are listed in Table 15.1.

DARK ADAPTATION

Dark adaptation is the process by which the photoreceptor cells of the retina (rods and cones) become increasingly sensitive to the detection of a small flash of light with time in the dark. Sensitivity is a measure of how intense the stimulus must be for detection; the more light required, the lower the sensitivity. (The threshold is the inverse of the sensitivity; a decrease in function is associated with lower sensitivity and higher threshold.)

The Goldmann-Weekers adaptometer has been the classic device for measuring dark adaptation. However, many automated static perimeters can be used to measure dark adaptation, provided that the background light can be turned off.

To measure the dark-adaptation curve, the patient first looks at a very bright light for a few minutes (to "bleach" the photoreceptors), and then is placed in total darkness. The intensity required to see a small spot of light at a specific retinal site (typically 10–20° from the fovea, the area of the highest rod concentration) is measured as a function of time. A dark-adaptation curve is generated in this way, over a 30- to 40-min period. The dark-adaptation curve (Fig. 15.1) has two branches because of the differing adaptation rates of cones and rods (Table 15.1). The cones are initially more sensitive than the rods, so the early portion of the curve is determined by cone adaptation. Cones reach their maximal sensitivity at about 5 min in the dark, after which the level of retinal sensitivity plateaus for 2 or 3 min. Then the rods become more sensitive than the cones (the rod–cone break), and continue to increase in sensitivity until they reach their final maximal sensitivity (1000 times more sensitive than the cones) at about 30 min. Levels of final dark adaptation are often expressed in log units of change from normal; for example, a patient with a 2 log unit decrease in dark-adapted sensitivity requires 100 times

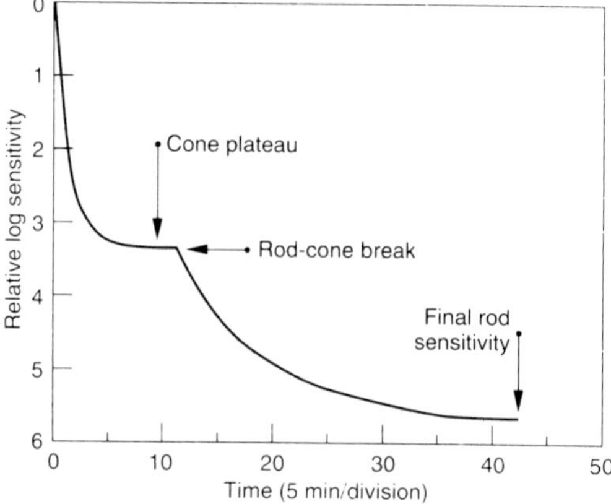

Figure 15.1. A normal dark adaptation curve. The cones adapt more rapidly than the rods. The cones reach full adaptation by about 5 minutes (cone plateau) and dominate the first phase of the graph. By about 10 minutes, the rods become more sensitive than the cones, and the rod–cone break occurs. Thereafter, rod sensitivity is predominant. Final maximal rod sensitivity is achieved by 40 minutes. (Reprinted with permission from J. S. Sunness, Clinical retinal function testing. *Focal Points: Clinical Modules for Ophthalmologists*, IX(1), American Academy of Ophthalmology, San Francisco, 1991.)

more light to see the stimulus. (A decibel is 0.1 log units.)

Often, the aspect of interest in dark adaptation is the final sensitivity level achieved, rather than the specific time course of adaptation. In many cases, such as in retinitis pigmentosa, more information may be derived from simply patching an eye for 30 to 45 min, and then performing dark-adapted static perimetry to determine the final dark-adapted sensitivity at a number of retinal locations. This affords both a measurement of dark adaptation and a measure of how widespread the disease is throughout the retina.

In conditions in which rods and cones are differentially involved, the dark-adaptation curve will show which system is affected. In typical congenital stationary night blindness, for example, there is no rod portion of the curve, and the sensitivity remains at the level of the cone plateau.[6] The dark-adaptation curve in this case is useful for distinguishing depressed sensitivity due to a nonspecific involvement of the retina from a specific rod disorder. In rod monochromatism, in which no functioning cones are present, the dark-adaptation curve shows an absence of the cone branch.

Until recently, delays in dark adaptation were not frequently reported. Classically, the rare condition of fundus albipunctatus has been the main example of delayed dark adaptation, with marked delays in both the rod and cone branches of the dark-adaptation curve. Final normal sensitivity may not be achieved for 3 hours or more[25,33] (Fig. 15.2). Recently, a number of other genetic disorders have been found to be associated with delayed dark adaptation. This includes some patients with Stargardt disease,[12] cone–rod dystrophy,[13] and retinitis pigmentosa.[24]

Additional studies can shed light on the site of the possible defect in eyes with problems with dark adaptation. For example, using retinal densitometry, Carr[6] investigated the amount of rhodopsin (rod pigment) and the kinetics of rhodopsin recovery following exposure to a bleaching light, as they relate to dark-adaptation rates measured psychophysically. He found that the amount and kinetics of rhodopsin were normal in typical congenital stationary blindness. This then implicated the neural transmission in the outer retina as responsible for night blindness. In contrast, patients with fundus albipunctatus show delayed

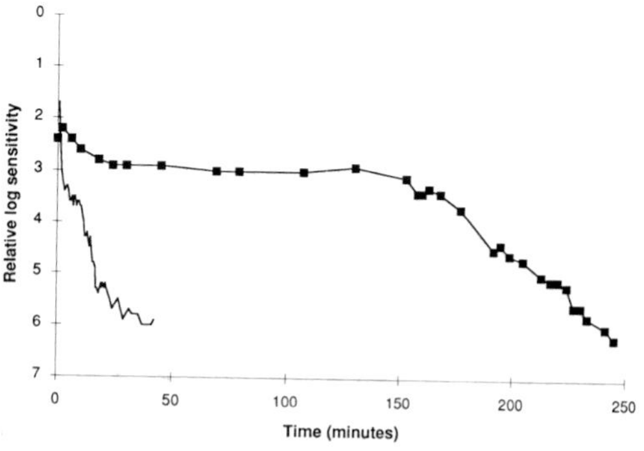

Figure 15.2. Markedly prolonged dark adaptation in fundus albipunctatus. The curve without symbols to the left is a normal dark adaptation curve. The curve with square symbols to the right is the dark adaptation curve of a patient with fundus albipunctatus.

photopigment recovery from a bleach, thus implicating a defect within the photopigment system itself as the cause of the prolonged dark adaptation. Readers interested in a more complete discussion of the categories of congenital stationary night blindness are referred to Carr's works,[6,7] and to the section on these diseases in Chapter 22.

Dark adaptation, in terms of both its time course and its final sensitivity, has also been found to be affected in some common retinal disorders. For example, many patients with even early age-related macular degeneration complain of difficulties adapting to the dark. When formal dark-adapted testing is performed, there may be a decrease in the final sensitivity level and an actual small delay in dark adaptation. The decreased sensitivity and prolongation of dark adaptation have been shown to be predictive of the subsequent development of advanced age-related macular degeneration.[10,37,38] This work suggests that dark-adapted sensitivity measures may yield insight into the risk of developing further visual loss in other retinal diseases as well.

A great deal of information can be obtained by comparing the dark-adapted sensitivity to stimuli of different colors.[27] The rods are about 2 log units more sensitive to blue-green light (500 nm) than to red light (650 nm), and the cones are about equally sensitive to blue-green and red, with the rods and cones having about equal sensitivity to red in the fully dark-adapted state. Normally, the rods mediate retinal sensitivity except in the fovea, so outside the fovea the blue–green stimulus is seen at significantly lower intensity levels than the red. If the rods are defective in a given region and the cones mediate sensitivity, one will find that the blue–green stimulus is no longer seen at a lower intensity than the red in that region. If both rods and cones are defective, the overall level of sensitivity to red will decrease, and there will still be evidence of rods mediating the blue–green sensitivity. This distinction has been used clinically to divide patients with retinitis pigmentosa (RP) into two groups.[27] In type 1, or diffuse RP, the rods throughout the retina are affected early and the cones later become involved. Patients characteristically have long histories of night blindness and show cones mediating detection on two-color dark-adapted perimetry. Patients with type 2, or regional RP, do not develop early night blindness. Early in the disease, their rods appear to function throughout the retina. As the disease progresses, they develop localized areas of involvement of both rods and cones. These patients show a pattern of rods mediating detection on two-color dark-adapted perimetry.

VISUAL FIELD TESTING (PERIMETRY)

Most investigators are familiar with standard visual fields, such as kinetic perimetry using a Goldmann perimeter, and static perimetry using a Humphrey perimeter. The methods are not described in detail here; the interested reader is referred to works on this topic.[19,42]

Visual fields measure the area of seeing retina (and optic nerve pathway integrity). In diseases such as retinitis pigmentosa, the visual field is arguably the most important measure of the progression of the disorder and of the patient's degree of disability. The patient is well served by the Goldmann perimeter or the full-field Humphrey perimeter to assess visual function; the Goldmann is able to test the full extent of the field, and the Humphrey is limited to 60°. Investigators have assessed the natural course of RP using changes in visual field area.[3,26] Massof et al. found that the decrease in visual field area is proportional to the remaining visual field area. His findings suggest that the critical age, the age when visual field starts to decline, is different for different genetic subtypes. However, once the decrease begins, the rate of decay seems to be the same for all the genetic forms and the sporadic form of RP.[26]

Measuring the Central Field; Macular Perimetry

Many genetic retinal disorders, such as Stargardt disease and cone dystrophy, affect the macula, and disease progression must be monitored by observing progression of blind spots (scotomas) near or involving the fovea. This is particularly true since the ophthalmoscopically observed macular lesion may not give an adequate estimate of the degree of involvement.[34]

Until recently, testing of the central visual field was daunting. Standard central visual field testing, whether by an automated perimeter or with a tangent screen, is likely to be inaccurate. Patients with central scotomas generally adopt an eccentric site of fixation, so that the zero degree point at the center of the field may be aligned with an eccentric retinal site rather than the macula. In addition, patients with central scotomas often have instability of fixation, so that the size of the mapped scotoma may be incorrect. These two sources of error are often present together, so that neither the location nor the size of the scotoma may be accurate.

Fundus perimetry relies on the ability to simultaneously visualize the retina and the location of the stimulus on it during testing. A number of different fundus perimeters have been used in the past. The current and most effective fundus perimeter is the scanning laser ophthalmoscope (SLO). This instrument uses a narrow laser beam of infrared light to scan and image the retina, and a narrow beam of red (helium neon laser) light to present the stimuli on the retina. The red laser can be controlled so that different intensities may be delivered for each pixel in the field. The SLO can present any stimulus that computer graphics can create, so spots of light, letters and words, and different patterns can be displayed. The fundus image is viewed on a monitor, and it is possible to see the stimulus and its position on the retina. One can then observe where the patient fixates, and whether fixation moves during testing. Sunness and co-workers have developed a technique for macular perimetry on the SLO that corrects for eye movements during the testing and provides a retinally correct display of the results on a fundus image.[39] The SLO technique allows for preplanning a grid of points to test, and randomizing the order. The investigator chooses two retinal landmarks (such as vessel bifurcations) and clicks on one of these to present each stimulus. The stimulus is then moved to a corrected position, based on the movement of the landmark that has taken place. In future years, the same retinal locations can be tested even if fixation has changed, since the technique specifies stimulus position by its relationship to retinal landmarks, rather than by the location of fixation. This will allow for longitudinal testing to map progression and therapeutic efficacy.[39] With this technique, one can better understand the visual difficulties of patients with tiny central seeing islands surrounded by an absolute scotoma in Stargardt disease, cone dystrophy, and other bulls-eye macular disorders (Fig. 15.3*A*,*B*).

When the SLO technique was used, central scotomas were mapped and fixation was studied in eyes with Stargardt disease and compared to eyes with the geographic atrophy form of advanced age-related macular degeneration and comparable visual acuity. Age-related geographic atrophy of the macula causes circumscribed areas of loss of retinal pigment epithelium and the area of atrophy enlarges over time. Geographic atrophy causes an absolute scotoma in affected areas of the macula.[35] In patients with geographic atrophy and foveal involvement, fixation is essentially always just at the edge of the scotoma (presumably because this is the site closest to the fovea and thus has the best acuity).[34] In eyes with Stargardt disease and visual acuity of 20/80 to 20/200, there was also an atrophic region with a corresponding central absolute scotoma. In contrast to geographic atrophy, fixation in eyes with Stargardt disease and a central scotoma was located not at the edge of the absolute scotoma, but rather at a position several degrees above the edge on normal-appearing retina.[34] The intervening retina detected stimuli, though it may have had a mild relative scotoma (Fig. 15.3*C*). These findings suggest that the areas with decreased function were not limited to the atrophic areas seen on fundus examination, but included less clinically involved retina. Similarly, the measured visual acuity may be less than might be predicted by fundus appearance alone.[34] The SLO can help give insight into the pattern of fixation that a patient has adopted, so that the physician and low-vision specialist can help the patient utilize the remaining vision optimally.

THE ELECTRORETINOGRAM

The electroretinogram (ERG) is an electrical mass response of the entire retina. Widespread

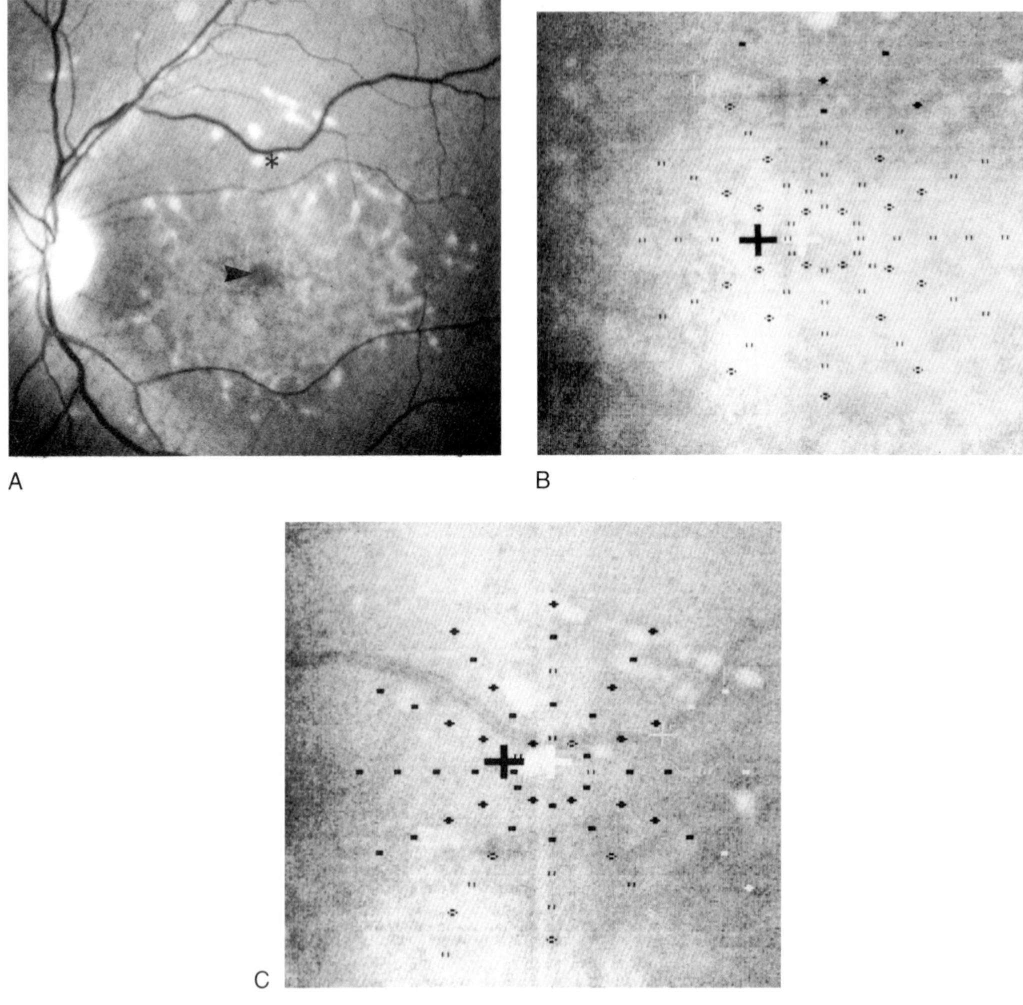

Figure 15.3. Scanning laser ophthalmoscope macular perimetry in an eye with fundus flavimaculatus (Stargardt's disease) from Sunness et al., ref. 34. (**A**) Fundus photograph showing an atrophic macular lesion and flecks surrounding this. There is a very small spared area centrally (arrowhead). Fixation is placed either in this center or superiorly, just near the superior arcade vessel, at a distance from the edge of the atrophic lesion (asterisk). (**B**) Scanning laser ophthalmoscope perimetry of the eye in (**A**). The white fixation cross was seen and fixated centrally in the spared area indicated by the arrowhead in (**A**). (The black cross is generated by the computer and is not displayed to the patient.) This area was totally surrounded by an area of dense scotoma extending to an eccentricity of 3° degrees (900 μm) superiorly and to at least 5° (1500 μm) in all other directions. The unfilled symbols show areas of dense scotoma; the solid symbols show areas of seeing retina. Letters of 20/60 in size were read in this fixation site. (**C**) Scanning laser ophthalmoscope perimetry of eye in (**A**). The symbols are the same as in (**B**). For a good portion of the test, the patient used a second fixation site—near the arcade vessel—corresponding to the site marked with an asterisk in (**A**). In this site, letters of 20/160 could be read. This site is not at the margin of the dense scotoma but at a distance from it.

retinal disease must be present to cause a significant ERG abnormality. To ensure uniform illumination of the retina, a bowl that diffusely illuminates the entire retina (a Ganzfeld, or full-field stimulus) must be used. The ERG can distinguish between rod and cone function, and between inner retinal (bipolar cell) and outer retinal (photoreceptor) disease. It is not affected by isolated ganglion cell or optic nerve damage.

The pupils are dilated. The eyes are patched for 30 or more minutes of dark adaptation. The ERG testing conditions are designed to separate rod from cone function (Table 15.1). Specifically, rods are very sensitive in the dark and to blue stimuli but they cannot follow a rapidly flashing stimulus, and they become saturated in bright light. In contrast, cones can follow rapidly flashing stimuli and retain sensitivity in the light. To measure rod function, a dark-adapted ERG is performed with a flash of light in the dark. Blue light or dim white light flashes can be used to isolate the rod component, but even a bright flash in the dark reflects primarily rod activity. To measure cone function, either a light-adapted (photopic) ERG with a bright flash of light, or a flicker ERG, typically using a 30 Hz flicker frequency of the stimulating light, is performed in the presence of background illumination. A contact lens electrode is used to measure the electrical events occurring in the eye in response to the stimulus. The waveform of voltage is measured as a function of time. The voltages measured over time may be displayed on an oscilloscope and photographed. Alternatively, computer-controlled systems are now widely used to present stimuli and record the electrical responses so that these may be printed and stored for analysis at a later time. A standard for ERG testing has been published in an effort to have comparable responses recorded in different laboratories across the world.[22] The standards recommend measuring five responses. A dim white or blue light in the dark-adapted state (1) and a bright flash in the dark-adapted state (2) primarily measure rod activity. Oscillatory potentials (3) are a measure of inner retinal (amacrine cell) activity and are extracted from the ascending portion of the response to (2). A flickering light (4) and a flash on a light background (5) are used to measure cone function.

The dark-adapted flash and the flicker are described in detail in this chapter. Typical normal waveforms for the dark-adapted and flicker ERG are shown in Figs. 15.4 and 15.5. Clinically, we generally evaluate the *a* and *b* waves, although these waves are actually composites of three different cellular responses.[18] The negative *a* wave represents outer retinal function, and the *b* wave reflects inner retinal (primarily bipolar cell, through the conduction of Müller

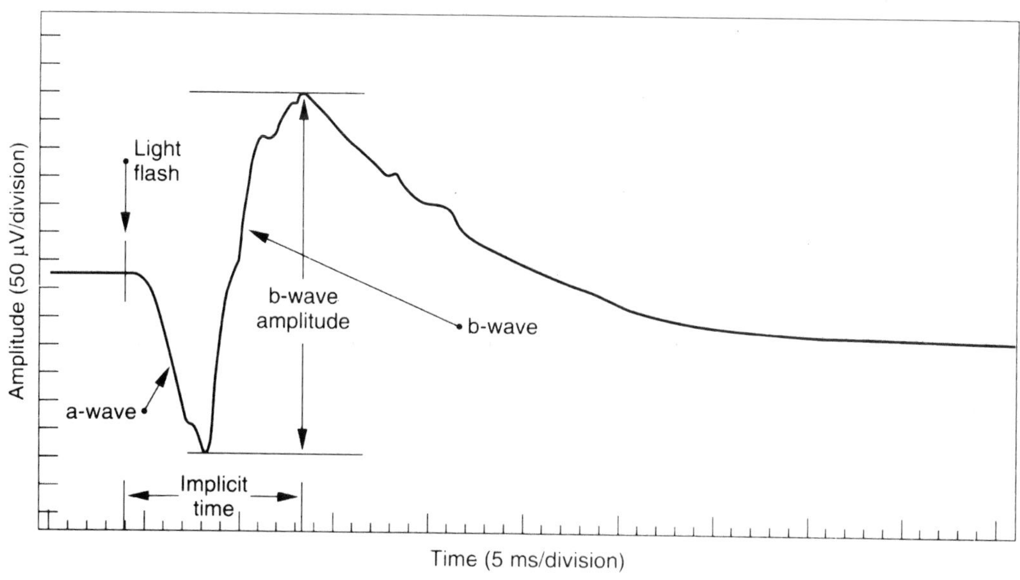

Figure 15.4. The dark-adapted electroretinogram to a bright flash. The *a* wave, *b* wave, and oscillatory potentials are shown. *b*-Wave amplitude is measured from the trough of the *a* wave to the peak of the *b* wave. *b*-Wave implicit time is measured from the onset of the light flash to the peak of the *b* wave. (Reprinted with permission from J. S. Sunness, Clinical retinal function testing. *Focal Points: Clinical Modules for Ophthalmologists*, IX(1), San Francisco, American Academy of Ophthalmology, 1991.)

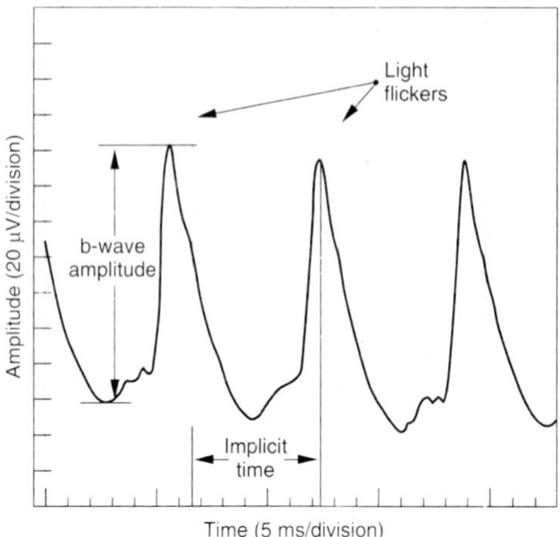

Figure 15.5. The flicker electroretinogram (ERG) in response to a 30-Hz stimulus. *b*-Wave amplitude and implicit time are defined in the same manner as for the single-flash ERG (**A**). (Reprinted with permission from J. S. Sunness, Clinical retinal function testing. In *Focal Points: Clinical Modules for Ophthalmologists*, IX(1), American Academy of Ophthalmology, 1991.)

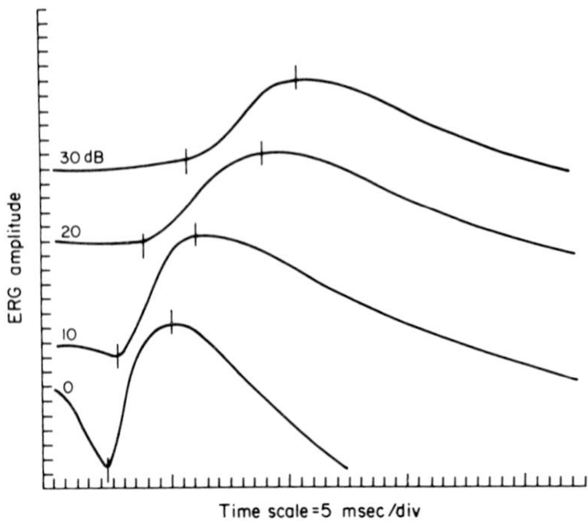

Figure 15.6. The dark-adapted electroretinogram in response to flashes of different stimulus intensity. The decibel (dB) level is the magnitude in decibels of the neutral density filter used, so that a 30-dB stimulus is 3 log units less intense than the 0-dB stimulus. As the stimulus intensity increases, the *a* wave becomes more prominent and the implicit time (time from stimulus onset to the peak of the *b* wave becomes shorter).

cells) function. The oscillatory potentials appear on the ascending limb of the *b* wave when a bright flash is used, and may reflect amacrine cell activity. The implicit time (time from onset of stimulus to peak of *b* wave), and amplitude of the *b* wave (measured from trough of the *a* wave to the peak of the *b* wave) are measured from each waveform. In our laboratory, the dark adapted *b* wave has a normal amplitude $\leq$300 μV and an implicit time of about 50 ms. The shape of the waveform changes with stimulus intensity (Fig. 15.6). At low-intensity levels, the *a* wave is smaller and the implicit time of the response is longer. An intensity-response function (Fig. 15.7), showing the dependence of the *b* wave amplitude of the response on stimulus intensity, may be evaluated to learn more, for example, about whether the changes in the ERG are due to loss of photoreceptors or a decrease in their sensitivity.[29] Ischemic change in the retina may lead to changes in the intensity-response function and in changes in the implicit time of the response.[23] An intensity-response function of the *a* wave has been used to study rod phototransduction in retinitis pigmentosa.[21]

The flicker ERG has a normal amplitude of about 100 μV and an implicit time of about 30 ms. By inspecting the tracing, one can roughly determine if a flicker response is delayed. Normally, the *b* wave peaks just before the next flash (i.e., before the next vertical line); a *b* wave coming after the vertical line is a delayed response.

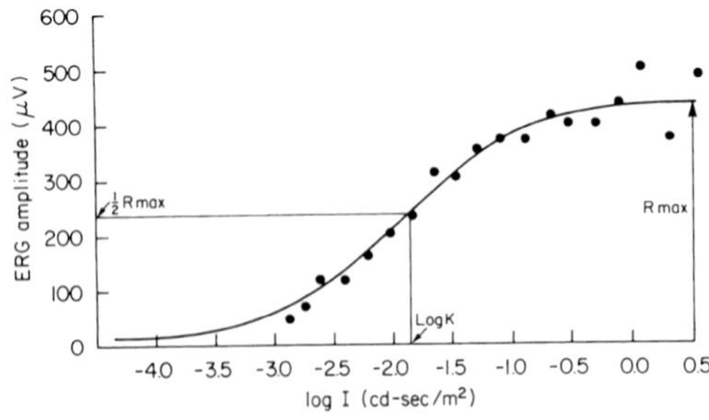

Figure 15.7. The electroretinogram *b*-wave intensity response function. The ERG is measured over a range of stimulus intensities. The data are then fit to a Naka–Rushton equation,[29] and the s-shaped curve is obtained. One can extract R_{max}, the maximal stimulus intensity, log *K* (also called log sigma), the intensity at which the response is half the maximal response, and a slope parameter. Log *K* reflects retinal sensitivity and may reflect changes caused by ischemia and other pathologic processes.

The use of the ERG has come to be associated with the workup of patients with retinal degenerations, and especially with RP, in which the ERG response is often unrecordable except with special averaging techniques. Natural history studies of RP have followed the decrease in ERG amplitude over time.[3] A recent treatment trial of RP showed that patients who were treated with vitamin A had less progressive reduction in ERG amplitude than patients who did not receive vitamin A.[2] There was a trend to a reduced loss of visual field in treated patients. The significance of the results of this study has been disputed, in part because of the very small ERG amplitudes and signal-averaging techniques on which the study relied.[28]

The usefulness of the ERG is certainly not limited to RP, and in most typical cases of RP the ERG is not necessary for diagnosis. The ERG can be helpful in many other clinical situations, as discussed in the paragraphs that follow.

Diffuse Versus Localized Retinal Disease

The ERG is a summated response of the whole retina, so that a disease confined to the macula will only cause at most a small decrease in ERG amplitude. Even though the cone density is very high in the fovea, this high density is confined to a very small retinal area, so that about 95% of the cones are located outside the foveal region. In cone dystrophy, a diffuse retinal disease with prominent macular manifestations, there are significant abnormalities in the photopic and flicker ERG, whereas a localized macular process would not have a significant ERG abnormality. On the other hand, the ERG often does not correlate with the visual acuity; a patient with a diffuse disease such as retinitis pigmentosa that has not yet severely affected the macular region may have 20/20 visual acuity and a nonrecordable ERG.

Rod Versus Cone Involvement

The different components of the ERG allow the separate evaluation of rod and cone functions, therefore allowing the assessment of the integrity of each system. For example, in cone dystrophy the flicker or photopic ERG is significantly reduced, whereas the dark-adapted ERG may be near normal (Fig. 15.8). In contrast, in typical congenital stationary night blindness, the dark-adapted ERG is abnormal, with a normal light-adapted or flicker ERG, although there are variations of this pattern. In retinal degenerations involving both systems, dark-adapted, photopic, and flicker ERGs are abnormal.

Outer Versus Inner Retinal Involvement

The *a* wave reflects outer retinal function, and the *b* wave reflects inner retinal function. The ERG waveform may reflect the abnormalities in the involved retinal layers. For example, a central retinal artery occlusion affects the inner retina and causes a loss of the *b* wave but leaves the *a* wave intact. (It then appears as a giant negative *a* wave since the opposing *b* wave is absent.) If both inner and outer retina are in-

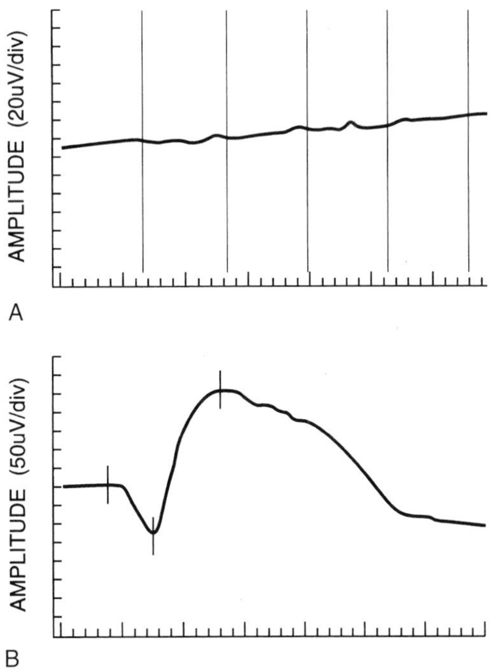

Figure 15.8. Electroretinogram (ERG) in cone dystrophy. (**A**) The flicker ERG response is severely reduced, reflecting the cone involvement. (**B**) The dark-adapted response to a bright flash is normal, reflecting the basically intact rod system.

volved, such as in an ophthalmic artery occlusion, loss of both *a* and *b* waves occurs.

Other conditions, such as X-linked juvenile retinoschisis and some forms of congenital night blindness, may have a loss of *b* wave amplitude as compared with the *a* wave.

Retinal Versus Central Nervous System Pathology

The ERG as described thus far is purely a retinal response and provides an objective measure of retinal function. If the optic nerve or central visual pathways are damaged while the retina is normal, the ERG will be normal. A normal ERG may also provide confirmatory evidence for cases of hysteria or malingering. But, again, it is not sensitive to isolated macular defects, so it cannot help distinguish between a localized macular lesion and an optic nerve or other neural defect. An abnormal ERG thus provides evidence of retinal dysfunction, but a normal ERG cannot rule out a localized retinal disorder. (See the discussion of the focal and multifocal ERG below.)

Using the ERG in Infants or in Patients Who Cannot Give Subjective Responses

When subjective measures of visual function cannot be used, as in infants or mentally retarded patients, the ERG, along with the flash visual evoked response, may provide helpful objective evidence of the presence of retinal function.

Using the ERG When the Retina Cannot Be Visualized

The ERG may also help in the assessment of the potential for retinal functional viability in eyes with a dense cataract or vitreous hemorrhage.

Focal, Multifocal, and Pattern ERG Testing

The focal ERG is a measurement of the electrical response of the eye to stimulation of a localized area of retina by a flickering light. A surrounding ring of bright light prevents the flickering light from stimulating other retinal areas, so that unlike the standard ERG, the focal ERG is not a mass response of the eye. The pupil is dilated, and a contact lens electrode is used to record the response. The electrical responses are very small (less than 1 μV). The Maculascope (Doran Instruments, Littleton, MA) incorporates the stimulating device into a direct ophthalmoscope so that the area being stimulated can be directly viewed, whereas the LKC system (Gaithersburg, MD) uses a monocular indirect ophthalmoscope. Other devices allowing for retinal viewing during stimulation have also been used for focal recording. The focal ERG is used to measure macular function, as its amplitude falls off rapidly outside the macula. The focal ERG is abnormal in the presence of almost any macular disease with visual acuity of 20/40 or less, but it is not specific for particular diseases.[11] Its clinical usefulness has not yet been established. Miyake has described a group of patients with a hereditary bilateral macular dystrophy associated with decreased central vision. This condition is characterized by an abnormal focal ERG in the presence of a normal Ganzfeld ERG.[30] Miyake categorizes these patients as having a specific cone defect limited to the macula. However, the focal ERG is also reduced due to involvement of the macula by processes not specific for cone disorders.

The multifocal ERG uses different sequences of stimuli to a number of retinal areas, and simultaneously records ERGs from these areas. In this way, a map of the retina to about 50° can be constructed. Good mapping of decreased function in some retinal diseases has been published, although normal data, reproducibility, and reliability of measurements have not. This is an exciting instrument that may play an important role in mapping retinal dysfunction in the future.[40]

The pattern ERG measures ganglion cell function. It uses a stimulus similar to the pattern visual evoked potential (VEP). Its clinical usefulness has not yet been established, but research on its use is ongoing in patients with glaucoma and ocular hypertension, and in a variety of diseases causing decrease in central vision.[1]

THE ELECTROOCULOGRAM

The electrooculogram (EOG) is a slow electrical mass response of the eye. It measures the changes (over a 30 min interval) in the electric potential of the eye caused by exposure to dark and to light. It is thought to reflect the metabolic integrity of the retinal pigment epithelium. The EOG is measured by applying skin electrodes near the inner and outer canthi and measuring the voltage difference between the anterior and posterior points of the globe by having the patient look in one direction and then in the other. The EOG is also a summated electrical potential of the eye, and Ganzfeld (full-field) illumination should be employed. In the LKC instrument, there is a central fixation target and two red light–emitting diodes (LEDs), one to the left and one to the right of the fixation target. During the test, the two LEDs alternately go on and off for about 15 sec for each minute, so that the subject shifts gaze from one LED to the other. The computer measures the difference in potential between the anterior and posterior aspect of each eye by adding the electrical potentials measured between the EOG electrodes when the eye is pointed in one direction and then in the other. After a few minutes of preadaptation to a background light, the light is turned off and measurement is done in the dark for about 15 min. The background light is then turned on again and the measurement in the light is done for another 15 min. Most ERG systems are suited for measuring EOGs. Computer-based systems can measure and record the response over time.

A typical EOG curve is shown in Fig. 15.9. The critical value is the Arden ratio, the ratio of the height of the light peak to the dark trough; it should be approximately 1.8 or more, depending on the laboratory.

In most disorders, the EOG parallels the ERG and is probably not required for evaluation. The prominent exception to this rule is in Best's vitelliform macular dystrophy, in which the EOG is abnormal and the ERG is normal (Fig. 15.10). Interestingly, in this disorder, while the ophthalmoscopic findings are often limited to the macular region, the EOG abnormality reflects the diffuse retinal pigment epithelial changes found on histopathology.[16] The EOG is also used for measuring the toxicity of chloroquine.

Devices for measuring focal EOGs have been used to try to emphasize the contribution of the central retina to the EOG response.[15] However, the EOG remains insensitive to many types of macular change.[36]

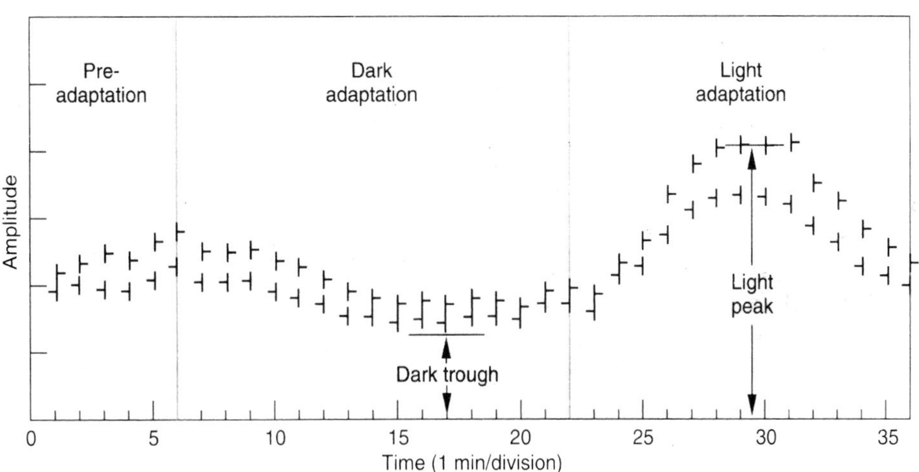

Figure 15.9. A normal electrooculogram curve of electrical potential versus time. Both eye areas plotted. The ratio of the light peak to the dark trough (Arden ratio) is measured from this curve as shown, and is 2.6. (Reprinted with permission from J. S. Sunness, Clinical retinal function testing. In *Focal Points: Clinical Modules for Ophthalmologists*, IX(1). American Academy of Ophthalmology, San Francisco, 1991.)

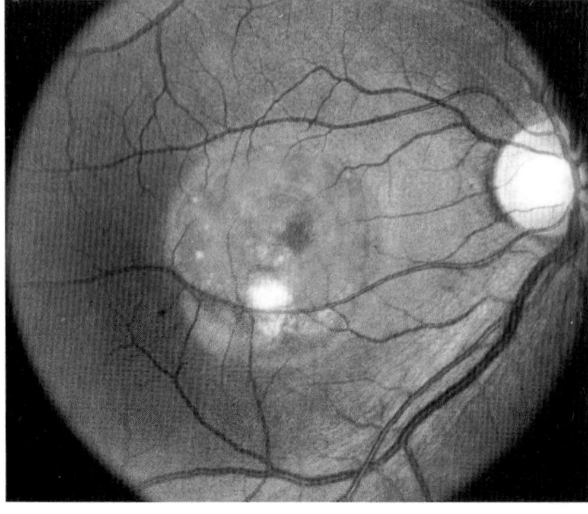

A

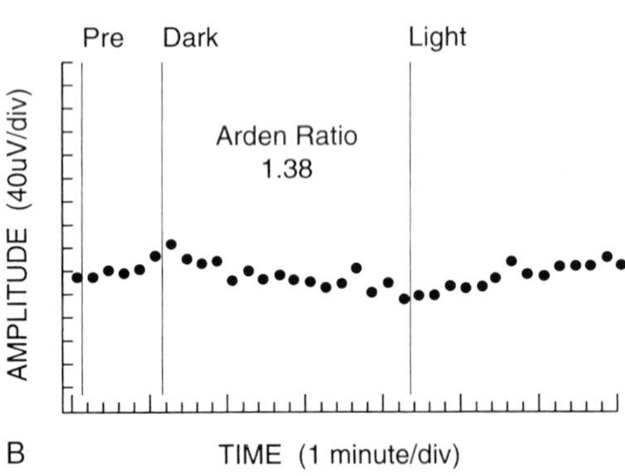

Figure 15.10. Electrooculogram (EOG) in Best's disease. (**A**) Fundus photograph showing a central vitelliform lesion typical of Best's disease. (**B**) EOG of eye shown in (**A**). The light peak is markedly reduced, with an Arden ratio of 1:38.

THE VISUAL EVOKED POTENTIAL

The VEP is the electrical activity generated in the occipital cortex in response to retinal stimulation. The test typically uses a patterned stimulus like a checkerboard to measure the response of the visual cortex. Squares of varying size are used, and the VEP can be recorded as a function of their size. Alternatively, the VEP may be recorded to a bright flash of light (bright-flash VEP). The patient must be wearing corrective lenses and the pupils are not dilated because good resolution of the stimulus is important. Scalp electrodes are used to measure and record the electrical response.

Measurement of the VEP requires a display that can generate alternating checkerboard squares with a range of sizes. Recording systems are necessary. Some computer-based testing systems combine ERG, EOG, and VEP recording capabilities.

The main clinical parameters evaluated in the VEP are the amplitude of, and the time to, the first positive peak, called P1 or P100, since it is seen about 100 ms following pattern alternation (Fig. 15.11). Signal averaging is required since the amplitude of the response may only be a few microvolts. The response may be delayed in conditions such as optic neuritis (Fig. 15.11B). A bright-flash VEP may be used if the ocular media are opaque and an assessment of the visual pathways is required.

The VEP provides an evaluation of the totality of the visual system from retina through primary visual cortex, but the response reflects mainly macular function, because the macula is geographically overrepresented on the occipital cortex. Although it does not provide specific information about retinal function, it may be useful as part of a retinal evaluation in two ways: If the pattern or bright-flash VEP is normal, it suggests integrity of the visual system (although there may still be peripheral field defects, for example). This may be useful in situations in which the retina cannot be visualized and in cases of hysteria or malingering. If the retina appears normal and the ERG is normal, but the VEP is abnormal, one must consider an evaluation for optic nerve or higher center disease. Again, one must remember that a normal ERG does not rule out isolated macular pathology. The VEP may have characteristic amplitude and timing changes that may also help to evaluate the specific nature of the defect. Macular disorders tend to produce a decrease in VEP amplitude, or a change confined to the smaller check sizes, whereas optic nerve and higher center defects may produce a delayed response or a different pattern of change as a function of check size. More refined testing, using lateral scalp electrodes, can assess abnormal decussation patterns in albinism.

CONCLUSIONS

The visual function tests described have been of significant value in making diagnoses and quantifying the impact of a retinal disease on visual function. With time, these tests may

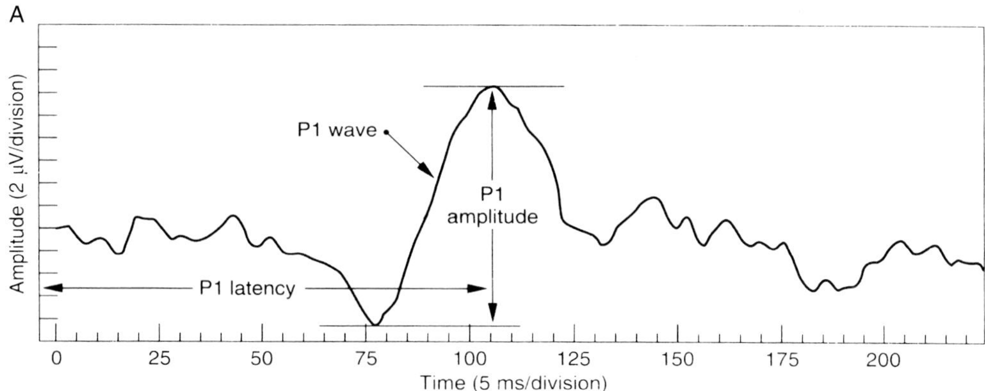

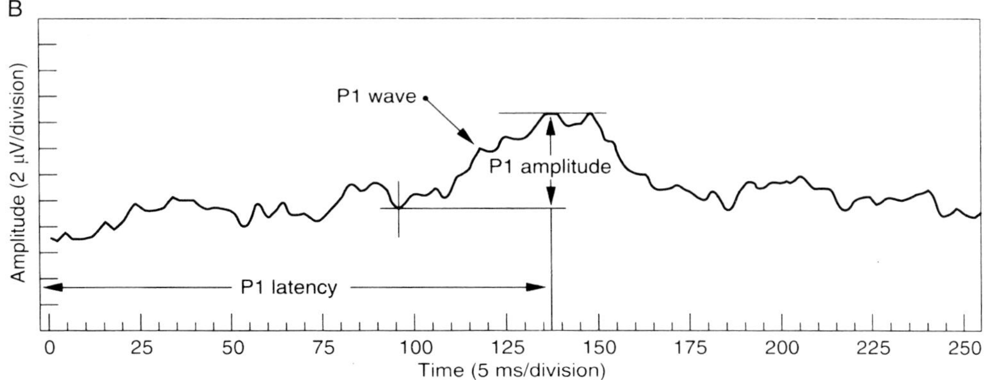

Figure 15.11. The visual evoked potential (VEP). (**A**) A normal VEP, showing the P1 (or P100) wave. P1 latency is measured from the time of pattern alternation to the time of peak of the P1 wave (107 ms in this case), and P1 amplitude is measured from the trough of the negative wave just before P1 (called N1) to the peak of the P1 wave. (**B**) A VEP recorded with stimulation of an eye with optic neuritis in a patient with multiple sclerosis. The P1 amplitude is decreased, and there is an increase in P1 latency to 137 ms. (Reprinted with permission of J. S. Sunness, Clinical retinal function testing. In *Focal Points: Clinical Modules for Ophthalmologists*, IX(1), San Francisco, American Academy of Ophthalmology, 1991.)

prove to be even more important because they may be good measures of both the efficacy and the toxicity of different proposed therapies. This determination will require critical assessments of the reproducibility and variability of such measures in normal patients over time. Thus visual function measures and other forms of assessment may advance understanding of visual physiology and help determine the function of various gene products in the retina.

Acknowledgements: This work was supported in part by National Eye Institute Research grant EY08552. The author would like to thank Ms. Stacy Cofield for collecting the electrophysiological data included, and Mr. Joseph Dieter for his help with the illustrations. Figures 15.1, 15.4, 15.5, 15.9, and 15.11 and Table 15.1 are reprinted with permission from J. S. Sunness, Clinical retinal function testing. In *Focal Points: Clinical Modules for Ophthalmologists*, IX(1), American Academy of Ophthalmology, 1991.

REFERENCES

1. Berninger T, Arden GB. The pattern electroretinogram. In *Principles and Practice of Clinical Electrophysiology of Vision*, J. R. Heckenlively and G. B. Arden, eds. St. Louis: Mosby Year-Book, 1991, pp. 291–300.
2. Berson EL, Rosner B, Sandberg MA et al. A randomized trial of vitamin A and vitamin E supplementation for retinitis pigmentosa. *Arch Ophthalmol* 1993;111:761–772.

3. Berson, EL, Sandberg MA, Rosner B et al. Natural course of retinitis pigmentosa over a three-year interval. *Am J Ophthalmol* 1985; 99:240–251.
4. Bird AC. Retinal photoceptor dystrophies. L. I. Edward Jackson Memorial Lecture. *Am J Ophthalmol* 1995;119:543–562.
5. Boynton RM. *Human Color Vision*. New York: Holt, Rinehart and Winston, 1979.
6. Carr RE. Congenital stationary nightblindness. *Trans Am Ophthalmol Soc* 1974;72:448–487.
7. Carr RE. Abnormalities of cone and rod function. In *Retina* S. J. Ryan, ed. St. Louis: Mosby Year-Book, 1994; pp. 502–514.
8. Carr RE, Siegel IM. *Electrodiagnostic Testing of the Visual System: A Clinical Guide*. Philadelphia: F.A. Davis Company, 1990.
9. Cornsweet TN. *Visual Perception*. New York: Academic Press, 1971.
10. Eisner A, Klein ML, Zilis JD et al. Visual function and the subsequent development of exudative age-related macular degeneration. *Invest Ophthalmol Vis Sci* 1992;33:3091–3102.
11. Fish GE, Birch DG. The focal electroretinogram in the clinical assessment of macular disease. *Ophthalmology* 1989;96:109–114.
12. Fishman GA, Farbman JS, Alexander KR. Delayed rod dark adaptation in patients with Stargardt's disease. *Ophthalmology* 1991;98: 957–962.
13. Fishman GA, Pulluru P, Alexander KR et al. Prolonged rod dark adaptation in patients with cone-rod dystrophy. *Am J Ophthalmol* 1994; 118:362–367.
14. Fishman GA, Sokol S. *Electrophysiologic Testing in Disorders of the Retina, Optic Nerve, and Visual Pathway*. Ophthalmology Monographs. San Francisco: American Academy of Ophthalmology, 1990.
15. Fishman GA, Young RSL, Schall SP et al. Electro-oculogram testing in fundus flavimaculatus. *Arch Ophthalmol* 1979;97:1896–1898.
16. Frangieh GT, Green WR, Fine SL. A histopathological study of Best's vitelliform dystrophy. *Arch Ophthalmol* 1982;100:1115–1121.
17. Fuller DG, Birch DG, eds. Assessment of visual function for the clinician. *Ophthalmol Clin N Am* Saunders, 1989;2.
18. Granit R. The components of the retinal action potential and their relation to the discharge in the optic nerve. *J Physiol (London)* 1933;77:207–240.
19. Harrington DO. *The Visual Fields: A Textbook and Atlas of Clinical Perimetry*, 5th ed. St. Louis: Mosby Year-Book, 1981.
20. Heckenlively JR, Arden GB: *Principles and Practice of Clinical Electrophysiology of Vision*. St. Louis: Mosby Year-Book, 1991.
21. Hood DC, Birch DG. Rod phototransduction in retinitis pigmentosa: Estimation and interpretation of parameters derived from the rod a-wave. *Invest Ophthalmol Vis Sci* 1994;35:2948–2961.
22. Marmor MF, Zrenner E. Standard for clinical electroretinography (1994 update). *Doc Ophthalmol* 89:199–210, 1995.
23. Johnson MA, Marcus S, Elman MJ et al. Neovascularization in central retinal vein occlusion: Electroretinographic findings. *Arch Ophthalmol* 1988;106:348–352.
24. Kemp CM, Jacobson SG, Roman AJ et al. Abnormal rod dark adaptation in autosomal dominant retinitis pigmentosa with proline-23-histidine rhodopsin mutation. *Am J Ophthalmol* 1992;113:165–174.
25. Marmor MF. Fundus albipunctatus: A clinical study of the fundus lesions, the physiologic defect, and vitamin A metabolism. *Doc Ophthalmol* 1977;43:277–302.
26. Massof RW, Dagnelie G, Benzschawel T et al. First order dynamics of visual field loss in retinitis pigmentosa. *Clin Vis Sci* 1990;5:1–26.
27. Massof RW, Finkelstein D. Two forms of autosomal dominant primary retinitis pigmentosa. *Doc Ophthalmol* 1981;51:289–346.
28. Massof RW, Finkelstein D. Supplemental vitamin A retards loss of ERG amplitude in retinitis pigmentosa. *Arch Ophthalmol* 1993;111: 751–754.
29. Massof RW, Wu L, Finkelstein D et al. Properties of electroretinographic intensity-response functions in retinitis pigmentosa. *Doc Ophthalmol* 1984;57:279–296.
30. Miyake Y, Ichikawa K, Shiose Y et al. Hereditary macular dystrophy without visible fundus abnormality. *Am J Ophthalmol* 1989;108:292–299.
31. Newman EA, Odette LL. Model of electroretinogram b-wave generation: A test of the K^+ hypothesis. *J Neurophysiol* 1984;51:164–182.
32. Pokorny J, Smith VC, Verriest G et al. *Congenital and Acquired Color Vision Defects*. New York: Grune & Stratton, 1979.
33. Sunness JS. Visual function evaluation of a patient with congenital nightblindness and white spots in the fundus. *Optical Society of America Technical Digest, Noninvasive Assessment of the Visual System*, 1992; pp. TuB1-1–TuB1-4.
34. Sunness JS, Applegate CA, Haselwood D, Rubin GS. Fixation patterns and reading rates in eyes

with central scotomas from advanced atrophic age-related macular degeneration and Stargardt's disease. *Ophthalmology*, 1996;103: 1458–1466.

35. Sunness JS, Johnson MA, Massof RW et al. Retinal sensitivity over drusen and nondrusen areas. A study using fundus perimetry. *Arch Ophthalmol* 1988;106:1081–1084.
36. Sunness JS, Massof RW. The focal electro-oculogram in age-related macular degeneration. *Am J Optom Physiol Opt* 1986;63:7–11.
37. Sunness JS, Massof RW, Johnson MA et al. Diminished foveal sensitivity may predict the development of advanced age-related macular degeneration. *Ophthalmology* 1989;96:375–381.
38. Sunness JS, Massof RW, Johnson MA et al. Peripheral retinal function in age-related macular degeneration. *Arch Ophthalmol* 1985;103: 811–816.
39. Sunness JS, Schuchard R, Shen N et al. Landmark-driven fundus perimetry using the scanning laser ophthalmoscope (SLO). *Invest Ophthalmol Vis Sci* 1995;36:1863–1874.
40. Sutter EE, Tran D. The field topography of ERG components in man—I. The photopic luminance response. *Vision Res* 1992;32:433–446.
41. Teller DY. Linking propositions. *Vision Res* 1984;24:1233–1246.
42. Walsh TJ, ed. *Visual Fields: Examination and Interpretation.* Ophthalmology monograph #3. San Francisco: American Academy of Ophthalmology, 1990.

16

Disorders of Color Vision

SAMIR S. DEEB
ARNO G. MOTULSKY

Color vision and its mechanism have intrigued and puzzled scientists for several hundred years. An important part of the puzzle was uncovered in the seventeenth century by Sir Isaac Newton, who demonstrated that light was a mixture of different-colored rays and that rays reflected from objects had the power to elicit color sensation in the retina. The color objects appear to have is therefore determined by the subsets of rays they reflect.

HISTORICAL

The existence of individuals with severe color vision defects has been known for several centuries, but the first published reports were from the eighteenth century.[31] Milder anomalies in color vision have been known for over 100 years. Two centuries ago the chemist John Dalton described his own red–green color blindness,[13] and since then the term "daltonism" has been commonly used as a name for "color blindness." Dalton is credited with the first in-depth analysis of color blindness. He proposed that his color blindness resulted from having a vitreous humor that was tinted blue and absorbed light of longer wavelengths. He donated his eyes after death in order to confirm his hypothesis. Examination of Dalton's vitreous humor found no support for his hypothesis to explain color blindness. Alternative explanations for color blindness had been proposed at that time. One involved defects in the visual center of the brain. We know now that color vision is mediated by three classes of retinal photoreceptors tuned to different parts of the visible spectrum, and that color vision defects are due to either loss or modification of the pigments in one or more of these photoreceptors. Amazingly, explanations similar to these were circulating at the end of the eighteenth century (see Gouras,[29] for a review). The three-receptor theory of color vision was proposed by Giros von Gentilly and Thomas Young. Based on Dalton's description of the solar spectrum as having lacked red color, Young postulated that Dalton lacked the red photoreceptors and therefore would be classified as a protanope.

The type and molecular basis for Dalton's color vision defect was recently determined.[38] Fragments from one of Dalton's eyes had been preserved. DNA analysis of the X-linked red and green pigment genes revealed that, contrary to Young's conclusion, he was a deuteranope, missing the gene encoding the green-sensitive pigment.

Pedigrees of "color-blindness" extending over several generations were reported,[37] long before the rediscovery of Mendel's laws. Very early in the history of human genetics, the American pioneer of fruit fly genetics, Wilson in 1911, suggested X-linked recessive inheritance as the explanation for the transmission of color blindness. *Color blindness*, or more correctly, *color vision defects*, therefore represents one of the first human traits shown to follow Mendelian inheritance.

COLOR VISION AND ITS ASSESSMENT

Visible colors represent the range of electromagnetic radiation extending from about 400 nm (violet) to 700 nm (red). Visible radiation of a particular wavelength (monochromatic light) under well-defined conditions has a characteristic color for observers with normal color vision. Most naturally occurring colors or hues may be produced by mixtures of monochromatic light. Newton already noticed this phenomenon in that the human eye could not distinguish between a mixture of red and green light and the sensation produced by pure yellow light that had a refractive angle intermediate between red and green. During the nineteenth century the trichromatic theory of color perception was placed on a firm basis.[335,55,109] It was shown that most colors can be matched by a mixture of three primary lights. Each set of three primaries has to include a long-wave, an intermediate-wave, and a short-wave light. Equal portions of these lights produce the perception of white. Color vision, therefore, was shown to be a system with only three perceptual dimensions.

Psychophysical methods of assessment of the color vision status are based on color-matching ability. They are exquisitely sensitive and are used to differentiate the various classes and subclasses of color vision defects, and even to measure subtle variations in color discrimination ability among individuals with normal color vision (see review by Ruddock[82]).

Clinically used tests are simplified versions of the psychophysical methods (see review by Birch[6]) and are generally based on pigment colors. They are used in screening for individuals with color vision deficiency and in grading them as having slight, moderate, or severe defects. Therefore, these tests are designed to place subjects into the protan, deutan, or tritan series but not to subclassify them into dichromats and anomalous trichromats. Subclassification requires the use of spectral tests (anomaloscopy). The most commonly used tests are briefly described as follows.

Pseudoisochromatic plates are the most widely used tests for screening of color vision defects. The figures to be discriminated on these plates appear in shades of different chromatic quality. The tests usually use patterns of variously colored printed dots, which usually are shaped as numbers. The subject is asked to read or trace a shape or number. The charts are so designed that persons with color vision defects will miss shapes or numbers and see different shapes than persons with normal color vision. The most widely used varieties are the Ishihara charts and the American Optical H-R-R (Hardy-Rand-Ritter) polychromatic plates. Distinction between deutan and protan abnormalities is usually possible using these charts, but subclassification is difficult, as severe anomalous trichromats cannot often be differentiated from dichromats.

The Farnsworth–Munsell 100 Hue Color arrangement test[24] has been widely used to identify and grade the severity of color vision deficiencies. In this test, an observer is asked to arrange a series of 85 color chips in their natural order of hue. Depending on the mistakes made, a standardized score is calculated and recorded on a special chart. Characteristic patterns for protans, deutans, and tritans are obtained, but differentiation between protanomaly and protanopia is difficult.

Anomaloscopy has been used widely and is based on color matching. Lord Rayleigh[81] devised a simple test system to classify individuals with red–green color vision abnormalities. The observer views a pure yellow light (589–590 nm) on one half of a screen while the other half of the screen projects a mixture of red (650 nm) and green (545–550 nm) lights. The brightness or intensity of the yellow light as well as the proportion of the green and red lights are adjusted by the subject until both hemifields appear identical in color and brightness. The most frequently used instrument is the Nagel anomaloscope. The range, referred to as the Rayleigh match range, of accepted matches of mixtures of green and red light against yellow is recorded, as is the midpoint of such matches.

Figure 16.1 shows typical findings for normal and various color defective persons and indicates the wide variation in severity of the color vision defects represented by the width of the Rayleigh match range. In addition, subtle variations in the width of the Rayleigh match range have also been observed among individuals classified as having normal color vision. Studies during the past few years have focused on correlating the genotype at the red/green gene locus with the color vision phenotype.

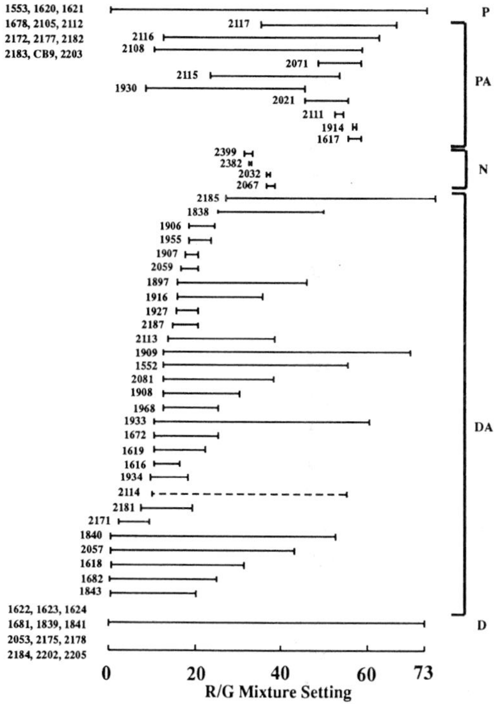

Figure 16.1. Anomaloscopic Rayleigh match ranges of protan, deutan, and normal subjects. Horizontal bars represent the range of red/green (R/G) mixture settings that each subject matched to the standard yellow light. Numbers to the left of the bars are for subject identification. The dotted bar is an approximation of the color match range of subject 2114, who had unreliable color match reports. P =protanopic; PA = protanomaly; D = deuteranopia; DA = deuteranomaly; N = normal. (Figure from S. S. Deeb et al., ref 15.)

CLASSIFICATION, FREQUENCY, AND INHERITANCE OF CONGENITAL COLOR VISION DEFECTS

In accordance with the trichromatic theory of color vision, individuals with normal color vision can match the color of a test light of any wavelength composition by mixing the right proportions of three primaries, such as red, green, and blue, or by mixing two of the primaries and adding the third to the test light. They are referred to as having trichromatic color vision. Individuals who lack functional red or green cones but retain blue cone function are known as protanopes (P) or deuteranopes (D), respectively. They are able to match the color of a test light by mixing two primaries only and, therefore, have dichromatic color vision. Dichromacy occurs in approximately 2% of Caucasian males, but it appears to be a common form of color vision among nonprimate mammals (reviewed in Jacobs[44]). Individuals with only blue functional cones are rare and are classified as having monochromatic vision.

A milder form of defective color vision among humans is anomalous trichromacy, which occurs in approximately ~5% of males of European origin (Table 16.1). Anomalous trichromats are believed to have three classes of photoreceptors, one of which has an anomalous spectral sensitivity curve. Protanomalous (PA) males (~1%) have normal blue-sensitive and green-sensitive cones but also anomalous red-sensitive cones with a spectral sensitivity that is shifted significantly toward that of the green-sensitive cone. Deuteranomalous (DA) individuals (~5%) have normal blue-sensitive and red-sensitive cones together with anomalous green-sensitive cones with a spectral sensitivity that is shifted significantly toward that of the red-sensitive cones.[80] It is interesting to note that the incidence of all forms of red–green color vision defects among Japanese males is 4.9% (with 95% confidence limits of 1.9).[40,75] The lower frequency relative to Caucasians is mainly due to a lower frequency (~2%) of deuteranomaly.

Color vision defects are frequently observed in several very rare cone dystrophies. In achromatopsia, there may be complete absence of cone responses, causing very poor or no color

Table 16.1 Classification and Frequency of Color Vision Defects

Type	Inheritance	Frequency[a]	Symptoms
Red–Green Defects	X-linked Recessive		
Protanopia, red–green		~1%	Severe color confusion
Deuteranopia		~1%	Severe red–green color confusion
Protanomaly		~1%	Mild red–green color confusion
Deuteranomaly		~5%	Mild red–green color confusion
Blue–Yellow Defects	Autosomal Dominant	~0.2%	Blue–yellow color confusion
Tritanopia			
Tritanomaly[b]	Autosomal dominant	?	
Achromatopsias			
Typical rod monochromacy	Autosomal recessive	~0.003%	Onset in infancy; low visual acuity
Atypical rod monochromacy (cones present but nonfunctional)	Autosomal recessive	Very rare	Pendular nystagmus, photophobia
Blue cone monochromacy	X-linked recessive	Rare	No ocular findings

[a]Among Caucasians.
[b]Distinction between tritanopia and tritanomaly not fully clarified.

discrimination, associated with low visual acuity, photophobia, and pendular nystagmus (Table 16.1). Onset is usually in infancy. Three principal classes have been identified (reviewed in references 63, 79, and 82): (*1*) Typical complete achromatopsia in which there are no or very few cones (rod monochromacy). This is inherited as an autosomal recessive trait. (2) Atypical rod monochromacy with present but non-functioning cone pigments. This defect is also inherited as autosomal recessive. (3) Blue-cone monochromacy, or X-linked incomplete achromotopsia,[66,67] where both red and green cones are nonfunctional, whereas blue-cone function is preserved. Many patients with these cone dystrophies also develop electroretinographically detectable rod abnormalities that are associated with symptoms of night blindness.[66]

PRACTICAL IMPLICATIONS OF COLOR VISION DEFECTS

Approximately 8%–10% (mostly males) of European extraction and 5% of males in other parts of the world have color vision defects and therefore live in a different perceptual world than those with normal color vision. The color perception of color-defective observers has been studied in a few individuals who for unknown reasons were color defective in one eye only. One otherwise healthy young woman was deuteranopic in the left eye and color-normal in the right eye (see Kalmus[48]). Her color vision defective eye had only three color sensations: gray, yellow, and blue and lacked any green and red sensations. Her normal eye gave normal color vision. Color perception of dichromatic deuteranopes in general conform to this general pattern. To a deuteranope, a rainbow looks mostly yellow and blue with a faint red stripe. On the other hand, dichromatic protanopia appears as a more severe defect than deuteranopia. Protanopes confuse not only red, yellow, and green like deuteranopes but also deep red, dark brown, or even black, and have particular problems with red color perception. A ripe red fruit might be considered black by a protanope. Color perception defects in anomalous trichromats are milder than in dichromats. Green and red are not absent but appear less intense. Color-defective persons, including dichromats, usually have no problem with the naming of colors. Apparently there are enough differences in color sensation to allow the denotation of the appropriate color as taught by parents and teachers.

It has been claimed by anecdotal evidence that color-defective observers can detect camouflaged objects better than normal observers.[47] This advantage would be useful under military conditions and could have played a role in the evolution of color vision.[1] A recent study suggests that dichromats, in fact, perform better than normal trichromats under experimental conditions where texture was camouflaged by color.[64]

Color vision is important in certain tasks and occupations. A questionnaire was designed to investigate whether color-defective individuals were aware of their defect and if they experienced any difficulties with everyday tasks and occupations that involved color.[86] About 90% of dichromats and up to two-thirds of anomalous trichromats reported difficulties. Half the dichromats reported confusion of colors of traffic lights, one-third found it difficult to distinguish traffic lights from street lighting, and one-fifth had difficulty detecting rear brake lights. It is therefore noteworthy that rear-end collisions, particularly under conditions of poor visibility, were slightly more common among protan drivers who have more problems with perception of red rear warning lights.[90] Although dichromats have problems with colors of traffic lights, they are able to distinguish between green and yellow lights because green appears white and yellow, yellow. The yellow light appears to be darker than it is. When it comes to recognizing stop signs, dichromats may have trouble noticing them if they happen to be placed against a backdrop of green foliage.

It is extremely important to identify color-defective children as early as possible in order to prevent learning disadvantages due to the increasing use of color in a variety of educational tools. Simple psychophysical or molecular genetic tests have not yet been developed to identify color-defective vision in children. Substantial numbers of dichromats reported that their defect influenced their choice of career and that they had been excluded from certain occupations. The ability of deutan to perform color-dependent tasks that are critical to air traffic controllers was investigated.[51,52] It was shown that mild deutan color vision defectives performed adequately, but moderately and severely defective subjects did not.

Voke,[91] Fletcher and Voke,[26] and Rosenthal and Phillips[81a] have written in detail on the subject of color vision defects in relation to various industrial and professional occupations. Currier[12] presented an interesting account of the experiences of a deuteranope in everyday life and in the medical profession.

THE GENETICS OF VARIATION IN RED–GREEN COLOR VISION

Photoreceptors and Photopigments

The human retina contains two classes of photoreceptor cells—rods and cones. Rods are responsible for vision in dim light, and cones are responsible for vision in bright light and for color vision. Human color vision is due to the absorption of light by three classes of cone photoreceptors, the short-wave-sensitive (blue), middle-wave-sensitive (green) and long-wave-sensitive (red) cones that have overlapping sensitivity curves with maxima at ~560, ~530, and ~420 nm, respectively.[14,61] Neural comparisons of quantal catches by the three cone classes give the sensation of color. The ratio between quantal catches by the three photoreceptors, which varies with wavelength of light (Fig. 16.2), is interpreted by the brain as a color along the spectrum. Because three classes of photoreceptors are used, humans, Old World monkeys, and a limited number of New World monkeys have full trichromatic color vision. There are approximately twice as many red as green cones in the human retina, with considerable variation in this ratio among individuals;[93] Blue cones constitute 10%–20% of the total number of cones.[11] Each cone contains only one of the photopigments. The photopigments are composed of a protein moiety called *opsin,* which is covalently linked to the chromophore *cis*-retinal, a derivative of vitamin A. The various opsins share varying degrees of homology. The red and green opsins are far more closely related to each other (96% amino acid identity) than to the blue and the red pigment rhodopsin (40%–45% identity). A charac-

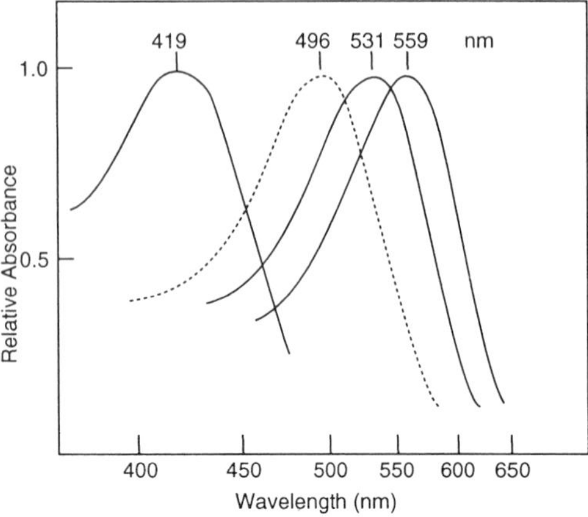

Figure 16.2. Absorption spectra of the four human photoreceptors. The dotted line is for rhodopsin and the solid lines are for the blue (l max = 419 nm), the green (l max = 531 nm), and the red (l max = 559 nm) cones. These curves are based on microspectrophotometric measurements of individual cones from human retinas. (Adapted from J. D. Mollon, ref. 61.)

teristic structural motif of this family of photopigments is the heptahelical transmembrane bundle within which the chromophore is held[8] (Fig. 16.3). The photopigments are embedded in the multiply folded membranes of the cone outer segments. The seven transmembrane segments are believed to be largely alpha-helical in character (Fig. 16.4).[36] The visual pigments belong to an evolutionarily related superfamily of heptahelical transmembrane receptors that includes the adrenergic, serotonergic, dopaminergic, muscarinic, and olfactory chemoreceptors (reviewed by Dohlman et al.[17]).

The absorption of a single photon of light causes the isomerization of the retinal chromophore of photopigments from the 11-*cis* to the all-*trans* configuration. This isomerization results in the formation of an activated photopigment that triggers the signal amplification cascade.[27,28,87] The first step in this cascade involves activation of transducin, which in turn activates a c-GMP (cyclic-guanosine 5′-monophosphate) phosphodiesterase. The resultant de-

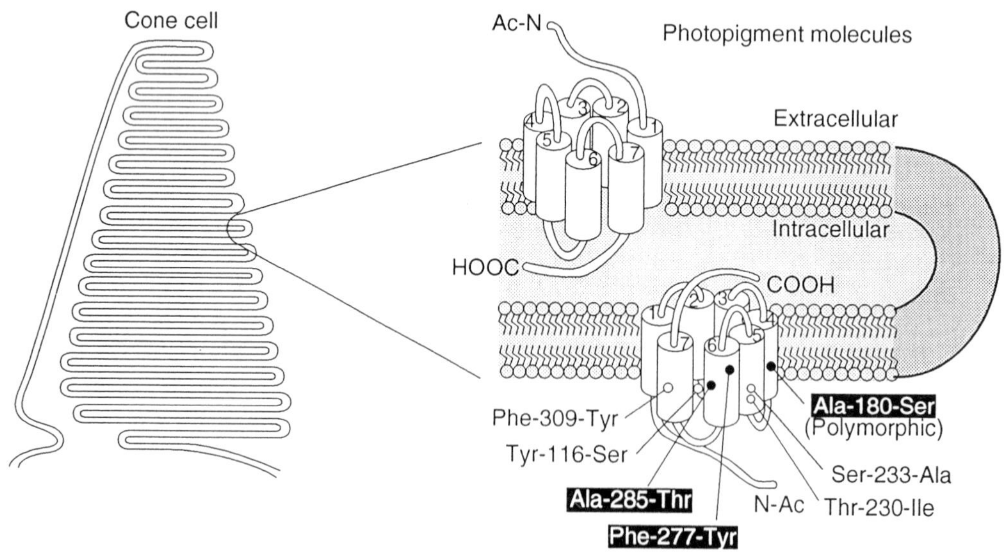

Figure 16.3. Diagram of a photopigment molecule embedded within the photoreceptor outer segment membrane. Diagram of photopigment molecules embedded within the membrane of cone outer segment. The cylinders represent the 7-a helices that form a bundle that holds the chromophore 11-*cis*-retinal. The difference in spectral sensitivity between the red and green pigments depends to a large extent on amino acid residues at positions 180, 277, and 285 and, to a lesser extent, on positions 116, 230, 233, and 309. Amino acids to the left of residue numbers are found in the green pigment and those to the right are found in the red pigment. (Adapted from J. D. Mollon, ref. 62.)

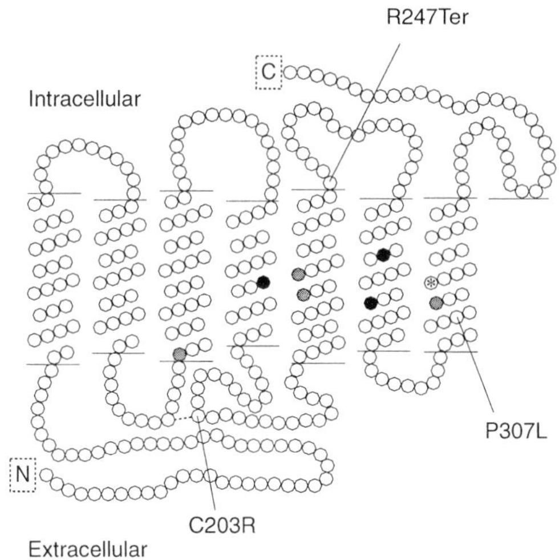

Figure 16.4. Schematic representation of the red/green pigments showing location of the seven amino acids involved in spectral tuning as well as of three point mutations. The seven a-helical segments are shown embedded within the plasma membrane. N and C denote amino- and carboxy-termini, respectively. The three amino acid residues at positions 180, 277, and 285 (filled with black) play a major role in spectral differences between the red and green pigments, whereas those at positions 116, 230, 233, and 309 filled (with a cross-hatched pattern) play a minor role. The residue marked with an asterisk is the lysine at position 312, to which the chromophore 11-*cis* retinal is linked. The three amino acid substitutions that result in loss of function were observed among individuals with blue cone monochromacy, and one of which (C203R) was also observed in all three green pigment genes of a deuteranomalous male and in 1%–2% of males (who have other normal green pigment genes) with normal color vision.

crease in c-GMP level triggers closure of c-GMP-gated membrane cation channels and hyperpolarization of the photoreceptor cell.

Spectral Tuning of the Photopigments

Each photopigment contains the chromophore 11-*cis*-retinal covalently linked to a lysine residue on the opsin by means of a protonated Schiff base. Despite having an identical chromophore, these pigments have very different absorption spectra. Therefore, differences in spectral characteristics of the photopigments are dictated by the interaction of amino acid residues at key positions in the opsin proteins. This is referred to as spectral tuning of the chromophore by the opsin. Residues within the membrane bilayer that interact directly with the chromophore retinal, as well as those that indirectly influence the structure of the pocket within which the chromophore is embedded, are likely to play inportant roles in tuning the absorption spectrum of the photopigment. Substitution of nonhydroxyl-bearing by hydroxyl-bearing residues has been proposed as a mechanism of spectral tuning,[49] the latter being associated with a spectral red shift.

The red and green photopigments differ in at most 15 of a total of 364 amino acid residues.[68] The presence of hydroxyl-bearing versus nonpolar residues constitutes the difference at eight amino acid residues at positions 65, 116, 180, 230, 233, 277, 285, and 309. All but residue 116 are located in the transmembrane pocket and are therefore likely to interact directly with the chromophore and influence its absorption spectrum. Comparing differences in amino acid sequence to spectral characteristics of pigments of the blind fish *Astyanax fasciatus*, Yokoyama and Yokoyama[108] suggested that amino acid residues at positions 180, 277, and 285 play a major role in determining the spectral difference (30 nm) between the human red and green visual pigments. The amino acid at each of these three positions is hydroxyl bearing in the red pigment and nonhydroxyl bearing in the green pigment. A year later, based on a comparative study of the sequence and spectral characteristics of the color vision pigments of Old and New World monkeys, Neitz et al.[73] confirmed the importance of these three residues in spectral tuning. Evidence for the contribution of residue 233 was derived from comparison of primate pigments.[39,100]

Spectral characteristics of the visual pigments were initially determined by retinal reflectance densitometry,[59] microspectrophotometry of individual human cones,[61] and electroretinography.[72,73] Direct measurements of absorption spectra of pigments expressed in tissue culture cells confirmed and refined the earlier results obtained by electroretinography and microspectrophotometry of cone cells. The human red pigment variants bearing either Ser or Ala at position 180 were shown to differ in their wavelength of maximal absorption (λ_{max}) by approximately 5 nm (Ser at 180 = 557 nm; Ala at 180 = 552 nm).[57] Furthermore, substitutions at positions 277 and 285 resulted in shifts in absorption maxima of 7 and 14 nm, respectively.[69] In addition, substitution at positions 116, 230, 233, and 309 produced small spectral shifts.[3,58] No change was observed on substitution at position 65.[3] In conclusion, differences at only seven amino acid positions (116, 180, 230, 233, 277, 285, and 309) are responsible for the difference in spectral characteristics between the human red and green visual pigments (Figs. 16.3 and 16.4). Residues at positions 180, 277, and 285 contribute the majority of the difference in absorption. These results are consistent with the studies of Winderickx et al.[102] and Deeb et al.[15] on genotype–phenotype relationships in normal and defective red–green color vision.

The Red and Green Pigment Genes of Individuals with Normal Color Vision

The genes that encode rhodopsin and the blue visual pigments are located on the long arms of human chromosomes 3 and 7, respectively. These genes have remarkably similar structures that are comprised of five exons encoding polypeptides of 348 amino acids. In humans, great apes, and Old World Monkeys the red and green pigment genes, which are located in close proximity to each other on the long arm of the X-chromosome (Xq28), are almost identical in structure, each having six exons instead of five, and they encode proteins with 364 amino acids (Fig. 16.5). The red and green pigment genes are arranged in a head-to-tail tandem array comprised of one red pigment gene located upstream (5′) of one or more green pigment genes (Fig. 16.6A).[25,68,92] The number of green pigment genes per X chromosome is highly variable. A higher mean of the number of green pigment genes per array was observed among U.S. Caucasians (mean of 2) than among Africans or Japanese (mean of 1).[19,45] This difference in the number of green pigment genes may have some bearing on the frequency of deuteranomaly, which is twice as high among Caucasians as among Africans and Japanese. Nathans and colleagues[69] proposed that the high degree of homology (even in introns) among the repeating units of the red and green pigment genes in the array has predisposed the locus to relatively frequent unequal (illegitimate) recombination. The observed copy number polymorphism in the green pigment gene could be the result of unequal recombination in the red–green intergenic region (Fig. 16.6B).

In most New World primates, a single gene on the X chromosome is present, and it encodes a red-to-green pigment. The gene duplication event that gave rise to the red and green pigment genes of the New World primates must have occurred after separation of the New and Old World lineages. It is interesting to note that despite the presence of only the blue and red–green pigment genes in the New World

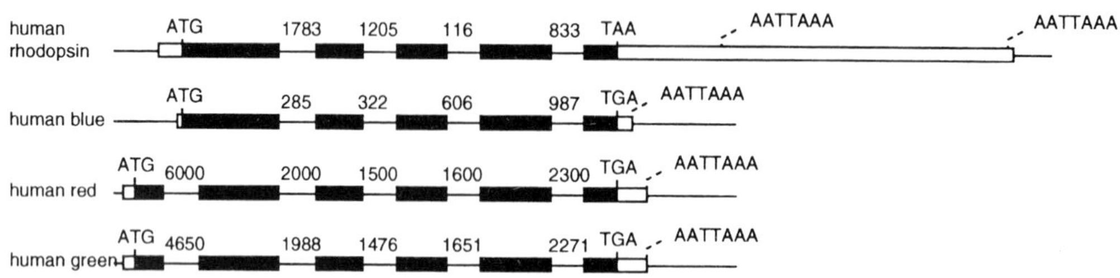

Figure 16.5. Comparison of the structure of the human visual pigment genes. Coding sequences of the genes are denoted by boxes and noncoding regions by lines (not to scale). Open boxes represent untranslated regions and filled boxes denote the coding regions. The length of introns in number of base pairs is shown. Also indicated are the initiation and termination codons and the polyadenylation signal sequences. (Adapted from M. Applebury and P. A. Hargrave, ref. 2.)

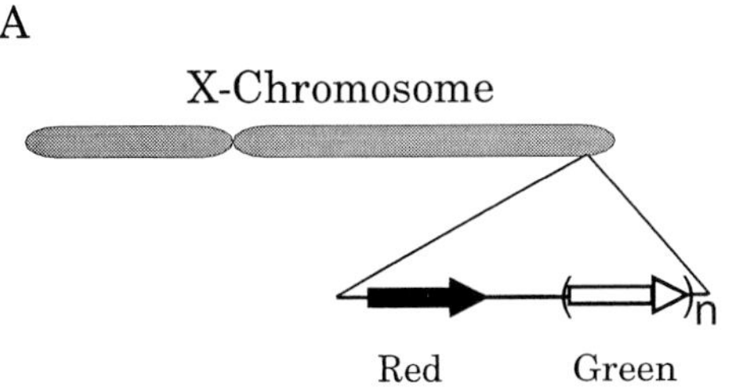

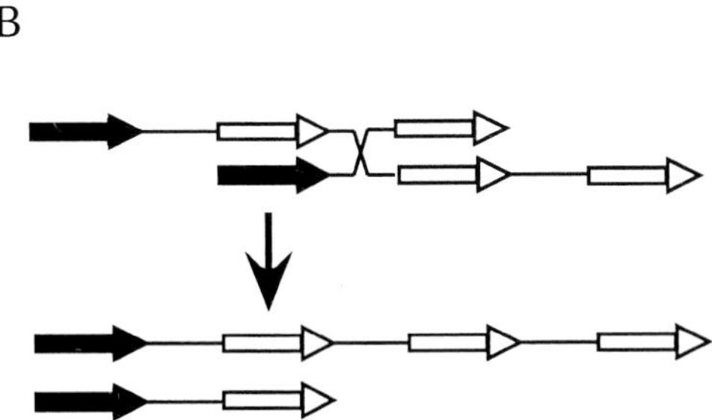

Figure 16.6. Numerical polymorphism in the number of green pigment genes. (**A**) Diagram of chromosome X showing the location (Xq28) of the red–green gene array that differ in the number of green opsin genes. Filled arrows denote red opsin genes and open arrows denote green opsin genes. Thin lines represent intergenic regions. (**B**) Unequal recombination within the homologous intergenic regions as a mechanism of generating polymorphism in the number of green pigment genes in an array.

primates, a limited degree of trichromatic color vision has been observed in females who are heterozygotes for two alleles of the single X-chromosome–linked pigment gene that encode pigments of different absorption maxima. Recently, Jacobs et al.[44a] showed that one genus of New World monkeys (*Alouatta,* the howler monkey) has two X-linked photopigment genes, probably due to an independent gene duplication, and have full trichromatic color vision.

The Serine/Alanine Polymorphism at Position 180

Subtle variation in color perception in the red–green region of the spectrum has been observed among individuals considered to have normal color vision. Rayleigh color matches of male subjects with normal color vision fell into two main groups.[21,22,70,71] Females with normal color vision showed a third and larger group with intermediate values of match midpoints.[70] A similar independently described Rayleigh match variability fitted transmission by X-linked inheritance in families.[93] These observations pointed to the presence of two common spectrally different forms of the red pigment gene on the X chromosome. Assuming the occurrence of random X-chromosome inactivation, females who are heterozygous for these two forms would be expected to have patches of cones containing either one or the other of the pigment forms and therefore would show a color match distribution intermediate between those of the two homozygotes.

We discovered a common single amino acid polymorphism (62% Ser, 38% Ala) at residue 180 of the red photopigment in the Caucasian population. Approximately 15% of males had Ser instead of Ala in some of their green pigment genes.[102] Because this amino acid was known to play a role in spectral tuning of the red and green pigment, we hypothesized that this polymorphism may account for some of the variations observed in both normal and defective color vision. Fifty Causacian males with normal color vision were tested for the hypothesis that the two major groups in the distribution of color matching could be explained by the above Ser/Ala polymorphism. The frequency distributions of Rayleigh match midpoints and of the deduced amino acid sequence of the red photopigment (Fig. 16.7) show that higher sensitivity to red light (i.e., requirement of less red in the mixture of red and green to match the standard yellow light) was highly correlated with the presence of Ser at position 180.[102] Therefore, these males have a different perception of red light than those having alanine at this site. Later on, Sanocki et al.[83,84] showed that the Ser/Ala polymorphism at position 180 of the red pigment gene underlies variation in color matching among individuals with color vision deficiencies.

Females having both the Ala and Ser alleles would be expected to have two types of red-sensitive photoreceptors due to X-chromosome inactivation and thus have the potential for tetrachromatic vision. This is analogous to the situ-

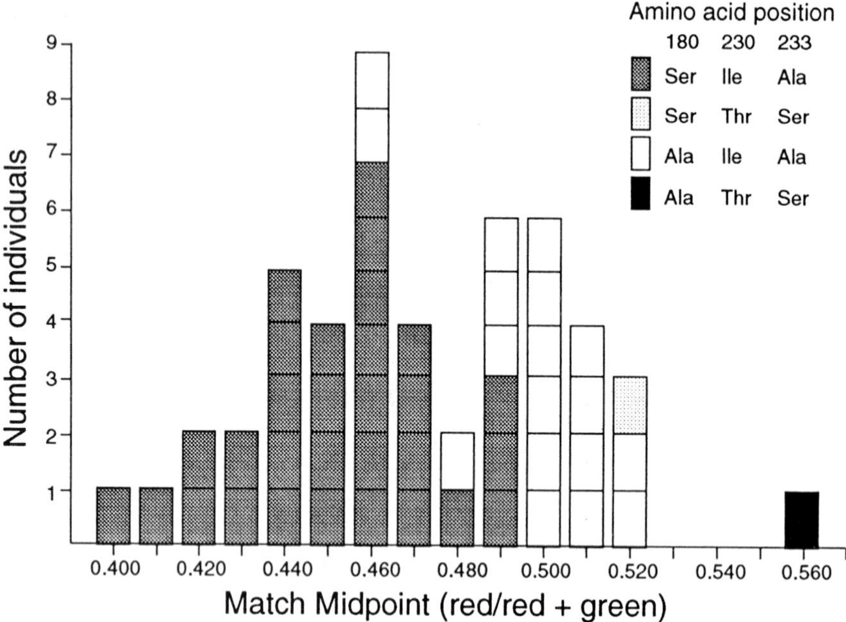

Figure 16.7. Frequency distribution of Rayleigh match midpoints and the presence of serine or alanine at position 180 of the red pigment. Male subjects with serine (Ser) at position 180 of the red pigment required less red in the mixture of red and green to match the standard yellow light than did those who had alanine (Ala). The two individuals who had threonine (Thr) and Ser at position 230 and 233 in place of isoleucine (Ile) and Ala, respectively required more red light than individuals with the same amino acid at position 180. (Figure from J. Winderickx et al., ref. 104.)

ation in the New World monkeys, which have only a single X-chromosome-encoded pigment gene with several alleles, where females heterozygous for two alleles of this gene achieve trichromacy, whereas males and homozygous females test as dichromats.[42] The frequency of the Ser/Ala polymorphism in the red gene among Afro-Americans was 80%/20% and among Japanese 84%/16% (unpublished personal observations).

Merbs and Nathans[57] and Asenjo and Oprian[3] determined the absorption spectra of recombinant human red pigments that differed in sequence by having only Ser or Ala at position 180. The absorption maximum of the red pigment with Ser at position 180 was approximately 5 nm longer than that with Ala.

Gene Arrays in Males with Defective Red–Green Color Vision

Unequal Recombination Between the Red and Green Pigment Genes Leads to Color Vision Defects. The relatively common (8% of Caucasian males) red–green color vision defects in which the red- or the green-sensitive cones are affected are inherited as X-linked recessive traits. These defects are associated with loss of either the red or the green photopigments or with the formation of a pigment with shifted absorption maximum. Unequal homologous recombination, to which the locus is highly predisposed, is the driving force behind both the loss of pigment genes and the formation of hybrid pigment genes that encode pigments with shifted absorption maxima. The X-linked mode of inheritance, lack of selection against individuals with defective color vision, and the high frequency of illegitimate recombination between the red and green pigment genes are believed to be responsible for the high frequency of these defects among males.

Deletion of green pigment genes results from unequal recombination or crossing over events that occur within the intergenic regions (which are highly homologous in sequence to

A. Deletion of the green pigment gene

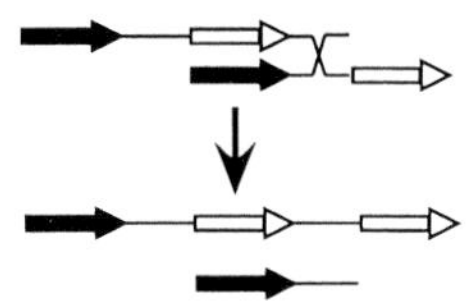

B. Formation of hybrid pigment genes

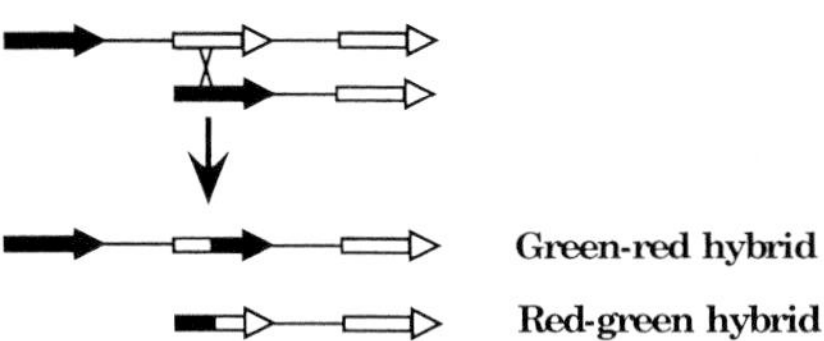

Figure 16.8. Unequal crossing over leading to deletion of the green pigment gene or formation of hybrid genes. Solid arrows = red pigment genes; open arrows = green pigment genes. Arrays with a single red pigment gene are associated with deutan color vision defects and those containing 5′ red–green 3′ hybrid genes are associated with protan color vision defects. Arrays comprised of a 5′ green–red 3′ hybrid in addition to normal red and green pigment genes are associated with either normal of deutan color vision.

one another) of the red–green gene locus (Fig. 16.8A). Hybrid genes are the result of unequal recombination events that occur within the red and green pigment genes themselves, as illustrated in Figure 16.8B. These events have introduced into the population a variety of chimeric pigments with different absorption maxima, depending on the point of fusion between the red and green pigment genes.

The exonic distribution of the seven amino acid residues that determine the difference (30 nm) in absorption maxima between the red and green pigments is shown in Figure 16.9. Note that exon 5, which contains positions 277, 285, and 309, contributes the majority (21 nm) of this difference in absorption maxima. Therefore any crossover in or 5′ of intron 4 will result in two hybrid pigments that have intermediate absorption maxima between the red and green pigment genes but, more importantly, will convert a red pigment into a green-like pigment and vice versa (Fig. 16.9). The structure of hybrid genes observed among color-deficient individuals and the absorption maxima of the encoded pigments are shown in Figure 16.10. The absorption maxima of these chimeric pigments were determined after expression of the

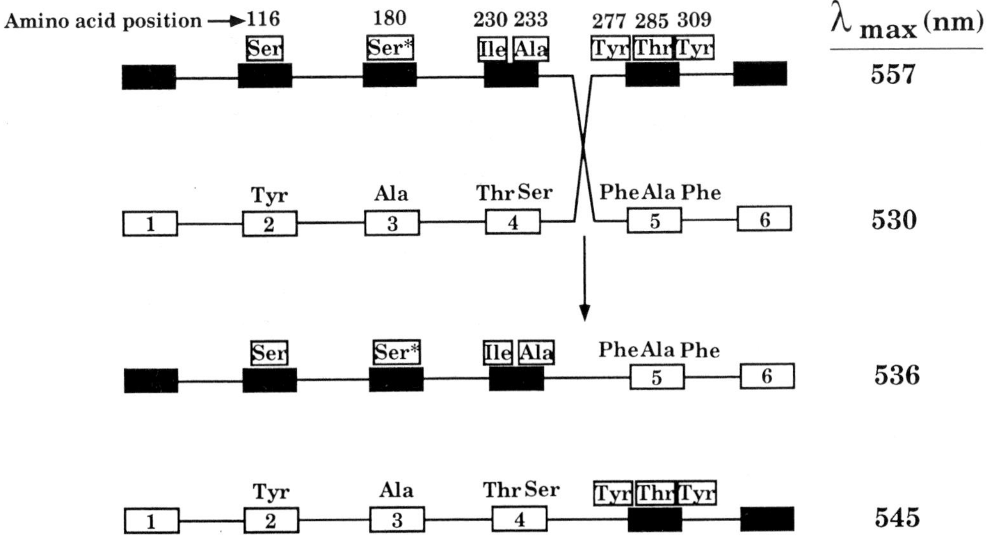

Figure 16.9. Unequal crossing over between the X-chromosome-linked red and green pigment genes. Open and filled rectangles represent exons derived from the green and red pigment genes, respectively. The seven amino acid residues that differentiate between the red and green pigments are indicated above the exons. The absorption maxima (λ_{max}) in nanometers (nm) are indicated for the normal and hybrid pigments.[56]

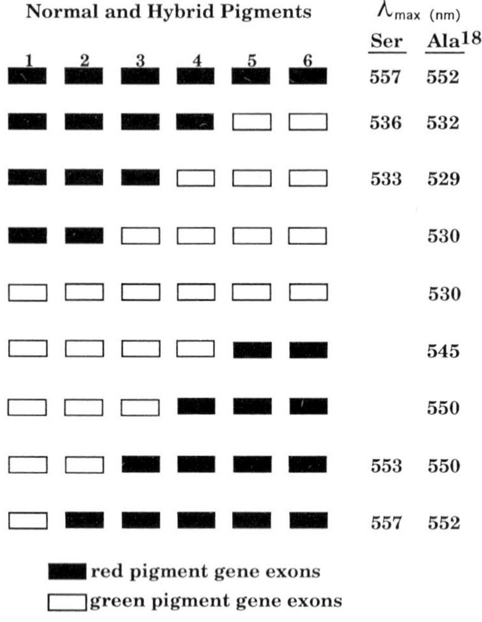

Figure 16.10. Absorption maxima of red/green hybrid pigments. Solid and open rectangles represent exons (numbers on top) of the red and green pigment genes, respectively. The absorption maxima of the encoded pigments are according to Merbs and Nathans, refs. 56, 57. The two columns on the right indicate absorption maxima (λ_{max}) of the pigment with either Ser or Ala at the polymorphic position 180. The pigments in the first and fifth rows represent normal red and green pigments; other rows represent red–green and green–red hybrid pigments.

proteins in tissue culture cells and the pigments reconstituted with the chromophore 11-*cis*-retinal.[3,56] Because introns are much longer than exons, recombination events are more likely to occur in introns. Note that recombinations in intron 5 would not result in a hybrid encoding a new pigment, as the exons 6 of the red and green pigment genes are identical in sequence.

5′ Red–green 3′ and 5′ green–red 3′ hybrid genes were first discovered in arrays of individuals with defective red–green color vision.[15,68] Subsequently, a small fraction of individuals with normal color vision (Fig. 16.11A) was observed to have, in addition to normal red and green pigment genes, 5′ green–red 3′ hybrid genes.[15,74] The significance of hybrid genes in determining the color vision phenotype will be discussed below in conjunction with expression of red and green pigment genes in the retina.

Gene Arrays in Protans and Deutans

Protanopic subjects have no functional red cones and are considered to be dichromats since they have only blue-sensitive and green-sensitive cones. Protanomalous subjects have an anomalous red pigment together with a normal green pigment and are referred to as anomalous trichromats. Deuteranopic individuals have no functional green-sensitive cones (dichromats), and deuteranomalous individu-

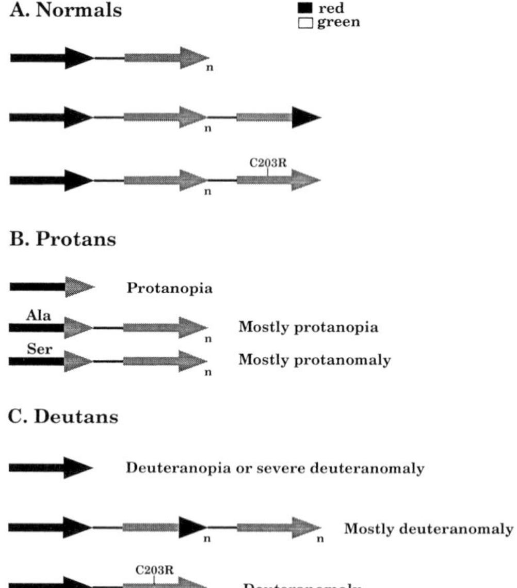

Figure 16.11. Gene arrays associated with normal, protan, and deutan color vision. (**A**) Arrays of individuals with normal color vision occasionally contain either green–red hybrid genes or green pigment genes with the Cys to Arg mutation at position 203. However, these anomalous pigments are most likely not expressed in sufficient amounts to influence color vision. They are arbitrarily drawn in the distal 3′ position to indicate minimal expression. (**B**) The presence of Ala or Ser at position 180 of the red pigment influences the severity of color vision defect. If Ala is present, then the hybrid and normal green pigment may have identical absorption maxima and the carrier would be expected to test as a dichromat. On the other hand, the presence of Ser allows a separation of 5 nm in absorption maxima between the two encoded pigments and the carrier would be expected to test as an anomalous trichromat. (**C**) In most cases, deuteranomaly results from the preferential expression of the green–red hybrid pigment that occupies the proximal position relative to the normal green pigment gene, and rarely from the presence of the Cys to Arg mutation in the green pigment gene(s).

als have an anomalous green pigment together with a normal red pigment (anomalous trichromats). The frequency of protanopia, protanomaly, and deuteranopia is about 1% each in Europeans, whereas that of deuteranomaly is around 4%–5%. Considerable variation in the severity of anomalous trichromacy has been observed.

Nathans and colleagues[69] were the first to examine the X-chromosome-linked red and green pigment gene arrays of 25 individuals with red–green color defects. Using Southern blot analysis, which detects major gene rearrangements, they found that among individuals with protan defects, protanopia (dichromacy) was associated with gene arrays comprised of a 5′ red–green 3′ hybrid gene found singly or together with normal green pigment genes, and protanomaly was associated with gene arrays comprised of a 5′ red–green 3′ hybrid together with a normal green pigment gene (Fig. 16.11B). Among deutans, deuteranopia (dichromacy) was associated with gene arrays comprised either of a single red pigment gene or a red pigment gene together with a 5′ green–red 3′ hybrid gene, whereas deuteranomaly was associated with gene arrays comprised of a normal red pigment gene, a 5′ green–red 3′ hybrid gene, in the absence or presence of a normal green pigment gene (Fig. 16.11C). Subsequently, we determined the gross structure of the X-linked red–green pigment gene locus among a group of 64 males who had defective red–green color vision.[15] The results of quantitative Southern blot analysis were basically in agreement with those of Nathans and colleagues[69] in that the majority of color vision defects were associated with either deletion of the green pigment gene or the formation of 5′ red–green 3′ or 3′ green–red 5′ hybrids (reviewed in Motulsky and Deeb[65]).

By determining the points of fusion in hybrid genes, we showed that exon 5 plays a major role in determining spectral sensitivity of the photopigments.[15] For example, a recombination in intron 4, which results in the replacement of exon 5 of the red pigment gene with that of the green pigment gene, produced a hybrid pigment that was sufficiently green-like in its spectral properties so that the subjects performed as protans. The significant role of exon 5 of the red opsin gene was predicted, as it contains two of the three amino acid residues (at positions 277 and 285) thought to account for the major difference in spectral properties between the red and green photopigments (Fig. 16.9).[58,72,73] Details of the methodologies employed to determine the gross structure of the gene arrays as well as the point of fusion are described in several publications.[15,65,69]

In addition to the mechanism of unequal recombination, we found that another cause of color vision deficiency was the presence of a point mutation in all three of the green pigment genes of one of the 64 color-defective individuals, leading to the substitution of arginine for the highly conserved serine at position 203 (Fig. 16.11C).[104] We subsequently found this mutation to be as common as 2% among color-normal Caucasian males (Fig. 16.11A). The presence of this mutation in one of the two to three green pigment genes in these individuals had no phenotypic consequences, presumably because the mutant green pigment gene is not in position to be expressed (see below). This mutation was also discovered as the cause of inactivation of the single 5′ red-green 3′ hybrid gene in arrays of 15 probands with blue cone monochromacy.[67] Thus, the presumably unexpressed green pigment genes with the Cys 203 Arg mutations act as a reservoir for gene arrays, produced by unequal crossing over, that cause color vision defects and possibly disorders involving cone degeneration.

Predicting Severity of Red–Green Color Vison Defects from the Genotype. Knowing the gross features of the X-linked red–green gene array allowed classification of color-defective individuals only as either protans or deutans but could not strictly predict the severity (dichromacy versus trichromacy) of the color vision defect. For example, males who have one 5′ red–green 3′ hybrid gene in addition to one or more green pigment genes tested as either protanopes (dichromats) or protanomals (anomalous trichromats) (Fig. 16.11B), and deutan individuals who had a 5′ green–red 3′ hybrid gene in addition to normal red and green pigment genes tested as either deuteranopes (dichromats) or deuteranomals (anomalous trichromats) (Fig. 16.11C). These apparent discrepancies may be related to the phenomena discussed in the paragraphs that follow.

1. *Pigment spectral separation and pigment density*. We hypothesized that if the absorption maxima of the hybrid and normal pigments encoded by the genes of color-defective individuals have identical absorption maxima, the individual will test as a dichromat, whereas if the encoded pigments differ, even by a few nanometers, then the individual will test as an anomalous trichromat. Furthermore, we predicted that the Ser–Ala polymorphism at position 180 of the red pigment gene would be the major determinant of the difference between the normal and hybrid pigment absorbance. For example, if both the red–green hybrid and green pigment have Ala, there would be no difference in absorption between them and the subject would test as a protanope. On the other hand, if the hybrid had Ser and the nomal green had Ala, then the pigments would differ by about 5 nm in absorption maxima and the subject would test as a protanomal (Fig. 16.11B). A similar argument would hold for deutans who have a normal red and green–red hybrid pigments.

We tested the hypothesis that chromatic discrimination in such color-defective individuals depends on the difference between spectra of the normal and hybrid pigments in the array.[16] Sequences of the normal and hybrid pigments were determined in 19 protan and 19 deutan male subjects, and the wavelength of maximum absorption of each pigment was inferred from the data of Merbs and Nathans.[56] Eight of nine protanopes had spectrally identical red–green hybrid and normal green pigments. Only six of ten protanomalous subjects had pigments that differed in absorption maxima. However, the four-protanomalous subjects with identical pigments had a markedly wider (more severe color vision defect) mean match range (41.5 units) than that (9.3 units) of the six subjects who had different pigments. Spectrally identical pigments were found in the array of the two deuteranopes as well as in seven of the seventeen deuteranomalous subjects.

Using pseudoisochromatic plates to assess severity of color vision defects among males, Neitz et al.[74a] found in general that the severity of deuteranomaly was directly proportional to the separation in λ_{max} of the pigments that contribute to color vision which, among deuteranomals, are the red and the green–red pigments.

Thus, the correspondence between match range and the difference in spectra between hybrid and normal pigments was strong in protans and weak in deutans, and the majority of exceptions involved subjects who had a narrower match range than predicted from spectral differences. The most puzzling cases we encountered were subjects (3 of 10) who have only a single pigment gene and yet tested as severely anomalous trichromats instead of dichromats. Therefore, factors other than sequence of the pigments may influence the width of the Rayleigh match. Recent evidence suggests that difference in effective optical density of the pigments in cone populations in the same retina that synthesize the same pigment is sufficient to yield some red–green color discrimination.[34] Cones with a higher density of pigment have a broader absorption spectrum than those with lower density. This would explain how a single genotype can be associated with two phenotypes.

2. *Selective gene expression in the retina*. We had previously observed that the frequency of hybrid red–green pigment genes among Caucasians, and more so among African Americans, was respectively two and five times greater than that of phenotypic color vision defects.[9,45] We hypothesized that some individuals with hybrid genes have normal color vision. This was proven by finding that 4 of 129 male Caucasian subjects with 5′ green–red 3′ hybrid pigment genes along with normal red and green pigment genes had normal color vision as determined by anomaloscopy.[15] Furthermore, the majority (80%) of deuteranomalous individuals have hybrid genes in addition to normal red and green pigment genes.[15] Normal color vision would be expected if all three types of genes were expressed in the retina. The hypothesis that not all opsin genes in an array are expressed in the retina in a sufficient number of cones to influence color vision was advanced to explain these observations. We suggested that in deuteranomalous individuals the red and hybrid were expressed but not the normal green pigment genes, whereas in normal individuals the normal red and green, but not hybrid genes are expressed.

We tested the foregoing hypothesis by comparing the pigment gene sequences in genomic DNA with the corresponding mRNA sequences expressed in postmortem retinas. Advantage was taken of a relatively common but silent polymorphism (A versus C at the third position of codon 283) in exon 5 of the green pigment gene. The two alleles can be differentiated by polymerase chain reaction (PCR) amplification followed by digestion with EcoO109I. Analysis in ten male subjects who had two or more green pigment genes in their genomic DNA showed clearly that, whenever the two alleles of exon 5 were present in genomic DNA, only one was represented in expressed retinal mRNA,[103] indicating the expression of only a single green opsin gene. In another set of 51 unselected postmortem retinae, three male donors had gene arrays comprised of one red, one 5′ green–red 3′ hybrid, and one normal green pigment gene. We found that one of these expressed mRNA transcripts encoded by the normal red and the 5′ green–red 3′ hybrid but not the normal green pigment gene, and presumably had deuteranomalous color vision. The other two expressed the normal red and green pigment genes but not the green–red hybrid, and presumably had normal color vision.[103,106]

The model illustrated in Figure 16.12 was proposed to explain such selective expression in the retina.[103,106] In this model, a locus control region (LCR), is postulated to regulate expression of the opsin genes of the array in a position-dependent manner. Thus, if the LCR forms a stable transcriptionlly active complex with the red opsin gene promoter, a red-sensitive cone will result. If the LCR forms a stable complex with the proximal green pigment gene promoter instead, a green-sensitive cone is formed. Transcriptionally active complexes between the LCR and promoters of pigment genes located downstream of the two proximal pigment genes are much less favored. We therefore suggest that only the two most proximal pigment genes of an array are expressed in sufficient cones to influence color vision as measured anomaloscopically.

The concept of a LCR was first suggested for the regulatory sequences 5′ upstream of the β-globin gene locus. The globin LCR was shown to be essential for developmental

A. **Expression of the red pigment gene results in formation of a red cone.**

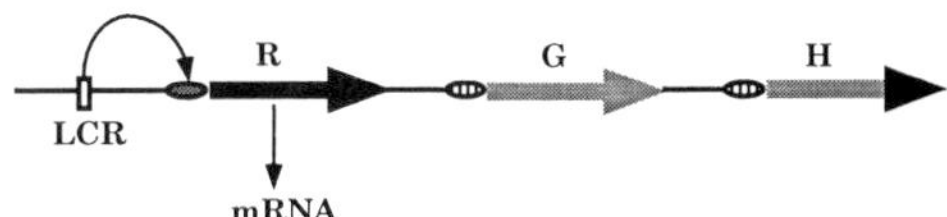

B. **Expression of the green pigment gene gives rise to a green cone which confers normal color vision.**

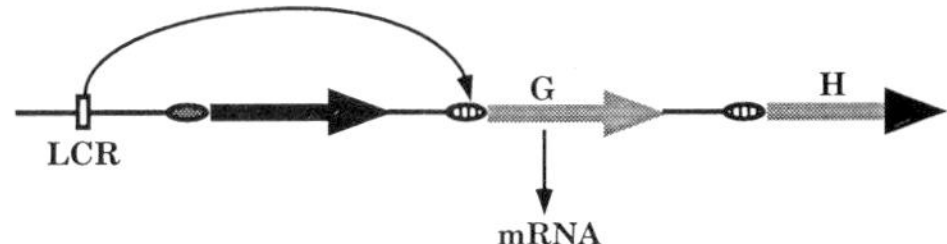

C. **Expression of the hybrid pigment gene instead of the normal green gives rise to an anomalous "red-like" cone, resulting in deuteranomaly.**

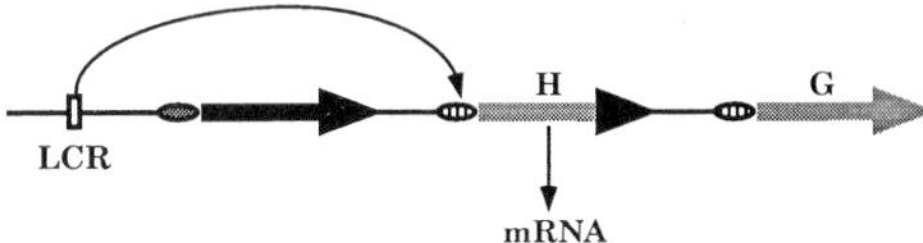

Figure 16.12. Model for selective expression in the X-linked red–green pigment gene complex. Numbers denote visual length in kilobase pairs. (**A**) A red cone is formed if by chance the locus control region (LCR) binds permanently to the red (R) pigment gene promoter (mediated by DNA binding proteins) and turns on expression of only the red pigment gene. (**B**) A green cone is formed if the LCR happens to bind permanently to the proximal green pigment gene promoter and turns on its expression. Distal green pigment gene promoters are not activated presumably due to the low probability of coupling to the LCR. (Adapted from J. Winderickx et al., ref. 102.)

switching of expression from fetal to adult globin genes, and that the order of the genes comprising this locus is important for such a transcriptional switch.[4,23,33,77,85] Strong evidence for such an LCR at the red–green opsin locus has been provided by Nathans and colleagues,[66,67] who found that blue cone monochromacy, a disorder in which both red and green cone functions are absent (see below), is often associated with deletion of a regulatory sequence located 3.8–4.3 kb upstream of the transcription initiation site of the red pigment gene and 43 kb upstream of that of the proximal green pigment gene. They subsequently showed that a region between −3.1 and −3.7 kb of the red pigment gene is required for cone-specific expression of the β-galactosidase reporter gene in transgenic mice.[95]

Female Heterozygotes for Red–Green Color Vision Deficiency

Because the total frequency of color vision defects among European populations is 8%, approximately 15%–16% of the female population will be heterozygotes for one or another red–green color vision defect. The majority of such heterozygotes (7%–10%) are heterozygotes for deuteranomaly, as this abnormality is the most frequent defect. Some heterozygotes have been found to exhibit a mild version (detected by psychophysical testing) of the typical color vision defects exhibited by color-deficient males. This is explained by the random inactivation in any given cell of either the paternal or maternal X chromosomes during early development. The pattern of inactivation is preserved throughout development, resulting in patches of somatic cells that are functionally hemizygous. Therefore, the retinae of heterozygous females would be expected to contain patches of photoreceptors that express the normal red–green gene array and others to express the abnormal gene array. There is good experimental evidence that heterozygotes are mosaics for normal and abnormal color vision in their retinae. By shining a very narrow beam of red or green light into the retinae of female heterozygotes for X-linked color vision defects, patches of defective color perception were found.[7,30] In other experiments, heterozygotes made more errors than controls when asked to identify the color of briefly presented stimuli under conditions that did not allow any eye movement.[10]

The majority of heterozygotes for color vision deficiencies are classified as having normal color vision by the standard clinical tests. Occasionally, heterozygous females exhibit the typical color vision deficiency. This is most likely due to the presence of a small proportion of females with extremely skewed X inactivation who by chance have inactivated most of their normal X chromosome and thus express the mutant X chromosome.[41,53] Skewed X inactivation appears to be more common in one member of identical female twin pairs,[46] and six pairs of heterozygote female identical twins discordant for color vision have been reported.[76,78] The expected skewed inactivation of one X chromosome has been directly demonstrated in one of these twin pairs.[46] Furthermore, two of five Dionne identical quintuplet girls were color blind[94] as was one of three identical Japanese female triplets.[107]

Electroretinography has been successful in identifying a large number of both protan and deutan heterozygotes by the ratio of sensitivity to short (480 nm) and long (620 nm) wavelengths of light.[32]

Females who are compound heterozygotes for two abnormal red–green gene arrays have been observed. Heterozygotes for both deuteranomaly and deuteranopia manifest with deuteranomaly[5,47,75] and protanope/protanomalous heterozygotes manifest with protanomaly. The milder phenotype is dominant over the more severe one. This is expected as the retinae of such individuals will have normal red, normal green, and red–green hybrid photoreceptors. Examples of genotypes and phenotypes of heterozygous females are given in Figure 16.13.

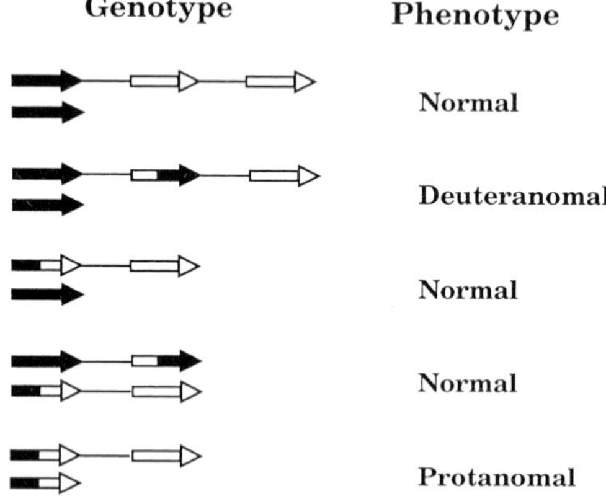

Figure 16.13. Phenotypes of female heterozygote carriers of gene arrays associated with red–green color vision defects. Shown are red (filled arrows)/green (open arrows) gene arrays on the pair of X chromosomes of females who are heterozygotes for arrays that are associated with defective color vision. Gene arrays comprised of a single gene are generally associated with a more severe color vision defect. Note that the phenotype of heterozygote carriers is dictated by the array associated with the milder defect. Compound heterozygotes for arrays associated with deutan and protan defects (second pair from bottom) have normal color vision.

In contrast, compound heterozygotes for both a deutan and protan defect will not present with color vision defects.[75,105] This finding is not surprising, as normal alleles for red and green pigments are present in addition to the defective in both the protan and deutan genes. Compound heterozygosity for protanopia/deuteranomaly and protanomaly/deuteranomaly was studied in one large family by molecular techniques and showed no color vision abnormalities (Fig. 16.13).[18]

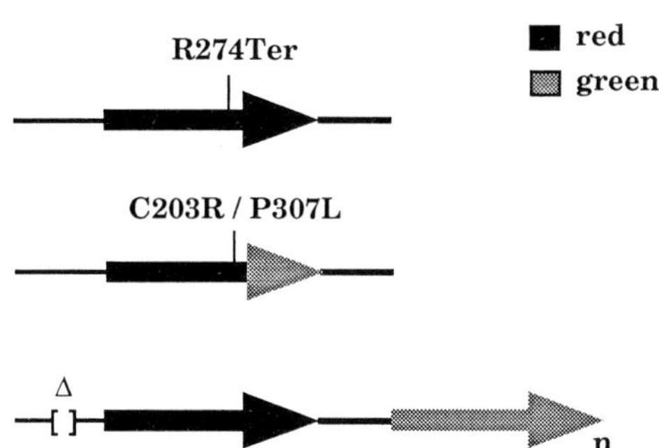

Figure 16.14. The molecular basis of blue cone monochromacy. Three mechanisms of generating red–green pigment gene arrays found in blue cone monochromats. Deletion of the green pigment gene followed by a chain termination or nonsense mutation (R247ter) in the coding sequence of the red pigment gene leading to the synthesis of a truncated and nonfunctional protein. Unequal recombination between a mutant (C203R or P307L) green pigment gene of one array and the red pigment gene of a normal array, one of the products of which is a gene array with a single nonfunctional red–green hybrid gene. Deletion of the locus control region (demarcated by brackets) prevents expression of both red and green visual pigment genes.

THE MOLECULAR BASIS OF BLUE CONE MONOCHROMACY

Blue cone monochromacy (BCM) is rare disorder (less than 1 in 100,000) in which both red and green cone sensitivities are absent.[80] The physiologic functions of both rods and blue cones are preserved. Significant linkage of BCM to the red–green pigment gene locus was established.[54] This led Nathans and colleagues[66] to analyze the red–green locus in individuals with BCM. Their studies on thirty-three unrelated subjects with BCM have uncovered three mechanisms for generating this phenotype.[67] One, found in six affected individuals, involved deletion of the locus control region (see above), the major switch for the whole visual pigment gene array, located 3.4 kb 5′ upstream of the transcription of initiation site of the red pigment gene (Fig. 16.12). The second involved unequal homologous recombination between a normal red and a mutant green pigment gene to form hybrid genes that encoded nonfunctional pigment (Fig. 16.14). The green portion of the hybrid gene had, in fourteen affected subjects, the same Cys203 Arg mutation found to be relatively common in Causasian males.[67,71] One subject had a Pro3071Leu instead of the Cys203Arg substitution in the single 5′ red–green 3′ hybrid gene. The third mechanism involved deletion of the green pigment genes and a point mutation (either the Cys203Arg or a R247ter) in the remaining red pigment gene, found in two of the subjects (see Fig. 16.4 for position of these mutations). Progressive central retinal dystrophy has been reported in some patients with BCM,[66] indicating that cone degeneration may result from the accumulation of an abnormally assembled photopigment in analogy with the mutations in rhodopsin found to underlie autosomal dominant retinitis pigmentosa.[20]

THE MOLECULAR BASIS OF TRITANOPIA

Tritanopia is a rare autosomal dominant[98] disorder characterized by selective loss of the shortwave or blue photoreceptor function and greatly diminished or absent chromatic discrimination in the blue region of the spectrum. A survey in the Netherlands indicates that its frequency in the population may be as high as 1 in 500.[89] Three missense mutations in the blue pigment gene, located on chromosome 7,[68] have been shown to cause tritanopia: Gly79-Arg in two Japanese subjects, Ser214Pro in two Caucasian subjects, and Pro264Ser in three Caucasian subjects.[96,97] The three mutant alleles cosegregate with tritanopia in an autosomal dominant fashion; however, incomplete penetrance was observed in association with the Gly-79Arg substitution. The mutations affect residues located in the second, fifth, and sixth transmembrane α-helical segments of the blue pigment. The dominant mode of inheritance suggests that accumulation of a defective pigment within photoreceptors causes either loss of function or cell death, reminiscent of the mutations in the rhodopsin and peripherin genes that cause a subset of autosomal dominant retinitis pigmentosa. Tritanopia has also been observed in association with some disorders of vision such as autosomal dominant juvenile optic atrophy.[50,60]

Acknowledgments: The preparation of this chapter was supported by National Institutes of Health grant EY 08395.

REFERENCES

1. Adam A. A further query on color blindness and natural selection. *Soc Biol* 1969;16: 197–202.
2. Applebury M, Hargrave PA. Molecular biology of the visual pigments. *Vision Res* 1986;26: 1881–1895.
3. Asenjo AB, Rim J, Oprian DD. Molecular determinants of human red/green color discrimination. *Neuron* 1994;12:1131–1138.
4. Behringer RR, Ryan TM, Palmiter RD, Brinster RL, Townes TM. (1990) Human d to B-global gene switching in transgenic mice. *Genes Dev* 1990;4:380–389.
5. Birch J. Congenital protan and deutan defects in women. In *Color vision deficiencies*, vol. IX. B. Drum and G. Verriest, eds. Dordrecht, Netherlands: Kluwer Academic Publishers, 1989, pp. 101–106.
6. Birch J. (1991) Colour vision tests: General classification. In *The Perception of Color Vision*, P. Gouras, ed. *Vision and Visual Dysfunctions*, vol. 7. Boca Raton: CRC Press, pp. 215–231.
7. Born G, Grutzner P, Hemminger H. Evidenz fur eine Mosaikstruktur der Netzhaut bei Konduktorinnen fur dichromasie. *Hum Genet* 1976;32:189–196.
8. Caron MC, Lefkowtiz RJ. Model systems for the study of seven-transmembrane-segment receptors. *Annu Rev Biochem* 1991;60:653–688.
9. Cicerone CM, Nerger JL. The relative numbers of long-wavelength-sensitive and middle-wavelength-sensitive cones in the human fovea centralis. *Vision Res* 1989;19:115–128.
10. Cohn SA, Emmerich DS, Carlson EA. Differences in the responses of heterozygous carriers of colorblindness and normal controls to briefly presented stimuli. *Vision Res* 1989;29:255–262.
11. Curcio CA, Allen KA, Sloan KR, Lerea CL, Hurley JB, Klock IB, Milam AH. Distribution and morphology of human cone photoreceptors stained with anti-blue opsin. *J Comp Neurol* 1991;312:610–624.
12. Currier RD. A two-and-a-half color rainbow. *Arch Neurol* 1994;51:1090–1992.
13. Dalton J. Extraordinary facts relating to the vision of colours, with observations. *Mem Lit Philos Soc Lond* 1798;5:28–45.
14. Dartnall HJA, Bowmaker JK, Mollon JD. Human visual pigments: Microspectrophotometric results from the eyes of seven persons. *Proc R Soc Lond* Ser B 1983;220:115–130.
15. Deeb SS, Lindsey DT, Hibiya Y, Sanocki E, Winderickx J, Teller DY, Motulsky AG. Genotype-phenotype relationships in human red/green color vision defects: Molecular and psychophysical studies. *Am J Hum Genet* 1992; 51:687–700.
16. Deeb, SS, Jorgensen, AL, Battisti L, Iwasaki L, Motulsky AG. Sequence divergence of the red and green visual pigments in the Great Apes and Man. *Proc Natl Acad Sci USA* 1994;91: 7262–7266.
17. Dohlman G, Thorner J, Caron M, Lefkowitz R. Model systems for the study of seven-transmembrane-segment receptors. *Annu Rev Biochem* 1992;60:653–688.
18. Drummond-Borg M, Deeb S, Motulsky AG. Molecular basis of abnormal red-green color vision: A family with three types of color vision defects. *Am J Hum Genet* 1988;43:675–683.
19. Drummond-Borg M, Deeb S, Motulsky AG. Molecular patterns of X chromosome-linked color vision genes among 134 men of European ancestry. *Proc Natl Acad Sci USA* 1989;86: 983–987.
20. Dryja TP, McGee TL, Hahn LB, Cowley GS, Ollson JE, Reichel E, Sandberg MA, Berson EL. Mutations within the rhodopsin gene in patients with autosomal dominant retinitis pigmentosa. *N Engl J Med* 1990;323:1302–1307.
21. Eisner A, MacLeod DIA. Flicker photometric study of chromatic adaptation: Selective sup-

pression of cone inputs by colored backgrounds. *J Optom Soc Am* 1981;71:705–717.

22. Elsner AE, Burns SA. Classes of color normal observers. *J Opt Soc Am* 1987;4:123.
23. Enver T, Raich N, Ebens AJ, Papayannopoulou T, Constantini F, Stamatoyannopoulos G. Developmental regulation of human fetal-to-adult globin gene switching in transgenic mice. *Nature* 1990;344:309–313.
24. Farnsworth D. (1957) *Farnsworth-Munsell 100 Hue Test for the Examination of Color Discrimination Manual.* Baltomore: Munsell Color Co., Inc.
25. Feil R, Aubourg P, Heilig R, Mandel JL. A 195-kb cosmid walk encompassing the human Xq28 color vision pigment genes. *Genomics* 1990;6:367–373.
26. Fletcher R, Voke J. *Defective colour vision fundamentals, diagnosis and management.* Boston: Adam Hilger Ltd., 1991.
27. Fung BK-K, Hurley JB, Stryer L. Flow of information in the light-triggered cyclic nucleotide cascade of vision. *Proc Natl Acad Sci USA* 1981;78:152–156.
28. Fung BK-K, Stryer L. Photolyzed rhodopsin catalyzes the exchange of GTP for bound GDP in retinal rod outer segments. *Proc Natl Acad Sci USA* 1980;77:2500–2504.
29. Gouras P. The history of colour vision. In *The Perception of Colour Vision,* P. Gouras, ed. *Vision and Visual Dysfunctions,* Vol. 6. Boca Raton: CRC Press, 1992, pp. 1–9.
30. Grutzner P, Born G, Hemminger HJ. Colored stimuli within the central visual field of carriers of dichromatism. *Mod Prob Ophthalmol* 1976; 17:147–150.
31. Halbertsma KTA. *A History of the Theory of Colour.* Amsterdam: Swets and Zitlinger, 1949.
32. Hanazaki H, Tanabe J, Kawasaki K. Electroretinographic findings in congenital red-green color deficiency. In *Color Vision Deficiencies,* Y. Otha, ed. Berkeley: Kugler & Ghedini Publications, 1990, p. 71.
33. Hanscombe O, Whyatt D, Fraser P, Yannoutsos N, Greaves D, Dillon N, Grosveld F. Importance of globin gene order to correct developmental expression. *Genes Dev* 1991; 5:1387–1394.
34. He JC, Shevell SK. Variation in color matching and discrimination among deuteranomalous trichromats: Theoretical implications of small differences in photopigments. *Vision Res* 1995; 35:2579–2588.
35. Helmholtz HLF von. On the theory of compound colours. *Philosophical Magazine* (Series 4) 1852;4:519–534.
36. Henderson R. The purple membrane from Halobacterium holobium. *Annu Rev Biophys Bioeng* 1977;6:87–109.
37. Horner JF. Die Erblichkeit des Daltonismus. Amtl Ber Verwalt Med Kantons Zurich, 1876;108.
38. Hunt DM, Dulai KS, Bowmaker JK, Mollon JD. The chemistry of John Dalton's color blindness. *Science* 1995;267:984–988.
39. Ibbotson RE, Hunt DM, Bowmaker JK, Mollon JD. Sequence divergence and copy number of the middle- and long-wave photopigments in Old World monkeys. *Proc R Soc Lond B,* 1984;47:145–154.
40. Ichikawa H, Majima A. Genealogical studies on interesting families of defective colour vison discovered by a mass examination in Japan and Formosa. *Mod Prob Ophthalmol* 1974;13: 265–271.
41. Ingerslev J, Schwartz M, Lamm LU, Kruse TA, Bukh A, Stenberg S. Female haemophilia A in a family with seeming extreme bidirectional lyonization tendency: Abnormal premature X-chromosome inactivation? *Clin Genet* 1989; 35:41–48.
42. Jacobs GH, Neitz J. Inheritance of color vision in a New World monkey (*Saimiri sciureus*). *Proc Natl Acad Sci USA* 1987;84:2545–2549.
43. Jacobs J, Neitz J. Electrophysiological estimates of individual variation in the L/M cone ratio. In B. Drum, ed. *Color Vision Deficiencies XI.* Proc Int Symp on Color Vision Deficiencies, Sydney: 1991. Kluwer, P 1993, pp. 107–112.
44. Jacobs J. Variation in color vision in non-human primates. The perception of colour vision. In *Vision and Visual Dysfunctions,* Vol. 7, P. Gouras, ed. Boca Raton: CRC Press, 1991, pp. 199–211.

44a. Jacobs, GH, Neitz M, Deegan F, Neitz, J. Trichromatic color vision among New World monkeys. *Nature* 1996;382:156–158.

45. Jorgensen AL, Deeb S, Motulsky AG. Molecular genetics of X chromosome-linked color vision among populations of African and Japanese ancestry: High frequency of a shortened red pigment gene among Afro-Americans. *Proc Natl Acad Sci USA* 1990;87:6512–6516.
46. Jorgensen AL, Philip J, Raskind WH, Matsushita M, Christensen B, Dreyer V, Motulsky AG. Different patterns of X inactivation in MZ

twin discordant for red-green color-vision deficiency. *Am J Hum Genet* 1992;51:291–298.

47. Judd DB. Color blindness and the detection of camouflage. *Science* 1943;97:544.
48. Kalmus H. *Diagnosis and Genetics of Defective Colour Vision*. Oxford: Pergamon Press, 1965.
49. Kosower EM. Assignment of groups responsible for the "opsin shift" and light absorptions of rhodopsin and red, green, and blue iodopsins (cone pigments). *Proc Natl Acad Sci USA* 1988;85:1076–1080.
50. Krill AE, Smith VC, Pokorny J. Further studies supporting the identity of congenital tritanopia and hereditary dominant optic atrophy. *Invest Ophthalmol* 1971;10:457–465.
51. Kuyk TK, Veres JG III, Lahey MA, Clark DJ. The ability of protan color defectives to perform color-dependent air traffic control tasks. *Am J Optom Physiol Optom* 1986;63:582–586.
52. Kuyk TK, Veres JG III, Lahey MA, Clark DJ. The ability of protan color defectives to perform color-dependent air traffic control tasks. *Am J Optom Physiol Optom* 1987;64:2–10.
53. Lascari AD, Hoak JC, Taylor JC. Christmas disease in a girl. *Am J Dis Child* 1969;117:585.
54. Lewis RA, Holcomb JD, Bromley WC, Wilson MC, Roderick TH, Hejtmancik JF. Mapping X-linked ophthalmic diseases. III. Provisional assignment of the locus for blue cone monochromacy to Xq28. *Arch Ophthalmol* 1987;105:1055–1059.
55. Maxwell JC. On colour vision. *Proc R Inst Great Britain* 1872;6:260–271.
56. Merbs SL, Nathans J. Absorption spectra of the hybrid pigments responsible for anomalous color vision. *Science* 1992b;258:464–466.
57. Merbs SL, Nathans J. Absorption spectra of human cone pigments. *Nature* 1992a;356:433–435.
58. Merbs SL, Nathans J. Role of hydroxyl-bearing amino acids in differentially tuning the absorption spectra of the human red and green cone pigments. *Photochem Photobiol* 1993;58:869–881.
59. Mitchell DE, Rushton WAH. The red/green pigments of normal vision. *Vision Res* 1971;11:1045–1056.
60. Miyake Y, Yagasaki K, Ichikawa H. Differential diagnosis of congenital tritanopia and dominantly inherited juvenile optic atrophy. *Arch Ophthalmol* 1985;103:1496–1501.
61. Mollon JD. Color vision. *Annu Rev Psychol* 1982;33:41–85.
62. Mollon JD. Mixing genes and mixing colors. *Current Biol* 1993;3:82–85.
63. Moore AT. Cone and cone-rod dystrophies. *J Med Genet* 1992;29:289–290.
64. Morgan MJ, Adam A, Mollon JD. Dichromats detect colour camouflaged objects that are not detected by trichomats. *Proc R Soc Lond (Biol)* 1992;248:291–295.
65. Motulsky AG, Deeb S. Color vision and its genetic defects. In *The Metabolic and Molecular Bases of Inherited Disease. Seventh Edition.* CR Scriver, AL Beaudet, WS Sly, and D. Valle, eds. Vol. III, McGraw-Hill, NY, 1995, pp. 4275–4296.
66. Nathans J, Davenport CM, Maumenee IH, Heijtmancik JF, Litt M, Lovrien E, Weleber R, Bachynski B, Zwas F, Klingman R, Fishman G. Molecular genetics of blue cone monochromacy. *Science* 1990;245:831–838.
67. Nathans J, Maumenee IH, Zrenner E, Sadowski B, Sharpe LT, Lewis RA et al. Genetic heterogeneity among blue-cone monochromats. *Am J Hum Genet* 1993;53:987–1000.
68. Nathans J, Thomas D, Hogness DS. Molecular genetics of human color vision: The genes encoding blue, green and red pigments. *Science* 1986a;232:193–202.
69. Nathans J, Piantanida TP, Eddy RL, Shows TB, Hogness DS. Molecular genetics of inherited variation in human color vision. *Science* 1986;232:203–210.
70. Neitz J, Jacobs GH. Polymorphism of the long-wavelength cone in normal human color vision. *Nature* 1986;323:623–625.
71. Neitz J, Jacobs GH. Polymorphism in normal human color vision and its mechanism. *Vision Res* 1990;30:621–636.
72. Neitz J, Neitz M, Jacobs GH. Analysis of fusion gene and encoded photopigment of colour-blind humans. *Nature* 1989;342:679–682.
73. Neitz M, Neitz J, Jacobs GH. Spectral tuning of pigments underlying red-green color vision. *Science* 1991;252:971–974.
74. Neitz M, Neitz J. Numbers and ratios of visual pigment genes for normal red-green color vision. *Science* 1995;267:1013–1016.

74a. Neitz J, Neitz M, Kainz PM. Visual pigment gene structure and the severity of color vision defects. *Science* 1996;274:801–804.

75. Nemoto H, Murao M. A genetic study of colorblindness. *Jpn J Hum Genet* 1961;6:165–173.
76. Nettleship E. Some unusual pedigrees of color blindness. *Trans Ophthalmol Soc UK* 1912;32:309.
77. Peterson KR, Stamatoyannopoulos G. Role of gene order in developmental control of human

g- and b-globin gene expression. *Mol Cell Biol* 1993;13:4836–4843.

78. Philip J, Vogelius-Anderson CH, Dreyer V, Freiesleben E, Gurtler H, Haughe M, Kissmeyer-Nielsen F, et al. Color vision deficiency in one of two presumably monozygotic twins with secondary amenoorhoea. *Ann Hum Genet* 1969;33:185–195.
79. Piantanida T. Genetics of inherited colour vision deficiencies. In *Inherited and Acquired Colour Vision Deficiencies.* DH Foster, ed. *Vision and Visual Dysfunction Vol. 7,* Boca Raton: CRC Press 1991, pp. 88–144.
80. Pokorny J, Smith VC, Verriest G. Congenital color defects. In *Congenital and Acquired Color Vision Defects,* J. Pokorny, V.C. Smith, G. Verriest, A.J.L.G. Pinckers, eds. New York: Grune and Stratton, 1979, p. 183.
81. Rayleigh (Lord). Experiments on color vision. *Nature* 1881;25:64–66.

81a. Rosenthal O, Phillips RH. *Coping with Color-Blindness.* Garden City, NY: Avery Publishing Group, 1997.

82. Ruddock KH. Psychophysics of inherited colour vision deficiencies. In *The Perception of Color Vision,* P. Gouras, ed. *Vision and Visual Dysfunctions, Vol. 7.* Boca Raton: CRC Press, 1991, pp. 4–31.
83. Sanocki E, Lindsey DT, Winderickx J, Teller DY, Deeb SS, Motulsky AG. Serine/alanine amino acid polymorphism of the L and M cone pigments: Effects on Rayleigh matches among deuteranopes, protanopes, and color normal observers. *Vision Res* 1993;33:2139–2152.
84. Sanocki E, Shevell SK, Winderickx J. Serine/Alanine amino acid polymorphism of the L-cone pigment assessed by dual Rayleigh-type color matches. *Vision Res* 1994;34:377–382.
85. Stamatoyannopoulos G. Human hemoglobin switching. *Science* 1991;252:383.
86. Steward JM, Cole BL. What do color vision defectives say about everyday tasks? *Optom Vis Sci* 1989;66:288–295.
87. Stocks P, Karn MN. A biometric investigation of twins and their brothers and sisters. *Ann Eugenics* 1933;5:17.
88. Stryer L. Visual excitation and recovery. *J Biol Chem* 1991;266:1071–1074.
89. Van Heel, Wen LN, Van Norren D. Frequency of tritan disturbances in population study. In: G. Verriest, ed. *Color vision deficiencies* 1980;5:256–260, Bristol, England: Hilger.
90. Verriest G, Neubauer O, Marre M, Uvijls A. New investigations on the relationships between congenital colour vision defects and road traffic safety. In *Colour vision deficiencies, Vol. V,* G. Verriest, ed. Bristol, England: Hilger, 1980, pp. 331–342.
91. Voke J. *Color Vision Testing in Specific Industries and Professions.* London: Keeler, 1980.
92. Vollrath D, Nathans J, Davis RW. Tandem array of human visual pigment genes at Xq28. *Science* 1988;240:1669–1672.
93. Waaler GHM. Heredity of two types of colour normal vision. *Nature* 1967;215:406.
94. Walls GL. Peculiar color blindness in peculiar people. *Arch Ophthalmol* 1959;62:13–32.
95. Wang Y, Macke JP, Merbs SL, Zack D, Klaunberg B, Bennet J, Gearhart J, Nathans J. A locus control region adjacent to the human red and green visual pigment genes. *Neuron* 1992;9:429–440.
96. Weitz CJ, Miyake Y, Shinzato K, Montag E, Zrenner E, Went LN, Nathans J. Human tritanopia associated with two amino acid substitutions in the blue sensitive opsin. *Am J Hum Genet* 1992a;50:496–507.
97. Weitz CJ, Went L, Nathans J. Human tritanopia associated with a third amino acid substitution in the blue-sensitive visual pigment. *Am J Hum Genet* 1992b;51:444–446.
98. Went LN, Pronk N. The genetics of tritan disturbances. *Hum Genet* 1985;69:255–262.
99. Wesner MF, Pokorny J, Shevell SK, Smith VC. Foveal cone detection statistics in color normals and dichromats. *Vision Res* 1991;31: 1021–1037.
100. Williams AJ, Hunt DM, Bowmaker JK, Mollon JD. The polymorphic pigments of the marmoset: Spectral tuning and genetic basis. *EMBO J* 1992;1:2039–2045.
101. Wilson EB. The sex chromosomes. *Arch Mikrosk Anat Enwicklungsmech* 1911;77:249.
102. Winderickx J, Lindsey DT, Sanocki E, Teller DY, Motulsky AG, Deeb SS. A Ser/Ala polymorphism in the red photopigment underlies variation in color matching among color-normal individuals. *Nature* 1992a;356:431–433.
103. Winderickx J, Battisti L, Motulsky AG, Deeb SS. Selective expression of the human X-linked green pigment genes. *Proc Natl Acad Sci USA* 1992c;89:9710–9714.
104. Winderickx J, Sanocki E, Lindsey DT, Teller DY, Motulsky AG, Deeb SS. Defective color vison associated with a missense (Cys-203-Arg) mutation in the human green visual pigment gene. *Nature Genet* 1992b;1:251–256.
105. Yagasaki Y, Jacobson SG. Cone-rod dystrophy. Phenotypic diversity by retinal function testing. *Arch Ophthalmol* 1989;107:701.

106. Yamaguchi T, Motulsky AG, Deeb, SS. Visual pigment gene structure and expression in human retinae. *Hum Mol Genet* 1997;6:981–990.
107. Yokota A, Shin Y, Kimura J, Senos T, Seki R, Tsubota K. Congenital deuteranomaly in one of three MZ triplets. In *Color Vision Defects*, Y. Ohta, ed. Tokyo: Kuguler 7 Ghedini, 1990.
108. Yokoyama S, Yokoyama R. Convergent evolution of the red- and green-like visual pigment genes in fish, *Astyanax fasciatus*, and human. *Proc Natl Acad Sci USA* 1990;87:9315–9318.
109. Young T. On the theory of light and colours. *Phil Trans R Soc Lond* 1802;92:12–48.

17

Retinitis Pigmentosa

ALAN C. BIRD

Investigative activity into the pathogenesis of retinal dystrophies has been highly productive over the last two decades, and yet from the early part of this century until about 20 years ago there was little advance in the understanding of retinal dystrophies. Renewed interest was heralded by the advent of electrophysiology. At the outset of the current era of research, it was realized that retinal photoreceptor dystrophies comprise a variety of disparate genetically determined conditions, and that to achieve any success in research it was important to identify single nosological entities or at least to divide the whole into purer samples of disease. That they differed one from another in their mode of inheritance, their pattern of visual loss, and their ophthalmoscopic appearances was evident, but no reliable system of classification existed, and the significance of the varied attributes of the pathogenesis of disease was unknown. It was possible to subdivide photoreceptor dystrophies into broad groups depending on their clinical features. Some cause symptoms early in the course of disease, indicating primary loss of rod function, and examination reveals defective vision in the mid zone of the visual field and morphological changes in the postequatorial fundus. Most of the diseases in this category are known collectively as *retinitis pigmentosa*. Other disorders involving loss of cone function and morphological changes in the central fundus are known as *macular* or *cone* dystrophies. This subdivision into "peripheral degenerations," in which the rods may be the primary target of disease, and "central degenerations," in which the cones may be the cells initially affected, is superficially attractive. However, the function of both rod and cone systems is compromised in most, if not all, progressive disorders, even in the early stages of disease. The receptor dystrophies, therefore, comprise a spectrum of disease ranging from predominant rod dystrophies to predominant cone dystrophies, with disorders intermediate between the two in which there is varying involvement of the rod and cone systems.

The discovery in 1989 that the gene responsible for retinitis pigmentosa (RP) in one large Irish family was on the long arm of chromosome 3,[118] and in the following year that a point mutation in the rhodopsin gene was responsible for disease in a proportion of subjects in North America with autosomal disease[38] provided a major impetus to research. During the last 5 years six genes have been implicated in retinal degeneration—rhodopsin, peripherin/"retinal degeneration slow" (RDS), tissue inhibitor of metalloproteinase (TIMP)-3, geronyl–geronyl transferase, ornithine amino acid-transferase, and -phosphodiesterase and in some, many different mutations have been identified with variable phenotypes. Furthermore, 20 other loci have been linked to retinal dystrophy, although the responsible genes have yet to be determined. It was hoped that knowledge of the function of the protein, and the putative dysfunction consequent on the mutation, would give some indication as to the pathogenesis of the disorders, and that this could be matched with the phenotype.

ROD STRUCTURE AND FUNCTION

Histopathological studies show primary loss of photoreceptor cells with variable loss of inner retina.[50] The recent demonstration of aberrant photoreceptor cell axons extending into the inner retina is intriguing, although the functional consequences are unknown.[103] Lipofuscin accumulation in the retinal pigment epithelium may or may not be excessive.[163] It is generally believed that most disorders within retinitis pigmentosa are due to a primary defect in rod photoreceptor cells. Other cellular changes are thought to be secondary events. Therefore, it follows that a mutation in a gene encoding a protein that is peculiar to rods or important to rod function may cause demise of rods and, consequently, retinitis pigmentosa. A great deal of information is available concerning the proteins involved in rod phototransduction and these have been well summarized.[55,136] In the dark-adapted state the cyclic guanosine monophosphate (cGMP)-gated cation channels are open, and a dark current is maintained by the sodium/potassium exchanger. Photoactivation is initiated by absorption of photons by rhodopsin converting it to R* in which 11-*cis* retinal is converted to the all-*trans* isomer. The conformational change of the rhodopsin molecule triggers a reaction involving transducin and phosphodiesterase, which causes a reduction of the level of cGMP by converting it to 5′ GMP. This causes an increase in the proportion of the cation channels to be closed and consequent hyperpolarization of the photoreceptor cell. The reaction is modulated by many other proteins such as rhodopsin kinase, recoverin, and arrestin, and by the cytoplasmic level of calcium, which itself is subject to complex regulatory mechanisms. Two structural proteins are known to be important to the physical stability of the rod, namely ROM1 (rod outer segment membrane protein 1) and peripherin/RDS. Mutations in any of the genes coding for these proteins represent candidate genes for retinitis pigmentosa. The normal function of the rod photoreceptor also depends on the retinal pigment epithelium, which is responsible for recycling outer segment constituents, and on the production of growth factors, which govern its cyclic activity. On a theoretical basis, disturbance of these functions may also cause demise of rods, as is evident in the Royal College of Surgeons (RCS)-rat, in which the primary disorder resides in the retinal pigment epithelium.

CLINICAL ASPECTS

Clinical Genetics

The initial subdivision of retinitis pigmentosa was achieved on the basis of inheritance, about 60% having autosomal recessive disease, 10%–25% autosomal dominant, and 5%–18% X linked.[76]

Functional Deficits

Visual Loss

In general the first symptom is difficulty with night vision, followed by loss of peripheral visual field occurring at variable intervals thereafter. There is great variation in the age of onset of symptoms, as well as speed of progress between families and even within families. It is usual for X-linked and autosomal recessive disease to be severe, and autosomal dominant disease is often mild. However, in some patients with assumed recessive disease, the disorder may have a benign course. Loss of scotopic function is most often detected first between 10° and 40° from fixation, and with time this spreads, so that in the late stages the remaining visual field is limited to the central few degrees and the temporal periphery.

To gain a better understanding of these disorders, attempts were made to subdivide the retinal dystrophies into purer samples of disease on the basis of functional loss. Two broad categories of autosomal dominant retinitis pigmentosa have been identified that are designated *type I* or "diffuse," and *type II* or "regional" forms.[87,107,112] The functional characteristics are consistent within families, indicating genetic heterogeneity. In families with diffuse retinitis pigmentosa, affected members show widespread loss of rod function with relatively well-preserved cone function at some stage in the evolution of their disease. In contrast, those with regional retinitis pigmentosa show variation in the state of rod and cone function, with severe losses of both systems in some regions and near normal function in others. In regional retinitis pigmentosa loss of rhodopsin accounts for the reduction of sensitivity, but in diffuse retinitis pigmentosa there is more rhodopsin than would be predicted if reduced light absorption by visual pigment were responsible for sensitivity loss. These findings suggest that in regional retinitis pigmentosa loss of rod function is due to photoreceptor cell death, short outer segments, or a combination of the two, whereas in diffuse retinitis pigmentosa this cannot be the case. Usually these two subtypes can be distinguished clinically by history alone. In the diffuse form, night blindness is consistently reported within the first decade of life, and symptoms of visual field loss by day follow some 20 years later. Pigmentation is often sparse until late in the disease, which may reflect the lack of cell death at least in the first few years of disease. In contrast, in the regional form, night blindness and trouble by day occur simultaneously, and the age of onset is variable, even within the same family. Pigmentation is seen much earlier in regional retinitis pigmentosa than in the diffuse form.

Other distinctive characteristics have also been recognized in autosomal disease. In some families there is slow recovery from bleach.[87,107,112] Cone adaptation and the early part of the recovery of rod sensitivity follow the normal time course, but the later phase of rod adaptation is markedly prolonged. The expressivity in some families is highly variable, such that about 70% of members with the abnormal gene have moderate to severe disease. The remainder are asymptomatic, with mild fundus abnormalities and electrophysiological changes indicating the presence of the abnormal gene.[120] In some families, there appears to be bimodal expression of disease.[41]

Specific clinical subtypes have also been recognized within autosomal recessive retinitis pigmentosa. Since its original description, Leber's congenital amaurosis has been considered a distinct category of disease.[99] In one study it appears to be a monofactorial autosomal recessive affection,[2] but in another several forms of the disease appeared to exist, some of which were indistinguishable from autosomal recessive retinitis pigmentosa of early onset.[69] In terms of pathogenesis some may represent severe forms of autosomal recessive disease, whereas those with poor vision from birth may have a maturation failure of the retina rather than degeneration of fully developed photoreceptor cells.

Electroretinographic Loss

Soon after the introduction of the electroretinogram (ERG) into clinical practice, its amplitude was found to be reduced in retinitis pigmentosa, and patients with relatively good visual function had unrecordable ERGs.[143] Riggs believed that receptor cell death alone was insufficient to account for the absence of the ERG[143] and suggested that peripheral receptor degeneration caused short-circuiting between the retina and the choroid so that potentials generated in the retina could not be recorded by a distant corneal electrode. However, it became evident that with better recording systems and averaging techniques, electroretinographic potentials could be recorded in many cases.[68] It was concluded that the reduction of the ERG in retinitis pigmentosa is due to retinal dysfunction alone.

Using a homogeneous light stimulus and an adapting background illumination, qualitative analyses of the ERG in different forms of retinitis pigmentosa have been undertaken. It has been postulated that diminution of the electroretinographic potential in the presence of normal latency implies a reduced population of normal receptors, whereas a prolonged implicit time implies widespread receptor dysfunction.[12] The ERG varies in different forms of retinitis pigmentosa. For example, in patients of a single pedigree with dominantly inherited disease the rod ERG component was reduced in amplitude and in latency, whereas the cone component was normal. In another family with dominantly inherited retinitis pigmentosa with reduced penetrance, the cone responses were also abnormal.[10] This finding supports the concept that the difference in penetrance signifies distinct forms of autosomal dominant retinitis pigmentosa, and the difference in the influence of the diseases on retinal function implies the presence of different pathogenetic mechanisms within this genetic group of retinitis pigmentosa. In X-linked disease, both cone and rod responses are delayed and reduced.[11]

Fundus Appearance

In most cases the earliest changes correspond to the area of functional loss and are seen as discoloration of the retinal pigment epithelium, which often appears gray with pale deposits at the level of the outer retina. At this stage fluorescein angiography demonstrates loss of pigment epithelial melanin. With time there is migration of pigmented cells into the inner retina. The cells often migrate to blood vessels[103] forming the "typical bone-corpuscle" pigmentation (Fig. 17.1). Loss of inner retina with optic disc pallor and narrowing of the retinal blood is a late phenomenon and is inconsistent even in advanced disease. Macular edema is a common complication and retinal telangiectasis is well reported.

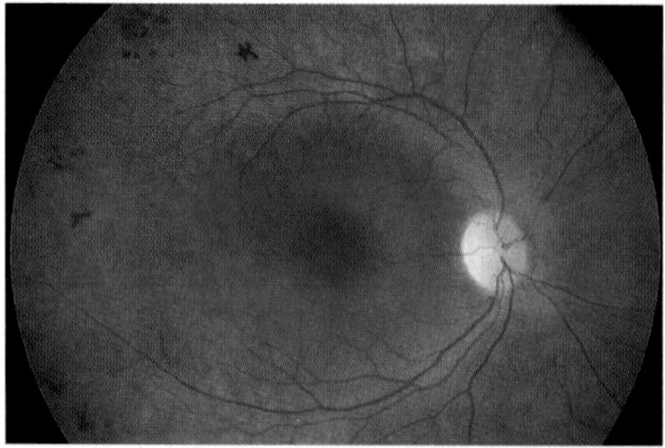

Figure 17.1. Retinitis pigmentosa. The optic nerve is waxy pale, the retinal vessels are attenuated, and there is midperipheral retinal atrophy and atrophy of the retinal pigment epithelium with bony spicule pigment clumping.

Autosomal dominant disease has been described in which the distribution is different from the usual pattern of preferential involvement in the midperiphery throughout 360° of the fundus. Sector retinitis pigmentosa is characterized by retinal atrophy restricted to part of the fundus, and gross field loss is confined to the area of visual field corresponding to the involved retina.[60] The lower half of the fundus is usually affected with loss of visual function in the upper field, but rarely does the disease affect only the superior, nasal, or temporal fundus. In most reported cases with limited sector involvement the inheritance is autosomal dominant, and the distribution of disease was common to affected members of the family.[95] However, a similar pattern of disease also appears in patients with relatives who have involvement of the whole fundus, and some are heterozygous for X-linked retinitis pigmentosa.[20] In typical sector retinitis pigmentosa, rod and cone ERGs show mild reduction in amplitude with normal cone implicit times.[13] This pattern of disease is common to all affected members within a family irrespective of age, suggesting that the disease, in contrast to other forms of autosomal dominant retinitis pigmentosa, is nonprogressive or progresses very slowly. Retinitis pigmentosa has also been described with preservation of the retinal pigment epithelium adjacent to the retinal arterioles, and, unlike many patients with retinitis pigmentosa, they are consistently hypermetropic.[65] Paravenous pigmented chorioretinal atrophy has been discribed in several reports in which there is atrophy of the retinal pigment epithelium underlying the retinal veins, which usually extends from the optic disc with pigment around the retinal veins. In most cases the disorder is described as an isolated phenomenon that may be inflammatory in origin.[51,128] However, reports exist with familial involvement, namely a mother and son, a father and son, and three brothers.[101,154,165] It has been shown to be very variable in its severity within a family such that the presence of affected relatives cannot be excluded without undertaking a family survey. Most authors take the view that this condition may be genetically determined but that phenocopies exist. Rapid progression, slow progression, and stable visual function have been described. The disorder may also be asymmetrical.

Well-defined atrophy radiating from the optic disc but not following the blood vessels was first described in an Icelandic family and was called "choroiditis striata," although in a further report on the same family the term "helicoid peripapillary chorioretinal degeneration" was used.[161,162] Several reports have followed that appear to concern families exclusively from Iceland and Switzerland, implying the possibility that only two families exist.[21,52,109,147] The disorder is believed to be slowly progressive, the visual loss is variable, and it is associated with refractive error, which is often the reason for ascertainment.

No good explanation exists for the variation of distribution of disease. In most forms of retinitis pigmentosa the functional loss appears to start from 15° to 20° from fixation, but in some it appears first in the far periphery and in others in a restricted band at 10° of eccentricity. No unique physiological attribute is known that would predict one pattern or another. It is to be hoped that knowledge of the mutations causing these different patterns will allow concepts to be formulated. It is tempting to ascribe the inferior involvement to higher lighting levels of the inferior retina than the superior retina.[66]

A further variant comprises night blindness and variably reduced visual acuity associated with restricted pigmentation in the ocular fundus, cystoid macular changes resembling macular schisis, and distinctive electroretinographic abnormalities.[111] The scotopic ERG is unrecordable, maximal stimulus evokes a large response with very prolonged implicit time of the b-wave, photopic and scotopic responses are of similar magnitude, and the response is much larger when produced by short- than by long-wavelength light. The last attribute is known as the enhanced-cone response. At least in some respects this disorder resembles the Goldmann-Favre syndrome[46]; it is not yet clear if this represents a single disorder with variable expressivity.

A unique fundus appearance was reported by Bietti in three patients, two of whom were brothers, who had crystals in the retina and in the peripheral cornea.[18] There is progressive atrophy of the retina with prominent loss of the pigment epithelium and inner choroid. As the atrophy supervenes, the intraretinal crystals disappear. The pattern of retinal functional loss is similar to that of retinitis pigmentosa, with the initial symptoms usually appearing in the third or fourth decade of life. Autosomal recessive inheritance was established in this condition by Hu,[71] although crystals have been described in patients heterozygous for the abnormal gene.[139] Patients with a similar fundus appearance but without corneal changes have been described and are considered to represent the same disorder. No systemic biochemical disorder has been identified, although the corneal crystals resemble cholesterol or cholesterol ester, suggesting that Bietti crystalline dystrophy may be due to a systemic abnormality of lipid metabolism. This conclusion was supported by the finding of crystals in lymphocytes.[183]

As early as 1914, Diem reported abnormal fundus reflexes in females heterozygous for X-linked retinitis pigmentosa,[34] but during subsequent years similar phenomena were reported in other genetic forms of the disease and were referred to as "tapetal reflexes."[44] An abnormal tapetal reflex has been reported to be the most common expression of the heterozygous state in X-linked disease.[94] However, Schappert-Kimmijser could identify this abnormal reflex in females of only one family out of eight and concluded that although this sign is useful when present, its absence does not indicate a normal genotype.[151] Attempts have been made to subdivide X-linked retinitis pigmentosa on the basis of differential affection of heterozygotes.[92,116] However, subsequent experience showed that considerable intrafamilial variation in the severity of the disease in heterozygotes implies little justification for separating X-linked retinitis pigmentosa (RP) into different categories on the basis of the severity of the disease in women.[20] Recently, two different clinical profiles in X-linked disease have been defined as a function of age and mode of onset. The first clinical form has very early onset with severe myopia, whereas the second form starts later with night blindness and mild or no refractive error. The first appeared to be associated with the centromeric gene locus (RP2) and the second with the telemeric locus (RP3),[82] although this remains to be confirmed.

Unilateral disease was reported as early as 1865,[134] and the ophthalmoscopic observations were corroborated by histological examination 25 years later.[33] However, the commonly held view is that there is no good evidence that unilateral disease represents a heritable condition,[54] and that the disease is due to vascular disease, trauma, "diffuse unilateral subacute neuroretinitis," or "acute zonal occult outer retinopathy."[24,56,57] In no case of unilateral disease has a family history of eye disease been identified: the parents of one patient were, however, consanguineous.[31]

MOLECULAR BIOLOGY

The first retinitis pigmentosa gene to be localized was one for X-linked retinitis pigmentosa using a probe L1.28[17] that maps to the short arm near the centromere at Xp11. This is now known as RP2. Subsequently, further loci were identified that were telomeric to the first. One was sited between OTC and CYBR in Xp21.1,[32,129,132] which was termed RP3, and one in Xp22.13-p22.11 (RP 15).[115] The possiblity of more than one abnormal allele at each locus has not been excluded. The identification of a deletion at Xp21 in a child (BB) with retinitis pigmentosa, Duchenne muscular dystrophy, and X-linked chronic granulomatous disease[53] indicated a potential site for the causative gene for RP3 at a site telomeric to OTC. Recently several mutations in gene RPGR have been found in patients with X-linked retinitis pigmentosa.[119] The function of this gene, and its relevance to retinal function, are unknown. As yet, the proportion of families with RP3 having mutations within this gene is not evident. Interestingly, it is close to OTC and is not within the BB deletion, indicating that the form of the disease in the child with this deletion is different from that seen in some families with RP3.

In 1989, a locus for autosomal dominant retinitis pigmentosa was identified on the long arm of chromosome 3.[118] Three candidate genes exist close to the proposed site, and within a short time a proline–histidine mutation was detected at codon 23 of the rhodopsin molecule in a proportion of patients with autosomal dominant retinitis pigmentosa in North Amerca.[38] Since then many genomic defects have been detected in the rhodopsin gene, and it appears that it accounts for about 30% of autosomal dominant retinitis pigmentosa.[36,37,74,157] Most mutations appear to be peculiar to a single family, although some, for example at codon 347, have been found in many parts of the world. The proline–histidine mutation at codon 23 was identified in a proportion of apparently unrelated subjects in the United States, but not in other countries, suggesting that they may all belong to one large pedigree.

In several families with autosomal dominant retinitis pigmentosa, the locus on the long arm of chromosome 3 was excluded, confirming heterogeneity of dominant disease, and it has now been shown that genes other than that for rhodopsin may be responsible for autosomal dominant disease. One of these is the gene for the glycoprotein peripherin/RDS[45,80] which is of particular interest, because it is a mutation in this gene that is responsible for the retinal degeneraton in the *rds*-mouse.[29,166] Peripherin/RDS is localized to the outer segment disc membranes of both rods and cones, and is thought to be essential for the assembly, orientation, and physical stability of the outer segment discs of the retinal photoreceptors.[4,30,169]

Recently mutations have been identified as responsible for recessive disease. A stop sequence at codon 249 in exon 4 of the rhodopsin gene caused no symptoms or fundus changes in the heterozygous state, although the ERG potentials were reduced to 50% of normal.[146] Patients homozygous for the mutation had retinitis pigmentosa. A missense mutation at codon 150 has also been associated with autosomal recessive retinitis pigmentosa.[96] Mutations in the gene coding for the β-subunit of phosphodiesterase (-PDE) have also been recorded as causing autosomal recessive retinitis pigmentosa.[117] Five different mutations were found in the first five of the 22 exons, and one case appeared to be heterozygous for two different mutations, which is termed a *compound heterozygous state.* These findings are of particular interest given that a mutation in the *-pde* gene is responsible for retinal degeneration in the *rds*-mouse.

Recently it has been shown that two distinct and unlinked genetic abnormalities may cause retinal dystrophies.[79] In three families it was shown that being heterozygous for specific mutations, in either peripherin/*RDS* or *ROM1* did not produce disease, but possession of both mutant genes was associated with retinitis pigmentosa. This was termed *digenic inheritance* and may produce pedigrees that appear to be autosomal dominant but with less than 100% penetrance, or recessive disease.

PATHOGENESIS OF PHOTORECEPTOR DYSTROPHIES

General Considerations

The initial subdivision of retinal dystrophies was achieved on the basis of its inheritance and its morphological and functional attributes. As a consequence of identifying the responsible mutations, or at least the causative gene, it is now possible to attempt correlation of these characteristics to putative disease mechanisms and to generate hypotheses that are amenable to testing in the laboratory. There is every prospect that our understanding of the pathogenetic mechanisms will increase in the next few years, particularly if there is continued and, if possible, increasing collaboration between clinicians and basic scientists. This requires better knowledge of the precise function of the proteins involved, the nature of dysfunction likely to arise from mutations, and observation of the consequences in humans and in transgenic animals.

Hereditary disorders are caused by defects in the genetic code, which, in turn, result in an abnormal amino acid composition of specific proteins. If a mutant gene codes for a protein the activity of which is confined to a single cell type, the primary effect will be localized to that cell, and secondary effects may occur in other cells. For example, the mutation may either reside in the photoreceptor cell giving rise to the observed degeneration or it may be expressed in a support tissue, leading to similar consequences. The recognition that a disease affecting the retinal pigment epithelium is due to mutations in the peripherin/*RDS* gene, which is expressed in photoreceptor cells, has already induced a change in our appreciation of potential disease processes. Alternatively, a systemic metabolic abnormality may result in the degeneration of a specific cell type, such as visual cells, by depriving those cells of vital metabolites.

In autosomal recessive conditions, the disease exists in the homozygous state, in which both alleles are abnormal. The assumption is that the product of a single normal gene is sufficient to maintain normal cellular function. In autosomal dominant disease the abnormality is produced in the heterozygous state. The disease may be due to the product of the abnormal gene disrupting cell function or to a shortage of product from a single normal gene. The first is shown by the observation that mice transfected with a mutant rhodopsin gene develop retinal degeneration.[130] The second possibility is illustrated in the *rds*-mouse in which transgenic rescue has been achieved by insertion of a normal peripherin gene on a rhodopsin promoter.[168] Retinal changes in the heterozygous *rds*-mouse are compatible with this concept.[64]

Some observations on the behavior of the abnormal protein made in the laboratory illustrate cellular handling of abnormal gene products. Abnormal mRNA may not leave the nucleus so that translation does not occur. After translation, it has been shown that abnormal proteins may not pass from the rough endoplasmic reticulum to the Golgi apparatus, and that this depends on the influence of the mutation on molecular folding.[105] Those proteins that do not pass on may be destroyed or may accumulate in the rough endoplasmic reticulum, and this accumulation, in turn, may interfere with cell function.[23,91,104] From these considerations it is predictable that the nature of cell dysfunction would depend on the site of expression of the abnormal protein. For example, if the protein is not expressed in the outer segment, only the product of one gene would be available and disease may be a consequence of reduced quantities of rhodopsin, so-called haplotype insufficiency. In contrast, if the abnormal protein were incorporated into the outer segment it might generate dysfunction.

The fate of protein produced by rhodopsin genes with mutations found in human retinitis pigmentosa has been investigated.[85,158,160] COS and 293S cells were transfected with various mutant rhodopsin genes. The abnormal proteins could be divided into distinct classes according to their behavior when compared with normal. Class I mutant protein behaved like wild-type protein in that it was expressed on the plasma membrane and bound 11-*cis*-retinal, creating a chromophore with an absorbance spectrum similar to that of rhodopsin. Class II mutations showed little if any ability to form a pigment when exposed to 11-*cis*-retinal, to inefficient transport to the plasma membrane, and to low levels of cell surface localization. However, in no instance was expression on the plasma membrane absent. In a similar experiment, mutant rhodopsin was prepared by site-directed mutagenesis, and COS cells were transfected and incubated in the presence of 11-*cis* retinal. There was no binding of 11-*cis* retinal with the 68-72 deletion. Binding did occur with Thr-58-Arg, 137-Leu, and Arg-135-Trp mutations, giving rise to a pigment with a max of 500 n · ms. Although light caused conversion to meta-rhodopsin II. When incubated with guanosine diphosphate (GDP) and transducin there was defective activation.

Several of the mutations were identical to those found in forms of retinitis pigmentosa in which the functional deficit has been characterized. Pro-347-Leu was designated as biochemical class I, and the same mutation in humans causes diffuse retinitis pigmentosa. The mutations Pro-23-His, Thr-58-Arg, and Gly-106-Trp were designated as biochemical class II, and in humans are associated with regional retinitis pigmentosa with altitudinal distribution of disease and slow recovery from strong light adaptation. These findings give some credence to the clinical relevance of these findings.

It cannot be assumed that the distribution of protein in cell culture reflects expression in the retina. Some information now exists concerning in vivo expression. A mouse with a naturally occurring mutation (Gln344ter), which truncates the last five amino acids from the C-terminal, has significant expression of the mutant protein on the plasma membrane of the photoreceptor cell rather than having it exclusively in the outer segment.[159]

The identification of mutations in the rhodopsin and peripherin genes allows investigation of pathogenetic mechanisms involved. It is fortunate that much was known concerning the structure and function of both proteins prior to discovery of the mutations.

Rhodopsin Mutations

Attempts have been made to correlate the phenotype with specific mutations. Severity of disease has been reported to be determined to some extent by the location of the mutation in the gene.[148] Patients with mutations coding for amino acids in the intradiscal domain or low-numbered condons had milder disease than those with altered cytoplasmic domain or higher-numbered codons. Mutations altering the transmembrane domains had intermediate severity.

Qualitative differences in phenotype have also been demonstrated with different mutations.[47–49,88–90,93,133,140,155] In three mutations, pro347leu, lys296glu (the binding site for retinal), and an isoleucine deletion at codon 255 or 256, functional loss compatible with diffuse (type I) autosomal dominant retinitis pigmentosa was identified. With all three mutations poor night vision was consistently present in early life, and rod ERGs were severely reduced or unmeasurable. In patients with measurable visual function, psychophysical testing showed rod function to be severely affected throughout the retina with threshold elevations of more than 3 log units, whereas loss of cone function was less widespread and less severe than loss of rod function. In one of the most severe disorders (Lys-296-Glu), there was little visual function after 30 years of age in most affected family members. With the isoleucine deletion at codon 256, cone function was limited to the central 10° by 25 years of age, but little further loss occurred thereafter. Cone function was retained over most of the visual field until middle life with the 347 mutation despite widespread and severe early loss of rod function. The functional abnormality in families with mutations Thr17Arg, Pro23His, Thr58Arg, Gly106Arg, and Gua182Ade is qualitatively different with altitudinal distribution of disease, and this attribute appears to be constant within the families. Rod sensitivity is severely depressed in the superior field but is nearly normal in the inferior field. Loss of cone sensitivity closely follows that of the rods. In this respect the pattern of disease resembles regional (type II) retinitis pigmentosa. An additional striking finding in these families with sector type retinitis pigmentosa is a characteristic abnormality in one component of the kinetics of dark adaptation following exposure to a bright light. Prior to bleaching, measurements made in the relatively intact portion of the visual field show mild threshold elevations of approximately 1 log unit. Following light adaptation there is a marked delay in the recovery of sensitivity. The initial portion of recovery mediated by cones and rods is normal. However after 1 h, when recovery of sensitivity in the normal subjects was complete, these patients showed residual threshold elevations of 1–2 log units from the prebleach values. Even after nearly 2 h thresholds were still elevated by more than 1.0 log unit. In two subjects it was found that the time course of this recovery of sensitivty was at least 80–120 h.[121] Using a model based on primate data of rod outer segment length and turnover, it has been calculated that the delayed phase of the recovery of rod sensitivty following strong light adaptation could be due in part to the formation of new disc membranes with a normal concentration of rhodopsin rather than in situ regeneration of photopigment. The model requires that the outer segments are short as a result of retinitis pigmentosa and that a major portion of the outer segment is shed following strong light adaptation.

These findings show that there are both quantitative and qualitative differences in the retinitis pigmentosa consequent to different mutations in the rhodopsin gene. Also important is the demonstration for the first time that some forms of retinitis pigmentosa are due to defects of metabolic systems that are limited to rod photoreceptors, and yet it is evident that loss of photopic function is consistently found in these disorders.

The basic membrane topography of the rhodopsin molecule is known, but details of structural reorganization during photostimulation and consequent alterations in receptor unmasking are less well understood. Therefore, at present it is not possible to predict with confidence the subtle alterations in function consequent to specific changes in amino acids. The rhodopsin molecule consists of 348 amino acid residues with two aspargine-linked oligosaccharide side chains. Peptide folding results in seven predominantly α-helices being embedded in the outer segment disc bilayer, with interconnecting hydrophilic segments protruding from the membranous surface.[1,62] A lysine residue (296) situated at the midpoint of the seventh helix is the attachment site for the 11-*cis* retinal chromophore. This 11-*cis* retinal also interacts with the other helices and as all seven are aligned in a plane perpendicular to the disc surface, they effectively form a cage around the chromophore. Photon absorption by 11-*cis* retinal causes isomerization of the chromophore to the all-*trans* form with simultaneous rearrangement of the helices. This conformational change in rhodopsin exposes a binding site (residues 231–252) for the G protein, transducin, on the cytoplasmic surface. This is the first step in signal amplification and activation of the enzymic cascade leading to visual transduction. On the cytoplasmic surface, the carboxy terminal contains many serines and threonines, which subsequent to formation of R* are phosphorylated by a rhodopsin kinase. The ensuing binding of arrestin to phosphorylated rhodopsin blocks the further activation of transducin, which is one of the termination steps in visual transduction.

With some mutations the available information about its influence on function allows speculation as to the possible disease mechanisms if the gene product is expressed in the outer segment. It has been shown in vitro that rhodopsin with a mutation at codon 296, which determines the binding site for retinal, would prevent binding with 11-*cis* retinal and that the opsin reacts constantly with transducin. It would be predicted from this observation that the retina may act as if it were in constant lighting and would not dark adapt. Similarly, the mutant protein Ala292Glu activates opsin in vitro and is associated with stationary night blindness. The mutant with Gly90Asp in the second transmembrane segment of rhodopsin, which causes retinitis pigmentosa also constitutively activates transducin.[138,144,145] It has been postulated that the constitutively activating mutations operate by a common molecular mechanism, disrupting a salt bridge between Lys296 and the Schiff base counterion, Glu 113. These observations would explain insensitivity to light. However, in a mouse transfected with mutant rhodopsin (Lys296Glu), the mutant opsin was found to be invariably phosphorylated and stably bound to arrestin.[102] Light-independent activation of transducin was demonstrated only after the removal of arrestin and dephosphorylation of mutant opsin. This observation throws some doubt on the suggestion that these mutations cause constant activation of transducin in vivo, and leaves open the question of why degeneration occurs.

Physical instability of the molecule would occur if glycosylation on the *N*-terminal or the disulfide bond between the cysteine residues 110 and 187 were abnormal.[35,83,84] Disruption of this conserved disulfide bond by Cys187Tyr mutation causes early and severe autosomal dominant retinitis pigmentosa.[141] Transduction efficiency may be reduced by mutations near the c-terminal causing a reduction of sensitivity due to a reduced signal. A great deal of work is in progress attempting to identify the functional abnormalities likely to result from mutations found in humans,[3,19,42,119a,142,177,190] which will broaden the scope for formulating pathogenetic concepts. It is also hoped that studies on transgenic mice will give additional information as to the pathogenesis of disease. To date such studies have shown differential affection of rod and cone photoreceptors which simulates human disease, although qualitative differences in disease have yet to be shown with various mutations.

Peripherin/*RDS* Mutations

Even more striking is the identification that both retinitis pigmentosa and macular dystrophy may be due to mutations in the *RDS* gene.[45,80,81,127,178,180,184,185] The retinitis pigmentosa is of early onset and is not obviously different from that seen with rhodopsin mutations, with one exception in which the disease simulated retinitis punctata albescens. Two families with a form of macular dystrophy have been shown to have a tryptophan substitution for arginine at codon 172, and another family with an almost identical disease has a glutamine substitution at the same codon. A mutation resulting in a stop codon at position 258 has been identified in a family with a retinal degeneration similar in appearance to adult vitelliform macular dystrophy, and a mutation at codon 168 causes a pattern dystrophy. The variability of phenotype caused by mutations at different codons suggests that the functional significance of certain amino acids to cones and rods may be different.

The current knowledge of the putative function of peripherin/*RDS* provides a potential explanation for diseases being different with different mutations in the peripherin/*RDS* gene. Peripherin/*RDS*, has an amino acid sequence of 346 amino acids with four transmembrane hydrophobic domains and two putative *N*-linked glycosylation sites.[4,30,166,167,169] One of these is conserved across four species and is thought to be important to the protein's function in stabilizing photoreceptor outer segment membranes. Immunohistochemical studies have shown that the protein is limited to the edges of outer segment discs of both rods and cones, and the general belief is that peripherin/*RDS* is important in closing outer segment discs. It has been shown that peripherin/*RDS* may bind noncovalently to rom1, a protein structurally related to peripherin/*RDS*. Rom1 also has been localized to the disc rims of rod outer segments but has not been identified in cones.[8] It has been proposed that the formation and stability of the bend in the disc membrane in rods is dependent on the association between peripherin/*RDS* and rom1. However, the absence of rom1 in cones implies that differences exist between the precise mechanisms by which the outer segment membranes are stabilized in the two classes of photoreceptor. In rods the association between the two proteins may be important, whereas in cones peripherin/*RDS* may bind to a different membrane protein or act alone. If the binding sites are different in rods and cones, constancy of one amino acid of the peripherin/*RDS* molecule may be important to rods only, and a mutation causing an abnormality at this site would cause a dystrophy falling within the category of retinitis pigmentosa, in which the rod is the target cell of disease with relative preservation of cones. Conversely, a different mutation on the peripherin/*RDS* gene may disrupt either the metabolism or structure of cones alone, causing macular dystrophy of both rods and cones. It appears that the presence of arginine at 172 is important to the structure and function of cones but not rods.[180] However, recently it has been shown that the influence on photoreceptor function is qualitatively similar in patients with either central or peripheral degenerations with peripherin/*RDS* mutations,[86] implying that the difference in disease is not absolute. This conclusion is supported by the observation of pattern dystrophy and retinitis pigmentosa in the same family.[178]

The disorders associated with a stop sequence at codon 258 and the mutation at codon 167 are superficially different from the others with mutations in the peripherin/*RDS* gene in that there is little evidence of functional loss, and the changes in the ocular fundus are apparently at the level of the retinal pigment epithelium. It is possible that these mutations produce metabolic changes similar to those seen in the mouse heterozygous for the mutant gene in which there is a 10 kB insert in the gene at codon 238. In the homozygous *rds*-mouse (*rds*/*rds*) a relatively high molecular weight mRNA is produced, demonstrating that the whole insert is transcribed. However, it is unlikely that the mutant protein is expressed, as the mRNA does not appear to leave the nucleus. Consequently, outer segment discs are not formed, the disc membrane being discharged as small vesicles into the subretinal space.[27,75,150,172] Predictably, only half the normal amount of protein would be available in the heterozygous state (*rds*/+) as a result of expression of a single normal gene. The photoreceptor outer segments develop but contain long lengths of disc membrane,[149] a situation compatible with there being less than the normal quantity of protein. However the ERG is well preserved, and 50% of the photoreceptors survive after 18 months of life, which is close to the life expectancy of the mouse. The outer segments appear to be unstable, and the retinal pigment epithelium contains large and abnormal phagosomes. Such a situation may exist in some patients with adult vitelliform macular degeneration and pattern dystrophies, since the mutations are close. As in the heterozygous *rds*-mouse it is likely that the photoreceptors receive only half the normal quantity of peripherin/rds, and that the abnormal protein does not pass into the outer segment. If the homology is close, it would be understandable that excessive shedding of the photoreceptor outer segments over many years would cause change in the retinal pigment epithelium, but little photoreceptor dysfunction. If this reasoning is correct, a primary photoreceptor disease causes changes that are recognizable clinically only at the level of the retinal pigment epithelium.

Determination of Severity of Disease

Although there are both quantitative and qualitative differences in functional loss between families that may be explained by the different function of proteins encoded by the mutant genes, the severity of disease also varies considerably within families. In many inherited diseases recent studies have elucidated some of the mechanisms whereby variation of phenotype may be caused. For example, in dystrophia myotonica the disease results from the insertion of a nucleotide repeat sequence (cytosine, thymine, guanine—(CTG) in the dystrophia myotonica gene.[22,73,110] The repeat becomes longer in subsequent generations, causing the disease to become more severe. Furthermore, the disease is more severe if inherited from the mother and not the father.[63,97] It appears that the influence of paternal genes may differ from maternal genes in determining some phenotypic characteristics such as placental and fetal size by mechanisms of genomic imprinting and allelic competition.[122,182] This may explain the observation that a mutation inherited from the mother will give rise to the Prader–Willi syndrome, whereas an identical mutation derived from the father results in Angelman syndrome.[108,126] It is also recognized that the expression of one gene may be modulated by another. It is recognized that the heterozygous state of hemoglobin-S gives rise to little disease, but another mutation on the allelic hemoglobin gene—such that either hemoglobin-C, -D, Punjab, O-Arab, or -E is produced—a distinctive phenotype arises.[153] This condition is generally referred to as the *compound heterozygous state.* Digenic inheritance, in which disease is produced by two mutations on different and unlinked genes, may also produce apparent dominant disease with incomplete penetrance or recessive disease.[79] However, this does not account for the phenotype in two families described recently in which there appears to be a negative correlation between the severity of the disease in the parent and the offspring.[41] This could be explained by a common genetic variant that protects from disease such as occurs in sickle cell disease with hereditary persistent high fetal hemoglobin, particularly if such a variant were allelic with the causative gene.[28,70,164] How many of these mechanisms are important in determining the severity of retinal degeneration is not known, but predictably they will be sought in the near future.

Cause of Cell Death

There has been increasing evidence that the metabolic defect caused by the mutation does not cause cell death directly, at least in some disorders, in both humans and animals. This is evident with respect to cone loss in patients with retinitis pigmentosa due to mutations in the rhodopsin gene. A similar situation exists in mice transfected with a mutant rhodopsin gene.[125,130] and in the setter, which has progressive atrophy of both the rod and cone photoreceptors, although cone-pde (phosphodiesterase) activity is normal.[156] This is also illustrated by loss of photoreceptors in the RCS-rat, in which the primary defect is in the retinal pigment epithelium.[123] Of great interest is a chimera created of an albino mouse transfected with a mutant rhodopsin gene and of a wild-type pigmented mouse. Although there was regional distribution of pigmented and nonpigmented cells, the photoreceptor cell death was diffuse rather than regional, implying that the cells containing the mutant and wild-type rhodopsin genes degenerated simultaneously.[72] The only recorded variation between animals was that the proportions of mutant to wild-type populations determined the speed of degeneration. Atrophy was faster in animals in which the chimera consisted of more than 50% of mutant cell as judged by skin pigmentation when compared with animals with less than 50%.

This dilemma may be explained by the observation that cell loss is due to apoptosis. Apoptosis (as opposed to necrosis), or programmed cell death, is a genetically encoded potential of all cells, and it is an essential part of embryonic development. It has been well recorded in many tissues of both vertebrates and invertebrates as a cause of cell loss.[131,137,170,186,187] It may also represent the mechanism of cell turnover and of removal of cells that are infected by virus or that harbor mutations. It is characterized morphologically by disintegration of the nucleolus and generalized condensation of the chromatin. This is associated with incision of most of the nuclear DNA into short but well-organized chains of nucleosomes in multiples of 200 base pairs by an endogenous nonlysosomal nuclease.[186a] These DNA fragments can be identified by gel electrophoresis of a pooled DNA or in situ.[58] After death, a cell is engulfed and quickly degraded by a neighboring cell. In contrast to necrosis, the process affects individual cells within a tissue, its neighbors remaining healthy, and takes place in the absence of inflammation. There is increasing evidence from work on a nematode, *Caenorhabditis elegans,* that apoptosis is regulated by a group of genes, some of which induce (*ced 1, 3, 4*), and others which inhibit (*ced 2, 9*) cell death.[39,67] It is the expression of these genes that governs the production of endonucleases. A homologue to *ced 9, bcl 2* has been identified in vertebrates.[176,189] It had been shown that *bcl 2* inhibited cell death in vertebrates, including humans,[175] and subsequently that *bcl 2* and *ced 9* had considerable structural and functional similarities.[174] The engulfment of the apoptotic cells is also dependent on a further series of genes.[40] For degradation to occur, engulfing cells must recognize, phagocytose, and digest the corpses of dying cells. The factors that govern expression of the genes that induce or suppress apoptosis are as yet unknown.

Apoptosis has been shown to be the cause of cell death in all animals with genetically determined retinal degeneration examined to date, whether naturally occurring or induced by transfection by mutant genes.[25,106,135,171] Thus it appears that cell loss is not a direct consequence of the intrinsic metabolic defect but is due to a change in the metabolic environment of the tissue that influences those genes that govern apoptosis.

CLINICAL MANAGEMENT

There are few forms of retinal dystrophy for which treatment will modify the course of the primary disorder,[26,59,61,77,78,124,173,179] and clearly it is important to identify these disorders. A-betalipoproteinemia can be diagnosed on the basis of the clinical presentation of malabsorption in infancy, and low levels of cholesterol and betalipoproteinemia in blood. The diagnosis of gyrate atrophy of the retina and choroid can be established by recognizing the typical fundus appearance and demonstrating raised blood ornithine and low or absent cellular orthinine aminotransferase activity. Refsum syndrome usually presents with visual loss alone, other deficits appearing some years later. This accounts for the very long delays in making the diagnosis after presentation to ophthalmologists. Most patients have symptoms by 30 years of age and present to the ophthalmologist by 40 years of age. The only other physical deficits likely to be present in early disease are anosmia, hearing loss, and short terminal phalanges of the thumbs, but many patients will have visual loss alone. It is justified to exclude the condition by measuring plasma levels of phytanic acid in patients having symptoms in the first 30 years of life and without evidence of dominant or X-linked inheritance.

In a large study it appears that long-term administration of vitamin A may influence the course of the disorder,[14–16] although this conclusion has not been universally accepted.[113,114] Macular edema and cataract as secondary consequences of retinitis pigmentosa may be amenable to therapy.

In the absence of specific treatment by which the course of the disorder can be modified, patients can reasonably expect accurate advice concerning the genetic implications of the disease and of the visual prognosis. Genetic counseling demands that the inheritance be defined. When transmission can be identified through several generations, the recognition of X-linked or autosomal dominant inheritance is usually simple. As with other disorders, parental consanguinity may indicate the possibility of autosomal recessive inheritance. The inheritance may be evident if the pattern of disease is distinctive and indicative of a single nosological entity with known inheritance. Such a situation is illustrated by choroideremia and gyrate atrophy, which are X-linked and autosomal recessive, respectively. If there is doubt as to inheritance, the genetic status may be established by detailed inquiry of the family by which affected relatives previously unknown to the patient are identified. This is particularly the case in X-linked disease. Further genetic information may be obtained by examining asymptomatic relatives, which may reveal females heterozygous for X-linked disease or evidence of dominant disease if the disorder is mild or has variable expressivity.

When researchers are faced with a sporadic case without distinctive changes, the problem of identifying the genetic form of the disease may be more difficult. Until fairly recently it was commonly assumed that patients with retinitis pigmentosa and no known affected relative had autosomal recessive disease. However, the excess of males over females in this group implies that a number have X-linked disease.[76] Failure to recognize X-linked disease would occur if heterozygous females are asymptomatic and affected male relatives are not known to the proband. Alternatively, the disease may be autosomal dominant as a result of a new mutation, although this is probably uncommon. If a mutation is identified that is known to cause a specific form of retinal dystrophy, the problem may be solved. Finally the possibility of a phenocopy cannot be ignored although in a large series of such cases there is good evidence that such cases are rarely diagnosed as retinitis pigmentosa.[76]

Experience shows that uncertainties are bound to occur, however thorough the enquiry into the family and clinical examination. Difficulty is encountered in females at 50% risk of being heterozygous for X-linked retinitis pigmentosa if the disease is one without a tapetal reflex in the heterozygous state. A similar situation exists with incomplete penetrance of an autosomal dominant mutation, in which there may be no phenotypic expression. In both situations the genetic counselor is in a position to give bad news if the phenotype is recognized, but not good news since the presence of the abnormal gene cannot be excluded by clinical examination. This problem has been solved in a few families in which the locus of the abnormal gene has been identified and the likelihood of the abnormal gene assessed by haplotype analysis.[41,90] Knowledge of the responsible genes and the relevant mutations would give greater accuracy to this analysis. The recent identification of an abnormal gene causing one form of X-linked disease is of paramount importance to clinical management.[119] It may allow confirmation of X-linked disease when this is suspected but unproven on the basis of the family history, and in a family with a known mutation the identification of the heterozygous state can be made with confidence.

To date the considerable advances in research have not led to any treatment by which the basic disease process can be modified, although the impact on clinical management is already evident. Genetic counseling in a family is undoubtedly simplified if the mutation is known. The distribution of the abnormal gene in a family can be documented with almost 100% certainty, and the genetic status of a subject can be established at any age and at any stage of evolution of disease. Furthermore, advice on visual prognosis may be made on a firmer basis if single nosological entities are identified by genomic studies.

These discoveries allow certain management options with respect to the family as a whole. Selective termination of pregnancy may be requested by patients in a small number of conditions in which the disease is severe. Selective implantation of normal embryos following in vitro fertilization is also now feasible. These management techniques have been initiated in severe diseases such as cystic fibrosis. Population screening has also been initiated for cystic fibrosis, by which it is proposed to identify the distribution of the mutant genes within the population.[181] It is not clear if this would be feasible or desirable for retinal dystrophies; to some extent this would depend on the number of genes involved.

Potential for Therapy

Various approaches to treatment have been investigated over the last few years. These include replacement of the defective cells such as retinal pigment epithelium and photoreceptor cells.[5,98,152,188] It has been shown that retinal pigment epithelium survives as a monolayer when inserted into the subretinal space, and that in the RCS-rat the photoreceptor cells overlying the donor cells survive better than cells elsewhere. Fetal photoreceptor cells have also been inserted into the subretinal space in dystrophic animals and animals with photoreceptor loss due to light exposure. The cells survive and have limited functional capability. They express photopigment, and neural connections are formed. However, the cells do not have normal morphology and their visual potential has not been proven. The techniques of grafting retinal pigment epithelium and photoreceptor cells are still in their infancy, but these forms of management may one day be feasible.

In both *rd*- and *rds*-mice, transfection of the fertilized ovum with the appropriate wild-type gene causes photoreceptor rescue for weeks in the case of the *rd* mouse and months in the *rds* mouse.[100] However, there are major differences between insertion of genes into the fertilized ovum of animals and into nondividing photoreceptor cells in humans. Attempts to transfect mature photoreceptor cells has had limited success using adenovirus to introduce reporter genes with rhodopsin promoters.[9] However, the expression occurred only in a very limited number of cells, and the expression was not long-lasting.

An alternative approach to treatment involves the injection of growth factors into the eye, and this has been shown to result in long-term survival of photoreceptors in the RCS-rat.[43] The mechanism by which this occurs is not certain, but it is possible that it influences apoptosis.[6,7] If this were shown to be the case, the application would become widespread such that at least some cells may be induced to survive.

If any treatment becomes available by which functional loss may be modified in retinal dystrophies, it is likely that it will be specific to a disease or diseases identified by the target cell involved, the causative gene, or the mutation within that gene. Therefore, foreknowledge of the genetic defect in a subject would be necessary.

CONCLUSIONS

The management of retinal dystrophies now requires a team of workers in a variety of disciplines. Advice is dependent on establishing the ophthalmic diagnosis in the first instance, which may involve clinical, psychophysical, and electrophysiological evaluation. The inheritance can only be established if the family is well known to the patient. The pedigree may be constructed by the patient on the basis of memory or inquiries within the family. Failing this, the help of genetic services may be needed to search other sources of information such as registers of births, marriages, and deaths, and census or parish records. Examination of relatives at risk of having the abnormal gene but who are asymptomatic is often helpful. In addition, the mutation may be sought by molecular biologists.

Ideally, this bank of information should be available to all ophthalmic practitioners in the form of a genetic register, which would contain the full pedigree with names of affected individuals in previous generations, the precise diagnosis, and the mutation. It is hoped that treatment will become available with time. It is likely that any one therapy will be limited to certain categories of disease identified by the causative genes or their specific mutation. Therefore, it would only be possible to take full advantage of the advances if a comprehensive register of disease existed. Compiling such a register will require time and should not wait until the cures are shown to be feasible.

REFERENCES

1. Albert A, Litman B. Independent structural domains in the membrane protein bovine rhodopsin. *Biochemistry* 1978;17:3893–3900.
2. Alstrom C, Olson O, Heredo-retinopathia congenitalis monohybrida recessive autosomalis. *Hereditas* 1957;43:1–178.
3. Anukanth A, Khorana H. Structure and function in rhodopsin. Requirements of a specific structure for the intradiscal domain. *J Biol Chem* 1994;269:19738–19744.
4. Arokawa K, Molday M, Molday R, Williams D. Localization of peripherin/rds in the disk membranes of cone and rod photoreceptors; Relationship to disk membrane morphogenesis and retinal degeneration. *J Cell Biol* 1992; 116:659–667.
5. Banerjee R, Lund R. A role for microglia in the maintenance of photoreceptors in retinal transplants lacking pigment epithelium. *J Neurocytol* 1992;21:235–243.
6. Barres B, Hart I, Coles H, Burne, J, Voyvodic J, Richardson W, et al. Cell death and control of cell survival in the oligodendrocyte lineage. *Cell* 1992;70:31–46.
7. Barres B, Hart I, Coles H, Burne J, Voyvodic J, Richardson W, et al. Cell death in the oligodendrocyte lineage. *J Neurobiol* 1992;23: 1221–1230.
8. Bascom R, Manara S, Collins L, Molday R, Kalnins V, McInnes R. Cloning of the cDNA for a novel photoreceptor membrane (rom-1) identifies a disk rim protein family implicated in human retinopathies. *Neuron* 1992;8:1171–1184.
9. Bennett J, Wilson J, Sun D, Forbes B, Maguire A. Adenovirus vector-mediated in vivo gene transfer into adult murine retina. *Invest Ophthalmol Visual Sci* 1994;35:2535–2542.
10. Berson E, Gouras P, Gunkel R, Myrianthopoulos N. Dominant retinitis pigmentosa with reduced penetrance. *Arch Ophthalmol* 1969; 81:226–235.
11. Berson E, Gouras P, Gunkel R, Myrianthopoulos N. Rod and cone responses in sex-linked retinitis pigmentosa. *Arch Ophthalmol* 1969; 81:215–225.
12. Berson E, Gouras P, Hoff M. Temporal aspects of the electroretinogram. *Arch Ophthalmol* 1969;81:207–214.

13. Berson E, Howard J. Temporal aspects of the electroretinogram in sector retinitis pigmentosa. *Arch Ophthalmol* 1971;48:653–665.
14. Berson E, Rosner B, Sandberg M, Hayes K, Nicholson B, Weigel-Franco C, et al. A randomized trial of vitamin A and vitamin E supplementation for retinitis pigmentosa. *Arch Ophthalmol* 1993;111:761–772.
15. Berson E, Rosner B, Sandberg M, Hayes K, Nicholson B, Weigel-Franco C, et al. Vitamin A supplementation and retinitis pigmentosa. *Arch Ophthalmol* 1993;111:1456–1458.
16. Berson E, Rosner B, Sandberg M, Hayes K, Nicholson B, Weigel-Franco C, et al. A randomized trial of vitamin A and vitamin E supplementation for retinitis pigmentosa. *Arch Ophthalmol* 1993;111:1463–1466.
17. Bhattacharya S, Wright A, Clayton J, Price W, Phillips C, McKeown C. Close genetic linkage between X-linked retinitis pigmentosa and a restriction fragments length polymoretinitis pigmentosahism identified by recombinant DNA probe L128. *Nature* 1984;309:253–255.
18. Bietti G. Über famili res Vorkommen von "retinitis punctata albescens" (verbunden mit "dystrophia marginalis cristallinea cornea"), glitzern des Glascöretinitis pigmentosaers und anderen degenerativen Augenveränderungen. *Klin Monastbl Augenheilkd* 1937;99:737–756.
19. Birch D, Hood D, Nusinowitz S, Pepperberg D. Abnormal activation and inactivation mechanisms of rod transduction in patients with autosomal dominant retinitis pigmentosa and the pro-23-his mutation. *Invest Ophthalmol Visual Sci* 1995;36:1603–1614.
20. Bird A. X-linked retinitis pigmentosa. *Br J Ophthalmol* 1975;59:177–199.
21. Brazitikos P, Safran A. Helicoid peripapillary chorioretinal degeneration. *Am J Ophthalmol* 1990;109:290–294.
22. Brook J, McCurach M, Harley H, Buckler A, Church D, Aburatani H, et al. Molecular basis of myotonic dystrophy: Expansion of trinucleotide (CTG) repeat at the 3′ end of a transcript encoding a protein kinase member. *Cell* 1992;68:799–808.
23. Carlson J, Rogers B, Sifers R, Hawkins H, Finegold M, Woo S. Multiple tissues express alpha 1-antitrypsin in transgenic mice and man. *J Clin Invest* 1988;82:26–36.
24. Carr R, Siegel I. Unilateral retinitis pigmentosa. *Arch Ophthalmol* 1973;90:21–22.
25. Chang G, Hao Y, Wong F. Apoptosis: Final common pathway of photoreceptor death in rd, rds, and rhodopsin mutant mice. *Neuron* 1993;11:595–605.
26. Claridge K, Gibberd F, Sidey M. Refsum disease: The presentation and ophthalmic aspects of Refsum disease in a series of 23 patients. *Eye* 1992;6:371–375.
27. Cohen A, Some cytological and initial biochemical observations on photoreceptors in retinas of rds mice. *Invest Ophthalmol Visual Sci* 1983;24:832–843.
28. Conley C, Weatherall D, Richardson S, Shephard M, Charache S. Hereditary persistance of fetal haemogobin: A study of 79 affected persons in 15 negro families in Baltimore. *Blood* 1963;21:261–281.
29. Connell G, Bascom R, Molday L, Reid D, McInnes RR, Molday RS. Photoreceptor peripherin is the normal product of the gene responsible for retinal degeneration in the rds mouse. *Proc Natl Acad Sci USA* 1991;88: 723–726.
30. Connell G, Molday RS. Molecular cloning, primary structure and orientation of the vertebrate photoreceptor cell protein peripherin in the rod disc membrane. *Biochemistry* 1990;29:4691–4698.
31. Cordier J, Reny A, Seigneur J-B. Rétinite pigmentaire unilatérale. *Bull Soc Ophthalmol Fr* 1966;66:224–227.
32. Denton M, Chen J-D, Serravalle S, Colley P, Halliday FB, Donald J. Analysis of linkage relationships of X-linked retinitis pigmentosa with the following Xp loci: L128, OTC, 754, XJ11, pERT 87 and C7. *Hum Genet* 1988;78:60–64.
33. Deutschman R. Einseitige typische retinitis pigmentosa mit pathologisch anatomischem Befund. *Beitr Augenheilkd* 1891;1:69–80.
34. Diem M. Retinitis punctata albescens et pigmentosa. *Klin Monatsbl Augenheilkd* 1914; 53:371–379.
35. Doi T, Molday R, Khorana H. Role of the intradiscal domain in rhodopsin assembly and function. *Proc Natl Acad Sci USA* 1990; 87:4991–4995.
36. Dryja T, Hahn LB, Cowley G, McGee T, Berson E. Mutation spectrum of the rhodopsin gene among patients with autosomal dominant retinitis pigmentosa. *Proc Natl Acad Sci USA* 1991;88:9370–9374.
37. Dryja T, McGee T, Hahn L, Cowley G, Olsson J, Reichel E, et al. Mutations within the rhodopsin gene in patients with autosomal dominant retinitis pigmentosa. *N Engl J Med* 1990;323:1302–1307.
38. Dryja T, McGee T, Reichel E, Hahn LB, Cowley G, Yandell D, et al. A point mutation of the rhodopsin gene in one form of retinitis pigmentosa. *Nature* 1990;343:364–366.

39. Ellis R, Horvitz H. Two C elegans genes control the programmed deaths of specific cells in the pharynx. *Development* 1991;112:591–603.
40. Ellis R, Jacobson D, Horvitz H. Genes required for the engulfment of cell corpses during programmed cell death in Caenorhabditis elegans. *Genetics* 1991;129:79–94.
41. Evans K, Al-Maghtheh M, Fitzke F, Moore A, Jay M, Inglehearn C, et al. Bimodal expressivity in autosomal dominant retinitis pigmentosa genetically linked to chromosome 19q. *Br J Ophthalmol* 1995;79:841–846.
42. Fahmy K, Siebert F, Sakmar T. A mutant rhodopsin photoproduct with a protonated Schiff base displays an active-state conformation: A Fourier-transform infrared spectroscopy study. *Biochemistry* 1994;33:13,700–13,705.
43. Faktorovich E, Steinberg R, Yasumura D, Matthes M, LaVail M. Photoreceptor degeneration in inherited retinal dystrophy delayed by basic fibroblast growth factor. *Nature* 1990; 347:83–86.
44. Falls H, Cotterman C. Choroido-retinal degeneration. A sex-linked form in which heterozygous women exhibit a tapetal-like reflex. *Arch Ophthalmol* 1948;40:685–703.
45. Farrar G, Kenna P, Jordan S, Kumar-Singh R, Humphries M, Sharp E, et al. A three-base-pair deletion in the peripherin-RDS gene in one form of retinitis pigmentosa. *Nature* 1991;354:478–480.
46. Favre M. A propos de deux cas de dégénérescence hyaloido-rétinienne. *Ophthalmologica* 1958;135:337–341.
47. Fishman G, Stone E, Gilbert L, Kenna P, Sheffield V. Ocular findings associated with a rhodopsin gene codon 58 transversion mutation in autosomal dominant retinitis pigmentosa. *Arch Ophthalmol* 1991;109:1387–1393.
48. Fishman G, Stone E, Sheffield V, Gilbert L, Kimura A. Ocular findings associated with rhodopsin gene codon 17 and codon 182 transition mutations in dominant retinitis pigmentosa. *Arch Ophthalmol* 1992;110:54–62.
49. Fishman G, Vandenberg K, Stone E, Gilbert L, Alexander KR, Sheffield V. Ocular findings associated with rhodopsin gene codon 267 and codon 190 mutations in dominant retinitis pigmentosa. *Arch Ophthalmmol* 1992;110:1582–1588.
50. Flannery J, Farber D, Bird A, Bok D. Degenerative changes in a retina affected with autosomal dominant retinitis pigmentosa. *Invest Ophthalmol Visual Sci* 1989;30:191–211.
51. Foxman S, Heckenlively J, Sinclair S. Rubeola retinopathy and pigmented paravenous retinochoroidal atrophy. *Am J Ophthalmol* 1985; 99:605–606.
52. Franceschetti A. A curious affection of the ocular fundus. Helicoid peripapillary chorioretinal degeneration. Its relation to pigmented paravenous chorioretinal degeneration. *Doc Ophthalmol* 1962;16:108–109.
53. Franche U, Ochs H, DeMartinville B, Giacalone J, Lindergren V, Disteche C. Minor Xp21 chromosome deletion in a male associated with expression of Duchenne muscular dystrophy and McLeod syndrome. *Am J Hum Genet* 1985;37:250–267.
54. François J, Verriest G. Rétinopathie pigmentaire unilatérale. *Ophthalmologica* 1952; 124:65–88.
55. Fung B. K-K Transducin: Structure, function and role in phototransduction. *Prog Retinal Res* 1987;6:151–177.
56. Gass J. Acute zonal occult outer retinopathy. *J Clin Neurophthalmol* 1993;13:79–97.
57. Gass J, Gilbert WR, Guerry R, Scelfo R. Diffuse unilateral subacute neuroetinitis. *Ophthalmology* 1978;85:521–545.
58. Gavrieli Y, Sherman Y, Ben-Sasson S. Identification of programmed cell death in situ via specific labeling of nuclear DNA fragmentation. *J Cell Biol* 1992;119:493–501.
59. Gibberd F, Billimoria J, Page N, Retsas S. Heredopathia atactica polyneuritiformis (Refsum's disease) treated by diet and plasma-exchange. *Lancet* 1979;2:575–578.
60. Haase W, Hellner K. Über familiäre bilaterale sektorenförmige Retinopathia pigmentosa. *Klin Monatsbl Augenheilkd* 1965;147:365–375.
61. Hansen E, Bachen N, Flage T. Refsum's disease. Eye manifestations in a patient treated with low phytol low phytanic acid diet. *Acta Ophthalmol* 1979;57:899–913.
62. Hargrave P. Rhodopsin chemistry, structure and topography. *Prog Retinal Res* 1982;1:1–51.
63. Harley H, Rundle S, MacMillan J, Myring J, Brook J, Crow S, et al. Size of the unstable repeat sequence in relation to phenotype and parental transmission in myotonic dystrophy. *Am J Hum Genet* 1993;52:1164–1174.
64. Hawkins R, Jansen H, Sanyal S. Development and degeneration of retina in rds mutant mice: Photoreceptor abnormalities in the heterozygotes. *Exp Eye Res* 1985;41:701–720.
65. Heckenlively J. Preserved para-arteriole retinal pigment epithelium (PPRPE) in retinitis pigmentosa. *Br J Ophthalmol* 1982;66:26–31.

66. Heckenlively J, Rodriguez J, Daiger S. Autosomal dominant sectoral retinitis pigmentosa. Two families with transversion mutation in codon 23 of rhodopsin. *Arch Ophthalmol* 1991;109:84–91.
67. Hengartner M, Ellis R, Horvitz H. *Caenorhabditis elegans* gene ced-9 protects cells from programmed cell death. *Nature* 1992;356: 494–499.
68. Henkes H, van der Tweel L, van der Gon J. Selective amplication of the electroretinogram. *Ophthalmologica* 1956;132:140–150.
69. Henkes H, Verduin P. Dysgenesis or abiotrophy? A differentiation with the help of the electroretinogram (ERG) and electroculogram (EOG) in Leber's congenital amaurosis. *Ophthalmologica* 1963;145:144–160.
70. Herman E, Conley C. Hereditary persistance of foetal haemoglobin A family study. *Am J Med* 1960;29:9–17.
71. Hu DN. Ophthalmic genetics in China. *Ophthalmic Paediatr Genet* 1983;2:39–45.
72. Huang P, Gaitan A, Hao Y, Petters R, Wong F. Cellular interactions implicated in the mechanism of photoreceptor degeneration in transgenic mice expressing a mutant rhodopsin gene. *Proc Natl Acad Sci USA* 1993;90:8484–8488.
73. Hunter A, Tsilfidis C, Mettler G, Jacob P, Mahadevan M, Surh L, et al. The correlation of age of onset with CTG trinucleotide repeat amplification in myotonic dystrophy. *J Med Genet* 1992;29:774–779.
74. Inglehearn C, Keen T, Bashir R, Jay M, Fitzke F, Bird A, et al. A completed screen for mutations on the rhodopsin gene in a panel of patients with autosomal dominant retinitis pigmentosa. *Hum Mol Genet* 1992;1:41–45.
75. Jansen H, Sanyal S. Development and degeneration of retina in rds mutant mice: Electron microscopy. *J Comp Neurol* 1984; 224:71–84.
76. Jay M. On the hereditary of retinitis pigmentosa. *Br J Ophthalmol* 1982;7:405–416.
77. Kaiser-Kupfer M, Caruso R, Valle D. Gyrate atrophy of the choroid and retina. Long-term reduction of ornithine slows retinal degeneration. *Arch Ophthalmol* 1991;109:1539–1548.
78. Kaiser-Kupfer M, deMonasterio F, Valle D. Gyrate atrophy of the choroid and retina: Improved of visual function by reduction of plasma ornithine by diet. *Science* 1980; 210:1128–1131.
79. Kajiwara K, Berson E, Dryja T. Digenic retinitis pigmentosa due to mutations at the unlinked peripherin/RDS and ROM 1 loci. *Science* 1994;264:1604–1608.
80. Kajiwara K, Hahn L, Mukai S, Travis G, Berson E, Dryja T. Mutations in the human retinal degeneration slow gene in autosomal dominant retinitis pigmentosa. *Nature* 1991;354:480–483.
81. Kajiwara K, Sandberg M, Berson E, Dryja T. A null mutation in the human peripherin/RDS gene in a family with autosomal dominant retinitis punctata albescens. *Natur Genet* 1993; 3:208–212.
82. Kaplan J, Pelet A, Martin C, Delrieu O, Ayme S, Bonneau D, et al. Phenotype-genotype correlations in X linked retinitis pigmentosa. *J Med Genet* 1992;29:615–623.
83. Karnik S, Khoranna H. Assembly and functional rhodopsin requires a disulphide bond between cysteine residues 110 and 187. *J Biol Chem* 1990;265:17520–17524.
84. Karnik S, Sakmar T, Chen H, Khorana H. Cysteine residues 110 and 187 are essential for the formation of correct structure in bovine rhodopsin. *Proc Natl Acad Sci USA* 1988; 85:8459–8463.
85. Kaushal S, Khorana H. Structure and function in rhodopsin 7. Point mutations associated with autosomal dominant retinitis pigmentosa. *Biochemistry* 1994;33:6121–6128.
86. Kemp C, Jacobson S, Cideciyan A, Kimura A, Sheffield V, Stone E. RDS gene mutations causing retinitis pigmentosa or macular degeneration lead to the same abnormality in photoreceptor function. *Invest. Ophthalmol Visual Sci* 1994;35:3154–3162.
87. Kemp C, Jacobson S, Faulkner D. Two types of visual disfunction in autosomal dominant retinitis pigmentosa. *Invest Ophthalmol Visual Sci* 1988;29:1235–1241.
88. Kemp C, Jacobson S, Roman A, Sung C, Nathans J. Abnormal rod adaptation in autosomal dominant retinitis pigmentosa with Pro-23-His rhodopsin mutation. *Am J Ophthalmol* 1992;113:165–174.
89. Kim R, Al-Maghtheh M, Fitzke F, Arden G, Jay M, Bhattacharya S, et al. Dominant retinitis pigmentosa associated with two rhodopsin mutations. *Arch Ophthalmol* 1993;111:1518–1524.
90. Kim R, Dollfus H, Keen T, Fitzke F, Arden G, Bhattacharya S, et al. Autosomal dominant pattern dystrophy of the retina associated with a 4 bp insertion at codon 140 in the RDS/peripherin gene. *Arch Ophthalmol* 1995;113: 451–453.

91. Klausner R, Sitia R. Protein degradation in the endoplamic reticulum. *Cell* 1990;62:611–614.
92. Kobayashi V. Genetic study on retinitis pigmentosa. *Jpn J Ophthalmol* 1960;7:82–88.
93. Kranich H, Bartowski S, Denton M, Krey S, Dickinson P, Duvigneau C, et al. Autosomal dominant "sector" retinitis pigmentosa due to a point mutation predicting an Asn-15-Ser substitution of rhodopsin. *Hum Mol Genet* 1993;2:813–814.
94. Krill A. X-chromosomal linked diseases affecting the eye: Status of the heterozygote female. *Trans Am Ophthalmol Soc* 1969;67:535–608.
95. Krill A, Archer D, Martin D. Sector retinitis pigmentosa. *Am J Ophthalmol* 1970;69: 977–987.
96. Kumaramanickavel G, Maw M, Denton M, John S, Srimakumari C, Orth U, et al. Missense mutation (E150K) of rhodopsin in a family with autosomal recessive retinitis pigmentosa. *Nature Genet* 1994;8:10–11.
97. Lavedan C, Hofmann-Radvanyi H, Shelbourne P, Rabes J, Duros C, Savoy D, et al. Myotonic dystrophy: Size- and sex-dependent dynamics of CTG meiotic instability, and somatic mosaicism. *Am J Hum Genet* 1993; 52:875–883.
98. Lazar E, Cerro MD. A new procedure for multiple intraretinal transplantation into mammalian eyes. *J Neurosci Meth* 1992;43:157–169.
99. Leber T. Über anomale Formen der retinitis pigmentosa. *Graefes Arch Clin Exp Ophthalmol* 1871;17:314–341.
100. Lem J, Flannery J, Li T, Applebury M, Farber D, Simon M. Retinal degeneration is rescued in transgenic rd mice by expression of the cGMP phosphodiesterase beta subunit. *Proc Natl Acad Sci USA* 1992;89:4422–4426.
101. Lessel M, Thaler A, Heilig P. ERG and EOG in progressive paravenous retinochoroidal atrophy. *Doc Ophthalmol* 1986;62:25–30.
102. Li T, Franson W, Gordon J, Berson E, Dryja T. Constitutive activation of phototransduction by K296E opsin is not a cause of photoreceptor degeneration. *Proc Natl Acad Sci USA* 1995;92:3551–3555.
103. Li Z, Kljavin I, Milam A. Rod photoreceptor neurite sprouting in retinitis pigmentosa. *J Neurosci* 1995;15:5429–5438.
104. Lippincott-Shwartz J, Bonifacio J, Yuan L, Klausner R. Degradation from the endoplasmic reticulum: Disposing of newly synthesised protein. *Cell* 1988;54:209–220.
105. Lodish H. Transport of secretory and membrane glycoproteins form the rough endoplasmic reticulum to the Golgi. *J Biol Chem* 1988;263:2107–2110.
106. Lolley R, Rong H, Craft C. Linkage of photoreceptor degeneration by apoptosis with inherited defect in phototransduction. *Invest Ophthalmol Visual Sci* 1994;35:358–362.
107. Lyness A, Ernst W, Quinlan M, Clover G, Arden G, Carter R, et al. A clinical, psychophysical, and electroretinographic survey of patients with autosomal dominant retinitis pigmentosa. *Br J Ophthalmol* 1985;69:326–339.
108. Magenis R, Toth-Fejel S, Allen L, Black M, Brown N, Budden S, et al. Comparison of the 15q deletions in Prader-Willi and Angelman syndromes: Specific regions, extent of deletions, parental origin and clinical consequences. *Am J Med Genet* 1990;35:333–336.
109. Magnusson L. Atrophia areata, a variant of peripapillary chorioretinal degeneration. *Acta Ophthalmol* (Copenh.) 1981;59:659–664.
110. Mahadevan M, Tsilfidis C, Sabourin L, Shutler G, Amemiya C, Jansen G, et al. Myotonic dystrophy mutation: An unstable CTG repeat in the 3′ untranslated region of the gene *Science* 1992;255:1253–1255.
111. Marmor M, Jacobson S, Foerster M, Kellner U, Weleber R. RG Diagnostic findings of a new syndrome with night blindness, maculopathy, and enhanced s-cone sensitivity. *Am J Ophthalmol* 1990;110:124–134.
112. Massof R, Finkelstein D. Two forms of autosomal dominant primary retinitis pigmentosa. *Doc Ophthalmol* 1981;51:289–346.
113. Massoff R, Finkelstein D. Editorial; Supplemental vitamin A retards loss of ERG amplitude in retinitis pigmentosa. *Arch Ophthalmol* 1993;111:751–754.
114. Massoff R, Finkelstein D. Vitamin A supplementation and retinitis pigmentosa. *Arch Ophthalmol* 1993;111:1458–1459.
115. McGuire R, Sullivan L, Blanton S, Church M, Heckenlively J, Daiger S. X-linked dominant cone-rod degeneration: Linkage mapping of a new locus for retinitis pigmentosa (RP 15) to Xp22.13-p22.11. *Am J Hum Genet* 1995;57: 87–94.
116. McKenzie D. The inheritance of retinitis pigmentosa in one family. *Trans Ophthalmol Soc NZ* 1951;5:79–82.
117. McLaughlin M, Sandberg M, Berson E, Dryja T. Recessive mutations in the gene encoding the beta subunit of phosphodiesterase in patients with retinitis pigmentosa. *Nature Genet* 1993;4:130–134.
118. McWilliams P, Farrar G, Kenna, P, Bradley

D. Humphries M, Sharp E, et al. Autosomal dominant retinitis pigmentosa (ADRP). Localization of an ADRP gene to the long arm of chromosome 3. *Genomics* 1989;5:619–622.

119. Meindl A, Dry K, Hermann K, Manson F, Ciccodicola A, Edgar A, et al. A gene (RRP1) with homology to the RCC1 family of guanine neucleotide exchange factors in mutated in X-linked retinitis pigmentosa (RP3). *Nature Genet* in press.
120. Moore A, Fitzke F, Jay M, Inglehearn F, Keen T, Bhattacharya S, et al. Autosomal dominant retinitis pigmentosa with apparent incomplete penetrance: A clinical, electrophysiological, psychophysical and molecular biological study. *Br J Ophthalmol* 1933;77:473–479.
121. Moore A, Fitzke F, Kemp C, Arden G, Bird A. Abnormal dark adaptation kinetics in autosomal dominant sector retinitis pigmentosa due to rod opsin mutation. *Br J Ophthalmol* 1992;76:465–469.
122. Moore T, Haig D. Genomic imprinting in mammalian development: A parental tug of war. *Trend Genet* 1991;7:45–49.
123. Mullen R, Lavail M. Inherited retinal dystrophy: Primary defect in pigment epithelium determined with experimental rat chimeras. *Science* 1976;192:799–801.
124. Muller D, Lloyd J, Bird A. Long-term management of Abetalipoproteinaemia. Possible role for vitamin E. *Arch Dis Child* 1977;52: 209–214.
125. Naash M, Hollyfield J, Ubaidi Ma, Baehr W. Simulation of human autosomal dominant retinitis pigmentosa in transgenic mice expressing a mutated murine opsin gene. *Proc Natl Acad Sci USA* 1993;90:5499–5503.
126. Nicholls R, Knoll J, Butler M, Karam S, Lalande M. Genetic imprinting suggested by maternal heterosomy in non-deletion Prader-Willi syndrome. *Nature* 1989;342:281–285.
127. Nichols B, Sheffield V, Vandenburgh K, Drack A, Kimura A, Stone E. Butterfly-shaped pigment dystrophy of the fovea caused by a point mutation in codon 167 of the RDS gene. *Nature Genet* 1993;3:202–207.
128. Noble K, Carr R. Pigmented paravenous chorio-retinal atrophy. *Am J Ophthalmol* 1983;90:338–344.
129. Nussbaum R, Lewis R, Lesko J, Ferrell R. Mapping ophthalmological disease II. Linkage of relationship of X-linked retinitis pigmentosa to X chromosome short arm markers. *Hum Genet* 1985;70:45–50.
130. Olsson J, Gordon J, Pawlyk B, Roof D, Hayes A, Molday R, et al. Transgenic mice with a rhodopsin mutation (Pro23His): A mouse model of autosomal dominant retinitis pigmentosa. *Neuron* 1992;9:815–830.
131. Oppenheim R. Cell death during development of the nervous system. *Annu Rev Neurosci* 1991;14:453–501.
132. Ott J, Bhattacharya S, Chen J, Denton M, Donald J, Dubay C, et al. Localizing multiple X chromosome-linked retinitis pigmentosa loci using multilocus homogeneity tests. *Proc Natl Acad Sci USA* 1990;87:701–704.
133. Owens S, Fitzke F, Inglehearn C, Jay M, Keen T, Arden G, et al. Occular manifestations in autosomal dominant retinitis pigmentosa with a Lys-296-Glu rhodopsin mutation at the retinal binding site. *Br J Ophthalmol* 1994; 78:153–158.
134. Pedralgia C. Klinische Beobachtungen Retinitis pigmentosa. *Klin Monatsbl Augenheilkd* 1865;3:114–117.
135. Portera-Cailliau C, Sung C, Nathans J, Adler R. Apoptotic photoreceptor cell death in mouse models of retinitis pigmentosa. *Proc Natl Acad Sci USA* 1994;91:974–978.
136. Pugh E, Lamb T. Amplification and kinetics of the activation steps in phototransduction. *Biochim Biophys Acta* 1993;1141:111–149.
137. Raff M. Social controls on cell survival and cell death. *Nature* 1992;356:397–400.
138. Rao V, Cohen G, Oprian D. Rhodopsin mutation G90D and a molecular mechanism for congenital night blindness. *Nature* 1994;367: 639–642.
139. Richards B, Brodstein D, Nussbaum J, Ferencz J, Maeda K, Weiss L. Autosomal dominant crystaline dystrophy. *Ophthalmology* 1991;98: 658–665.
140. Richards J, Kuo C, Boehnke M, Sieving P. Rhodopsin Thr58Arg mutation in a family with autosomal dominant retinitis pigmentosa. *Ophthalmology* 1991;98:1797–1805.
141. Richards J, Scott K, Sieving P. Disruption of conserved rhodopsin disulfide bond by Cys187Tyr mutation causes early and severe autosomal dominant retinitis pigmentosa. *Ophthalmology* 1995;102:669–677.
142. Ridge K, Zhang C, Khorana H. Mapping of the amino acids in the cytoplasmic loop connecting helices C and D in rhodopsin. Chemical reactivity in the dark state following single cysteine replacements. *Biochemistry* 1995;34:8804–8811.

143. Riggs L. Electroretinography in cases of night blindness. *Am J Ophthalmol* 1954;38:70–78.
144. Robinson P, Buczylko J, Ohguro H, Palczewski K. Opsins with mutations at the site of chromophore attachment constitutively activate transducin but are not phosphorylated by rhodopsin kinase. *Proc Natl Acad Sci USA* 1994;91:5411–5415.
145. Robinson P, Cohen G, Zhukovsky E, Oprian DD. Constitutively active mutants of rhodopsin. *Neuron* 1992;9:719–725.
146. Rosenfield P, Cowley G, McGee T, Sandberg M, Berson E, Dryja T. A null mutation in the rhodopsin gene causes rod photoreceptor dysfunction and autosomal recessive retinitis pigmentosa. *Nature Genet* 1992;1:209–213.
147. Rubino A. Su una paraticolarae anomalia bilaterale alle e simmetica dello stratato pigmento retinico. *Bull Oculusta* 1940;19:318.
148. Sandberg M, Weigel-DiFranco C, Dryja T, Berson E. Clinical expression correlates with location of rhodopsin mutation in dominant retinitis pigmentosa. *Invest Ophthalmol Visual Sci* 1995;36:1934–1942.
149. Sanyal S, Hawkins R. Development and degeneration of retina in rds mutant mice. Altered disc shedding pattern in the albino heterozygotes and its relation to light exposure. *Vision Res* 1987;28:1171–1178.
150. Sanyal S, Jansen H. Absence of receptor outer segments in the retina of rds mutant mice. *Neurosci Lett* 1992;21:23–26.
151. Schappert-Kimmijser J. Les dégénérescences tapéto-rétiniennes du type X chromosomal aux Pays-Bas. *Bull Mem Soc Fr Ophthalmol* 1963; 76:122–129.
152. Schuschereba S, Silverman M. Retinal cell and photoreceptor transplantation between adult New Zealand red rabbit retinas. *Exp Neurol* 1992;115:95–99.
153. Serjeant G. *Sickle Cell Disease*. Oxford: Oxford University Press, 1985, p. 8.
154. Skalka H. Hereditary pigmented paravenous retinochoroidal atrophy. *Am J Ophthalmol* 1979;87:286–291.
155. Stone E, Kimura A, Nichols B, Khadivi P, Fishman G, Sheffield V. Regional distribution of retinal degeneration in patients with the proline to histidine mutation in codon 23 of the rhodopsin gene. *Ophthalmology* 1991;98: 1806–1813.
156. Suber M, Pittler S, Qin N, Wright G, Holcombe V, Lee R, et al. Hurwitz Irish setter dogs affected with rod/cone dysplasia contain a nonsense mutation in the rod cGMP phosphodiesterase subunit gene. *Proc Natl Acad Sci USA* 1993;90:3968–3972.
157. Sung C, Davenport C, Hennessey J, Maumenee I, Jacobson S, Heckenlively J, et al. Rhodopsin mutations in autosomal dominant retinitis pigmentosa. *Proc Natl Acad Sci USA* 1991;88:6481–6485.
158. Sung C, Davenport C, Nathans J. Rhodopsin mutations responsible for autosomal dominant retinitis pigmentosa. Clustering of functional classes along the polypeptide chain. *J Biol Chem* 1993;15:26,645–26,649.
159. Sung C, Makino C, Baylor D, Nathans J. A rhodopsin gene mutation responsible for autosomal dominant retinitis pigmentosa results in a protein that is defective in localization to the photoreceptor outer segment. *J Neurosci* 1994;14:5818–5833.
160. Sung C, Schneider B, Agerwal N, Papermaster D, Nathans J. Functional heterogeneity on mutant rhodopsins responsible for autosomal retinitis pigmentosa. *Proc Natl Acad Sci USA* 1991;88:8840–8844.
161. Sveinsson K. Choroiditis areata. *Acta Ophthalmol* (Copenh) 1939;17:73–79.
162. Sveinsson K. Helicoid peripapillary chorioretinal degeneration. *Acta Ophthalmol* (Copenh) 1979;57:69–75.
163. Szarmier R, Berson E, Klein R, Myers S. Sex-linked retinitis pigmentosa: Ultrastructure of photoreceptors and pigment epithelium. *Invest Ophthalmol Visual Sci* 1971;18:145–160.
164. Talbot J, Bird A, Serjeant G. Retinal changes in sickle cell/hereditary persistence of foetal haemoglobin syndrome. *Br J Ophthalmol* 1983;67:777–778.
165. Traboulsi E, Maumenee I. Hereditary pigmented paravenous chorioretinal atrophy. *Arch Ophthalmol* 1986;104:1636–1640.
166. Travis G, Brennan M, Danielson P, Kozak C, Sutcliffe J. Identification of a photoreceptor-specific mRNA encoded by the gene responsible for retinal degeneration slow (rds). *Nature* 1989;338:70–73.
167. Travis G, Christerson L, Danielson P, Klisak J, Sparkes R, Hahn L. The human retinal degeneration slow (RDS) gene: Chromosome assignment and structure of the mRNA. *Genomics* 1991;10:733–739.
168. Travis G, Lloyd M, Bok D. Complete reversal of photoreceptor dysplasia in transgenic retinal degeneration slow (rds) mice. *Neuron* 1992; 9:113–120.

169. Travis G, Sutcliffe J, Bok D. The retinal degeneration slow (rds) gene product is a photoreceptor disc membrane associated glycoprotein. *Neuron* 1991;6:61–70.
170. Truman J, Schwartz L. Steroid regulation of neuronal death in the moth nervous system. *J Neurosci* 1984;4:274–280.
171. Tso M, Zhang C, Abler A, Chang C, Wong F, Chang G, et al. Apoptosis leads to photoreceptor degeneration in inherited retinal dystrophy of RCS rat. *Invest Ophthalmol Visual Sci* 1994;35:2693–2699.
172. Usukura J, Bok D. Changes in the localization and content of opsin during retinal development in the rds mutant mouse: Immunocytochemistry and immunoassay. *Exp Eye Res* 1987;45:501–515.
173. Vannas-Sulonen K, Simell O, Sipila I. Gyrate atrophy of the choroid and retina; The ocular disease progresses in juvenile patients despite normal or near normal plasma ornithine concentration. *Ophthalmology* 1987;94:1428–1433.
174. Vaux D. Toward an understanding of the molecular mechanisms of physiological cell death. *Proc Natl Acad Sci USA* 1993;90:786–789.
175. Vaux D, Cory S, Adams J. Bcl-2 gene promotes heamopoetic cell survival and promotes cooperates with c-myc to immortanize pre-B cells. *Nature* 1988;335:4440–442.
176. Vaux D, Weissman I. Neither macromolecular synthesis nor myc is required for cell death via the mechanism that can be controlled by Bcl-2. *Mol Cell Biol* 1993;13:7000–7005.
177. Weiss E, Osawa S, Shi W, Dickerson C. Effects of carboxyl-terminal truncation on the stability and G protein-coupling activity of bovine rhodopsin. *Biochemistry* 1994;33:7587–7593.
178. Weleber R, Carr R, Murphey W, Sheffield V, Stone E. Phenotypic variation including retinitis pigmentosa, pattern dystrophy, and fundus flavimaculatus in a single family with a deletion of codon 153 or 154 of the peripherin/RDS gene. *Arch Ophthalmol* 1993;111:1531–1542.
179. Weleber R, Kennaway N, Buist N. Clinical trial of vitamin B6 for gyrate atrophy of the choroid and retina. *Ophthalmology* 1981;88:316–324.
180. Wells J, Wroblewski J, Keen J, Inglehearn C, Jubb C, Eckstein A, et al. Mutations in the human retinal degeneration slow (rds) gene can cause either retinitis pigmentosa or macular dystrophy. *Nature Genet* 1993;3:213–217.
181. Williamson R. Universal community carrier screening for cystic fibrosis? *Nature Genet* 1993;3:195–201.
182. Willison K. Opposite imprinting of the mouse Igf2 and Igf2r genes. *Trends Genet* 1991;7:107–109.
183. Wilson D, Weleber R, Klein M, Welch R, Green W. Bietti's crystalline dystrophy: A clinicopathologic correlative study. *Arch Ophthalmol* 1989;107:213–221.
184. Wrobleski J, Wells J, Eckstein A, Fitzke F, Jubb C, Keen J, et al. Macular dystrophy associated with mutations at codon 172 in the human retinal degeneration slow (RDS) gene. *Ophthalmology* 1994;101:12–22.
185. Wrobleski J, Wells J, Eckstein A, Fitzke F, Jubb C, Keen T, et al. Ocular findings associated with a three-base pair deletion in the peripherin-RDS gene in autosomal dominant retinitis pigmentosa. *Br J Ophthalmol* 1994;78:83–86.
186. Wyllie A. Glucocorticoid-induced thymocyte apoptosis is associated with endogenous endonuclease activation. *Nature* 1980;284:555–556.
187. Wyllie A, Kerr J, Currie A. Cell death: The significance of apoptosis. *Int Rev Cytol* 1980;68:251–306.
188. Yamaguchi K, Yamaguchi K, Young R, Gaur V, Greven C, Slusher M, et al. Vitreoretinal surgical technique for transplanting retinal pigment epithelium in rabbit retina. *Jpn J Ophthalmol* 1992;36:142–150.
189. Zhong L, Sarafian T, Kane D, Charles A, Mah S, Edwards R, et al. Bredesen bcl-2 inhibits death of central neural cells induced by multiple agents. *Proc Natl Acad Sci USA* 1993;90:4533–4537.
190. Zvyaga T, Min K, Beck M, Sakmar T. Movement of the retinylidene Schiff base counterion in rhodopsin by one helix turn reverses the pH dependence of the metarhodopsin I to metarhodopsin II transition. *J Biol Chem* 1993;268:4661–4667.

18

Juvenile Retinoschisis

PAUL A. SIEVING

Juvenile retinoschisis is an X-linked vitreoretinal dystrophy that manifests early in life. The formation of intraretinal cysts in the macula impairs visual acuity and, in some affected males, the peripheral retina splits into sheets of tissue and causes substantial visual field loss. The first published description of affected males may have been by Haas, who in 1898[21] observed a "spoke-wheel" pattern (Fig. 18.1) of macular cysts in two men. Wilczek introduced the term *retinoschisis* in 1935.[43] The male predominance was suggested when Mann and MacRae in 1938[27] described peripheral retinal degeneration that they termed *congenital vascular veils in the vitreous* in two brothers and in a third unrelated male. This appearance results from a splitting of the inner aspect of the retina through the nerve fiber layer, with subsequent elevation of this thin sheet of tissue to "float" in the vitreous cavity (Fig. 18.2). Additional cases were reported by Sorsby et al.[37] of eight affected males in three generations of an X-linked recessive pedigree, several of whom had retinal detachments. The first major American description was in 1961 by Gieser and Falls,[17] who termed this *hereditary retinoschisis.* Eight of nine affected males in this large pedigree showed macular changes, and many had peripheral retinal "veils" and vascular sheathing. One female carrier also showed macular cystic changes but exhibited no peripheral retinal pathology. Such descriptions of changes in female carriers are quite uncommon. Other descriptions of this disease have highlighted the variable clinical manifestation, and a variety of names have been used to describe the condition, including *neural retinal disease in males,* which identifies the retinal involvement and the X-chromosomal nature of the disease[39]; *anterior dialysis of the retina,* which highlights the intraretinal splitting in the periphery[3]; and *congenital vascular veils in the vitreous,* which results from elevation of the inner-retinal sheath into the vitreous cavity.[27] The current terminology of *sex-linked juvenile retinoschisis* was first applied by Deutman in 1971,[12] and this term has generally been followed in recent years.

CLINICAL MANIFESTATIONS

Retinoschisis (RS) affects males nearly exclusively, with carrier females nearly never exhibiting fundus changes or visual symptoms. Affected males typically come to medical attention in early grade school years due to reduced acuity, which can range from minimally reduced to severe loss. These children rarely complain of night blindness or peripheral vision loss. Visual acuity typically stabilizes during late grade school and teenage years in af-

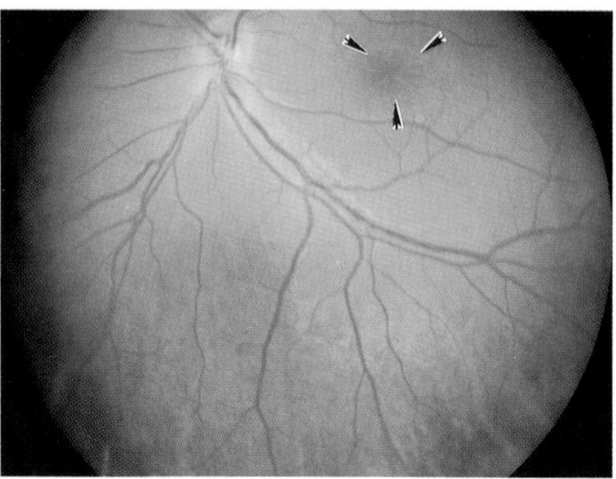

Figure 18.1. Fundus photograph of a male with juvenile retinoschisis shows spoke-wheel pattern of foveal cysts covering an area of about 1 disc diameter. The disease in this family results from a frameshift at residue 193 from an insertion in the XLRS1 gene.

fected males and thereafter remains constant into middle age. Progressive macular atrophy begins in late middle age and progresses toward legal blindness of 20/200 acuity in most males in later age. Typically, the macula exhibits linear cystic structures that extend from the fovea in a spoke-wheel pattern for approximately 1–1.5 disc diameter (DD). This is nearly pathognomonic of juvenile X-linked retinoschisis (see Fig. 18.1). The macula in some affected males shows many parafoveal cysts in no particular configuration; these can subsequently coalesce into a larger pattern that leads to central macular atrophy (see Fig. 18.4).

Retinoschisis is highly penetrant, with upwards to 95% of affected males showing some degree of foveal schisis. These changes can be quite subtle, however, and even an experienced clinical observer may fail to identify these schisis cavities as the cause of the reduced acuity. The frequency of peripheral retinoschisis may be as high as 50%, although this is probably somewhat lower based on our experience of examining males in 40 different families with this condition.

In mild cases, the parafoveal spoke-wheel intraretinal cysts are observed only by careful ophthalmoscopy and are not evident on fluorescein angiography (FA). However, some older affected males exhibit macular atrophy of the retinal pigment epithelium, which causes hyperfluorescent window defects on FA (Fig. 18.3). Some younger affected males have a golden macular sheen that can be confused with the "beaten-bronze" appearance in some Stargardt maculopathy. In such cases, both the electroretinogram (ERG) and an FA are essential for diagnosis (Fig. 18.4). The ERG shows an electronegative pattern in retinoschisis, and the FA will not exhibit the dark choroid sign that is typically present in Stargardt maculopathy. The macula in some cases of RS exhibit

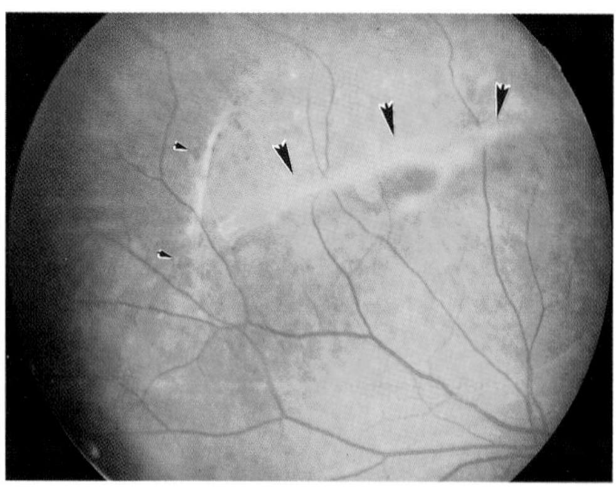

Figure 18.2. Fundus photograph of the peripheral retina of a male with retinoschisis shows the inner retinal layer elevated into the vitreous (large arrows) and hiding the blood vessels. Several partial-thickness retinal holes are present (small arrows).

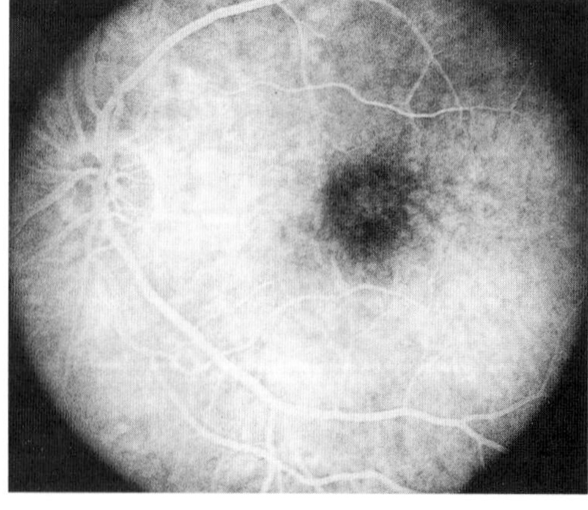

Figure 18.3. Fundus fluorescein angiogram shows hyperfluorescent "blush" from partial window defect in the fovea due to changes in the retinal pigment epithelium caused by disease from an Arg213Trp mutation in the XLRS1 gene.

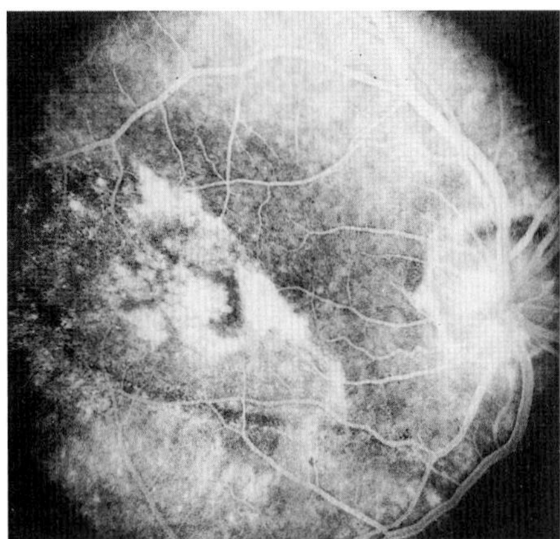

Figure 18.4. Fundus fluorescein angiogram shows extensive disruption and injury to the reginal pigment epithelium in the macula caused by disease from a Gly70Ser mutation in the XLRS1 gene.

the Mizuo–Nakamura phenomenon, in which a golden-yellow sheen is seen when light adapted, but that disappears when dark adapted.[11]

The peripheral retina also is subject to schisis and can split through the nerve fiber layer that lies at the inner surface of the retina. This disrupts transmission of visual signals and causes an absolute scotoma in the involved areas. The inferotemporal retinal area is most commonly involved.[7,34]

In our experience, many affected males have been mistaken for having amblyopia rather than being properly diagnosed with retinal disease. This was particularly striking in a large retinoschisis family in which the trait was passed into two half-sibships through marriage of an affected male to two different women. Affected grandsons in the one sibship were identified as having retinoschisis, along with the grandfather, who suffered retinal detachment in one eye. However, six affected grandsons in the second sibship were all misdiagnosed as having amblyopia. Subsequent genetic marker haplotyping identified all of these affected grandsons as having inherited the grandfather's affected X chromosome.

There is debate as to whether retinoschisis is congenital or is acquired after birth. The youngest affected male we have examined was 9 months old and came to the parents' attention due to leukocoria caused by bullous retinal detachments in both eyes. Surgical repair by scleral buckling can be beneficial in young patients with rhegmatogenous or exudative retinal detachment, although these eyes are at risk for subsequent proliferative vitreoretinopathy.[33] Other cases during infancy are described with peripheral bullous elevation of the inner retinal layer accompanied with vitreous hemorrhage.[16] Surgical repair is quite difficult in such cases and is not expected to improve the vision prognosis if separation of the neural retinal layers interrupts neural signal transmission.

Carrier females rarely show macular or retinal changes, and neither their central or peripheral vision is affected. In this regard, the female carriers are unlike many of the other X-linked conditions in which lyonization of the disease gene causes observable fundus pathology, as in X-linked ocular albinism, X-linked retinoschisis, and choroideremia. Gieser and Falls[17] and Wu et al.[44] each observed a macular cyst in one eye of a female carrier, and Forsius et al.[14] identified an affected woman who was apparently homozygous as the offspring of an affected male and his second cousin. The affected female studied by Wu et al.[44] had an electronegative ERG response to a bright flash, with the a-wave larger than the b-wave, as is typical for affected males. Because affected females are quite uncommon, such cases warrant careful consideration for a condition that might mimic retinoschisis.

VISION FUNCTION TESTS

Visual acuity normally is somewhat reduced and can be diminished to 20/200 or less even by grade school years. Peripheral visual fields typically remain full or nearly full except in areas of peripheral retinoschisis in which the splitting through the nerve fiber layer disrupts visual signal transmission and causes an absolute scotoma. Color vision remains normal or can have mild tritanopic defects that accompany the parafoveal pathology. Symptoms rarely include complaints of night blindness, and formal testing of rod absolute thresholds typically shows sensitivities that are normal or within 1 log unit of normal.

The electroretinogram is the single most useful test for confirming a diagnosis of juvenile retinoschisis. The textbook description of ERG change in retinoschisis is an electronegative response caused by normal amplitude of the negative a-wave (leading wave of the ERG) but reduction of the positive b-wave (which follows the a-wave).[32] The rod photoreceptors generate the dark-adapted a-wave, whereas the b-wave originates from activity of the second-order neurons, which are the bipolar cells that lie postsynaptic to the rods (Fig. 18.5). Classically, the b-wave origin is described as resulting from potassium released by depolarizing bipolar cells.[24] The Müller cells internalize this potassium excess and thereby depolarize and cause a transretinal positive voltage that is called the *b-wave*.[29] However, some investigators believe that the b-wave originates directly from the bipolar cells and does not involve Müller cell depolarization. A deeply "electronegative" pattern results from the a-wave pulling the response and an absence of any positive b-wave following it. Other diseases can cause an electronegative pattern, including congenital stationary night blindness,[5] but this condition always causes night blindness, whereas nyctalopia is rarely a complaint in retinoschisis.

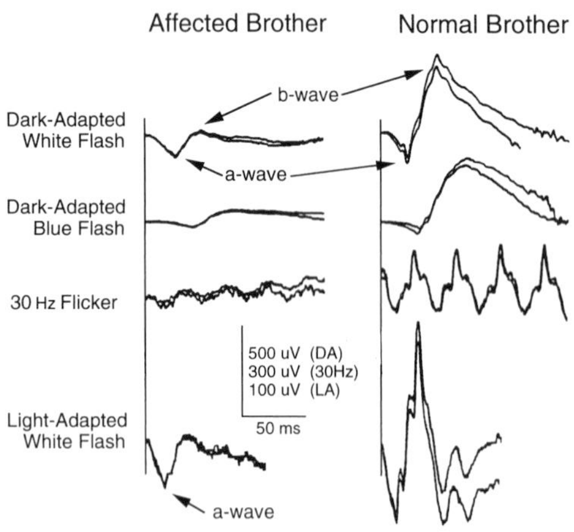

Figure 18.5. Electroretinogram shows reduction of the b-wave in the retinoschisis-affected brother compared with his unaffected brother for both the dark-adapted response from the rod system and from the light-adapted response of the cone system. The 30 Hz flicker responses from the cone system are also reduced.

ASSOCIATED CONDITIONS

Juvenile retinoschisis appears to be an isolated ocular condition without other systemic involvement. No cases have been reported with a contiguous gene syndrome or a deletion that might cause systemic abnormalities due to involvement of a neighboring gene. Both the hypophosphatemic rickets gene[38] and X-linked liver phosphorylase kinease deficiency gene[40] are in the genetic vicinity of retinoschisis, but no RS patients have been identified with combined disease.

DIFFERENTIAL DIAGNOSIS

Clinical diagnosis of retinoschisis normally proceeds smoothly after identification of the nearly pathognomonic parafoveal intraretinal cysts. Finding an "electronegative" ERG response then solidifies the diagnosis. Among the conditions that may mimic RS is Goldmann–Favre, which can show cystic maculopathy, although it is autosomal recessive and thus can affect both men and women. Peripheral retinal lattice degeneration occurs, but vitreous veils are not present, and, unlike juvenile retinoschisis, nyctalopia is a prominent symptom.[13] The ERG is severely reduced. Wagner's vitreoretinal dystrophy is an autosomal dominant trait associated with vitreous syneresis causing pigmentary clumping in the macula, but vitreous veils rarely occur; unlike retinoschisis, cataracts commonly develop during teenage years in Wagner syndrome and progress significantly by the fourth decade.[26] Neither Goldmann–Favre nor Wagner syndrome has the electronegative response pattern on the electroretinogram.

In retinoschisis, leukocoria from retinal detachment at a young age can mimic retinoblastoma. Many RS-affected males exhibit macular atrophy in later age, and these cases may be confused with age-related macular degeneration (AMD), although AMD rarely causes the peripheral retinoschisis, vascular sheathing, or extensive pigment epithelial changes that are found in juvenile retinoschisis. Nicotinic acid maculopathy[15] can cause atypical cystoid maculopathy that can resolve on discontinuing the drug.

Retinoschisis can also mimic Stargardt maculopathy, retinal dialysis, and some forms of cone or cone–rod dystrophies. The most useful adjunct in clinical diagnosis comes from identifying disease segregating in X-linked recessive fashion in relatives. Female carriers of retinoschisis rarely show parafoveal cysts, and if these are found, one should suspect other conditions. One example is termed *familial foveal retinoschisis,* which is an autosomal recessive trait. Lewis et al.[25] described three sisters of a nonconsanguineous marriage of ophthalmoscopically normal parents. The foveal dysmorphology was indistinguishable from RS, although no peripheral retinal abnormalities were noted. Cibis[9] reported a case of peripheral retinoschisis in two 19-year-old females who were monozygotic twins. However, all such conditions of foveal or peripheral retinoschisis are very much less frequent than X-linked juvenile retinoschisis.

HISTOPATHOLOGY

Only a few retinal histopathology studies are available for retinoschisis. Yanoff et al.[45] reported histopathology of an eye thought to have a solid retinal detachment of the inferotemporal aspect and enucleated for the possibility of retinoblastoma. Splitting was found through the nerve fiber layer, with areas of isolated schisis cavities that had not become confluent. A full-thickness retinal hole was found, with several larger holes present in the inner wall aspect of these cysts. The mass that had led to enucleation consisted of fibrous tissue with macrophage invasion. The retinal pigment epithelium underlying the involved neural retinal area showed numerous tiny nodules of hyperplasia. A second report by Condon et al.[10] found splitting through the nerve fiber layer and ganglion cell layer in three RS eyes. This is different from typical senile retinoschisis, in which splitting occurs in the outer retina through the outer nuclear and plexiform layers. Of particular interest were fine filaments measuring up to 20 nm in diameter within the amorphous material in the extracellular space adjacent to the schisis cavities. The larger filaments had striations with a 5 nm periodicity. No filaments were apparent within the schisis cavities themselves. These filaments merged with the Müller cell plasma membrane, and it was thought that this might represent an extrusion from the Müller cells. Similar filaments have also been reported associated with typical cystoid degeneration and with senile outer retinal retinoschisis.[19,20] Thus, it is not known whether the filaments in juvenile retinoschisis result from the novel pathophysiology of this disease. Condon et al.[10] also observed focal degeneration of the retinal pigment epithelium in areas where there was extensive disruption of photoreceptor cells. Mild photoreceptor cell disruption was observed elsewhere in the retina in areas of intact pigment epithelium, leading to the conclusion that the retinal pigment epithelium (RPE) changes were secondary degeneration.

PATHOPHYSIOLOGY

Müller cells are believed to be involved in the pathophysiology of juvenile retinoschisis. This supposition comes principally from three observations: First, the retinal splitting in juvenile retinoschisis occurs through the nerve fiber–ganglion cell layer.[45] The primary cell in this region is the Müller cell, a glial cell that traverses the entire retinal thickness. A splitting in this location suggests involvement of an adhesion molecule or a matrix molecule. Second, the reduced b-wave of the electroretinogram points toward primary involvement of Müller cells. The b-wave origin has classically been described as resulting from Müller cell depolarization subsequent to these cells processing the increased extracellular potassium load that results from light activation of the depolarizing of the bipolar cells. Even in eyes that have clinically minimal peripheral retinoschisis, the b-wave can be substantially diminished, suggesting that potassium processing by Müller cells is deficient, even at a stage prior to mechanical disruption of these cells. Third, the retinas in some RS cases exhibit a Mizuo–Nakamura phenomenon in which the macula undergoes a color change from normal in the dark-adapted state to a golden macular sheen shortly after the onset of light.[11] A similar retinal discoloration has been observed experimentally in laboratory cat and animal studies on leakage of potassium from an intraretinal microelectrode tip. Because Müller cells are involved in potassium extracellular homeostasis, this raises the possibility that Müller cells are involved in the pathophysiology.

The scotopic threshold response (STR) of the electroretinogram is also significantly reduced in juvenile retinoschisis. The STR originates in the proximal retina due to potassium release by amacrine cells and a subsequent depolarization of the Müller cells from this excess potassium. One study has suggested that the STR is the most sensitive ERG component for identifying juvenile retinoschisis.[28] Despite this sensitivity, female carriers exhibited no change in the STR compared to normals. A caution is necessary regarding ERG diagnosis of retinoschisis, however, since in our experience, many males with retinoschisis exhibit only minimal changes in the b-wave to maximal ERG stimuli, which is a condition typically used in clinical diagnostic laboratories. The b-wave reductions are best observed at lower flash intensities that are not always used in clinical laboratories.

Not all work leads to the conclusion that Müller cells are the primary site of defect in retinoschisis. Some evidence suggests that female RS carriers may exhibit subtle vision abnormalities in a condition called *suppressive rod–cone interaction.* Rods, which normally function in dim light, can influence the sensitivity of the cones near cone thresholds through an interaction that is thought to occur in the outer retina through horizontal cells.[18] Arden et al.[4] found an absence of this normal rod–cone interaction in 11 obligate carriers in eight retinoschisis families by measuring cone threshold to a flickering dim red light while stimulating rod vision with a blue background. Arden and colleagues suggest that the pathophysiology in retinoschisis may extend to the outer retinal neurons, which is somewhat at conflict with prevailing ideas that retinoschisis is primarily a Müller glial cell abnormality at the inner retinal surface. A separate group studied rod–cone interaction in one RS-affected male and did not find any abnormality,[1] and this conflict in the results has not fully been resolved.

CURRENT STATUS OF GENE IDENTIFICATION

On clinical grounds, juvenile retinoschisis is an X-chromosomal disease, by virtue of its familial inheritance pattern. The first reported genetic linkage for retinoschisis was with the Xg blood group by Ives et al.[22] The first molecular linkage for RS was with the anonymous marker RC8 on the short arm of the X chromosome, which demonstrated a recombination fraction of only 15% and thereby mapped retinoschisis to Xp22.1–22.3 on the short are of the X chromosome.[42]

Several subsequent studies used RFLP (restriction fragment length polymorphism) markers to define the genetic flanking interval for retinoschisis as lying between DXS41-RS-DXS43-XTER.[2] Sieving et al.[36] found no evidence for genetic heterogeneity in RS, and it appears that RS represents a single-gene disease. In the 1990s a new category of molecular DNA markers became available that utilized the technique of polymerase chain reaction (PCR), and subsequent studies provided fine mapping of the RS interval.[6,30,41] Mapping (as of 1996) placed retinoschisis within a physical interval of about 900 kb between markers Xp_{ter}-DXS418-RS-DXS999-Xp_{cen}.[31] The RS gene was cloned in fall 1997 and was designated XLRS1.[35] Preliminary characterization indicates six exons coding for 224 aminoacid residues and a C-terminal domain similar to discoidin, which in other proteins can mediate cell–cell adhesion. The retinal localization and function of the XLRS1 protein remain to be elucidated. It will be interesting to learn whether XLRS1 affects Müller cell function and the mechanism by which the ERG b-wave is suppressed in this disease.

MANAGEMENT

At present, there is no treatment for the parafoveal cystic degeneration in retinoschisis that causes reduced acuity. Visual acuity typically is subnormal and is reduced to a level that threatens the prospect for obtaining a driver's license in these teenage males. The patients should be counseled that the acuity typically stabilizes by the teenage years and remains fairly constant throughout middle age but can then deteriorate to legal blindness in later middle age and beyond. Although peripheral retinoschisis does not typically lead to retinal detachment, when this occurs, it frequently is severe and prognosis for surgical stabilization is difficult, although this should be attempted. To prevent extension of bullous peripheral retinoschisis toward the macula, photocoagulation has been tried by Castier et al.,[8] but they advise against this approach because of the poor outcomes in 28 RS eyes they treated and because the peripheral retinoschisis can spontaneously regress with age.

If rhegmatogenous or exudative retinal detachment results in young RS males, these eyes may benefit from surgical repair by scleral buckling, although these eyes are at risk for subsequent proliferative vitreoretinopathy.[33] Other RS males are described during infancy with peripheral bullous elevation of the inner retinal layer accompanied with vitreous hemorrhage.[16] Surgical repair is quite difficult in such cases and is not expected to improve the vision prognosis if separation of the neural retinal layers interrupts neural signal transmission.

Genetic counseling should be directed along the lines of classical X-linked recessive inheritance patterns. Unfortunately, carriers are identified only by their obligate status within a pedigree, and females at risk for carrier status cannot be identified clinically by ophthalmologic examination, by visual functional testing, or by electroretinogram testing. Haplotype analysis of the X-chromosomal region Xp22.2 has been done in selected families by linkage analysis.[23] However, molecular identification of female carriers will now become straightforward, a benefit of the recent cloning of the RS gene.

Acknowledgments: This work was supported by NIH grant RO1EY10259 and The Foundation Fighting Blindness, Hunt Valley, Maryland.

REFERENCES

1. Alexander KR, Fishman GA. Rod influence on cone flicker detection. *Vision Res* 1986; 26:827.
2. Alitalo T, Kurse TA, de la Chapelle A. Refined localization of the gene causing X-linked juvenile retinoschisis. *Genomics* 1991;9:505–510.
3. Anderson JR. Anterior dialysis of the retina: disinsertion or avulsion at ora serrata. *Br J Ophthalmol* 1932;16:641–670; 705–727.
4. Arden GB, Gorin MB, Polkinghorne PJ, Jay M, bird AC. Detection of the carrier state of X-linked retinoschisis. *Am J Ophthalmol* 1988; 105:590–595.
5. Bornschein H, Schubert G. Das photopische flimmer-elektroretinogramm des menschen. *Z Biol* 1953;106:229–238.
6. Brown D, Barker D, Litt M. Dinucleotide repeat polymorphisms at the DXS365, DXS443 and DXS451 loci. *Hum Mol Genet* 1992;1:213.
7. Burns RP, Lovrien EW, Cibis AB. Juvenile sex-linked retinoschisis: Clinical and genetic studies. *Trans Am Acad Ophthalmol Otolaryngol* 1971; 75:1011–1021.
8. Castier P, Turut P, Francois P, Woillez JP. La photocoagulation dans le retinoschisis heredofamilial lie au sexe. *Bull Soc Ophtalmol Fr* 1990;90:149–152.
9. Cibis PA. Retinoschisis-retinal cysts. *Trans Am Ophthalmol Soc* 1965;53:417–453.
10. Condon GP, Brownstein S, Wang N-S, Kearns JAF, Ewing CC. Congenital hereditary (juvenile X-linked) retinoschisis: histopathologic and ultrastructural findings in three eyes. *Arch Ophthalmol* 1986;104:576–583.
11. de Jong PTVM, Zrenner E, van Meel GJ, Keunen JEE, van Norren D. Mizuo Phenomenon in X-linked retinoschisis: Pathogenesis of the Mizuo Phenomenon. *Arch Ophthalmol* 1991; 109:1104–1108.
12. Deutman AF. Sex-linked juvenile retinoschisis. In *The Hereditary Dystrophies of the Posterior Pole of the Eye,* A. F. Deutman, ed. Assen, The Netherlands: Van Gorcum Press, 1971, pp. 48–98.
13. Feiler-Ofry V, Adams A, Regenbogen L, Godel V, Stein R. Hereditary vitreoretinal degenera-

tion and night blindness. *Am J Ophthalmol* 1969;67:553–558.
14. Forsius H, Ericksson A, Nuutila A, Vainio-Mattila B. Geschlechtsgebundene, erbliche Retinoschisis in zwei Familien in Finnland. *Klin Monatsbl Augenheilkd* 1963;143:806–816.
15. Gass JDM. Nicotinic acid maculopathy. *Am J Ophthalmol* 1973;76:500–510.
16. George NDL, Yates JRW, Moore AT. X-linked retinoschisis. *Br J Ophthalmol* 1995;79: 679–702.
17. Gieser EP, Falls HF. Hereditary retinoschisis. *Am J Ophthalmol* 1961;51:1193–1200.
18. Goldberg SH, Frumkes TE, Nygaard RW. Inhibitory influence of unstimulated rods in the human retina. Evidence provided by examining cone flicker. *Science* 1983;221:180–182.
19. Gottinger W. *Senile Retinoschisis.* Stuttgart, Germany: Georg Thieme Verlag, 1978.
20. Gottinger W. Formation of basement membranes and collagenous fibrils in peripheral cystoid degeneration and retinoschisis. *Dev Ophthalmol* 1981:2363–2368.
21. Haas J. Ueber dat Zusammenvorkommen von veränderungen der retina und choroidea. *Arch Augenheilkd* 1898;37:343–348.
22. Ives EJ, Ewing CC, Innes R. X-linked juvenile retinoschisis and Xg linkage in five families. *Am J Hum Genet* 1970;22:17A–18A.
23. Kaplan J, Pelet A, Hentati H, Jeanpeirre M, Briard ML. Contribution to carrier detection in X-linked retinoschisis. *J Med Genet* 1991;28: 383–388.
24. Karwoski CJ, Proenza LM. Relationship between Muller cell responses, a local transretinal potential, and potassium flux. *J Neurophysiol* 1977;40:244–259.
25. Lewis RA, Lee GB, Martonyi CL, Barnett JM, Falls HF. Familial foveal retinoschisis. *Arch Ophthalmol* 1977;95:1190–1196.
26. Liberfarb RM, Hirose T. The Wegner-Stickler syndrome. *Birth Defects Orig Art Ser* 1982; 18:525–538.
27. Mann I, MacRae A. Congenital vascular veils in the vitreous. *Br J Ophthalmol* 1938;22:1–10.
28. Murayama K, Kuo C, Sieving PA. Abnormal threshold ERG response in X-linked juvenile retinoschisis, evidence for a proximal retinal origin of the human STR. *Clin Vis Sci* 1991;6: 317–322.
29. Newman EA, Frambach DA, Odette LL. Control of extracellular potassium levels by retinal glial cell K^+ siphoning. *Science* 1984;225:1174–1175.
30. Oudet C, Weber C, Kaplan J, Segues B, Croquette M-F, Roman EO, Hanauer A. Characterisation of a highly polymorphic microsatellite at the *DXS207* locus: Confirmation of very close linkage to the retinoschisis disease gene. *J Med Genet* 1993;30:300–303.
31. Pawar H, Bingham EL, Hiriyanna K, Segal M, Richards JE, Sieving PA. X-linked juvenile retinoschisis: Localization between (DXS1195, DXS418) and AFM291 wf5 on a single YAC. *Hum Hered* 1996;46:329–335.
32. Peachey NS, Fishman GA, Derlacki DJ, Brigell MG. Psychophysical and electroretinographic findings in X-linked juvenile retinoschisis. *Arch Ophthalmol* 1987;105:513–516.
33. Regillo CD, Tasman WS, Brown GC. Surgical management of complications associated with X-linked retinoschisis. *Arch Ophthalmol* 1993; 111:1080–1086.
34. Sarin LK, Green WR, Dailey EG. Congenital vascular veils and hereditary retinoschisis. *Am J Ophthalmol* 1964;57:793–796.
35. Sauer CG, Gehrig A, Warneke-Wittstock R, Marquardy A, Ewing CC, Gibson A, Lorenz B, Jurklies B, Weber BHF. Positional cloning of the gene associated with X-linked juvenile retinoschisis. *Nature Genet* 1997; 17:164–170.
36. Sieving PA, Bingham EL, Roth MS, Young MR, Boehnke M, Kuo CY, Ginsburg D. Linkage relationship of X-linked juvenile retinoschisis with Xp22.1–p22.3 probes. *Am J Hum Genet* 1990; 47:616–621.
37. Sorsby A, Klein M, Gann JH, Siggins G. Unusual retinal detachment, possibly sex-linked. *Br J Ophthalmol* 1951;35:1–10.
38. The HYP Consortium. A gene (PEX) with homologies to endopeptidases is mutated in patients with X-linked hypophosphatemic rickets. *Nature Genet* 1995;11:130–136.
39. Thomson E. Memorandum regarding a family in which neuroretinal disease of an unusual kind occurred only in males. *Br J Ophthalmol* 1932;16:681–686.
40. van den Berg IET, van Buerden EACM, Malingre HEM, Ploos van Amstel HK, Poll-The BT, Smeitink JAM, Lamers WH, Berger R. X-linked liver phosphorylase kinase deficiency is associated with mutations in the human liver phosphorylase kinase alpha subunit. *Am J Hum Genet* 1995;56:381–387.
41. Weber BHF, Janocha S, Vogt G, Sander S, Ewing CC, Roesch M, Gibson A. X-linked juvenile retinoschisis (RS) maps between DXS987

and DXS443. *Cytogenet Cell Genet* 1995;69: 35–37.
42. Wieacker P, Wienker TF, Dallapiccola B, Bender K, Davies K, Ropers H. Linkage relationships between retinoschisis, Xg and a cloned DNA sequence from the distal short arm of the X chromosome. *Hum Genet* 1983;64:143–145.
43. Wilczek M. Ein der netzhautspaltung(retinoschisis) mit einer offnung. *Z Augenheilkd* 1935;85:108–116.
44. Wu G, Cotlier E, Brodie S. A carrier state of X-linked juvenile retinoschisis. *Ophthalmic Paediatr Genet* 1985;5:13–17.
45. Yanoff M, Rahnek EK, Zimmerman LE. Histopathology of juvenile retinoschisis. *Arch Ophthalmol* 1968;79:49–53.

19

Cone Dystrophies

ELIAS I. TRABOULSI

Cone dystrophies may be divided into those with stationary and those with progressive cone dysfunction (Table 19.1). Stationary disorders include normal variation in color vision, anomalous trichromacy, dichromacy, and complete achromatopsia or rod monochromacy. Although incomplete achromatopsia or blue cone monochromacy was initially thought to be a static disorder, patients have been found to develop progressive macular degeneration in middle and old age.[40]

The progressive cone dysfunction syndromes or cone dystrophies are characterized by the clinical triad of photophobia, abnormal color vision or dyschromatopsia, and reduced central vision. Progressive cone dysfunction syndromes have been further classified into pure cone degenerations, and cone-rod degenerations, or into diffuse and regional cone degenerations. Atypical cone degenerative disorders include benign concentric annular dystrophy, cone dystrophy with supernormal electroretinogram (ERG), and occult macular degeneration. Cone-rod degeneration also occurs in a number of systemic conditions such as Bardet-Biedl syndrome, fucosidosis, neuronal ceroid lipofuscinosis, infantile phytanic acid storage disease, methylmalonic aciduria with homocystinuria, and in other rare conditions. Finally, toxicity from some medications such as digoxin and chloroquine may result in a macular degeneration and cone dysfunction. Toxic retinopathies are not covered in this chapter, which deals mostly with the inherited cone and cone-rod dystrophies and degenerations. The stationary cone dysfunction syndromes are covered in Chapter 16 by Samir Deeb in this text. The ceroid ipofuscinoses, infantile phytanic acid storage disease, and Bardet-Biedl syndrome are discussed in Chapter 32 by Traboulsi et al. and Chapter 33 by Weleber.

ROD MONOCHROMACY (ACHROMATOPSIA)

Patients with this rare autosomal recessive disease have a total absence of color discrimination, reduced central visual acuity to 20/200 or less, photodysphoria or discomfort in daylight or in bright light, and nystagmus that appears in the first 4 weeks of life.[35] Rod monochromacy occurs worldwide and has a prevalence of 3 per 100,000.[54] It may be more common among Moroccan, Iraqi, and Iranian Jews.[58] The first description of the disease in 1684 is attributed to Daubeney.[14] The largest reported family is from the Island of Fuur in the Limfjord in the north of Denmark,[24] but the disease is most common among the Pingelapese people of the eastern Caroline Islands.[7]

Table 19.1. Classification of Cone Dysfunction Syndromes

Stationary Disorders	***Cone-Rod Degeneration in Systemic Disorders***
Normal variation in color vision	Bardet-Biedl syndrome
Anomalous trichromacy	Fucosidosis
Dichromacy	Neuronal ceroid lipofuscinosis
Rod monochromacy (complete achromatopsia)	Infantile phytanic acid storage disease
Progressive Disorders	Hereditary ataxias
Blue cone monochromacy (incomplete achromatopsia)	Methylmalonic aciduria with homocystinuria
Pure cone degenerations	Congenital amaurosis with hypertrichosis
Autosomal dominant	Aplasia cutis congenita, high myopia, and cone-rod dysfunction
X-linked recessive	Cone-rod dystrophy and amelogenesis imperfecta
Cone-rod degenerations	***Toxic Cone-Rod Degenerations***
Benign concentric annular dystrophy (AD)	Chloroquine
Cone dystrophy with supernormal ERG	Digoxin
Occult macular degeneration (AD)	

Patients with rod monochromacy are severely photophobic and exhibit significant blepharospasm. They avoid bright lights and prefer to stay indoors. The amplitude of the nystagmus that appears in the first few weeks of life decreases with age and in dim illumination.

Visual acuity is 20/200 and remains stable throughout life. Most patients develop compound myopic astigmatism with an oblique axis. All patients have paradoxical pupillary responses such as those initially observed in congenital stationary night blindness.[3] A paradoxical pupillary response is detected in the following manner: after the pupil is light adapted, the lights are turned off, and the pupil is observed to initially constrict to a minimal diameter after 1–2 seconds, following which it dilates.[35]

The fundus of patients with rod monochromacy is normal except for an occasional attenuation of the foveal reflex and the progressive development of a myopic conus. Histologic studies reveal a fovea without thickening and abnormal or absent cones.[13,17,19] Color vision is severely impaired.

Herring demonstrated in 1891 that the photopic luminosity curve of patients with achromatopsia was identical to the scotopic curve of normal individuals. The scotopic ERG waveform is normal, whereas the photopic is nonrecordable. There is no Purkinje phenomenon, and the Stiles-Crawford phenomenon cannot be demonstrated.

The gene for rod monochromacy was presumed to be on chromosome 14 because of one published report of a 20-year-old woman with achromatopsia, short stature, developmental delay, premature puberty, small hands and feet, recurrent miscarriages, and a karyotype of 45,XX,rob(14;14). All portions of the abnormal chromosome 14 in this patient were maternally inherited (so-called maternal isodisomy).[42] Arbour and co-workers,[1a] however, mapped the gene to the pericentral region of chromosome 2 in an inbred Iranian Jewish family.

CONE AND CONE-ROD DEGENERATIONS

The differentiation between pure cone dystrophies and cone-rod degenerations has become blurred with the realization that, in most instances, some degree of rod dysfunction develops as the disease progresses, regardless of mode of inheritance of genetic locus. We shall continue to use the term *cone dystrophy* for retinal diseases with predominant cone dysfunction with late onset and mild rod involvement, and *cone-rod degeneration* for retinal dystrophies with early onset cone dysfunction followed shortly thereafter by significant rod disease. Patients with cone dystrophies have progressive loss of visual acuity, photophobia, and defective color vision. Unlike patients with retinitis pigmentosa, those with cone dystrophy rarely lose peripheral vision and they are not night blind. There is a prominent variability in the severity of the disease among family members and between families, regardless of mode inheritance or genetic locus.

The prevalence of cone-rod dystrophies is unknown, but many young patients diagnosed with cone dystrophy may actually have early stages of cone-rod dystrophy. In one study, 41% of 278 patients with retinal dystrophy had a cone-rod type of deficit, based on rod-threshold measurements.[23] Cone-rod dystrophies are characterized by initial loss of visual acuity and color vision, and subsequent progressive peripheral visual field loss. Macular atrophic and pigmentary changes are detected first (Fig. 19.1). Peripheral pigmentary abnormalities that may resemble those of classic retinitis pigmentosa occur later in the course of the disease.[20] Young patients are generally diagnosed with cone dystrophy, whereas older ones receive a label of retinitis pigmentosa if the full extent of the phenotype is not appreciated in one family, or if they have not been examined and electrophysiologic studies obtained at a younger age. The diagnosis is generally made on the basis of marked reduction or absence of cone electroretinographic responses in the presence of quantitatively less reduction in rod responses. A wide range of clinical phenotypes are associated with this pattern of electroretinographic responses; this has led investigators to classify cone-rod dystrophies on the basis of fundus appearance,[21] visual field defects,[31] electroretinographic responses,[51] and dark-adapted static threshold profiles.[57]

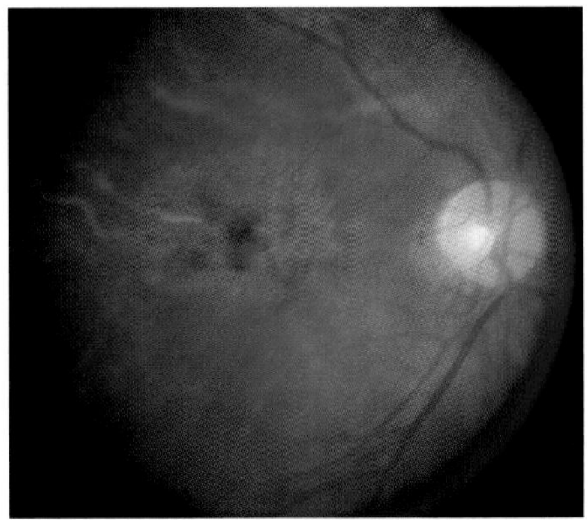

Figure 19.1. Macular atrophic changes in a patient with cone-rod dystrophy.

The cone-rod dystrophies are genetically heterogeneous with simplex cases as well as cases with autosomal dominant, autosomal recessive, and X-linked patterns of inheritance.[39] Individual cases with chromosomal abnormalities have suggested loci for the disease on chromosome 18q21.1,[55] and on chromosome 17q in a patient with cone-rod dystrophy and neurofibromatosis 1.[33]

Krill et al.[32] published several large pedigrees of families with cone dystrophy. Other reports include those of Berson et al.,[6] Davis and Hollenhorst,[9] and Sloan and Brown.[48] Went et al.[56] described an autosomal dominant cone dystrophy in seven generations of a Dutch family. The patients started losing vision after the age of 20 years. Loss of blue cone function was the earliest abnormality followed by changes in visual acuity, visual fields, or fluorescein angiography.

IDENTIFIED GENETIC LOCI FOR CONE AND CONE-ROD DYSTROPHIES (Table 19.2)

Chromosome 6q25-q26

Tranebjaerg et al.[52] described a 6-year-old mentally retarded boy with cone dystrophy, facial dysmorphism, and other malformations. He had a translocation involving chromosomes 1 and 6, t(1;6)(q44;q27), suggesting the presence of a locus for cone dystrophy on chromosome 6q.

Chromosome 17p3-p12 (CORD5 and CORD6)

Balciuniene and co-workers[2] mapped a gene for a progressive cone-rod dystrophy (CORD5) to 17p13-p12 in a five-generation family. Multipoint analysis gave a maximum lod score

Table 19.2. Genetic Map of the Cone Dystrophies and Cone-Rod Degenerations

Type of Cone Dystrophy	Genetic Locus	Reference
Cone dystrophy with dysmorphism	6q25-q26	52
Rod monochromacy (achromatopsia)	2p11-q12	1a
Autosomal dominant cone degeneration (CORD5)	17p13-p12	2, 50
Autosomal dominant cone rod degeneration (CORD6)	17p13-p12	27a
Cone-rod dystrophy with dysmorphism	18q21.1-q21.3	55
Cone-rod dystrophy 2 (CORD2)	19q13.1-q13.2	12
X-linked cone dystrophy (COD1)	Xp11.1-Xp21.1	4, 5, 25
Blue cone monochromacy	Xq28	36

of 7.72 at the marker D17S938. There was a recombination between the disease gene and the one encoding recoverin, excluding the latter as a candidate local gene.

Kelsell and co-workers[27a] mapped the gene for a cone-rod dystrophy occurring in a large British family to the same 17p12-p13 region but numbered this as CORD6. These authors remarked that this region of the genome was rich in genes that result in retinal dystrophies when mutated. These include Leber's congenital amaurosis, central areolar choroidal dystrophy, and dominant cone dystrophy. Patients with CORD6 type of cone-rod dystrophy had early onset of central vision, usually before 7 years of age. Peripheral visual field defects occurred later in life.

Small and Gehrs[49] studied a single large family from Eastern Tennessee with autosomal dominant cone degeneration. Seventy-three individuals were examined, of whom 34 were affected. Symptoms began in the first or second decades of life and progressed slowly. Early onset of symptoms usually correlated with a more severe clinical course. Twenty-six of the 34 patients complained of photophobia, glare, and hemeralopia. Visual acuity varied from 20/20 to 5/200 with a median of 20/70. Color vision was mildly to moderately impaired in 24 patients and was normal in three. Younger patients had fine macular granularity, whereas older ones had central atrophy. Full-field ERGs showed selective diminution in the b-wave of the photopic response. Two older individuals also had diminution of the b-wave under scotopic conditions. Focal ERGs of the macula were abnormally low, or the foveal/parafoveal ratio was reduced in all patients. Clinical severity of the disease varied widely. The diagnosis of affected individuals relied on a combination of clinical and psychophysical abnormalities; the latter, especially an abnormal foveal/parafoveal ERG ratio, were important in the diagnosis of mild cases.

The gene responsible for the disease in this family was mapped to the region of chromosome 17p where the candidate genes for recoverin, β-arrestin-2, and guanylate cyclase reside.[50] The authors did not report the results of analysis of any of these three genes in this particular family.

Chromosome 17q

Kylstra and Aylsworth[33] reported a patient with cone-rod retinal dystrophy and neurofibromatosis type 1. This association suggests a possible locus for cone-rod dystrophy close to NF1 on 17q.

Chromosome 18q21.1-q21.3 (CORD1)

Warburg et al.[55] reported the case of a 20-year-old mentally retarded man with hypogonadism, central postsynaptic hearing impairment, and a cone-rod dystrophy of childhood onset. This patient had a chromosomal deletion of the 18q21.1-qter segment. Three patients with more distal deletions on chromosome 18 did not present retinal dystrophies. This led Warburg and co-workers[55] to propose that a locus for cone-rod dystrophy is located in the segment 18q21.1-q21.3.

Chromosome 19q13.1-q13.2 (CORD2)

Evans and co-workers[12] mapped one gene for autosomal dominant cone-rod dystrophy to chromosome 19q. The phenotype associated with this locus did not appear to fit well with ones that were previously described. These investigators[11] studied 34 affected and 22 unaffected individuals in four generations of one family. Patients lost visual acuity in the first decade of life. The onset of night blindness occurred after 20 years of age, and there was little remaining visual function after the age of 50 years. Macular and, later, peripheral retinal fundus changes were present. Visual field defects included central scotomas, pseudoaltitudinal field defects, and, in more advanced cases, diffuse loss. Electrophysiologic testing before the age of 26 years showed more marked loss of cone than rod function.

X-Linked Progressive Cone Dystrophy (COD1)

Only a few families with X-linked progressive cone dystrophy have been described to date.[22,25,28,43–45] Although the COD1 locus was placed in the Xp21.1-p11.3 region (closely linked to the DXS84 locus in band Xp21.1) by two groups of investigators,[4,5] Hong et al.[25] mapped the gene in one family to Xp11.3 They raise the possibility of genetic heterogeneity of the disease, with two genes in adjacent chromosomal regions, or the possibility that the disease in some of the families is due to mutations in the X-linked retinitis pigmentosa genes RP2 or RP3. Hong et al.[25] do, however, consider their family to have the same disorder as that in other published pedigrees because of the overlap in clinical features between patients and families.

Affected males have progressive deterioration of visual acuity starting in the teens, enlarging central scotomas in the late teens and twenties, and moderate to high myopia. Photophobia is a universal complaint. There is no nystagmus. Color vision is impaired with eventual loss of all color discrimination. Ophthalmoscopic macular changes vary from granularity of the retinal pigment epithelium to bull's eye lesions and geographic atrophy in older patients. There is good correlation between the degree of visual dysfunction, age, and severity of macular and retinal degenerative changes. Some patients have a tapetallike sheen and a Mizuo phenomenon.[22] Female carriers may be clinically asymptomatic, or may be photophobic under normal daylight conditions, with mild impairment of visual acuity and color vision.[22,25,28,43–45] Older female carriers in the family reported by Hong et al.[25] had drusen or mottling of the retinal pigment epithelium in the temporal aspect of the macula.

There is wide variability in the clinical phenotype and in the cone and rod responses in all families.[22,25,28,43–45] Although the cones are more severely affected, rod dysfunction is present to a variable extent in most patients. The proband in the family reported by Hong et al.[25] had more severely reduced rod than cone responses at an early age, indicating that both rods and cones are vulnerable to the COD1 mutation.

ATYPICAL CONE DYSTROPHIES

Benign Concentric Macular Dystrophy

Deutman[10] described four members of a family with an autosomal dominant macular dystrophy characterized by a ringlike depigmentation around the fovea (Fig. 19.2) and associated with unusually good visual acuity, even in the oldest individual (20/60). Patients did not have the typical symptoms associated with cone dystrophy. A 10-year follow-up study of this family was reported by van den Biesen et al.[53] In some patients, visual acuity, night vision, and color vision had deteriorated. The macular dystrophy had progressed and there were ophthalmoscopic changes in the fundus periphery, including bone corpusclelike pigmentation in two patients. Electrophysiologic examination showed increasing photoreceptor dysfunction, with equal involvement of the rod and cone systems. Hence, this family may be better classified as having a mild form of autosomal dominant cone-rod degeneration.

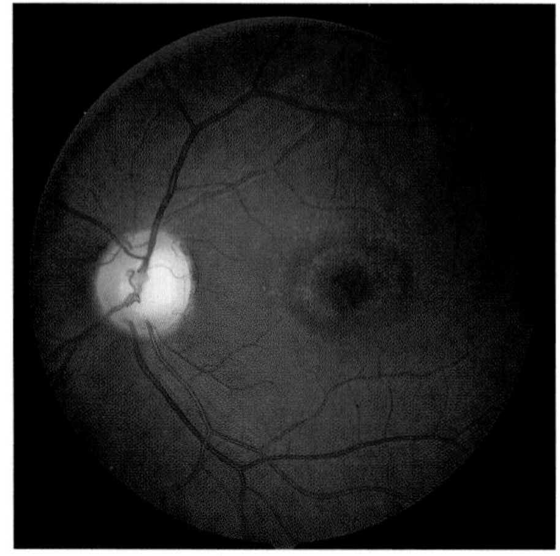

A

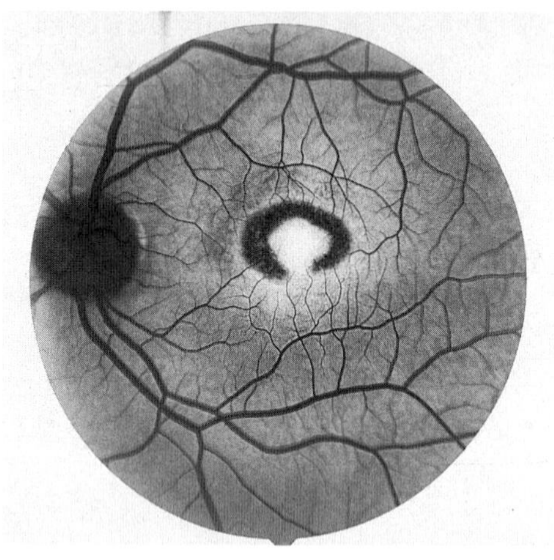

B

Figure 19.2. Fundus photograph (**A**) and fluorescein angiogram (**B**) of presumed benign concentric macular dystrophy in an asymptomatic 30-year-old black man. Visual acuity was 20/30 in each eye. Color vision, electroretinography, and electrooculography were normal. No progression was noted over 2 years of observation. (Courtesy of Dr. David O. Mazur.)

Cone Dystrophy with Supernormal ERG

Patients with this presumably distinct condition have signs and symptoms of rod and cone dysfunction such as night blindness, loss of visual acuity and color vision, and photophobia. They have severely abnormal cone-mediated electroretinographic responses, but supernormal rod-mediated responses, despite elevated rod dark adaptation thresholds.[1,15,18] The rod b-wave amplitudes are absent or small at dimmer stimulus intensities, and much greater than normal at the highest stimulus intensity, resulting in a stimulus-response curve with a steep slope. Gouras et al.[18] postulated that the electrophysiologic findings in this type of retinal dystrophy may be the result of a defect in the retinal enzyme cyclic nucleotide phosphodiesterase.

Occult Macular Dystrophy

Patients with this disease, first described by Miyake and co-workers,[38] have a normal fundus and no abnormalities on fluorescein angiography. A progressive decline in visual acuity occurs with age. The diagnosis lies in demonstrating normal full-field cone and rod ERGs with abnormal focal macular cone electroretinographic responses. In a follow-up report of 13 familial and sporadic cases, Miyake et al.[37] report that the fundus appearance is normal except in the oldest patient, who, at the age of 65 years, had a bull's eye maculopathy. The pedigrees in Miyake's series are compatible with autosomal dominant inheritance. Visual acuity ranged from 20/20 to 20/200. All patients had a color vision defect along either the red-green or blue-yellow axis. Young patients had cone sensitivity loss in the macular area, whereas older patients had both cone and rod sensitivity loss in the macula. Miyake et al.[37] believe that this condition is a form of central cone dystrophy.

CONE DEGENERATION IN SYSTEMIC DISEASE

Bardet-Biedl Syndrome

The distinctive features of the retinal dystrophy in Bardet-Biedl syndrome are the relatively fast progression of visual loss in the teenage years and the relative absence of significant pigment proliferative changes in the fundus until late stages of the disease.[29] The earliest ophthalmoscopic alterations appear as atrophic changes in the macular and peripapillary areas (Fig. 19.3).[8] The electroretinographic pattern of cone-rod dysfunction in some patients has led

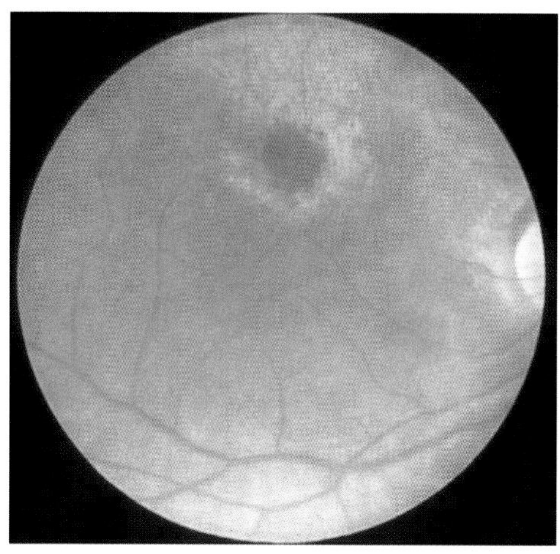

Figure 19.3. Posterior pole of patient with Bardet-Biedl syndrome. Note atrophic changes in macular and peripapillary area.

authors to call the retinal dystrophy in Bardet-Biedl syndrome a cone-rod retinal degeneration.

Amaurosis Congenita, Cone-Rod Type, with Congenital Hypertrichosis

Jalili[26] reported two female cousins with a severe type of congenital cone-rod retinal dystrophy and excessive body hair. Both patients were significantly photophobic but not night blind. There was trichomegaly with bushy eyebrows, synophrys, and excessive facial and body hair. The patients were not mentally retarded. Photophobia may be a prominent symptom of Leber's congenital amaurosis. It is not clear whether the syndrome reported by Jalili[26] is distinct, or whether the two patients in his article had Leber's congenital amaurosis and coincidental hypertrichosis.

Aplasia Cutis Congenita, High Myopia, and Cone-Rod Dysfunction

Gershoni-Baruch and Leibo[16] reported a brother and sister with aplasia cutis congenita of the midline of the scalp vertex, high myopia, congenital nystagmus, and cone-rod dysfunction. The patients had a tendency to develop permanent atrophic linear or macular cutaneous scars following minor trauma to the forearms, hands, and lower legs. Leung et al.[34] had previously described two sibs with aplasia cutis congenita of the scalp associated with myopia, keratoconus, nystagmus, atrophic irides, and atrophic pigment epithelium. There is significant overlap in the clinical features of patients in these two families with those of patients with the similarly autosomal recessive Knobloch syndrome, in which patients may have encephaloceles, scalp defects, high myopia, and a very strong predisposition for retinal detachment.[30,41,46,47]

Cone-Rod Dystrophy and Amelogenesis Imperfecta

Jalili and Smith[27] reported 29 individuals from a highly inbred Arab family from the Gaza Strip, with a combination of cone-rod dystrophy and amelogenesis imperfecta. All affected individuals had photophobia and nystagmus, starting in the first 2 years of life. Patients had no perception of color, but they were not night blind. The teeth of all affected individuals were abnormally shaped and discolored as soon as they erupted.

REFERENCES

1. Alexander K, Fishman G. Super normal scotopic ERG in cone dystrophy. *Br J Ophthalmol* 1984;68:69–78.

1a. Arbour NC, Zlotogora J, Knowlton RG, Merin S, Rosenmann A, Kanis AB, Rokhlina T, Stone EM, Sheffield VC. Homozygosity mapping of achromatopsia to chromosome 2 using DNA pooling. *Hum Mol Genet* 1997;6:689–694.

2. Balciuniene J, Johansson K, Sandgren O, Wachtmeister L, Holmgren G, Forsman K. A gene for autosomal dominant cone-rod dystrophy maps to chromosome 17p12-p13. *Genomics* 1995;30:281–286.

3. Barricks M, Flynn J, Kushner B. Paradoxical pupillary responses in congenital stationary night blindness. *Am J Ophthalmol* 1977;95: 1800–1804.

4. Bartley J, Gies C, Jacobson D. Cone dystrophy (X-linked) (COD1) maps between DXS7 (L1.28) and DXS206 (Xj1.1) and is linked to

DXS84 (754). *Cytogenet Cell Genet* 1989;51: 959.

5. Bergen AA, Meire F, ten Brink J, Schuurman EJ, van Ommen GJ, Delleman JW. Additional evidence for a gene locus for progressive cone dystrophy with late rod involvement in Xp21.1-p11.3. *Genomics* 1993;18(2):463–464.
6. Berson E, Gouras P, Gunkel R. Progressive cone degeneration, dominantly inherited. *Arch Ophthalmol* 1968;80:77–83.
7. Brody J, Hussels I, Brink E, Torres J. Hereditary blindness among Pingelapese people of eastern Caroline Islands. *Lancet* 1970;i:1253–1257.
8. Campo R, Aaberg T. Ocular and systemic features of the Barget-Biedl syndrome. *Am J Ophthalmol* 1982;92:750–756.
9. Davis C, Hollenhorst R. Hereditary degeneration of the macula (occurring in five generations). *Am J Ophthalmol* 1955;39:637–643.
10. Deutman A. Benign concentric annular macular dystrophy. *Am J Ophthalmol* 1974;78:384–396.
11. Evans K, Duvall-Young J, Fitzke F, Arden G, Bhattacharya S, Bird A. Chromosome 19q cone-rod retinal dystrophy: Ocular phenotype. *Arch Ophthalmol* 1995;113:195–201.
12. Evans K, Fryer A, Inglehearn C, Duvall-Young J, Whittaker J, Gregory C, et al. Genetic linkage of cone-rod retinal dystrophy to chromosome 19q and evidence for segregation distortion. *Nature Genet* 1994;6:210–213.
13. Falls H, Wolter J, Alpern M. Typical total monochromacy—A histological and psychophysical report. *Arch Ophthalmol* 1965;74: 610–616.
14. Franceschetti A, Francois J, Babel J. *Chorioretinal Heredodegenerations.* Springfield, IL: Charles C. Thomas, 1974.
15. Francois J, De Rouck A, Verriest G, De Laey J, Cambie E. Progressive generalized cone dysfunction. *Ophthalmologica* 1974;169:255–284.
16. Gershoni-Baruch R, Leibo R. Aplasia cutis congenita, high myopia, and cone-rod dysfunction in two sibs: A new autosomal recessive disorder. *Am J Med Genet* 1996;61:42–44.
17. Glickstein M, Heath G. Receptors in the monochromat. *Vision Res* 1975;15:633–636.
18. Gouras P, Eggers H, MacKay C. Cone dystrophy, nyctalopia and supernormal rod responses: A new retinal degeneration. *Arch Ophthalmol* 1983;101:718–724.
19. Harrison R, Hoefnagel D, Hayward J. Congenital total color blindness: A clinicopathological report. *Arch Ophthalmol* 1960;64:685–692.
20. Heckenlively J. RP cone-rod degeneration. *Trans Am Ophthalmol Soc* 1987;85:438–470.
21. Heckenlively J, Martin D, Rosales T. Telangiectasia and optic atrophy in cone-rod degenerations. *Arch Ophthalmol* 1981;99:1983–1991.
22. Heckenlively J, Weleber R. X-linked recessive cone dystrophy with tapetal sheen: A newly recognized entity with Mizuo-Nakamura phenomenon. *Arch Ophthalmol* 1986;104:1322–1328.
23. Heckenlively J, Yoser S, Friedman L, Oversier J. Clinical findings and common symptoms in retinitis pigmentosa. *Am J Ophthalmol* 1988; 105:504–511.
24. Holm E, Lodberg C. Family with total colorblindness. *Acta Ophthalmol (Copenh)* 1940;18: 224–258.
25. Hong HK, Ferrell RE, Gorin MB. Clinical diversity and chromosomal localization of X-linked cone dystrophy (COD1). *Am J Hum Genet* 1994;55(6):1173–1181.
26. Jalili I. Cone-rod congenital amaurosis with congenital hypertrichosis: An autosomal recessive condition. *J Med Genet* 1989;26: 504–510.
27. Jalili I, Smith N. A progressive cone-rod dystrophy and amelogenesis: A new syndrome. *J Med Genet* 1988;25:738–740.

27a. Kelsell RE, Evans K, Gregory CY, et al. Localization of a gene for dominant cone rod dystrophy (CORD6) to chromosome 17p. *Hum Mol Genet* 1997;6:597–600.

28. Keunen J, van Everdignen J, Went L, Oosterhuis J, van Norren D. Color matching and foveal densitometry in patients and carriers of an X-linked progressive cone dystrophy. *Arch Ophthalmol* 1990;108:1713–1719.
29. Klein D, Ammannn F. The syndrome of Laurence-Moon-Bardet-Biedl and allied diseases in Switzerland: Clinical, genetic and epidemiologic studies. *J Neurol Sci* 1969;9:479–513.
30. Knobloch W, Layer I. Retinal detachment and encephalocele. *J Pediatr Ophthalmol* 1971;8: 181–184.
31. Krauss H, Heckenlively J. Visual field changes in cone-rod degenerations. *Arch Ophthalmol* 1982;100:1784–1790.
32. Krill A, Deutman A, Fishman G. The cone degenerations. *Doc Ophthalmol* 1973;35:1–80.
33. Kylstra J, Aylsworth A. Cone-rod retinal dystrophy in a patient with neurofibromatosis type I. *Can J Ophthalmol* 1993;28:79–80.
34. Leung R, Beer W, Mehta H. Aplasia cutis congenita presenting as a familial triad of atrophic alopecia, ocular defects and a peculiar scarring

tendency of the skin. *Br J Dermatol* 1988; 118:715–720.
35. Lewis R. *Juvenile Hereditary Macular Dystrophies.* New York, Raven Press, 1988.
36. Lewis R, Holcomb J, Bromley W, Wilson M, Roderick T, Hejtmancik J. Mapping X-linked ophthalmic diseases. III. Provisional assignment of the locus for blue cone monochromacy to Xq28. *Arch Ophthalmol* 1987;105:1055–1059.
37. Miyake Y, Horiguchi M, Tomita N, Kondo M, Tanikawa A, Takahashi H, et al. Occult macular dystrophy. *Am J Ophthalmol* 1996;122:644–653.
38. Miyake Y, Ichikawa K, Shiose Y, Kawase K. Hereditary macular dystrophy without visible fundus abnormality. *Am J Ophthalmol* 1989; 108:292–299.
39. Moore A. Cone and cone-rod dystrophies. *J Med Genet* 1992;29:289–290.
40. Nathans J, Davenport C, Maumenee I, Lewis R, Hejtmancik J, Litt M, et al. Molecular genetics of human blue cone monochromacy. *Science* 1989;245:831–838.
41. Passos-Bueno M, Marie S, Monteiro M, Neustein I, Whittle M, Vainzof M, et al. Knobloch syndrome in a large Brazilian family: Confirmation of autosomal recessive inheritance. *Am J Med Genet* 1994;52: 170–173.
42. Pentao L, Lewis R, Ledbetter D, Patel P, Lupski J. Maternal uniparental isodisomy of chromosome 14: Association with autosomal recessive rod monochromacy. *Am J Hum Genet* 1992;50:690–699.
43. Pinckers A. X-linked progressive cone dystrophy. *Doc Ophthalmol* 1982;33:399–403.
44. Pinckers A, Groothuizen G, Timmermann G, Deutman A. Sex-difference in progressive cone dystrophy. II. *Ophthalmic Paediatr Genet* 1981;1:25–36.
45. Pinckers A, Timmerman G. Sex-difference in progressive cone dystrophy. I. *Ophthalmic Paediatr Genet* 1981;1:17–23.
46. Seaver L, Leonard J, Spark R, Smith B, Hoyme H. Congenital scalp defects and vitreoretinal degeneration: Redefining the Knobloch syndrome. *Am J Med Genet* 1993;46:203–208.
47. Sertie A, Quimby M, Moreira E, Murray J, Zatz M, Antonarakis S, et al. A gene which causes severe ocular alterations and occipital encephalocele (Knobloch syndrome) is mapped to 21q22.3. *Hum Mol Genet* 1996;5: 843–847.
48. Sloan L, Brown D. Progressive retinal degeneration with selective involvement of the cone mechanism. *Am J Ophthalmol* 1962;54:629–641.
49. Small K, Gehrs K. Clinical study of a large family with autosomal dominant progressive cone degeneration. *Am J Ophthalmol* 1996; 121:1–12.
50. Small K, Syrquin M, Mullen L, Gehrs K. Mapping of autosomal dominant cone degeneration to chromosome 17p. *Am J Ophthalmol* 1996;121:13–18.
51. Szlyk J, Fishman G, Alexander K, Peachy N, Derlacki D. Clinical subtypes of cone-rod dystrophy. *Arch Ophthalmol* 1993;107:781–788.
52. Tranebjaerg L, Sjo O, Warburg M. Retinal cone dysfunction in mental retardation associated with a balanced translocation 1;6 (q44-q27). *Ophthalmic Genet* 1986;7:167–173.
53. van den Biesen P, Deutman A, Pinckers A. Evolution of benign concentric annular macular dystrophy. *Am J Ophthalmol* 1985;100:73.
54. Verriest G. Les deficiences de la vision des couleurs. *Bull Soc Fr Ophtalmol* 1969;69: 901–927.
55. Warburg M, Sjo O, Tranebjaerg L, Fledelius H. Deletion mapping of a retinal cone rod dystrophy, assignment to 18q21.1. *Am J Med Genet* 1991;39:288–293.
56. Went LN, van Schooneveld MJ, Oosterhuis JA. Late onset dominant cone dystrophy with early blue cone involvement. *J Med Genet* 1992;29: 295–298.
57. Yagasaki K, Jacobson SG. Cone-rod dystrophy. Phenotypic diversity by retinal function testing. *Arch Ophthalmol* 1989;107:701–708.
58. Zlotogora J. Hereditary disorders among Iranian Jews. *Am J Med Genet* 1995;58:32–37.

20

North Carolina Macular Dystrophy

KENT W. SMALL

Once considered an extremely obscure disease, North Carolina macular dystrophy turns out to be a much more common condition that had been reported under several aliases. This macular dystrophy was first reported in 1971 by Lefler, Wadsworth, and Sidbury[8] as "dominant macular degeneration and amino aciduria" and became known as the "Lefler-Wadsworth-Sidbury syndrome." The aminoaciduria was subsequently found to be unrelated to the macular degeneration and therefore was of unclear significance.[2] The same family from the mountains of North Carolina was studied further and the condition was published as "dominant progressive foveal dystrophy." A branch of this family had moved to the Midwest and was ascertained by University of Iowa investigators approximately 10 years ago.[5] This branch of the family was published as a distinct clinical entity referred to as "central areolar pigment epithelial dystrophy" (CAPED). The genealogical tie to the original family was unknown to the original authors of this CAPED family.[12] Another group of family members had moved to Chicago and the same disease was published in that branch of the pedigree as a distinct clinical entity called "central pigment epithelial and choroidal degeneration."[9] Again, this branch of the family and the genealogical tie to the North Carolina family were not known at the time of that publication by the original authors. Finally, Gass[3] described this disease in his atlas, dubbing it "North Carolina macular dystrophy" and, in effect, naming it after the state in which it was originally described. More recently, in 1991, the Human Genome Organization (HUGO) assigned it the symbol MCDR1 to the gene causing the clinical diseases (*MC* = macular, *D* = dystrophy, *R* = subtype retina, *1* = first macular dystrophy mapped).[14]

After extensive genealogical work expanding the original pedigree, the family was now found to consist of over 5000 members scattered across the United States. There is a founder effect according to the family history of "three Irish brothers" moving into the mountains of North Carolina in the early 1800s. Closer examination of genealogical records indicates that this family has lived in the Carolinas since 1715. In the family, 285 members, of whom 193 are affected, have been examined to date.

CLINICAL FINDINGS

North Carolina macular dystrophy (NCMD) is a congenital autosomal dominant trait.[1–3,5–12] All evidence suggests that it is completely penetrant. The condition is presumed to be present at birth since a 3-month-old has been observed with the most severe manifestation of the disease. NCMD is generally considered to be

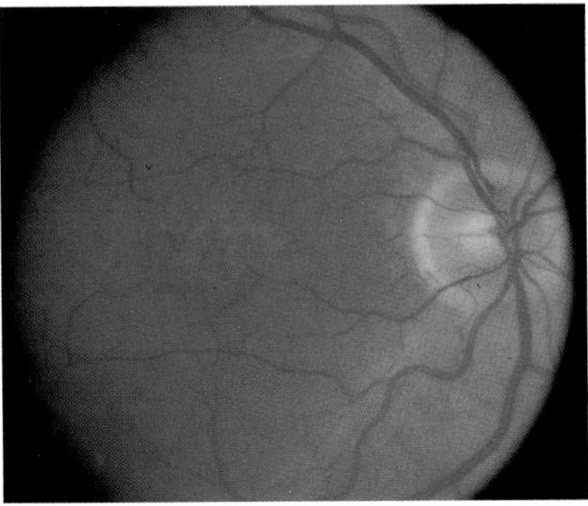

Figure 20.1. Right fundus of a 50-year-old man with grade I macular dystrophy. There is a small amount of subretinal blood from presumed choroidal neovascularization.

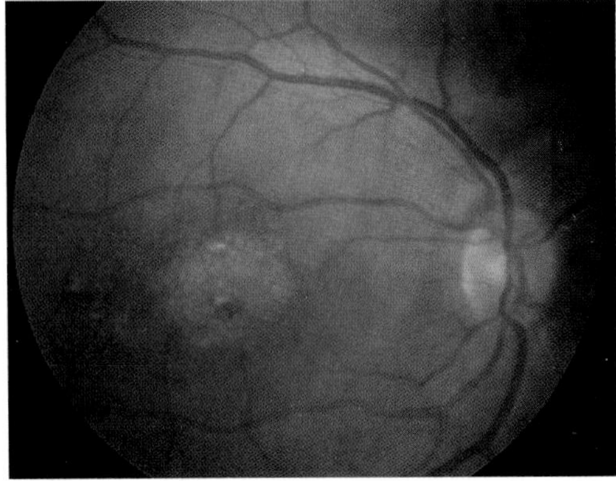

Figure 20.3. Right fundus of a 29-year-old man with grade II macular dystrophy, 20/20 acuity, and confluent drusen.

nonprogressive except for the development of choroidal neovascular membranes in some patients. Visual acuity ranges from 20/20 to 20/400 with a median of 20/60.

The ophthalmoscopic findings are also highly variable and are always much more dramatic than one would predict from the relatively good visual acuity level. Patients may have only a few drusen in the central macular region (grade I; Figs. 20.1, 20.2), confluent drusen confined to the central macular region (grade II; Figs. 20.3–20.6), or a severe macular coloboma/staphyloma (grade III; Figs. 20.7–20.10) involving three to four disc areas of the central macular region. These macular lesions have sharp, well-delineated subretinal scar tissue, which is presumably due to recurrent remissions and relapses of asymptomatic choroidal neovascular membranes. Patients with these macular lesions use the nasal edge of the lesion for fixation. This results in a positive angle kappa. Grade II lesions seem to be the most likely to develop choroidal neovascular mem-

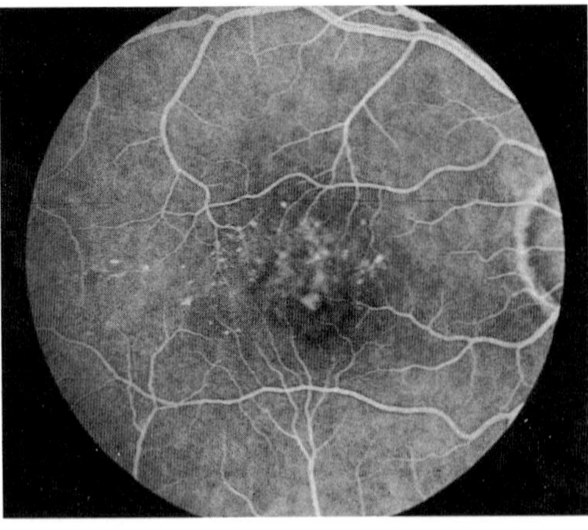

Figure 20.2. Fluorescein angiogram corresponding to Figure 20.1. There is fluorescein leakage near subretinal blood and window defects corresponding to drusen.

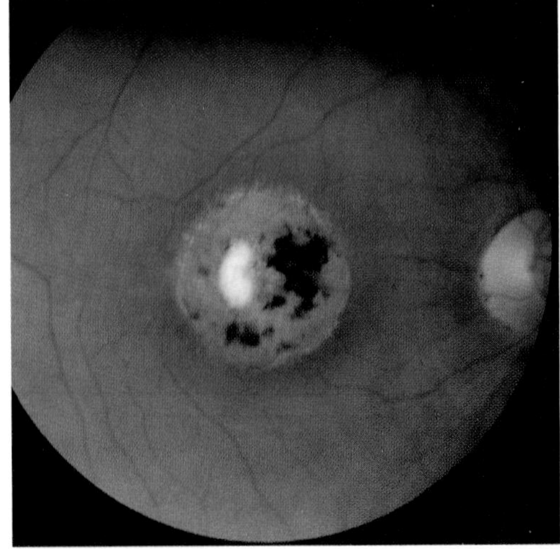

Figure 20.4. Right fundus of a 36-year-old woman with 20/60 vision.

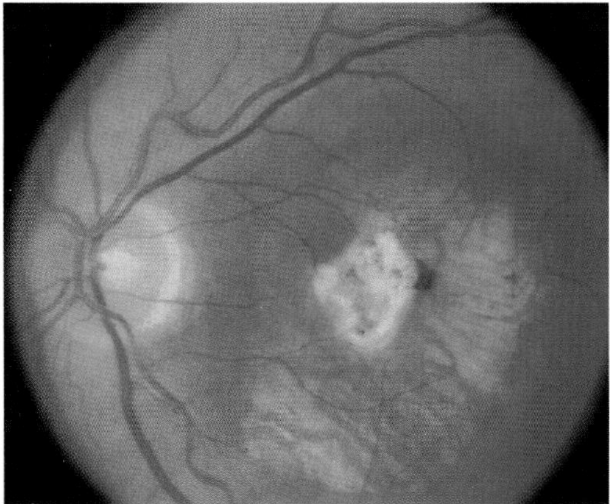

Figure 20.5. Left fundus of a patient whose right fundus is shown in Figures 20.1 and 20.2. Vision is 20/400. There are grade II dystrophic lesions and subretinal neovascularization.

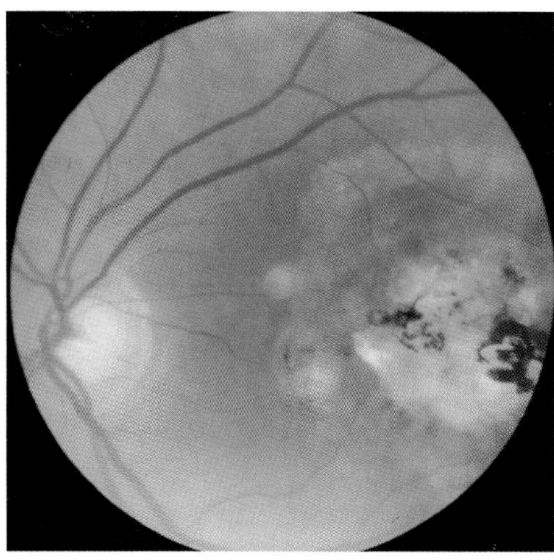

Figure 20.7. Right fundus of a 64-year-old woman with 20/40 vision and grade III dystrophic lesions.

branes, and patients with grade II lesions are at greatest risk for severe visual loss. Fortunately, choroidal neovascularization usually occurs in only one eye of any individual patient. Otherwise, as with most macular dystrophies, the ophthalmoscopic findings are fairly symmetric. Electrophysiologic studies were performed on some of these patients 20 years ago by Frank et al.[2] and by Lefler et al.[8] and were normal. Color vision is also normal.

There are many clinical similarities between age-related macular degeneration and NCMD. Drusen, choroidal neovascular membranes, and peripheral retinal drusen are striking features of both. The normal electrophysiologic test results, as well as normal color vision, also help distinguish (age-related macular degeneration) (ARMD) and NCMD from other maculopathies. One of the major differences between NCMD phenotype and ARMD is the age of onset of the disease.

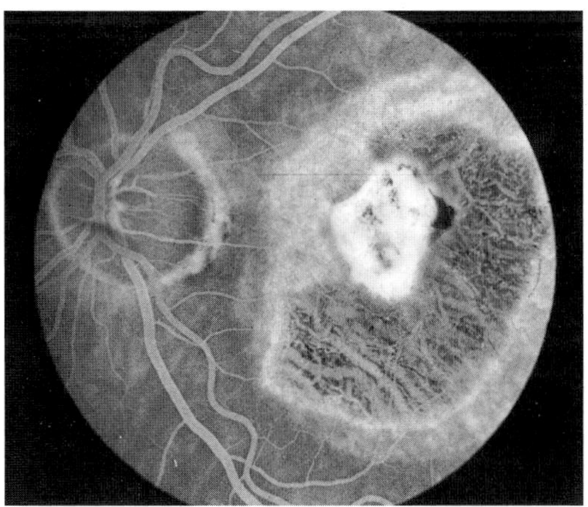

Figure 20.6. Fluorescein angiogram of eye depicted in Figure 20.5. There is a subretinal disciform scar with surrounding loss of choriocapillaris.

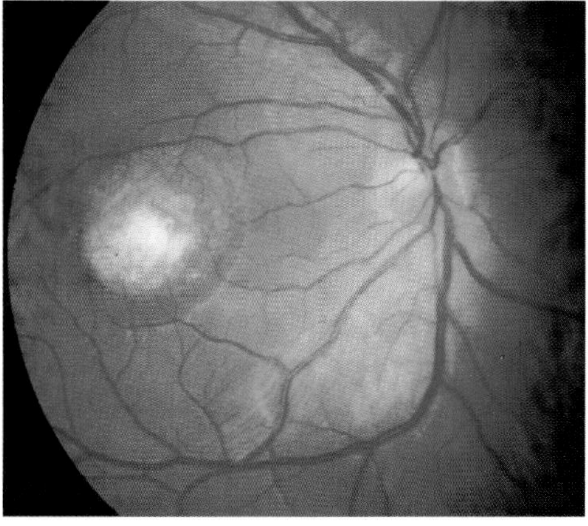

Figure 20.8. Right fundus of a 21-year-old man with grade III coloboma and 20/40 vision.

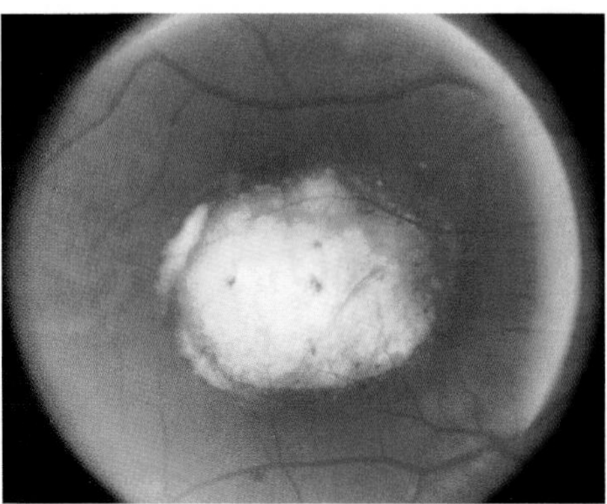

Figure 20.9. Right fundus of 29-year-old woman with 20/40 vision and grade III dystrophic lesion.

GENETICS

The original goal for studying this family was to map the gene responsible and by so doing, hopefully gain some insight into macular function and dysfunction as well as possible relationships with ARMD.[4,7,16] The initial studies were conducted using restriction fragment length polymorphism (RFLP) markers until microsatellite markers were developed by Weber and May,[16] making the screening of the human genome much more efficient.[13] Shortly thereafter, NCMD became the first ophthalmic disease to be mapped using the microsatellite class of markers.[14] Initially, the linked markers were crudely localized with somatic cell hybrid panels to chromosome 6q16-6q21.[14] Subsequently, as more markers have become available through the Cooperative Human Linkage Center (CHLC), Genome DataBase (GDB), and Centre d'Etude du Polymorphisme Humain (CEPH), tight flanking markers have been defined down to approximately 1 cM genetic distance.

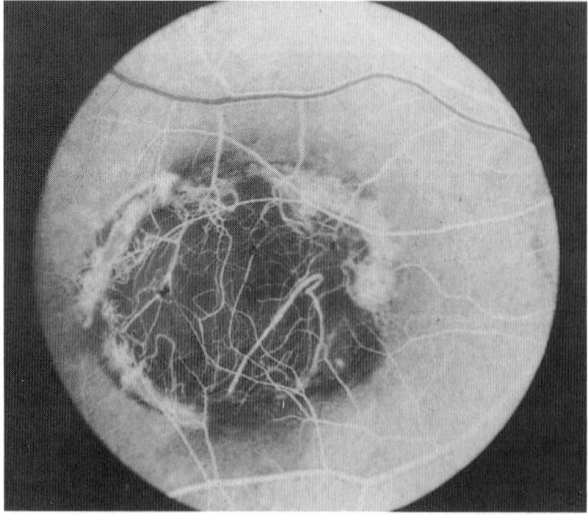

Figure 20.10. Fluorescein angiogram of the retina shown in Figure 20.9.

Because of its large size, the North American family offered an unusual opportunity to study non-Mendelian influences on the ocular phenotype. A curious "parent of origin effect" was found. An affected female was found to transmit the disease twice as often to her offspring as an affected male. Affected men and women had equal numbers of offspring. These findings suggest that an egg carrying the affected allele was somehow more likely to be fertilized than an egg carrying the unaffected allele or, conversely, that an affected sperm was less likely to fertilize an egg than a sperm with an unaffected allele. The exact molecular mechanism for this parental effect remains to be defined.

FAMILIES WITH THE NORTH CAROLINA MACULAR DYSTROPHY PHENOTYPE

There are eight genealogically distinct families with the NCMD phenotype. A moderate-sized Caucasian family from rural Texas was recently ascertained with the same phenotype and tight linkage to the MCDR1 region on chromosome 6. Haplotype analysis shows the same alleles as those in the original NCMD family. This suggests that the Texas family probably descends from a common founder of the North Carolina family. Because the alleles are shared for markers that are several centimorgans away, this would even suggest that the common founder of NCMD and this Texas family are relatively few generations apart.

A Mayan Indian family from Belize, Central America, was recently ascertained with the NCMD phenotype. This family was of sufficient size to perform linkage analysis and indeed showed tight linkage to the MCDR1 locus. The affected haplotype associated in this family, however, is distinct from that of the North Carolina and Texas families. This suggests that this family either represents a new spontaneous mutation in MCDR1, or that there was a common founder to both branches, several generations ago, such that crossovers have occurred.

A small Caucasian family with NCMD from Washington, D.C., was not large enough to permit linkage analysis to chromosome 6q markers. Patients from that family did, however, have the same affected haplotype as that of the NCMD family. After a more detailed genealogical search, it became evident that they were descendants from the original NCMD family.

Leveille and co-workers[9] reported a black family from Chicago with the NCMD phenotype. Linkage analysis was not possible because of the small family size. Patients, however, also have the exact same affected haplotype as that of the North Carolina family. Careful genealogical search in the family going back eight generations did not show such an overlap with the North Carolina family. The investigation of a Wisconsin family that was ascertained by Dr. Klein (University of Wisconsin, Madison) and of a West Virginia family by Dr. Flaxel (University of West Virginia, Morgantown) (personal communications) yielded similar results. There is another family with NCMD in France that maps to the MCDR1 locus.[15a]

To date, there is no clear evidence of genetic heterogeneity in NCMD. The Mayan Indian family in Belize and the French family seem to represent either new spontaneous mutations in MCDR1 or may have a common founder with the American families, but they are separated by enough generations such that ancestral crossovers occurred.

REFERENCES

1. Fetkenhour CL, Gurney N, Dobbie GJ, Choromokos E. Central areolar pigment epithelial dystrophy. *Am J Ophthalmol* 1976;8:745–753.
2. Frank HR, Landers MB III, Williams RJ, Sidbury JB. A new dominant progressive foveal dystrophy. *Am J Ophthalmol* 1974;78:903–916.
3. Gass JDM. *Stereoscopic Atlas of Macular Diseases*, 3rd ed. St. Louis: C. V. Mosby, 1987: 98–99.
4. Haynes CS, Pericak-Vance MA, Hung W-Y, Deutsch DB, Roses AR. PEDIGENE—A computerized data collection and analysis system for genetic laboratories. *Am J Hum Genet* 1988;43:A146.
5. Hermsen VM, Judisch GF. Central areolar pigment epithelial dystrophy. *Ophthalmologica* 1984;189:69–72.
6. Klein R, Bresnick G. An inherited central retinal pigment epithelial dystophy. *Birth Defects Orig Art Ser* 1982;19:281–296.
7. Lathrop GM, Lalouel JM, Julier C, Ott J. Strategies for multilocus linkage analysis in humans. *Proc Natl Acad Sci USA* 1984;81:3443–3446.
8. Lefler WH, Wadsworth JAC, Sidbury JB. Hereditary macular degeneration and aminoaciduria. *Am J Ophthalmol* 1971;71:224–230.
9. Leveille AS, Morse PH, Kiernan JP. Autosomal dominant central pigment epithelial and choroidal degeneration. *Ophthalmology* 1982;89: 1407–1413.
10. Small KW. North Carolina macular dystrophy, revisited. *Ophthalmology* 1989;96:1747–1754.
11. Small KW, Killian J, McLean WL. North Carolina dominant progressive foveal dystrophy, how progressive is it? *Br J Ophthalmol* 1991;75: 401–406.
12. Small KW, Hermsen V, Gurney N, Fetkenhou C, Folk J. North Carolina macular dystrophy (NCMD) and central areolar pigment epithelial dystrophy (CAPED), one family, one disease. *Arch Ophthamol* (in press).
13. Small KW, Weber JL, Pericak-Vance MA, Vance J, Hung W-Y, Roses AD. Exclusion map of North Carolina macular dystrophy using RFLPs and microsatellites. *Genomics* 1991;11: 763–766.
14. Small KW, Weber JL, Lennon F, Vance J, Roses AD, Pericak-Vance MA. North Carolina macular dystrophy maps to chromosome 6. *Genomics* 1992;13:681–685.
15. Small KW, Weber J, Roses AD, Pericak-Vance P. North Carolina macular dystrophy (MCDR1). A review and refined mapping to 6q14-q16.2. *Ophthalmic Paediatr Genet* 1993; 14:143–150.

15a. Small KW, Puech B, Mullen L, Yelchits S. North Carolina Macular Dystrophy phenotype in France maps to the MCDR1 locus. *Mol Vis* 1997;3:1–6.

16. Weber JL, May PE. Abundant class of human polymorphisms which can be typed using the polymerase chain reaction. *Am J Hum Genet* 1989;44:388–396.

21

Leber's Congenital Amaurosis, Stargardt Disease, and Pattern Dystrophies

ROBERT K. KOENEKOOP
ELIAS I. TRABOULSI

Leber's congenital amaurosis (LCA) was first described by Theodor Leber in 1869 as a form of congenital blindness with severely reduced vision before the age of 1 year, nystagmus, poor pupillary reaction, tapetoretinal degeneration, and an autosomal recessive inheritance pattern.[45] In 1954, Franceshetti[19] added a severely attenuated or abolished electroretinogram (ERG) to this constellation of clinical findings. LCA accounts for almost 20% of blind children in The Netherlands.[72] It is thought to be a common cause of blindness in children around the world with an estimated prevalence of 3 cases for every 100,000 normally sighted children.[47]

CLINICAL FEATURES AND EVOLUTION

The appearance of the retina is highly variable, ranging from normal to a retinitis pigmentosa-like (RP) picture with intraretinal bone spicules, vascular attenuation, and optic disc pallor.[23] Other reported ophthalmoscopic findings include salt-and-pepper changes,[72] chorioretinal atrophy,[72] macular colobomas,[46,51] a retinitis punctata albescens-like appearance (Fig. 21.1),[14] disc edema,[18] and a nummular pigmentary pattern (Fig. 21.2).[73] Thus the diagnosis of LCA cannot be based on ophthalmoscopic appearance alone. Some children with LCA perform the oculodigital maneuver[35]: by pressing on their eyes, these blind children presumably induce phosphenes or patterns of light (Fig. 21.3). Some patients with LCA are very light sensitive.[45] This photoaversion may be so prominent that initial diagnostic considerations may include achromatopsia; an ERG that shows markedly reduced or nonrecordable photopic and scotopic responses clinches the diagnosis of LCA.[82] Other ocular abnormalities include high hyperopia, high myopia, cataracts, keratoglobus, and keratoconus.

Some systemic and neurologic diseases may lead to ocular phenotypes identical to LCA. Some patients have polycystic kidney disease,[6] renal aplasia,[74] or osteopetrosis.[38] Rarely do patients have central nervous system abnormalities such as mental retardation, seizures, or hydrocephalus.[35]

In a retrospective study of 43 patients with LCA, Schroeder and co-workers[73] found a visual acuity range of 20/200 to light perception, with a majority of patients having an acuity less than 20/400. Refractive errors ranged from −5.50 to +15.00, with 75% of patients being

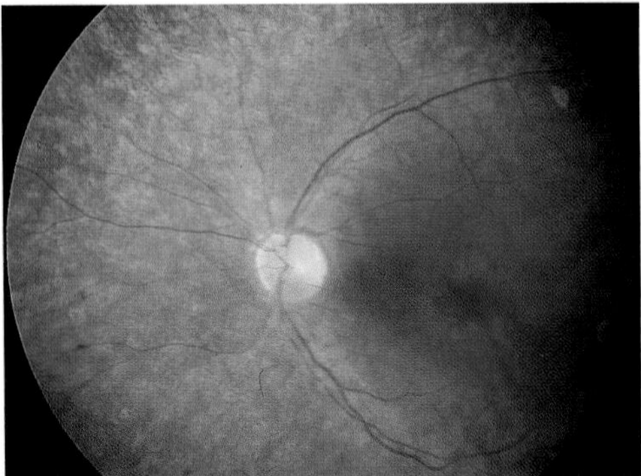

Figure 21.1. A 20-year-old woman with Leber's congenital amaurosis. The macula and fundus periphery have a mottled appearance; the retinal vessels are attenuated.

hyperopic. These authors noted that the most common retinal appearance was that of a RP picture in 20 patients; they found a normal-appearing retina in 5 cases, salt-and-pepper changes in 3, chorioretinal atrophy in 6, macular colobomas in 2, a "retinitis punctata albescenslike picture" in 2, a "marbleized fundus" in 1, and a nummular pigmentary pattern in 2 cases. They also found systemic abnormalities in about 25% of their patients, the most common being mental retardation in 10, followed by cystic renal disease in 3, skeletal problems in 3, hydrocephalus in 2, seizures in 1, decreased hearing in 1, and cleft palate in 1 patient.

There is marked phenotypic and probable genetic heterogeneity in patients with LCA. In an effort to provide some order in this hetero-

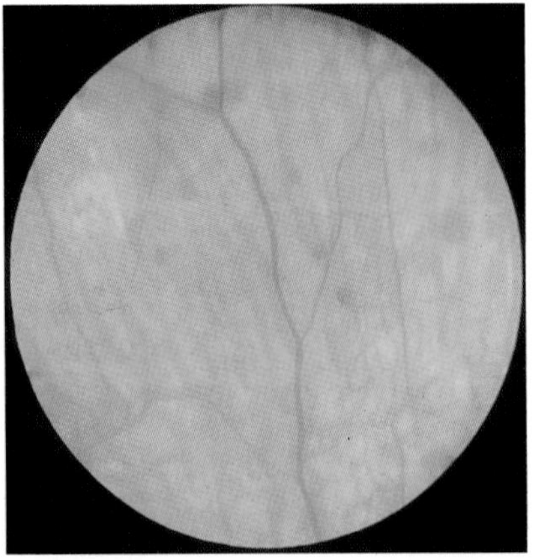

Figure 21.2. Peripheral nummular pattern of pigmentation in a patient with Leber's congenital amaurosis. (Courtesy of Dr. Irene H. Maumenee.)

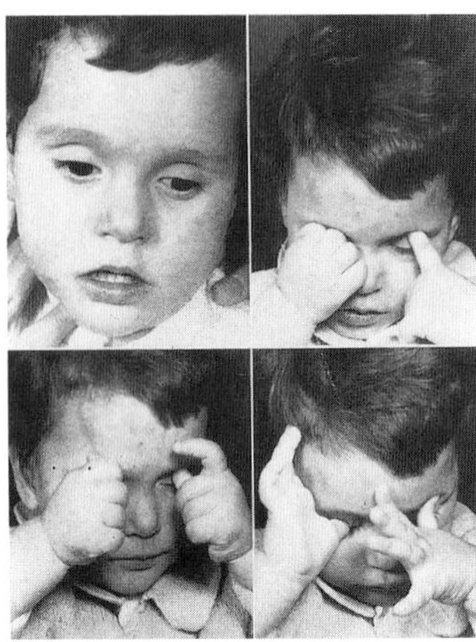

Figure 21.3. Oculodigital sign in a patient with Leber's congenital amaurosis.

geneous group of diseases, Heckenlively[30] proposed a classification scheme that is based on the age of visual loss, the severity of visual loss, and the presence or absence of systemic abnormalities. He proposed four groups. Group 1 includes patients with "uncomplicated LCA"; these patients have congenital blindness, an extinguished ERG, sluggish pupillary responses to light, searching nystagmus, and a hyperopia greater than 5 diopters (D). Group 2 includes patients with "complicated LCA"; these patients have the same clinical features as group 1 except high hyperopia. In addition, they have associated neurological or systemic abnormalities. Syndromes that meet the criteria for group 2 include the cerebrohepatorenal syndrome of Zellweger, the Senior-Loken syndrome of renal and retinal aplasia, and the Saldino-Mainzer syndrome with renal and retinal abnormalities and cone-shaped epiphyses of the hands. Group 3, also called "juvenile RP," includes children who demonstrate signs of visual impairment within the first several years of life and who develop severe visual loss and retinal degeneration by age 6 years. Initial visual acuity is often around 20/100 and progressively deteriorates, leading to blindness by the third decade. Group 4, or "early-onset RP," is similar to the classical adult-onset RP, but the disease starts at a much younger age. Visual difficulties commence with impaired dark adaptation, night blindness, and midperipheral visual field loss. As the disease progresses, patients lose far-peripheral field and eventually central vision as well.

Although LCA has been equated with congenital RP[45] and subclassified under the large RP family of diseases, the clinical course of its classical uncomplicated form appears to be completely different from other forms of RP. Heher and co-workers[31] studied the natural history of 22 patients with uncomplicated LCA. They found that visual acuity ranged from 20/100 to no light perception at the initial visit. These authors also found that 6 very young patients had normal retinal examinations. After the age of 3 years, all patients had a variety of abnormal ophthalmoscopic findings. Eighteen patients developed progressive retinal and/or retinal pigment epithelial degeneration, but visual acuity remained stable throughout the study period. Three patients with macular colobomata and one with keratoconus developed progressive loss of vision. The findings of Heher and co-workers[31] suggest that uncomplicated LCA may be a developmental retinal dystrophy that commences in utero and becomes apparent immediately at birth. Different levels of visual function may be attained, depending on the degree of retinal development. These levels appear to be maintained throughout life unless macular colobomas or keratoconus develop. Patients with the latter abnormalities may have different genetic forms of LCA.

LCA can be a difficult diagnosis to make. Because of the variability in fundus appearance, visual acuity, and associated systemic abnormalities. The ERG is pivotal in establishing the diagnosis. The differential diagnosis of congenital blindness of retinal origin includes LCA, achromatopsia, albinism, aniridia, congenital stationary night blindness, macular coloboma, infectious chorioretinitis, and Bardet-Biedl syndrome.

Three systemic diseases with early onset blindness and a potentially extinguished ERG are abetalipoproteinemia, infantile phytanic acid storage disease (Refsum disease), and neuronal ceroid lipofuscinosis. Some of these are potentially treatable metabolic diseases that should be ruled out by serum assays or by conjunctival biopsy.

HISTOPATHOLOGICAL STUDIES

There are six pathological reports of enucleated eyes with LCA. Sorsby and Williams[77] reported a case where the entire retina was diffusely atrophied and disorganized at all levels, making it impossible to hypothesize about the original insult.

Kroll and Kuwabara[42] described a 35-year-old with LCA whose retina was entirely devoid of rods. Cone remnants were present but lacked an outer segment and had short inner segments with small, poorly oriented mitochondria. The retinal pigment epithelium was reduced in height and was full of abnormal, large, round inclusion bodies.

Gillespie[28] described the histopathologic findings of the eye of a 40-year-old with LCA. He found an intact retinal pigment epithelium, but the retina was completely devoid of rods and cones that were replaced by a layer of cuboidal-shaped cells. These cells may represent primitive undifferentiated photoreceptor cells.

Mizuno et al.[56] reported the pathology of an enucleated eye of a blind baby with an extinguished ERG. They found immature and undifferentiated photoreceptor and retinal pigment epithelial layers.[56] Photoreceptor cell bodies were larger and more oval than usual and their nuclei resembled those of the neuroblastic layer of the human embryo. The pigment epithelium was intact and regular, but its poor differentiation was evident.

Noble and Carr[62] reported an 8-month-old child with psychomotor retardation, blindness, an extinguished ERG, optic atrophy, and a normal-appearing retina. At autopsy, the brain had multiple defects, and the eye showed a decrease in the number of ganglion cells, with degeneration and vacuolization of the remaining cells. The inner segments of the rods and cones were normal, and the outer segments were shortened.

Finally, Horsten[34] reported a 20-year-old patient with congenital blindness and an extinguished ERG who had an entirely normal layer of rods and cones. The ganglion cells were slightly abnormal.

Again, pathological reports illustrate the variability of LCA, suggesting the original insult of disease to be in photoreceptors in some cases and in the retinal pigment epithelium in others.

GENETICS

Autosomal recessive inheritance is by far the most common pattern in LCA. Leber[45] noted consanguinity in 25% of cases. The parents had normal eye examinations. About 20% of Leber's affected subjects had blind siblings with an identical disease. There is evidence of genetic heterogeneity, however, with one report of parents with LCA who married and produced normal-seeing children who are presumably double heterozygotes.[77] A rare form of autosomal dominant LCA has been described,[77] and confirmed by Reiss et al.[67]

MOLECULAR GENETIC STUDIES

The molecules of the rod and cone phototransduction cascade and the genes encoding these molecules are important candidate genes for LCA because of its clinical similarity to RP. Five rod phototransduction or related molecules and their genes have been implicated in the pathogenesis of RP: rhodopsin,[12] peripherin/retinal degeneration slow (RDS),[15] β-cyclic guanosine monophosphate (GMP) phosphodiesterase,[54] rod cyclic GMP-gated channel protein,[53] and rod outer membrane protein-1 (ROM-1).[71]

Patients with LCA have been screened for causative mutations in the genes encoding rhodopsin,[49] the rhodopsin promoter region,[49] the β-subunit of cyclic GMP phosphodiesterase (PDE),[67] the γ-subunit of rod cyclic PDE,[29] the cyclic GMP-gated channel protein,[53] recoverin,[11] and peripherin/RDS.[15] No disease-causing pathological mutations were found in any of these studies.

In addition to mutation analysis, linkage analysis has been done on the PDE-β subunit (PDEB) gene and the recoverin gene in families with LCA. Two intragenic dinucleotide repeat polymorphisms (CA repeats) were found in the PDEB gene and linkage was excluded in 13 LCA families.[67] Another intragenic dinucleotide repeat polymorphism in the recoverin gene allowed the exclusion of linkage between recoverin and the LCA phenotype in 10 of 20 affected families that showed significant linkage to chromosome 17, the location of the recoverin locus.[5] In another study utilizing microsatelite markers, Camuzat et al.[5] established significant linkage of LCA to 17p13.1. Furthermore, these authors showed that LCA families with a North African Maghrebian origin linked to this locus, whereas families from the European mainland did not, illustrating genetic heterogeneity. Robitaille et al.[69] excluded the 17p13 locus in a large family with LCA belonging to the order of River Brethren, also originating from the mainland of Europe.[69] Koenekoop et al.[40] excluded the candidate gene pigment epithelium derived factor (PEDF), a new pigment epithelial gene also located at position 17p13.1. Exclusion was based on a combination of mutation analysis and intragenic restriction fragment length polymorphism (RFLP) linkage analysis in 15 families with LCA from around the world, including the Mediterranean basin.

Recently, Perrault et al.[65a] reported pathological mutations in the retinal-specific guanylate cyclase gene (RETGC, or GDB symbol GUC2D) in North African patients with LCA. Homozygous missense and frameshift mutations were found which presumably led to an impaired production of cGMP in the phototransduction cascade and permanent closure of the photoreceptor cation channels. In another study, Loyer et al.[48a] found several compound heterozygous missense mutations in LCA patients from Greece and North America, in addition to a homozygous deletion-insertion mutation from North Africa.

A second gene for LCA has also been reported. Interestingly, this is the first gene for a human retinal dystrophy which is specific for the retinal pigment epithelium (RPE). A frameshift and a nonsense mutation were found in the gene RPE65 in a sib-pair with LCA by Marlhens et al.[51a] A number of other mutations were reported by Gu et al.[28a] The gene is located on chromosome 1p31 and the protein product of RPE65 is almost certainly involved in retinoid metabolism.

STARGARDT DISEASE AND FUNDUS FLAVIMACULATUS

Introduction and History

Stargardt disease and fundus flavimaculatus are names given to one nosologic entity that is a hereditary retinal pigment epithelial storage disease characterized by bilateral progressive loss of central visual acuity. The onset of the disease is variable, but symptoms usually become apparent in the first two decades. Fundus appearance is heterogeneous as well, ranging from subtle signs of maculopathy in most patients, to choroidal atrophy in some, with or without macular or extramacular yellow subretinal flecks.

In 1909, the German ophthalmologist Karl Stargardt[78] described a juvenile macular dystrophy in seven patients from two separate families. The patients presented in the first or second decade of life with a reduction in central visual acuity and often normal-appearing maculae. Eventually, progressive atrophic macular lesions developed, with further loss of central vision. In 1963, Franceschetti[20] proposed the name "fundus flavimaculatus" for "that peculiar affection not unlike the white dots of retinitis punctata albescens, which is characterized by somewhat larger white spots of round or irregular form" (Fig. 21.4). In the same year, he recognized that patients with fundus flavimaculatus develop macular lesions similar to those of Stargardt disease.[21,22] Forty-five years after the original description, Rosehr[70] reexamined the family originally described by Stargardt and discovered further deterioration of vision and the development of yellow subretinal flecks in the macula, beyond the arcades, and nasal to the optic disc.

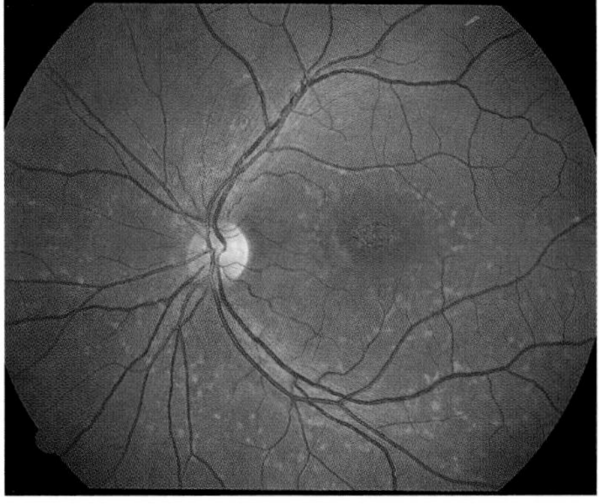

Figure 21.4. Fish-tail flecks in a patient with Stargardt disease/fundus flavimaculatus.

Most investigators[4,7,41,63,87] agree with Franceschetti[20–22] that based on clinical, electrophysiological, and psychophysical findings, Stargardt macular dystrophy and fundus flavimaculatus are different clinical manifestations of the same disease that we will refer to as Stargardt disease in this chapter.

Clinical Features and Evolution

Stargardt disease is a bilateral and progressive macular dystrophy with blurring of central vision as the common presenting complaint. Some asymptomatic patients are discovered on routine examination. In Stargardt's[78] original report, patients became symptomatic between ages 8 and 16 years, but many subsequent studies have shown the age of onset to be more variable. For Blacharski's[4] 41 patients the age of onset ranged from age 5 to 64 years, and for Noble and Carr's[63] 67 patients this range was from the first to the fifth decades. Of 55 patients who were symptomatic in the latter study, 18 patients presented in the first decade, 17 in the second decade, 11 in the third decade, 6 in the fourth decade, and 3 in the fifth decade. This implies that 60% of patients have the onset of disease in their first two decades, and 20% do not experience decreased vision until the fifth decade.

All races can be afflicted by this disease and both sexes are equally affected.[4,7,22,41,63] The prevalence of Stargardt disease is estimated to be between 1 in 8,000–10,000.[4]

Even patients with 20/20 vision complain of a change in quality of central vision. Night blindness is a rare complaint,[22] as is photophobia.[4] When specifically asked, patients admit they prefer more subdued lighting.[4]

All patients who present with visual complaints have evidence of macular disease, although the retinal findings can be extremely subtle. The macular changes are variable and progressive, and range from a "broadening of the foveal reflex," fine granularity of the central pigment epithelium, a bull's-eye maculopathy, focal or multifocal pigment epithelial and/or choroidal atrophy, to a "beaten metal or bronze" appearance of the central macula. With disease progression, the atrophic changes in the macula increase and may become so extensive and well demarcated that the disease resembles central areolar choroidal atrophy (Fig. 21.5). Although central visual loss is progressive, and at times rapid, it does not correlate with the changing macular appearance. Peripheral vision is preserved in most patients.

The most characteristic retinal findings are the soft yellow–white subretinal flecks. They may surround the fovea like a crown (Fig. 21.6), or appear more widespread within the macula or outside the arcades and nasal to the disc. The flecks vary in color from white to yellowish-white to deep yellow, and are only rarely seen with hyperpigmented borders. The shape of the flecks is variable as well, from small and round to irregular, or linear, fishtaillike, angular, or even stellate. In the periphery the flecks become more confluent and assume a reticular pattern. The number of flecks is not stable, and they can be evanescent, appearing or disappearing.

Peripheral retinal findings include pigment patches or frank bone spicules resembling retinitis pigmentosa. Local areas of atrophy can be seen, similar to the punched-out lesions in

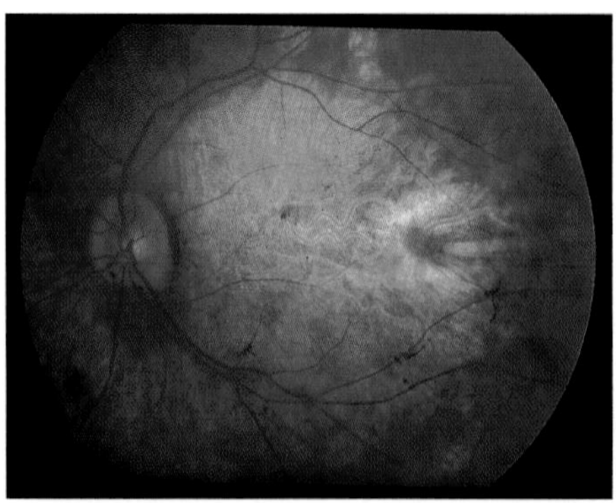

Figure 21.5. Extensive macular and posterior pole lesions in a 50-year-old man with Stargardt disease.

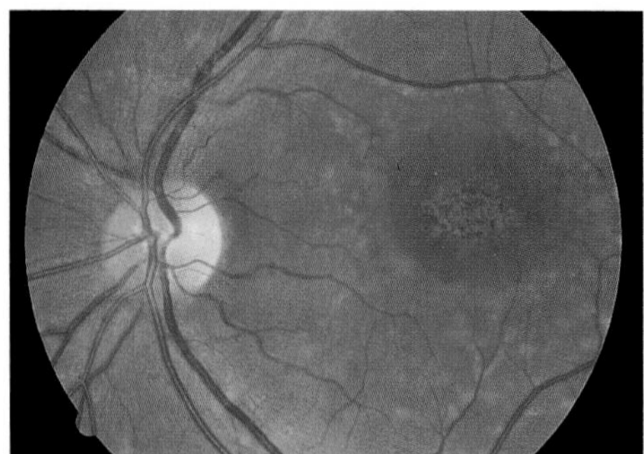

Figure 21.6. Crownlike pattern of flecks in a patient with fundus flavimaculatus/Stargardt disease.

presumed ocular histoplasmosis syndrome. The retinal vessels are of normal caliber throughout the disease process, and this represents an important distinguishing feature from cone degenerations. The optic nerve head can develop temporal pallor that corresponds to the macular atrophy.

Visual Testing and Diagnostic Procedures

The majority of patients have vision between 20/40 and 20/400. Of the 67 patients in the series published by Noble and Carr,[63] 21 had 20/40 or better vision, 11 between 20/50 and 20/80, 32 between 20/100 and 20/400, and 3 less than 20/400. Although there are no characteristic color defects in Stargardt disease, mild red–green axes of confusion can be detected on Farnsworth 100-hue color vision testing. In the Noble and Carr series,[63] 17 of 40 patients had mild red–green defects on American Optical Hardy-Rand-Rittler plates.

The most common abnormality noted by Goldmann perimetry is a central scotoma that is present in most patients with a visual acuity below 20/40.[4] Paracentral scotomas are common as well,[4] but ring scotomas are very rare,[65] and so is peripheral field constriction.[4]

Electroretinographic findings in Stargardt disease are not diagnostic and cannot separate Stargardt disease from fundus flavimaculatus as previously suggested,[43] nor can they facilitate staging of disease.[17] Numerous studies have shown that the ERG is often abnormal in patients with Stargardt disease, especially the photopic portion.[4,17,39,43,63] The majority of patients have a moderately reduced photopic ERG and a nearly normal scotopic tracing. The electrooculogram (EOG) is reported to be abnormal in 75%–80% of cases.[7] Dark adaptation final thresholds are generally normal or slightly elevated, but there may be substantial delay in reaching them.[7,41]

Fluorescein angiography plays an important role in establishing the diagnosis of Stargardt disease and in excluding differential diagnostic possibilities. The perifoveal window defects that correspond to dropped out retinal pigment epithelial cells, and the "silent" choroid sign (Fig. 21.7) are classical features of this disease. The characteristic flecks represent enlarged pigment epithelial cells packed with a lipofuscinlike material,[13] and they may hypo- or hyperfluoresce and have an irregular patchy pattern on fluorescein angiography. More flecks are apparent on angiography than on clinical examination. It is believed that the silent choroid is the result of diffuse storage or deposition of material at the level of the retinal pigment epithelium.[13,39] An angiographically dark choroid is a unique feature of Stargardt disease and is present in 50%–88% of patients.[24] Early in the disease process, a ring of patchy transmission defects is often evident around the fovea resulting in a bull's-eye lesion. In later stages, with centrifugal spread of disease and atrophy, the area of hyperfluorescence is evident with easier visualization of the large choroidal vessels.

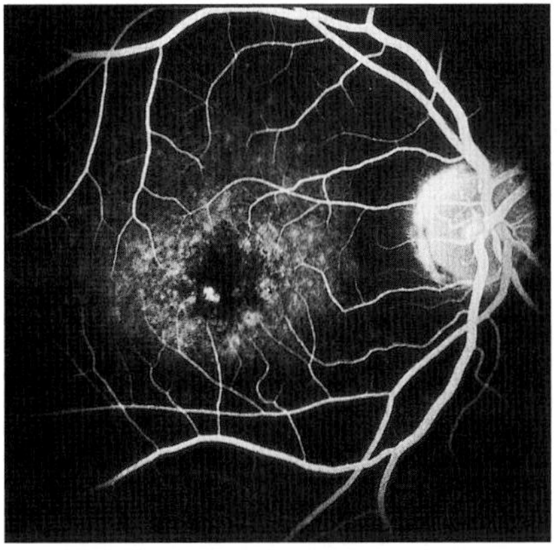

Figure 21.7. Fluorescein angiogram showing characteristic silent choroid sign in a patient with Stargardt disease.

Histopathology

Stargardt disease appears to be a retinal pigment epithelial storage disease, with the intraepithelial accumulation of a lipofuscinlike substance representing the characteristic retinal flecks. This accumulation leads to pigment epithelial cell destruction and dropout, with subsequent death of the overlying photoreceptors, giving rise to transmission defects on angiography and macular atrophy.

The first clinicopathological correlation of Stargardt disease was by Klein and Krill.[39] They showed distended pigment epithelial cells packed with periodic acid–Schiff (PAS)-positive granules, displacement of the nuclei from the base to the center of the cell, a condensation of pigment in a linear fashion on the apical surface of the cell, and marked variation in cell size. Eagle et al.[13] reported that there was massive intracellular accumulation of a lipofuscinlike substance in retinal pigment epithelial cells, some of which were 10 times larger than surrounding cells.

Birnbach and co-workers[3] confirmed the accumulation of lipofuscin in RPE cells, and noted in their pathological study a striking centripetal gradient of increased swelling and accumulation of storage material in the RPE cells from the periphery to the center of the fovea. The RPE in the far periphery was nearly normal, whereas RPE cells in the equatorial region were engorged with pigment and had lost their cohesiveness with neighboring cells and the underlying Bruch's membrane. Their surface membranes were extremely fragile, and some cells had lysed. The photoreceptors were also progressively more severely affected from the periphery to the macula and often contained lipofuscin granules as well.

Lopez and co-workers[48] reported the ocular histopathological findings in a patient with dominant, late-onset Stargardt disease with similar findings, including the centrifugal decrease in severity of disease.

Genetics

The Stargardt phenotype is genetically heterogeneous. At least five genes are implicated in the pathophysiology of this disease by linkage and candidate gene analyses. Three genes that may cause Stargardt disease are now known, the remaining three are implicated through linkage studies. Weleber and co-workers[86] identified a three base pair deletion in the peripherin/RDS gene in some patients with a Stargardt-like phenotype. Heher and Johns[32] described a family with a mitochondrial DNA mutation at position 15,257 and retinal flecks similar to those of Stargardt disease; other members of the same family had Leber's hereditary optic neuropathy.

Stone and co-workers[81] reported linkage of a dominant Stargardt phenotype to markers on the proximal long arm of chromosome 6. The disease-causing gene is not yet known but lies in a 18 cM interval between markers D6S313 and D6S252. The peak lod score of 6.2 centered on marker D6S280. Affected family members noted onset of central visual loss between 5 and 23 years of age; visual acuity decreased to 20/200 or worse by age 30 years. Retinal flecks and central atrophy of the macula were evident, but there was no silent choroid on fluorescein angiography.

In another large pedigree, Zhang and associates[89] linked a dominant Stargardt-like phenotype to markers on chromosome 13q34. The gene is located in a 8 cM interval between markers D13S159 and D13S158/D13S174. Affected individuals reported onset of symptoms between the ages 5 and 46 years and visual acuity ranged from 20/40 to 20/400. Retinal findings included retinal flecks and central macular and choroidal atrophy. Fluorescein angiograms were not done but some patients had markedly reduced scotopic ERGs.

A recessive form of Stargardt disease was mapped to chromosome 1p21-p13 by Kaplan and colleagues[36] using eight multiplex recessive pedigrees. The gene lies between D1S424 and D1S236, with a peak lod score of 12.66 over marker D1S435. Patients had loss of central vision at the age of 7–12 years, with obvious maculopathy and retinal flecks, silent choroid on angiography, and normal or reduced photopic electroretinographic responses.

The Stargardt gene on chromosome 1p was recently identified by Allikmets et al.[1a] as the rod-specific ABC gene (ATP binding cassette protein). Multiple homozygous missense, nonsense, and frameshift mutations have been reported in patients with both Stargardt disease and fundus flavimaculatus.[37] The ABC gene is expressed exclusively in the neurosensory retina, and, interestingly, in situ hybridization localized the ABC transcripts to the rod photoreceptor cells only.[81a]

Differential Diagnosis

Partly because of its phenotypic variability, but also because of its rapidly changing fundus appearance, Stargardt disease may be a difficult diagnosis to make under certain circumstances. In particular, progressive cone degenerations and central areolar choroidal atrophy, but other diseases as well, must be diligently ruled out. Central areolar choroidal atrophy can have an identical appearance to advanced macular atrophy in Stargardt disease, although the onset of choroidal atrophy comes in later adulthood and lacks the retinal flecks and the dark choroid on angiography. Cone degenerations may be the most difficult to distinguish from Stargardt disease, but patients with cone degenerations often have nystagmus, arteriolar narrowing, profound color and photopic ERG abnormalities, and no flecks. Chloroquine toxicity may appear very similar but can be distinguished by history. In fundus albipunctatus, the white subretinal round dots are evenly spaced, and there are no pigment disturbances; night blindness is common and the disease is stationary. Familial drusen are round and discrete and may coalesce and fluoresce uniformly on angiography. Finally, Kandori's flecked retina has irregular flecks in the midperiphery and equator but spares the posterior pole; pigmentary changes and night blindness are commonly present in this rare disease.

BEST VITELLIFORM MACULAR DYSTROPHY

Clinical Features and Natural History

Best disease, or vitelliform macular dystrophy, is named after the German ophthalmologist Friedrich Best,[2] who published the first pedigree with this entity in 1905. The first detailed description was given by Adams[1] in 1883. The disease is a peculiar juvenile macular dystrophy with autosomal dominant inheritance characterized by the subretinal accumulation of yellowish material in the macular area. It is slowly progressive and eventually results in atrophy of the retinal pigment epithelium and photoreceptors, severely impairing central vision. The underlying biochemical defect is not yet known.

Best disease is highly variable in its clinical expression and often has an asymmetric presentation. It may commence shortly after birth, or decades later. The classic vitelliform lesion is an egg-yellow, round, raised, macular lesion measuring 0.5–3.0 disc diameters in size (Fig. 21.8). This lesion is not always present, however, and the macular findings range from a tiny yellow dot, multiple vitelliform or atrophic lesions (Fig. 21.9), or a toxoplasmosislike chorioretinal scar. The characteristic foveal "egg yolk" is rarely present at birth; it usually begins to evolve between the ages of 5 and 10 years. Patients may complain of blurred vision, uncorrectable poor acuity, or metamorphopsia. Despite some dramatic fundus changes, 75% of patients have a visual acuity better than 20/40. Attempts have been made to classify the natural evolution of Best disease.[9,10,58] Difficulties have been encountered, partly because the disease is variable in its expressivity. The earliest visible lesion appears to be a yellow subfoveal pigment disturbance, so-called previtelliform stage. Angiography may reveal a subtle window defect.

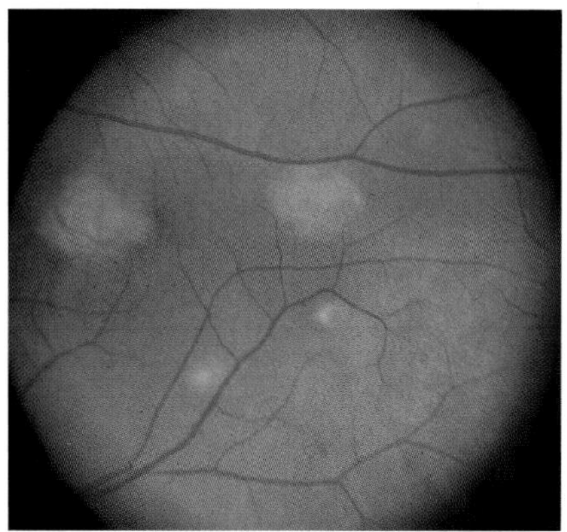

Figure 21.9. Multiple vitelliform lesions in a patient with Best disease. (Courtesy of Dr. Irene H. Maumenee.)

The vitelliform lesion appears at a later stage and has been described as an intact "egg yolk." The yellow-orange cyst reaches a size of about 1 disc diameter and may remain intact for many years with maintenance of good visual function. When the cyst breaks up, it takes the appearance of a "scrambled egg" (Fig. 21.10), with slight reduction in vision. If layering of the subretinal material occurs, the lesion is described as a "pseudohypopyon." If the yellow material is resorbed, it may be replaced by

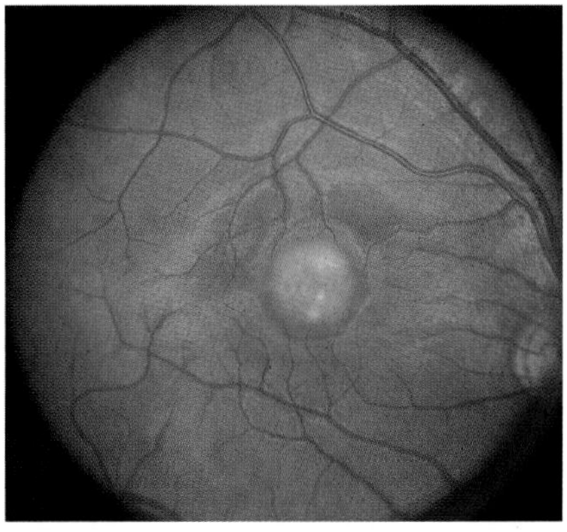

Figure 21.8. Characteristic "egg yolk" lesion in a patient with Best disease.

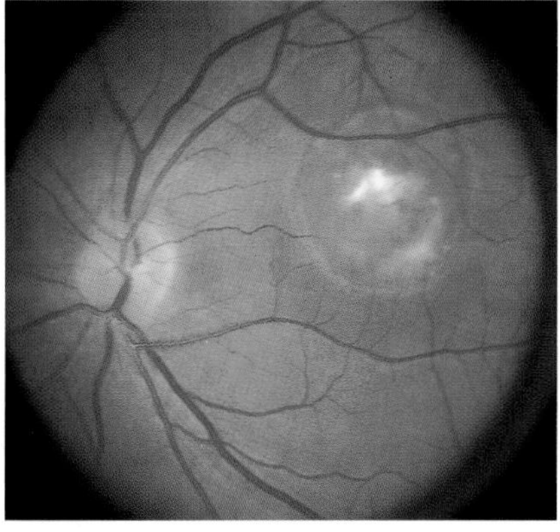

Figure 21.10. "Scrambled egg" appearance of macular lesion in a patient with Best disease. (Courtesy of Dr. Irene H. Maumenee.)

an area of pigment epithelial or a subretinal neovascular membrane may develop leading to a disciform scar. Deutman[9,10] classified the evolution of Best disease into the following seven stages (modified by Mohler and Fine[58]):

Stage 1. Normal fundus, abnormal EOG

Stage 2. Previtelliform stage (RPE mottling, yellow foveal dot)

Stage 3. Vitelliform stage (classic "egg yolk" lesion)

Stage 4. "Scrambled egg" stage

Stage 5. "Cyst" stage

Stage 6. "Pseudohypopyon" stage

Stage 7. Cicatricial stage

Extrafoveal lesions may be present. these include clusters of drusen and/or extrafoveal vitelliform cysts. Although the egg yolk lesion is classic for Best disease, patients may have other fundus manifestations ranging from small strophic foveal lesions reminiscent of pattern dystrophy to choroidal sclerosis, geographic atrophy, and small pisciform deposits reminiscent of fundus flavimaculatus.

It is impossible to predict visual acuity from the appearance of the macula. The patient's vision is often considerably better than expected. Visual loss can be substantial, however, but is often asymmetric. Reduced vision is most often due to atrophic changes in the macula with resultant loss of rod and cone function (Fig. 21.11). Subretinal membranes,[56] and rarely retinal holes,[64] may lead to rapid loss of vision.

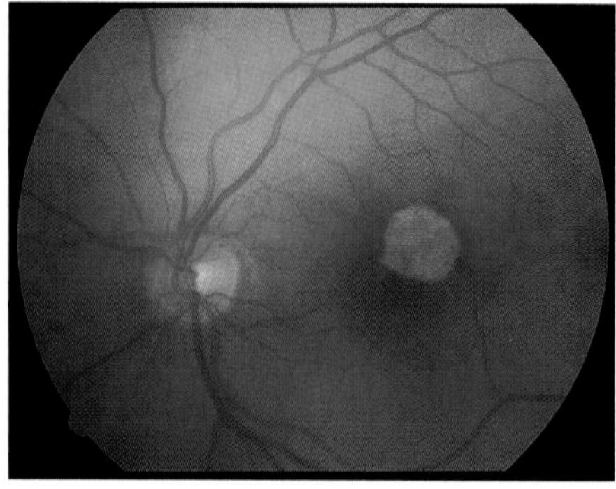

Figure 21.11. Atrophic macular appearance in a 75-year-old man with Best disease. Visual acuity is 20/60.

Diagnostic Procedures

Visual fields may show subtle central sensitivity losses. Color vision can be affected. Nagel anomaloscopy may reveal a red-green dyschromatopsia. There may be a tritan axis of confusion on the Farnsworth-Munsell 100-hue test. Dark adaptation and electroretinography, including oscillatory potentials, are completely normal. EOG is always abnormal. The EOG measures the electrical potential across the retinal pigment epithelium. The Arden ratio represents the light peak divided by the dark trough and is normally greater or equal than 2. The Arden ratio is often less than 1.5 in patients with Best disease, or asymptomatic carriers of the Best gene. Pattern dystrophies and some cases of Stargardt disease share with Best disease the combination of a normal ERG and an abnormal EOG. Inner retinal function has been assessed using pattern ERG (PERG); five of nine patients with Best disease and good visual acuity had abnormal PERGs.[66] Horiguchi and co-workers[33] also found abnormal local macular ERG values in patients with Best and normal visual acuity. Finally, Massof and co-workers[52] reported abnormal flicker fusion threshold intensities in Best patients; these findings may be interpreted as abnormal elevations in the foveal cone thresholds or loss of cone temporal resolution or both. The latter three studies present evidence that Best disease affects the inner neurosensory retina in the foveal area at a time when Snellen visual acuity is still normal or near normal.

Pathology

Light and transmission electron microscopic studies in an 80-year-old patient with well-documented Best disease disclosed striking abnormalities of the retinal pigment epithelium (RPE), photoreceptors, and sub-RPE area.[25] The RPE cells were diffusely flattened, with displacement of their nuclei toward the apex, and diffuse deposition of abnormal lipofuscin and pleomorphic melanolipofuscin granules. A PAS-positive, fine granular material was deposited in the inner segments of the degenerating photoreceptors and Müller cells and an abnormal fibrillar material was found underneath the abnormal RPE cells.[25] Other light microscopic studies in young patients have also shown diffuse RPE abnormalities with collection of lipofuscinlike material in and under the RPE cells. The material was most prominent in the macular area but was also present in the periphery.[85]

Genetics

Best disease is transmitted as an autosomal dominant trait with decreased penetrance and high phenotypical variability. In 1992, Stone and associates[80] reported linkage of the Best disease phenotype to chromosome 11q13. The maximum lod score of 9.3 was found in the interval between markers INT2 and D11S871. One subsequent study of other families found no evidence of locus heterogeneity.[83] Another study, however, excluded linkage to the 11q13 locus in one family, illustrating genetic heterogeneity.[50] Rod outer membrane protein (ROM-1) is a retinal candidate gene in the 11q13 location, but a number of studies have failed to find mutations within the coding sequence of this gene in patients with Best disease, and a recombination event has excluded ROM-1 as the disease-causing gene in this condition.[61,79] There is one report of nonpenetrance with one person who has inherited the Best disease haplotype, but repeated fundus and EOG exams failed to show signs of clinical disease.[84]

Clinical and Genetic Heterogeneity

There are several variants of Best disease. Multiple vitelliform lesions may occur. Atypical vitelliform macular dystrophy differs from typical Best disease in that the vitelliform lesions are smaller, the EOG is sometimes normal, and the disease-causing gene is linked to the GPT-1 marker on chromosome 8q24.[16] A mitochondrial myopathy with vitelliform lesions has been described.[57] Lachapelle et al.[44] described a family with atypical Best disease and autosomal dominant inheritance. Fundus features and EOGs were typical of Best disease, but there were markedly reduced scotopic ERG amplitudes and oscillatory potentials (OP-3 and OP-4).[44] Finally, an adult vitelliform macular dystrophy has been described with a premature stop codon mutation (codon 258) in the peripherin/RDS gene.[88] Thus, there are at least four genes that are capable of causing a vitelliform dystrophy phenotype.

PATTERN DYSTROPHIES

Introduction and History

The pattern dystrophies of the RPE are a group of inherited dystrophies that share in common the presence of yellow, orange or gray deposits under the RPE in a variety of "patterns," without significant visual loss. Gass[26] divided the pattern dystrophies into four principal groups based on their fundus appearance: adult-onset foveomacular dystrophy, butterfly dystrophy, reticular dystrophy, and fundus pulverulentus.

Clinical Features and Diagnostics

The four pattern dystrophies share in common their asymptomatic detection on routine examination. Patients occasionally complain of mild metamorphopsia, or mild central visual loss to the level of 20/25 to 20/40, despite the presence of fundus lesions since early life. Slow progression of the visual loss is the rule, as are the slow changes in the fundus. Most patients maintain good vision in at least one eye until late in life. Visual fields are normal, except for a slightly diminished central sensitivity. Color vision, dark adaptation, and electroretinography are all completely normal. Electrooculography is moderately to severely abnormal in all four types of pattern dystrophies.[8,26,27,75,76] Fluorescein angiography is very helpful and shows hypofluorescence corresponding to the hyperpigmented "figure," with surrounding hyperfluorescence.

Adult-onset foveomacular dystrophy was described by Gass[26] in 1974 and is characterized by solitary, yellow, round, slightly elevated, foveal lesions, one-third to one disc diameter in size. The lesion often contains a central pigmented spot. Small yellow flecks may or may not be present in the surrounding macula.[26] The central foveal lesion may fade over time and leave an atrophic area.

Butterfly dystrophy was first described by Deutman[8] et al. in 1970. It is characterized by a bilaterally symmetric "winged" pigmented pattern in the fovea, with a yellow or gray colored central deposit.

Reticular dystrophy was first reported by Sjögren[75] in 1950. Patients have a coarse, knotted fishnet pattern of pigment that starts in the fovea but extends into the periphery. Initially, there is only a central pigmented spot in the fovea, the size of a disc. Gradually, the network develops, and extends to the midperiphery, but not past the equator. Later in life, the hyperpigmented bands fade, leaving yellow white linear arrays.

Fundus pulverulentus was named as such by Slezak and Hommer[76] in 1969. In this condition, there is prominent, coarse, punctate mottling of the RPE within the central macular area.

Pathology

The histopathology has only been described in adult-onset foveomacular dystrophy.[26] There are hyperplastic RPE cells with intra- and extracellular melanin and lipofuscin. The characteristic yellow lesion is composed of a collagenous, granular, PAS-positive deposit located between the RPE and the underlying Bruch's membrane.

Genetics

Most cases of pattern dystrophy are inherited as autosomal dominant except for the reticular form, which is transmitted as autosomal recessive. Butterfly dystrophy can be caused by mutations in the peripherin/RDS gene: a point mutation in codon 167 in one family,[59] a two base pair deletion in another,[60] and a four base pair insertion in a third family[37] have been reported. In a four generation family, a Pro-216-Ser missense mutation of the peripherin/RDS gene was found in patients who had both retinitis pigmentosa and pattern dystrophy.[68]

REFERENCES

1. Adams JE. Case showing peculiar changes in the macula. *Trans Ophthalmol Soc UK* 1883; 3:113.

1a. Allikmets R, Singh N, Sun H, et al. A photoreceptor cell-specific ATP-binding transporter gene (ABCR) is mutated in recessive Stargardt macular dystrophy. *Nature Genet* 1997;15: 236–246.

2. Best F. Uber eine hereditare Maculaaffektion: Beitrage zur Vererbungslehre. *Z Augenheilkd* 1905;13:199.

3. Birnbach CD, Jarvelainen M, Possin DE, Milam AH. Histopathology and immunocytochemistry of the neurosensory retina in fundus flavimaculatus. *Ophthalmology* 1994; 101:1211–1219.

4. Blacharski PA. Fundus flavimaculatus. In *Retinal Dystrophies and Degenerations,* D. A. Newsome, ed. New York: Raven Press, 1988:135–159.

5. Camuzat A, Dollfus H, Rozet JM, et al. A gene for Leber's congenital amaurosis maps to chromosome 17p. *Hum Mol Genet* 1995;4(8):1447–1452.

6. Dekaban A. Hereditary syndrome of congenital retinal blindness (Leber), polycystic kidneys, and maldevelopment of the brain. *Am J Ophthalmol* 1969;68:1029–1037.

7. Deutman AF. Stargardt's disease. In *The Hereditary Dystrophies of the Posterior Pole of the Eye,* A. F. Deutman, ed. Assen, The Netherlands: Van Gorcum Comp. N.V., 1971: 100–171.

8. Deutman AF, Bommestein van JD, Henkes HE, et al. Butterfly-shaped pigment dystrophy of the fovea. *Arch Ophthalmol* 1970;83: 558–569.

9. Deutman AF. Hereditary dystrophies of the central retina and choroid. In *Perspectives in Ophthalmology,* vol. 2, J. E. Winkelman and R. A. Crone, eds. Amsterdam: Excerpta Medica, 1970.

10. Deutman AF. *The Hereditary Dystrophies of the Posterior Pole of the Eye.* Assen, The Netherlands: Van Gorcum Comp. N.V., 1971.

11. Dollfus H. Exclusion of the recoverin gene as the candidate gene in Leber's congenital amaurosis. *Invest Ophthalmol Vis Sci* 1993; 34:1462.

12. Dryja TP, McGee TL, Reichel E, et al. A point mutation of the rhodopsin gene in one form of retinitis pigmentosa. *Nature* 1990;343: 364–366.
13. Eagle RC, Lucier AC, Bernardino VB, Yanoff M. Retinal pigment epithelial abnormalities in fundus flavimaculatus. *Ophthalmology* 1980; 87:1189–1200.
14. Edwards WC, Price WD, MacDonald R Jr. Congenital amaurosis of retinal origin (Leber) *Am J Ophthalmol* 1971;72:724–728.
15. Farrar GJ, Kenna, P, Jordan SA, et al. A three-base-pair deletion in the peripherin-RDS gene in one form of retinitis pigmentosa. *Nature* 1991;354:478–480.
16. Ferrell RE, Hittner HM, Antoszyk JH. *Am J Hum Genet* 1983;35:78–84.
17. Fishman GA. Fundus flavimaculatus. A clinical classification. *Arch Ophthalmol* 1976;94:2061–2067.
18. Flynn JT, Cullen RF. Disc oedema in congenital amaurosis of Leber. *Br J Ophthalmol* 1975;59:497–502.
19. Franceschetti A. L'importance diagnostique de l'ERG dans les dégénérescences tapétorétiniennes avec retrecissement du champ visuel et héméralopie. *Confin Neurol* 1954; 14:184–186.
20. Franceschetti A. Uber tapeto-retinale Degeneration im Kindersalter. In *Eintwickelung und Fortschritt in der Augenheilkunde*, H. Sautter, ed. Stuttgart: Ferdinand Enke Verlag, 1963: 107–120.
21. Franceschetti A. La rétinopathie ponctuée albecente. *Bull Mem Soc Fr Ophtalmol* 1963; 76:15–19.
22. Franceschetti A, Francois J. Fundus flavimaculatus. *Arch Ophthalmol* 1965;25:505–530.
23. Francois J. Leber's congenital tapeto-retinal degeneration. *Int Ophthalmol Clin.* 1968;8: 929–947.
24. Francois P, Turut P, Puech B, Hache JC. Maladie de Stargardt et fundus flavimaculatus. *Arch Ophthalmol* 1975;35:817–846.
25. Frangieh G and Green W, Fine SL. A histopathologic study of Best's macular dystrophy. *Arch Ophthalmol* 1982;100:1115–1121.
26. Gass JD. A clinicopathologic study of a peculiar foveomacular dystrophy. *Trans Am Ophthalmol Soc* 1974;72:140–156.
27. Gass JD. *A Stereoscopic Atlas of Macular Disease: Diagnosis and Treatment.* St. Louis: C. V. Mosby Co., 1987.
28. Gillespie F.D. Congenital amaurosis of Leber. Am J Ophthalmol 1966;61:874.
28a. Gu S, Thompson DA, Srikumari CRS, et al. Mutations in the RPE65 cause autosomal recessive childhood-onset severe retinal dystrophy. *Nat Genet* 1997;17:194–197.
29. Hahn L, Berson EL, Dryja TP. Evaluation of the gene encoding the gamma subunit of rod phosphodiesterase in retinitis pigmentosa. *Invest Opthalmol Vis Sci* 1994;35:1077–1082.
30. Heckenlively J. *Retinitis Pigmentosa.* Philadelphia: J. B. Lippincott, 1988:269.
31. Heher KL, Traboulsi, EI Maumenee IH. The natural history of Leber's congenital amaurosis. *Ophthalmology* 1992;99:241–245.
32. Heher KL, Johns DR. A maculopathy associated with the 15257 mitochondrial DNA mutation. *Arch Ophthalmol* 1993; 111:1495–1499.
33. Horiguchi MY, Miyake K, Yagasaki K. Local macular ERG in patients with Best's disease. *Doc Ophthalmol* 1986;63:325–331.
34. Horsten GP. Development of the ERG in relation to the histological differentiation of the retina of man and animals. Arch Ophthalmol 1960;63:232–242.
35. Jan JE, Freeman RD, McCormick AQ, et al. Eye pressing by visually impaired children. *Dev Med Child Neurol* 1983;25:755–762.
36. Kaplan J, Gerber S, Larget-Piet D, et al. A gene for Stargardt's disease (fundus flavimaculatus) maps to the short arm of chromosome 1. *Nature Genet* 1993;5:308–311.
37. Keen TJ, Inglehearn, CF, Kim R, et al. Retinal pattern dystrophy associated with a 4 bp insertion at codon 140 in the peripherin/RDS gene. Hum Mol Genet 1994;3:367–368.
38. Keith C. Retinal atrophy in osteopetrosis. Arch Ophthalmol 1968;79:234–241.
39. Klein BA, Krill AE. Fundus flavimaculatus: Clinical, functional, and histopathological observations. *Am J Ophthalmol* 1967;64:3–23.
40. Koenekoop RK, Tombran-Tink J, Loyer M, Davidson J, Wise L, Traboulsi E, Maumenee I. Pigment epithelium derived factor (PEDF) does not cause Leber's congenital amaurosis: A mutation and linkage exclusion analysis with a report of four new intragenic polymorphisms. Genomics (submitted).
41. Krill AE. Fundus flavimaculatus. In *Hereditary Retinal and Choroidal Diseases*, vol. II. *Clinical Characteristics.* Hagerstown, MD: Harper & Row, 1970:749–787.
42. Kroll AJ, Kuwabara T. Electron microscopy of a retinal abiotrophy. *Arch Ophthalmol* 1964; 71:683.
43. Lachapelle P, Little JM, Roy MS. The electroretinogram in Stargardt's disease and fundus

flavimaculatus. *Doc Ophthalmol* 1990;73: 395–404.

44. Lachapelle P, Quigley MG, Polomeno RC, Little JM. Abnormal dark adapted electroretinogram in Best's vitelliform macular degeneration. *Can J Ophthalmol* 1985;23:279–284.
45. Leber T. Uber Retinitis pigmentosa und angeborene Amaurose. *Albrecht von Graefes Arch Klin Ophthalmol* 1869;15:1–25.
46. Leighton DA, Harris R. Retinal aplasia in association with macular coloboma, keratoconus and cataract. *Clin Genet* 1973;4:270.
47. Lewis RA. Juvenile hereditary macular dystrophies. In *Retinal Dystrophies and Degenerations,* D. Newsome, ed. New York: Raven Press, 1988.
48. Lopez PF, Maumenee IH, Cruz Z de la, Green WR. Autosomal dominant fundus flavimaculatus. *Ophthalmology* 1990;97:798–809.

48a. Loyer M, ElHilali H, Peschlow A, et al. Mutations in the gene for retinal guanylate cyclase in patients with Leber's congenital amaurosis. *Invest Ophthalmol Vis Sci* 1977;38(4):S680.

49. Macke JP, Davenport CM, Jacobson SG, et al. Identification of novel rhodopsin mutations responsible for retinitis pigmentosa: Implications for the structure and function of rhodopsin. *Am J Hum Genet* 1993;53:80–89.
50. Mansergh F, Kenna P, Rudolph G, et al. Evidence for genetic heterogeneity in Best's vitelliform macular dystrophy. *J Med Genet* 1995; 32:855–858.
51. Margolis S, Scher BM, Carr RE. Macular colobomas in Leber's congenital amaurosis. *Am J Ophthalmol* 1977;83:27–31.

51a. Marlhens F, Bareil C, Griffoin JM, et al. Mutations in the RPE65 cause Leber's congenital amaurosis. *Nature Genet* 1997;17:139–141.

52. Massof RW, Fleischman JA, Fine SL, Yoder F. Flicker fusion thresholds in Best's macular dystrophy. *Arch Ophthalmol* 1977;95(6): 991–994.
53. McGee T, Lin D, Berson EL, et al. Defects in the rod cGMP gated channel gene in with patients with retinitis pigmentosa. *Invest Ophthalmol Vis Sci* 1994;35:1716.
54. McLaughlin M, Sandberg MA, Berson EL, Dryja TP. Recessive mutations in the gene encoding the B subunit of rod phosphodiesterase in patients with RP. *Nature Genet* 1993;4: 130–133.
55. Miller SA, Bresnick GH, Chandra SR. Choroidal neovascular membrane in Best's vitelliform macular dystrophy. *Am J Ophthalmol* 1976;82: 252–255.
56. Mizuno K, Takei Y, Sears ML, et al. Leber's congenital amaurosis. *Am J Ophthalmol* 1977; 83:32–42.
57. Modi G, Heckman JM, Saffer D. Vitelliform macular degeneration associated with mitochondrial myopathy. *Br Ophthalmol* 1992;76: 58–60.
58. Mohler C, Fine S. Long term evaluation of patients with Best's vitelliform dystrophy. *Ophthalmology* 1981;88:688–691.
59. Nichols BE, Sheffield VC, Vandenburgh K, et al. Butterfly-shaped pigment dystrophy of the fovea caused by a point mutation in codon 167 of the RDS gene. *Nature Genet* 1993;3: 202–207.
60. Nichols BE, Drack AV, Vandenburgh K, et al. A 2 base pair deletion in the RDS gene associated with butterfly shaped pigment dystrophy of the fovea. *Hum Mol Genet* 1993; 2:601–603.
61. Nichols BE, Bascom R, Litt M, et al. Refining the locus for Best's vitelliform macular dystrophy and mutation analysis of the candidate gene ROM-1. *Am J Hum Genet* 1994;54: 95–103.
62. Noble K, Carr RE. Leber's congenital amaurosis. A retrospective study of 33 cases and a histopathological study of one case. *Arch Ophthalmol* 1978;96:818–821.
63. Noble KG, Carr RE. Stargardt's disease and fundus flavimaculatus. *Arch Ophthalmol* 1979; 97:1281–1285.
64. Noble KG, Chang S. Adult vitelliform macular degeneration progressing to full thickness macular hole. *Arch Ophthalmol* 1991;109:325.
65. Passmore JA, Robertson DM. Ring scotomata in fundus flavimaculatus. *Am J Ophthalmol* 1975;80:907–912.

65a. Perrault I, Rozet JM, Calvas P, et al. Retinal-specific guanylate cyclase gene mutations in Leber's congenital amaurosis. *Nature Genet* 1997;14:461–464.

66. Power WJ, Coleman K, Curtin DM, Mooney DJ. The pattern ERG in Best's disease. *Doc Ophthalmol* 1990;76:279–284.
67. Reiss O, Weber B, Noeremolle A, et al. Linkage studies and mutation analysis of the PDEB gene in 23 families with Leber's congenital amaurosis. *Hum Mutat* 1992;1:478–485.
68. Richards SC, Creel DJ. Pattern dystrophy and retinitis pigmentosa caused by a peripherin/ RDS mutation. *Retina* 1995;15:68–72.
69. Robitaille JM, Palincsar LK, Zhu D, Maumenee IH. Linkage analysis in an Amish family with Leber's congenital amaurosis. *Invest Ophthalmol Vis Sci* 1996;37(3):S998.

70. Rosehr K. Uber den weiteren Verlauf der von Stargardt und Behr beschriebenen familiaren Degeneration der Makula. *Klin Monatsbl Augenheilkd* 1954;124:171–179.
71. Sakuma H, Inana G, Murakami A, et al. A heterozygous putative null mutation in ROM-1 without a mutation in peripherin in a family with RP. *Genomics* 1995;27:384–386.
72. Schappert-Kimmijser J, Henkes HE, van den Bosch J. Amaurosis congenita (Leber). *Arch Ophthalmol* 1959;137:420.
73. Schroeder R, Mets MB, Maumenee IH. Leber's congenital amaurosis. Retrospective review of 43 cases and a new fundus finding in two cases. *Arch Ophthalmol* 1987;105: 356–359.
74. Senior B. Familial renal-retinal dystrophy. *Am J Dischild* 1973;125:442–447.
75. Sjögren H. Dystrophia reticularis laminae pigmentosae retinae: Earlier not described hereditary eye disease. *Acta Ophthalmol* (Copenh) 1950;28:279–295.
76. Slezak H, Hommer K. Fundus pulverulentus. *Graefes Arch Clin Exp Ophthalmol* 1969;178: 176–182.
77. Sorsby A, Williams CE. Retinal aplasia as a clinical entity. *Br Med J* 1869;I:293.
78. Stargardt K. Uber familiare, progressive Degeneration in der Makulagegend des Auge. *Graefes Arch Clin Exp Opthalmol* 1909;71: 534–550.
79. Stohr H, Weber B. A recombination even excludes the ROM-1 locus from the Best's vitelliform macular dystrophy region. *Hum Genet* 1995;95:219–222.
80. Stone EM, Nichols BE, Streb LM, et al. Genetic linkage of vitelliform macular degeneration (Best's disease) to chromosome 11q13. *Nature Genet* 1992;1:246–250.
81. Stone EM, Nichols BE, Kimura AE, Weingeist TA, Drack A, Sheffield VC. Clinical features of a Stargardt's-like dominant progressive macular dystrophy with genetic linkage to chromosome 6q. *Arch Ophthalmol* 1994;112:765–772.
81a. Sun H, Nathans J. Stargardt's ABCR is localized to the disc membrane of retinal rod outer segments. *Nature Genet* 1997;17:15–16.
82. Traboulsi EI, Maumenee IH. Photoaversion in Leber's congenital amaurosis. *Ophthalmol Genet* 1995;16:27–30.
83. Weber BH, Walker D, Muller B, Mar L. Best's vitelliform dystrophy maps between D11S903 and PYGM: No evidence for locus heterogeneity. *Genomics* 1994;20:267–274.
84. Weber BH, Walker D, Müller B. Molecular evidence for non-penetrance in Best's disease. *J Med Genet* 1994;31:388–392.
85. Weingeist TA, Kobrin JL, Watzke RC. Histopathology of Best's macular dystrophy. *Arch Ophthalmol* 1982;100:1108–1114.
86. Weleber RG, Carr RE, Murphey WH, Sheffield VC, Stone EM. Phenotypic variation including retinitis pigmentosa, pattern dystrophy, and fundus flavimaculatus in a single family with a deletion of codon 153 or 154 of the peripherin/RDS gene. *Arch Ophthalmol* 1993;111:1531–1542.
87. Weleber RG. Stargardt's macular dystrophy (editorial). *Arch Ophthalmol* 1994;112:752–754.
88. Wells J, Wroblewski J, Keen T, et al. Mutations in the retinal degeneration slow (RDS) gene can cause either retinitis pigmentosa or macular dystrophy. *Nature Genet* 1993;3:213–218.
89. Zhang K, Bither PP, Park R, Donoso LA, Seidman CE. A dominant Stargardt's dystrophy locus maps to chromosome 13q34. *Arch Ophthalmol* 1994;112:759–764.

22

Congenital Stationary Night Blindness

JOHN HECKENLIVELY

Congenital stationary night blindness (CSNB) is the name given to a set of diseases defined by their congenital (or early-onset) night blindness, and by the documentation of lack of a progressive retinal degeneration.

In his review of CSNB, Carr cites that the earliest documented familial case of congenital stationary night blindness was reported by Cunier in 1838[8,9]—a seven-generation family named Nougaret. Jean Nougaret was born in 1637 in Southern France. Nettleship described nine generations of this autosomal dominant CSNB family encompassing 2121 individuals, 135 of whom were affected.[32] The X-linked recessive form was recognized by Donders[10] in the 1850s, while Gassler[17] is credited with identifying an autosomal recessive form of CSNB in 1925.

A number of different types of CSNB have been described over the years. Our understanding of this group of disorders evolved from a variety of electrophysiological, clinical, and genetic studies. As currently understood, a classification of CSNB is given in Table 22.1. This classification is based primarily on electroretinographic (ERG) findings and Mendelian inheritance type.[22] Molecular genetic findings in these conditions will clarify our understanding of rod system abnormalities and will lead to a better classification system (Table 22.2).

The term "hemeralopia" is used in the older medical literature and refers to seeing well in the day; this term was replaced in more recent writings by "night blindness."

ELECTRORETINOGRAPHIC CHANGES IN CSNB

Two types of electroretinographic (ERG) patterns were originally described in patients with CSNB. In type I, or the Nougaret type of CSNB scotopic ERG waveform, there is a reduced response that does not increase in darkness. In type II, or the Schubert–Bornschein type of waveform, patients have a striking absence of the b-wave on the dark-adapted, bright-flash ERG. The abnormal tracing has been termed a *negative waveform* (Fig. 22.1).[3,36] Patients with CSNB also have reduced photopic ERGs. Heckenlively et al.[20] and LaChapelle et al.[24] separately reported that patients with CSNB have missing oscillatory potentials in the photopic and bright-flash, dark-adapted ERGs (Fig. 22.1).

Miyake et al.[27] found that patients with CSNB and negative waveforms could be further subdivided into two types, complete and incomplete, based on a number of abnormalities (Table 22.3). Both types are inherited in an X-linked recessive manner and linkage studies have placed the genes in the same region (Table

Table 22.1. Clinical Classification of Congenital Stationary Night Blindness (CSNB)

CSNB with normal fundus appearance (autosomal dominant, autosomal recessive, X-linked recessive)
CSNB with absent scotopic electroretinogram (ERG) (Riggs type; type I)
CSNB with negative ERG (Schubert–Bornschein type, type II)
Complete
Incomplete
CSNB with abnormal fundi
Oguchi disease
Fundus albipunctatus
Flecked retina of Kandori

From Carr, ref 8.

22.2). Patients with incomplete CSNB have some rod function as recorded by the rod-isolated ERG and psychophysical testing. Patients with the complete form of X-linked CSNB, on the other hand, have very poor to flat rod ERGs. The photopic ERG tends to be more abnormal in the incomplete type and the diagnosis may be confused with that of cone dystrophy, in which patients have stable but abnormal rod isolated ERGs. Further studies by Miyake showed that the 30 Hz flicker response was unusually suppressed in incomplete CSNB, and that it increased rapidly after light adaptation (Fig. 22.2).[28,29]

The electroretinographic differences between the complete and incomplete types of CSNB have been further delineated by studies of the scotopic threshold response (STR). There is no STR in the complete type of CSNB, whereas this response is clearly recordable in the incomplete type, indicating different rod system abnormalities between the two types. In a personal communication, Miyake stated that patients with the complete type of CSNB appear to have a defect of the "on" response of the rod bipolar cells, whereas patients with the incomplete type may have a problem related to the "off" response of the same cells.

Weleber[43] reported a patient with the Forsius–Eriksson type of ocular albinism (Åland eye disease, another X-linked recessive disor-

Table 22.2. Summary of Genetic Studies in Congenital Stationary Night Blindness (CSNB)

Chromosome Location	Study	Authors
Typical CSNB		
Xp11.3	Eight multigeneration families, seven with complete CSNB. lod 7.35, with marker DXS7, $\theta = 0.00$.	Musarella et al.[31]
Xp11.4–p11.23	Five-generation family with Åland eye Disease, CSNB type 2, linked to PFC(cA) $Z_{max} = 3.56$, $\theta = 0.00$.	Glass et al.[18]
	Recombinant CSNB type 2 pedigree, one recombinant event suggests that one gene is proximal to MAOB and linked to DXS255.	Bergen et al.[5]
Xp21.1	Dutch family with linkage in region of RP3.	Bergen et al.[6]
Autosomal Dominant CSNB		
4p16.3	Missense mutation in rod cGMP phosphodiesterase β-subunit gene.	Gal et al.[15]
3q21–q24	Mutations in codons 90 and 292 of rhodopsin gene.	Sieving et al.,[39] Dryja et al.[11]
	Mutation in α-subunit of rod cGMP PDE.	Dryja et al.[12]
Oguchi Disease		
2q37.1	Homozygous deletions of the arrestin gene have been identified in five unrelated Japanese patients with Oguchi disease	Fuchs et al.[13]

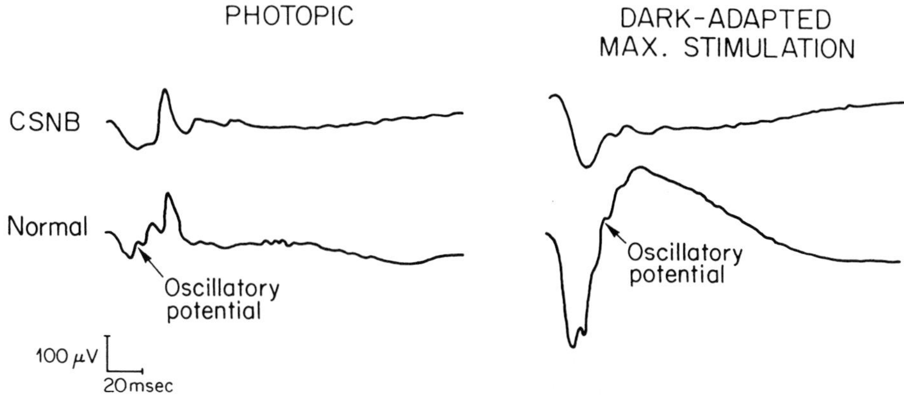

Figure 22.1. Photopic and bright-flash dark-adapted electroretinograms from a patient with complete X-linked recessive congenital stationary night blindness and from a normal control showing the loss of the oscillatory potentials and the negative waveform in the affected individual.

der) who also had incomplete CSNB. Weleber raised the issue of whether Åland eye disease and incomplete CSNB are one and the same disorder. Rosenberg et al.[35] reported a six-generation Danish family with Åland eye disease whose main features were congenital nystagmus and subnormal vision. Most patients had myopia, and the ERG showed negative waveforms and poor scotopic and flicker ERGs. Further clinical studies of CSNB have been performed in large families from Canada and Wales.[19,34]

CLINICAL FINDINGS IN X-LINKED CSNB

Patients with complete X-linked CSNB usually have high myopia with a tigroid-appearing fundus and "tilted" myopic discs. It is not clear whether the discs are tilted or whether their temporal edges are atrophic (Fig. 22.3). Fluorescein angiography reveals that papillary vessels are present at the edge of the disc, where axons would have been present if the disc were round, suggesting that some atrophy may have occurred at an earlier age.[20] The patients' best corrected visual acuity is typically in the 20/40 to 20/50 range, but varies from 20/25 and 20/200. Some patients have mild nystagmus. Individuals with incomplete X-linked CSNB tend to be mildly myopic, but their vision is in the same range as those with the complete form, and they may have nystagmus.

FUNDUS ALBIPUNCTATUS

Lauber is credited with the first description of fundus albipunctatus, an autosomal recessive disorder.[25] Patients with this disorder have dis-

Table 22.3. Criteria for Distinguishing Incomplete and Complete Congenital Stationary Night Blindness (CSNB)

Parameter	Incomplete CSNB	Complete CSNB
Photopic ERG	Very small amplitude	Reduced amplitude
Rod-isolated ERG	Reduced amplitude	Flat
30-Hz flicker ERG	Small amplitude	Relatively normal
Light-adapted flicker ERG	Grows 2–3X normal over 10 min. Has bimodal apex	No change in size
200 ms flash	On-response bipolar defect	Off-response bipolar defect

ERG = electroretinogram.

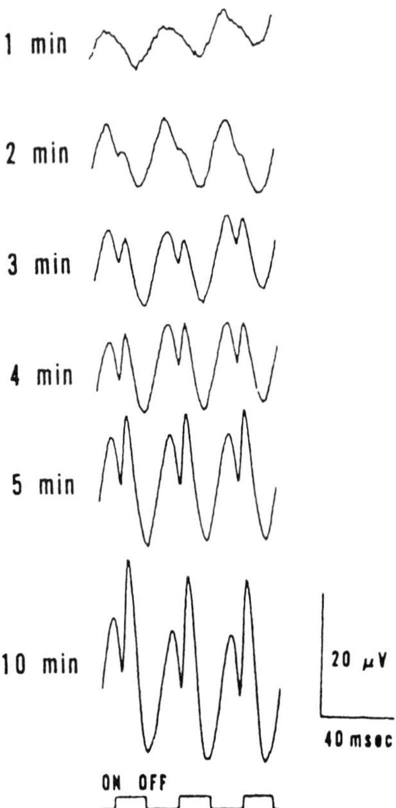

Figure 22.2. Changes in the 30 Hz flicker electroretinogram during light adaptation in incomplete congenital stationary night blindness (CSNB) demonstrating a marked increase in amplitude and development of a bimodal notch in the waveform characteristic of this form of CSNB. (From Miyake et al. *Invest Ophthalmol Visual Sci* 1987;28:1816–1823. Used by permission.)

tinctive white-to-yellow round flecks scattered in a radial pattern from the fovea throughout the retina, sparing the macula region (Fig. 22.4). Krill gives an extensive description of the disease in his textbook on hereditary retinal dystrophies and places it in the group of "flecked" retinal diseases.[23] There is a characteristic initial poor dark-adapted rod response on ERG testing, but the response improves with prolonged dark adaptation. Fundus albipunctatus is considered to be a form of CSNB because of the stationary nature of disease and the associated night blindness. It should be noted that long-term follow-up has not been published on this group of patients to validate that the disease is truly stationary over the life of the patient. Patients with retinitis punctata albescens (RPA) have similar ophthalmoscopic findings as fundus albipunctatus, but ERG changes and visual field loss are similar to those of patients with retinitis pigmentosa; hence this disease is not classified under CSNB.

OGUCHI DISEASE

Before World War I Oguchi reported a peculiar form of CSNB characterized by a mottled gray-white discoloration of the retina that gives a metallic sheen to the eye grounds.[33] The maculae are abnormally dark against the rest of the fundus. Mizuo observed that the unusual fundus color disappears after dark adaptation.[30] The mottled appearance reappears after light adaptation. This disease is inherited in an autosomal recessive fashion. Takagi and Kawakami reported three new patients and reviewed another 56; they found a history of consanguity in 62% of cases.[40] Fuchs and co-workers found homozygous deletions of the arrestin gene in five unrelated Japanese patients.[13]

Psychophysical testing shows that a prolonged dark adaptation period of 4 h results in improvement of rod thresholds to a normal level (it takes a normal individual 30 min to achieve good levels of sensitivity). Electroretinographic cone responses are normal, whereas rod responses are very abnormal.

FLECKED RETINA OF KANDORI

This rare condition was described by Kandori in four patients, one of whom had consanguineous parents.[21] The fundus appearance is characterized by deep gray-yellow irregular subretinal deposits (termed "flecks," but different from those seen in other retinal diseases). The psychophysical dark adaptation thresholds are delayed but become normal after about 40 min. Likewise, the ERG scotopic responses are delayed but the b-wave amplitudes are reported to become normal with time.

VISUAL PIGMENT KINETIC STUDIES

In several reports, Carr was able to demonstrate that patients with CSNB type I have

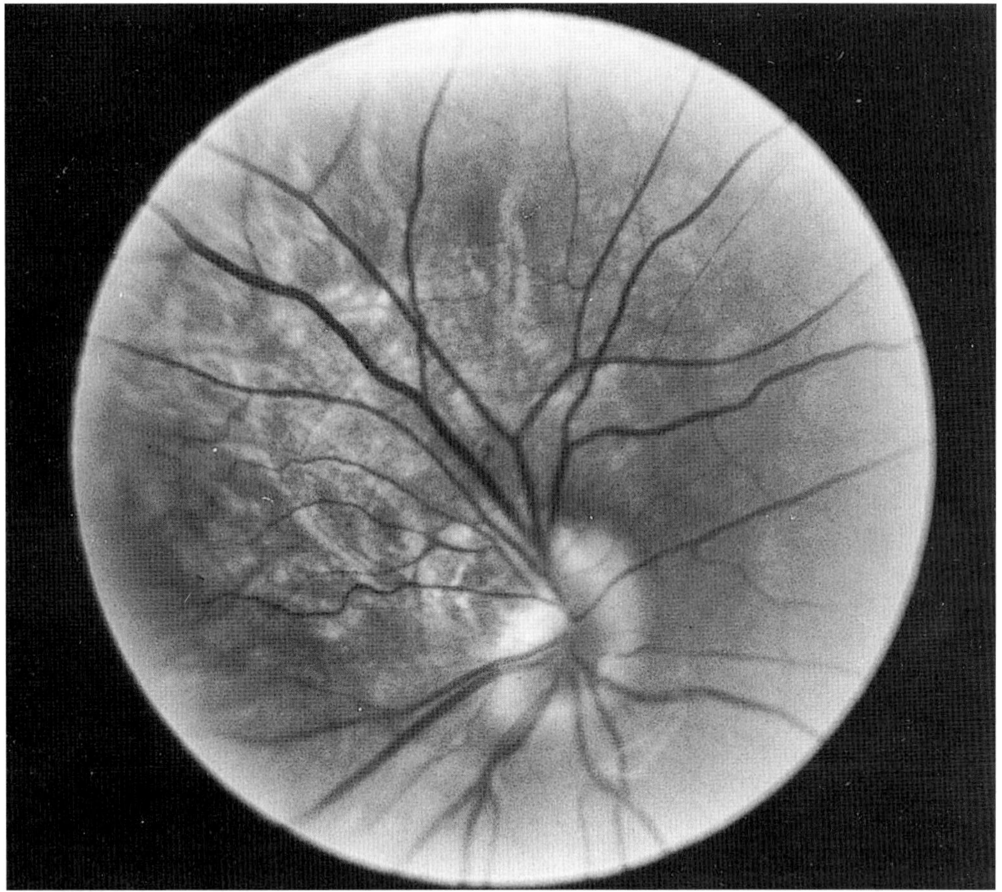

Figure 22.3. Fundus photograph of the left eye of 16-year-old boy with complete X-linked recessive congenital stationary night blindness (CSNB), demonstrating a typical tigroid fundus and "tilted" disc.

normal visual pigment kinetics, suggesting that the ERG abnormalities were due to transmission defects in the inner segments of the rods, or between the rod and the bipolar cell.[8] Patients with type II CSNB also have normal visual pigment kinetics and a-waves, but psychophysical studies suggest that the defect lies in the interplexiform layer.[38] Histologic studies of types I and II CSNB have revealed no retinal abnormalities. The ocular histology of the Appaloosa horse with type II ERG is also normal.[41,42,44]

Siegel et al.[38] studied one patient with autosomal recessive CSNB who had been investigated 23 years previously; his rod thresholds had remained the same, but cone sensitivity had decreased.

MAPPING STUDIES

With autosomal dominant and recessive forms of CSNB, and possibly three X-linked forms, molecular genetic correlation with the phenotypes in families with clear modes of inheritance will greatly clarify our understanding of these nonprogressive forms of retinal dystrophies with nyctalopia. To date, the genes for all three X-linked forms of CSNB have been localized to the proximal end of the short arm of the X chromosome, suggesting that they may be allelic. The gene for complete CSNB was mapped between DXS7 and DXS426,[1,4,14] whereas the one for incomplete CSNB was localized proximal to MAOB in a Dutch family by a single key recombination event.[5] The

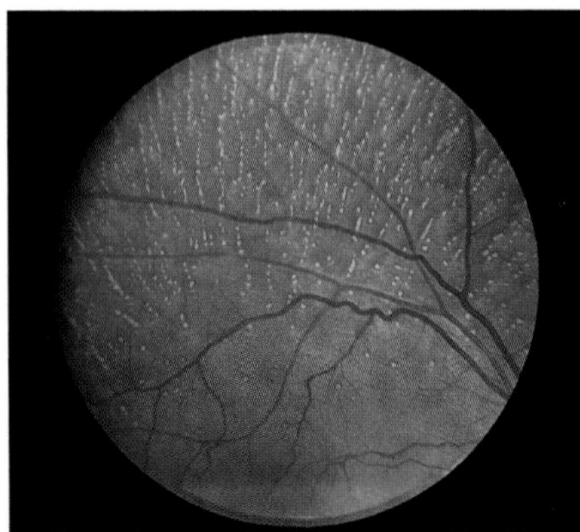

Figure 22.4. Widely distributed white retinal dots in both eyes of a 61-year-old woman. After dark adaptation, the rod-isolated electroretinogram was nonrecordable at 10 min, delayed and subnormal at 60 min, and delayed with normal amplitudes at 135 min. The final rod threshold was 4.2 log units elevated at 45 min and 3.25 units elevated at 150 min.

Åland eye disease gene has been mapped between DXS7 and DXS255.[2,18,37] Bergen et al.[6] described a Dutch family with linkage to Xp21.1 near RP3, distinctly away from previous linkage data.

Autosomal dominant CSNB has been attributed to three different types of mutations, two of them in genes where mutations have been classically associated with retinitis pigmentosa. Gal et al. described a heterozygous missense mutation in the rod cGMP (cyclic guanosine monophosphate) phosphodiesterase gene,[15,16] while Sieving et al.[39] and Dryja et al.[11] reported mutations at codon 90 and 292 of rhodopsin. Most recently Dryja and colleagues[12] found a missense mutation in the α-subunit of rod transducin in affected descendants of Jean Nougaret.

REFERENCES

1. Aldred MA, Dry KL, Sharp DM, van Dorp DB, Brown J, Hardwick LJ, Lester HD, Pryde FE, Teague PW, Jay M, Bird AC, Jay B, and Wright AF. Linkage analysis in X-linked congenital stationary night blindness. *Genomics* 1992;14: 99–104.
2. Alitalo T, Kruse TA, Forsius H, Eriksson AW, del Chappel A. Localization of the Åland island eye disease locus to the pericentromeric region of the human X-chromosome by linkage analysis. *Am J Hum Genet* 1991;48:31–38.
3. Auerbach E, Godel V, Rowe H. An electrophysiologic and psychophysical study of two forms of congenital stationary night blindness. *Invest Ophthalmol Visual Sci* 1969;8:332–345.
4. Bech-Hansen NT, Moore BJ, Pearce WG. Mapping a locus of X-linked congenital stationary night blindness (CSNB) proximal to DXS7. *Genomics* 1992;12:409–411.
5. Bergen AAB, Kestelyn Ph. Leys M, Meire F. Identification of a key recombinant which assigns the incomplete congenital stationary night blindness gene proximal to MAOB. *J Med Genet* 1994;31:580–582.
6. Bergen AAB, Brink JB, Riemslag F, Schuurman EJM, Tijmes N. Localization of a novel X-linked congenital stationary night blindness locus: close linkage to the RP3 type retinitis pigmentosa gene region. *Hum Mol Genet* 1995;4:931–935.
7. Carr RE, Gouras P. Oguchi's disease. *Arch Ophthalmol* 1965;73:646–656.
8. Carr, RE. Congenital stationary night blindness. In *Principles and Practice of Clinical Electrophysiology of Vision*, J. R. Heckenlively and G. B. Arden, eds. St. Louis: Mosby-Yearbook, 1991, pp. 713–720.
9. Cunier R. Histoire d'une hemerglopie, hereditaire depuis des siecles dans un famille de la commune de Vendemaian, pres de Montpellier. *Ann Soc Med Gand* 1838;4:385.
10. Donders FC. Torpeur de la retine congenitale hereditaire. *Ann Ocul (Paris)* 1855;34:270.
11. Dryja TP, Berson EL, Rao VR, Oprian DD. Heterozygous missense mutation in the rhodopsin gene as a cause of congenital stationary night blindness. *Nature Genet* 1993;4:280–283.
12. Dryja TP, Hahn LB, Reboul T, Arnaud B. Missense mutation in the gene encoding the alpha subunit of rod transducin in the Nougaret form of congenital stationary night blindness. *Nature Genet* 1996;13:358–365.
13. Fuchs S, Nakazawa M, Maw M, Tamai M, Oguchi Y, Gal A. A homozygous 1-base pair deletion in the arrestin gene is a frequent cause of Oguchi disease in Japanese. *Nature Genet* 1995;10:360–362.
14. Gal A, Scinzel A, Orth U, Fraser NA, Mollica F, Craig IW, Kruse T, Machler M, Neugehauer M, and Bleeker-Wagemakers EM. Gene of X-chromosomal congenital stationary night blindness if closely linked to DXS7 on Xp. *Hum Genet* 1989;81:315–318.

15. Gal A, Orth U, Baehr W, Schwinger E, Rosenberg T. Heterozygous missense mutation in the rod cGMP phosphodiesterase subunit gene in autosomal dominant congenital stationary night blindness. *Nature Genet* 1994;7:64–68.
16. Gal A, Xu S, Piczenik Y, Eiberg H, Duvigneau C, Schwinger E, Rosenberg T. Gene for autosomal dominant congenital stationary night blindness maps to the same region as the gene for the beta-subunit of rod photreceptor cGMP phosphodiesterase (PDEB) in chromosome 4p16.3. *Hum Mol Genet* 1994;3:323–325.
17. Gassler VJ. Ueber eine jetztnich bekannte rezessive Verkn_pfung von hochgradiger Myopie mit angeborener Hemeralopie (thesis), Zurich, 1925.
18. Glass IA, Good P, Coleman MP, Fullwood P, Giles MG, Nemeth AH, Davies KE, Willshaw HA, Fielder A, Kilpatrick M, Farndon PA. *J Med Genet* 1993;30:1044–1050.
19. Hawksworth NR, Headland S, Good P, Thomas NST, Clarke A. Åland island eye disease: Clinical and electrophysiological studies in a Welsh family. *Br J Ophthalmol* 1995;79:424–430.
20. Heckenlively JR, Martin DA, Rosenbaum AL. Loss of ERG oscillatory potentials, optic atrophy and dysplasia in CSNB. *Am J Ophthalmol* 1983;96:525–534.
21. Kandori F. Very rare cases of congenital nonprogressive night blindness with fleck retina. *Jpn J Ophthalmol* 1959;13:384–386.
22. Krill AE. Congenital stationary night blindness. In *Hereditary Retinal and Choroidal Diseases,* A. E. Krill and D. B. Archer, eds. New York: Harper & Row, 1977, pp. 391–420.
23. Krill AE. Fleck retina diseases, In *Hereditary and Retinal and Choroidal Diseases,* A. E. Krill and D. B. Archer, eds. New York: Harper & Row, 1977, p. 739.
24. LaChapelle P, Little JM, Polomeno RC. The photopic electroretinogram in congenital stationary night blindness with myopia. *Invest Ophthalmol Vis Sci* 1983;24:442–450.
25. Lauber H. Die sogenannte retinitis punctata albescens. *Klin Monatsbl Augenheilkd* 1910; 48:133–148.
26. McKusick VA. Online *Mendelian Inheritance in Man,* OMIM Center for Medical Genetics, Johns Hopkins University (Baltimore, MD) and National Center for Biotechnology Information, National Library of Medicine (Bethesda, MD), 1997. World Wide Web URL: http://www.nebi.nlm.nih.gov/omim/.
27. Miyake Y, Yagasaki K, Horiguichi M, Kawase Y, Kanda T. Congenital stationary night blindness with negative electroretinogram. A new classification. *Arch Ophthalmol* 1986;104:1013–1020.
28. Miyake Y, Horiguchi M, Ota I, Shiroyama N. Characteristic ERG flicker anomaly in incomplete congenital stationary night blindness. *Invest Ophthalmol Visual Sci* 1987;28:1816–1823.
29. Miyake Y. Incomplete-type congenital stationary night blindness. In *Principles and Practice of Clinical Electrophysiology of Vision,* J. R. Heckenlively and G. B. Arden, eds. St. Louis: Mosby-Year Book, 1991, pp. 721–725.
30. Mizuo G. On a new discovery in the dark adaptation of Oguchi's disease. *Acta Soc Ophthalmol Jpn* 1913;17:1148–1150.
31. Musarella MA, Weleber RG, Murphey WH, Young RSL, Anson-Cartwright, Mets M, Kraft SP, Polemeno R, Litt M, Worton RG. Assignment of the gene for complete X-linked congenital stationary night blindness (CSNB1) to Xp11.3. *Genomics* 1989;5:727–737.
32. Nettleship, E. A history of congenital stationary night blindness in nine consecutive generations. *Trans Ophthalmol Soc UK* 1907;27:269–293.
33. Oguchi C. Ueber die eigenartige Hemeralopie mit diffuser weissgraulicher Verfargung des Augenhintergrundes. *Graefes Arch Clin Ophthalmol* 1912;81:109–117.
34. Pearch WG, Reedyk M, Coupland SG. Variable expressivity in X-linked congenital stationary night blindness. *Can J Ophthalmol* 1990;25: 3–10.
35. Rosenberg T, Schwartz M, Simonsen SE. Åland Eye Disease (Forsius-Eriksson-Miyake syndrome) with probability established in a Danish family. *Acta Ophthalmol* 1990;68:281–291.
36. Schubert G, Bornschein H. Beitrag zur Analyse des menschlichen electroretinogram. *Ophthalmologica* 1952;123:396–413.
37. Schwartz M, Rosenberg T. Åland island eye disease: Linkage data. *Genomics* 1991;10:327–332.
38. Siegel IM, Greenstein VC, Seiple W, Carr RE. Cone function in congenital nyctalopia. *Doc Ophthalmol* 1987;65:307–318.
39. Sieving PA, Richard JE, Bingham EL, Naarendorp F. Dominant congenital complete nyctalopia and Gly90Asp rhodopsin mutation. *Invest Ophthalmol Visual Sci* (Suppl) 1992;33:1397.
40. Takagi R, Kawakami R. Uber da Wesen der Oguchischer Krankheit. *Klin Monatsbl Augenheilkd* 1924;72:349–371.
41. Vaghefi A, Vaghefi HA, Green WR, Kelley JS, Sloan LL, Hoover RE, Patz A. Correlation of clinicopathologic findings in a patient. *Arch Ophthalmol* 1978;96:2097.

42. Watanabe I, Taniguchi Y, Morioka K, Kato M. Congenital stationary nightblindness with myopia: A clinico-pathologic study. *Doc Ophthalmol* 1986;63:55.
43. Weleber RG, Pillers DA, Powell BR, et al. Åland Island eye disease (Forsius–Eriksson syndrome) associated with contiguous deletion syndrome at Xp21. Similarity to incomplete congenital stationary night blindness. *Arch Ophthalmol* 1989;107:1170–1179.
44. Witzel DA, Smith EL, Wilson RD, Aquirre GD: Congenital stationary nightblindness: An animal model. *Invest Ophthalmol Visual Sci* 1978; 17:788.

23

Choroideremia

IAN M. MACDONALD

Choroideremia (CHM) is an X-linked progressive chorioretinal degeneration. Mauthner first described the disorder in 1871 and coined the term *choroideremia* as he believed the condition represented a congenital absence of the choroid. The disorder intrigued a number of notable ophthalmologists, including Sir Duke-Elder who could not explain why the eye should maintain its normal physiology in the face of extensive chorioretinal atrophy.[11] The lack of histopathological material from patients with this condition limited many theoretical explanations. Mann considered that choroideremia might have resulted from abnormal development: either of the vascular tree of ciliary arteries from the ophthalmic arteries or the retinal pigment epithelium (RPE) from the optic cup.[29] Careful clinical observations by Pameyer and co-workers disputed these theories, and they proposed that the disorder was primarily an abiotrophy of the RPE with a secondary degeneration of the choriocapillaris and outer retinal layers.[39] Pameyer pointed out that the disorder was not a dysplasia or a dystrophy, but in fact, a degeneration. The authors also reviewed many of the important findings of an earlier study by McCulloch and McCulloch.[31] The McCullochs had studied a large Canadian kindred and provided an extensive inventory of the clinical features of the disorder in 33 males and 53 carriers. They correctly concluded that the theory of congenital absence of the choroid was impossible without histopathologic evidence that was then unavailable. They also disputed the suggestion of Verhoeff that choroideremia was a form of retinitis pigmentosa (RP).[58] They succinctly expressed that affected males and carrier females had clinical features distinct from those of classical RP and that the two diagnoses were separate.

CLINICAL MANIFESTATIONS

Choroideremia primarily affects males. Night blindness and progressive loss of peripheral vision become evident by the second and third decade of life in most patients. In some cases, these symptoms appear in the first decade of life. Patients complain first of night blindness. In general, and after a period of thirty-five years from the onset of symptoms, males with choroideremia will be significantly limited in terms of peripheral field.[31] The early findings in a male with choroideremia are very similar to those of carrier females. Areas of RPE disruption are first noted in the mid-peripheral fundus. Chorioretinal atrophy becomes more maked and there is progression from loss of choriocapillaris, to the exposure of choroidal vessels, and finally to denuded large areas of bare sclera between the macula and the ora serrata (Fig. 23.1). Small amounts of intraretinal pigment may be seen in a random distribution, but the pigment is not dispersed as bone spicules such as those seen in RP. In all cases, central visual acuity is well maintained until quite late in the course of the disease despite substantial loss of peripheral vision. By contrast, many patients with RP have a parallel decrease in visual acuity and peripheral field.

Female carriers of choroideremia can be identified clinically by the presence of patchy areas of retinal pigment epithelial atrophy (Fig. 23.2). Although earlier reports did not consider these findings to be progressive,[31] subsequent observations documented mild progression.[14,24] Ophthalmologists may be reluctant to assign carrier status to a girl in a family with choroideremia unless her father was affected. As she becomes older, clinical findings may be more evident. Fluorescein angiography has been advocated by van Dorp and van Balen as a supplemental examination in the investigation of female carriers.[57] In a case reported by them, the intravenous fluorescein angiogram was more predictive of carrier status than the clinical examination. There are reports of occasional female patients who are fully affected by choroideremia.[16] Harris and Miller reported a female CHM carrier with constricted visual fields, an extinguished ERG, and significant elevation of the cone and rod thresholds on dark adaptation.[20] Burke and colleagues described a CHM carrier with fundus and fluorescein angiographic findings identical to those of an affected male. Nonrandom inactivation of the normal X-chromosome, the Lyon hypothesis, has traditionally been used to explain the clinical findings in affected females. This hypothesis has not satisfied some authors.[16,20] The similarity of the distribution of findings in males and carriers and the rare occurrence of female cases suggest that gene dosage could equally be very important in controlling the manifestations of this disorder. Haploinsufficiency of the CHM gene product would explain the findings in carrier females, but would not explain the lack of findings in the normal hemizygous male with only one copy of the CHM gene product.

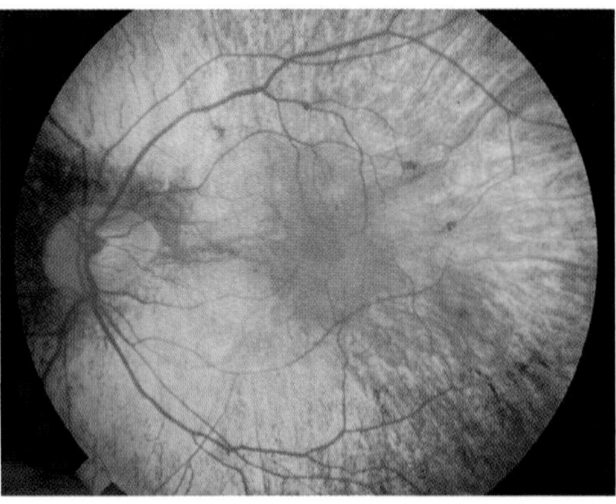

Figure 23.1. Fundus photograph of a male choroideremia patient with extensive chorioretinal atrophy and preservation of the central macula.

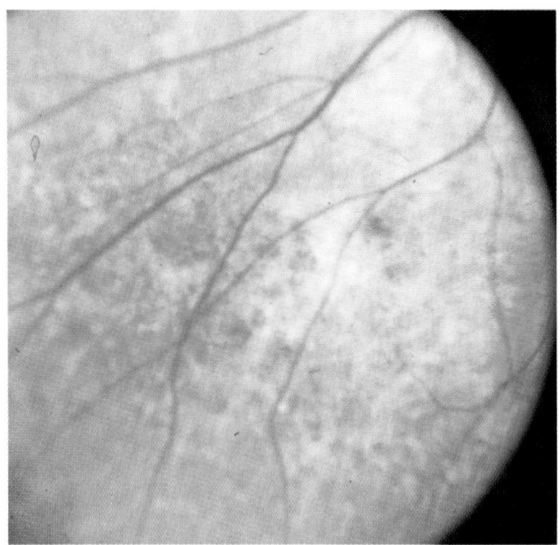

Figure 23.2. Fundus photograph of a choroideremia (CHM) carrier with areas of retinal pigment epithelial thinning and atrophy.

VISUAL FUNCTION TESTS

Color vision is normal in choroideremia.[39] Myopia is found more commonly in affected males than in the general population, but glaucoma is uncommon.[24] Visual fields in affected males show significant loss with preservation of the central 5 degrees until late in life.[39] There is no correlation between specific mutations in the CHM gene and the rate of progression of visual field loss.[43] Carriers do not in general have visual field defects, except perhaps enlargement of the blind spot.[39]

The electroretinogram (ERG) and electrooculogram (EOG) do not add to the clinical examination and the family history in establishing a diagnosis of choroideremia. The ERG is abnormal in males and will show progressive deterioration.[48] François stated that the ERG and EOG were normal CHM carriers.[15] Lachapelle and Little have noted that in some carriers of choroideremia, there is an abnormal light-adaptation effect where the photopic (cone) ERG recorded at the onset of the light-adaptation process is significantly smaller than normal, while that obtained at the end of light adaptation is normal.[26] The most significant ERG modifications affect OP4, the largest oscillatory potential of the cone ERG. Pinckers and colleagues reported that the EOG in CHM carriers did not differ significantly from controls.[40] In a study of 26 obligate carriers of choroideremia by Sieving and colleagues using three tests, a blue flash, a dark-adapted white flash, and a white 30 Hz flicker, no single test was abnormal in all carriers and no carrier had abnormal amplitudes on all three tests.[48] Whereas the ERG was normal in most cases, 25 of the 26 obligate carriers could be identified by fundus examination. Clinical examination therefore provides the best evidence of carrier status.

ASSOCIATED CONDITIONS

Choroideremia is usually not associated with nonocular systemic disorders. Van den Bosch reported a syndrome of choroideremia, mental retardation, acrokeratosis verruciformis, recurrent bronchial and skin infections in three generations of a Dutch pedigree. He considered that the disorder likely represented a *complex of genes on the X chromosome.* A submicroscopic deletion at the CHM locus has been postulated to explain the coincident finding of choroideremia and hypopituitarism in two unrelated Caucasian patients.[32]

Although catalogued as a discrete disorder, choroideremia and deafness (MIM 303110) likely represent a contiguous gene syndrome. DFN3, X-linked deafness with perilymphatic gusher, is a distinct genetic disorder and maps to the same region as choroideremia.[33] The gene for this disorder, *POU3F4* has recently been isolated.[9]

DIFFERENTIAL DIAGNOSIS

If a patient has classical clinical signs of chorioretinal atrophy and a family history of an X-linked disorder, the diagnosis of choroideremia can be made with some certainty. Both choroideremia and RP exhibit X-linked inheritance. The end stages of RP with widespread chorioretinal atrophy may be confused with the end stages of choroideremia. The cardinal features of RP: posterior subcapsular cataracts, retinal vessel attenuation, waxy pallor of the optic disc, occasional optic nerve head drusen, bone spicule pigment dispersion into the retina, and vitreous cells, are all not seen in choroideremia.

Mapping data for X-linked RP clearly defines two loci on the short arm of the X chromosome at Xp11 (RP2)[59] and Xp21 (RP3).[35] Choroideremia maps to Xq21 by linkage analysis,[27,36] deletion[4,42] and translocation patients.[34]

Gyrate atrophy of the choroid and retina may present with signs and symptoms similar to those of choroideremia.[21] Patients with gyrate atrophy have symptoms of nyctalopia and peripheral field loss by the first decade of life.[23] They have axial myopia, which is also seen in choroideremia.[24] In gyrate atrophy, abruptly defined circinate areas of chorioretinal atrophy begin in the periphery and coalesce with time. As with choroideremia, the symptoms and signs are confined to the eye. Gyrate atrophy is differentiated from choroideremia as an autosomal recessive trait with associated serum hyperonithinemia[50] due to deficiency of ornithine aminotransferase.[52] Choroideremia is not associated with abnormal levels of any of the serum amino acids.

The older literature referred to diffuse choroidal sclerosis and high myopia as entities that could be confused with choroideremia.[31] The chorioretinal atrophy in high myopia is centered on the disc and macula, unlike that in choroideremia, which begins in the peripheral fundus. There are some forms of heritable choroidal atrophy (diffuse choroidal atrophy, diffuse choriocapillaris atrophy, generalized choroidal sclerosis) that mimic choroideremia but follow an autosomal dominant pattern of inheritance.[21]

HISTOPATHOLOGY

Ghosh and McCulloch reported light and electron microscopic findings of eyes from two males, aged 65 and 71 with advanced clinical signs of choroideremia.[18] The principal findings were extensive loss of photoreceptor outer segments, broadening of Bruch's membrane and the basement membrane of the retinal pigment epithelium, thickening of the internal elastic lamina, and formation of an epiretinal membrane. In a histopathologic study of a 66-year-old male with choroideremia, Cameron and colleagues noted that there was fragmentation of Bruch's membrane. Also, the basement membrane between pericytes and endothelial cells was fragmented, and the basement membrane of the vascular endothelium of uveal vessels was attenuated.[3] Atrophy of RPE and overlying retina in the posterior segment, and thinning of the iris pigment epithelium and atrophy of the dilator muscle in the anterior segment were thought to be secondary effects.[3] These investigators hypothesized that the primary defect is located in the vessels of the uveal tract and that the other findings were secondary. Fluorescein angiography of CHM carriers by Forsius and colleagues showed that the choroidal circulation was affected.[14] Instead of an initial appearance of the choroidal flush, the choroidal circulation was delayed such that the retinal and choroidal circulation appeared to fill simultaneously. In more severely affected females or males, filling of the retinal circulation preceded that of the choroidal circulation.

In a younger patient, a 19-year-old male with choroideremia, preretinal gliosis was not yet evident. There were areas of relatively preserved RPE and overlying retina, and the underlying choriocapillaris was intact. Affected areas showed loss of choriocapillaris with overlying loss of Bruch's membrane, RPE, and retina. Occasional retinal rosettes were noted. Macrophages with pigment and rod-like profiles were noted in both the RPE and the retina.[41]

Three eyes from female carriers of choroideremia have been reported. In the first case studied by Krill, areas of RPE atrophy or areas of pigment clumping were noted, suggesting that the primary defect in CHM was at the level of the RPE.[25] A second study of a female carrier's eye by Ghosh and co-workers suggested that the defect was at the retina–RPE interface, as the RPE was relatively normal.[19] The most recent report by Flannery and colleagues showed that the RPE was abnormal throughout the retina, not simply in areas in which the overlying photoreceptors were abnormal.[13] In contrast, the choriocapillaris was normal only in areas where the retina appeared normal, and was atrophic in areas where the photoreceptors were abnormal. The RPE showed variability in the amount of pigmentation and thickness. There were areas of sharp demarcation between normal-appearing RPE and retina, and areas lacking RPE and outer segments. Bruch's membrane was thickened throughout the retina. The histopathologic changes noted in the carrier eye parallel the geographic distribution of clinical findings, being concentrated in the mid-peripheral fundus. In a light microscopic study of a CHM carrier female eye from our center, thinning of the RPE was noted in the mid-peripheral fundus (Fig. 23.3).[28] Remarkable pleiomorphism of the RPE layer was seen with scanning electron microscopy. The normal ordered array of RPE cells had been replaced by cells of varying shape and size (Fig. 23.4).

LINKAGE AND ISOLATION OF THE GENE

Choroideremia is one of a few examples where the technique of positional cloning has resulted in the isolation of a gene. This approach first maps the location of the gene using linkage analysis. Early linkage studies suggested that choroideremia was not linked to the Xg blood group.[38] With the advent of DNA-based technology, restriction fragment length polymor-

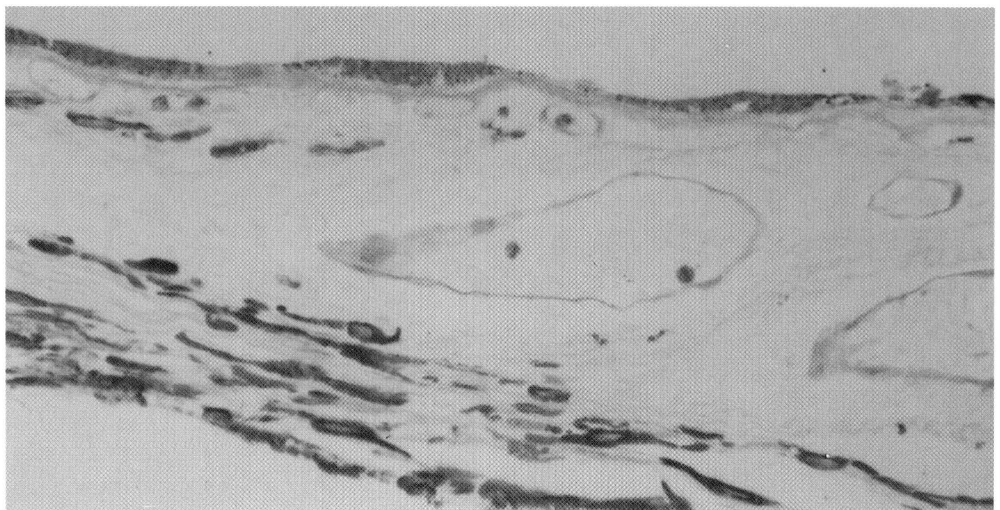

Figure 23.3. Light microscopy of an eye from a 89-year-old female carrier of choroideremia (CHM) with the areas of retinal pigment epithelial thinning and relative hypocellularity of the choroid in the mid-periphery (stained with hematoxylin, eosin ×425).

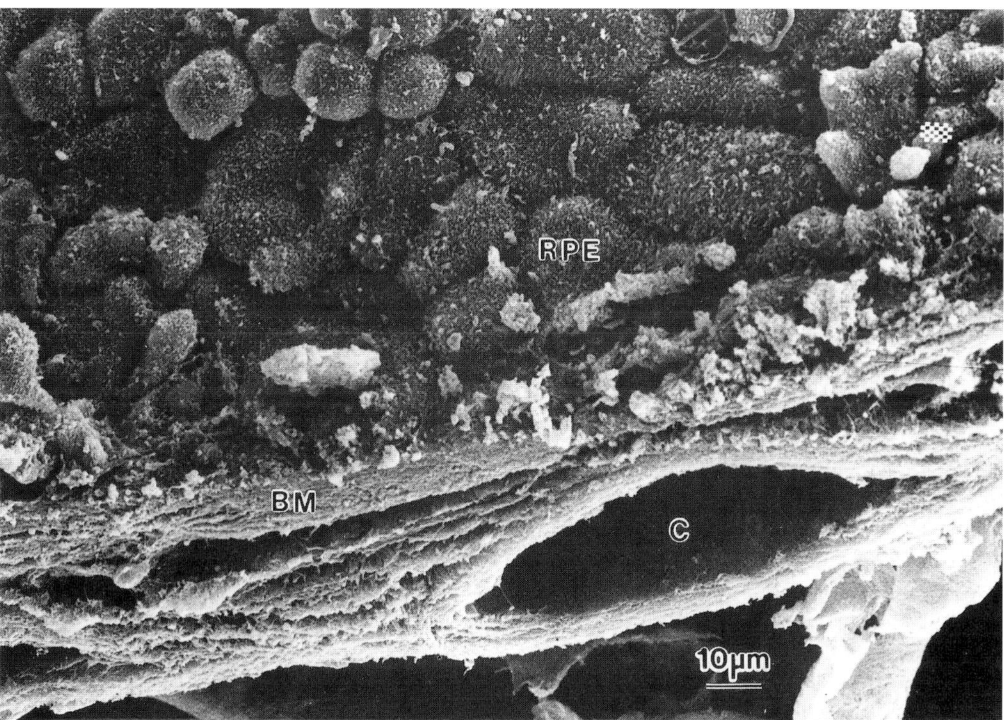

Figure 23.4. Scanning electron micrograph of a cross-section from the mid-periphery of the eye of the female choroideremia (CHM) carrier in Fig. 23.4 showing marked differences in size and shape of RPE cells (RPE, retinal pigment epithelium; BM, basement membrane; C, choriocapillaris).

phic (RFLP) markers became available to map the location of the choroideremia gene. The first published studies using RFLPs defined a map location in a broad region: Xq12-21.[27,37]

An interstitial deletion of Xq21 [del(X) (q21.1::q21.33] in a young boy with choroideremia, mental retardation, cleft lip and palate, and agenesis of the corpus callosum further narrowed the locus for choroideremia.[42] The mother and sister were both phenotypically normal, but both had fundus findings of the carrier state of choroideremia, most marked in the mid-periphery. Another case of an interstitial deletion of Xq21.1 was found in a male with choroideremia and mental retardation.[22] In this case the mother and the sister also carried the deleted chromosome and had fundus findings consistent with the carrier state of choroideremia. In two families reported by Nussbaum and co-workers, choroideremia segregated with mental retardation and deafness.[36] In one of these families there was a visible deletion of Xq21 and in the other a deletion could not be confirmed by cytogenetics. These families afforded the possibility of isolating sequences that were deleted in these patients and that contained the gene for choroideremia. In some submicroscopic deletion cases where choroideremia was the only clinical manifestation, the marker DXS165 was found to be deleted.[4] Using this marker as a starting point, Cremers and co-workers[5] defined four breakpoints in patients with classical choroideremia and microdeletions, and they characterized the breakpoint in a female choroideremia patient with an (X;13)(q21.2;p12) translocation.[49] From a region of approximately 45 kb, containing most of the deletions, Cremers and co-workers derived a single copy sequence which was conserved across species and revealed a message with Northern analysis.[6] This clone was then used to isolate 8 overlapping cDNAs comprising a 4.5 kb segment with an open reading frame (ORF). Surprisingly, this candidate gene was expressed in retina, choroid, RPE, and also lymphocytes—an unexpected result for a disorder that was thought only to affect the eye.

The choroideremia gene comprises 15 exons spanning approximately 150 kb.[53] The ORF was disrupted in ten male CHM patients with known cytogenetic deletions and one female CHM patient with a balanced translocation at the choroideremia locus.[56] Schwartz and colleagues searched for mutations in twelve Danish patients with choroideremia by PCR-single strand conformation polymorphism (PCR-SSCP) analysis and found six different mutations.[44] All mutations were predicted to result in translation of an mRNA that would result in a truncated gene product or no gene product at all. It was later stated that all mutations in the CHM gene in families of European origin create stop codons in the coding sequence of the gene and result in a truncated protein product.[54] To date, this is apparently the case for most cases of choroideremia except in one case reported by Donnelly and colleagues where a missense mutation was found.[10]

BIOCHEMISTRY

The CHM gene encodes the Rab escort protein-1 (REP-1) of geranylgeranyl transferase (GGT).[46] The escort protein, previously termed *component A*, presents the Rab protein to the catalytic site of the enzyme. The enzyme adds geranylgeranyl (20 carbon) groups to two cysteines of the carboxy-terminus of Rab proteins.[45] Recently, Seabra and colleagues, using recombinant REP-1, showed that in vitro REP-1 participated in the prenylation of a novel specific Rab protein (Rab27).[47] Normally Rab 27 is present in the membrane fractions from cells. In CHM patients, up to 70% of Rab27 was found in the cytosol in the unprenylated state. It was further demonstrated by immunohistochemistry that Rab27 was normally expressed in the RPE and choroid. REP-1 presumably binds preferentially to certain Rabs, such as Rab 27, and acts as a molecular "chaperone" to target these Rabs to their final destination in the cell membrane.[12] The actual pathogenesis of the chorioretinal degeneration that occurs in choroideremia must still be determined. Now that its biochemistry is better understood, attempts might be made for a treatment.

The clinical effect of the lack of the normal gene product (REP-1) is seen only in the eye; other tissues appear not to be affected. A theoretical explanation for the ocular specificity of the disorder was not plausible until the discovery of the choroideremia-like (CHML) gene, which encodes REP-2.[8] It has been suggested that the presence of REP-2 in tissues other than the eye is sufficient to maintain normal function in those tissues. Mutations in the CHML gene may cause other disorders. CHML was viewed as a possible candidate gene for Usher syndrome (USH2A);[7] however, PCR-SSCP analysis in ten Dutch families and nine Danish families did not detect a mutation.[52]

MANAGEMENT

At present there is no treatment for choroideremia. Patients with choroideremia may benefit from career counseling and referral to agencies and patient support groups who deal with the blind. Patients and families need support and an identifiable source for information on this disorder. They need help in coping with the diagnosis and answering questions about the future course of the disease. In some cases, genetic counseling may be requested by the family.

Although prenatal diagnosis of this condition is available, patients and families differ in their attitude toward screening and diagnostic testing. From personal experience, some individuals have requested termination of a male fetus when molecular testing could not determine if the fetus was affected. Others have shown no intention of undergoing prenatal testing or screening to determine if they were carriers. This variability would appear at first to be in direct correlation with how severely the disorder has affected a close male relative. In a survey of Finnish CHM patients by Furu and co-workers there was surprisingly no correlation between the severity of CHM and the acceptance of termination of pregnancy.[17] Only 30% indicated that they would hypothetically opt for abortion if offered prenatal diagnosis.

Acknowledgments: The light micrograph was provided with the assistance of David Addison, University of Ottawa. The scanning micrograph was prepared with the technical assistance of Nancy Nesslinger and Ming Chen, University of Alberta. Clinical photographs were from a personal collection and a patient of John Parker, Toronto. I also acknowledge the constant support and interest of families with choroideremia whom I have seen throughout my research and clinical career.

REFERENCES

1. Ayazi S. Choroideremia, obesity, and congenital deafness. *Am J Ophthalmol* 1981;92:63–69.
2. Burke MJ, Choromokos EA, Bibler L, Sanitato JJ. Choroideremia in a genotypically normal female. A case report. *Ophthalmic Pediatr Genet* 1985;6:163–168.
3. Cameron JD, Fine BS, Shapiro I. Histopathologic observations in choroideremia with emphasis on vascular changes of the uveal tract. *Ophthalmology* 1987;94:187–196.
4. Cremers FPM, Brunsmann F, van de Pol TJR, Pawlowitzki IH, Paulsen K, Wieringa B, Ropers HH. Deletion of the DXS165 locus in patients with classical choroideremia. *Clin Genet* 1987; 32:421–423.
5. Cremers FPM, van de Pol DJR, Wieringa B, Collins FS, Sankila E-M, Siu VM, Flintoff WF, Brunsmann F, Blonden LAJ, Ropers HH. Chromosomal jumping from the DXS165 locus allows molecular characterization of four microdeletions and a *de novo* chromosome X/13 translocation associated with choroideremia. *Proc Natl Acad Sci USA* 1989;86:7510–7514.
6. Cremers FPM, van de Pol TJR, van Kerkhoff LPM, et al. Cloning of a gene that is rearranged in patients with choroideremia. *Nature* 1990; 347:674–677.
7. Cremers FPM, Molloy CM, van de Pol TJR, van den Hurk JAJM, Bach I, Geurts van Kessel AHM, Ropers HH. An autosomal homologue of the choroideremia gene colocalizes with the Usher syndrome type II locus on the distal part of chromosome 1q. *Hum Mol Genet* 1992; 1:71–75.
8. Cremers FPM, Armstrong SA, Seabra MC, Brown MS, Goldstein JL. REP-2, a Rab escort protein encoded by the choroideremia-like gene. *J Biol Chem* 1994;269:2111–2117.
9. de Kok YJM, van der Maarel SM, Bitner-Glindzicz M, Huber I, Monaco AP, Malcom S, Pembrey ME, Ropers HH, Cremers FPM. Association between X-linked mixed deafness and mutations in the POU domain gene *POU3F4*. *Science* 1995;267:685–688.

10. Donnelly P, Menet H, Fouanon C, Herbert O, Moisan JP, Le Roux MG, Pascal O. Missense mutation in the choroideremia gene. *Hum Mutat* 1994;3:1017.
11. Duke-Elder S. *Text-book of Ophthalmology*, Vol. II. p. 1329–1330 London: Kimpton, 1938.
12. Fischer von Mollard G, Stahl B, Li C, Sÿdhof TC, Jahn R: Rab proteins in regulated exocytosis. *TIBS* 1994;19:164–168.
13. Flannery JG, Bird AC, Farber DB, Weleber RG, Bok D. A histopathologic study of a choroideremia carrier. *Invest Ophthalmol Visual Sci* 1990;31:229–236.
14. Forsius H, HyvŠrinen L, Nieminen H, Flower R. Fluorescein and indocyanine green fluorescence angiography in study of affected males and in female carriers with choroideremia. A preliminary report. *Acta Ophthalmol (Copenh)* 1977; 55:459–470.
15. François J. Importance of electrophysiology in ophthalmogenetics. *Ophthalmologica* 1984;188: 14–27.
16. Fraser GR, Friedmann AI. Choroideremia in a female. *Br Med J* 1968;2:732–734.
17. Furu T, KŠŠriŠinen H, Sankila E-M, Norio R. Attitudes towards prenatal diagnosis and selective abortion among patients with retinitis pigmentosa or choroideremia as well as among their relatives. *Clin Genet* 1993;43:160–165.
18. Ghosh M, McCulloch JC. Pathological findings from two cases of choroideremia. *Can J Ophthalmol* 1980;15:147–153.
19. Ghosh M, McCulloch C, Parker JA. Pathological study in a female carrier of choroideremia. *Can J Ophthalmol* 1988;23:181–186.
20. Harris GS, Miller JR. Choroideremia. Visual defects in a heterozygote. *Arch Ophthalmol* 1968;80:423–429.
21. Hayasaka S, Shoji K, Kanno C-I, Oura K, Mizuno K. Differential diagnosis of diffuse choroidal atrophies. Diffuse choriocapillaris atrophy, choroideremia, and gyrate atrophy of the choroid and retina. *Retina* 1985;5:30–37.
22. Hodgson SV, Robertson ME, Fear CN, Goodship J, Malcolm S, Jay B, Bobrow M, Pembrey ME. Prenatal diagnosis of X-linked choroideremia with mental retardation, associated with a cytologically detectable X-chromosome deletion. *Hum Genet* 1987;75:286–290.
23. Kaiser-Kupfer MI, Caruso RC, Valle D. Gyrate atrophy of the choroid and retina. Long-term reduction of ornithine slows retinal degeneration. *Arch Ophthalmol* 1991;109:1539–1548.
24. KŠrnŠ J. Choroideremia. *Acta Ophthalmologica* 1986;176(suppl):1–68.
25. Krill AE. Hereditary Retinal and Choroidal Diseases, vol 2, New York: Harper & Row, 1977: 1036–1037.
26. Lachapelle P, Little JM. Abnormal light-adaptation of the electroretinogram in some carriers of choroideremia. *Clin Vision Sci* 1992; 7:403–411.
27. Lewis RA, Nussbaum RL, Ferrell R. Mapping X-linked ophthalmic diseases. Provisional assignment of the locus for choroideremia to Xq13-q24. *Ophthalmology* 1985;92:800–880.
28. MacDonald IM, Chen MH, Addison DJ, Mielke BW, Nesslinger NJ. Histopathology of the retinal pigment epithelium of a female carrier of choroideremia. *Can J Ophthalmol* 1997;32: 329–333.
29. Mann I. Developmental Abnormalities of the Eye. p. 196. London: Cambridge University Press, 1937.
30. Mauthner H. Ein fall von choroideremia. *Naturwiss Med Verein* 1871;2:191 (cited by Bedell AJ. Choroideremia. *Arch Ophthalmol* 1937;17:444–467).
31. McCulloch C, McCulloch RJP. A hereditary and clinical study of choroideremia. *Trans Am Acad Ophthalmol Otolaryngol* 1948;52:160–190.
32. Menon RK, Ball WS, Sperling MA. Choroideremia and hypopituitarism: an association. *Am J Med Genet* 1989;34:511–513.
33. Merry DE, Lesko JG, Sosnoski DM, Lewis RA, Lubinsky M, Trask B, van den Engh G, Collins FS, Nussbaum RI. Choroideremia and deafness with stapes fixation: a contiguous gene deletion syndrome in Xq21. *Am J Hum Genet* 1989; 45:530–540.
34. Merry DE, Lesko JG, Siu V, Flintoff WF, Collins E, Lewis RA, Nussbaum RL. DXS165 detects a translocation breakpoint in a woman with choroideremia and a *de novo* X;13 translocation. *Genomics* 1990;6:609–615.
35. Musarella MA, Anson-Cartwright L, Leal SM, Gilbert LD, Worton RG, Fishman GA, Ott J. Multipoint linkage analysis and heterogeneity testing in 20 X-linked retinitis pigmentosa families. *Genomics* 1990;8:286–296.
36. Nussbaum RL, Lesko JG, Lewis RA, Ledbetter SA, Ledbetter DH. Isolation of anonymous DNA sequences from within a submicroscopic X chromosomal deletion in a patient with choroideremia, deafness, and mental retardation. *Proc Natl Acad Sci USA* 1987;84:6521–6525.
37. Nussbaum RL, Lewis RA, Lesko JG, Ferrell R. Choroideremia is linked to the restriction fragment length polymorphism *DXYS1* at Xq13-21. *Am J Hum Genet* 1985;37:473–481.

38. Other A. Choroideremia and the Xg blood group. *Acta Ophthalmol (Copenh)* 1968;46:79–82.
39. Pameyer JK, Waardenburg PJ, Henkes HE. Choroideremia. *Br J Ophthalmol* 1960;44:724–738.
40. Pinckers A, van Aarem A, Brink H. The electro-oculogram in heterozygote carriers of Usher syndrome, retinitis pigmentosa, neuronal ceroid lipofuscinosis, Senior syndrome and choroideremia. *Ophthalmic Genet* 1994;15:25–30.
41. Rodrigues MM, Ballintine EJ, Wiggert BN, Lee L, Fletcher RT, Chader GJ. Choroideremia: A clinical, electron microscopic, and biochemical report. *Ophthalmology* 1984;91:873–883.
42. Rosenberg T, Schwartz M, Niebuhr E, Yang H-M, Sardemann H, Anderson O, Launsteen C. Choroideremia in interstitial deletion of the X chromosome. *Ophthalmic Pediatr Genet* 1986; 7:205–210.
43. Rosenberg T, Schwartz M. Age differences of visual field impairment and mutation spectrum in Danish choroideremia patients. *Acta Ophthalmol (Copenh)* 1994;72:678–682.
44. Schwartz M, Rosenberg T, van den Hurk JAJM, van de Pol DJR, Cremers FPM. Identification of mutations in Danish choroideremia families. *Hum Mutat* 1993;2:43–47.
45. Seabra MC, Brown MS, Slaughter CA, Sÿdhof TC, Goldstein JL. Purification of component A of Rab geranylgeranyl transferase: possible identity with the choroideremia gene product. *Cell* 1992;70:1049–1057.
46. Seabra MC, Brown MS, Goldstein JL. Retinal degeneration in choroideremia: deficiency of Rab geranylgeranyl transferase. *Science* 1993; 259:377–381.
47. Seabra MC, Ho YK, Anant JS. Deficient geranylgeranylation of Ram/Rab27 in choroideremia. *J Biol Chem* 1995;270:24420–24427.
48. Sieving PA, Niffenegger JH, Berson EL. Electroretinographic findings in selected pedigrees with choroideremia. *Am J Ophthalmol* 1986; 101:361–367.
49. Siu VM, Gonder JR, Jung JH, Sergovich FR, Flintoff WF. Choroideremia associated with an X-autosomal translocation. *Hum Genet* 1990; 84:459–464.
50. Takki K, Simell O. Genetic aspects in gyrate atrophy of the choroid and retina with hyperornithinemia. *Br J Ophthalmol* 1974; 58:907–916.
51. Valle D, Kaiser-Kupfer MI, Del Valle LA. Gyrate atrophy of the choroid and retina: deficiency of ornithine aminotransferase in transformed lymphocytes. *Proc Natl Acad Sci USA* 1974; 11:5159–5161.
52. van Bokhoven H, van Genderen C, Molloy CM, van de Pol DJR, Cremers CWRJ, van Aarem A, Schwartz M, Rosenberg T, Geurts van Kessel AHM, Ropers HH, Cremers FPM. Mapping of the choroideremia-like (CHML) gene at 1q42-qter and mutation analysis in patients with Usher syndrome type II. *Genomics* 1994;19: 385–387.
53. van Bokhoven H, van den Hurk JAJM, Bogerd L, Philippe C, Gilgenkrantz S, de Jong P, Ropers H-H, Cremers FPM. Cloning and characterization of the human choroideremia gene. *Hum Mol Genet* 1994;3:1041–1046.
54. van Bokhoven H, Schwartz M, Andréasson S, van den Hurk JAJM, Bogerd L, Jay M, Rÿther K, Jay B, Pawlowitzki IH, Sankila E-M, Wright A, Ropers H-H, Rosenberg T, Cremers FPM. Mutation spectrum in the CHM gene of Danish and Swedish choroideremia patients. *Hum Mol Genet* 1994;3:1047–1051.
55. van den Bosch J. A new syndrome in three generations of a Dutch family. *Ophthalmologica* 1959;137:422–423.
56. van den Hurk JAJM, van de Pol TJR, Molloy CM, Brunsmann F, Rÿther K, Zrenner E, Pinckers AJLG, Pawlowitzki IH, Blecker-Wagermakers EM, Wieringa B, Ropers H-H, Cremers FPM. Detection and characterization of point mutations in the choroideremia candidate gene by PCR-SSCP analysis and direct DNA sequencing. *Am J Hum Genet* 1992;50:1195–1202.
57. van Dorp DB, van Balen ATM. Fluorescein angiography in potential carriers for choroideremia. *Ophthalmic Pediatr Genet* 1985;5:25–30.
58. Verhoeff FH. Retinitis pigmentosa with widespread gliosis—so-called choroideremia. *Arch Ophthalmol* 1942;27:688–691.
59. Wright AF, Bhattacharya SS, Aldred MA, Jay M, Carothers AD, Thomas NST, Bird AC, Jay B, Evans HJ. Genetic localization of the RP2 type of X linked retinitis pigmentosa in a large kindred. *J Med Genet* 1991;28:453–457.

24

Genetics of Age-Related Maculopathy

MICHAEL B. GORIN

Age-related maculopathy (ARM) is one of the leading causes of untreatable visual loss in the elderly population in the United States and most developed countries. Also known as age-related macular degeneration and senile macular degeneration, age-related maculopathy[74] encompasses a broad spectrum of macular changes and complications. The term *age-related maculopathy* is preferable in genetic discussions of this condition because we must consider the status of the disease in eyes that have not experienced a decline in visual acuity or significant degeneration. ARM includes the entire spectrum of the disease process including retinal pigment epithelial (RPE) and/or choroidal atrophy and the disruption of the macula by the sequelae of subretinal neovascular membranes. In the section addressing the definition of ARM, it should become clear that even ARM is an inadequate term to describe the group of conditions that have previously been clinically defined as age-related macular degeneration.

ARM is a heterogeneous collection of disorders and the familial nature of these conditions has been repeatedly acknowledged.[45,49,65,73,153] Until recently, the majority of ARM research has focused on the histopathology and biochemical derangements, and the evaluation of environmental and dietary risk factors.[2,4,12,30,42,54,84,86,102,105,147] However, the development of new molecular genetic tools and new computational methods has allowed the genetics of ARM to be reconsidered. There has also been a fundamental change in our perception of complex genetic disorders, which includes a better understanding of the interaction of genes and exogenous factors. In this chapter we reevaluate the clinical definition of ARM, the evidence that ARM is a collection of genetic disorders, the relationship of ARM to other hereditary macular dystrophies, the strategies for identifying genes that contribute to ARM, and the promise of current and future genetic studies of ARM.

EPIDEMIOLOGY

The prevalence of ARM is highly dependent on the definition of the condition, how it is classified and graded, and the population under consideration. The Framingham Eye Study evaluated 2631 persons between the ages of 52 and 85 years using ophthalmology residents to document macular lesions.[96] ARM as defined by macular changes and a visual acuity of 20/30 or worse was diagnosed in 5.7% of the entire sample population with a prevalence of 1.2% for the 52- to 64-year-old group, rising to 19.7% for individuals between the ages of 75 and 85 years.[76] In contrast, when only macular

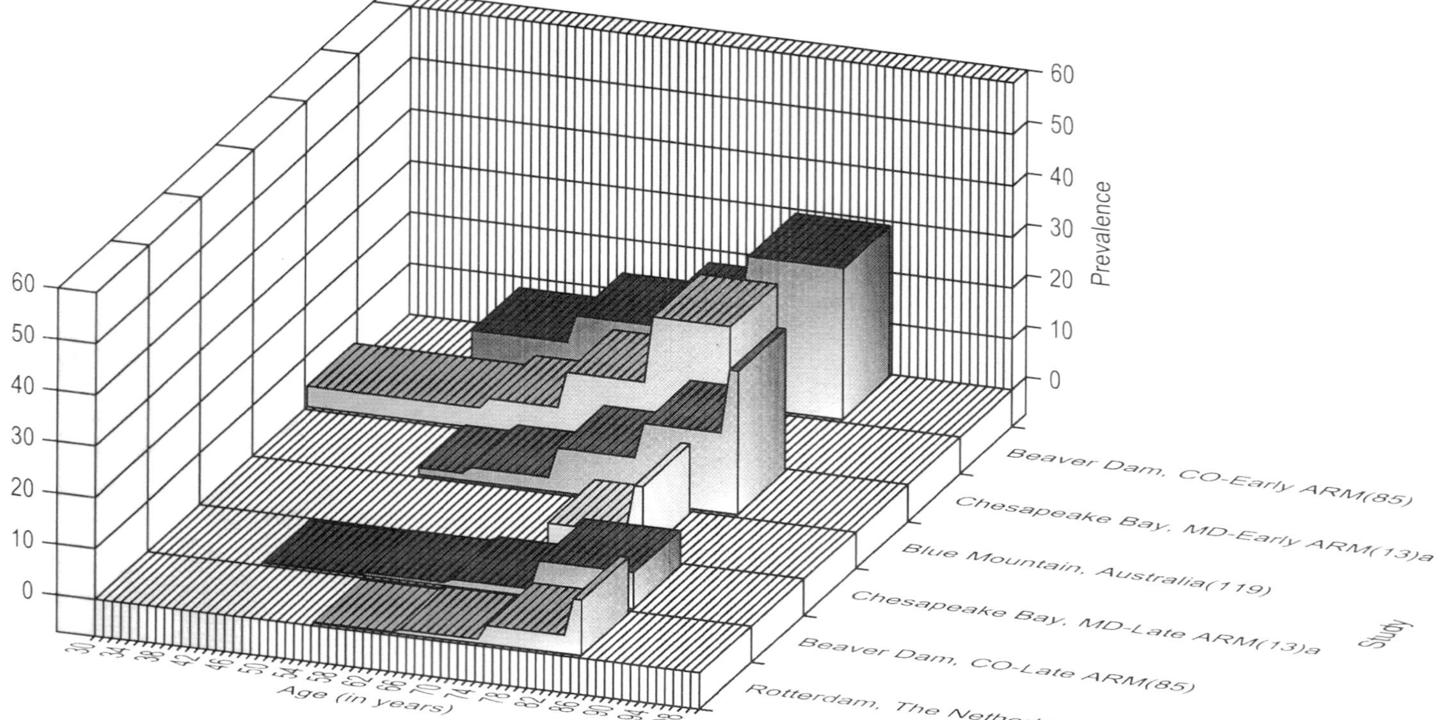

Figure 24.1. Prevalence of age-related maculopathy (ARM) in men and women based on the Wisconsin age-related maculopathy grading system criteria. a = Early ARM refers to soft drusen, men only studied.

changes were considered independently of visual acuity, the prevalence of moderate to severe abnormalities was 18% in those 52–64 years and increased to 36% in those between the ages of 75 and 85 years.[158] The National Health and Nutrition Examination Survey (1971–1972)[46,81] defined ARM in terms of macular degeneration and visual acuity of 20/25 or worse. In that study, a 0.3% prevalence of ARM was present in those between 25 and 34 years. The prevalence rose to 3% for those between 55 and 64 years and up to 8.5% for persons between 65 and 74 years. Comparable results were found in a population survey of individuals aged 65 years and older in New Zealand,[106] Iceland,[75] rural England,[51] and Denmark,[171] and in two studies of an Australian population over the age of 50 years.[119,120] In a survey of 1019 individuals over the age of 50 years (up to age 98) from various regions in China, Wu[187] reported a prevalence of ARM rising from 7.7% in those 50–59 to 22.5% for those aged 70–98 with an overall prevalence of 10.6%. The most extensive epidemiologic surveys of ARM were the Beaver Dam Eye Study,[85] which surveyed 4926 individuals between the ages of 43 and 86 years and the Rotterdam study[174] of 6251 subjects who were over 55. The clinical findings were graded from standardized photographs using the Wisconsin grading system. Visual acuity was not included in the grading system. The overall prevalence of advanced age-related maculopathy in the Beaver Dam population was 1.6%. Exudative lesions were present in at least one eye of 1.2% of the participants and geographic atrophy in 0.6% of cases. This was comparable to the 1.5% prevalence of advanced ARM in those over 52 years of age in the Framingham Eye Study and comparable to the prevalence of ARM in the Chesapeake Bay watermen study.[13] The age-dependent prevalence rates for ARM reported by these major studies are displayed in Figure 24.1. Despite the different criteria used by each of these studies, the age-dependent rates of ARM prevalence are remarkably similar. This suggests that all of these studies are identifying comparable disease processes. The markedly higher prevalences of early ARM changes in younger age groups in the Beaver Dam study in comparison to the ARM prevalences in the other studies suggest that the perception of ARM as a disease occurring primarily after the age of 50 years is distorted by the inclusion of visual acuity loss.

In the Framingham study (Fig. 24.2), approximately 90% of the ARM was reportedly of the "dry or atrophic" form with the remainder representing "wet or exudative disease." This is roughly comparable to the distribution of ARM reported in the Danish population by Vinding,[172] who observed 78.6% of individuals with ARM to have the atrophic form of the disease while 21.4% of the individuals had the exudative form. In contrast, the study by Wu[187] identified exudative forms of ARM in only 4% of the ARM cases. It is unknown if this marked disparity in the prevalences of endstage forms of ARM is a reflection of environmental or genetic differences between different populations.

A DEFINITION OF ARM

Most epidemiologic and case studies of ARM employ a broad definition that may or may not include the presence of drusen,[14,25,42,70,83,130,139,141,143,172] vision loss,[12] and endstage disease. Properly defining ARM is essential to understanding this condition as a genetic disorder. The name itself—age-related macular degeneration or age-related maculopathy—is a starting point for establishing a suitable definition of ARM. Age of onset has long been a part of the definition of ARM and has been used to delineate age-related macular disease from the juvenile, hereditary macular dystrophies.[80] Some authors have used a sharp cutoff such as the onset of symptoms after the age of 50 years,[12] while others have viewed ARM as part of a continuum that includes the juvenile hereditary dystrophies.[49,56,160] The use of an age-dependent criterion becomes more difficult when one considers the onset with respect to clinical findings or based on vision loss. It is not unusual to observe large amounts of drusen and pigment epithelial changes consistent with ARM in an individual in their forties or fifties, who may not experience vision loss for a decade or longer. Many subjects who are seen at the time they experience vision loss in their sixties

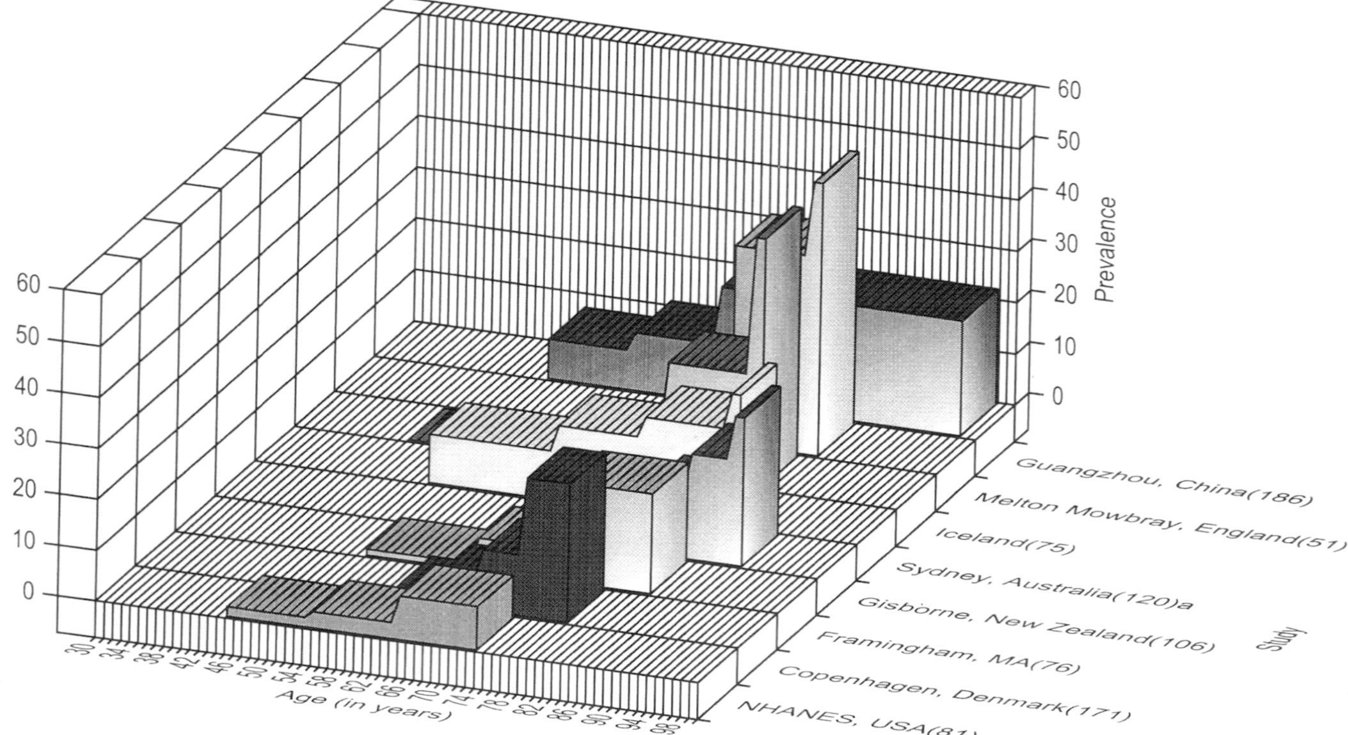

Figure 24.2. Prevalence of age-related maculopathy in men and women based on the Framingham Eye Study or similar criteria. a = Self-report only, records checked by an ophthalmologist.

or seventies report decreased ability to adapt to rapid changes in light levels for more than 10 years preceding any decline in visual acuity. Given the longstanding and progressive nature of ARM, it makes little sense to state that the person does not have the condition until vision loss is documented. Although population-based studies of ARM demonstrate a strong age-dependent prevalence, the age of onset cannot be fixed at an arbitrary cutoff in order to distinguish ARM from other hereditary macular disorders.

A more compelling example of the difficulties of using a specific age threshold for defining ARM is seen when families with several ARM-affected individuals are screened for other at-risk family members. When family members are not selected on the basis of visual acuity loss, it becomes clear that within some families, probands with late age of onset macular degeneration may have family members with significant macular pathology in their thirties and forties. Conversely, we investigated families with autosomal dominant retinal degenerations due to peripherin mutations in which the majority of affected individuals demonstrated abnormalities from childhood or early adulthood. Yet within these families there were also affected family members who have had good vision into late adulthood and some of the older affected individuals had been diagnosed initially as having age-related macular degeneration.[56] Thus, the revised definition of ARM must consider the possibility that this macular degeneration, although predominantly of late onset, may be manifested by signs and/or symptoms in younger individuals.

Having now suggested that diagnosis of age-related maculopathy should not be constrained by age-dependent criteria or specific levels of visual acuity, we must consider those clinical features that have been used to define this condition. We can turn to the name of the disorder to appreciate that historically the clinical features have been focused on those within the macular region of the retina and pigment epithelium. Drusen, geographic atrophy, pigment epithelial detachments, pigment epithelial figures, and subretinal neovascular membranes (and their sequelae) are all major features used to describe ARM. However, all of these features can also be found in other conditions. Soft, hard, and basal laminar drusen are often considered to be pathognomonic for ARM and yet it is well-recognized that other specific disorders may have deposits that are virtually indistinguishable from drusen associated with ARM, including Sorsby fundus dystrophy,[131] North Carolina macular dystrophy,[154,155] type II membranous glomerulonephritis,[99] pseudoxanthoma elasticum,[36] peripherin mutations,[56,79,183,186] familial drusen (Doyne honeycomb dystrophy,[38] and Malattia Leventinese[66]).

Pigment epithelial figures, which represent focal lesions in the pigment epithelium with both hypo- and hyperpigmentation, can be observed in quiescent central serous retinopathy. Subretinal neovascular membranes have been reported in a large number of acquired and hereditary disorders including pattern dystrophies,[40] angioid streaks, degenerative myopia, trauma, ocular histoplasmosis syndrome, inner punctate choroidopathy, juxtafoveolar telangiectasia, and postinflammatory conditions.[48] There are numerous causes of geographic RPE atrophy including photic damage, toxic causes, chronic macular edema or retinal detachment. However, once we have excluded all of the known infectious, toxic, or environmental insults to the macula, are all of the remaining conditions causing macular degeneration the result of ARM? To a large extent the diagnosis of ARM relies on the exclusion of these other causes of macular pathology. These macular findings are part of the constellation of ARM but cannot be considered pathognomonic. In fact, a small percentage of patients are inaccurately diagnosed as having ARM and are actually variants of "juvenile" hereditary dystrophies.[160]

It is increasingly clear that for some individuals, ARM does not exclusively affect the macular region of the eye. Lewis et al.[97] reported a strong association of extramacular drusen and reticular degeneration of the peripheral pigment epithelium (RDPE)[98,163] with macular findings of ARM. In a number of the ARM families that we have studied, one or more members may have advanced complications of macular degeneration such as serous pigment epithelial detachments or subretinal neovascular membranes in association with extensive reticular degeneration of the peripheral retinal pigment epithelium with numerous extramacular drusen. Other members of the family (usually younger) may show nearly comparable levels of peripheral RPE changes with only minimal drusen or RPE disturbances in the macula. The concordance of these peripheral features of ARM within our ARM families is as high as that of the macular pathology. Given the strong association of RDPE and extramacular drusen with ARM, it is logical to conclude that these family members are also at serious risk for developing the complications of ARM, even in the absence of obvious macular drusen. For this reason, photographic grading of ARM solely on the basis of macular views (such as in the Wisconsin grading system[83]) may be valuable in establishing the concordance of macular features of ARM among family members but provides an incomplete ascertainment of affected individuals.

Using the macular degeneration associated with specific peripherin mutations as an analogy for ARM, the age of onset of signs and/or symptoms may cover a large range as well as a range of phenotypes. Within a single family, one may observe affected individuals with classic drusen, others with atrophic macular degeneration and others with peripheral vision loss similar to that seen in retinitis pigmentosa.[56,79] There is also the potential that at least some of the same genes that confer susceptibility to an individual to develop ARM may be associated with a range of clinical features that do not necessarily restrict the retinal pathology to the macula.

A working clinical definition of ARM is that of a group of conditions that affect the long-term integrity and health of the retina and create an age-dependent predisposition of the macula to undergo degenerative changes that include the accumulation of drusen, pigment epithelial detachments, pigment epithelial atrophy (with or without the loss of corresponding choriocapillaris), and/or the development of subretinal or choroidal neovascular membranes. This definition does not exclude the early onset of RPE changes or even the loss of vision during early adulthood. Similarly, it does not require the loss of visual acuity or specific visual symptoms to establish the diagnosis. ARM, unlike other hereditary retinal degenerations such as retinitis pigmentosa, cone-rod, or cone dystrophies, does not appear to involve primary photoreceptor death but rather the disruption of coordinated function of the retina, RPE, and choroid. Retinal atrophy and photoreceptor degeneration appear to be secondary complications of ARM. ARM can progress through several common pathways that can cause vision loss either secondary to RPE atrophy and/or to disruption of the retinal architecture by choroidal neovascular membranes, fibrovascular scarring, subretinal fluid, and/or hemorrhage.

This definition of ARM does not exclude the potential contribution of environmental factors to progressive retinal degenerative changes. However, it distinguishes ARM from such specific environmental insults as intraoperative photic injury, trauma, infections, or drug toxicities that can directly cause macular degeneration. A corollary of this ARM definition is that ARM is a collection of conditions for which genetic susceptibility is one of the primary determinants of increased risk to an individual and family.

As there are a wide variety of clinical presentations and patterns of ARM, it is unlikely that ARM represents a homogeneous group of genetic conditions. Therefore, are the most common forms of ARM merely allelic variants for other forms of the rarer, hereditary "juvenile" macular degenerations? Until the molecular genetics of ARM are defined, this question must be left unanswered. Like retinitis pigmentosa, we must consider the possibility that multiple genes may contribute to the susceptibility of developing ARM. In some instances, alterations in different genes may be responsible for common phenotypes. In addition, we must recognize that even for a specific genetic constitution, a variety of clinical features and degrees of severity (expressivity) may be present. Finally, we must consider the interaction of multiple genes that may give rise to ARM and that ARM should be considered a complex genetic disorder, much like hypertension, glaucoma, or myopia.

EVIDENCE FOR THE GENETIC ETIOLOGY OF ARM

The familial nature of ARM was suggested by François,[45] who cited case reports of families dating back to the 1920s with classical ARM or central areolar choroidal atrophy. He concluded that both autosomal dominant and recessive inheritance patterns accounted for the disciform diseases, and that those with choroidal atrophy were genetically distinct. Epidemiologic studies have consistently shown that a positive family history is a major risk factor for developing ARM.[64,73,96] Hyman et al.'s[73] case-control study indicated that first-degree relatives of ARM patients had a 2.9-fold increased risk of developing ARM compared to a control population. Gass[49] retrospectively evaluated 200 patients with ARM and observed that 38 of his ARM patients had a positive family history. For five probands, a parent and at least one additional sibling were reportedly affected. Sixteen of the individuals reported that one parent was affected, and both parents of one individual were affected with ARM. In one family there were three affected siblings and an affected maternal grandmother, suggesting incomplete penetrance or reduced expressivity. In 10 of the 38 cases, Gass[49] was able to confirm the family histories from medical records or by direct examination. The prevalence of 19% positive family history in this retrospective study is in close agreement with the 21.6% prevalence reported by Hyman et al.[73] in their case-control study. In a case-control, prospective study of patients evaluated in a university ophthalmology clinic, Soubrane et al.[157] observed that 10% of 352 ARM patients reported having other affected family members.

In total, 24 of the 38 familial ARM cases reviewed by Gass[49] had at least one affected family member in the previous generation. This strongly suggests that autosomal dominant inheritance is relatively common. Of the 15 families described by Heinrich,[65] 4 (27%) were considered to have autosomal dominant ARM. Nearly one-third of the familial ARM cases reported by Hyman et al.[73] identified an ARM-affected parent. Meyers[115] reported that 10% of the monozygotic or dizygotic twin pairs that he evaluated for ARM had at least one parent with ARM. In the first 45 ARM families that we obtained for genetic studies, 53% were strongly suggestive of autosomal dominant inheritance, and an additional 33% provided historical data supporting autosomal dominant inheritance.[55] Because these families were recruited on the basis of having at least two living ARM-affected individuals, there may be a strong bias that would select for autosomal dominant pedigrees, as the probands were aware of other affected family members at the time they were contacted. Other studies[9,157] have suggested that autosomal recessive forms of ARM may be more common, but incomplete penetrance, variable expressivity, and limited ascertainment of the older generation could account for a portion of these "autosomal recessive" families.

These studies can only approximate the genetic contribution to ARM because of the reliance on unsubstantiated, historical data. Historical recall can cause inaccurate and biased ascertainment of familial involvement. Verification of the diagnosis in family members, particularly in a deceased generation, is often difficult. In population studies, probands are more likely to underreport ARM as they may be unaware of affected family members who have not yet experienced vision loss. In the case-control study by Hyman et al.,[73] senile macular degeneration was reported by ophthalmologists or optometrists in 19.9% of brothers and sisters of patients with ARM compared to 11.3% of self-reported siblings. An even higher percentage (29%) of siblings who were examined from ARM families with nontwin affected sibpairs were identified as having ARM.[115] Thus, a substantial number of individuals were unaware of having ARM despite having been diagnosed by an eye care specialist. A similar discrepancy between self-reporting of ARM by subjects and the results of clinical examinations was established in the Beaver Dam study.[101] The late onset of the diseases tends to cause underreporting of the condition in parents if they died at relatively young ages. The problems of historical recall of ARM among family members may account for why at least one cross-sectional study of ARM failed to detect a significant risk associated with a positive family history.[52] Despite these limitations, the majority of these population and case-control studies support the fact that a significant percentage of ARM can be considered a familial disorder.

Autosomal dominant and recessive inheritance are not the only inheritance patterns that must be considered. Pseudodominant inheritance can occur if the gene frequency is very high in the population. As noted later in this chapter, mitochondrial genes have been implicated in some forms of macular and retinal degeneration, and a number of genes involved in retinal function and disease have been localized on the X chromosome. Mitochondrial inheritance would not alter the distribution of ARM between the males and females but would cause a skew in the gender distribution of ARM affected parents. To date, no epidemiologic studies have addressed this question. One would need to account for the fact that traditionally women tend to live longer than men, which might artifactually make ARM seem more prevalent in women. Some epidemiologic studies have reported a higher prevalence of ARM in women,[96,157] but these findings are not consistent.[46,106,171] At present there is insufficient evidence to support the possibility of an X-linked dominant gene contributing to ARM development resulting in a higher prevalence of ARM in women.

Ethnic and racial variations in allele frequencies have been observed for a number of genetic conditions. For genetic disorders such as thalassemia, sickle cell disease, Tay-Sachs disease, and other lysosomal storage diseases, the higher prevalence in specific groups can be attributed to founder effects, rather than environmental or socioeconomic differences. There are several studies that suggest that ARM is less common in the black population,[23,60,156] but this was not supported by the National Health and Nutrition Examination Survey.[46] Allele frequency studies will be necessary to establish if the racial differences of ARM prevalences are valid and attributable to genetic disequilibrium or to the protective effects of ocular pigmentation.[4,166,181]

Despite distinct subgroups of ARM patients with positive family histories for more than one generation, the majority of ARM cases reported are sporadic or involve only affected sibships. Autosomal recessive inheritance could play a role in these cases, although incomplete penetrance and variable expressivity of an autosomal dominant pattern could also account for a large percentage of these cases. There also remains the possibility that some of these sporadic cases represent acquired macular degeneration from nongenetic factors.

Only two controlled genetic epidemiologic studies of ARM have been conducted to attempt to reduce the bias of family selection and historical data. The study of the Beaver Dam population[64] used comparisons of graded photographs of siblings within the community to assess the genetic relatedness of macular features of ARM. The gradings and comparisons were of individual eyes and not of individuals (in sibships). To obtain the maximal amount of information and avoid the problems caused by combining the analyses of both eyes, the segregation models were tested using data sets from the right and left eyes separately. The majority of the siblings had none or relatively mild amounts of macular changes, but the distribution of pathology was not clearly stated. The age dependence of the ARM was carefully considered and included in the model in order to account for differences in the severity of macular pathology among siblings of disparate ages. The analysis strongly supports an autosomal dominant model with a major gene effect compared to other genetic, mixed, and nongenetic models.

In a separate population-based epidemiologic study, Klaver et al.[79a] observed a relative risk for siblings (mean age of 75 years) of those with late ARM to also develop late ARM of 12.4 (95% confidence interval: 2.7–57.4). For large drusen, the relative risk in these siblings was 3.6 (95% confidence interval: 1.5–8.6). This relative risk is comparable to that seen for type I diabetes mellitus, which has been associated with less than 10 genetic loci and has been evaluated successfully by affected sibpair linkage studies.[30a]

Segregation analysis cannot distinguish how many genes may affect the macular features among all of the different families but does address the number of genes that are likely to account for the features within a family. This study and the Framingham study both relied exclusively on macular features, and thus also provide the strongest evidence of the concordance of macular changes, particularly the quality and quantity of drusen, within families. Specific differences in the characteristics of drusen with respect to fluorescein uptake,[10,14,132] choroidal perfusion,[21,131] and risks for developing neovascular membranes or geographic atrophy[10,14,49,70,129,130,141,142] have been described, but the relevance and concordance of the specific drusen characteristics in familial cases of ARM have not been established.

De la Paz et al.[32a] recently examined the clinical features of ARM in several pedigrees with multiply affected individuals. They observed considerable variability in the findings and severity of ARM among individuals within a family using a photographic grading system. These differences may be partly the result of varying ages among the family members but could also reflect true phenotypic variability. One can conclude that either multiple genes and/or factors contribute to the phenotype of ARM as well as that the current classification of ARM phenotypes may have limited relevance in genetic studies. This latter issue is perhaps reinforced by the observation of extreme phenotypic variability among individuals with mutations in the Stargardt-related ABCR gene that have been attributed to ARM.[29]

Independent support for an autosomal dominant model of ARM involving a single major gene also comes from the examination of siblings, twins, and other family members with ARM. These clinical comparisons provide valuable insights into the concordance or heterogeneity of clinical findings of ARM within and between families. The concordance of ARM in monozygotic twins was noted in the retrospective studies by Gass[49] and by François.[45] There have been several clinical descriptions of monozygotic cases of ARM.[34,113,114] In these cases, all of the affected individuals developed subretinal neovascular membranes within 16 months of their sibling. More recently, larger series of monozygotic and dizygotic twin studies of ARM have been done[82,115] which confirmed zygosity by genetic testing. Meyers[115] reported concordance of ARM in 23 of 23 monozygotic and 2 of 8 dizygotic twin pairs; this included 1 dizygotic pair that was discordant for basal laminar drusen. Klein et al.[82] noted that 8 of the 9 monozygotic twin pairs had similar fundus appearances and severities of visual impairment. In the ninth pair, one twin had advanced exudative age-related macular degeneration with vision loss in one eye, while the other had large, confluent drusen and good visual function in both eyes. Like Klein et al.[82] and other investigators,[105,115] we have observed occasional cases of monozygotic twins who have similar features of ARM but differ significantly with respect to visual loss and macular pathology because of the stochastic onset of subretinal neovascular membranes. This degree of discordance is also seen in comparisons of both eyes of individuals with ARM at different stages of the disease. When one takes into account the difference in ages of affected siblings within ARM families, the similarities in the clinical findings of ARM are comparable with those of affected monozygotic twins. This suggests that, within a family, the complexity of the genetics of ARM is relatively low. If multiple genes were responsible for the clinical phenotype then we would predict that siblings would have much less clinical concordance than that seen between monozygotic twins.

In some families, the majority of ARM-affected individuals progress with subretinal neovascular membranes while other families predominantly experience progressive geographic atrophy. Reticular degeneration of the pigment epithelium and extramacular drusen are prominent features in some families. These peripheral changes are present even in young at-risk adults and can precede clinical features in the macula. In other families, peripheral changes are minimal or inconsistent. Finally the quality, quantity, and distribution of drusen in the macula show fairly consistent patterns within families, unless there is disruption of the macula by geographic atrophy or subretinal neovascular membranes. However, much greater diversity of drusen characteristics is observed among ARM families than among members within a family, although this has been disputed recently by de la Paz et al.[32a]

We can no longer perceive genetic diseases in terms of classical Mendelian, single-gene disorders that have distinctive clinical features.

Modern ophthalmic genetics has expanded this limited view, particularly from studies of retinal degenerations. We recognize the potential for variable phenotypes from a single mutation (i.e., peripherin), variable expressivity (i.e., Best disease), and incomplete penetrance. Linkage studies have established the genetic heterogeneity of disorders with distinctive phenotypes (i.e., Bardet-Biedl syndrome)[19,89,151] and North Carolina macular dystrophy,[69] as well as for relatively common phenotypes such as for retinitis pigmentosa[72] and Stargardt disease.[50,161,188] The recent demonstration of digenic inheritance for retinitis pigmentosa[77] is an example of the interaction of multiple genes to create a disease. From these examples, we can appreciate that the genetics of ARM may be far more complex than that suggested by epidemiologic studies, segregation analyses, and twin studies. Similarly, we can begin to consider how the genetics of ARM can potentially interact with exogenous factors such as light exposure and diet.

RELATIONSHIP OF GENETIC SUSCEPTIBILITY AND DIETARY AND ENVIRONMENTAL FACTORS

The interaction of genetics and exogenous factors in ocular disease has received relatively little attention. The studies of damage to the retina from ambient light in different albino mouse strains[92,93] clearly illustrate how genetic factors can alter tissue vulnerability. We can also look to nonocular genetic conditions to appreciate the crucial roles that environment or diet have on the biological impact of an altered gene. For example, glucose 6-phosphate dehydrogenase deficiency is a relatively common enzyme deficiency that is manifested by mild anemia in most affected individuals. However, in the presence of certain medications or the ingestion of fava beans, a severe hemolytic anemia can be precipitated.[111] At least two forms of non-insulin-dependent diabetes with early onset have been shown to have autosomal dominant inheritance. For one of these conditions, individuals with maturity-onset diabetes of the young (MODY) can exhibit varying degrees of insulin resistance that make them highly susceptible to developing diabetes. The clinical course of this hereditary form of diabetes mellitus, like the other types of diabetes, can be greatly affected by diet. Sickle cell disease or trait, which is relatively common in the African and Afro-American population, places the affected individuals at risk for the precipitation of sickling crises either spontaneously or in response to exogenous conditions. Patients with xeroderma pigmentosum are extremely susceptible to developing skin cancer in response to light exposure because of defects in the DNA repair pathways. These systemic conditions illustrate the complex interplay of genetics and environmental and/or dietary factors that can affect the expression of genetic conditions. It is important to recognize that a genetic approach to ARM does not lessen the importance of understanding the contributions of diet and light exposure. However, we may be unable to appreciate the effects of exogenous factors until we can effectively clarify the genetic heterogeneity in individuals who are at risk to develop ARM.

Recently two epidemiologic studies have implicated dietary carotenoids in the development of age-related macular degeneration. Seddon et al.[147] reported that individuals with high intakes of carotenoids, specifically lutein and zeaxanthin, were found to have a 43% lower risk for macular degeneration than those with the lowest intakes of these compounds. However, a subsequent study by Mares-Perlman et al.[104] failed to confirm the association of these particular carotenoids but found that individuals with low serum levels of lycopene were twice as likely to have macular degeneration. In a creative combination of genetics and physiology, Hammond et al.[62] investigated the variation in macular pigment densities between 10 pairs of monozygotic twins. Significant differences in the macular pigments were observed in 5 of the 10 pairs of twins and these variations were moderately related to differences in the intake of dietary fat. However, all of the subjects were between 19 and 22 years and none had any vision problems. No ophthalmic examination was performed, except for color testing, which was normal. The authors concluded that the large variations between identical twins indicate that the amounts of macular pigment were determined by exogenous factors and not strictly by heredity. However, from a genetic perspective, these results could also be interpreted as evidence that the macular pigments have little to do with the etiology of ARM, given the extraordinary concordance of ARM observed in other monozygotic twin studies. Future studies of dietary and environmental factors affecting ARM will increasingly incorporate genetic considerations into research designs and analyses.

MOLECULAR AND CELL BIOLOGY OF ARM IN THE CONTEXT OF GENETICS

Whether one employs random genome-wide searches for genetic linkage of ARM or a more focused, hypothesis-driven selection of genetic markers, the identification of genes related to ARM involves testing of candidate genes. Candidate genes are implicated in the pathogenesis of a disease based on their position to the disease locus (as determined by linkage studies) and/or their role in the biology of the condition. The identification of opsin as one of the genes responsible for retinitis pigmentosa was a combination of the knowledge that *(1)* a retinitis pigmentosa family had been linked to a region in close proximity to opsin on chromosome 3[110] and that *(2)* opsin plays a crucial role in the function of the photoreceptors that degenerate in retinitis pigmentosa. More recently, mutations in the TIMP-3 gene, which encodes for an inhibitor of the metalloproteinases, were found in two families with Sorsby fundus dystrophy.[176] This was the result of mapping studies and that this gene could affect the maintenance of the basement membrane, which had been implicated as a potential site of damage. It is worthwhile to briefly review our current knowledge of the biology of ARM so that we can consider which genes and pathways might be implicated in this disease process.

Studies of the clinical features, histopathology, and biochemistry of ARM have suggested a number of target areas that could contribute to the development of drusen and degenerative changes in the retina, RPE, and choroid. The retina has been .implicated primarily on the basis of recent genetic studies that have shown that mutations in peripherin (a photoreceptor-specific protein) can give rise to macular changes that are clinically and histologically indistinguishable from the classical descriptions of ARM.[47,56] The majority of individuals with ARM do not show changes in the function of the retina until there are clinically evident changes at the level of thė pigment epithelium or Bruch's membrane. It is possible that alterations in photoreceptor-specific genes, such as opsin and peripherin, could have subtle effects on the metabolism, structure, and shedding of the outer segments that gradually cause a deterioration in the maintenance of this cell layer by the pigment epithelium. Recently, mutations in the ABCR gene, which is expressed specifically in photoreceptors, have been shown to be responsible for autosomal recessive Stargardt disease[2b] and other amino acid variants in this gene have also been implicated in ARM.[2a] Both cellular and mitochondrial genes[88,107,122,137] have been implicated in retinal and macular degenerations. It is not surprising that mitochondrial genes involved in oxidative phosphorylation would be critical in the preservation of the retina and optic nerve, given the enormous metabolic activity required by the retina to sustain the phototransduction cascade and renew the constantly shed outer segments of the rod and cone photoreceptors.

Deficiencies in specific, essential polyunsaturated fatty acids have been demonstrated to affect photoreceptor function in human infants[68,167] as well as in animal models.[17,18,28,100] The susceptibility of these lipids to peroxidation by free radicals and the mechanisms by which the eye processes the oxidation products may play an important role in the aging process in the eye.[126] Specific differences in the lipid compositions of the macula compared to the retinal periphery could perhaps account for some of the regional specificities of ARM.[170]

The photoreceptors and pigment epithelium both contribute to the composition and maintenance of the interphotoreceptor matrix. Within this intercellular compartment, there is a rich mixure of glycosaminoglycans, proteolipids, and other constituents that comprise the cone and rod matrix sheaths.[78,90,94,138] The retinal degenerations that have been reported in association with specific mucopolysaccharidoses, such as MPSI, II, III, and VII, correlate with enzyme deficiencies that would affect the major mucopolysaccharides found in the interphotoreceptor space.[95] Peripherin, a key membrane protein in the photoreceptor outer segments that has already been implicated in retinal degenerations, is a glycoprotein.[27] The isomerization of retinol in the RPE and its transport to the photoreceptors by transport proteins such as the interphotoreceptor binding protein have been postulated as crucial steps for the function and maintenance of the retina. An RPE-specific gene, RPE-65, has been implicated in an early-onset, severe retinal dystrophy[60a] and mutations within a cellular retinaldehyde-binding protein in the pigment epithelium have been shown to cause an autosomal recessive retinal degeneration with macular dystrophy.[108a] Alterations in the rod and cone interphotoreceptor matrices may be responsible for the retinal degenerations in some disorders. It is certainly reasonable to consider that even mild abnormalities in retinol transport, the composition of the interphotoreceptor matrix, and outer segment maintenance, shedding, recognition, and phagocytosis could lead to long-term degenerative changes.

In addition to its role in the synthesis of the interphotoreceptor matrix and the phagocytosis and process of the rod and cone outer segments, the RPE is crucial to maintaining fluid and small molecular and ionic transport across the interphotoreceptor compartment and across Bruch's membrane. To accomplish these tasks, the RPE must maintain a highly polarized configuration with specialized apical and basal membranes. The RPE has long been implicated in the pathogenesis of ARM because of the changes it undergoes and the development of drusen either along the basal surface of the RPE or within Bruch's membrane. Thus, genes that are either constitutive or specific to the RPE and whose protein products participate in the intracellular pathways responsible for protein and lipid processing, mainteinance of RPE polarity, and/or RPE phagocytosis could contribute to ARM.

The RPE is responsible in part for the synthesis and maintenance of Bruch's membrane, which is a multilayered extracellular matrix containing two basement membranes. The integrity of Bruch's membrane and its ability to allow for the transport of fluid, nutrients, and secreted molecules have also been implicated in the pathogenesis of ARM. Some have suggested that accumulation of lipid materials within Bruch's membrane impairs this transport and leads to drusen and pigment epithelial detachments.[10,21,131] Progressive breaks in Bruch's membrane are thought to contribute to the development of subretinal neovascular membranes that arise from the choriocapillaris.[140,142] Additional evidence implicating basement membranes, connective tissue, and Bruch's membrane also comes from the association of ARM with degenerative changes in skin[11] and from degenerative changes in the eye associated with pseudoxanthoma elasticum, Ehlers-Danlos syndrome, and type II membranous glomerulonephritis. Those who have suggested that zinc deficiency may contribute to ARM[124] have cited the critical role of zinc and other metal ions as cofactors in collagen synthesis and basement membrane metabolism. More recently, the role of the TIMP-3 gene in the pathogenesis of Sorsby fundus dystrophy[176] has also implicated genes involved in connective and basement membrane synthesis and turnover.

Finally, one must consider the potential contribution of the choriocapillaris to the pathogenesis of ARM. This highly specialized vascular bed is not only essential for the transport of oxygen, nutrients, metabolic byproducts, and retinol to and from the pigment epithelium, but it also is responsible for the synthesis and maintenance of the outer half of Bruch's membrane. Subretinal neovascular membranes, which are a major complication of ARM, develop from the capillary beds of the choroid. Alterations in the choriocapillaris have been correlated with the development of ARM based on fluorescein angiographic studies.[57,131] Two forms of hereditary macular dystrophy—central areolar choroidal sclerosis and choroideremia—provide clinical evidence that the loss of the choriocapillaris can occur concomitantly with RPE atrophy, and not necessarily as a late-stage outcome of the degenerative process. There has been relatively little study of the role of the choriocapillaris in the development of ARM, but it is a potentially critical part of the biological pathway that maintains the retina.

There has been a tendency for some investigators to become fixated on cell-specific or tissue-specific genes. However, the evidence from studies of gyrate atrophy,[118] choroideremia,[145,169] and Sorsby fundus dystrophy[176] indicates that genes that are expressed constitutively or are present in multiple tissues in the body can lead to ocular-specific degeneration. Presumably this is because the highly specialized functions of the photoreceptors or pigment epithelium depend on common metabolic pathways. Although the evaluation of photoreceptor-specific genes such as opsin and peripherin are reasonable starting points of a candidate gene-based search for ARM-related genes, it will take a genome-wide endeavor to uncover all of the potential loci that may contribute to the etiology of ARM.

THE DESIGN OF GENETIC RESEARCH FOR ARM

The investigation of the genetics of ARM requires the integration of multiple strategies and approaches. These approaches include segregation analysis to model the contribution of inheritance to the development of ARM, family studies of ARM and other hereditary dystrophies, as well as nonparametric linkage studies that address the heterogeneity and complexity of inheritance as it pertains to ARM. We must consider the potential genetic contribution of candidate genes that have been implicated by the biology of ARM, as well as genes that have not yet been isolated or characterized. The following section addresses the major types of genetic studies as they pertain to ARM. No single approach is sufficient, and each strategy provides support for the others.

Segregation Analysis

Segregation analysis explores the genetic epidemiology of a disorder by examining the prevalence of a condition among family members of an affected individual (or proband) in comparison to a control population or families with an unaffected proband. The approach allows one to test specific hypotheses as to the extent that a given genetic, nongenetic, or mixed model can account for the distribution of affected individuals. In practice, the complexity of the genetic models that can be effectively tested is limited by the increasing number of variables that must be calculated to fit into the model. Factors such as environmental effects, age dependence, penetrance, gene frequency, and mode of inheritance can all be considered. Data collection is rarely ideal and many of the assumptions and methods have been developed to overcome the known limitations and bias of the data. Data of family members based on historical recall of the proband or another family member are usually readily accessible but often unreliable. Individuals with ARM are often undiagnosed (or even uninformed) regarding their condition and family members may have incomplete or inaccurate information. In other cases, individuals diagnosed with ARM are more likely to be aware of other family members having the disorder than individuals who are unaffected by the condition. I have encountered a number of occasions in family studies in which a specific family member was reported to have ARM according to several family members and yet the individual lacked any signs or symptoms of the condition or had an unrelated condition such as diabetic retinopathy or a macular branch vein occlusion.

Until recently, segregation analysis was the only means of identifying a genetic effect for a complex disorder. Although the approach is useful for risk analysis, it provides no insight into the actual genes or number of genes that contribute to disease susceptibility. This fundamental limitation is perhaps the major reason why detailed segregation studies are not a major focus of future ARM genetic research.

Parametric Linkage Studies of ARM Families and Other Macular Dystrophies

Linkage analysis exploits the rearrangements that occur between paired chromosomes during meiosis to determine the likelihood that two or more markers (or traits or disease) are in proximity to each other based on the observed and expected frequencies that they would remain together or be separated. The closer the two markers are to one another, the less likely they are going to be separated by recombination events. Although the overall frequency of recombination events in a cell is relatively constant, the distributions of those events along a chromosome are not completely random. Thus the frequency of a recombination event between two markers in a given region of a chromosome will be a function of the physical distance between these markers; however, the relationship is not exactly linear.

In parametric linkage analysis, the mode of inheritance is specified as well as the gene frequency, penetrance, and certainty of diagnosis. For classical linkage analysis, large pedigrees are ideal because one can avoid the problem of many phenotypes resulting from different genes. It is essential to not mix families whose conditions are caused by different genes. Depending on the degree of confidence to which one can assign affected or unaffected status to different individuals within a family, one can obtain sufficient power to detect linkage in a moderately sized family. Autosomal dominant ARM families have long been reported and these families are used with standard genotyping methods and linkage analysis to identify one or more of the genes that are involved in ARM. The challenge is to find a large enough family with ARM-affected living individuals in two or more generations given the late onset of the condition. One must also address the possibilities that *(1)* an individual who has married into the pedigree may also have a predisposition for developing ARM, *(2)* the diagnosis may not be able to be established with certainty in the younger generations, *(3)* some individuals may have the genetic susceptibility without clinical signs or symptoms (incomplete penetrance), and *(4)* the pathology may be incorrectly ascribed to ARM (phenocopy). Despite these difficulties, large families are occasionally found. There are select populations such as the Bedouin tribes,[19,89,151] the Amish,[116,128] and others[35,53,117,135] that have remained genetically isolated and with well-established lines of descent. By identifying one or more ARM-related genes in these families, we can then estimate the extent to which these genes contribute to ARM in smaller families from a more heterogeneous population.

In our initial discussion of the relationship of ARM with other hereditary "juvenile" macular dystrophies, it was noted that there is considerable clinical overlap with a number of these syndromes. Table 24.1 lists some of these dystrophies and the linkage data or genes. It is possible that a percentage of familial ARM cases are the result of alterations in genes that have been either linked to these dystrophies or established definitively as having mutations responsible for these conditions. Classical linkage analysis of all of the hereditary macular dystrophies and the identification of the causative genes are highly relevant to genetic studies of ARM. The genetic loci or specific genes that are implicated in other macular or retinal dystrophies can serve as candidates for nonparametric linkage studies or candidate screening approaches for large numbers of small ARM families or individuals.

Linkage Disequilibrium

Linkage disequilibrium is another method of identifying the close association of a DNA marker with a disease or trait. If one evaluates a group of individuals or families that come from a limited geographic area or are derived from an isolated ethnic or religious group, and the disease is suspected to be the result of genetic alterations that have been transmitted by a limited set of ancestors, then one can test the hypothesis that those individuals affected by the disorder will have a more limited or skewed distribution of the alleles associated with the tightly linked marker than would be observed in a normal, unaffected population. The closer the disease is associated with the marker, the higher the degree of linkage disequilibrium. The fewer the number of ancestral mutations, the more likely that disequilibrium will be detected. For ARM, which is likely to be extremely heterogeneous, the only situations in which linkage disequilibrium is likely to be an effective tool are when extended families or genetically isolated populations are available.[103,121,125,127] This approach is important in that it allows for refinement or narrowing of the

Table 24.1. Macular, Cone, and Cone-Rod Dystrophies

Dystrophy	Locus	Marker(s)	Gene	Ref.
Autosomal dominant (AD) Drusen-Malattia Leventinese	2p16-21	D2S378		66
Sorsby fundus dystrophy	22q13-qter	D22S275, D22S274	TIMP-3 gene	176, 177
Best vitelliform dystrophy	11q13	INT2, D11S871, ROM-1 excluded		58, 159, 162
North Carolina dystrophy	6q14-q16.2			155
North Carolina-like dystrophy	? excluded from MCDR1 locus			69
Atypical vitelliform macular dystrophy (VMD-1)	8q24.2-qter	Glutamate pyruvate transaminase (GPT)		41
Macular dystrophy/retinitis pigmentosa (RP) (AD)	6p21.2-cen	Peripherin/RDS		56, 79, 182, 183, 186
AD cystoid macular dystrophy	7p15-p21	D7S493, D7S435, D7S526		87
X-linked retinoschisis	Xp22.2-p22.1	DXS43, DXS207, DXS987, DXS443		3, 6, 7, 133, 143a
Autosomal recessive Stargardt	1p21-p13	D1S435, D1S415	ABCR gene	2b, 50
AD Stargardt	13q34	D13S154, D13S158		188
AD Stargardt-like dystrophy	6q	D6S313, D6S252		161
Fleck retina	Ring 17			20
AD cone-rod dystrophy	18q21	Deletion mapping		175
AD cone-rod dystrophy	19q13.1-q13.2	D19S47		37
X-linked progressive cone dystrophy	Xp21-p11.1			5, 71, 112
Macular pattern dystrophy (associated with diabetes and deafness)	Mitochondrial genome		Leucine transfer RNA	107
Vitelliform macular degeneration (associated with mitochondrial myopathy)	Mitochondrial genome			122

region containing a disease gene by comparing individuals from families that are so distinctly related that the ancestral origins may date back many generations.

Nonparametric Linkage Studies

In the last decade, nonparametric linkage analyses have been developed that avoid many of the limitations of classical linkage analysis and thus are suitable for the investigation of complex genetic disorders. Originally known as sib pair analysis,[91,164] and later expanded to include other family members (the affected-pedigree-member method),[178] these nonparametric linkage studies test the hypothesis that if two or more members of a family share the same condition, then it is likely that they share one or more regions of the genome containing genes responsible for conferring disease susceptibility. If one examines many small families, a nonrandom association of these regions with the disease will gradually be established. The mode of inheritance (i.e., recessive, dominant, or X linked) does not need to be specified and gene interactions (such as the digenic inheritance reported for several retinitis pigmentosa families) do not confound the analysis.[16,108,179] The issues of variable expressivity and incomplete penetrance are eliminated as one only compares the genetic information of clearly affected individuals. However, the wonderful freedom of the nonparametric methods from the difficulties of classical (parametric) linkage methods comes at a significant price. Affected-pedigree-member analyses[178–180] require considerably larger numbers of families and individuals than in classical family linkage analysis as they have less power to detect linkage. If multiple genes are involved with ARM, then even more families need to be compared. Unaffected individuals within a family contribute a limited amount of genetic information if the clinical status is in doubt because of incomplete penetrance or minimal expressivity. Finally, these methods rely on our ability to infer whether two or more individuals share a common region of DNA by descent (identity-by-descent) when they have the same alleles for a given marker (identity-by-state). If a particular allele for a specific DNA marker is very rare in the general population, and two family members share that allele, then they very likely acquired the allele from a common ancestor. In contrast, if the marker allele is very common in the population, then the fact that two siblings share this allele is not as convincing. Some adjustments can be made if the genotypes of the parents are known, but given the older age of most ARM patients the parents are usually not available. In the absence of the parental DNA information, we must rely on either inferred information from other siblings or on observed allele frequencies in the general population. Errors in observed allele frequencies can greatly affect the likelihood that an observed identity-by-state reflects a true identity-by-descent, thus altering the value of the statistic that is calculated as a measure of the likelihood of a particular marker being linked to the disease compared to a nonlinked model. The current versions of the affected-pedigree-member programs are capable of using the genetic information from other family members to better approximate the probabilities of identity-by-descent.[144]

Extensive simulation studies with actual ARM families demonstrate that when the affected-pedigree-member method is applied to genotypings using current microsatellite repeats and polymerase chain amplification, there is sufficient power to detect linkage of a DNA marker with a major ARM locus greater than 90% of the time given a sample size of 75 families using 2.2 individuals per family, markers spaced every 10 cM, and a p value of 0.05.[55] In order to detect linkage with higher p values, more informative markers and families are necessary. The certainty of detecting linkage also increases as more tightly spaced markers are genotyped. If several genes contribute to the disease then many more families may be required. The enormous effort required to conduct tightly spaced genotyping across the entire genomes of hundreds of individuals has led us to develop a staged strategy for genotyping.[16] By initially scanning the genome with widely spaced markers, one selects those regions containing loci that have even weak evidence of linkage based on the statistics calculated by the affected-pedigree-member methods. By selecting a relatively low screening value for this statistic, there is a high probability of not overlooking a true positively linked marker. Unfortunately, the majority of the markers that will be selected for additional testing will be "false positives." However, by performing additional genotyping with flanking markers and by using more families, these false-negative regions are excluded, and the regions that are associated with ARM susceptibility can be confirmed. By selecting optimal thresholds for each level of screening, the total number of genotypings that are required can be significantly reduced and the power of the effort is increased.

A genome-wide mapping effort is underway in our laboratory using polymerase chain amplification of microsatellite markers. We have initially focused on genetic markers that have been linked to known retinal or macular dystrophies, photoreceptor-specific genes, or basement membrane-specific genes. Given the potential for significant artifact and false-positive loci based on a low cutoff value for the statistics, each marker that yields a positive linkage statistic requires multiple flanking markers to confirm the association of the region with ARM. In this fashion, the TIMP-3 locus has been excluded as a major contributer in our ARM families despite the initially promising statistic value. At least three additional loci have been selected from the first genotyping pass and are currently in the second stages of genotype screening. Even with current technologies, it will take several more years and many more families to confidently assign the location of one or more ARM-susceptibility genes by nonparametric methods.

Candidate Gene Screening

Based on the results of classical linkage analysis of macular dystrophy families and from the genes suggested by mapping using the affected-pedigree-member approach, specific genes are likely to be implicated in the pathogenesis of ARM. The confirmation of these candidate genes will require the identification of nucleotide alterations that clearly segregate with individuals at risk for ARM and can account for an alteration in the expression or function of the encoded protein product for that gene. The nucleotide sequences comprising the final RNA transcript that serve as the template for protein synthesis are distributed in the genome as small blocks called exons. Typically, the exons of genes are screened for mutations that will either terminate protein synthesis or cause a change in the amino acid sequence. Such exon screening has been extremely effective for identifying opsin and peripherin mutations in retinitis pigmentosa. In ARM, the challenge is greater since the disorder could also be the result of an altered expression of a normal protein and nucleotide changes in the promoter or enhancer regions of the gene may also be relevant. Until specific nucleotide alterations can be demonstrated to reliably segregate with the disease phenotype and are shown to cause predictable changes in protein expression or structure, the primary evidence that a gene is related to the development of ARM will be based on linkage studies and/or disequilibrium analyses.

The selection of candidate genes for ARM is based on several different criteria. The colocalization of specific genes with genetic markers that have been linked to ARM susceptibility is a logical outgrowth of all of the genetic linkage studies of ARM. As more genes and genetic markers are identified for a growing number of the traditional hereditary macular dystrophies such as Best disease, adult foveomacular dystrophy, Stargardt disease, and dominant drusen, these will become appropriate candidates for evaluation of ARM-susceptibility loci. Candidate genes can also be selected by inference from the participation of their protein products in the pathogenesis of ARM. However, it should be clear from the brief review of the molecular and cellular biology of ARM, that there is a wide range of cell-specific, tissue-specific, and constitutive metabolic processes that have been implicated in ARM. It is debatable if evaluating each of these genes (of which only a subset has been cloned or mapped) is a more effective approach than conducting a genomewide search with anonymous DNA markers. Perhaps the greatest limitation of attempting to directly screen candidate genes is that most genes are not highly polymorphic, and thus a linkage strategy would be difficult unless more informative markers are known to be associated with the gene. In contrast, the microsatellite DNA markers currently used for genetic linkage studies are highly polymorphic and informative, and are ideal for identifying regions of the genome which are associated with familial ARM.

Without polymorphisms or the ability to perform linkage analysis with specific candidate genes, one is forced to directly screen for nucleotide alterations in the gene that are presumably limited to the exon regions. Direct mutation screening, although limited somewhat by the sensitivity of the detection method, does have the advantage that a large number of independent, affected individuals can be evaluated without regard to other family members. Such approaches have been successful for a subset of autosomal dominant retinitis pigmentosa patients identified with opsin or peripherin mutations and for some autosomal recessive retinitis pigmentosa patients with mutations in the phosphodiesterase β-subunit[109] or the cGMP-gated channel.[134] A similar screening of a large cohort of ARM patients for peripherin mutations identified only a small set of cases with mutations (Stone, personal communication). Based on the similarities between Sorsby's fundus dystrophy and ARM, Weber et al.[177] and Stone (personal communication) screened a group of ARM patients for potential changes in the TIMP-3 coding regions. No mutations were identified, although there still remains the possibility that this gene could be modified in the promoter or intron regions. In the past, exhaustive direct screening was impractical, due to the size of many genes, the need to screen many exons, and the inability of screening methods to identify all possible mutations. However, 51 exons of the ABCR gene were successfully screened in several hundred ARM, Stargardt, and normal subjects to identify potential ARM-related nucleotide alterations.[2a] This report of ARM-related mutations in the ABCR gene has provided renewed support for the candidate gene approach.

Additional genetic studies will be necessary to establish that these variants segregate with ARM within families to confirm that the alterations are causal for the disease. It is difficult to assess the overall success of this population-based, candidate gene screening strategy as most investigators only publish the results of successful searches for mutations of specific genes.

Animal Studies

Animal models have played a central role in the molecular genetics of retinal degenerations and other ocular disorders. The rd and rds mouse were responsible for the elucidation of the cGMP-dependent phosphodiesterase β-subunit and peripherin, genes that contribute to human retinal degenerations.[109] Mouse mutants such as *small eye,*[136] *albino,*[61] *pink-eye,*[15] and *splotch*[33] have been instrumental in the discovery of the genes for aniridia, tyrosinase-negative albinisim, type II oculocutaneous albinism, Prader-Willi syndrome, and Waardenburg syndrome, respectively. A growing list of human genetic diseases has been characterized through appropriate mouse models.[146] More recently, genes that contribute to complex genetic disorders such as diabetes,[150] obesity,[189] and hypertension[29] have been identified from rodent studies. Unfortunately, there are few comparable examples for ARM in well-characterized animal strains. Aging changes, including the formation of drusen, have been reported in Japanese quail,[44] rhesus macaque monkeys (*Macaca mulatta*),[31,32,123,126,168] and cynomolgus macaque monkeys (*Macaca fascicularis*).[39] The rhesus macaque monkeys develop vision loss, disciform lesions, and macular atrophy in the later stages of the condition, not unlike human disease,[31] whereas the end-stage aging changes in the cynomolgus macaques are typically atrophic.[39] The genetics of drusen formation have been partially explored in an isolated rhesus macaque colony in Cayo Santiago. Hereditary patterns are present within different social groups and along matriarchial lines.[32] However, formal segregation analysis or molecular genetic linkage analyses have not been reported. Molecular genetic studies of this colony could offer significant insights into at least one of the major genes that contributes to ARM in the human population.

Deposits similar to drusen have been reported in the eyes of cats with Chediak-Higashi syndrome, a form of oculocutaneous albinism that is also seen in humans.[26] It is unlikely that the gene responsible for this form of oculocutaneous albinism, which is also associated with immune deficiency, plays a critical role in the development of ARM. However, there is strong evidence from human epidemiologic studies that ocular pigmentation is a risk factor for ARM development.[173,181] The relevance of ocular pigmentation to ARM may require the investigation of other hypopigmented mouse mutants in order to understand the impact of pigment synthesis on retinal metabolism and function.

THE POTENTIAL BENEFITS OF GENETIC RESEARCH FOR ARM

The importance of understanding the interplay of genetics and exogenous factors cannot be overstated as we seek strategies to retard or halt the progression of ARM. Large clinical studies that attempt to determine the potential benefits of therapy such as specific vitamin or mineral supplements may fail to identify a significant effect if the benefits are limited to a small subset of the ARM population. The admixture of individuals who are genetically at risk for developing ARM, but have minimal macular features, with individuals who have lower risks of developing ARM can greatly alter the detection power of the study and the ability to extend those results to the general population. This is potentially an issue for the Age-Related Eye Disease Study, which includes a number of individuals who are self-selected to participate and have minimal macular pathology. A number of these individuals volunteer for this study because of their awareness of ARM in other family members and consequently may not be representative of a "normal" or unaffected population. By relying solely on the photographic grading of macular pathology, a certain percentage of individuals will be overlooked who have an increased risk for developing ARM as determined by peripheral retinal findings and positive family histories. These individuals will be randomized to both arms of the clinical trial and will not compromise the study results, but the effective power of the study is less than what would have been achieved if these individuals had not been mixed with those who are truly at lower risk for developing ARM. Any treatment benefits identified in this group of subjects will need to account for this potential bias before the results can be applied to the general public.

The identification of alterations in specific genes associated with ARM susceptibility will provide invaluable insights into the metabolic pathways that are involved in ARM. Current treatments for ARM are primarily directed to limiting the damage and visual loss from subretinal neovascular membranes[12,149,185] but do not halt the progressive nature of the underlying condition. There has been a growing effort to understand the causes of ARM and develop strategies to slow the progression of ARM.[8,22,148,184]

The observation that some mutations of the TIMP-3 gene can cause Sorsby fundus dystrophy raises the possibility that this gene may be involved in more common forms of ARM. This relationship would justify the investigation of a whole new class of drugs that have been developed to inhibit the metalloproteinases associated with other systemic diseases.[67] Drugs such as thalidomide that are potent inhibitors of neovascularization are now being tested to slow the progression or reduce the recurrence of subretinal neovascular membranes. More effective drugs that can block the initiation of the neovascularization process and maintain the integrity of Bruch's membrane could play an important role in the prevention of vision loss. Prophylactic photocoagulation of the macula was first advocated in 1979[24] and has recently been reconsidered specifically for the resorption of soft drusen.[43,63,152,185] Clinical and investigative trials are currently attempting to determine whether the resorption of drusen is associated with a lowered risk of neovascular membranes or geographic atrophy. If these studies demonstrate a clinical benefit, then the diagnosis and management of ARM will shift away from acute intervention for sudden vision loss to the recognition of individuals with treatable forms of ARM prior to vision changes. Genetic testing would aid in the identification of the individuals who have the greatest risk of ARM and are the most likely to benefit from these interventions.

The prevalence and relatively late onset of ARM in the population make the likelihood of direct gene therapy very limited. The primary goals of ARM therapy must be retardation of ARM progression and the preservation of sight rather than the rescue of retinal function or acute surgical interventions. Modern medicine is turning increasingly to diet, lifestyle modification, and medications to minimize the deleterious effects of hypertension, hypercholesterolemia, and other systemic disorders. We are beginning to recognize the importance of focused surveillance for individuals at risk for specific forms of cancer to allow for early detection and more successful treatment. The first chemopreventive trials for breast cancer and prostate cancer are now underway.[1,59] These strategies will also be the foundation for the future management of ARM and allow a larger percentage of our population to face their advancing years without the fear of legal blindness.

Acknowledgments: This work was supported in part by Pennsylvania Lions Sight Conservation and Eye Research Foundation, Inc., The Eye & Ear Foundation of Pittsburgh, and National Eye Institute grant EY09859 (M.B.G.).

The author acknowledges the efforts of Ms. Tammy Mah, who assisted in the editing of this manuscript and preparing the figure summarizing the ARM prevalence studies.

REFERENCES

1. Alberts DS, Garcia DJ. An overview of clinical cancer chemoprevention studies with emphasis on positive phase III studies (review). *J Nutr* 1995;125(3 suppl):692S–697S.
2. Alexander LJ. The prevalence of macular drusen in a population of patients with known insulin-dependent diabetes mellitus. *J Am Optom Assoc* 1985;56(10):806–810.

2a. Allikmets R, Shroyer N, Singh N, et al. Mutation of the Stargardt disease gene (ABCR) in age-related macular degeneration. *Science* 1997;277:1805–1807.

2b. Allikmets R, Singh N, Sun H, et al. A photoreceptor cell-specific ATP-binding transporter gene (ABCR) is mutated in recessive Stargardt macular dystrophy. *Nature Genetic* 1997;15:236–245.

3. Alitalo T, Kruse TA, de la Chapelle A. Refined localization of the gene causing X-linked juvenile retinoschisis. *Genomics* 1991;9(3):505–510.
4. Anonymous. Risk factors for neovascular age-related macular degeneration. The Eye Disease Case-Control Study Group. *Arch Ophthalmol* 1992;110(12):1701–1708.
5. Bergen AA, Meire F, ten Brink J, Schuurman EJ, van Ommen G, Delleman JW. Additional evidence for a gene locus for progressive cone dystrophy with late rod involvement in Xp21.1-p11.3. *Genomics* 1993;18(2):463–464.
6. Bergen AA, ten Brink J, Bleeker-Wagemakers LM, van Schooneveld MJ. Refinement of the chromosomal position of the X linked juvenile retinoschisis gene. *J Med Genet* 1994;31(12):972–975.
7. Bergen AA, van Schooneveld MJ, Orth U, Bleeker-Wagemakers EM, Gal A. Multipoint linkage analysis in X-linked juvenile retinoschisis. *Clin Genet* 1993;43(3):113–116.
8. Berson EL, Rosner B, Sandberg MA, Hayes KC, Nicholson BW, Weigel DC, Willett W. A randomized trial of vitamin A and vitamin E supplementation for retinitis pigmentosa (see comments). *Arch Ophthalmol* 1993;111(6):761–772.
9. Bhatt S, Warren C, Yang H, Bu X, Cantor R, Kenney MC, Nesburn A, Raffel LJ. Age related macular degeneration—Evidence of a major gene. *Am J Hum Genet* 1994;55(3):A146.
10. Bird AC. Bruch's membrane change with age (review). *Br J Ophthalmol* 1992;76(3):166–168.
11. Blumenkranz MS, Russell SR, Robey MG, Kott BR, Penneys N. Risk factors in age-related maculopathy complicated by choroidal neovascularization. *Ophthalmology* 1986;93(5):552–558.
12. Bressler N, Bressler S, Fine S. Age-related macular degeneration. *Surv Ophthalmol* 1988;32(6):375–413.
13. Bressler NM, Bressler SB, West SK, Fine SL, Taylor HR. The grading and prevalence of macular degeneration in Chesapeake Bay watermen. *Arch Ophthalmol* 1989;107(6):847–852.

14. Bressler SB, Maguire MG, Bressler NM, Fine SL. Relationship of drusen and abnormalities of the retinal pigment epithelium to the prognosis of neovascular macular degeneration. The Macular Photocoagulation Study Group. *Arch Ophthalmol* 1990;108(10):1442–1447.
15. Brilliant MY. The mouse pink-eyed dilution locus: A model for aspects of Prader-Willi syndrome, Angelman syndrome, and a form of hypomelanosis of Ito (review). *Mammal Genome* 1992;3(4):187–191.
16. Brown DL, Gorin MB, Weeks DE. Efficient strategies for genomic searching using the affected-pedigree-member method of linkage analysis. *Am J Hum Genet* 1994;54(3):544–552.
17. Bush RA, Malnoe A, Reme CE, Williams TP. Dietary deficiency of N-3 fatty acids alters rhodopsin content and function in the rat retina. *Invest Ophthalmol Vis Sci* 1994;35(1):91–100.
18. Bush RA, Reme CE, Malnoe A. Light damage in the rat retina: The effect of dietary deprivation of N-3 fatty acids on acute structure alterations. *Exp Eye Res* 1991;53(6):741–752.
19. Carmi R, Rokhlina T, Kwitek BA, Elbedour K, Nishimura D, Stone EM, Sheffield VC. Use of a DNA pooling strategy to identify a human obesity syndrome locus on chromosome 15. *Hum Mol Genet* 1995;4(1):9–13.
20. Charles S, Moore A, Davison B, Dyson H, Wilatt L. Flecked retina associated with ring 17 chromosome. *Br J Ophthalmol* 1991;75:125–127.
21. Chen JC, Fitzke FW, Pauleikhoff D, Bird AC. Functional loss in age-related Bruch's membrane change with choroidal perfusion defect. *Invest Ophthalmol Vis Sci* 1992;33(2):334–340.
22. Christen WJ. Antioxidants and eye disease (review). *Am J Med* 1994;97(3A).
23. Chumbley LC. Impressions of eye diseases among Rhodesian blacks in Mashonaland. *S Afr Med J* 1977;52(8):316–318.
24. Cleasby GW, Nakanishi AS, Norris JL. Prophylactic photocoagulation of the fellow eye in exudative senile maculopathy. A preliminary report. *Mod Probl Ophthalmol* 1979;20(141):141–147.
25. Cohen SY, Meunier I, Soubrane G, Glacet BA, Coscas GJ. Visual function and course of basal laminar drusen combined with vitelliform macular detachment. *Br J Ophthalmol* 1994;78(6):437–440.
26. Collier LL, King EJ, Prieur DJ. Age-related changes of the retinal pigment epithelium of cats with Chediak-Higashi syndrome. *Invest Ophthalmol Vis Sci* 1986;27(5):702–707.
27. Connell G, Molday RS. Molecular cloning, primary structure, and orientation of the vertebrate photoreceptor protein peripherin in the rod outer segment disk membrane. *Biochemistry* 1990;29:4691–4698.
28. Connor WE, Neuringer M, Reisbick S. Essential fatty acids: The importance of n-3 fatty acids in the retina and brain (review). *Nutr Rev* 1992;50:21–29.
29. Corvol P, Jeunemaitre X, Charru A, Kotelevtsev Y, Soubrier F. Role of the renin-angiotensin system in blood pressure regulation and in human hypertension: New insights from molecular genetics (review). *Recent Prog Horm Res* 1995;50(287):287–308.
30. Cruickshanks KJ, Klein R, Klein BE. Sunlight and age-related macular degeneration. The Beaver Dam Eye Study. *Arch Ophthalmol* 1993;111(4):514–518.
30a. Davies JL, Kawaguchi Y, Bennett ST, et al. A genome-wide search for human type 1 diabetes susceptibility genes (see comments). *Nature* 1994;371(6493):130–136.
31. Dawson WW, Engel HM, Hope GM, Kessler MJ, Ulshafer RJ. Adult-onset macular degeneration in the Cayo Santiago macaques. *PR Health Sci J* 1989;8(1):111–115.
32. Dawson WW, Ulshafer RJ, Engel HM, Hope GM, Kessler MJ. Macular disease in related rhesus monkeys. *Doc Ophthalmol* 1989;71(3):253–263.
32a. de la Paz M, Pericak-Vance M, Haines J, Seddon J. Phenotypic heterogeneity in families with age-related macular degeneration. *Am J Ophthalmol* 1997;124:331–343.
33. Delezoide AL, Vekemans M. Waardenburg syndrome in man and splotch mutants in the mouse: A paradigm of the usefulness of linkage and synteny homologies in mouse and man for the genetic analysis of human congenital malformations (review). *Biomed Pharmacother* 1994;48(8–9):335–339.
34. Dosso AA, Bovet J. Monozygotic twin brothers with age-related macular degeneration. *Ophthalmologica* 1992;205(1):24–28.
35. Eiberg H, Nielsen IM. Linkage studies of cholestasis familiaris groenlandica/Byler-like disease with polymorphic protein and blood group markers. *Hum Hered* 1993;43(4):250–256.
36. Erkkila H, Raitta C, Niemi KM. Ocular findings in four siblings with pseudoxanthoma

elasticum. *Acta Ophthalmol (Copenh)* 1983; 61(4):589–599.

37. Evans K, Fryer A, Inglehearn C, Duvall YJ, Whittaker JL, Gregory CY, Butler R, Ebenezer N, Hunt DM, Bhattacharya S. Genetic linkage of cone-rod retinal dystrophy to chromosome 19q and evidence for segregation distortion. *Nature Genet* 1994;6(2):210–213.
38. Farkas T, Krill A, Sylvester V, Archer D. Familial and secondary drusen: Histologic and functional correlations. *Trans Am Acad Ophthalmol Otol* 1971;75:333–343.
39. Feeney BL, Malinow R, Klein ML, Neuringer M. Maculopathy in cynomolgus monkeys. A correlated fluorescein angiographic and ultrastructural study. *Arch Ophthalmol* 1981; 99(4):664–672.
40. Feist RM, White MJ, Skalka H, Stone EM. Choroidal neovascularization in a patient with adult foveomacular dystrophy and a mutation in the retinal degeneration slow gene (Pro 210 Arg) (letter). *Am J Ophthalmol* 1994; 118(2):259–260.
41. Ferrell R, Hittner H, Antoszyk J. Linkage of atypical vitelliform macular dystrophy (VMD-1) to the soluble glutamate pyruvate transaminase (GPT-1) locus. *Am J Hum Genet* 1983; 35:78–84.
42. Ferris FLI. Senile macular degeneration: Review of epidemiologic features (review). *Am J Epidemiol* 1983;118(2):132–151.
43. Figueroa MS, Regueras A, Bertrand J. Laser photocoagulation to treat macular soft drusen in age-related macular degeneration. *Retina* 1994;14(5):391–396.
44. Fite KV, Bengston CL, Cousins F. Drusen-like deposits in the outer retina of Japanese quail. *Exp Eye Res* 1994;59(4):417–424.
45. François J. The inheritance of senile macule degeneration [French]. *Ophthalmologica* 1977;175(2):67–72.
46. Ganley J, Roberts J. Eye conditions and related need for medical care among persons 1–74 years of age, United States 1971–72. Washington, D.C.: DHHS publication no. 83-1678, 1983, *Vital Health Statistics*, series 11, no. 228.
47. Gass J. A clinicopathologic study of a peculiar foveomacular dystrophy. *Trans Am Ophthalmol Soc* 1974;72:139–56.
48. Gass J. *Stereoscopic Atlas of Macular Diseases*. St. Louis: C. B. Mosby, 1987.
49. Gass JDM. Drusen and disciform macular detachment and degeneration. *Arch Ophthalmol* 1973;90:206–217.
50. Gerber S, Rozet JM, Bonneau D, Souied E, Camuzat A, Dufier JL, Amalric P, Weissenbach J, Munnich A, Kaplan J. A gene for late-onset fundus flavimaculatus with macular dystrophy maps to chromosome 1p13. *Am J Hum Genet* 1995;56(2):396–399.
51. Gibson JM, Rosenthal AR, Lavery S. A study of the prevalence of eye disease in the elderly in an English community. *Trans Ophthalmol Soc UK* 1985;104:196–203.
52. Gibson JM, Shaw DE, Rosenthal AR. Senile cataract and senile macular degeneration: An investigation into possible risk factors. *Trans Ophthalmol Soc UK* 1986;105(4):463–468.
53. Glaser B, Chiu KC, Anker R, Nestorowicz A, Landau H, Ben BH, Shlomai Z, Kaiser N, Thornton PS, Stanley CA, et al. Familial hyperinsulinism maps to chromosome 11p14-15.1, 30 cM centromeric to the insulin gene. *Nature Genet* 1994;7(2):185–188.
54. Goldberg J, Flowerdew G, Smith E, Brody JA, Tso MO. Factors associated with age-related macular degeneration. An analysis of data from the first National Health and Nutrition Examination Survey. *Am J Epidemiol* 1988; 128(4):700–710.
55. Gorin M, Sarneso C, Paul T, Ngo J, Weeks D. The genetics of age-related maculopathy. In *Retinal Degeneration*, J. Hollyfield, R. Anderson, and M. La Vail, eds. New York: Plenum Press, 1993:35–47.
56. Gorin MB, Jackson KE, Ferrell RE, Sheffield VC, Jacobson SG, Gass JD, Mitchell E, Stone EM. A peripherin/retinal degeneration slow mutation (Pro-210-Arg) associated with macular and peripheral retinal degeneration. *Ophthalmology* 1995;102(2):246–255.
57. Gottsch JD, Bynoe LA, Harlan JB, Rencs EV, Green WR. Light-induced deposits in Bruch's membrane of protoporphyric mice. *Arch Ophthalmol* 1993;111(1):126–129.
58. Graff C, Forsman K, Larsson C, Nordstrom S, Lind L, Johansson K, Sandgren O, Weissenbach J, Holmgren G, Gustavson KH, et al. Fine mapping of Best's macular dystrophy localizes the gene in close proximity to but distinct from the D11S480/ROM1 loci. *Genomics* 1994;24(3):425–434.
59. Greenwald P. Chemoprevention research at the U.S. National Cancer Institute (review). *Milit Med* 1994;159(7):505–512.
60. Gregor Z, Joffe L. Senile macular changes in the black African. *Br J Ophthalmol* 1978; 62(8):547–550.

60a. Gu S-M, Thompson E, Srikumari C, et al.

Mutations in RPE65 cause autosomal recessive childhood-onset severe retinal dystrophy. *Nature Genet* 1997;17(2):194–197.

61. Halaban R, Moellmann G. White mutants in mice shedding light on humans [Review]. *J Invest Dermatol* 1993;Suppl 176S–185S.
62. Hammond BR, Fuld K, Curran-Celentano J. Macular pigment density in monozygotic twins. *Invest Ophthalmol Vis Sci* 1995;36(12): 2531–2541.
63. Haut J, Renard Y, Kraiem S, Bensoussan C, Moulin F. Preventive treatment using laser of age-related macular degeneration of the contralateral eye after age-related macular degeneration on the first eye (review) [French]. *J Fr Ophtalmol* 1991;14(8–9):473–476.
64. Heiba IM, Elston RC, Klein BE, Klein R. Sibling correlations and segregation analysis of age-related maculopathy: The Beaver Dam Eye Study. *Genet Epidemiol* 1994;11(1): 51–67.
65. Heinrich P. Senile degeneration of the macula. *Klin Monatsbl Augenheilkd* 1973;162: 3–26.
66. Heon E, Piguet B, Munier F, Sneed SR, Morgan CM, Forni S, Grasiano P, Schorderet D, Taylor CM, Streb LM, Wiles CD, Nishimura DY, Sheffield VC, Stone EM. Linkage of autosomal dominant radial drusen (Malattia Leventinese) to chromosome 2p16-21. *Arch Ophthalmol* 1996;114:193–198.
67. Hodgson J. Remodeling MMPIs. *Bio/Technology* 1995;13:554–557.
68. Uauy DR, Birch EE, Birch DG, Hoffman DR. Significance of omega 3 fatty acids for retinal and brain development of preterm and term infants. *World Rev Nutr Diet* 1994; 75(52):52–62.
69. Holz FG, Evans K, Gregory CY, Bhattacharya S, Bird AC. Autosomal dominant macular dystrophy simulating North Carolina macular dystrophy. *Arch Ophthalmol* 1995;113(2): 178–184.
70. Holz FG, Wolfensberger TJ, Piguet B, Gross JM, Wells JA, Minassian DC, Chisholm IH, Bird AC. Bilateral macular drusen in age-related macular degeneration. Prognosis and risk factors. *Ophthalmology* 1994;101(9): 1522–1528.
71. Hong HK, Ferrell RE, Gorin MB. Clinical diversity and chromosomal localization of X-linked cone dystrophy (COD1). *Am J Hum Genet* 1994;55(6):1173–1181.
72. Humphries P, Farrar GJ, Kenna P, McWilliam P. Retinitis pigmentosa: Genetic mapping in X-linked and autosomal forms of the disease. *Clin Genet* 1990;38:1–13.
73. Hyman LG, Lilienfeld AM, Ferris FLI, Fine SL. Senile macular degeneration: A case-control study. *Am J Epidemiol* 1983;118(2): 213–227.
74. Jampolsky A. Senile accommodative degeneration (SAD). *Am J Ophthalmol* 1991;111:510.
75. Jonasson F, Thordarson K. Prevalence of ocular disease and blindness in a rural area in the eastern region of Iceland during 1980 through 1984. *Acta Ophthalmol (Copenh) Suppl* 1987;182:40–43.
76. Kahn HA, Leibowitz HM, Ganley JP, Kini MM, Colton T, Nickerson RS, Dawber TR. The Framingham Eye Study. I. Outline and major prevalence findings. *Am J Epidemiol* 1977;106(1):17–32.
77. Kajiwara K, Berson EL, Dryja TP. Digenic retinitis pigmentosa due to mutations at the unlinked peripherin/RDS and ROM1 loci. *Science* 1994;264(5165):1604–1608.
78. Keegan WA, McKechnie NM, Converse CA, Foulds WS. D-[3H]-galactose incorporation in the bovine retina: Specific uptake and transport of the radiolabel in cones. *Exp Eye Res* 1985;40(4):619–628.
79. Kemp CM, Jacobson SG, Cideciyan AV, Kimura AE, Sheffield VC, Stone EM. RDS gene mutations causing retinitis pigmentosa or macular degeneration lead to the same abnormality in photoreceptor function. *Invest Ophthalmol Vis Sci* 1994;35(8):3154–3162.

79a. Klaver C, Wolfs R, van Duijn C, Hofman A, de Jong P. Familial aggregation of age-related macular degeneration in the Rotterdam Study. *Invest Ophthalmol Vis Sci* 1997;38(4): S967.

80. Klein B. Some aspects of classification and differential diagnosis of senile macular degeneration. *Am J Ophthalmol* 1964;58:927–939.
81. Klein B, Klein R. Cataracts and macular degeneration in older Americans. *Arch Ophthalmol* 1982;100:571–573.
82. Klein ML, Mauldin WM, Stoumbos VD. Heredity and age-related macular degeneration. Observations in monozygotic twins. *Arch Ophthalmol* 1994;112(7):932–937.
83. Klein R, Davis MD, Magli YL, Segal P, Klein BE, Hubbard L. The Wisconsin age-related maculopathy grading system. *Ophthalmology* 1991;98(7):1128–1134.
84. Klein R, Klein BE, Franke T. The relationship of cardiovascular disease and its risk factors to age-related maculopathy. The Beaver Dam

Eye Study (see comments). *Ophthalmology* 1993;100(3):406–414.

85. Klein R, Klein BE, Linton KL. Prevalence of age-related maculopathy. The Beaver Dam Eye Study. *Ophthalmology* 1992;99(6):933–943.
86. Klein R, Klein BE, Linton KL, DeMets DL. The Beaver Dam Study: The relation of age-related maculopathy to smoking. *Am J Epidemiol* 1993;137(2):190–200.
87. Kremer H, Pinckers A, van den Helm B, Deutman AF, Ropers HH, Mariman EC. Localization of the gene for dominant cystoid macular dystrophy on chromosome 7p. *Hum Mol Genet* 1994;3(2):299–302.
88. Kuriyama M, Umezaki H, Fukuda Y, Osame M, Koike K, Tateishi J, Igata A. Mitochondrial encephalomyopathy with lactate-pyruvate elevation and brain infarctions. *Neurology* 1984;34(1):72–77.
89. Kwitek BA, Carmi R, Duyk GM, Buetow KH, Elbedour K, Parvari R, Yandava CN, Stone EM, Sheffield VC. Linkage of Bardet-Biedl syndrome to chromosome 16q and evidence for non-allelic genetic heterogeneity. *Nature Genet* 1993;5(4):392–396.
90. Landers RA, Hollyfield JG. Proteoglycans in the mouse interphotoreceptor matrix. VI. Evidence for photoreceptor synthesis of chondroitin sulfate proteoglycan using genetically fractionated retinas. *Exp Eye Res* 1992;55(2): 345–356.
91. Lange K. The affected sib-pair method using identity by state relations. *Am J Hum Genet* 1986;39:148–150.
92. LaVail MM, Gorrin GM, Repaci MA. Strain differences in sensitivity to light-induced photoreceptor degeneration in albino mice. *Curr. Eye Res.* 1987;6(6):825–834.
93. LaVail MM, Gorrin GM, Repaci MA, Thomas LA, Ginsberg HM. Genetic regulation of light damage to photoreceptors. *Invest Ophthalmol Vis Sci* 1987;28(7):1043–1048.
94. Lazarus HS, Hageman GS. Xyloside-induced disruption of interphotoreceptor matrix proteoglycans results in retinal detachment. *Invest Ophthalmol Vis Sci* 1992;33(2):364–376.
95. Lazarus HS, Sly WS, Kyle JW, Hageman GS. Photoreceptor degeneration and altered distribution of interphotoreceptor matrix proteoglycans in the mucopolysaccharidosis VII mouse. *Exp Eye Res* 1993;56(5):531–541.
96. Leibowitz HM, Krueger DE, Maunder LR, Milton RC, Kini MM, Kahn HA, Nickerson RJ, Pool J, Colton TL, Ganley JP, Loewenstein JI, Dawber TR. The Framingham Eye Study monograph: An ophthalmological and epidemiological study of cataract, glaucoma, diabetic retinopathy, macular degeneration, and visual acuity in a general population of 2631 adults, 1973–1975. *Surv Ophthalmol* 1980;24(suppl):335–610.
97. Lewis H, Straatsma BR, Foos RY. Chorioretinal juncture. Multiple extramacular drusen. *Ophthalmology* 1986;93(8):1098–1112.
98. Lewis H, Straatsma BR, Foos RY, Lightfoot DO. Reticular degeneration of the pigment epithelium. *Ophthalmology* 1985;92(11): 1485–1495.
99. Leys A, Vanrenterghem Y, Van DB, Snyers B, Pirson Y, Leys M. Fundus changes in membranoproliferative glomerulonephritis type II. A fluorescein angiographic study of 23 patients. *Graefes Arch Clin Exp Ophthalmol* 1991;229(5):406–410.
100. Lin DS, Anderson GJ, Connor WE, Neuringer M. Effect of dietary N-3 fatty acids upon the phospholipid molecular species of the monkey retina. *Invest Ophthalmol Vis Sci* 1994;35(3):794–803.
101. Linton KL, Klein BE, Klein R. The validity of self-reported and surrogate-reported cataract and age-related macular degeneration in the Beaver Dam Eye Study. *Am J Epidemiol* 1991;134(12):1438–1446.
102. Mainster MA. Light and macular degeneration: A biophysical and clinical perspective. *Eye* 1987;1:304–310.
103. Malmgren H, Gustavson KH, Oudet C, Holmgren G, Pettersson U, Dahl N. Strong founder effect for the fragile X syndrome in Sweden. *Eur J Hum Genet* 1994;2(2):103–9.
104. Mares-Perlman JA, Brady WE, Klein R, Klein BEK, Bowen P, Stacewicz-Sapuntazakis M, Palta M. Serum antioxidants and age-related macular degeneration in a population-based case-control study. *Arch Ophthalmol* 1995; 113:1518–1523.
105. Marshall J. Radiation and the aging eye. *Ophthalmol Physiol Optom* 1985;5(3):241–263.
106. Martinez G, Campbell A. Prevalence of ocular disease in a population study of subjects 65 years old and older. *Am J Ophthalmol* 1982; 94(2):181–189.
107. Massin P, Guillausseau P-J, Vialettes B, Paquis V, Orsini F, Grimaldi AD, Gaudric A. Macular pattern dystrophy associated with a mutation of mitochondrial DNA. *Am J Ophthalmol* 1995;120(2):247–248.
108. Matise TC, Weeks DE. Detecting hetero-

geneity with the affected-pedigree-member (APM) method. *Genet Epidemiol* 1993;10(6): 401–406.

108a. Maw M, Kennedy B, Knight A, et al. Mutation of the gene encoding cellular retinaldehyde-binding protein in autosomal recessive retinitis pigmentosa. *Nature Genet* 1997;17(2): 198–205.

109. McLaughlin ME, Sandberg MA, Berson EL, Dryja TP. Recessive mutations in the gene encoding the beta-subunit of rod phosphodiesterase in patients with retinitis pigmentosa. *Nature Genet* 1993;4(2):130–134.

110. McWilliams P, Farrar GJ, Kenna P, Bradley DG, Humphries M, Shapr EM, McConnell DJ, Lawler M, Sheils D, Ryan C, Stevens K, Daiger SP, Humphries P. Autosomal dominant retinitis pigmentosa (ADRP): Localization of an ADRP gene to the long arm of chromosome 3. *Genomics* 1989;5:619–622.

111. Mehta AB. Glucose-6-phosphate dehydrogenase deficiency (review). *Postgrad Med J* 1994;70(830):871–877.

112. Meire FM, Bergen AA, De Rouck A, Leys M, Delleman JW. X linked progressive cone dystrophy. Localisation of the gene locus to Xp21-p11.1 by linkage analysis. *Br J Ophthalmol* 1994;78(2):103–108.

113. Melrose MA, Magargal LE, Lucier AC. Identical twins with subretinal neovascularization complicating senile macular degeneration. *Ophthalmic Surg* 1985;16(10):648–651.

114. Meyers S, Zachary A. Monozygotic twins with age-related macular degeneration. *Arch Ophthalmol* 1988;106:651–653.

115. Meyers SM. A twin study on age-related macular degeneration. *Trans Am Ophthalmol Soc* 1994;92(775):775–843.

116. Mirow AL, Kristbjanarson H, Egeland JA, Shilling P, Helgason T, Gillin JC, Hirsch S, Kelsoe JR. A linkage study of distal chromosome 5q and bipolar disorder. *Biol Psychiatry* 1994;36(4):223–229.

117. Mitchell BD, Kammerer CM, Hixson JE, Atwood LD, Hackleman S, Blangero J, Haffner SM, Stern MP, MacCluer JW. Evidence for a major gene affecting postchallenge insulin levels in Mexican-Americans. *Diabetes* 1995; 44(3):284–289.

118. Mitchell G, Brody L, Looney J, Steel G, Suchanek M, Dowling C, Der Kaloustian V, Kaiser-Kupfer M, Valle D. An initiator codon mutation in ornithine δ-aminotransferase causing gyrate atrophy of the choroid and retina. *J Clin Invest* 1988;81:630–633.

119. Mitchell P, Smith W, Attebo K, Wang JJ. Prevalence of age-related maculopathy in Australia: The Blue Mountains Eye Study. *Ophthalmology* 1995;102(10):1450–1460.

120. Mitchell RA. Prevalence of age related macular degeneration in persons aged 50 years and over resident in Australia. *J Epidemiol Commun Health* 1993;47(1):42–45.

121. Mitchison HM, O'Rawe AM, Taschner PE, Sandkuijl LA, Santavuori P, de Vos N, Breuning MH, Mole SE, Gardiner RM, Jarvela IE. Batten disease gene, CLN3: Linkage disequilibrium mapping in the Finnish population, and analysis of European haplotypes. *Am J Hum Genet* 1995;56(3):654–662.

122. Modi G, Heckman JM, Saffer D. Vitelliform macular degeneration associated with mitochondrial myopathy. *Br J Ophthalmol* 1992; 76(1):58–60.

123. Monaco WA, Wormington CM. The rhesus monkey as an animal model for age-related macuopathy. *Optom Vis Sci* 1990;67(7): 532–537.

134. Newsome D, Swartz M, Leon N, Elston R, Miller E. Oral zinc in macular degeneration. *Arch Ophthalmol* 1988;106:192–198.

125. Nikali K, Suomalainen A, Terwilliger J, Koskinen T, Weissenbach J, Peltonen L. Random search for shared chromosomal regions in four affected individuals: The assignment of a new hereditary ataxia locus. *Am J Hum Genet* 1995;56(5):1088–1095.

126. Olin KL, Morse LS, Murphy C, Paul MJ, Line S, Bellhorn RW, Hjelmeland LM, Keen CL. Trace element status and free radical defense in elderly rhesus macaques (*Macaca mulatta*) with macular drusen. *Proc Soc Exp Biol Med* 1995;208(4):370–377.

127. Oudet C, von Koskull H, Nordstrom AM, Peippo M, Mandel JL. Striking founder effect for the fragile X syndrome in Finland. *Eur J Hum Genet* 1993;1(3):181–189.

128. Pakstis AJ, Kidd JR, Castiglione CM, Kidd KK. Status of the search for a major genetic locus for affective disorder in the Old Order Amish. *Hum Genet* 1991;87(4):475–483.

129. Pauleikhoff D. [Drusen in Bruch's membrane. Their significance for the pathogenesis and therapy of age-associated macular degeneration (review) [German]. *Ophthalmologe* 1992;89(5):363–386.

130. Pauleikhoff D, Barondes MJ, Minassian D, Chisholm IH, Bird AC. Drusen as risk factors in age-related macular disease. *Am J Ophthalmol* 1990;109(1):38–43.

131. Pauleikhoff D, Chen JC, Chisholm IH, Bird AC. Choroidal perfusion abnormality with age-related Bruch's membrane change. *Am J Ophthalmol* 1990;109(2):211–217.
132. Pauleikhoff D, Zuels S, Sheraidah GS, Marshall J, Wessing A, Bird AC. Correlation between biochemical composition and fluorescein binding of deposits in Bruch's membrane. *Ophthalmology* 1992;99(10):1548–1553.
133. Pawar H, Bingham EL, Lunetta KL, Segal M, Richards JE, Boehnke M, Sieving PA. Refined genetic mapping of juvenile X-linked retinoschisis. *Hum Hered* 1995;45(4):206–210.
134. Peng Y-W, Finn JT, Li J, Dryja TP, McGee TL, Hahn LB, Berson EL, Yau KW. Putative functional defects in rod cGMP-gated channel mutants implicated in retinitis pigmentosa. *Invest Ophthalmol Vis Sci* 1995; 36(4):S919.
135. Prochazka M, Lillioja S, Tait JF, Knowler WC, Mott DM, Spraul M, Bennett PH, Bogardus C. Linkage of chromosomal markers on 4q with a putative gene determining maximal insulin action in Pima Indians. *Diabetes* 1993;42(4):514–519.
136. Quiring R, Walldorf U, Kloter U, Gehring WJ. Homology of the eyeless gene of *Drosophila* to the Small eye gene in mice and aniridia in humans (see comments). *Science* 1994;265(5173):785–789.
137. Rummelt V, Folberg R, Ionasescu V, Yi H, Moore KC. Ocular pathology of MELAS syndrome with mitochondrial DNA nucleotide 3243 point mutation. *Ophthalmology* 1993; 100(12):1757–1766.
138. Sameshima M, Uehara F, Ohba N. Specialization of the interphotoreceptor matrices around cone and rod photoreceptor cells in the monkey retina, as revealed by lectin cytochemistry. *Exp Eye Res* 1987;45(6):845–863.
139. Sarks JP, Sarks SH, Killingsworth MC. Evolution of soft drusen in age-related macular degeneration. *Eye* 1994;8(3):269–283.
140. Sarks S. Aging and degeneration in the macular region: A clinicopathological study. *Br J Ophthalmol* 1976;60:324–341.
141. Sarks S. Drusen in patients predisposing to geographic atrophy of the retinal pigment epithelium. *Aust J Ophthalmol* 1982;10(2): 91–97.
142. Sarks S, Van Driel D, Maxwell L, Killingsworth M. Softening of drusen and subretinal neovascularization. *Trans Ophthalmol Soc UK* 1980;100:414–422.
143. Sarks SH. Drusen and their relationship to senile macular degeneration. *Aust J Ophthalmol* 1980;8(2):117–130.
143a. Sauer C, Gehrig A, Warneke-Wittstock R, et al. Positional cloning of the gene associated with X-linked juvenile retinoschisis. *Nature Genet* 1997;17(2):164–170.
144. Schroeder M, Brown DL, Weeks DE. Improved programs for the affected-pedigree-member method of linkage analysis. *Genet Epidemiol* 1994;11(1):69–74.
145. Seabra M, Brown M, Goldstein J. Retinal degeneration in choroideremia: Deficiency of rab geranylgeranyl transferase. *Science* 1993; 259:377–381.
146. Searle AG, Edwards JH, Hall JG. Mouse homologues of human hereditary disease. *J Med Genet* 1994;31:1–19.
147. Seddon JM, Ajani UA, Sperduto RD, Hiller R, Blair N, Burton TC, Farber MD, Gragoudas ES, Haller J, Miller DT, et al. Dietary carotenoids, vitamins A, C, and E, and advanced age-related macular degeneration. Eye Disease Case-Control Study Group (see comments). *JAMA* 1994;272(18):1413–1420.
148. Seddon JM, Hennekens CH. Vitamins, minerals, and macular degeneration. Promising but unproven hypotheses (editorial; comment). *Arch Ophthalmol* 1994;112(2):176–179.
149. Segato T, Midena E, Blarzino MC. Age-related macular degeneration (review). *Aging* 1993;5(3):165–176.
150. Shafrir E. Animal models of non-insulin-dependent diabetes (review). *Diabetes Metab Rev* 1992;8(3):179–208.
151. Sheffield VC, Carmi R, Kwitek BA, Rokhlina T, Nishimura D, Duyk GM, Elbedour K, Sunden SL, Stone EM. Identification of a Bardet-Biedl syndrome locus on chromosome 3 and evaluation of an efficient approach to homozygosity mapping. *Hum Mol Genet* 1994; 3(8):1331–1335.
152. Sigelman J. Foveal drusen resorption one year after perifoveal laser photocoagulation. *Ophthalmology* 1991;98(9):1379–1383.
153. Singerman LJ, Berkow JW, Patz A. Dominant slowly progressive macular dystrophy. *Am J Ophthalmol* 1977;83(5):680–693.
154. Small KW, Hermsen V, Gurney N, Fetkenhour CL, Folk JC. North Carolina macular dystrophy and central areolar pigment epithelial dystrophy. One family, one disease. *Arch Ophthalmol* 1992;110(4):515–518.
155. Small KW, Weber J, Roses A, Pericak VP.

North Carolina macular dystrophy (MCDR1). A review and refined mapping to 6q14-q16.2 (see comments) (review). *Ophthalmic Paediatr Genet* 1993;14(4):143–150.
156. Sommer A, Tielsch JM, Katz J, Quigley HA, Gottsch JD, Javitt JC, Martone JF, Royall RM, Witt KA, Ezrine S. Racial differences in the cause-specific prevalence of blindness in east Baltimore (see comments). *N Engl J Med* 1991;325(20):1412–1417.
157. Soubrane G, Souied E, Kaplan J, Oubraham H, Coscas G. Prevalence of familial cases with age related maculopathy. *Invest Ophthalmol Vis Sci* 1995;36(4):S1001.
158. Sperduto R, Seigel D. Senile lens and senile macular changes in a population-based sample. *Am J Ophthalmol* 1980;90:86–91.
159. Stohr H, Weber BH. A recombination event excludes the ROM1 locus from the Best's vitelliform macular dystrophy region. *Hum Genet* 1995;95(2):219–222.
160. Stone E, Sheffield V. The molecular genetic approach to macular degeneration. In *Molecular Genetics of Inherited Eye Disorders,* vol 2, *Modern Genetics,* A. Wright and B. Jay, eds, and H. Evans, series ed. Switzerland: Harwood Academic Publishers, 1994.
161. Stone EM, Nichols BE, Kimura AE, Weingeist TA, Drack A, Sheffield VC. Clinical features of a Stargardt-like dominant progressive macular dystrophy with genetic linkage to chromosome 6q (see comments). *Arch Ophthalmol* 1994;112(6):765–772.
162. Stone EM, Nichols BE, Streb L, Kimura AE, Sheffield VC. Genetic linkage of vitelliform macular degeneration (Best's disease) to chromosome 11q13. *Nature Genet* 1992;1: 246–250.
163. Straatsma BR, Lewis H, Foos RY, Evans R. Fluorescein angiography in reticular degeneration of the pigment epithelium. *Am J Ophthalmol* 1985;100(1):202–208.
164. Suarez B, Van Eerdewegh P. A comparison of three affected-sib-pair scoring methods to detect HLA-linked disease susceptibility genes. *Am J Med Genet* 1984;18:135–146.
165. Sverrisson T, Gottfredsdottir MS, Stefansson E. Age-related macular degeneration in monozygotic twins and their spouses. *Invest Ophthalmol Vis Sci* 1995;36(4):S10.
166. Tso MO. Pathogenetic factors of aging macular degeneration. *Ophthalmology* 1985;92(5): 628–635.
167. Uauy DR, Mena P, Hoffman DR. Essential fatty acid metabolism and requirements for LBW infants (review). *Acta Paediatr Suppl* 1994;405(78):78–85.
168. Ulshafer RJ, Engel HM, Dawson WW, Allen CB, Kessler MJ. Macular degeneration in a community of rhesus monkeys. Ultrastructural observations. *Retina* 1987;7(3):198–203.
169. van Bokhoven H, van den Hurk JA, Bogerd L, Philippe C, Gilgenkrantz S, de Jong P, Ropers HH, Cremers FP. Cloning and characterization of the human choroideremia gene. *Hum Mol Genet* 1994;3(7):1041–1046.
170. van Kuijk F, Buck P. Fatty acid composition of the human macula and peripheral retina. *Invest Ophthalmol Vis Sci* 1992;33(13):3493–3496.
171. Vinding T. Age-related macular degeneration. Macular changes, prevalence and sex ratio. An epidemiological study of 1000 aged individuals. *Acta Ophthalmol* 1989;67(6):609–616.
172. Vinding T. Occurrence of drusen, pigmentary changes and exudative changes in the macula with reference to age-related macular degeneration. An epidemiological study of 1000 aged individuals. *Acta Ophthalmol* 1990; 68(4):410–414.
173. Vinding T. Pigmentation of the eye and hair in relation to age-related macular degeneration. *Acta Ophthalmol* 1990;68:53–58.
174. Vingerling JR, Dielemans I, Hofman A, Grobbee DE, Hijmering M, Kramer CF, de Jong PT. The prevalence of age-related maculopathy in the Rotterdam Study. *Ophthalmology* 1995;102(2):205–210.
175. Warburg M, Sjo O, Tranebjaerg L, Fledelius HC. Deletion mapping of a retinal cone-rod dystrophy: Assignment to 18q211. *Am J Med Genet* 1991;39(3):288–293.
176. Weber BH, Vogt G, Pruett RC, Stohr H, Felbor U. Mutations in the tissue inhibitor of metalloproteinases-3 (TIMP3) in patients with Sorsby's fundus dystrophy. *Nature Genet* 1994;8(4):352–356.
177. Weber BHF, Felbor U, Schneider U, Doepner D. Mutational analysis of TIMP3 in Sorsby's fundus dystrophy (SFD) and age-related macular dystrophy (AMD). *Invest Ophthalmol Vis Sci* 1995;36(4):S1064.
178. Weeks D, Lange K. The affected-pedigree-member method of linkage analysis. *Am J Hum Genet* 1988;42:315–326.
179. Weeks DE, Harby LD. The affected-pedigree-member method: Power to detect linkage. *Hum Hered* 1995;45(1):13–24.
180. Weeks DE, Lange K. A multilocus extension

of the affected-pedigree-member method of linkage analysis (review). *Am J Hum Genet* 1992;50(4):859–868.

181. Weiter JJ, Delori FC, Wing GL, Fitch KA. Relationship of senile macular degeneration to ocular pigmentation. *Am J Ophthalmol* 1985;99(2):185–187.
182. Weleber RG, Carr RE, Murphey WH, Sheffield VC, Stone EM. Phenotypic variation including retinitis pigmentosa, pattern dystrophy, and fundus flavimaculatus in a single family with a deletion of codon 153 or 154 of the peripherin/RDS gene. *Arch Ophthalmol* 1993;111(11):1531–1542.
183. Wells J, Wroblewski J, Keen J, Inglehearn C, Jubb C, Eckstein A, Jay M, Arden G, Bhattacharya S, Fitzke F, et al. Mutations in the human retinal degeneration slow (RDS) gene can cause either retinitis pigmentosa or macular dystrophy (see comments). *Nature Genet* 1993;3(3):213–218.
184. West S, Vitale S, Hallfrisch J, Munoz B, Muller D, Bressler S, Bressler NM. Are antioxidants or supplements protective for age-related macular degeneration? (see comments). *Arch Ophthalmol* 1994;112(2): 222–227.
185. Wetzig PC. Photocoagulation of drusen-related degeneration: A long-term outcome. *Trans Am Ophthalmol Soc* 1994;92(299): 299–303.
186. Wroblewski JJ, Wells JA III, Eckstein A, Fitzke F, Jubb C, Keen TJ, Inglehearn C, Bhattacharya SS, Arden GB, Jay MR, et al. Macular dystrophy associated with mutations at codon 172 in the human retinal degeneration slow gene. *Ophthalmology* 1994;101(1):12–22.
187. Wu L. Study of aging macular degeneration in China. *Jpn J Ophthalmol* 1987; 31:349–367.
188. Zhang K, Bither PP, Park R, Donoso LA, Seidman JG, Seidman CE. A dominant Stargardt's macular dystrophy locus maps to chromosome 13q34 (see comments). *Arch Ophthalmol* 1994;112(6):759–764.
189. Zhang Y, Proenca R, Maffei M, Barone M, Leopold L, Friedman JM. Positional cloning of the mouse obese gene and its human homologue [published erratum appears in *Nature* 1995; 374(6521):479]. *Nature* 1994; 372(6505):425–432.

25

Hereditary Vitreoretinopathies

DANIEL F. ROSBERGER
MORTON F. GOLDBERG

The hereditary vitreoretinopathies are a group of inherited disorders characterized by degenerative changes in the vitreous and retina. This chapter discusses snowflake degeneration; familial exudative vitreoretinopathy; Goldmann-Favre syndrome; autosomal dominant vitreoretinochoroidopathy; X-linked congenital retinoschisis; Wagner disease; Stickler syndrome; a syndrome of myelinated nerve fibers, vitreoretinopathy, and skeletal malformations; and the Knobloch syndrome. Until recently, little was known about the molecular genetics of these disorders, and it was necessary to rely on clinical characteristics and electrophysiologic and psychophysical testing to establish a diagnosis. Given the variability of penetrance and expressivity, it was often difficult to make a diagnosis—especially in mild or atypical cases. As we see in Table 25.1, much is still unknown about the precise molecular biology of these disorders. However, it is likely that genetic testing will soon improve our ability to provide accurate diagnoses.

SNOWFLAKE DEGENERATION

Historical Perspective

Snowflake degeneration was first described in 1974 by Hirose et al.,[62] who reported three generations of a single family. It is a rare, autosomal dominant degeneration characterized by small, yellow-white, opacities seen in the peripheral retina. To date there have only been a few pedigrees reported.[27,49,50,62,65,109,117] Although it has been questioned whether or not snowflake degeneration is a variant of retinitis pigmentosa,[27] the presence of characteristic clinical and functional features suggests strongly that it is, in fact, a distinct entity.

Clinical Features

In the original article describing the syndrome, Hirose et al.[62] proposed a four-stage schema for snowflake degeneration. In stage 1, white without pressure is a constant feature in the peripheral retina and is accompanied by small, punctate yellow opacities. Fundus biomicroscopy may reveal early fibrillar degeneration of the vitreous. In stage 2, numerous yellow-white granular or crystalline-appearing "snowflake" deposits are seen to thicken the midperipheral and peripheral retina. They are 100–200 μm in size and may have a predilection for the inferior retina. The posterior border of the lesions may be less distinct than anteriorly, and postequatorial snowflakes are commonly oriented radially along retinal vessels. Fibrillar condensation of the vitreous is more readily apparent than in stage 1 and may be appreciated with direct

Table 25.1 Hereditary Vitreoretinopathies

Name	Inheritance Pattern	Chromosomal Pattern	Gene Product
Snowflake degeneration	AD	Unknown	Unknown
Familial exudative vitreoretinopathy	AD	11q13-23	Unknown
Autosomal dominant vitreoretinochoroidopathy	AD	Unknown	Unknown
Goldmann-Favre syndrome	AR	Unknown	Unknown
X-linked congenital retinoschisis	XR	Xp22.1-22.3	Unknown
Wagner disease	AD	5q13-14	Unknown
Stickler syndrome	AD	12q1.23-3.21	Procollagen II
Syndrome of myelinated nerve fibers, vitreoretinopathy, and skeletal malformations	AD/XD	Unknown	Unknown
Knobloch syndrome	AR	21q22.3	Unknown

AD = autosomal dominant; AR = autosomal recessive; XD = X dominant; XR = X recessive.

ophthalmoscopy. In stage 3, the changes become more advanced, with prominent lens changes, peripheral pigment deposition and clumping, and vascular sheathing. Fibrillar strands of condensed vitreous are evident with the indirect ophthalmoscope. In stage 4, the snowflake deposits are less well identified, peripheral retinal vessels appear obliterated, and there are round-to-oval pigment deposits. Retinal neovascularization has been reported in some patients,[49,109] and retinal tears and detachment are common in advanced cases, sometimes leading to severe visual loss.[62,49,109]

Gheiler et al.[49] described four patients with peripheral retinal neovascularization adjacent to areas of snowflake deposits and vascular sheathing among 36 members of one family. Fluorescein angiography may reveal areas of capillary nonperfusion bordering abnormal retinal vessels. Robertson et al.[117] have reported a more benign variant that may be stable over longer periods. It is characterized by stage 2 retinal changes with numerous discrete snowflake deposits in the equatorial retina. These deposits are not necessarily associated with vitreous liquefaction, traction, peripheral retinal pigmentation, or retinal breaks. In some cases there was no apparent progression for as long as 5 years. A case of a 9-year-old son and his mother, having the same degree of involvement, suggests that snowflake degeneration can be a relatively benign, stationary process. Pollack et al.[109] have suggested that vitreous changes may occur at an early stage in the absence of any demonstrable retinal pathology.

Electrophysiologic and Psychophysiologic Testing

Limited data are available, but retinal function appears to be progressively affected in snowflake degeneration. Marked abnormalities have been seen in the later stages. Abnormal retinal function may also be seen in patients with minimal fundus changes.[62,65] Goldmann perimetry may show peripheral defects not necessarily corresponding to ophthalmoscopically visible lesions. These defects may be more pronounced in the superior visual field, perhaps corresponding to the predilection for the snowflake lesions inferiorly.[117]

Dark adaptation demonstrated elevated rod thresholds in the later stages. All patients studied by Hirose,[65] regardless of stage, showed decreased amplitudes in the scotopic b-wave elicited by dim white light, and some patients had decreased amplitudes of photopic b-wave and photopic flicker responses. No patient had a nonrecordable electroretinogram (ERG). The electrooculogram was abnormal in only a few patients. Four patients studied by Pollack et al.[109] had normal ERGs.

These abnormalities are milder than most progressive primary retinal dystrophies and suggest that snowflake degeneration is in fact, distinct from retinitis pigmentosa.

Differential Diagnosis

The differential diagnosis for snowflake degeneration includes other hereditary vitreoretinopathies with overlapping characteristics as well as disorders with peripheral punctate lesions.

Peripheral white spots seen in fundus albipunctatus and retinitis punctata albescens can be distinguished ophthalmoscopically from snowflake degeneration. These disorders do not have the white without pressure or vitreous changes that characterize snowflake degeneration. Also, pigment deposition and retinal detachment are not present in either fundus albipunctus or retinitis punctata albescens.

Birdshot retinochoroidopathy has yellow-white peripheral lesions, but they are located deeper in the retina, sometimes oriented radially, and they can be present more posteriorly. There are no vitreous cells or macular edema seen in snowflake degeneration, unlike birdshot retinochoroidopathy.

Goldmann-Favre syndrome can be differentiated from snowflake degeneration by the presence of nonrecordable electroretinograms and the presence of retinoschisis, neither of which characterizes snowflake degeneration. In Wagner disease the earliest changes occur in the deep retina and choroid, whereas in snowflake degeneration early changes are confined to the vitreous and superficial retina.

Genetics

Snowflake degeneration is inherited as an autosomal dominant trait with variable phenotypic expressivity. Little is known about the molecular biology of the disease.

Treatment

The main focus of treatment for snowflake degeneration is aimed at the complication of retinal detachment, which is frequently seen in advanced stages. The incidence of retinal detachment is not known, but it is believed to be high and associated with a poor success rate following reattachment surgery.[49,50,62,109,117] This has prompted the recommendation to prophylactically surround all retinal breaks with photocoagulation.[109] When detachments do occur, they may be treated with standard scleral buckling procedures; however, given the high failure rate and the continuing vitreous traction present in this disorder, pars plana vitrectomy may be appropriate in some cases. The role of scatter laser photocoagulation for peripheral neovascularization associated with capillary nonperfusion is not well defined but may be considered.

Because of the relatively mild initial course compared with other vitreoretinopathies, and the fact that phenotypic expression may not occur in some cases until the third decade of life, patients in affected families should be closely observed and should not be considered disease free even with a benign-appearing fundus.

FAMILIAL EXUDATIVE VITREORETINOPATHY

Historic Perspective

Familial exudative vitreoretinopathy (FEVR) was first described by Criswick and Schepens in 1969.[30] They described six patients from two families with temporal abnormalities of the vitreous and retina that resembled retinopathy of prematurity (ROP), but none of the patients had a history of gestational prematurity or supplemental oxygen exposure. In 1971, Gow and Oliver, described a large family and defined the clinical staging still generally in use.[54] They also confirmed that FEVR was inherited as an autosomal dominant trait. Fluorescein angiography studies by Canny and Oliver demonstrated marked pheripheral retinal capillary nonperfusion similar to that seen in ROP.[24] Subsequent reports by Laqua[77] and Nijhuis et al.[97] added additional features. As originally described by Criswick and Schepens, FEVR was inexorably progressive; however, later studies by several investigators[99,130] have demonstrated that perhaps the majority of cases remain stable.

Clinical Features

The clinical manifestations of FEVR vary greatly among individuals, with some manifesting only minor peripheral abnormalities of the vasculature and others showing complex total retinal detachment. Characteristically, the disorder is bilateral, although asymmetry is common. Patients may present early in childhood with findings identical to ROP but without any history of premature birth or exposure to supplemental oxygen. It is usually possible to elicit a family history or find subtle peripheral retinal vascular changes in family members that will identify the dominant inheritance. Children may present with decreased visual acuity, and sometimes, if sufficiently severe, with secondary nystagmus. They also may be noted to have an ocular deviation either from true stabismus or from pseudostrabismus secondary to temporal dragging of the macula and a large positive angle kappa. Amblyopia in the more severely affected eye is not uncommon.

The staging of FEVR was proposed by Gow and Oliver[54] and modified slightly by Laqua[77] to include angiographic findings. In stage 1, patients are largely asymptomatic and usually maintain good central visual acuity. White with and without pressure can be seen in the temporal periphery, often with associated vitreous membranes and, sometimes, mild vitreoretinal traction. Peripheral retinal nonperfusion and areas of frankly avascular retina peripheral to the abrupt termination of retinal vessels may be present. Although it is markedly more common temporally, the zone of avascular retina may extend circumferentially for up to 360°. Miyakubo et al.[93] have described a temporal wedge-shaped avascular zone with the apex toward the macula, with a corresponding V-shaped area of chorioretinal atrophy or retinal opacification. Peripheral cystoid degeneration is common. Yellow, refractile, intraretinal deposits, ranging in size from 100 to 500 μm, have been described.[39] Additionally, areas of finely dispersed pigmentation in areas of predominantly avascular retina,[139] as well as areas of central and peripheral pigment clumping, have been noted.

Fluorescein angiography[24,77,97] with sweep views of the retinal periphery may reveal areas of capillary nonperfusion. Angiography is most sensitive in the temporal periphery, where areas of nonperfusion are most prominent. Termination of retinal capillaries, forming a scalloped border with associated angiographic leakage, may be seen. Fluorescein angiography may highlight the abnormal straightening of the retinal vessels and arteriovenous shunts at the margin of the vascularized and nonvascularized retina. Occasionally, small hemorrhages and microaneurysms may be seen, as can mildly dilated perifoveal capillaries, which can leak slightly in the later phases of the angiogram.

Stage 2 is characterized by the development of exudative and proliferative changes, which may resemble the cicatricial phase of ROP. Peripheral retinal neovascularization, which is most prominent temporally, is seen. Subretinal and intraretinal exudation may be prominent in this stage. There is a characteristic finding of a temporal fibrovascular mass fed by large arteriovenous shunt vessels at the border of the avascular retina. Thickly condensed vitreous membranes may overlie the fibrovascular proliferation, and adjacent reactive pigmentary changes have been described. When the fibrous component contracts, there can be significant retinal traction, which can cause optic disc dragging and macular heterotopia with accompanying true and pseudostrabismus. Traction on the retinal microvasculature can stimulate perifoveal leakage and cystoid edema as well as significant transudation. In occasional cases, isolated traction retinal detachment may occur.

Fluorescein angiography shows clearly the extent of the fibrovascular proliferation and accompanying dye leakage. Areas of retinal neovascularization may resemble the "sea-fan" of sickle-cell retinopathy or of incontinentia pigmenti.

The blinding complications of FEVR are present in stage 3. For the most part, these are secondary to the cicatrization of the temporal fibrovascular proliferative mass. As the mass contracts, it exerts traction on the retina, causing an expanding retinal detachment. This may initially be limited to a localized traction detachment; however, often it may progress with the development of retinal breaks to a complex combined traction and rhegmatogenous retinal detachment, sometimes with falciform folds. Vitreoretinal adhesions with development of fibrous tissue at the temporal equator can be seen in almost half of affected eyes.[92] Vitreous hemorrhage may occur secondary to bleeding from neovascular tissue or as a result of tearing of retinal vessels at the time of detachment.

Massive intraretinal and subretinal exudation, mimicking Coats disease, may occur. In the later phases of the disease, anterior segment changes, including neovascularization of the iris and angle with resultant neovascular glaucoma, may be seen. Cataracts, posterior synechiae, iris atrophy, and band keratopathy may also be present.

Electrophysiologic and Psychophysical Testing

Limited electrophysiologic and psychophysical studies have been performed on patients with FEVR. Visual fields appear to be moderately constricted peripherally, with changes more prominent nasally corresponding to the temporal avascular retina. Mild abnormalities in color vision have been reported.[139] Electroretinography, photopic and scotopic, is characteristically normal.[39,77] However, Ohkubo[101] reported mildly depressed ERG findings in two patients with advanced disease and noted that depressed ERG results are statistically related to more advanced fundus findings and worse visual acuity. Electrooculography has been reported to be subnormal in at least 40% of patients with attached retinas.[101,139] Dark adaptation is usually unaffected.[139]

Differential Diagnosis

Familial exudative vitreoretinopathy most closely resembles retinopathy of prematurity (ROP) clinically, but FEVR patients lack the characteristic history of gestational prematurity, low birth weight, and/or supplmental oxygen exposure. Conversely, it is usually possible to establish an inheritance pattern in patients with phenotypic FEVR (either dominant, in the majority of cases; X-linked in fewer pedigrees), which is absent in ROP. In contrast to ROP, FEVR is more generally bilateral, albeit with possible asymmetry, and more frequently demonstrates intraretinal lipid. Massive subretinal lipid may be present with FEVR. Patients with ROP are more frequently myopic.

The subretinal lipid can sometimes resemble Coats disease; however, FEVR lacks the characteristic telangiectatic vessels necessary for the diagnosis of Coats disease. In autosomal dominant FEVR, males and females are affected equally. Other diseases that appear to have subretinal exudation, including ocular toxocariasis, retinoblastoma, and retinal angiomatosis, must also be excluded.

Peripheral neovascularization can also be seen in sickle cell retinopathy, incontinentia pigmenti, and Eales disease. These, however, only occasionally present a diagnostic dilemma.

In addition to ROP, disorders that cause optic disc dragging and macular heterotopia must be excluded. These include persistent hyperplastic primary vitreous (PHPV) and Norrie disease. Unlike FEVR, PHPV is almost always unilateral. Furthermore, patients more frequently show the disease at birth, and the affected eye is usually microphthalmic. Interestingly, an X-linked form of FEVR has recently been described, which appears to share the locus with the gene for Norrie disease.[28,47,122]

Genetics

Familial exudative vitreoretinopathy is almost always inherited as an autosomal dominant trait with nearly 100% penetrance.[99] There is, however, tremendous variability in the phenotypic expression, with some asymptomatic individuals detected only because another more significantly affected family member is being investigated. Sporadic cases of FEVR have been reported[93,98] and may represent new somatic or germ-line mutations.

Recently, Li and co-workers, studying a large German kindred, have localized the gene for autosomal dominant FEVR to the long arm of chromosome 11.[78] Additional studies of two separate families using five markers from 11q13 to 11q23 revealed pairwise linkage data providing no evidence for genetic heterogeneity. The highest compiled two point lod score was obtained for the disease locus versus the D11S533 marker.[79] The exact location of the gene for autosomal dominant FEVR and the identity of the gene product are still unknown.

The primary pathogenesis of the disorder is still unclear. Criswick and Schepens[30] stressed the importance of the abnormal vitreoretinal interaction; others have argued the primacy of the retinal vascular maldevelopment.[97,99] Peripheral retinal ischemia could cause the release of angiogenic factors similar to what is presumed to occur in other proliferative retinopathies. The pathogenesis for the vascular occlusion is the subject of debate. Chaudhuri et al.[26] reported absent platelet aggregation with arachidonic acid in all affected members of two families. In addition, one severely affected patient demonstrated reduced platelet aggregation with collagen and epinephrine as well. In contrast, Laqua[77] found no platelet abnormalities in one thoroughly investigated patient. Similar additional studies by Friedrich et al.[45] failed to confirm Chaudhuri's findings but did note an abnormal bleeding time. Another study[16] of an additional kindred also failed to find any hematological defect in either the six affected members or any of the unaffected members. In particular, no abnormalities of arachidonic acid–induced platelet aggregation were noted.

Available histopathology is of limited value because all eyes evaluated to date have been end stage. No specimens reflecting early or mild disease have been studied. Brockhurst et al.[17] described two eyes enucleated from twins with presumed FEVR. A total retinal detachment was present in both specimens, with prominent preretinal and vitreous membranes firmly adherent to the retina and resulting retinal folds. Nicholson and Galvis[96] reported nine affected members of a Colombian family. One eye of an affected patient was enucleated for neovascular glaucoma and showed a focal, nodular zone of fibrovascular proliferation histopathologically. This was asociated with necrosis and acute inflammatory changes with dense preretinal fibrous organization in the temporal preequatorial retina. They postulated that such a nidus may be responsible for the temporal retinal dragging and falciform retinal folds sometimes seen in FEVR. Boldrey et al.[13] also reported two cases enucleated for neovascular glaucoma. Similarly, these eyes had total retinal detachments with peripheral retinal vascular proliferation and a fibrovascular preretinal membrane.

A disease phenotypically identical to autosomal dominant FEVR has been recently described with an X-linked inheritance pattern.[108] In fact, one of the original kindreds reported by Criswick and Schepens is consistent with either autosomal dominant or X-linked inheritance. Linkage studies of several families appear to suggest that the locus for X-linked FEVR maps in the vicinity of the Norrie disease gene locus.[28,47,122] Molecular analysis was performed on the Norrie gene locus in a four-generation kindred with X-linked FEVR and revealed a missense mutation resulting in neutral amino acid substitution (Leu124Phe) in all affected males but in none of the unaffected family members, nor in any of the controls.[28] This suggests that phenotypes for both X-linked FEVR and Norrie disease may result from mutations in the same gene.

Treatment

Management of FEVR involves identification of all, even asymptomatic, family members of affected individuals. Careful examination, possibly supplemented by fluorescein angiography, may be necessary to diagnose subtle disease in minimally affected patients. Once the gene for FEVR has been localized molecular genetic techniques may permit pre- and postnatal screening.

It is now clear that contrary to the initial description by Criswick and Schepens of a relentless progression,[30] the majority of patients remain stable.[99,130] Nonetheless, close observation and follow-up, to monitor for active proliferation, may be the most important aspect of clinical management. Prophylactic cryopexy or laser photocoagulation of avascular retina can probably be delayed until evidence of neovascular progression is noted. However, once progression is noted, peripheral retinal ablation should be initiated. Prompt application of retinal cryopexy has been shown to decrease the vascularity of the fibrovascular tissue and prevent the progression of disease to stage 3.[138]

Retinal detachments associated with FEVR are perhaps the most serious complication and are frequently complex and difficult to repair. In one large series reported by Miyakubo et al.,[92] retinal detachments secondary to traction were present in 17% of eyes, and rhegmatogenous detachments were present in 26%. The incidence of traction detachment was greatest in patients in their first decade of life and tended to be located in the temporal periphery.

Traction retinal detachments were likely to be stationary or only slightly progressive in this series. Rhegmatogenous detachments were most common in the second decade of life, but, when present in early childhood, patients had a poor prognosis,[140] often with redetachments requiring multiple surgical procedures.

Treatment of retinal detachments associated with FEVR must involve the release of vitreoretinal traction with scleral buckling that is often performed in conjunction with pars plana vitrectomy and membrane peeling.[129] Recently, Maguire and Trese[86] described a series of patients with favorable anatomic and functional results following lens-sparing vitrectomy in infants with FEVR.

With secondary anterior segment complications such as rubeosis iridis and neovascular glaucoma, an attempt should be made to induce regression of proliferative tissue with scatter laser photocoagulation or cryopexy. Clearly, aggressive correction of amblyopia is essential in infants, especially those with asymmetric involvement, Surgical realignment of eyes with strabismus should also be considered.

AUTOSOMAL DOMINANT VITREORETINOCHOROIDOPATHY

Historical Perspective

Autosomal dominant vitreoretinochoroidopathy (ADVIRC) was first described in 1982[72] and is characterized by the presence in the fundus of circumferential coarse peripheral pigmentary degeneration with a relatively discrete equatorial posterior border (Fig. 25.1), superficial yellow–white punctate retinal opacities, vitreous and vascular abnormalities, presenile cataracts, retinal neovascularization, breakdown of the blood–retina barrier, and choroidal atrophy. Only a few isolated kindreds of this rare dystrophy have been described.[10,52,57,72,134]

Clinical Features

It is difficult to determine the precise anatomic location of the initial pathology in ADVIRC. Abnormalities in the vitreous, retina, and choroid are present. The lenticular changes may be secondary to the other processes or may be an independent manifestation. The disease appears to be slowly progressive, with older patients manifesting more severe changes clinically and electrophysiologically. The age of patients described in the literature ranges from 7 to 88 years. An autosomal dominant pattern of inheritance has been easily identified in published kindreds.[10,52,57,72,134] Some patients with ADVIRC have been noted to be mildly or moderately myopic; however, pathologic myopia is not a feature of this disease. Occasionally, mild complaints of decreased night vision may be elicited, but nyctalopia is not a common or prominent feature. In contrast to some of the other hereditary vitreoretinopathies, patients generally maintain relatively good vision.

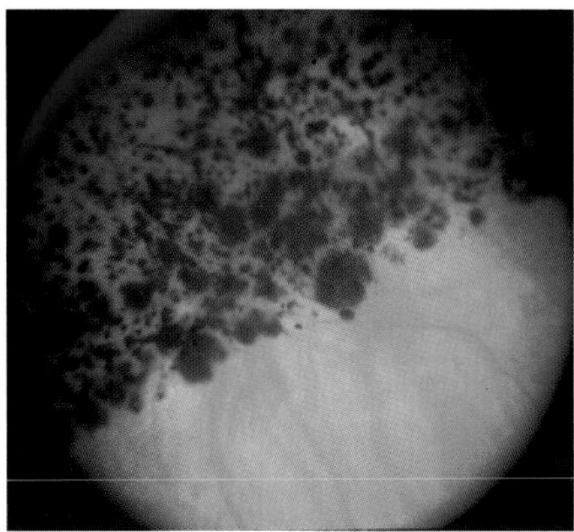

Figure 25.1. Demarcation between normal posterior and peripheral retina in a patient with autosomal-dominant vitreoretinochoroidopathy. (Reproduced with permission from ref. 134.)

Although there are overlapping features with other hereditary vitreoretinopathies, ADVIRC presents with a constellation of characteristic clinical findings.[10,52,57,72,134] These include vitreous liquefaction, which may be associated with fibrillar condensation. An "optically empty" vitreous is not seen. Perhaps pathognomonic for this condition is the coarse pigmentary degeneration extending for 360° from the ora serrata to the equatorial region, where there is a discrete posterior border. Punctate white or yellow opacities have been noted in the peripheral retina. Arteriolar narrowing and peripheral occlusion can be seen. Breakdown of the blood–

retina barrier is demonstrable in most cases[10,72] with fluorescein angiography and vitreous fluorophotometry. This breakdown may result in cystoid macular edema as well as vitreous cells. Presenile cataracts, which are a common finding, may be secondary to the retinal vascular incompetence. Retinal neovascularization and rarely vitreous homorrhage have been reported.[10,52,72] Retinal detachment does not appear to be an associated finding. Traboulsi and Payne[134] reported an 88-year-old patient who had developed a unilateral aphakic traumatic rhegmatogenous retinal detachment at age 53, which was successfully repaired. The same patient also suffered a spontaneous vitreous hemorrhage at age 75 years, which resolved spontaneously.

Extensive systemic evaluations have been performed on affected patients. Pediatric, orthodontic, craniofacial, skeletal, and audiometric examinations failed to reveal any consistent systemic abnormalities.

Electrophysiologic and Psychophysical Testing

The electroretinographic findings in ADVIRC can be summarized by noting that they are essentially normal in the younger patients and may be mildly depressed in older patients with more advanced disease. In the initial kindred described by Kaufman et al.,[72] four of the six affected family members had normal ERGs. One patient had a subnormal ERG with equally affected rod and cone responses, and the other patient had a subnormal ERG with rods and cones equally affected. In the second reported kindred,[10] four of the five affected patients had normal ERGs—the fifth patient refused evaluation, Han and Lewandowski[57] reported normal cone responses in four patients tested. Rod responses in this series were normal or mildly subnormal, except for one patient, a 53-year-old man, who had a reduced b-wave dark-adapted blue flash rod ERG.

Interestingly, in all four patients reported by Han and Lewandowski[57] there was a marked decrease in electrooculography. They reported Arden ratios of 1.1–1.5 (normal is greater than 1.8). They postulated that a diffuse disturbance of the photoreceptor–RPE complex may have been present prior to the development of more extensive photoreceptor functional loss.

Visual field testing has been reported as normal or mildly constricted[10,57,72,134] and may reflect the peripheral pigmentary degeneration noted in all cases. Vitreous fluorophotometry has demonstrated a breakdown of the blood–retina barrier and retinal vascular incompetence.[10,72] Fluorescein angiography may reveal dilation and leakage of posterior pole capillaries. Cystoid macular edema is often evident in the later frames. Retinal neovascularization in the posterior pole has also been observed.[10,72]

Histopathologic specimens of only two patients have been reported.[52,57a] Examination of an eye from an 88-year-old patient demonstrated disorganization of the peripheral retina with focal atrophic pigmentary changes. Altered RPE cells were noted surrounding the retinal vessels and lining the internal limiting membrane. A marked multifocal loss of photoreceptor cells was present at the equator, and an extensive membrane consisting of condensed vitreous with cellular debris and layers of Müller cells was demonstrated on the surface of the retina by electron microscopy and immunohistochemistry.[52] Similar findings of atrophic, disorganized peripheral retina replacement of peripheral vascular endothelium by presumed cells of RPE origin in eyes obtained from a 26-year-old woman[57a] suggest that histopathologic manifestations of ADVIRC may be of early onset with little subsequent progression.

Differential Diagnosis

Unlike Stickler syndrome, there have been no associated systemic abnormalities noted in patients with ADVIRC. Also patients with ADVIRC have not been seen to have an optically empty vitreous, high myopia, or retinal detachment.

Although the peripheral degeneration may be confused with some forms of retinitis pigmentosa, nyctalopia is not a prominent complaint, and electroretinography is usually normal or only slightly subnormal. Similarly, essentially normal ERGs would tend to exclude Goldmann-Favre disease and X-linked retinoschisis. The circumferential pigmentary degeneration with a sharply demarcated posterior border may be pathognomonic for ADVIRC and has not been described in snowflake degeneration, Wagner disease, or familial exudative vitreoretinopathy.

Genetics

As indicated by its name, ADVIRC is an autosomal dominantly inherited condition, although affected individuals may exhibit variable penetrance.[10,72,134] To date, nothing is known about the chromosomal location of the gene responsible for ADVIRC or about the gene product responsible for the phenotype characteristics.

Treatment

Because of the paucity of clinical experience, specific treatment recommendations are difficult to make with confidence. Many patients with ADVIRC develop presenile lenticular changes. In those patients for whom the cataract is felt to be responsible for the decline in visual acuity, cataract extraction is likely to be of benefit, as most patients seem to maintain good central vision.[10,72,134] In one case in the original kindred,[72] oral prednisone (40–60 mg daily) was tried in an attempt to decrease the associated cystoid macular edema. Although it was apparently effective, with improved visual acuity and a lessening of retinal thickening prednisone was discontinued secondary to systemic side effects. Without steroid treatment, visual acuity and edema returned to pretreatment level. Depot subtenons steroids were then employed (triamcinolone diacetate 20 mg) with improved visual acuity noted at 5 weeks. Clinically, however, no improvement in the macular edema was appreciated. It is unclear, therefore, whether steroid treatment is of benefit in the condition, but it is certainly not unreasonable to pursue a trial of oral prednisone in patients with prominent, symptomatic macular edema and no systemic contraindications. Acetazolamide has not yet been systemically evaluated in this disease.

Patients with ADVIRC may also lose vision from vitreous hemorrhage secondary to retinal neoascularization. Although it is evident that there are abnormalities in the retinal vasculature noted both by fluorescein angiography and vitreous fluorophotometry, overt retinal ischemia is not a conspicuous finding. Therefore, it is unclear whether there would be any indication for retinal ablation either with cryopexy or with scatter laser photocoagulation. One patient with vitreous hemorrhage 'reported by Traboulsi and Payne[134] had spontaneous resolution without intervention.

GOLDMANN-FAVRE SYNDROME

Historical Perspective

Goldmann-Favre syndrome was described independently in two adolescent siblings by Goldmann[53] in 1957 and Favre[38] in 1958 Ricci[113] reexamined the original patients and added an additional case, a woman in her fourth decade. The characteristic findings included a retinitis pigmentosa–like retinal degeneration with pigment clumping and central or peripheral retinoschisis.[38,53,113] Fibrillar degeneration and liquefaction of the vitreous, as well as complicated cataracts, were also described. It is an autosomal recessive disease with wide variation in the constellation of clinical findings.

Clinical Features

The clinical symptoms of the disease are primarily related to pigmentary degeneration, progressive cataracts, and central and peripheral retinoschisis, Early in the course of the disease, patients typically complain of bilateral progressive night blindness secondary to the peripheral pigmentary and retinal changes. Men and women appear to be affected equally. Central visual acuity may be affected by the central retinoschisis or by the macular cystoid changes that are frequently present. Patients are typically myopic and develop complicated lenticular changes. Patients have also been noted to have anterior chamber inflammation, and late-onset optic atrophy. Dendritic, whitish retinal vessels have been noted in the posterior pole and in areas of retinoschisis. They are helpful, when present, as a diagnostic sign. Retinal capillary abnormalities manifest as leakage on fluorescein angiography, have also been reported.[40] Similarly, perifoveal capillary incompetence can result in cystoid changes. In areas of peripheral retinoschisis, vascular occlusion has been observed, and may account for the dendritic appearance of the opaque blood vessels.

The macular lesions, which were originally described as resembling beaten copper,[38,53] may be continuous with the peripheral retinoschisis as microcystic changes develop. Vitreous liquefaction and fibrillar degeneration are usually observed, often with traction bands and posterior vitreous detachment.[25,38,40,42,43,48,53,113] Oval holes in the inner layer of the peripheral retinoschisis are a common finding. These are usually without consequence; however, retinal detachments, which may be difficult to repair, may also result.

Electrophysiologic and Psychophysical Testing

Electroretinography is usually profoundly abnormal[40,113]; however normal and near-normal results have been reported.[25] Often, rod-mediated responses are affected early in the syndrome,[43] with a nonrecordable ERG developing in the later phases.[40,42,113] The electrooculogram is usually flat or demonstrates a severely decreased light-to-dark ratio.[11,48]

Goldmann-Favre syndrome may be related to the enhanced S-cone syndrome.[68] Jacobson et al.[68] studied four patients with Goldmann-Favre syndrome with dark-adapted perimetry and noted that they all had severely reduced rod sensitivities and subnormal midspectral cone sensitivities. With S-cone perimetry, the patients had normal or subnormal S-cone function. There was higher sensitivity to S-cones relative to midspectral cones throughout the visual field.

Color vision has been reported to be abnormal, with blue-yellow defects noted on the Farnsworth-Munsell 100 hue test, and red–green defects seen with pseudoisochromatic plates.[11]

Visual fields may be abnormal, reflecting the absolute scotomas related to the peripheral retinoschisis.

Fluorescein angiography reveals areas of retinal capillary leakage and nonperfusion, with cystoid leakage present in the late frames.

Histopathologic examination from a full-thickness eye wall biopsy of a 27-year-old woman with Goldmann-Favre syndrome[105] has been performed. The 4 mm peripheral specimen was noted to have diffuse degenerative changes predominantly affecting the sensory retina, with the outer nuclear layer being attenuated and the photoreceptor outer segments being absent. The retinal pigment epithelium and choriocapillaris were largely spared. Based on these findings, it was postulated that a primary degeneration of the photoreceptors may be involved. Thickening of the retinal vasculature's basement membranes, as well as areas of vascular occlusion, were noted. A thick preretinal membrane composed of glial tissue was also reported.

Differential Diagnosis

Goldmann-Favre syndrome shares certain characteristics with congenital retinoschisis and Wagner disease. Goldmann-Favre syndrome may be differentiated on the basis of inheritance, as it is inherited as an autosomal recessive condition, whereas congenital retinoschisis is X linked, and Wagner disease is autosomal dominant. Nyctalopia, although a prominent early symptom in Goldmann-Favre syndrome, is not apparent in congenital retinoschisis or Wagner disease. Furthermore, the macular cystic changes in congenital retinoschisis are far more pronounced and lack the beaten-copper appearance of Goldmann-Favre syndrome. Electroretinography is generally more reduced in Goldmann-Favre syndrome than in Wagner disease, and the peripheral pigmentary changes in Goldmann-Favre syndrome, characterized by a bone corpuscle pattern, are not seen in Wagner disease.

Genetics

Goldmann-Favre syndrome is an exceedingly rare autosomal recessive condition with incomplete penetrance.[25,38,40,42,43,53,113] The genetics of the syndrome have yet to be determined in detail. Histopathology from one patient appears to suggest a primary sensory retinal defect; however, the specific abnormality awaits determination.[105] There is reason to believe that the Goldmann-Favre syndrome may share a common pattern of retinal dysfunction with the enhanced S-cone syndrome.[68] in which there is retinal degeneration associated with short wavelength (S-cone) hypersensitivity.

Treatment

Given that the prognosis for repair of retinal detachment associated with Goldmann-Favre is guarded, it may be reasonable to prophylactically seal full-thickness retinal tears or holes. Careful evaluation of family members is also suggested.

Retinal detachment, when present, can be usually managed with standard scleral buckling. In cases with significant traction or posterior retinal breaks vitrectomy may be the more appropriate intervention. Prophylactic treatment of outer layer breaks should probably be avoided, as this may precipitate a retinal detachment.

Recently, it was reported that immunosuppressive therapy with cyclosporin A may cause a regression in macular edema and flattening of the retinoschisis cavity,[48] but the effectiveness of cyclosporin A in this syndrome remains unclear.[84]

CONGENITAL X-LINKED RETINOSCHISIS

Historical Perspective

The first description of X-linked retinoschisis was made by Haas in 1898.[56] Early pedigrees established that this entity was found exclusively in males.[103,125,133] Over the years, many appellations have been applied to this condition; including *cystic disease of the retina in children, congenital vascular veils, juvenile retinoschisis* and *congenital cystic retinal detachment.* Jager applied the designation of retinoschisis in 1953.[69] (See also Chapter 18 by Sieving.)

Clinical Features

Congenital X-linked retinoschisis is a bilateral disease of young boys that may be clinically apparent at birth.[18,111,118] The clinical spectrum varies greatly among individuals and is related to abnormalities of the vitreous, macula, and retinal periphery. Invariably, both eyes are affected, and, although there may be asymmetry in involvement, as a rule both eyes are similarly affected.[128]

The characteristic foveal schisis (Fig. 25.2) is present in all cases[35–37] and may be the only sign of disease in half of all patients.[34,36] The splitting occurs at the level of the nerve fiber layer,[88,147] with radial plications of the retinal internal limiting membrane seen in some cases.[142] Approximately 50% of patients may also have peripheral nerve fiber layer retinoschisis as well, located most commonly inferotemporally.[23] These conditions only rarely extend to the ora serrata. The inner layer of the schisis is typically concave and immobile and may contain multiple holes.[76] Large blood vessels can often be observed in the inner schisis wall and may cross the schisis cavity.[58]

As in many of the hereditary vitreoretinopathies, vitreous abnormalities, including fibrillar degeneration, vitreous liquefaction, peripheral traction bands, and posterior vitreous detachment are frequently found.[119] Patients may present very early in life, and it appears that progression of the disease may be rapid in the

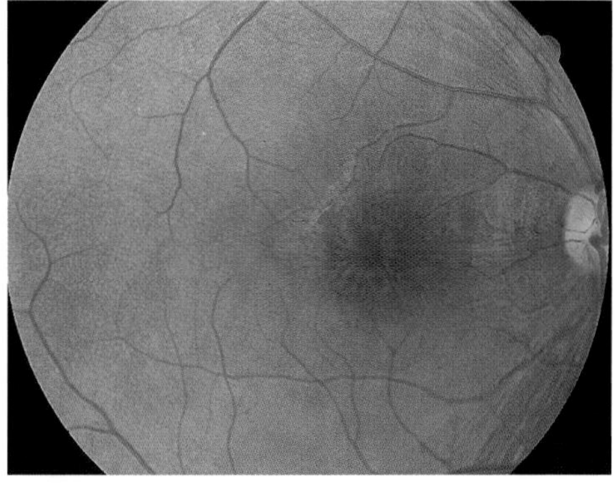

Figure 25.2. Characteristic macular spoke-wheel cystic changes in X-linked retinoschisis.

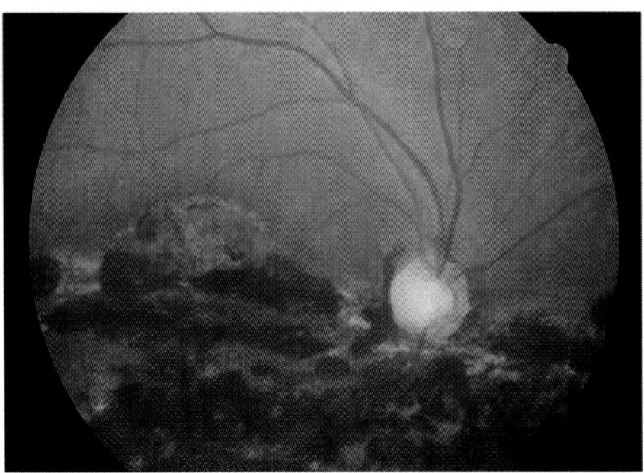

Figure 25.3. Extensive pigmentary changes in inferior half of right retina of a 60-year-old man with X-linked juvenile retinoschisis. Superior half of retina is normal.

first decade of life. Progression is noted by an increasing height of the schisis cavity, extensive peripheral chorioretinal atrophy and, in the macula, atrophy of the retinal pigment epithelium (RPE) underlying the cystic retina. In older patients, the stellate maculopathy characteristic of young patients may not be apparent, and the RPE changes may be the most prominent finding (Fig. 25.3).

Vitreous hemorrhage can occur secondary to unsupported retinal vessels bridging the schisis cavity and cause a sudden decrease in visual acuity. Sheathing of retinal vessels has also been reported.[55] The most serious complication of the retinal and vitreous changes in congenital X-linked retinoschisis is full-thickness rhegmatogenous retinal detachment, which may be quite difficult to repair.

Electrophysiologic and Psychophysical Testing

Results of ERG are related to progression of disease. There does, however, appear to be a preferential decrease in photopic voltages as opposed to scotopic voltages.[58] Early in the course of the disease, the a-wave is often normal or near normal but is associated with a markedly reduced b-wave.[66] This pattern is quite characteristic for X-linked congenital retinoschisis.[128] Given the divergence of a-wave and b-wave function and the importance of Müller cell contribution to the b-wave, it has been suggested that a primary Müller cell dysfunction may underlie the disorder.[104] Histopathologic and ultrastructural findings in three eyes were reported by Condon et al.,[29] and also suggest a defect in Müller cells. They found a periodic acid–Schiff (PAS) positive amorphous material within the retina adjacent to the schisis cavities. Ultrastructural examination revealed it to contain 11 nm extracellular filaments. Similar filaments were found in the vitreous. They hypothesized that the intraretinal filaments were produced by defective Müller cells and that their extracellular accumulation may lead to cellular degeneration and subsequent schisis formation. With late-stage disease, characterized by extensive retinal degeneration, the ERG may be extinguished.[33,34,132] Photoreceptor oscillatory potentials may be dramatically reduced.[60] Interestingly, although there is great variability among individuals with the disease, there is great electrophysiologic symmetry between the two eyes of an affected individual.[128]

The published results of electrooculography are not consistent. In one study, the electrooculogram was reported to be normal in over 90% of patients tested.[128] Another study reported abnormal tests, even with disease confined to the posterior pole.[142]

Visual evoked potentials (VEPs) are usually normal, even in cases with an abnormal ERG.[58] The macular VEP is, however, always abnormal[64] and underscores the universality of macular dysfunction in this disease.

Visual field abnormalities are related to areas of peripheral involvement, resulting in an absolute scotoma in regions of retinoschisis.[147] Results of flicker perimetry are usually abnormal, suggesting involvement of cone function.[66]

Color vision is usually interpreted as being within normal limits;[7,83] however, abnormalities including deuteranomalous and tritanopic defects have been reported.[61,100]

Multiple abnormalities have been reported on fluorescein angiography,[75] including prolonged transit time,[136] slow filling of dendritic vessels,[55] and peripheral capillary nonperfusion anterior to regions of schisis.[55] In general, although there have been isolated reports of faint staining,[100,115] the macular cystic spaces do not leak fluorescein in the late frames of the angiogram.[23,58,75,136] This differentiates X-linked congenital retinoschisis from other entities that manifest cystoid macular edema.

Differential Diagnosis

Congenital X-linked retinoschisis must be differentiated from acquired retinoschisis. In general, patients with acquired retinoschisis are older and are less likely to present with macular involvement. In addition, the characteristic combination of a maintained a-wave and depressed b-wave is absent in acquired disease.

There may be some overlap with the appearance of Goldmann-Favre disease; however, the ERG is usually extinguished in Goldmann-Favre disease. Whereas Goldmann-Favre disease is inherited as an autosomal recessive condition with male and females affected equally, X-linked retinoschisis is limited to males. Furthermore, nyctalopia is a more frequent and prominent complaint in Goldmann-Favre disease.

Cystoid macular edema (CME) can sometimes mimic the appearance of the macular changes in X-linked retinoschisis. Fluorescein angiography can usually differentiate these, as there is distinct leakage into the cystoid spaces of CME but rarely any leakage related to the "cystic" macula in retinoschisis.

Genetics

Congenital retinonschisis was early noted to be transmitted in an X-linked fashion.[7,14,56,103,125,133] Forsius et al.[41] have reported an unusual case of a homozygous woman with the disorder, a child of an affected father and his second cousin.

In 1970, Ives et al. demonstrated linkage of the gene for congenital retinoschisis to the distal Xg locus in five families studied.[67] Analysis of another family in 1976 was consistent with loose linkage between the loci for juvenile retinoschisis and the red cell antigen marker, Xga.[15] In 1983, Wieacker et al., using restriction fragment length polymorphisms (RFLPs), were able to localize the retinoschisis gene to the Xp21 segment on the distal end of the short arm of the X chromosome.[145] Alitalo and co-workers studied nine families with 24 affected males.[4] Using three polymorphic DNA probes, they were able to demonstrate close linkage to markers DXS41 and DXS16. Further work, in 1988,[3,31] placed the retinoschisis gene at Xp22 in the following order: Xpter-DXS85-DXS207-DXS43-retinoschisis-DXS41-DXS84-Xcen. Seven American families with 56 affected male members were studied by Sieving et al., who found an identical location for the retinoschisis locus at Xp22.1-p22.3[123] Alitalo et al.[5] refined the localization by demonstrating that the DXS274 marker is distal to the retinoschisis gene but proximal to DXS41, suggesting the following arrangement: Xpter-DXS16-DXS207-DXS43-retinoschisis-DXS274-DXS41-DXS92-Xcen. This arrangement implies a genetic distance between the closest markers on either side of the retinoschisis gene of approximately 7 cM. A French group,[102] using a highly polymorphic microsatellite at the DXS207 locus, were able to show that the DXS207-DXS43 cluster is located less than 2 cM telomeric to the retinoschisis locus. The gene was finally cloned in 1997 and was designated XLRS1.[119a] Its function is unknown.

The identification of the carrier state of X-linked congenital retinoschisis has important implications for genetic counseling. Carriers have not been reliably associated with any clinical abnormalities. Wu et al. reported a case with mild visual acuity and fundus changes in one eye of an obligate carrier.[146] More recently, genetic analyses of seven families by linkage studies were able to identify heterozygote carriers. These carriers were then noted to have peripheral retinal alterations similar to those seen in affected male family members.[71] Still, fundus abnormalities do not appear to be a sufficiently consistent finding to reliably identify carriers. Arden et al.[6] noted a lack of normal rod–cone interactions in carriers of the disease and suggested this as a method for identifying carriers. More recently, the use of RFLPs, representing five linked markers that extended between the DXS164 and the DXS85 loci, encompassing the retinoschisis locus, have been used to identify carrier females.[32,71]

Genetic counseling may also be facilitated by confirming the diagnosis in atypical cases. A Dutch group[141] reported the case of a deceased grandfather in whom the diagnosis of congenital X-linked retinoschisis was made posthumously by segregation analysis with DNA probes. Similarly, it is now theoretically possible to screen for the retinoschisis gene prenatally.[91]

Treatment

There is controversy concerning the treatment of retinoschisis. In cases where there is rapidly advancing schisis threatening the macula, laser photocoagulation to the outer lamina of the schisis cavity has been attempted with success[59] and with failure.[18] Brockhurst[18] reports attempting scatter laser photocoagulation to the outer schisis wall to halt the progression toward the macula. This resulted in outer layer holes, which resulted in retinal detachment. Alternatively, photocoagulation of intact retina posterior to the retinoschisis appears safe; however, its benefits are unclear.[135] Cryopexy[120] and scleral buckling[76] have also been attempted to prevent progression. In general, it is probably wise to avoid prophylactic therapy, and instead intervene only in the presence of a retinal detachment. The goal of therapy is closure of outer-layer or full-thickness retinal breaks. This is usually accomplished with scleral buckling procedures.[76,120] In the presence of significant traction either from proliferative vitreoretinopathy or the inherent vitreous degenerative changes sometimes seen, vitrectomy may be the procedure of choice. Similarly, vitrectomy may be appropriate for posteriorly located breaks. A recent series[112] indicates that with multiple procedures and using advanced vitreoretinal techniques, favorable anatomic and functional results are possible in treating severe, vision-threatening complication of X-linked congenital retinoschisis.

Vitreous hemorrhage may also complicate the course of the disease. Bleeding usually originates from unsupported vessels in the inner schisis layer. When satisfactory visualization permits, these vessels may be treated with laser photocoagulation at the slit lamp, aiming for the vessel in areas where the retina is flat. Alternatively, vitrectomy and endolaser may be necessary when hemorrhage obscures the view.

WAGNER DISEASE

Historical Perspective

Wagner disease was originally described in 1938[143] in thirteen members of a family from Zurich, Switzerland, with a constellation of clinical findings which included retinal, vitreous, and lenticular degeneration. This original family was restudied in 1960 by Bohringer, and in 1961 by Ricci. Many additional families have been studied since then; however, there is controversy whether, in fact, many of them actually had Wagner disease. Specifically, there was disagreement concerning whether Wagner disease is a separate entity from hereditary arthroophthalmopathy (Stickler syndrome) or whether the two conditions are related genetically and pathologically but differing only in severity.[51,80,81,82,89,90] Recently, however, the gene for Wagner disease was localized to the long arm of chromosome 5,[19] and Stickler syndrome has been shown to be caused by a mutation in the COL2A1 gene on chromosome 12,[44] proving them to be distinct.

Clinical Features

Patients with Wagner disease[143] have been described as having an optically empty vitreous cavity as a result of vitreous degeneration. Occasional vitreous strands have been noted (Fig. 25.4), and posterior vitreous detachment is probably common. A vitreous membrane originating from either a single point, multiple points, or a circumferential line near the equator has been described. Anteriorly, it attaches to the vitreous base. Posteriorly, the membrane drapes over the surface of the retina. Myopia in the range of 3 to 4 diopters appears characteristic.[12,89,114,143] Peripheral vascular sheathing with attenuation of retinal arterioles and perivascular pigmentary clumping mimicking retinitis pigmentosa may be prominent.[12,89,114,143] Pa-

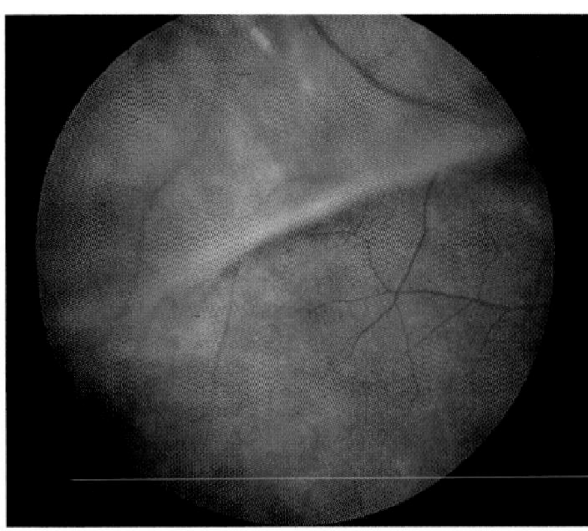

Figure 25.4. Peripheral vitreal condensation in a patient with Wagner syndrome. (Courtesy of Dr. Irene H. Maumenee.)

tients may occasionally complain of mild difficulties with night vision.

Wagner stressed the importance of the sclerosis and atrophy of the choroidal vessels and the associated chorioretinal degeneration. He also noted peripheral cystoid degeneration. Studies of five generations of the original pedigree indicate that retinal detachment is not a common feature of this disease.[12,54a,89,114,143]

Graemiger et al. reported on 28 affected individuals of 60 members of Wagner original pedigree.[54a] Chorioretinal atrophy and lenticular changes increased with age such that they were present in all patients older than 45 years of age. Only four patients had a history of a rhegmatogenous retinal detachment in one eye that occurred at a median age of 20 years. In contrast, 55% of patients older than 45 years had demonstrable peripheral retinal traction detachments. Glaucoma was present in 18% of eyes, with nearly half of these being neovascular.

Cataracts which often begin with dotlike opacities in the anterior and posterior cortex are usually present by the fourth decade of life[63] and often are visually significant. Visual acuity is generally well maintained in youth; however, lenticular changes, retinal degeneration, and posterior choroidal atrophy may lead to a progressive decrease in vision.[137] There are no associated systemic abnormalities.

Electrophysiologic and Psychophysical Testing

Electroretinography appears to be essentially normal in early stages of Wagner disease, with progressive rod and then cone dysfunction as the disease advances.[54a,63,106,107] The b-wave may be depressed with diminished oscillatory potentials. Electrooculography is depressed even in younger patients.[106,107] Dark adaptation is initially normal but may become depressed later in the course.[63]

Color vision has been reported to be normal.[85,106] Corresponding to the peripheral chorioretinal degeneration, peripheral constriction of the visual field and ring scotomas have been noted.[70,143]

Differential Diagnosis

The main differential diagnosis is between Wagner disease and Stickler syndrome. It is now clear that they represent two separate entities. Stickler syndrome shares many of the fundus abnormalities of Wagner disease, but the most important distinction is that Wagner disease is not associated with a significantly increased risk of rhegmatogenous retinal detachment. A careful family history can usually suffice to distinguish the two autosomal dominant conditions. Furthermore, patients with Wagner disease share none of the systemic abnormalities associated with Stickler syndrome. In addition, Stickler syndrome patients are generally highly myopic, whereas patients with Wagner disease have only mild refractive errors.

Another similar condition, erosive vitreoretinopathy, has recently been described.[19,20] This disease is characterized by vitreous degeneration, complicated retinal detachments, and an unusual progressive pigmentary retinopathy. Patients are generally not myopic and have none of the systemic features of Stickler syndrome.[20] Recent genetic studies have demonstrated that erosive vitreoretinopathy and Wagner disease are allelic disorders linked to chromosome 5q13-14 and are clearly distinct from Stickler syndrome.[19]

Patients with Goldmann-Favre syndrome have central and peripheral retinoschisis and more prominent complaints of nyctalopia. Goldmann-Favre syndrome is an autosomal recessive disorder and has a more severely affected ERG.

Genetics

Analysis of pedigrees with Wagner disease reveal an autosomal dominant pattern of inheritance,[12,114,143] with almost complete penetrance but variable expressivity.[85] Recently, 24 affected descendants of the original pedigree described by Wagner[143] were analyzed using a set of short tandem repeat polymorphisms distributed across the genome.[19] Significant linkage was demonstrated in each family between the Wagner disease phenotype and markers on the long arm of chromosome 5. Specifically, linkage was established within a 35 cM region, 5q13-14. Bowman and co-workers[19] postulated that Wagner disease and another hereditary vitreoretinopathy, erosive vitreoretinopathy, recently described[20] could originate from separate mutations in a single gene or two different but tightly linked genes. Two candidate genes (CRTL1 and CSPG2), which map to the long arm of chromosome 5 and whose products are involved with the extracellular matrices of cartilage and vascularized connective tissue, respectively, were identified for future investigation.

Eyes of two patients described by Wagner[143] have been studied histopathologically.[87] The retinas in both cases appeared relatively normal except for isolated areas of chorioretinal atrophy and retinoschisis involving the outer plexiform layer. A membrane of glial origin was attached to the retina as an equatorial band coursing anteriorly through the vitreous. Centrally it was adherent to the retina. Another study of two eyes noted a disorganized retina, an edematous choroid with thick-walled vessels, and infiltrating pigment cells.[2]

Treatment

Although the literature is ambiguous, it is likely that patients accurately diagnosed with Wagner disease do not have a substantially increased incidence of retinal detachment.[12,89,114,143] Therefore, asymptomatic, incidentally discovered retinal breaks probably should not be treated prophylactically unless they have associated vitreous traction. Similarly, symptomatic breaks should be handled as in the general population. presenile lenticular changes resulting in impaired visual acuity can be managed with standard cataract extraction. The mainstay of treatment remains appropriate genetic counseling, which will be faciltated by recent molecular genetic studies.[19]

STICKLER SYNDROME

Historical Perspective

Stickler syndrome was originally described in 1965 as a progressive hereditary arthroophthalmopathy.[126] It is inherited as an autosomal dominant trait with variable expressivity and nearly 100% penetrance. There has been controversy surrounding the relationship of Stickler syndrome to Wagner disease with the two, until recently, linked as part of a continuum (see the previous discussion of Wagner disease). The association, in Stickler syndrome, of defects including orofacial, skeletal, and ocular anomalies suggested an underlying abnormality of connective issue. Maumenee proposed that type II collagen, which is present in cartilage as well as secondary vitreous, might be involved.[89,90] In 1987, Francomano et al. provided evidence for close linkage of the gene for Stickler syndrome to the structural gene for type II collagen.[44] More recent work has identified specific abnormalities in the gene for type II procollagen in families with Stickler syndrome[1,21] and has excluded it as a candidate gene for Wagner disease.[46]

Clinical Features

The clinical features of Stickler syndrome may be categorized as ocular and nonocular. The ocular manifestations are similar to those of Wagner disease, making understandable the tendency to combine the two in older publications.

Patients with Stickler syndrome have an optically empty vitreous.[85,126] Often by the second decade, there has been fibrillar vitreous degeneration and liquefaction. Sheets of vitreous may

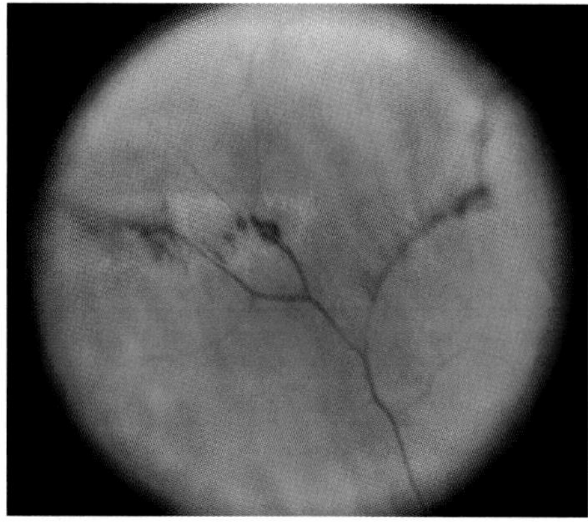

A

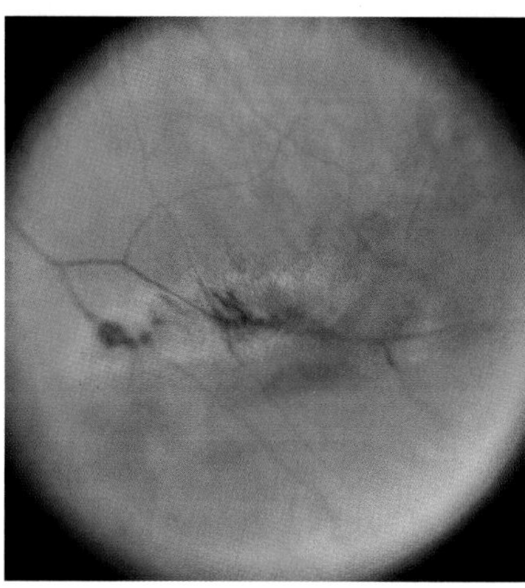

B

Figure 25.5. Radial perivascular lattice degeneration in patient with Stickler syndrome.

condense behind the lens, forming a veil.[85] Anterior vitreous membranes have been observed floating freely, often attached to equatorial retina or to radial perivascular and typical lattice degeneration (Fig. 25.5). Posterior membranes may be present on the surface of the retina, and posterior vitreous detachment is common.

Myopia in the range of 8–18 diopters is characteristic[126] and is associated with an increased axial length.[144] Staphylomata, choroidal neovascularization, and lacquer cracks are rarely observed. Progressive, presenile, lenticular changes with anterior and posterior cortical fleck and wedge-shaped opacities, similar to Wagner disease, are present in greater than half of patients.[121]

Glaucoma, with normal gonioscopic findings[90] or associated with uveitis secondary to chronic retinal detachment,[9] has been observed.

Initially, the fundus may have a tessellated appearance with circumferential hypopigmentation. There is pigment deposition circumferentially in the retinal periphery and in a radial perivascular distribution associated with chorioretinal atrophy.[63,126] This may resemble lattice degeneration. Retinal breaks may be observed in as many as three-quarters of patients. Most breaks occur in the superotemporal quadrant, The majority of patients having multiple breaks.[63] Giant tears, often located posteriorly, are common.[8] Hirose et al. report that by the second decade, retinal detachments are present in half of patients, and almost half are bilateral.[63]

Nonocular manifestations of Stickler syndrome[126,127,131] include hearing loss (Fig. 25.6); the Pierre-Robin anomalad of cleft palate, glossoptosis, and micrognathia; other orofacial abnormalities (Fig. 25.7); and musculoskeletal abnormalities, such as arthritis, marfanoid habitus, kyphosis, scoliosis, and arachnodactyly.

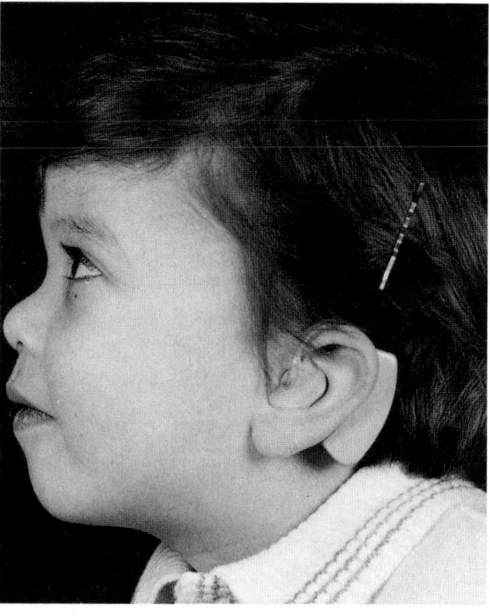

Figure 25.6. Young girl with Stickler syndrome wearing a hearing aid. Her ears are low set and there is a slight mandibular hypoplasia. (Courtesy of Drs. Irene Maumenee and Linn Murphree.)

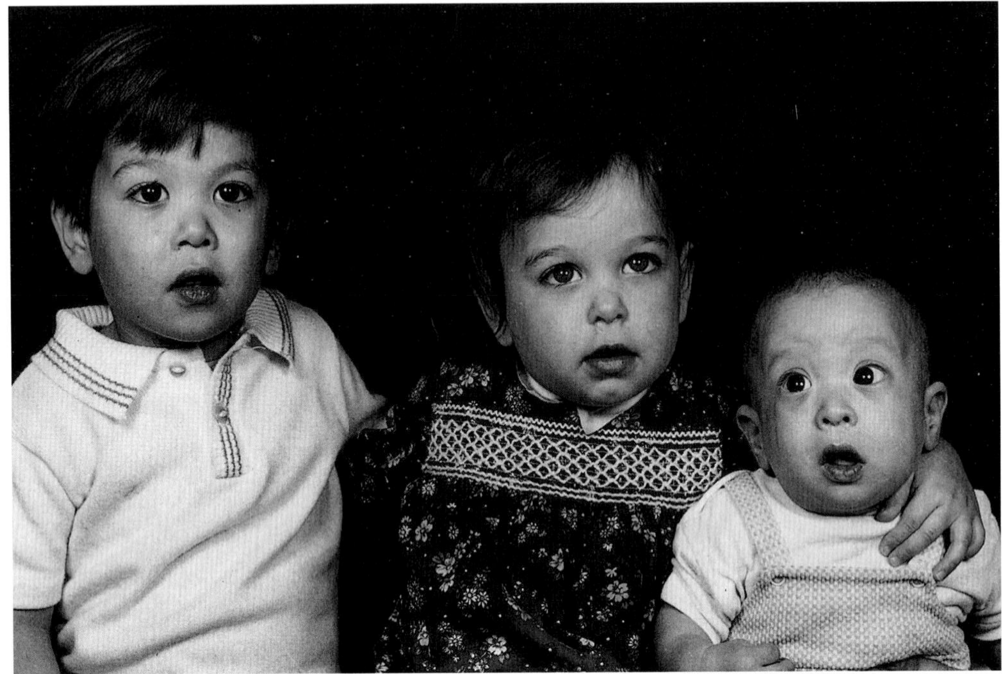

Figure 25.7. Three siblings with Stickler syndrome. The face is round and the nasal bridge is flat. (Courtesy of Drs. Irene Maumenee and Linn Murphree.)

Electrophysiologic and Psychophysical Testing

Electrophysiologic and psychophysical studies are essentially identical to those described in Wagner disease.

Differential Diagnosis

The important differential diagnosis is between Stickler syndrome and Wagner disease. The ocular findings in the two disorders are remarkably similar, with the exception of high myopia in Stickler syndrome and only mild refractive errors in Wagner disease. The distinction can be made on the basis of systemic findings and retinal detachment: Wagner disease has no consistent associated systemic abnormalities, and retinal detachment does not appear to be a part of this disorder. Shortly, molecular biologic techniques may permit prenatal genetic screening.[148]

Kniest syndrome may present with similar ocular findings to Stickler syndrome[90a]; however, patients with Kniest syndrome have dwarfism (Fig. 25.8), making the differential diagnosis difficult only neonatally.

Goldman-Favre syndrome may be differentiated on the basis of its autosomal recessive inheritance, more diffuse pigmentary changes, and markedly reduced ERGs.

Genetics

The constellation of ocular and systemic findings suggests a defect in type II collagen,[89,90] which is present in secondary vitreous as well as cartilage. In 1987, Francomano et al.[44] performed genetic linkage studies in two familes using RFLPs associated with the structural gene for type II collagen, COL2A1 on chromosome 12. Their findings suggested that the mutation causing Stickler syndrome affected the structural locus for type II collagen. The first specific Stickler mutation was reported in 1993.[1] Ahmad et al.[1] developed oligonucleotide primers to amplify and directly sequence eight of the first nine exons of COL2A1. They

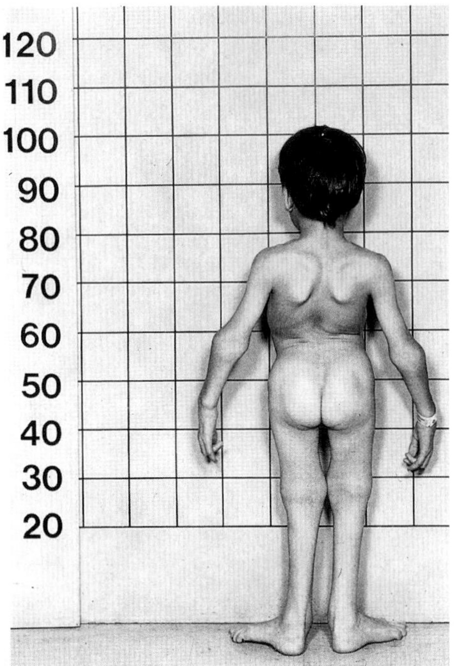

Figure 25.8. Patient with Kniest syndrome. He has short trunk dwarfism, scoliosis, and broad metaphyses.

found a single-base nonsense mutation converting the CGA codon for arginine at position 732 to TGA, a stop codon. Premature termination of the polypeptide chain prevents disulfide bonding of the three pro-alpha chains at the carboxy terminus, which is necessary for the formation of the procollagen triple helix. Therefore, procollagen will not fold properly and cannot assume its normal structural configuration.[110]

Brown et al.[21] reported a second mutation involving a frameshift mutation in exon 40 of COL2A1, involving four members of a family with Stickler syndrome. This mutation also results in truncation of the carboxy terminus of procollagen II. Ritvaniemi et al.[116] described an additional defect: a nonsense mutation in exon 43 of COL2A1, causing premature termination of the procollagen II sequence and Stickler syndrome in one affected family. It seems likely that there may be many mutations resulting in termination of translation of procollagen II that result in Stickler syndrome.

It is now possible to identify affected individuals prenatally. A recent report[148] in a family with several severely affected members describes DNA analysis of a chorionic villus sample, demonstrating that the fetus possessed the normal allele of COL2A1. The ability to detect Stickler syndrome in utero obviously will have an impact on genetic counseling.

There have also been reports suggesting genetic heterogeneity associated with the Stickler phenotype with genes other than COL2A1 implicated.[22,46,73,74,124] However, it is probably appropriate at this time to restrict the name *Stickler syndrome* to patients with the phenotype originally described who have a mutation in the procollagen II gene causing premature termination. Ideally, the original pedigree will be subjected to molecular genetic analysis.

Treatment

Patients at risk for the disorder must be carefully evaluated and followed for ocular signs of the syndrome. Systemic findings may precede the ocular manifestations. Since nearly half of all patients will eventually develop a retinal detachment, repeat ophthalmoscopic examinations are required. Multiple, bilateral, and frequently posterior, breaks are characteristic. Given the risk of retinal detachment, prophylactic treatment of breaks, although controversial, is probably warranted. This may be accomplished with either laser photocoagulation or cryotherapy, depending on the size, number, and location of the breaks. Because many breaks result from the abnormal vitreous traction present in this condition, the efficacy of retinopexy is unclear, and detachments are common despite seemingly adequate prophylactic therapy.[95] This has prompted some clinicians to suggest prophylactic encircling scleral buckling.[94] When detachments occur, they are often complicated and difficult to repair. When appropriate, vitreous traction may be relieved with scleral buckling procedures. In many cases, however, more advanced vitrectomy techniques are necessary.[8] Lenticular changes, when visually significant, should be managed with standard cataract extraction.

SYNDROME OF MYELINATED NERVE FIBERS, VITREORETINOPATHY, AND SKELETAL MALFORMATIONS

Recently, a new syndrome consisting of extensive myelination of the retinal nerve fiber layer, severe vitreoretinal degeneration, and limb-reduction abnormalities was described.[134a] A single family was reported with two affected members—a 37-year-old mother and her 10-year-old daughter. Both presented with ocular complaints of poor visual acuity in the count fingers range and nightblindness. On retinoscopy, severe myopia of between 10 and 19 diopters was present. Myelinated nerve fibers extended bilaterally from the optic nerves through the posterior pole temporally along the vascular arcades and involved the macula. Severe vitreous degeneration, with liquification, condensation, and strands, was noted in both patients. Peripherally, extensive chorioretinal atrophic changes and posterior subcapsular cataracts were present in the mother (Fig. 25.9) but not in her daughter. Electroretinography performed on the mother revealed markedly reduced photopic as well as scotopic responses, and Goldmann visual field testing revealedcecocentral scotomas and generalized constriction of all tested isopters. Additionally, the daughter had limb deformities with only one finger on each hand and one toe on each foot. based on this limited pedigree, the mode of inheritance is either autosomal dominant or X-linked dominant.

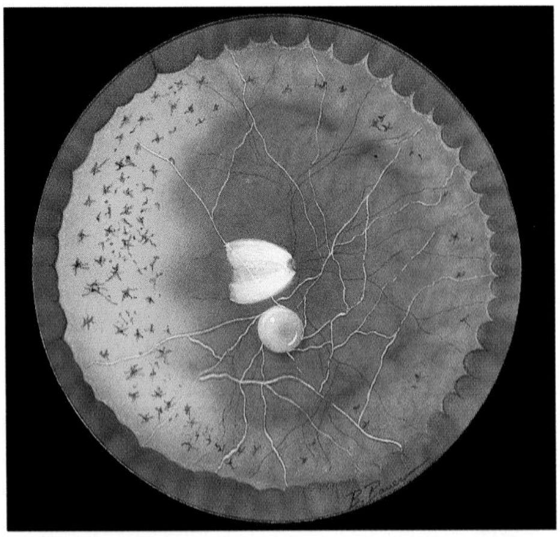

Figure 25.9. Artist's rendering of vitreoretinal changes in a patient with syndrome of myelinated nerve fibers, vitreoretinopathy, and skeletal abnormalities. (Reproduced with permission from ref. 134a.)

KNOBLOCH SYNDROME

Knobloch syndrome is an autosomal recessive condition characterized by high myopia, vitreoretinal degeneration with a high incidence of retinal detachment, macular abnormalities, and an occipital encephalocele.[30a,72a,103a,120a] The encephalocele may be subtle and appear as a soft round spot on the occiput. There is significant intra- and interfamilial variability, but the gene is fully penetrant in homozygotes. Some patients develop lens subluxation that may not be evident on initial examination (Maumenee IH, Traboulsi EI, personal communication). The gene for the Knobloch syndrome was mapped to 21q22.3 in a large Brazilian family.[121a]

Acknowledgments: Dr. Rosberger is the recipient of a 1994–1995 Heed Fellowship and a 1995–1996 Knapp Fellowship. This work was also supported in part by the Guerrieri Fund for Retinal Research, an unrestricted research grant from Research to Prevent Blindnes, Inc., New York.

REFERENCES

1. Ahmad NN, Ala-kokko L, Knowlton RG, Jimenez SA, Weaver EJ, Maguire JI, Tasman W, Prokop DJ. Stop codon in the procollagen II gene (COL2A1) in a family with the Stickler syndrome (arthro-ophthalmopathy). *Proc Natl Acad Sci USA*, 1991;88:6624–6627.
2. Alexander RL, Shea M. Wagner's disease. *Arch Ophthalmol* 1965;74:310–318.
3. Alitalo T, Forsius H, Karna J, Frants RR, Eriksson AW, Wood S, Kruse TA, de al Chapelle A. Linkage relationships and gene order around the locus for X-linked retinoschisis. *Am J Hum Genet* 1988;43:476–483.
4. Alitalo T, Karna J, Forsius H, de la Chapelle A. X-linked retinoschisis is closely linked to DXS41 and DXS16 but not DXS85. *Clin Genet* 1987;32:192–195.

5. Alitalo T, Kruse TA, de la Chapelle A. Refined localization of the gene causing X-linked juvenile retinoschisis. *Genomics* 1991;9:505–510.
6. Arden GB, Gorin MB, Polkinghorne PJ, Jay M, Bird AC. Detection of the carrier state of X-linked retinoschisis. *Am J Ophthalmol* 1988;105:590–595.
7. Bengtsson B, Linder B. Sex-linked hereditary juvenile retinoschisis: Presentation of two affected families. *Acta Ophthalmol* 1967;45: 411–423.
8. Billington BM, Leaver PK, Mcleod D. Management of retinal detachment in the Wagner-Stickler syndrome. *Trans Ophthalmol Soc UK* 1985;104:875–879.
9. Blair NP, Albert DM, Liberfarb RM, Hirose T. Hereditary progressive arthro-ophthalmopathy of Strickler. *Am J Ophthalmol* 1979; 88:876–888.
10. Blair NP, Goldberg MF, Fishman GA, Salzano T. Autosomal dominant vitreoretinochoroidopathy (ADVIRC). *Br J Ophthalmol* 1984;68:2–9.
11. Bloome MA, Garcia CA. *Manual of Retinal and Choroidal Dystrophies.* New York: Appleton-Century-Crofts, 1982.
12. Bohringer HR, Dieterle P, Landolt E. Zur Klinik und Pathologie der Degeneratio hyalloideo-retinalis hereditaria (Wagner). *Ophthalmologica* 1960;139:330–338.
13. Boldrey EE, Egbert P, Gass JD, Friberg T. The histopathology of familial exudative vitreoretinopathy. A report of two cases. *Arch Ophthalmol* 1985;103:238–241.
14. Boman H. Heilig P, Kolder HE, Giblett ER, Fialkow PJ. Hereditary retinoschisis linkage studies in a family and considerations in genetic counseling. *Can J Ophthalmol* 1976; 10:11–16.
15. Boman H, Hellig P, Kolder HE, Giblett ER, Fialkow PJ. Hereditary retinoschisis linkage studies in a family and considerations in genetic counseling. *Can J Ophthalmol* 1976; 11:11–16.
16. Bopp S, Wagner T, Laqua H. No disorder of arachidonic acid-induced thrombocyte aggregation in familial exudative vitreoretinopathy. *Klin Monatsbl Augenheilkd* 1989;194:13–15.
17. Brockhurst RJ, Albert DM, Zakov ZN. Pathologic findings in familial exudative vitreoretinopathy. *Arch Ophthalmol* 1981;99:2143–2146.
18. Brockhurst RJ. Photocoagulation in congenital retinoschisis. *Arch Ophthalmol* 1970;84: 158–165.
19. Brown DM, Graemiger RA, Hergersberg M, Schinzel A, Messmer EP, Niemeyer G, Schneeberger SA, Streb LM, Taylor CM, Kimura AE, Weingeist TA, Sheffield C, Stone EM. Genetic linkage of Wagner disease and erosive vitreoretinopathy to chromosome 5q13-14. *Arch Ophthalmol* 1995;113:671–675.
20. Brown DM, Kimura AE, Weingeist TA, Stone EM. Erosive vitreoretinopathy: A new clinical entity. *Ophthalmology* 1994;101:694–704.
21. Brown DM, Nichols BE, Weingeist TA, Sheffield VC, Kimura AE, Stone EM. Procollagen II gene mutation in Stickler syndrome. *Arch Ophthalmol* 1992;110:1589–1593.
22. Brunner HG, van Beersum SE, Warman ML, Olsen BR, Ropers HH, Mariman EC. A Stickler syndrome gene is linked to chromosome 6 near the COL11A2 gene. *Hum Mol Genet* 1994;3:1561–1564.
23. Burns RP, Lovrien EW, Cibis AB. Juvenile sex-linked retinoschisis: Clinical and genetic studies. *Trans Am Acad Ophthalmol Otolaryngol* 1971;75:1011–1021.
24. Canny CLB, Oliver GL. Fluorescein angiographic findings in familial exudative vitreoretinopathy. *Arch Ophthalmol* 1976;94:1114–1120.
25. Carr RE, Siegel JM. The vitreo-tapeto-retinal degenerations. *Arch Ophthalmol* 1970;84: 436–445.
26. Chaudhuri PP, Rosenthal AR, Goulstine DB, Rowlands D, Mitchell VE. Familial exudative vitreoretinopathy associated with familial thrombocytopathy. *Br J Ophthalmol* 1983; 167:755–758.
27. Chen CJ, Everett TK, Marascalco D. Snowflake degeneration: An independent entity or a variant of retinitis pigmentosa? *South Med J* 1986;79:1216–1223.
28. Chen ZY, Battinelli EM, Fielder A, Bundey S, Sims K, Breakefield XO, Craig IW. A mutation in the Norrie disease gene (NDP) associated with X-linked familial exudative vitreoretinopathy. *Nature Genet* 1993;5:180–183.
29. Condon GP, Brownstein S, Wang NS, Kearns JA, Ewing CC. Congenital hereditary (juvenile X-linked) retinoschisis. Histopathologic and ultrastructural findings in three eyes. *Arch Ophthalmol* 1986;104:576–583.
30. Criswick VG, Schepens CL. Familial exudative vitreoretinopathy. *Am J Ophthalmol* 1969;68:578–594.
30a. Czeizel A, Goblyos P, Kustos G, Mester E, Paraicz E. The second report of Knobloch

syndrome. *Am J Med Genet* 1992;42: 777–779.

31. Dahl N, Goonewardena P, Chotai J, Anvret M, Petersson U. DNA linkage analysis of X-linked retinoschisis. *Hum Genet* 1988;78: 228–232.
32. Dahl N, Pettersson U. Use of linked DNA probes for carrier detection and diagnosis of X-linked juvenile retinoschisis. *Arch Ophthalmol* 1988;106:1414–1416.
33. Denden A. X-Chromosomale vitreo-retinale Degeneration. ERG and EOG Untersuchungsergebnisse. *Klin Monatsbl Augenheilkd* 1975;166:355–343.
34. Deutman AF. *The Hereditary Dystrophies of the Posterior Pole of the Eye.* Assen, The Netherlands: Van Gorcum, 1971.
35. Deutman AF. Vitreoretinal dystrophies. In *Krill's Hereditary Retinal Choroidal Disease: Clinical Characteristics, Vol 2.* A.E. Krill, ed. Hagerstown, MD: Harper & Row 1977, pp. 1043–1108.
36. Ewing CC, Ives EJ. Juvenile hereditary retinoschisis. *Trans Ophthalmol Soc UK* 1969; 89:29–39.
37. Falls HF. Retinoschisis: Clinical description and course. In *Retinal Diseses.* S.J. Kumura and W.M. Caygilla, eds. Philadelphia, PA: Lea & Febiger, 1966, pp. 182–194.
38. Favre M. A propos de deux cas de degenerescence hyaloideo-retinienne. *Ophthalmologica* 1958;135:604–609.
39. Feldman EL, Norris JL, Cleasby GW. Autosomal dominant exudative vitreoretinopathy. *Arch Ophthalmol* 1983;101:1532–1535.
40. Fishman GA, Jampol LM, Goldberg MF. Diagnostic features of the Favre-Goldmann syndrome. *Br J Ophthalmol* 1976;60:345–353.
41. Forius H, Vainio-Mattila BA, Eriksson AW. X-linked hereditary retinoschisis. *Br J Ophthalmol* 1962;46:678–681.
42. Francois J, van Oye R. Degenerescence hyaloideo-tapeto-retinienne de Goldmann-Favre. *Ann Ocul* 1967;200:664–668.
43. Francois J, de Rouck A, Cambie E. Degenerescence hyaloideo-tapeto-retinienne de Goldmann-Favre *Ophthalmologica* 1974;168:81–96.
44. Francomano CA, Liberfarb RM, Hirose T, Maumenee IH, Streten EA, Meyers DA, Pyeritz RE. The Stickler syndrome: Evidence for close linkage to the structural gene for type II collagen. *Genomics* 1987;1:293–296.
45. Friedrich CA, Francis KA, Kim HC. Familial exudative vitreoretinopathy (FEVR) and platelet dysfunction. *Br J Ophthalmol* 1989;73:477–478.
46. Fryer AE, Upadhyaya M, Littler M, Bacon P, Watkins D, Tsipouras P, Harper PS. Exclusion of COL2A1 as a candidate gene in a family with Wagner-Stickler syndrome. *J Med Genet* 1990;27:91–93.
47. Fullwood P, Jones J, Bundey S, Dudgeon J, Fielder AR, Kilpatrick MW. X-linked exudative vitreoretinopathy: Clinical features and genetic linkage analysis. *Br J Ophthalmol* 1993;77:168–170.
48. Garweg J, Bohnke M, Mangold I. Treatment of Goldmann-Favre syndrome with cyclosporin A and bromocriptine. *Klin Monatsbl Augenheilkd* 1991;199:199–205.
49. Gheiler M, Pollack A, Uchenik D, Godel V, Oliver M. Hereditary snowflake vitreoretinal degeneration. *Birth Defects Orig Art Ser* 1982;18:577–580.
50. Girard P, Goichot L, Saragoussi JJ, Merad I, Forest A. Outcome of the unaffected eye in retinal detachment. Study of 1148 patients. *J Fr Ophthalmol* 1982;5:681–685.
51. Godel V, Nemet P, Lazar M. The Wagner-Stickler syndrome complex *Doc Ophthalmol* 1981;52:198–188.
52. Goldberg MF, Lee FL, Tso MO, Fishman GA. Histopathologic study of autosomal Dominant vitreoretinochoroidopathy. Peripheral annular pigmentary dystrophy of the retina. *Ophthalmology* 1989;96:1736–1746.
53. Goldmann H. Biomicroscopie du corps' vitre et du fond de l'oeil. *Bull Mem Soc Fr Ophtalmol* 1957;70:265–272.
54. Gow J, Oliver GL. Familial exudative vitreoretinopathy: an expanded view. *Arch Ophthalmol* 1971;86:150–155.

54a. Graemiger RA, Niemeyer G, Schneeberger SA, Messmer EP. Wagner vitreoretinal degeneration. Follow-up of of the original pedigree. *Ophthalmology* 1995;102: 1830–1839.

55. Green JL, Jampol LM. Vascular opacification and leakage in X-linked (juvenile) retinoschisis. *Br J Ophthalmol* 1979;63:368–373.
56. Haas J. Uber das Zusammenvorkommen von Varanderungen der Retina and Choroidea. *Arch Augenheilkd* 1898;37:343–348.
57. Han DP, Lewandowski MF. Electro-oculography in autosomal dominant vitreoretinochoroidopathy. *Arch Ophthalmol* 1992;110: 1563–1567.

57a. Han DP, Burke JM, Blair JR, Simons KB. Histopathologic study of autosomal dominant vitreoretinochoroidopathy in a 26-year-old woman. *Arch Ophthalmol* 1995;113:1561–1566.

58. Harris GS, Yeung JW. Maculopathy of sex-linked juvenile retinoschisis. *Can J Ophthalmol* 1976;11:1–10.
59. Harris GS. Retinoschisis: Pathogenesis and treatment. *Can J Ophthalmol* 1968;3:312–317.
60. Heilig P. Clinical and electroophthalmolic findings in x-chromosomal juvenile retinoschisis. *Fortschr Med* 1979;97:334.
61. Helve J. Colour vision in X-chromosomal juvenile retinoschisis. *Mad Probl Ophthalmol* 1972;11:122–129.
62. Hirose T, Lee KY, Schepens CL. Snowflake degeneration in hereditary vitreoretinal degeneration *Am J Ophthalmol* 1974;77:143–153.
63. Hirose T, Lee KY, Schepens CL. Wagner's hereditary vitreoretinal degeneration and retinal detachment. *Arch Ophthalmol* 1973;89:176–185.
64. Hirose T, Schepens CL, Brockhurst RJ, Wolfe E, Tolentino FI. Congenital retinoshisis with night blindness in two girls. *Ann Ophthalmol* 1980;12:848–856.
65. Hirose T, Wolfe E, Schepens CL. Retinal functions in snowflake degeneration. *Ann Ophthalmol* 1980;12:1135–1146.
66. Hirose T, Wolfe E, Hara A. Electrophysiological and psychophysical studies in congenital retinoschisis of x-linked recessive inheritance. *Doc Ophthalmol* 1977;13:173–184.
67. Ives EJ, Ewing CC, Innes R. X-linked juvenile retinoschisis and Xg linkage in five families. *Am J Hum Genet* 1970;22:17–18.
68. Jacobson SG, Roman AJ, Roman MI, Gass JD, Parker JA. Relatively enhanced S cone function in the Goldmann-Favre syndrome. *Am J Ophthalmol* 1991;111:446–453.
69. Jager GM. A hereditary retinal disease. *Trans Ophthalmol Soc UK* 1953;73:617–619.
70. Jansen MAA. Degeneratio hyloideo-retinalis hereditaria. *Ophthalmologica* 1962;144:458–464.
71. Kaplan J, Pelet A, Hentati H, Jeanpierre M, Briard ML, Journel Munnich A, Dufier JL. Contribution to carrier detection and genetic counseling in X-linked retinoschisis. *J Med Genet* 1991;28:383–388.
72. Kaufman SJ, Goldberg MF, Orth DH, Fishman GA, Tessler H, Mizuno K. Autosomal dominant vitreoretinochoroidopathy. *Arch Ophthalmol* 1982;100:272–278.

72a. Knobloch W, Layer I. Retinal detachment and encephalocele. *J Pediatr Ophthalmol* 1971;8:181–184.

73. Knowlton RG, Weaver EJ, Struyk AF, Knobloch WH, King RA, Norris K, Shamban A, Uitto J, Jimenez SA, Prockop DJ. Genetic linkage analysis of hereditary arthro-ophthalmopathy (Stickler syndrome) and the type II procollagen gene. *Am J Hum Genet* 1989;45:681–688.
74. Korkko J, Ritvaniemi P, Haataja L, Kaariainen H, Kivirikko KI, Prockop DJ, Ala-Kokko L. Mutation in type II procollagen (COL2A1) that substitutes aspartate for glycine alpha 1-67 and that causes cataracts and retinal detachment: evidence for molecular heterogeneity in the Wagner syndrome and the Stickler syndome (arthro-ophthalmopathy). *Am J Hum Genet* 1993;53:55–61.
75. Krause U, Vainio-Mattila BA, Eriksson AW, Forsius H. Fluorescein angiographic studies on X-chromosomal retinoschisis. *Acta Ophthalmol (Copenh)* 1970;48:794–807.
76. Krausher MF, Schepens CL, Kaplan JA, Freeman HM. Congenital retinoschisis. In *Contemporary Ophthalmology Honoring Sir Steward Duke-Elder,* J. G. Bellows, ed. Baltimore, MD: Williams and Wilkins, 1972, pp. 265–290.
77. Laqua H. Familial exudative vitreoretinopathy. *Graefes Klin Exp Ophthalmol* 1980;213:121–133.
78. Li Y, Furhmann C, Schwinger E, Cal A, Laqua H. The gene for autosomal dominant familial exudative vitreoretinopathy (Criswick-Schepens) on the long arm of chromosome 11. *Am J Ophthalmol* 1992;113:712–713.
79. Li Y, Muller B, Fuhrmann C, van Nouhuys CE, Laqua H, Humphries P, Schwinger E, Gal A. The autosomal dominant familial exudative vitreoretinopathy locus maps on 11q and is closely linked to D11S5333. *Am J Hum Genet* 1992;54:749–754.
80. Liberfarb RM, Hirose T, Holmes LB. The Wagner-Stickler syndrome—A genetic study. *Birth Defects Orig Art Ser* 1979;15:145–154.
81. Liberfarb RM, Hirose T, Holmes LB. The Wagner-Stickler syndrome—A study of 22 families. *J Pediatr* 1981;99:394–399.
82. Liberfarb RM, Hirose T. The Wagner-Stickler syndrome. *Birth Defects Orig Art Ser* 1982;18:525–538.
83. Lisch K. Idiopathische hereditare Retinoschisis. *Klin Monastbl Augenheilkd* 1968;153:204–210.

84. Lisch W. Bemerkungen zum Beitrag "Die Behandlung des Goldmann-Favre-Syndroms mit Cyclosporin A und Bromocriptin von" J. Garweg, M. Bohnke, J. Mangold. *Klin Monatsbl Augenheilkd* 1992;200:156.
85. Lisch W. Hereditary vitreoretinal degenerations. *Dev Ophthalmol* 1983;8:1–90.
86. Maguire AM, Trese MT. Visual results of lens-sparing vitreoretinal surgery in infants. *J Pediatr Ophthalmol Strabismus* 1993;30: 28–32.
87. Manschot WA. Pathology of hereditary conditions related to retinal detachment. *Ophthalmologica* 1971;162:223–234.
88. Manschot WA. Pathology of hereditary juvenile retinoschisis. *Arch Ophthalmol* 1972;88: 131–138.
89. Maumenee IH, Stoll HU, Mets BM. The Wagner syndrome versus hereditary arthroophthalmopathy. *Trans Am Ophthalmol Soc* 1982;80:349–465.
90. Maumenee IH. Vitreoretinal degeneration as a sign of generalized connective tissue diseases. *Am J Ophthalmol* 1979;88:432–449.
90a. Maumenee IH, Traboulsi EI. The ocular findings in Kniest dysplasia. *Am J Ophthalmol* 1985;100:155–160.
91. Michel-Awad A, Kaplan J, Briard ML, Turleau C, de Grouchy J, Munnich A, Dufier JL, Frezal J. Diagnostic antenatal de certaines maladies hereditaires cecitantes. *Ophtalmologie* 1990;4:237–239.
92. Miyakubo H, Hashimoto K, Inohara N. Retinal vascular pattern in familial exudative vitreoretinopathy *Ophthalmology* 1984;91: 1524–1530.
93. Miyakubo H, Inohara N, Hashimoto K. Retinal involvement in familiail exudative vitreoretinopathy. *Ophthalmologica* 1982;185: 125–135.
94. Monin C, Allagui M, Larricart P, Ameline B, Haut J. Prevention du decollement de retine non tramatique par cerclage chirurgical. A propos de vingt cas. *J Fr Ophtalmol* 1993; 16:247–253.
95. Monin C, Van Effenterre G, Andre-Sereys P, Haut J. Prophylaxie du decollament de retine de la maladie de Wagner-Stickler. Etude comparative des differentes methodes. A propos de vingt-deux cas. *J Fr Ophtalmol* 1994;17:167–174.
96. Nicholson DH, Galvis V. Criswick-Schepens syndrome (familial exudative vitreoretinopathy). Study of a Colombian kindred. *Arch Ophthalmol* 1984;102:1519–1522.
97. Nijihuis FA, Deutman AF, Aan de Kerk AL. Fluorescein angioraphy in mild stages of dominant exudative vitreoretinopathy. *Mod Probl Ophthalmol* 1979;83:234–241.
98. Nishimura M, Yamana T, Sugino M et al. Falciform retinal fold as a sign of familial exudative retinopathy. *Jpn J Ophthalmol* 1983;27:40–53.
99. Ober RR, Bird AC, Hamilton AM, Sehmi K. Autosomal dominant exudative vitreoretinopathy. *Br J Ophthalmol* 1980;64:112–120.
100. Odland M. Congenital retinoschisis. *Acta Ophthalmol (Copenh)* 1981;59:649–658.
101. Ohkubo H, Tanino T. Electrophysiological findings in familial exudative vitreoretinopathy. *Doc Ophthalmol* 1987;65:461–469.
102. Oudet C, Weber C, Kaplan J, Segues B, Croquette MF, Roman EO, Hanauer A. Characterisation of a highly polymorphic microsatellite at the DXS207 locus: Confirmation of very close linkage to the retinoschisis disease gene. *J Med Genet* 1993;30:300–303.
103. Pagenstecher HE. Uber eine unter dem Bilde der Netzhautablosung verlaufende, erbliche Erkrankung der Retina. *Graefes Arch Ophthalmol* 1913;86:457–462.
103a. Passos-Bueno M, Marie S, Monteiro M, Neustein I, Whittle M, Vainzof M, et al. Knobloch syndrome in a large Brazilian family: Confirmation of autosomal recessive inheritance. *Am J Med Genet* 1994;52:170–173.
104. Peachy NS, Fishman GA, Derlacki DJ, Brigell MG. Psychophysical and electroretinographic findings in X-linked juvenile retinoschisis. *Arch Ophthalmol* 1987;105:513–516.
105. Peyman GA, Fishman GA, Sanders DR, Vlchek J. Histopathology of Goldmann-Favre syndrome obtained by full-thickness eye-wall biopsy. *Ann Ophthalmol* 1977;9:479–484.
106. Pinckers A, Jansen LMMA. Wagner's syndrome (degeneratio hyloideo-retinalis hereditaria). *Doc Ophthalmol* 1974;37:245–259.
107. Pinckers AJLG. Le syndrome de Wagner, electro-oculographie et sens chromatique. *Ann Ocul* 1970;203:569–578.
108. Plager DA, Orgel IK, Ellis FD, Hartzer M, Trese MT, Shastry BS. X-linked recessive familial exudative vitreoretinopathy. *Am J Ophthalmol* 1992;114:145–148.
109. Pollack A, Uchenik D, Chemke J, Oliver M. Prophylactic laser photocoagulation in hereditary snowflake vitreoretinal degeneration: A family report. *Arch Ophthalmol* 1983;101: 1536–1539.

110. Prockop DJ. Mutations that alter the primary structure of type I collagen: Perils of a system for generating large structures by the principle of nucleated growth. *J Biol Chem* 1990; 265:15,349–15,352.
111. Prosper L. Congenital hereditary sex-linked retinoschisis. *J Pediatr Ophthalmol Strabismus* 1978;15:26–30.
112. Regillo CD, Tasman WS, Brown GC. Surgical management of complications associated with X-linked retinoschisis. *Arch Ophthalmol* 1993;111:1080–1086.
113. Ricci A. Clinique et transmission genetique des differentes formes de degenerescences vitreo-retiniennes. *Ophthalmologica* 1960; 139:338–343.
114. Ricci A. Clinique transmission hereditaire des degenerescences vitreo-retiniennes. *Ophthalmologica* 1961;139:338–343.
115. Richardson J. Juvenile retinoschisis, anterior retinal dialysis, and retinal detachment. *Br J Ophthalmol* 1973;57:34–40.
116. Ritvaniemi P, Hyland J, Ignatius J, Kivirikko KI, Prockop DJ, Ala-Kokko L. A fourth example suggests that premature termination codons in the COL2A1 gene are a common cause of the Stickler syndrome: Analysis of the COL2A1 gene by denaturing gradient gel electrophoresis. *Genomics* 1993;17:218–221.
117. Robertson DM, Link TP, and Rostvold JA. Snowflake degeneration of the retina. *Ophthalmology* 1982;89:1513–1517.
118. Sabates FN. Juvenile retinoschisis. *Am J Ophthalmol* 1966;62:683–688.
119. Sarin LK, Green WR, Dailey EG. Juvenile retinoschisis: Congenital vascular veils and hereditary retinoschisis. *Am J Ophthalmol* 1964;57:793–796.
119a. Sauer CG, Gehrig A, Warneke-Wittstock R, et al. Positional cloning of the gene associated with X-linked juvenile retinoschisis. *Nature Genet* 1997;17:164–170.
120a. Seaver L, Leonard J, Spark R, Smith B. Hoyme H. Congenital scalp defects and vitreoretinal degeneration: redefining the Knobloch syndrome. *Am J Med Genet* 1993;46:203–208.
121. Seery Cm, Pruett RC, Liberfarb RM, Cohen BZ. Distinctive cataract in the Stickler syndrome. *Am J Ophthalmol* 1990;110:143–148.
121a. Sertie A, Quimby M, Moreira E, Murray J, Zatz M, Antonarakis S, et al. A gene which causes severe ocular alterations and occipital encephalocele (Knobloch syndrome) is mapped to 21q22.3. *Hum Mol Genet* 1996;5:843–847.
122. Shastry BS, Trese MT. Mapping studies of an X-linked familial exudative vitreoretinopathy. *Biochem Biophys Res Commun* 1993; 193:599–603.
123. Sieving PA, Bingham EL, Roth MS, Young MR, Boehnke M, Kuo CY, Ginsburg O. Linkage relationship of X-linked juvenile retinoschisis with Xp22.1-p22.3 probes. *Am J Hum Genet* 1990;47:616–621.
124. Snead MP, Payne SJ, Barton DE, Yates JR, al-Imara L, Pope FM, Scott JD. Stickler syndrome: Correlation between vitreoretinal phenotypes and linkage to COL2A1. *Eye* 1994;8:609–614.
125. Sorsby A, Klein M, Gann JH, Siggens C. Unusual retinal detachment, possibly sex-linked. *Br J Ophthalmol* 1951;35:1–10.
126. Stickler GB, Belau PG, Farrell FG, Jones JD, Pugh DG, Steinberg AG, Ward LE. Hereditary progressive arthro-ophthalmopathy. *Mayo Clin Proc* 1965;40:433–447.
127. Stickler GB, Pugh DG. Hereditary progressive arthro-ophthalmopathy II. Additional observations on vertebral abnormalities, a hearing defect, and a report of a similar case. *Mayo Clin Proc* 1967;42:495–500.
128. Tanino T. Katsumi O. Hirose T. Electrophysiological similarities between two eyes with X-linked recessive retinoschisis. *Doc Ophthalmol* 1985;60:149–161.
129. Tano Y, Iked T. Treatment of familial exudative vitreoretinopathy with pars plana vitrectomy: *Ophthalmology* 1990;97:152.
130. Tasman W, Augsburger JJ, Shields JA, Caputo A, Annesley WH. Familial exudative vitreoretinopathy. *Trans Am Ophthalmol Soc* 1981; 79:211–255.
131. Temple IK. Stickler's syndrome. *J Med Genet* 1989;26:119–126.
132. Thaler A, Heilig P, Slezack H. Elektroretinogramm und Elektrookulogramm bei juveniler Retinoschisis. *Klin Monatstbl Augenheilkd* 1973;163:699–703.
133. Thomson E. Memorandum regarding a family in which neuroretinal disease of an unusual kind occurred only in males. *Br J Ophthalmol* 1932;16:681–686.
134. Traboulsi EI, Payne JW. Autosomal dominant vitreoretinochoidopathy. Report of the third family. *Arch Ophthalmol* 1993;111: 194–196.
134a. Traboulsi EI, Lim JL, Pyeritz R, Goldberg HK, Haller JA. A new syndrome of myelinated nerve fibers, vitreoretinopathy, and skeletal malformations. *Arch Ophthalmol* 1993; 111:1543–1545.

135. Turot P, Francois P, Castier P, Milazzo S. Analysis of results in the treatment of peripheral retinoschisis in sex-linked congenital retinoschisis. *Graefes Arch Clin Exp Ophthalmol* 1989;227:328–331.
136. Vainio-Mattila BA, Eriksson AW, Forsius H. X-chromosomal recessive retinoschisis in the region of Pori. An ophthalmogenetic analysis of 103 cases. *Acta Ophthalmol (Copenh)* 1969;47:1135–1148.
137. Van Nouhuys CE, Chorioretinal dysplasia in young subjects with Wagner's hereditary vitreoretinal degeneration. *Int Ophthalmol* 1981;3:67–77.
138. Van Nouhuys CE. Congenital retinal fold as a sign of dominant exudative vitreoretinopathy *Graefes Klin Exp Ophthalmol* 1981;217: 55–67.
139. Van Nouhuys CE. Dominant exudative vitreoretinopathy and other vascular developmental disorders of the periphral retina. *Doc Ophthalmol* 1982;54:1–414.
140. Van Nouhuys CE. Juvenile retinal detachment as a complication of familial exudative vitreoretinopathy. *Fortschr Ophthalmol* 1989;86:221–223.
141. van Schooneveld MJ, Bleeker-Wagemakers EM, Orth U, Neugebauer M, Hogenkamp T, Gal A. Posthumous diagnosis of X-linked retinoschisis using DNA analysis. *Ophthalmic Paediatr Genet* 1990;11:293–297.
142. Verdaguer JT. Juvenile retinoschisis. *Am J Ophthalmol* 1982;93:145–146.
143. Wagner H. Ein bisher unbekanntes Erbleiden des Auges (Degeneratio hyaloideretinalis hereditaria), beobachtet im Kanton Zurich. *Klin Monatsbl Augenheilkd* 1938;100:840–857.
144. Weingeist TA, Hermsen V, Hanson JW, Bumsted RM, Weinstein SL, Olin WH. Ocular and systemic manifestation of Stickler's syndrome. A preliminary report. *Birth Defects Orig Art Ser* 1982;18:539–560.
145. Wieacker P, Wienker TF, Dallapicola B et al. Linkage relationships between retinoschisis, Xg, and a cloned DNA sequence from the distal short arm of the X chromosome. *Hum Genet* 1983;64:141–145.
146. Wu G, Cotlier E, Brodie S. A carrier state of X-linked juvenile retinoschisis. *Ophthalmic Paediatr Genet* 1985;5:13–17.
147. Yanoff M, Rahn EK, Zimmerman LE. Histopathology of juvenile retinoschisis. *Arch Ophthalmol* 1968;79:49–53.
148. Zlotogora J, Granat M, Knowlton RG. Prenatal exclusion of Stickler syndrome. *Prenat Diagn* 1994;14:145–147.

26

Optic Atrophy

DAVID A. MACKEY

Optic atrophy is a clinical state in which there is pallor of the optic nerve due to loss of ganglion cell axons and supporting microvascular tissue. Optic neuropathy is a more general term, which includes the early phase of the disease, when optic atrophy may not yet be present. Optic atrophy may occur in a myriad of forms, ranging from an obvious loss of vision with a clinical diagnosis, to an incidentally identified optic atrophy where elucidating the history is difficult and no diagnosis is ever made. Optic atrophy may occur in either hereditary or nonhereditary diseases. Hereditary causes of optic atrophy may occur as a primary event or secondary to adjacent compression (as would occur with a hereditary tumor in neurofibromatosis) or degeneration (as occurs in the later stages of retinitis pigmentosa). Primary optic atrophy may occur as an isolated event or may be associated with other systemic manifestations.

Although each disease in this chapter may appear to be a distinct entity, diagnosing the cause of optic atrophy with certainty in any patient is difficult. Even with a strong family history of optic atrophy a patient may have an unrelated treatable tumor compressing the optic nerve. Thus, in most cases, neuroimaging is necessary.

In assessing a patient with optic atrophy a careful history is of particular importance. The onset of symptoms and associated phenomena may help with determining the age of onset and the nature of the visual loss. A thorough famiy history is very important and does not end with the first clinical consultation. Patients (or parents) should be asked to find out about anyone else in the extended family having any form of visual loss. Many causes of optic atrophy may not have been diagnosed correctly in the past: a great uncle who died of a brain tumor could easily be a person with optic atrophy who died from the complications of an exploratory craniotomy. History of the pregnancy, prematurity, and neonatal problems may suggest perinatal optic atrophy, which is often not hereditary. Associated neurological abnormalities and other problems with the patient may also lend a clue to the underlying cause. The past history of visual function may help define the onset of the disorder.

Examination will depend on the age of the patient. Visual acuity can be tested by the age appropriate method. Visual fields are difficult to assess in children under 10 years of age, but confrontation, tangent screen, and Goldmann fields can often be performed. In adults the traditional form of visual field assessment was the Goldmann field; however, there is now a large database on the use of automated perimetry, in particular with the Humphrey 30-2 visual field. A major problem with optic atrophy associated with a centrocecal scotoma is that it is difficult for the patient to maintain fixation. This will often show as a high negative error score or, if the scotoma is small, a high fixation loss score on automated perimetry. However, the same poor fixation is present, though often not detected, on Goldmann perimetry. Certain color vision abnormalities are often detected in the various forms of optic atrophy, these are, however, not as specific as with the inherited X-linked color vision defects. Although helpful, color vision abnormalities in a particular spectral axis are not always specific and will depend on the patient's ability and application to doing the test. Ishihara plates are designed to detect X-linked color abnormalities in the red-green axis, City University plates will detect a blue-yellow axis abnormality, as will the D15 Hue test, although both may not be as reliable as the Farnsworth-Munsell 100-hue test. Pupil responses, nystagmus, strabismus, and structural abnormalities of the eye may all be assessed.

Examination of the fundus, ideally by stereoscopic magnification, allows assessment of the optic disc for elevation or pallor, which may be diffuse or segmental. The appearance of the disc margin, cupping, size of the disc, retinal vessels around the disc, macular and peripheral retina are all important. Although marked optic atrophy with white discs is easily diagnosed, mild optic atrophy, with temporal pallor, may be very subtle and difficult to diagnose, even for the most experienced clinician. Investigations will, of course, be guided by the overall clinical picture and are discussed with the relevant diseases. At present, DNA testing for Leber's hereditary optic neuropathy is the only readily available diagnostic test. When further genes for the other optic atrophies are identified, other DNA tests will be useful. The primary investigation for the optic atrophy itself is neuroimaging. Even when the cause of optic atrophy appears obvious, it is wise to perform neuroimaging studies on virtually all patients to exclude a compressive lesion. A computed tomographic (CT) scan is usually adequate to exclude most treatable abnormalities, although magnetic resonance imaging (MRI) may give more information. If a person carries the gene for an optic atrophy, this does not guarantee that they will never get a brain tumor.

Table 26.1. Causes of Pediatric Optic Atrophy

Tumor	29%
Glioma	12%
Craniopharyngioma	6%
Other	11%
Postinflammatory	17%
Trauma	11%
No diagnosis	11%
Hereditary	9%
Autosomal dominant	6%
Leber's optic neuropathy	3%*
Perinatal disease	9%
Hydrocephalus (without tumor)	6%
Neurodegenerative disease	5%
Toxic/metabolic	1%
Miscellaneous	3%

* This study was done prior to the availability of DNA testing. (Modified from M. X. Repka and N. R. Miller. Optic atrophy in children. *Am J Ophthalmol* 1988;106: 191–193.)

The possible causes of optic atrophy will depend on the age of the patient. Taylor[50] gives a comprehensive diagram in his textbook. Repka and Miller[39] reviewed 218 children under 18 years referred to a tertiary neuroophthalmology center and found the causes of optic atrophy in Table 26.1.

LEBER'S HEREDITARY OPTIC NEUROPATHY (LHON)

This disease is discussed in Chapter 35.

AUTOSOMAL DOMINANT OPTIC ATROPHY (MIM 165500) (OPA1)

Autosomal dominant optic atrophy (ADOA) or Kjer optic atrophy is often reported as the most common form of hereditary optic atrophy (see Table 26.2). However, the recent developments in the molecular diagnosis of Leber's hereditary optic neuropathy (LHON) (see also Chapter 35) have greatly increased the number of LHON cases. In Australia it would appear that there are approximately equal numbers

Table 26.2. Hereditary Causes of Optic Atrophy

Primary Optic Atrophies
Leber's hereditary optic neuropathy (see Chapter 35)
Autosomal dominant optic atrophy
Autosomal recessive optic atrophy
Optic Atrophy Associated with Neurological Degeneration*
Wolfram
Behr
Friedreich ataxia
Olivopontocerebellar degeneration
Charcot-Marie-Tooth
Optic Atrophy Associated with Metabolic Diseases
Glucose-6-phosphate dehydrogenase deficiency
Adrenoleukodystrophy
Metachromatic leukodystrophy
Krabbe leukodystrophy
Menke
Schilder neuroaxonal dystrophy
Pelizaeus-Merzbacher disease
Zellweger syndrome
GM2 gangliosidoses
Tay-Sachs disease
Sandhoff disease
Neuronal ceroidal lipofuscinoses
Mucopolysaccharidoses
Myoclonic epilepsy and ragged red fiber disease
Leigh syndrome
Optic Atrophy Secondary to Eye Problems
Glaucoma primary and secondary
Retinal degenerations (retinitis pigmentosa, Leber's congenital amaurosis)
Optic Atrophy Secondary to Compression
Meningioma, optic nerve, and chiasmal glioma (neurofibromatosis)
Craniosynostoses (Crouzon, Apert)
Chondrodysplasia punctata (Conradi-Hunermann)
Osteopetrosis (Albers-Schonberg)

* McKusick[31] mentions almost 100 other optic atrophy associations, with allocated MIM numbers; however, these are usually single reports that may overlap the syndromes mentioned in this list.

of LHON and ADOA cases that each have a prevalence of around 1 in 100,000 and an equal number again of unexplained or miscellaneous optic atrophy cases. Snell[45] is generally credited with describing the first case of optic atrophy that was distinct from LHON. Iverson[20] reported a three-generation family with congenital optic atrophy. Kjer[25] described in detail 19 Danish families with approximately 1200 members, 200 of whom were affected by ADOA. ADOA has a variable phenotype with insidious onset in childhood. Acute visual loss is not described and the patient may not be diagnosed until a school eye examination. Caldwell et al.[6] separated ADOA into congenital and juvenile forms, and Stenddahl-Brodin et al.[46] described a family with late-onset ADOA. It is, however, often difficult to determine the age of onset of ADOA, as it may be very mild. Indeed, Kivlin et al.[24] found 6 patients where the diagnosis was uncertain, with 36 affected and 81 normal, when examining 123 family members of a large kindred. The spectrum of visual loss varies from 6/12 to 3/60.[22] However, pediatric ophthalmologists usually mention acuities ranging from 6/9 to 6/24, with 6/36 or worse being unusual.[51] This supports the idea that the visual acuity deteriorates as patients get older. Glaser[11] makes a similar extrapolation from Kjer's original data. There is usually a moderate centrocecal scotoma (Figs. 26.1–26.3). Color vision testing may shown a nonspecific defect, although

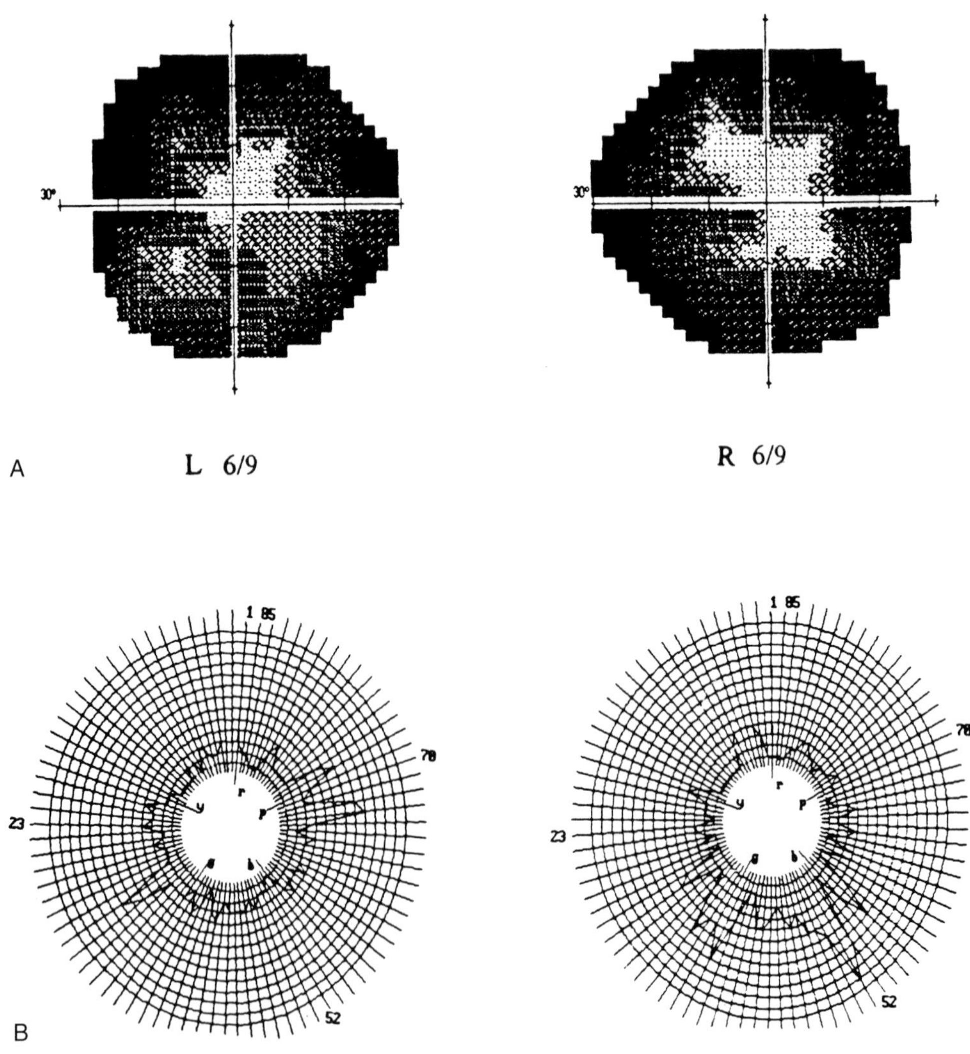

Figure 26.1. (**A**) Humphrey 30-2 visual fields on a 49-year-old woman with autosomal dominant optic atrophy, visual acuity 6/9 in each eye with temporal pallor of the optic nerve. The centrocecal scotoma shows an annular pattern. (**B**) The Farnsworth-Munsell 100-hue chart shows the moderately reduced color discrimination in the red-green axis in the right eye and the more classical blue-yellow axis in the left.

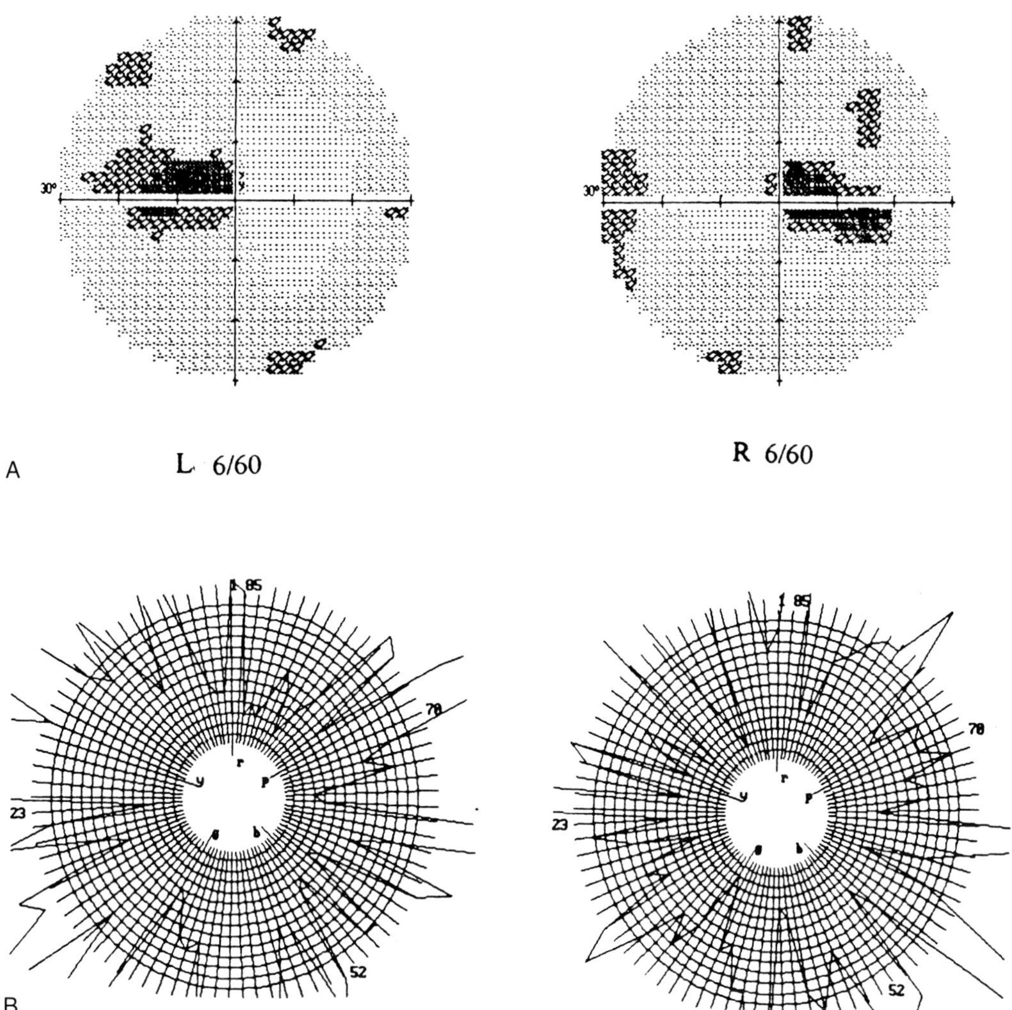

Figure 26.2. (**A**) Humphrey 30-2 visual fields on a 30-year-old woman with autosomal dominant optic atrophy, visual acuity 6/60 in each eye. The Humphrey field shows a small centrocecal scotoma. (**B**) The Farnsworth-Munsell 100-hue chart shows the generalized, poor color discrimination.

is more often a blue-yellow defect (Figs. 26.1–26.3). This was thought to be pathognomonic of Kjer-type optic atrophy,[44] although it may rarely be seen in other optic atrophies. Kjer[25] found that many of his patients had noticed no symptoms and were unaware of the familial nature of their disorder. Thus, in any suspected case of ADOA it is important to examine all the reportedly normal relatives, as they may well be mildly affected. Fundus examination usually reveals optic atrophy particularly in the temporal segment (Figs. 26.4, 26.5). This, however, may be subtle and difficult to diagnose. Flash electroretinogram (ERG) is normal, although Johnston et al.[22] did report a case where the scotopic ERG was reduced. Histopathologic reports are rare, although Johnston et al.[22] reported a case with diffuse atrophy of the ganglion cell layer of the retina and loss of myelin and nerve tissue within the optic nerve. Kjer et al.[26] reported ganglion cell loss in the retina and geniculate body, as well as axonal loss of both vestibuloauditory nerves. This suggests some primary retinal ganglion cell degenera-

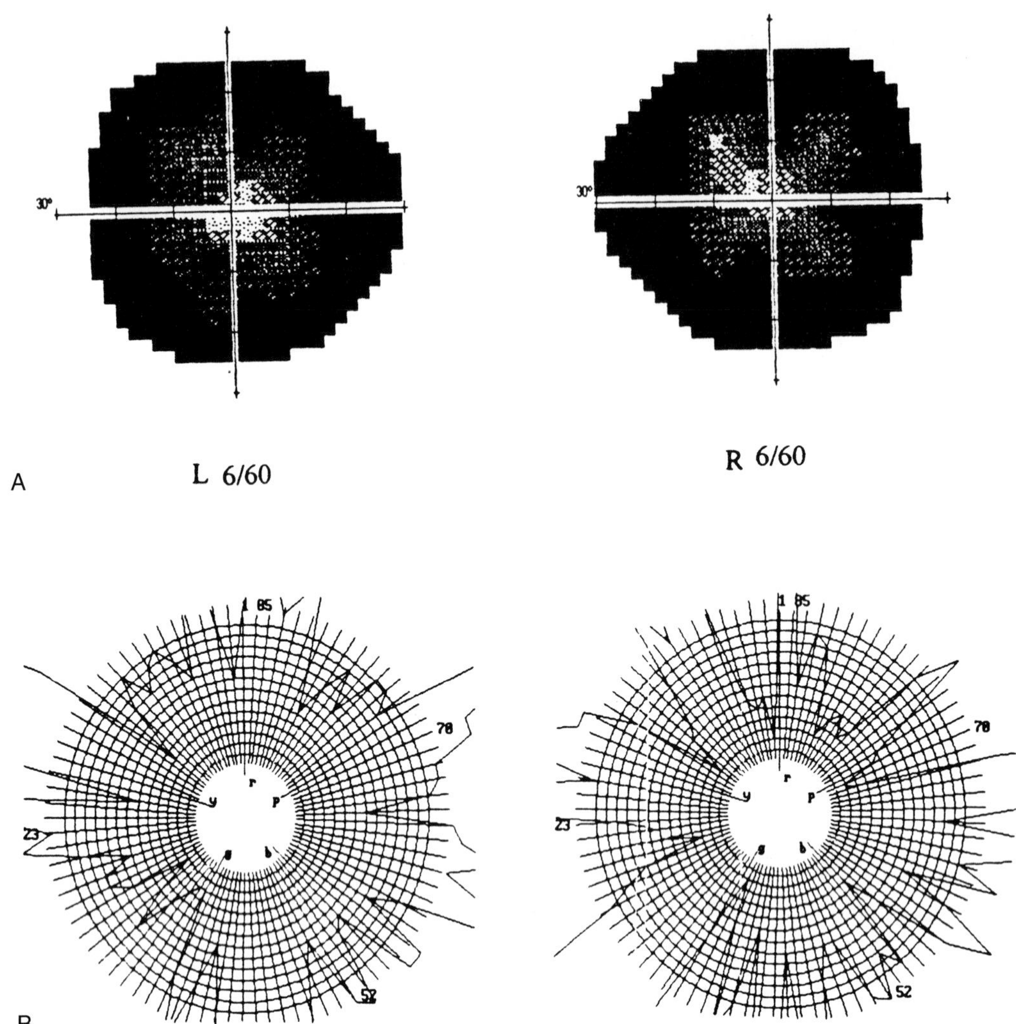

Figure 26.3. (**A**) Humphrey 30-2 visual fields on a 39-year-old man with autosomal dominant optic atrophy, visual acuity 6/60 in each eye. The Humphrey field shows a dense scotoma with a small central island of vision. (**B**) Farnsworth-Munsell 100-hue chart shows the generalized, poor color discrimination.

tion. Linkage analysis of three Danish pedigrees, using short tandem repeat polymorphisms, linked the OPA1 gene to chromosome 3q28-qter. This was between markers D3S1314 and D3S1265.[9] Other studies have confirmed this linkage and narrowed the interval, with no evidence of genetic heterogeneity in Cuban,[28a] French,[3a] British,[22a,53b] and American[3b] families. The "belly spot tail" (Bst) mouse has been proposed as an animal model because it has absent pupillary light responses.[39a] The gene maps mouse chromosome 16 in a region homologous to chromosome 3 in humans. However, further studies suggest that the OPA1 and Bst map to different regions.[39b] There is currently no treatment for ADOA. Most children have normal schooling, occasionally with assistance. Some patients may drive (although not always within the legal limits for visual acuity) and very few require aids beyond magnification of written text and assistance with colors. I could find no patient in Australia with ADOA who

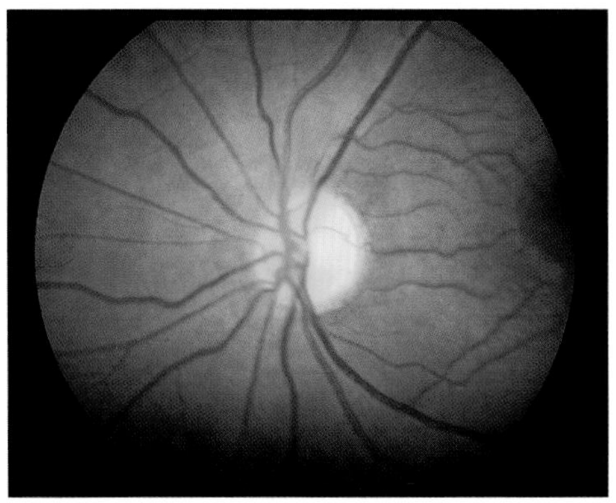

Figure 26.4. Fundus photograph showing diffuse optic atrophy in a 25-year-old patient with autosomal dominant optic atrophy and visual acuity of 6/36.

used a guide dog. The handicap of ADOA is usually less severe than LHON. Visual acuity in Kjer optic atrophy usually decreases by an average of one Snellin line per decade.[9a]

AUTOSOMAL RECESSIVE OPTIC ATROPHY (MIM 258500)

Autosomal recessive optic atrophy is difficult to distinguish from ADOA, but consanguineous families resembling Kjer optic atrophy have been described.[25] In addition, researchers in Australia and Europe have identified sibships of Leber-like optic atrophy which may be autosomal recessive in inheritance.

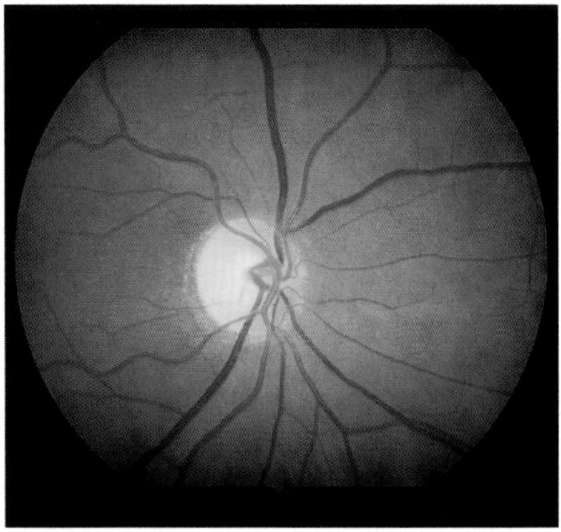

Figure 26.5. Fundus photograph showing diffuse optic atrophy in a 42-year-old woman with autosomal dominant optic atrophy and visual acuity of 6/60.

DIABETES INSIPIDUS, DIABETES MELLITUS, OPTIC ATROPHY, DEAFNESS SYNDROME (DIDMOAD), OR WOLFRAM SYNDROME (MIM 222300, 598500)

Wolfram syndrome is also known as diabetes insipidus, diabetes mellitus, optic atrophy, deafness. The association of juvenile diabetes mellitus and optic atrophy in 4/8 of a sibship was first described by Wolfram.[54] Tyrer[53] found affected individuals of a first cousin marriage and Ross et al.,[41] reviewing the literature, suggested that autosomal recessive inheritance of a gene with pleiotropic effects was involved. Gunn et al.[14] suggested that the frequency of DIDMOAD among patients with juvenile diabetes was between 1/148 and 1/175. Swift et al.[47] estimate the frequency of the heterozygous carrier state to be as high as 1%. Bundey et al.[4] suggested that DIDMOAD may be a mitochondrial disorder after reporting a patient with morphological and biochemical abnormalities of the mitochondria, but they did not find any abnormalities of the mitochondrial DNA (mtDNA). However, Rotig et al.[42] described a patient with a 7.6 kb heteroplasmic deletion of mtDNA. Pilz et al.[36] described a patient with optic atrophy, diabetes mellitus, sensorineural hearing loss, and grand mal seizures who also carried the 11778 mtDNA associated with LHON. The autosomal recessive form was linked to the short arm of chromosome 4. Using microsatellite repeats in 11 families, a lod score of 6.46 as obtained for marker D4S431, indicating strong linkage.[37] McKusick[31] feels that only insulin-dependent diabetes mellitus and bilateral progressive optic atrophy are necessary for a diagnosis of DIDMOAD. Diabetes mellitus is often detected first, and onset may be in childhood, adolescence, or adult life. Visual loss is usually severe. Peden et al.[35] described all five of his patients as being registered blind from primary optic atrophy. Lessell and Rosman[27] described anosmia, tonic pupils, and disc cupping. Swift et al.[47,48] also associated urinary tract atony, peripheral neuropathy, mental retardation, dementia, and psychiatric illness, and Rando et al.[38] added ataxia, nystagmus, and seizures. Page et al.[34] emphasized the importance of diagnosing diabetes insipidus, because all five of his cases had dilatation of the urinary tract, varying from mild hydroureter to severe hydronephrosis and this improved with treatment of the diabetes insipidus. Swift et al.[47,48] reported that 25% of homozygous patients had severe psychiatric illness resulting in hospitalization or suicide; heterozygous carriers were also at greater risk of severe psychiatric disturbance. Patients with diabetes mellitus and optic atrophy should be investigated regularly for diabetes insipidus. Diabetes insipidus may be confirmed by using a water deprivation test for 8 hours and measuring serum and urine osmolalities. Intravenous pyelogram, voiding cystourethrography, and ultrasound may reveal dilatation of the urinary tract. MDI studies may show widespread atrophic changes throughout the brain, some of which correlate with the major neurologic features of the syndrome.[38] Abnormal ERGs were described by Nimeyer and Marquardt.[33] Optic atrophy in children with diabetes may also occur because of the random overlap of two disorders, or be secondary to papilloedema. It may often be seen in severe proliferative diabetic retinopathy.

BEHR OPTIC ATROPHY (MIM 210000)

Behr[2] described an autosomal recessive disorder characterized by optic atrophy with visual loss, temporal field defects, and neurological abnormalities that included nystagmus, hyperreflexia, spasticity, ataxia, and mental retardation. The onset was in early infancy, with a period of progression followed by many years as a static condition. It is likely that cases described today as Behr syndrome are, in fact, a mixed group of disorders with early childhood spinocerebellar degeneration with evident optic atrophy and mental retardation.[19,52] Horoupian et al.[19] showed a pathological case with central atrophy of the optic nerves and total disarray of the normal laminar pattern of the lateral geniculate nucleus, dropout of neurons, and gliosis. Behr optic atrophy appears to be rare.

FRIEDREICH ATAXIA (MIM 229300)

Friedreich ataxia is a rare autosomal recessive spinocerebellar degeneration affecting the spinocerebellar and pyramidal tracts, the dorsal columns, the cerebellum, and the medulla. It is characterized by a preadolescent onset of incoordination of limb movements, dysarthria, nystagmus, reduced tendon reflexes, impaired position and vibration sense, scoliosis, and pes cavus. Sensorineural deafness, cardiac anormalities, and diabetes have also been described. Ophthalmic features include those related to cerebellar degeneration[23]: downbeat nystagmus, gaze paretic and rebound nystagmus, abnormal saccades, and poor fixation, as well as optic atrophy[28] and presymptomatic changes in the visual evoked responses.[7] It is slowly progressive, affecting an estimated 1 in 25,000. Optic atrophy does not feature prominently as a sign of Friedreich ataxia in neurology or genetics texts, although Friedreich ataxia is regularly listed in opthalmology texts as a cause of optic atrophy. Livingstone et al.[28] state that optic atrophy occurs frequently. Fourteen of their 21 patients had visual impairment and abnormal visual evoked potentials. The 6 who were symptomatic had severe optic atrophy, whereas the 8 asymptomatic patients had temporal pallor, mild visual loss 6/9–6/12, and normal Ishihara color vision. Cases of Friedreich ataxia with optic atrophy could be classified as Behr optic atrophy. The gene for Friedreich ataxia has been localized to 9p12-q13, mainly in families from Quebec, Acadians in Louisiana, and other populations of French ancestry. Sylvester[49] described a father and six out of nine offspring with Friedreich ataxia, optic atrophy, and nerve deafness (MIM 13660). Campuzano et al.[6a] identified the Frataxin gene, which has 6 exons and encodes a 210 amino acid protein. Point mutations were identified, but the majority of patients had a GAA triplet repeat expansion in the first intron. These ranged in size from 200 to 900 copies, with only 7–22 copies in normal controls. The length of repeat varied inversely with the age of onset of Friedreich ataxia.[8c,9b] Babcock et al.[1a] showed homology to the yeast Frataxin and indicated that Frataxin is a mitochondrial protein. Friedreich ataxia is associated with optic atrophy, cardiomyopathy, deafness, and diabetes mellitus, all of which are commonly found in mitochondrial disorders.[13a]

SPINOCEREBELLAR ATAXIA (SCA7), ALSO KNOWN AS OLIVOPONTOCEREBELLAR ATROPHY TYPE III (OPCA3) (MIM 164500)

Cerebellar ataxia II (also known as spinocerebellar ataxia or olivopontocerebellar atrophy type III) is a progressive autosomal dominant, adult-onset ataxia. It is characterized by ataxia, dysarthria, hyperreflexia, involuntary movements, and retinal degeneraton. Ophthalmological findings include ophthalmoplegia, nystagmus, optic atrophy, and a peripherally spreading macular degeneration. Retinal findings include a macular retinal pigment epithelial (RPE) atrophy with a sharp border.[43] Ophthalmic features of OPCA were first described by Froment et al.[10] Individuals in the older generations have a maculopathy and patients in younger generations have peripheral disease (Fig. 26.6). Visual loss results from the retinal degeneration. Onset usually occurs in middle age, but may start in adolescence, or even in infancy.[15,52a] The ophthalmoplegia is slowly progressive and of a supranuclear form, showing slow saccades and initially without ptosis.[21] CT scan reveals cerebellar and pontine atrophy. Presymptomatic visual evoked responses have been reported.[16] Pathology reveals cerebellar, pontine, and retinal ganglion cell degeneration. Abnormal large mitochondria with irregular cristae are also found on muscle biopsy.[8,12] David et al.[8a] found in 18 individuals from 5 families, a mean age of visual loss of 22 years (range 1–45 years), decreased vision in 83%, blindness in 28%, optic atrophy in 69%, pigmentary retinopathy in 43%, supranuclear ophthalmoplegia in 56%, and abnormal slow eye movements in 79%. The gene for spinocerebellar ataxia with pigmentary maculopathy (SCAII or ADCAII or OPCAIII) has been localized to chromosome 3p12-p21.1.[3,13,18b] Anticipation was observed and was greater in paternal transmission. Trottier et al.[52b] identified the 13 kD protein with triplet repeats in two SCA7 patients. (CAG)n repeats were found in all 8 members of 7 families tested ranging from 150 to 240 base pairs.[27a] The locus was refined[26a] and mapped to 13p13-p12.[8a,8b] The SCA7 gene, called ataxin-7, codes for a 892 amino acid protein with CAG repeats at codons 30–39, varying in size from 7 to 17 in normal and 38 to 130 in affected patients.

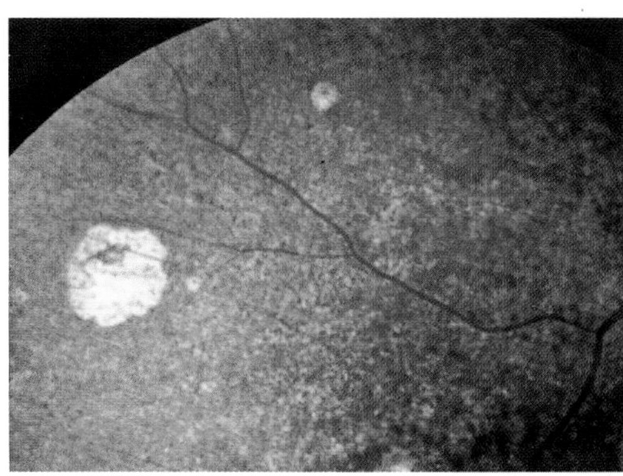

Figure 26.6. Peripheral fundus of a teenager with spinocerebellar ataxia with retinal degeneration. Note "salt-and-pepper" appearance and geographic areas of retinal pigment epithelial atrophy.

CHARCOT-MARIE-TOOTH DISEASE (CMT) (MIM 118200, 118300, 118301, 302801, 302900, 311070)

Charcot-Marie-Tooth disease is a sensorineural polyneuropathy with autosomal dominant and autosomal recessive forms being described. It is characterized by slowly progressive peroneal muscular atrophy with onset in late childhood. The motor neuropathy affecting the legs and small muscles of the feet and hands may accompany deafness and optic atrophy with loss of vision and a central scotoma.[5] An autosomal recessive variant of CMT with sensorineural deafness and optic atrophy was described by Rosenberg and Chutorian.[40] CMT may be divided into type I, with slow nerve conduction, and type II, with normal nerve conduction. Both dominant and recessive forms of each are seen.[17] Alajouanine et al.[1] described an original patient seen by Charcot in 1891 who had Argyll-Robertson pupils and blindness from optic atrophy, which began 40 years after the onset of the other signs of CMT. Autosomal dominant CMT has been linked to the myelin protein zero (MPZ; MIM 159440) located on chromosome 1q22.[18] Mutations of MPZ have also been associated with Dejerine-Sotas disease (MIM 145900). There is a second autosomal dominant locus (CMT1A) on chromosome 17p11.2.[32a,32b,53a] The autosomal dominant gene for the "trembler mutation" (*Tr*) mouse was homologous[53a] and identified as peripheral myelin protein-22 (PmP22). PmP22 maps to 17p11.2.[34a] The proposed mechanism of disease is thought to be duplications of the gene.[19a] X-linked form (CMTX1) with optic atrophy has been described.[18a] CMTX was linked to Xq13-Xq21[10a] and subsequently shown to be due to mutations in connexin-32. One family described with spastic paraplegia and RP was found to have mutation in the connexin-32 gene. McLeod et al.[32] reported an association between CMT and LHON. On reviewing this pedigree ("NSW1" with the 11778 mutation) 10 years later it was felt that this was just the coincidental overlap of two disease pedigrees, rather than a real association of CMT with LHON.[29] However, other CMT plus LHON families have been described.[3,30]

REFERENCES

1. Alajouanine T, Castaigne P, Cambier J, Escourolle R. Maladie de Charcot-Marie: Etude anatomo-clinique d'une observation suivie pendant 65 ans. *Presse Med* 1967; 75:2745–2750.

1a. Babcock M, de Silva D, Oaks R, Davis-Kaplan S, Jiralerspong S, Montermini L, Pandolfo M, Kaplan J. Regulation of mitochondrial iron accumulation by Yfh1p, a putative homolog of frataxin. *Science* 1997;276:1709–1712.

2. Behr C. Die komplizierte, hereditar-familiare Optikusatrophie des Kindesathers. *Klin Monatsbl Augenheilkd* 1909;47:138–160.

3. Benomar A, Krois L, Stevanin G, Caneel G, LeGuern E, David G, Ouhabi H, Martin JJ, Durr A, Zaim A, Ravise N, Busque C, Penet C, Van Regenmorter N, Weissenbach J, Yahyaoui M, Chkili T, Agid Y, Van Broeckhoven C, Brice A. The gene for autosomal dominant cerebellar ataxis with pigmentary macular dystrophy maps to chromosome 3p12-p21.1. *Nature Genet* 1995;10:84–88.

3a. Bonneau D, Souied E, Gerber S, Rozet J-M, D'Haens E, Journel H, Plessis G, Weissenbach J, Munnich A, Kaplan J. No evidence of genetic heterogeneity in dominant optic atrophy. *J Clin Genet* 1995;32:951–953.

3b. Brown J, Jr, Fingert JH, Taylor CM, Lake M, Sheffield VC, Stone EM. Clinical and genetic analysis of a family affected with dominant optic atrophy (OPA1). *Arch Ophthalmol* 1997;115:95–99.

4. Bundey S, Poulton K, Whitwell H, et al. Mitochondrial abnormalities in the DIDMOAD syndrome. *J Inheret Metab Dis* 1992;15: 315–319.

5. Burki E. Ophthalmologische Befunde bei der neuralen Muskelatrophie Charcot-Marie-Tooth, HMSN Typ 1. *Klin Monatsbl Augenheilkd* 1981;179:94.

6. Caldwell JBH, Howard RO, Riggs LA. Dominant juvenile optic atrophy. A study of two families and review of hereditary disease in childhood. *Arch Ophthalmol* 1971;85:133–147.

6a. Campuzano V, Montermini L, Molto MD, Pianese L, Cossee M, Cavalcanti F, Monros E, Rodius F, Duclos F, Monticelli A, Zara F, Canizares J, Koutnikova H, Bidichandani SI, Gellera C, Brice A, Trouillas P, De Michele G, Filla A, De Frutos R, Palau F, Patel PI, Di Donato S, Mandel JL, Cocozza S, Koenig M, Pandolfo M. Friedreich's ataxia: Autosomal recessive disease caused by an intronic GAA triplet repeat expansion. *Science* 1996;271: 1423–1427.

7. Carroll WM, Kriss A, Baraitser M, Barrett G, Halliday AM. The incidence and nature of visual pathway involvement in Friedreich's ataxia: A clinical and visual evoked potential study of 22 patients. *Brain* 1980;103:413–434.

8. Cooles P, Michaud R, Best PV. A dominantly inherited progressive disease in a black family characterized by cerebellar and retinal degeneration, external ophthalmoplegia and abnormal mitochondria. *J Neurol Sci* 1988;87: 275–288.

8a. David G, Abbas N, Stevanin G, Durr A, Yvert G, Cancel G, Weber C, Imbert G, Saudou F, Antoniou E, Drabkin H, Gemmill R, Giunti

P, Benomar A, Wood N, Ruberg M, Agid Y, Mandel JL, Brice A. Cloning of the SCA7 gene reveals a highly unstable CAG repeat expansion. Nature Genet 1997;17:65–70.

8b. David G, Giunti P, Abbas N, Coullin P, Stevanin G, Horta W, Gemmill R, Weissenbach J, Wood N, Cunha S, Drabkin H, Harding AE, Agid Y, Brice A. The gene for autosomal dominant cerebellar ataxia type II is located in a 5-cM region in 3p12-p13: Genetic and physical mapping of the SCA7 locus. *Am J Hum Genet* 1996;59:1328–1336.

8c. Durr A, Cossee M, Agid Y, Campuzano V, Mignard C, Penet C, Mandel JL, Brice A, Koenig M. Clinical and genetic abnormalities in patients with Friedreich's ataxia. *N Engl J Med* 1996;335:1169–1175.

9. Elberg H, Kjer B, Kjer P, Rosenberg T. Dominant optic atrophy (OPA1) mapped to chromosome 3q region. I. Linkage analysis. *Hum Mol Genet* 1994;3:977–980.

9a. Eliott D, Traboulsi EI, Maumenee IH. Visual prognosis in autosomal dominant optic atrophy (Kjer type). *Am J Ophthalmol* 1993;115: 360–367.

9b. Filla A, De Michele G, Cavalcanti F, Pianese L, Monticelli A, Campanella G, Cocozza S. The relationship between trinucleotide (GAA) repeat length and clinical features in Friedreich ataxia. *Am J Hum Genet* 1996;59:554–560.

10. Froment J, Bonnet P, Colrat A. Heredodegenerations retinienne et spinocerebelleuse variantes ophthalmoscopiques et neurologiques presentées par trois générations successives. *J Med Lyon* 1937;153–163.

10a. Gal A, Mucke J, Theile H, Wieacker PF, Ropers HH, Wienker TF. X-linked dominant Charcot-Marie-Tooth disease: Suggestion of linkage with a cloned DNA sequence from the proximal Xq. *Hum Genet* 1985;70:38–42.

11. Glaser JS. Topical diagnosis: Prechiasmal visual pathways. In *Duane's Clinical Ophthalmology*, Vol. 2, W. Tasman and E. A. Jaeger, eds. Philadelphia: J. B. Lippincott, 1989:27.

12. Gouw LG, Digre KB, Harris CP, et al. Autosomal dominant cerebellar ataxia with retinal degeneration: Clinical, neuropathologic and genetic analysis of a large kindred. *Neurology* 1994;44:1441–1447.

13. Gouw LG, Kaplan CD, Haines JH, Digre KB, Rutledge SL, Matilla A, Leppert M, Zoghbi Hy, Ptacck LJ. Retinal degeneration characterizes a spinocerebellar ataxis mapping to chromosome 3p. *Nature Genet* 1995;10: 89–93.

13a. Gray JV, Johnson KJ. Waiting for frataxin. *Nature Genet* 1997;16:323–325.

14. Gunn T, Bortolussi, Little JM, et al. Juvenile diabetes mellitus, optic atrophy, sensory nerve deafness and diabetes insipidus—A syndrome. *J Pediatr* 1976;89:565–570.

15. Halsey JH, Scott TR, Farmer TW. Adult hereditary cerebelloretinal degeneration. *Neurology* 1967;17:87–90.

16. Hammond EJ, Wilder BJ. Evoked potentials in olivopontocerebellar atrophy. *Arch Neurol* 1983;40:366–369.

17. Harding AE, Thomas PK. Genetic aspects of hereditary motor and sensory neuropathy (types I and II). *J Med Genet* 1980;17: 329–336.

18. Hayasaka K, Himoro M, Sato W, et al. Charcot-Marie-Tooth neuropathy type 1B is associated with mutations of the myelin p0 gene. *Nature Genet* 1993;5:31–34.

18a. Herringham WP. Muscular atrophy of the peroneal type affecting many members of a family. *Brain* 1889;11:230–236.

18b. Holmberg M, Johansson J, Forsgren L, Heijbel J, Sandgren O, Holmgren G. Localization of autosomal dominant cerebellar ataxia associated with retinal degeneration and anticipation to chromosome 3p12-p21.1. *Hum Mol Genet* 1995;1441–1445.

19. Horoupian DS, Zuker DK, Solomon M, et al. Behr syndrome; A clinicopathological report. *Neurology* 1979;29:323–327.

19a. Huxley C, Passage E, Manson A, Putzu G, Figarella-Branger D, Pellissier JF, Fontes M. Construction of a mouse model of Charcot-Marie-Tooth disease type 1A by pronuclear injection of human YAC DNA. *Hum Mol Genet* 1996;563–569.

20. Iverson HA. Hereditary optic atrophy. *Arch Ophthalmol* 1958;59:850–853.

21. Jampel RS, Okazaki H, Bernstein H. Ophthalmoplegia and retinal degeneration associated with spinocerebellar ataxia. *Arch Ophthalmol* 1961;66:247–259.

22. Johnston PB, Gaster RN, Smith VC, Tripathy RC. A clinicopathological study of autosomal dominant optic atrophy. *Am J Ophthalmol* 1979;88:868–875.

22a. Johnston RL, Burdon MA, Spalton DJ, Bryant SP, Behnam JT, Seller MJ. Dominant optic atrophy, Kjer type: Linkage analysis and clinical features in a large British pedigree. *Arch Ophthalmol* 1997;115:100–103.

23. Kirkhan TH, Guitton D, Katsarkis A, et al. Oculomotor abnormalities in Friedreich's ataxia. *Can J Neurol Sci* 1979;6:167–172.

24. Kivlin JD, Laurien EW, Bishop DT, Maumenee IH. Linkage analysis in dominant optic atrophy. *Am J Hum Genet* 1983;35:1190–1195.
25. Kjer P. Infantile optic atrophy with mode of inheritance. *Acta Ophthalmol (Copenh)* (Suppl) 1959;54:1–146.
26. Kjer P, Jensen OA, Klinken L. Histopathology of eye, optic nerve and brain in a case of dominant optic atrophy. *Acta Ophthalmol* 1983; 61:300.
26a. Krols L, Martin JJ, David G, Van Regemorter N, Benomar A, Lofgren A, Stevanin G, Durr A, Brice A, Van Broeckhoven C. Refinement of the locus for autosomal dominant cerebellar ataxia type II to chromosome 3p21.1-14.1. *Hum Genet* 1997;99:225–232.
27. Lessell S, Rosman NP. Juvenile diabetes mellitus and optic atrophy. *Arch Neurol* 1977; 34:759–765.
27a. Lindblad K, Savontaus ML, Stevanin G, Holmberg M, Digre K, Zander C, Ehrsson H, David G, Benomar A, Nikoskelainen E, Trottier Y, Holmgren G, Ptacek LJ, Anttinen A, Brice A, Schalling M. An expanded CAG repeat sequence in spinocerebellar ataxia type 7. Genome Res 1996;6:965–971.
28. Livingstone IR, Mastaglia FL, Edis R, Howe JW. Visual involvement in Friedreich's ataxia and hereditary spastic ataxia: A clinical and visual evoked response study. *Arch Neurol* 1981;38:75–79.
28a. Lunkes A, Hartung U, Magrino C, Rodriguez M, Palmero A, Rodriguez L, Heredero L, Weissenbach J, Weber J, Auburger G. Refinement of the OPA1 gene locus on chromosome 3q28-q29 to a region of 2-8 cM, in one Cuban pedigree with autosomal dominant optic atrophy type Kjer. *Am J Hum Genet* 1995;57:968–970.
29. Mackey DA. Three subgroups of patients with Leber hereditary optic neuropathy from the UK. *Eye* 1994;8:431–436.
30. McCluskey DJ, O'Connor PS, Sheehy JT. Leber's optic neuropathy and Charcot-Marie-Tooth disease. Report of a case. *J Clin Neuro-Ophthalmol* 1986;6:76–81.
31. McKusick VA. *Online Mendelian Inheritance in Man.* Baltimore: Johns Hopkins University Press, 1995; http://www3.ncbi.nlm.nih.gov/omim/.
32. McLeod JG, Low PA, Morgan Hughes JA. Charcot-Marie-Tooth disease with Leber optic atrophy. *Neurology* 1978;28:179–184.
32a. Middleton-Price HR, Harding AE, Monteiro CJ, Berciano J, Malcolm S. Linkage of hereditary motor and sensory neuropathy type I (HMSNI) to the pericentromeric region of chromosome 17 (abstract) *Cytogenet Cell Genet* 1989;51:1044.
32b. Nicholson GA, Mesterovic N, Ross DA, Block J, McLeod JG. Linkage of the gene for Charcot-Marie-Tooth neuropathy (abstract). *Cytogenet Cell Genet* 1989;51:1052–1053.
33. Niemeyer C, Marquardt JL. Wolfram-Tyer syndrome. *Invest Ophthalmol* 1972;11:617–624.
34. Page M, Asmal AC, Edwards CRW. Recessive inheritance of diabetes: The syndrome of diabetes insipidus, diabetes mellitus, optic atrophy and deafness. *Q J Med* 1976;45:505–520.
34a. Patel PI, Roa BB, Welcher AA, Schoener-Scott R, Trask BJ, Pentao L, Snipes GJ, Garcia CA, Francke U, Shooter EM, Lupski JR, Suter U. The gene for the peripheral myelin protein PMP-22 is a candidate for Charcot-Marie-Tooth disease type 1A. *Nature Genet* 1992;1:159–165.
35. Peden NR, Gay JD, Jung RT, et al. Wolfram (DIDMOAD) syndrome: A complex long-term problem in management. *Q J Med* 1986;58:167–180.
36. Pilz D, Quarrell OWJ, Jones EW. Mitochondrial mutation commonly associated with Leber's hereditary optic neuropathy observed in a patient with Wolfram syndrom (DIDMOAD). *J Med Genet* 1994;31:328–330.
37. Polymeropoulos MH, Swift RG, Swift M. Linkage of the gene for Wolfram syndrome to markers on the short arm of chromosome 4. *Nature Genet* 1994;8:95–97.
38. Rando TA, Horton JC, Layzer RB. Wolfram syndrome. Evidence of a diffuse neurodegenerative disease by magnetic resonance imaging. *Neurology* 1992;42;1220–1254.
39. Repka MX, Miller NR. Optic atrophy in children. *Am J Ophthalmol* 1988;106:191–193.
39a. Rice DS, Williams RW, Davisson MT, Harris B, Goldowitz D. A new mutant phenotype of retinal ganglion cell dysgenesis discovered in the mouse (abstract). *Soc Neurosci Abstr* 1993;19:51.
39b. Rice DS, Williams RW, Ward-Bailey P, Johnson KR, Harris BS, Davisson MT, Goldowitz D. Mapping the Bst mutation on mouse chromosome 16: A model for human optic atrophy. *Mammal Genome* 1995;6:546–548.
40. Rosenberg RN, Chutorian A. Familial opticoacoustic nerve degeneration and polyneuropathy. *Neurology,* 1967;17:827–832.

41. Ross FC, Fraser GR, Friedman AI. The association of juvenile diabetes mellitus and optic atrophy: Clinical and genetic aspects. *Q J Med* 1966;35:385–405.
42. Rotig A, Cormier V, Chatelain, P, et al. A deletion of mitochondrial DNA in an early case of early onset diabetes mellitus, optic atrophy and deafness (Wolfram syndrome, MIM222300). *J Clin Invest* 1993;91:1095–1098.
43. Ryan SJ, Knox DL, Green WB, Konigsmark BW. Olivopontocerebellar degeneration: Clinicopathologic correlation of the associated retinopathy. *Arch Ophthalmol* 1975;93:169–172.
44. Smith DP. Diagnostic criteria in dominantly inherited juvenile optic atrophy. *Am J Optom* 1971;49:183–194.
45. Snell S. Diseases of the optic nerve. I. Hereditary or congenital optic atrophy and allied cases. *Trans Ophthalmol Soc UK* 1897;17: 66–81.
46. Stenddahl-Brodin L, Moller E, Link H. Hereditary optic atrophy with probable association with a specific HLA haplotype. *J Neurol Sci* 1978;38:11–21.
47. Swift RG, Perkins DO, Chase CL, et al. Psychiatric disorders in 36 families with Wolfram syndrome. *Am J Psychiatry* 1991;148:775–779.
48. Swift RG, Sadler DB, Swift M. Psychiatric findings in Wolfram syndrome homozygotes. *Lancet* 1990;336;667–669.
49. Sylvester PE. Some unusual findings in a family with Friedreich's ataxia. *Arch Dis Child* 1958;33:217–221.
50. Taylor D. Optic neuropathies, In *Paediatric Ophthalmology*, D. Taylor, ed. London: Blackwell, 1990:699–701.
51. Taylor D. Optic neuropathies. In *Paediatric Ophthalmology*, D. Taylor, ed. London: Blackwell, 1990:473–488.
52. Thomas PK, Workman JM, Thage O. Behr's syndrome: A family exhibiting pseudodominant inheritance. *J Neurol Sci* 1984;64:137–148.
52a. Traboulsi EI, Maumenee IH, Green WR, Freimer ML, Moser H. Olivopontocerebellar atrophy with retinal degeneration. A clinical and ocular histopathologic study. *Arch Ophthalmol* 1988;106:801–806.
52b. Trottier Y, Lutz Y, Stevanin G, Imbert G, Devys D, Cancel G, Saudou F, Weber C, David G, Tora L, Agid Y, Brice A, Mandel JL. Polygluyamine expansion as a pathological epitope in Huntington's disease and four dominant cerebellar ataxias. *Nature* 1995;378: 403–406.
53. Tyrer J. A case of infantilism with goitre, diabetes mellitus, mental defect, and primary optic atrophy. *Med J Aust* 1943;11:398–401.
53a. Vance JM, Nicholson G, Yamaoka LH, Stajich J, Stewart CS, Speer C, Hung WY, Roses AD, Barker D, Gaskell PC, Pericak-Vance MA. Linkage of Charcot-Marie-Tooth neuropathy type 1a to chromosome 17 (abstract). *Cytogenet Cell Genet* 1989;51:1097–1098.
53b. Votruba M, Moore AT, Bhattacharya SS. Genetic refinement of dominant optic atrophy (OPA1) locus to within a 2 cM interval of chromosome 3q. *J Med Genet* 1997;34:117–121.
54. Wolfram DJ. Diabetes mellitus and simple optic atrophy among siblings. Report of 4 cases. *Mayo Clin Proc* 1938;13:715–718.

IV.

Disorders of Ocular Motility

27

The Genetics of Strabismus: Duane, Möbius, and Fibrosis Syndromes

ELIZABETH C. ENGLE

Strabismus is the pathological deviation of one eye with respect to the other, resulting in misalignment of the visual axes and loss of binocular fused vision.[142] Normal binocular vision depends on an extremely complex neuronal network of sensory, motor, and integrative pathways, and strabismus can result when these pathways are disturbed by any of a vast number of peripheral and central nervous system disorders.[3]

Although Hippocrates noted a familial tendency for strabismus,[162] the precise genetics of the various strabismic disorders have yet to be fully eluciated. This chapter discusses the genetics of isolated concomitant strabismus, Duane syndrome, Möbius syndrome, the fibrosis syndromes, and strabismus associated with neuromuscular diseases. There are, however, approximately 100 inherited disorders with associated strabismus. For many of these disorders, genetic information can be obtained by accessing the computer database OMIM (The Online Mendelian Inheritance in Man, part of The Human Genome Data Base Project, Johns Hopkins University, Baltimore MD) via The World Wide Web address http://gdbwww.gdb.org/omim/docs/omimtop.html and searching by the name of the disorder or by the key word "strabismus" (OMIM #185100).

STRABISMUS TERMINOLOGY

The term strabismus encompasses a variety of different disorders with the common feature of misalignment of the eyes. Strabismus may be evident in primary (straight ahead) gaze or only in eccentric vertical or horizontal gaze. It can be alternating, in which case either eye can be the fixating eye while the other is deviated, or monolateral, in which case only one eye fixates while the other is always deviated. Pure forms of strabismus include esotropia or convergent horizontal strabismus, exotropia or divergent horizontal strabismus, hypertropia or upward vertical strabismus, hypotropia or downward vertical strabismus, and incyclotropia and excyclotropia or torsional strabismus.[143] If latent, strabismus is termed "-phoria" rather than "-tropia," and becomes most evident with the interruption of binocular vision by occlusion of one eye.

Strabismus is either concomitant or incomitant. Concomitant strabismus occurs when the misalignment or the angle of deviation of the eyes remains constant independent of the direction of gaze. When concomitant strabismus results from a hyperopic refractive error and can be corrected by use of lenses it is "accommodative," when corrective lenses do not affect the strabismus it is "nonaccomodative." Strabismus is incomitant when the misalignment or the angle of deviation varies with gaze direction. This often results from mechanical dysfunction in the orbit or neuromuscular dysfunction at the level of the muscle, nerve, or brainstem.

ANATOMIC LOCALIZATION OF STRABISMUS

Orbit

The globe is suspended in the orbit by the extraocular muscles, connective tissue fascia, and fat. Because the bony orbits do not lie in the anterior-posterior plane but point outward at approximately a 23° angle and because the vertical recti and oblique muscles are not aligned with the primary visual axis when the eyes are in primary gaze, the action of the extraocular muscles depends somewhat on the position of the globe at the time of the action. Malformations, adhesions, or anomalous connective tissue septa between muscle and the orbital wall, anomalies of the trochlear apparatus or the check ligaments, infiltration of the oribital structures by connective tissue or tumor, and orbital trauma with muscle entrapment can all alter normal orbital development and mechanics and result in strabismus.

Extraocular Muscles

The visual system places unique demands on the extraocular muscles (EOMS) to perform a range of complex, integrated movements including tonic position-maintaining contractures, conjugate smooth pursuit and saccades, and dysconjugate vergence movements. It is likely because of these demands that EOMS are found to have unique developmental, morphological, and physiological properties when compared to other skeletal muscle groups. In humans, there are six EOMs that move the globe (four recti and two oblique) and one muscle that raises the eyelid (levator palpebrae superioris). Strabismus can result from dysfunction of any or all of the six muscles that move the globe, and can stem from maldevelopment, myopathies, dystrophies, metabolic disorders, or abnormalities at the neuromuscular junction. In addition, muscles can be missing, insert anomalously on the globe, or be replaced by fibrous or connective tissue bands.

Muscle Development

In a 1957 report of human EOM development, Gilbert[73] proposed that EOMs began to differentiate at the apex of the orbit and then proceeded in an anterior direction, reaching their final positions by 6 months. He reported that the EOMs arise from three independent but closely opposed mesodermal condensations; one premandibular and two maxillomandibular. The precursors of cranial nerve (CN) III-innervated muscles arise from prechordal mesoderm at the anterior end of the notochord at 25 days gestation to form the premandibular condensation which, at 29–33 days, differentiates into the superior, inferior, and medial recti and the inferior oblique muscles. The levator palpebrae superioris subsequently delaminates from the superior rectus beginning around 43–47 days. Gilbert[73] also reported that the two maxillomandibular condensations arise from mesenchymal cells lateral and adjacent to the developing premandibular condensations at about 29 to 33 days gestation, one becoming the lateral rectus and one the superior oblique muscle. Recent studies of avian eye muscle development have confirmed that the precursors of the muscles innervated by the oculomotor nerve are derived from prechordal mesoderm.[35,175] In addition, however, studies now suggest that the precursor cells of the lateral rectus and superior oblique are actually derived from paraxial somitomeric mesoderm that subsequently shifts rostrally and forms the mesenchymal condensation medial to the maxillomandibular lobe.[174,253]

A different theory of human eye muscle development has been proposed by Sevel.[215] He examined a series of human embryos and reportedly found a single mesenchymal condensation that differentiates into a superior and inferior mesodermal complex. He found that the superior rectus, superior oblique, and levator palpebrae superioris arise from the superior complex, the inferior rectus and inferior oblique arise from the inferior complex, and the medial and lateral recti arise from both. He observed that the muscles develop from mesoderm within the orbit and the origin, belly, and insertion of the muscle and the nerves develop contemporaneously along their whole axis, rather than beginning at the apex and growing anteriorly.[215,216] He agreed that the superior rectus and levator palpebrae superioris have a common epimysium and begin to separate from one another at 7 weeks.

Muscle Anatomy

The four rectus muscles originate from the annulus of Zinn at the posterior apex of the orbit, approach the globe from a posterior and medial angle, and insert on the globe anterior to its equator (Fig. 27.1). The lateral and medial recti are antagonists in the horzontal plane, abducting and adducting the eye, respectively. The superior and inferior recti are partial antagonists in the vertical plane. The superior rectus primarily elevates but also intorts and adducts the globe, and the inferior rectus primarily depresses but also extorts and adducts the globe. The oblique muscles differ from the recti by approaching the globe from an anterior and medial direction and inserting posterior to the equator. The superior and inferior obliques are partial antagonists and both have the greatest effect when the globe is adducted. The superior oblique muscle originates at the annulus of Zinn, its tendon passes through the trochlea in the superior and medial orbit, and inserts posterior-superior-temporally on the globe. It intorts, depresses, and abducts the globe. The inferior oblique arises from the medial orbital wall and inserts posterior, inferior and temporally on the globe, and it extorts, elevates, and abducts the globe.[142,192]

Muscle Morphology

Each EOM fiber has a long, tendonous origin and insertion of fibrous connective tissue.[48] A cross-section near the muscle insertion reveals

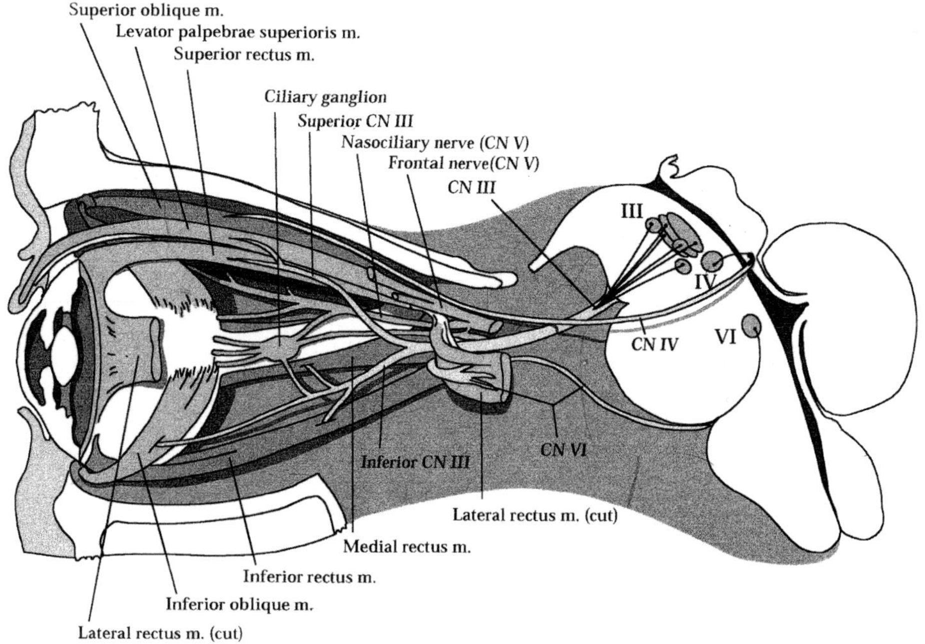

Figure 27.1. Lateral view of the brain stem and orbit showing the human extraocular motor system. The cranial nerve nuclei, extraocular muscles, and cranial nerves are shown. (Adapted with permission from the Ciba Collection of Medical Illustrations.)

a transition zone of mixed muscle and tendonous connective tissue of varying length. Cross-section of the muscle belly reveals rounder, smaller, and more variable myofibers than limb muscle, and greater amounts of perimysial and endomysial connective tissue. Unlike other skeletal muscle, the cross-section is not homogeneous but contains an orbital layer (adjacent to the orbit) and a global layer (adjacent to the globe). These layers differ from one another in muscle fiber types and richness of vascular supply.[48,191]

EOM fiber typing is more complicated and less well understood than that of limb skeletal muscle,[191,225] but its unique features probably underlie the muscle's capacity to perform uniquely fast and fatigue-resistant contractions. Spencer and Porter[225] describe six EOM fiber types based on location, mitochondrial content, and innervational pattern. These include singly innervated fast twitch, multiply innervated intermediate twitch, and multiply innervated slow nontwitch fibers. Contraction speed of a fiber is partially a function of its myosin heavy chain isoform; six different EOM isoforms have been identified[25] and at least one is unique to EOM.[256] Fatigue resistance of a fiber increases with increasing numbers of mitochondria; a subset of the singly innervated fibers has a very high mitochondria content and is among the most fatigue-resistant muscles known.

The motor units of EOMs are very small when compared to other skeletal muscle, often innervating only three to ten muscle fibers, and can fire very rapidly (approximately 600 Hz compared to approximately 200 Hz in extremity muscle).[205] In addition, EOM is the only known mammalian muscle to contain fibers innervatved by more than one motor unit (multiply innervated fibers). Researchers have identified antigenic differences between extremity muscle and EOM acetylcholine receptors at the neuromuscular junction,[119,178] and have demonstrated expression of an "embryonic" gamma subunit of the nicotinic acetylcholine receptor in adult EOM.[103]

The levator palpebrae superioris differs slightly in structure from the other EOM. Architecturally, it has no differentiation of orbital and global layers, and it lacks multiply innervated fibers.[193] It does, however, share many features with the six other EOMs and is innervated by CN III; ptosis and strabismus frequently occur together.

Muscle Pathology

The study of both normal and pathologic human EOM has been limited; EOM is rarely obtained at postmortem examination or biopsied at the time of orbital surgery. EOM cannot be interpreted using the standards applied to skeletal limb muscle; e.g., this would result in the misinterpretation of the normal small, round, variably sized fibers and increased connective tissue of EOM as "myopathic" muscle.[48,191] Some surgical biopsies interpreted as pathological "fibrosis" may actually be a sample of the normal connective tissue of the muscle's long fibrous tendon as it inserts on the globe. This sampling error was not infrequent in one large series.[155] In addition, the orbital and the global regions may differ in response to disease, yet they are not equally accessible to surgical biopsy.[48,53]

The response of developing EOM to injury is not known. The response of mature EOM, however, appears to be different and unique when compared to other skeletal muscle. Denervation of EOM in dog,[48] monkey,[194] and baboon[53] results in inflammatory, degenerative, and regenerative changes. These are the pathologic features found in limb muscle that has undergone myopathic, not neurogenic, injury. In Duchenne muscular dystrophy, which results in fibrosis and severe muscle wasting of all major muscle groups, the EOMs are spared from clinical[118] and pathological consequences of dystrophin loss.[126,196] This may be related to the observation that EOM is resistant to the myopathic damage normally caused by pharmacologically elevated calcium levels.[126]

Cranial Nerves and Nuclei

Development

During early fetal development, the nucleus and CN III arise from the mesencephalon, and the nuclei and CN IV, VI, and VII arise from the hindbrain.[124] Various regulatory genes have been implicated in both delineating and/or specifying hindbrain and midbrain development. The hindbrain develops in a segmental pattern of rhombomeres, with motor neurons and CN IV arising from rhombomere 1, of VI arising from rhombomeres 5 and 6, and of VII arising from rhombomeres 4 and 5.[124] The organization and development of the rhombomeres caudal to rhombomere 2 are believed to be influenced the Hox homeobox genes, which are expressed in overlapping domains extending along the anterior-posterior axis of the developing embryo and are postulated to determine the body's segmental organization. The development of the abducens nucleus, therefore, may be influenced by the expression of a subset of Hox genes. Although the oculomotor and trochlear motoneurons are rostral to Hox expression, putative regulatory genes such as non-Hox cluster homeobox genes (e.g., En-1 and En-2), Pou domain genes, Pax genes, and Wnt genes are expressed in this region.[68]

CN motor nuclei III, IV, and VI begin forming and emitting axons by gestational day 32 and continue to develop throughout the first trimester.[221] Gilbert[73] noted that the cranial nerves grow into the appropriate developing muscles between 31 and 33 days. Recent experimental work in the chick embryo has revealed that precise contacts between the abducens nerve and the precursor cells of the lateral rectus occur before either make contact with neural crest-derived periocular connective tissue.[253]

The primitive vascular plexus of the brain begins to develop at 24 days and the basilar artery differentiates by 29 days.[67] Initially, the posterior circulation, which supplies the developing mid- and hindbrain, is supplied by rostral to caudal flow through the basilar artery from the primitive trigeminal arteries. At 37–40 days of gestation the primitive trigeminal arteries regress and the first cervical intersegmental and vertebral arteries begin to provide the mature caudal to rostral flow.[17]

Anatomy

The oculomotor nucleus (III) is composed of contiguous subnuclei in the midbrain (Fig. 27.2). It projects uncrossed medial rectus, inferior rectus, inferior oblique, and pupillary constrictor fibers, crossed superior rectus fibers, and both crossed and uncrossed levator palpebrae superioris fibers within the oculomotor

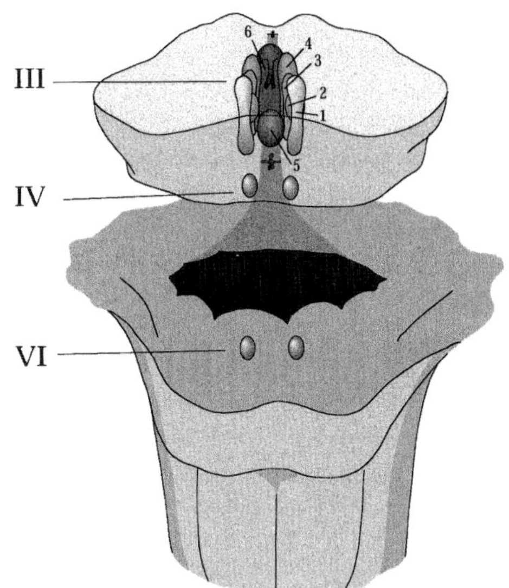

Figure 27.2. Anterior view of the human brain stem showing details of the cranial nerve nuclei that innervate the extraocular muscles. III = oculomotor nucleus, IV = trochlear nucleus, and VI = abducens nucleus. The oculomotor subnuclei are shown as follows, with the muscle they innervate in parentheses: 1 = ventral lateral (medial rectus); 2 = medial (superior rectus); 3 = intermediate lateral (inferior oblique); 4 = dorsal lateral (inferior rectus); 5 = central (levator); 6 = Edinger-Westphal (visceral motor).

nerve to the appropriate target muscles.[142] The trochlear (IV) nerve arises from its contralateral nucleus in the caudal midbrain, crosses in the tectum, exits the brain stem, and innervates the ipsilateral superior oblique. The abducens (VI) nerve arises from its ipsilateral nucleus in the pons and innervates the ipsilateral lateral rectus. Some neurons of the abducens nucleus and some medial rectus neurons in the contralateral oculomotor nucleus are connected via the medial longitudinal fasciculus (MLF). The EOMs are reciprocally innervated (i.e., the right lateral and right medial recti) such that when an agonist muscle contracts its antagonist relaxes, and are yoked in pairs (i.e., the right lateral rectus and left medial rectus), the eyes move together.[142]

Pathology

The cranial nerve nuclei can be congenitally aplastic or hypoplastic. The oculomotor, trochlear, or abducens nerves can be congenitally absent or can aberrantly innervate the EOMs, resulting in simple or complex strabismic disorders. Diffuse malformative, destructive, or degenerative processes of the brain stem can affect the cranial nerve nuclei, the gaze centers, and the medial longitudinal fasciculus.

Misexpression of the regulatory genes involved in midbrain and hindbrain development has been proposed as a theoretical etiology of some brain stem malformations. Knockouts of several of these genes in transgenic mice have resulted in intriguing phenotypes. Hox-A1 knockouts result in loss of some facial motoneurons,[27] Krox-20 knockouts result in loss of trigeminal and abducens motorneurons,[213] and Wnt-1 knockouts result in midbrain-anterior hindbrain defects and absence of oculomotor and trochlear motoneurons.[68] Engrailed-1 mutant mice with a homozygous targeted deletion have absence of most of the colliculi and cerebellum, absence of the third and fourth cranial nerves, and sternum, rib, and paw defects.[263] Genetic strabismic syndromes often occur in concert with additional defects. Some of these additional phenotypes have also been induced by misexpression of various homeobox genes in mice and include (*1*) abnormal eye opening at birth, craniofacial dysmorphisms and vertebral anomalies,[121] (*2*) cleft palate and abnormalities of craniofacial and tooth development,[209] (*3*) abnormalities of limb development,[232] and (*4*) absence of radius and ulna with severe kidney defects.[44]

The response of the brain stem to injury is dependent on when the development of injury occurs. In the first trimester, an insult is likely to result in brain stem malformation.[67,127] During this period, developing cranial nerve nuclei may be at selective risk for maldevelopment resulting from anoxic-ischemic damage. The nuclei are supplied by the developing basilar artery, and there is the risk of a perfusion defect at the time the direction of its flow reverses.[17] In the late second or third trimester, the developing brain stem becomes capable of responding to injury with gliosis, calcification, and neuronal depopulation.[127] Therefore, different mechanisms of injury may result in the same pathology if they occur at the same time in gestation, and one injury may result in different types of pathology when it occurs at different times in gestation.[127]

Supranuclear Etiologies

Supranuclear causes of strabismus include disturbances of cerebellar, vestibuloocular, thalamic, cortical white matter, and cortical neuronal function. Dysfunctions of the visual sensory system, including the retina, lateral geniculate, occipital cortex, integrative centers, and connecting axonal pathways, are implicated in many forms of concomitant strabismus.

CONCOMITANT STRABISMUS

Isolated Concomitant Strabismus

Isolated concomitant strabismus is the most common form of strabismus and includes congenital esotropia, accommodative esotropia, and exotropia. Congenital esotropia manifests between birth and 6 months of life as an esodeviation that is not corrected by hyperopic lenses and occurs in the absence of any neurologic abnormality. It may be accompanied by abnormal abduction, dysfunction of the oblique muscles, amblyopia, nystagmus, dissociated vertical and horizontal deviations (DVD, DHD), or torticollis.[93] Corrective surgery is recommended between 4 and 12 months for infants with congenital esotropia. Bimedial rectus recession results in satisfactory alignment in 80%–85% of patients. Accommodative esotropia is partially related to hyperopia and may be corrected solely by refractive lenses. It usually manifests between 6 months and 6 years, with most between 2 and 3 years of age. Because hyperopia itself can be familial (OMIM and ref. 187), some familial esotropia likely results from the inheritance of a primary accommodative error. Intermittent exotropia may be congenital or develop slowly during childhood.[143] It can be associated with myopia or can occur without a refractive error. In one study, nonstrabismic family members were found to share sensory abnormalities with strabismic probands, suggesting the sensory disturbance was the primary hereditary anomaly.[199]

Studies of isolated concomitant strabismus have not routinely analyzed data for each subtype, but typically group the disorders together. Population studies suggest that isolated concomitant strabimus affects 1%–5% of Americans and Europeans. It is somewhat more prevalent in females than in males, and in Caucasians than in blacks.[80,101,157,158,187] Population studies also show variability in the frequency of esotropia versus exotropia among different racial and ethnic groups. Esotropia is much more common than exotropia in the Caucasian population of the United States and Europe,[176,187] whereas exotropia is more frequent than esotropia in Japan and Indonesia and among the black populations of the United States and Africa.[187] In Hawaii, esotropia is more common in Caucasians, exotropia more common in Orientals, and the two forms are relatively equal in the mixed ethnic population.[109]

Family studies suggest that genetics influences the occurrence of concomitant strabismus.[51,143,157,162,212] Paul and Hardage[187] compiled a cohort of 7100 strabismic patients from 12 different published family studies and determined that 2171 (30.6%) of probands with strabismus had a family member or close relative with strabismus. Within each study the percent of probands with a positive family history ranged from 13%–65%. Families are usually concordant for either esotropia or exotropia, and many believe that the two forms result from the influence of separate genes. Families with both forms have been reported, however, any may reflect the presence of two relatively common genes or one gene with variable expressively.[159,212] Maumenee et al.[159] studied the families of 173 probands with congenital esotropia. In 113 families, only the proband was affected. In the remaining 60 families (35%), two or more members were affected. There were families with two or more siblings affected, with one parent and half the children affected, and with both parents and some or all children affected. The authors concluded that the inheritance of congenital esotropia best fits a Mendelian codominant model in which a homozygote for both relatively common alleles would have a high probability of being affected.

Paul and Hardage[187] also compiled 11 published strabismus twin studies comprising a combined total of 336 twin pairs. Of 206 monozygotic twin pairs, 73% were concordant for strabismus. Of 130 pairs of dizygotic twins, 35% were concordant for strabismus. These studies confirm that dizygotic twins have the same or a slightly higher prevalence of strabismus than is expected of siblings from the family studies. The much higher concordance between monozygotic twins supports a strong genetic component to concomitant strabismus.

Associated Concomitant Strabismus

Concomitant strabimus is a frequent component of genetic syndromes. It is found in association with trisomy of chromosomes 13, 18, and 21 and partial trisomy of 22. It is found with some deletions of chromosome 5 in cri-du-chat syndrome, and with some deletions of chromosome 15 in the Prader-Willi and Angelman syndromes. Strabismus is seen with some of the trinucleotide repeat expansion disorders, including fragile X and myotonic dystrophy. Both concomitant and incomitant strabismus can also be seen in association with multisystem disorders. Although the disease genes have been cloned for a few of these disorders, such as Marfan syndrome[46,112] and Crouzon disease,[113] the cause of strabismus in these disorders is not known. The occurrence of concomitant strabismus as a component of genetic syndromes that map to multiple chromosomal locations reinforces the concept that strabismus is a phenotype with marked genetic heterogeneity. The same phenotype can result from many different defects at many genetic locations.

INCOMITANT STRABISMUS

Duane Syndrome

Duane syndrome is a relatively rare but distinct form of strabismus, accounting for 1%–5% of all strabismus patients.[41,129] The disorder is defined by the combination of limited abduction, variably limited adduction, and retraction of the globe into the orbit with narrowing of the palpebral fissure on attempted adduction (Figs. 27.3A, B). Although narrowing of the palpebral fissure is generally felt to be a consequence of globe retraction resulting from cocontraction of the medial and lateral rectus, it has been reported to be present in cases without retraction and to be absent in cases with extreme

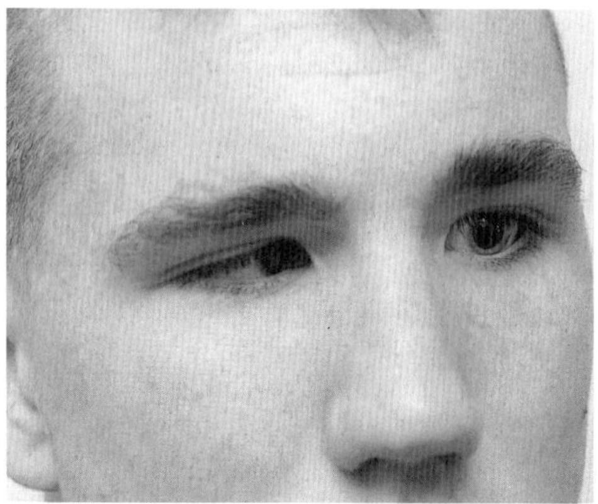

A

B

Figure 27.3. *A:* Sixteen-year-old man with left Duane syndrome. There is inability to abduct the left eye on attempted left gaze. *B:* Marked upshoot and retraction of the right globe on attempted left gaze in this young boy with Duane syndrome.

retraction.[45] Huber[106] has categorized individuals with Duane syndrome into three clinical groups: type I has poor abduction with slight limitation of adduction, type II has poor adduction with slight limitation of abduction, and type III has a combination of poor abduction and adduction. Globe retraction and palpebral fissure narrowing with adduction occur in all three categories. In one survey, type I accounted for 83%, type II for 11%, and type III for 2% of cases.[177]

Although this ocular movement disorder was described as early as 1900,[261] the syndrome was named for Alexander Duane[49] after he published his 1905 paper collating 54 cases. In his series, abduction was virtually absent in 41, adduction was abnormal in 52, oblique movements (upshoot, downshoot) occurred on attempted adduction in 31, and retraction was present in 52 of the 54 individuals. Many affected individuals had strabismus and abnormal head position in primary gaze. No one had accommodation or pupil abnormalities. Duane noted a preponderance of affected females and of unilateral left eye involvement. He did not mention the occurrence of associated malformations or affected family members.

Since Duane's original series, there have been multiple retrospective and prospective studies of Duane syndrome patients.[111,129,177,188,219] Although the syndrome is congenital and nonprogressive, only approximately one-third of cases are diagnosed in infancy. An additional one-third are diagnosed in childhood, and the remaining one-third in early to mid adult life.[188,219] Of affected individuals, 57%–65% are females, 80%–85% of cases are unilateral, and the left eye is affected in 65%–70% of unilateral cases. A significant proportion of individuals has strabismus; esotropia is more common in type 1 and exotropia in type II. Some individuals maintain a compensatory head turn to achieve single binocular vision. The vast majority of patients have good visual acuity and amblyopia occurs in only approximately 10% of patients.

Pathology and Pathogenesis

Early surgical and histopathologic studies of Duane syndrome[4,49,72] reported fibrosis, abnormal insertions, and adhesions of the lateral or medial rectus muscles, and led to the conclusion that this was a local, myogenic phenomenon. Subsequently, an electromyelogram (EMG) of the EOMs revealed the presence of electrically active medial and lateral recti and showed that the simultaneous cocontraction of both the medial and lateral recti resulted in globe retraction.[82,107] These findings suggested aberrant and paradoxical innervation of these muscles and supported a neurogenic etiology for Duane syndrome. Two careful postmortem examinations of isolated Duane syndrome with associated anomalies, one of bilateral type III[104] and one of unilateral type I,[165] have helped to explain the EMG findings. In both types, there was absence of the abducens nucleus and abducens nerve on the affected side(s), the oculomotor nuclei and nerves were normal, and the lateral rectus muscles were partially innervated by branches from the oculomotor nerves (Fig. 27.4).

These anatomic findings form the basis for the current belief that Duane syndrome is caused, at least in some cases, by a developmental neurological anomaly of the CN VI nucleus with primary or secondary aberrant innervation of the lateral rectus. Abnormal embryonic development might also explain the frequent association of Duane syndrome with other congenital anomalies of the skeletal, facial, and nervous systems. The differentiation of these structures coincides with the development of the cranial nerves and EOMs, all occurring between the fourth and eighth weeks of gestation. Genetic, inflammatory, toxic, traumatic, or vascular insults during this developmental period could potentially result in Duane syndrome with associated abnormalities.

The Hox and other related homeobox genes have been implicated in the normal segmentation of caudal somitomeres and spinal cord somites. As discussed previously, misexpression of Krox-20 in transgenic mice results in an absence of abducens motoneurons.[213] Abnormalities of these and related genes are interesting candidates for the etiology of both isolated Duane syndrome as well as Duane syndrome with associated anomalies.

In a comprehensive study of thalidomide embryopathy, Miller[163] reported that thalidomide is teratogenic to the developing embryo between 20 and 35 days gestation, and results in a spectrum of anomalies including maldevelopment of the extremities, craniofacial dysmorphisms, internal and external ear malformations with or without deafness, facial nerve palsy, various forms of strabismus, and abnormal tearing. Duane syndrome, isolated lateral rectus palsies, and gaze paresis can occur with exposure to thalidomide between 21 and 26 days gestation. Extremity anomalies range from thumb hypoplasia (22–27 days) to almost total absence of upper and lower extremities (24–33

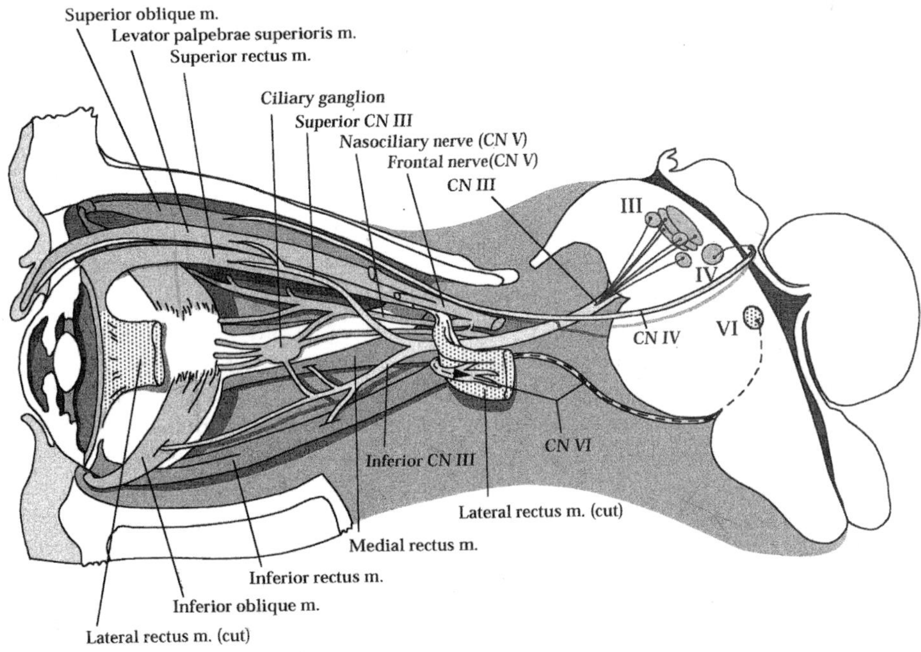

Figure 27.4. Lateral view of the brain stem and orbit showing the pathologic abnormalities in Duane syndrome. The dotted VI nerve nucleus and VI nerve are absent, and the shaded lateral rectus is abnormal.

days). Thalidomide exposure can mimic familial cases of Duane syndrome associated with upper extremity and thumb anomalies, hearing loss, or abnormal tearing. Miller[163] also identified individuals with thalidomide teratogenicity who had Duane syndrome and facial weakness, suggesting an etiologic overlap between the Möbius and Duane syndromes.

Genetics of Isolated Duane Syndrome

Although most cases of Duane syndrome are sporadic, studies have found that between 2% and 8% of probands have at least one family member with Duane syndrome.[72,129,177,188,223] Although one study found that none of 63 cases had an affected family member with Duane syndrome, it did find that 22% of the probands had close family members and 17.5% had distant relatives with other types of strabismus.[219] In addition, some individuals with Duane syndrome may have family members with normal eye movements but with one of the associated anomalies, which might result from segregation of a gene with variable expressivity.

There are families reported with isolated Duane syndrome in two and three generations.[76,129,136,223,252] Inheritance appears to be autosomal dominant with a greater frequency of affected females, and there is variability within families as to whether the disorder is left, right, or bilateral. One of the larger families with isolated Duane syndrome was reported by Goldfarb and Gannon[76]; a father, four of his nine children, and three of the six grandchildren born to affected parents had Duane syndrome. The syndrome was bilateral in all except one grandchild, who was affected only on the left side. In this family the syndrome may have been fully penetrant; 7 of 15 offspring born to an affected parent were affected, and no offspring born to an unaffected parent was affected. In other families, however, the syndrome is partially penetrant and there are individuals who are obligate carriers.[129,136] Laughlin[136] reported a three-generation family with Duane syndrome and variable expressivity; a mother had limited abduction and retraction with narrowing of the palpebral fissure on adduction, and her child had limited abduction but no retraction or palpebral fissure changes. There is a report of two sisters with "vertical Duane syndrome" in whom there was limitation of vertical gaze and globe retraction.[125]

There have been multiple twin studies of Duane syndrome. Two pairs of monozygotic twins were concordant for bilateral[100,177] and one pair for left-sided unilateral[66] Duane syndrome. One monozygotic pair was discordant for bilateral[202] and one for unilateral[254] Duane. There are two families in which the mother and both of her monozygotic twins were affected. In one family, the mother and one twin were affected on the right and the second twin was affected on the left,[161] and the second family, all three were affected on the left.[71]

Genetics of Duane Syndrome with Associated Anomalies

Duane syndrome frequently occurs in association with other congenital anomalies, particularly of the skeleton, ear, eye, and kidney. These associated findings are typically reported with sporadic cases of Duane syndrome, but they also occur together with Duane syndrome as familial malformation or genetic syndromes. These syndromes overlap, and most appear to be inherited with variable penetrance and expressivity.

Pfaffenbach et al.[188] studied 186 cases of Duane syndrome and found that 33% had at least one, 17% at least two, and 8% at least three additional congenital anomalies. The authors proposed that the incidence of associated anomalies may be even higher because 40% of the affected individuals did not undergo a general physical examination and fewer than 20% had spine radiographs or hearing examinations. Of those individuals who had a chest radiograph and full physical and otolaryngological examinations, 50% had at least one congenital anomaly.

In the Pfaffenbach et al.[188] series, skeletal deformities were noted on physical examination in 12% and by radiological examination in 18% of patients. Deformities included limb hypoplasia, polydactyly, hypoplastic or absent radius and thumb, foot anomalies, skull hypolasia and asymmetry, cleft palate, Klippel-Feil anomaly, scoliosis, spina bifida, and anomalous vertebrae, ribs, and scapulae. Additional ocular anomalies occurred in 19% of patients. Amblyopia accounted for 10% of these and is a complication of Duane syndrome rather than an associated finding. Additional ocular anomalies included nystagmus, ptosis, microphthalmia, coloboma, heterochromia iridis, and congenital cataract. Congenital ear anomalies were noted in 5% of patients and included malformed pinnae and/or inner ear and auricular appendages. Sensorineural deafness was present in 6.5%, genitourinary anomalies in 4%, and cardiac anomalies in 2% of patients.

Approximately 5% of patients had congenital central nervous system disorders including seizures, hypotonia, and congenital facial palsy. The first two findings suggest more diffuse brain or muscle disease, and the third demonstrates the overlap of Duane and Möbius syndromes. Two unrelated children have been reported with Duane syndrome, bland facial appearance, and paroxysmal gustatory-lacrimal reflex with profuse lacrimation associated with eating. One of these children had clinodactyly and one had external ear anomalies and congenital deafness.[197] Additional children have been reported with Duane syndrome and Marcus-Gunn jaw winking.[110] These associations suggest additional aberrant innervation.

Duane/Radial Dysplasia Syndrome. The familial association of Duane syndrome and radial ray dysplasia was first noted by Ferrell et al.[61] in 1966 in a report of a family with Holt-Oram and Duane syndromes. The association was first observed in the absence of cardiac defects by Temtamy et al.[233] in 1975 and by Okihiro et al.[180] in 1977. The association is referred to in the literature as Duane/radial dysplasia sydrome,[233] DR syndrome (acronym for Duane anomaly, deafness, radial dysplasia, renal dysplasia),[234] and Okihiro syndrome.[92] This syndrome has been reported in at least eight families and appears to be autosomal dominant with incomplete penetrance and variable expressivity.[12,33,61,92,151,160,180,233] The Duane syndrome anomaly can be unilateral or bilateral. The radial dysplasia can range from hypoplasia of the thenar eminence with or without thumb abduction and apposition weakness, hypoplasia or absence of the thumb, and hypoplasia or absence of the radial and ulnar bones to an absent forearm. Hearing loss, dysmorphic facies and cardiac, renal, and vertebral anomalies are variably expressed in some families.

Radiological studies of the upper extremities vary from atrophy of the thenar soft tissue to hypoplasia or absence of metacarpals and long bones with aberrant articulation. Electrical studies have shown markedly decreased or absent median nerve motor response with no electrical activity of the abductor pollicis brevis.[12,180] Vascular studies and surgical exploration of one case revealed a hypoplastic radial artery and an anomalous median nerve with two distinct recurrent motor branches to the thenar eminence. The proximal branch of the median nerve was not electrically excitable and was traced to the region of the thenar eminence normally occupied by the abductor pollicis brevis and the opponens pollicis.[12]

Duane/Holt-Oram Syndrome. The original family described by Ferrel et al.[61] consisted of four affected members in two generations. All four affected individuals had radial ray anomalies, two had the Duane anomaly, and one had an atrial septal defect (ASD). Holt-Oram syndrome is the association of a congenital cardiac anomaly [most commonly secondum ASD or ventricular septal defect (VSD)] with a spectrum of limb anomalies from absence or anomalous thumb to phocomelia or ectomelia. At least seven families with Holt-Oram have been linked to chromosome 12q21.3-q22.[13,235] None of the members of these linked families were reported to have Duane syndrome. Holt-Oram appears to be genetically heterogeneous, however, and several clinically indistinguishable familes are not linked to the 12q2 locus.[235] There is one report of a patient with Holt-Oram, strabismus, dysmorphisms, and cryptorchidism who has a 14q23-924.3 deletion syndrome,[243] and one report in abstract form of a patient with Holt-Oram and a chromosome 20 inversion with breakpoints at p13 and q13.2.[264] Chromosomes were normal in the Ferrell et al.[61] family, and it is unclear if this family had Duane/radial dysplasia syndrome and one affected member with incidental ASD or whether these two syndromes overlap genetically. It will be prudent to test Duane syndrome families for linkage to Holt-Oram loci.

Acro-Reno-Ocular Syndrome. The combination of Duane syndrome, radial ray anomalies, and kidney malformations has been reported in a three-generation family with normal chromosomal analysis.[83] Inheritance appears to be autosomal dominant with high penetrance and markedly variable expressivity. Six of seven affected members had thenar hypoplasia and thumb anomalies, six had malrotation, ectopia, or hypoplasia of a kidney or significant reflux, one had pulmonary stenosis, one had spina bifida occulta, and only one had the Duane anomaly with ptosis. This family overlaps with one of the Duane/radial dysplasia families[233] who has similar renal and limb anomalies, but also had several members with pectoral and upper limb muscle hypoplasia and had a higher penetrance of Duane syndrome.

Strabismus with Radial Anomalies. One family has been reported with esotropia/convergent squint, radial ray, hypoplasia, and mild facial dysmorphisms.[75] Although this family's syndrome is similar to the DR and the IVIC syndrome, the affected members did not have Duane anomaly, nor did any of them have auditory, cardiac, renal, or hematological abnormalities.

IVIC Oculo-Acoustic-Radial Syndrome. This syndrome, named for the institute of the original authors (Instituto Venezolano de Investiqaciones Científicas), has been described in three families who have a combination of eye movement abnomalities, radial ray defects, hearing impairment, and thrombocytopenia.[7,38,208] The disorder appears to be autosomal dominant with complete penetrance and variable expressivity. The original description was of 19 affected members of a Caucasian family from the Canary Islands.[7] The extraocular movement disorders in the affected individuals were congenital, nonprogressive, unilateral or bilateral, and included combinations of mild exotropia, narrowing of the palpebral fissure with abduction, significant limitations of horizontal gaze, and complete external ophthalmoplegia. Hypotropia was more common than hypertropia and no one had globe retraction. In the second reported family, one of the three affected members had strabismus,[208] and in the third family with two affected members, one had abduction limitation but there was no comment about globe retraction.[38] The radial ray defects were present in all members of all families with the exception of one member of the original family, and are similar but generally more severe than in the DR syndrome. In addition, several individuals had hypoplasia of the pectoral and deltoid muscles mimicking Poland syndrome (see description in the Möbius section). Some of the affected members of each family had sensorineural hearing loss. Therefore, this syndrome overlaps with DR, but affected members have variable complicated strabismus.

Chromosomal analyses were normal in the first and third families[7,38] and preliminary linkage analysis of the first family was not successful. In the second family, with a father and two children affected, chromosomal analysis of the father revealed a 5BDU induced fragile site {fra(10)(fq25)} in 30% of phytohemagglutinin-stimulated peripheral lymphocytes.

Duane Syndrome and Perceptive Deafness/ Oculo-Acoustic Syndrome. Sensorineural deafness was present in 6.5% of the Duane patients reported by Pfaffenbach et al.,[188] and is generally noted in 1%–10% of patients with Duane syndrome.[177,200,219] Kirkham[128,129] has described seven families with congenital Duane syndrome and perceptive deafness. In his original report, Kirkham[128] described a girl with left-sided ptosis, strabismus, left Duane anomaly, deafness, and mild mental retardation. Her maternal aunt had left Duane anomaly and deafness, and 20 of 34 relatives in five generations had perceptive deafness manifested in childhood or adolescence. If due to a single gene defect, this syndrome shows autosomal dominant inheritance with male to male transmission, high penetrance, and variable expression.

Duane Syndrome with Klippel-Feil Anomaly. Deformities of the cervical vertebrae and Klippel-Feil anomaly have been noted in 1%–6% of individuals with Duane syndrome.[129,177,219] Klippel-Feil anomaly consists of fused cervical vertebrae, cervical spine deformities, short neck with limited range of motion of the head and neck, and a low posterior hairline. The association of Duane and Klippel-Feil is typically sporadic, but there is one report of two sisters with Klippel-Feil of whom one also had Duane syndrome.[129] A balanced translocation between 5q11.2 and 17q23 has been found in one individual with Klippel-Feil syndrome without ocular anomalies.[179]

Wildervanck syndrome (cervico-oculo-acousticus syndrome) is the triad of Duane anomaly, Klippel-Feil anomaly, and perceptive deafness. Sporadic cases can be accompanied by craniofacial, chest, and limb anomalies. It has been described almost exclusively in females.[258] No clearly familial cases have been described, although one female proband with the triad had a paternal aunt with hearing loss.[129]

Duane Syndrome and Marfanoid Hypermobility. Two sisters have been described with Duane syndrome and marfanoid hypermobility whose father had a marfanoid habitus.[203] None had anomalies of the aorta or lens. The proband did not have homocystinuria, and analysis of skin fibroblasts revealed normal glycosylation and normal levels of fibronectin and collagen. Chromosomal analysis was normal. These patients do not have the full Marfan phenotype, which results from mutations of the 15q21.1 fibrillin gene.[46] These findings could result from a contiguous gene deletion syndrome including genes for Duane syndrome and collagen. The Marfan locus and other collagen loci remain candidate regions.

Duane Syndrome with Chromosomal Abnormalities

Duane Syndrome with Chromosome 4 Deletion. A 15-year-old boy with bilateral type I Duane syndrome, bilateral ptosis, and a mild learning disorder was found to have a deletion of 4q27-31.[29] The authors do not mention whether any family members have similar clinical or chromosomal findings. Families with Duane syndrome should be tested for linkage to this region of chromosome 4.

Duane and Bronchiootorenal (BOR) Syndromes on Chromosome 8. BOR syndrome, the association of preauricular pits, cervical fistulas or cysts, structural defect of the outer, middle, or inner ear (responsible for hearing loss), and renal anomalies, has been linked to chromosome 8q21-8q13.[135] Vincent et al.[248] described a patient with the association of the Duane anomaly, BOR, hydrocephalus, mild mental retardation, and trapezius aplasia who had a de novo 8q12.2-q21.2 deletion. The deletion in this patient likely interrupted several contiguous genes and has refined the localization of the BOR gene as well as suggested a candidate region for a Duane syndrome gene.

Duane Syndrome and Chromosome 22. The clinical and genetic findings of one family and two additional unrelated individuals suggest that there may be a Duane syndrome gene on chromosome 22. In 1977, Weleber et al.[255] described a girl with the Duane anomaly and the cat-eye syndrome. Chromosomal analysis revealed 47XX with an extra submetacentric chromosome thought to be derived from chromosome 22. In 1988, Kalpakian et al.[117] described a boy with the Duane anomaly, dysmorphic facial features, mental retardation, hearing loss, vertebral anomalies, and tetralogy of Fallot. Their chromosomal analysis revealed 46XY/47XY, +mar with the supernumerary chromosome present in 12.5% of blood lymphocytes and 100% fibroblasts also felt to be derived from chromosome 22. In 1993, Cullen et al.[37] reported a family in whom a daughter and son had the Duane anomaly, sensorineural deafness, preauricular skin tags, and renal agenesis. In addition, the daughter had primary amenorrhea secondary to absent uterus. The father had preauricular skin tags with normal extraocular movements, hearing, and kidneys. They all had normal vertebral and limb development and normal cardiac examinations. On chromosomal analysis, all three had a supernumerary bisatellited marker chromosome derived from the region of chromosome 22pter-q11. The mother had normal chromosomes and a normal examination.

Möbius Syndrome

In 1888, Möbius[167] described a man with congenital bilateral lateral rectus weakness, bilateral facial weakness, unilateral chest muscle malformation, and unilateral second and third finger syndactyly. The patient had bilateral lack of abduction, unilateral hypotropia, and convergence with attempted downgaze (Fig. 27.5). Upgaze, adduction, convergence, and pupillary response were normal. In a subsequent paper, Möbius[166] categorized the congenital and early childhood cranial nerve palsies into six groups; one category including the original and five additional sporadic cases of congenital abducens paralysis and facial paralysis. Therefore, even though similar cases had been published prior to 1888,[30,87,249] the syndrome was named for him.

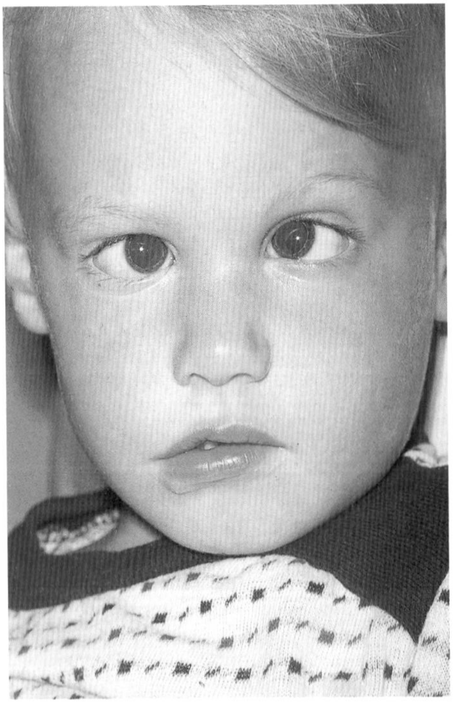

Figure 27.5. Möbius syndrome. Note bilateral facial palsy and esotropia from bilateral sixth cranial nerve palsy. (From Traboulsi and Maumenee,[242] with permission.)

Since the original papers, authors have used varying diagnostic criteria for Möbius syndrome. The three most commonly used minimal criteria are (*1*) congenital facial diplegia[10,94,134]; (*2*) congenital facial diplegia and unilateral or bilateral loss of abduction[244]; and (*3*) congenital facial diplegia, unilateral or bilateral loss of abduction, and congenital abnormalities of the extremities.[198] For this discussion of Möbius syndrome, the second defining criterion of facial and abduction weakness is required.

Möbius syndrome is nonprogressive and frequently occurs with additional anomalies. These include (*1*) additional cranial nerve anomalies such as external ophthalmoplegia, tongue hypoplasia or weakness, swallowing and respiratory difficulties, and deafness; (*2*) limb malformations such as hypoplasia, transverse terminal defects, syndactyly, brachydactyly, absent digits, talipes, and arthrogryposis multiplex congenita; (*3*) orofacial malformations such as cleft palate, bifid uvula, micrognathia, and ear deformities; (*4*) additional musculoskeletal malformations such as Poland and Klippel-Feil anomalies; (*5*) mental retardation; and (*6*) hypogonadotropic hypogonadism.

Temtamy and McKusick[234] classify Möbius with the group of "terminal transverse defects with orofacial malformations" (TTV-OFM). Gorlin et al.[78] classify Möbius as the most common of the six congenital oromandibular-limb hypogenesis syndromes. In addition to Möbius, these include Hanhart, hypoglossia-hypodactylia, glossopalatine ankylosis, limb deficiency-splenogonadal fusion, and Charlie M. syndromes. These syndromes consist of variable combinations of cranial nerve, craniofacial, and limb anomalies. Because of the frequency of associated anomalies with Möbius syndrome and the frequency of abduction and facial weakness in the associated syndromes, delineation between syndromes is often overlapping and ambiguous.

Pathology and Pathogenesis

Necropsy reports suggest that Möbius syndrome is not a single entity. In 1979, Towfighi et al.[240] categorized the published pathologic reports of 15 individuals with Möbius syndrome into four groups. Group I was characterized by hypoplasia or atrophy of cranial nerve nuclei, group II by possible primary peripheral nerve involvement, group III by focal necrosis in brain stem nuclei, and group IV by myopathic features. All 15 individuals were less than 6 years of age at the time of death and 12 were less than 6 months of age. Gestational histories did not suggest toxic, metabolic, infectious, or vascular insults. The vast majority had associated respiratory compromise and many of the infants were ventilator dependent throughout their short lives. Möbius syndrome with or without associated findings in an adult is likely to have more focal and less compromising pathology. It may be that neonates who die with Möbius syndrome have a severe form of the same disorder or it may be they have a different disorder compared to those individuals with Möbius syndrome who survive and have normal lower brain stem function. Necropsy studies reporting group I or group III changes are most frequent and are reviewed shortly. Although they are rarely reported, some cases may result from group II and IV changes reflecting a primary neuropathic or myogenic process.[189,242]

There are two affected infants who died recently and were reported to have group I neuropathologic changes. One infant had isolated Möbius,[77] and a second had Möbius and skeletal anomalies.[230] Both of these neonates had hypoplasia/agenesis of the CN VI and VII nuclei, supporting an etiologic event during the first trimester of gestation. Most recent neuropathologic studies, however, report group III changes, which suggest a late second or third trimester insult. Again, these reports are virtually all postmortem examinations of neonates, most of whom died of respiratory failure secondary to more diffuse brain stem dysfunction.[39,131,148,227,230,236,240,259] Several of the infants had external ophthalmoplegia rather than abduction weakness.[39,133,227,230,259] Neuronal depletion in the abducens and facial nuclei[39,60,148,236,240] and absence of the existing CN II and/or CN VII[39,227,236,240] frequently accompany the tegmental calcification. The facial and EOMs[240] and the vertebrobasilar vasculature[227] were each examined in one case and were normal.

Necropsy reports with group III changes of brain stem necrosis and calcification have been reported in infants with Möbius syndrome and hypoglossia.[148] craniofacial dysmorphisms,[39,60,148,227,236] limb anomalies,[39,70,148] Poland syndrome with limb anomalies,[148,227,236] and arthrogryposis.[133] In addition, neuroimaging of infants with Möbius,[79] and Möbius with limb defects[70] has revealed brain stem calcification, and one case of Möbius with arthrogryposis has revealed basal ganglia calcification.[230]

A first trimester genetic or vascular insult might account for group I pathology but would not account for isolated group III pathology. The developing brain stem responds to first trimester injuries typically with malformative changes, such as cranial nerve nuclear hypoplasia. The brain does not become capable of responding to injury with necrosis and gliosis until the late second trimester.[127] Therefore, cases with isolated group III pathology are unlikely to result froma first trimester insult. There are, however, two detailed pathologic reports of Möbius or Möbius-like syndromes with both early cranial nerve nuclear hypoplasia/dysgenesis and evidence of a later destructive process suggesting an early and ongoing insult.[39,127] Kinney et al.[127] documented these changes by three-dimensional computer reconstruction of the brain stem. They proposed that group I and group III injuries may represent a spectrum of the same disorder in which the pathology is determined by the timing of the injury during gestation. Therefore, in an ongoing injury beginning in the first trimester and extending into the third trimester, the malformative changes may not be detected because of the overlying destructive and calcified process.

Bouwes-Bavinck and Weaver[17] proposed an early vascular etiology for Möbius, Poland, and Klippel-Feil syndromes that could explain each of these syndromes individually and in combination, and subsequently many authors have attributed group III pathologic findings to such a vascular insult. The necrosis and calcification are typically bilaterally symmetric and focal, which could reflect a localized vascular insult or a particular susceptibility of the brainstem to hypoxic-ischemic damage. As reviewed in the introduction to this chapter, the subclavian, basilar, vertebral, and internal thoracic arteries undergo development and remodeling between the fourth and eighth weeks of gestation. During their own development, these vessels must supply the concomitantly developing cranial nerve nuclei, neck, pectoral muscles, and limb buds. Bouwes-Bavinck and Weaver[17] proposed that disruption of the developing vascular system could result in hypoxic-ischemic injury to these developing structures, and the location of the insult would determine the combination of organs affected. The vascular disruption could result from a myriad of underlying etiologies including genetic, infectious, inflammatory, and traumatic. There has been no pathologic evidence and little clinical evidence, however, for underlying infectious, inflammatory, or traumatic processes.

The segmental pattern of hindbrain development has been discussed previously. Similar to Duane syndrome, the localization of injury in Möbius syndrome to the pons, at times with involvement of the medulla, craniofacial bones, and limb buds, suggests the possibility of an underlying genetic defect similar to that seen with experimental misexpression of one of the homeobox genes. In addition, future pathologic studies of children and adults with Möbius syndrome associated with early teratogenic exposure[77,163] may offer us insight into brain stem development.

Möbius Syndrome Genetics

The incidence of familial Möbius syndrome depends on a given study's inclusion criteria. If isolated facial weakness is considered sufficient for the diagnosis, then the study will include the well-described entity of autosomal dominant isolated congenital facial diplegia,[10,94,156,245] which has been mapped by linkage analysis to chromosome 3.[131a] In 1939, Henderson[94] reviewed 61 individuals with Möbius syndrome using facial weakness as his inclusion criteria, and 11 of the individuals had isolated facial weakness. Four of the 61 patients had at least one affected family member, of which three were cases of isolated familial congenital facial diplegia. The fourth family was originally reported by Beetz[15] and was consanguineous with three siblings affected; one had a left exotropia and ptosis and one left lateral and medial rectus weakness. Similarly, Baraitser[10] conducted an 18-year retrospective study of Möbius syndrome with the inclusion criteria of congenital facial weakness. Of the 29 patients identified, 8 had died in the neonatal period, half because of respiratory or bulbar problems, and 15 were available for follow-up. Two of the 15 patients were found to have an affected relative. In the first family, two siblings had isolated facial weakness. In the second family, a sibling had facial weakness but no eye involvement and both the proband and sibling were rediagnosed with a progressive myopathic process.

MacDermot et al.[152] reviewed the familial cases of Möbius syndrome and divided the literature into five groups: (*1*) congenital facial nerve palsy without ocular involvement, (*2*) CN VI–VIII palsy with or without skeletal anomalies, (*3*) multiple cranial nerve palsies, (*4*) CN VI and VII palsies with or without other cranial nerve or skeletal involvement but with muscle aplasia and/or skeletal defects in relatives, and (*5*) cranial nerve palsies with neuromuscular disorders. Again, the only clearly consistent pattern of inheritance was families with autosomal dominant congenital facial weakness.

Some authors feel that familial cases of Möbius syndrome without limb anomalies are either autosomal dominant facial diplegia or misdiagnosed neuromuscular disorders, and that if a case of Möbius syndrome is associated with limb anomalies it is sporadic and the recurrence risk is nil.[10,94,95,148,152,198,231] There are, however, reports suggesting that genetic inheritance plays a role in Möbius syndrome with and without associated anomalies. These reports are reviewed in the paragraphs that follow.

Facial Diplegia with Linkage to Chromosome 3. Kremer et al.[131a] studied a Dutch family with incompletely penetrant autosomal dominant asymmetric bilateral facial weakness. Electrophysiologic studies of the facial muscle in an affected individual were considered compatible with a neuropathic lesion. None of the family members had abnormalities of eye movement. Using linkage analysis they have localized the disease gene to a 10 cM region at chromosome 3q21-22. They reported that a second family they studied with Möbius syndrome was not linked to the chromosome 3 locus but did not describe the family's clinical manifestations of the disorder.

Möbius Syndrome with Chromosomal Abnormalities. There are three reports of Möbius syndrome with chromosomal abnormalities. Together, these reports suggest that 13q12.2-13 is a good candidate region for a "Möbius syndrome" gene and that genes mapping to 1p22, 1p34, and 11p13 should also be considered possible candidates. The first report[265] is of a family with an autosomal dominant syndrome consisting of mild ptosis, facial weakness, hearing loss, mild mental retardation, and finger contractures. None of the affected members had abduction weakness or other abnormalities of eye movement. All seven affected individuals carry a chromosome 1 to 13 translocation t(1p34;13q13) and one unaffected individual who had several unaffected children did not carry the translocation. The second report[224] is a sporadic case of Möbius with bilateral abduction weakness, left-sided facial weakness, tongue weakness, and facial dysmorphisms in an individual with a de novo deletion of chromosome 13 (46XX, del(13)(q12.2)). In the third report,[47] the proband had abduction and facial weakness, hearing loss, bulbar dysfunction, profound developmental delay and hypotonia, craniofacial dysmorphism, skeletal deformities, and dextrocardia. The brother and father were unaffected. All three carried a chromosome 1 to 11 translocation t(1p22;11p13). As the translocation was found in unaffected as well as affected family members, the authors suggest that it may have either unmasked a genetic locus, contributed to an autosomal recessive disorder, or predisposed the affected individual to uniparental disomy.[47]

Möbius Syndrome in Two Family Members. There are at least five reported families in whom both a proband and an additional family member have abduction weakness and facial weakness. In two families there is vertical transmission from mother to son, consistent with autosomal dominant, X-linked, or even mitochondrial inheritance. In the first family the proband also has polydactyly and mental retardation,[99] and in the second family the proband also has craniofacial dysmorphisms.[152] There are three consanguineous families in which two or more siblings are affected. In all three families the parents were first cousins and the genetic etiology is likely to be autosomal recessive. In one, both siblings also have ptosis and high frequency hearing loss.[140] In the second, both siblings also have arthrogryposis and basal ganglia calcifications and one has a cardiac anomaly.[222] In the third family, all three affected children have additional ear deformities, two are mentally retarded, and two have skeletal anomalies.[15]

Proband with Möbius Syndrome and an Associated Anomaly/Family Member with an Associated Anomaly. It is not known if isolated limb defects or other associated anomalies in a family member of an individual with Möbius syndrome are coincidental or if they result from a genetic defect with variable expressivity. These cases are summarized below.

1. *With skeletal anomalies:* There are three reports of probands with abduction weakness, facial weakness, and skeletal anomalies who had vertically related family members with skeletal anomalies.[14,33,69] In one of these families additional family members also had facial weakness and/or anhydrosis.[14] In a fourth report,[165] the proband had abduction and facial weakness with a diminished gag reflex, a sister had skeletal anomalies, and the mother had facial weakness. There is a fifth report[115] of a proband with abduction and facial weakness, craniofacial dysmorphism, and mental retardation. The patient had two maternal cousins with mental retardation, one of whom also had craniofacial and limb anomalies.

Carey-Fineman-Ziter syndrome was first described in 1982 and has now been reported in four patients,[11,26,211] two of whom were identically affected siblings suggesting autosomal recessive inheritance. This syndrome includes the features of Möbius syndrome and consists of specific craniofacial dysmorphism, ptosis, abduction limitation, facial weakness, poor suck and swallow, hypoglossia, hypotonia, poor muscle mass, proximal weakness, bilateral pectoralis muscle hypoplasia, and skeletal malformations including club feet and brachydactyly.

Three of the four patients had short stature and two had strabismus in primary gaze. Two patients had muscle biopsies: one had slightly small fibers and a moderate increase in connective tissue, and the second had mild myopathic changes. Chromosomal studies have been normal.

2. *With Poland syndrome:* Poland anomaly is the absence of the pectoralis muscle(s), and Poland syndrome is the anomaly together with hand defects of the symbrachydactyly types.[233] When it occurs with Möbius syndrome it is referred to as the Poland-Möbius syndrome. Möbius syndrome has been reported with both the Poland anomaly[231] and the Poland syndrome.[164,201] The accompanying cranial nerve abnormalities vary. In one review of 34 individuals with Poland-Möbius syndrome,[95] 2 had isolated abduction weakness, 5 had isolated facial weakness, 11 had both abduction and facial weakness, 8 had more of an external ophthalmoplegia and facial weakness, and the remaining cases had lower brain stem dysfunction. There is a single report of a boy with Poland-Möbius syndrome whose mother has Poland syndrome.[201] A possible anatomic basis for this association has been discussed.

3. *With arthrogryposis:* Arthrogryposis is a consequence of a lack of sufficient prenatal movement resulting in joint contractures. It is etiologically diverse. Singh et al.[222] reported two siblings with Möbius syndrome and arthrogryposis. There is one report of a proband with Möbius syndrome and arthrogryposis whose sibling had arthrogryposis,[226] and a report of twins who died as neonates supposedly with Möbius syndrome (who actually had ophthalmoplegia) and arthrogryposis.[84]

4. *With mental retardation:* Approximately 10% of individuals with Möbius syndrome are mentally retarded.[228] There is one report of a proband with limitation of abduction, facial weakness, deafness, skeletal anomalies, and mental retardation who has a brother with esotropia and mental retardation and a sister with mental retardation.[228]

5. *With myopathic features:* The facial and abduction weakness of Möbius syndrome are congenital and therefore should rarely overlap with progressive neuromuscular disorders. There have been reports, however, of patients initially diagnosed with Möbius syndrome who have later been diagnosed with fascio-scapular-humeral muscular dystrophy (the patient had facial weakness only),[86] or myotonic dystrophy.[90] There is one report of a proband diagnosed with Möbius syndrome who actually had abduction and facial weakness, skeletal anomalies, and myopathic features and whose sister has facial weakness and other myopathic features.[10] Both siblings progressed and more likely had an undiagnosed neuromuscular disorder.

External Ophthalmoplegia and Facial Weakness. There are several reports of alleged Möbius syndrome in which the affected individual had external ophthalmoplegia (with or without ptosis) and facial weakness. Two of these families[132,140] were clinically indistinguishable from the families with autosomal dominant congenital external ophthalmoplegia linked to chromosome 12[57] and were probably misdiagnosed. There is one family in whom the proband has ptosis, external ophthalmoplegia, and club feet, and a cousin has limb anomalies.[144] The twins just discussed had arthrogryposis, external ophthalmolplegia, and absence of spontaneous respirations.[84]

Sporadic Möbius syndrome and hypogonadotropic hypogonadism were first reported by Olson et al.[181] in 1970. They described an 18-year-old man with the complex of eye movement and pupil abnormalities, ptosis, facial weakness, hypoactive deep tendon reflexes, peripheral weakness, and absent puberty. EMG suggested motor neuron disease, muscle biopsy revealed minimal changes consistent with denervation, and endocrine evaluation revealed hypogonadotropic hypogonadism. Subsequently, five additional unrelated patients have been described in the literature.[2,18,123,148,204] All six had hypogonadotropic hypogonadism and normal chromosomes. All patients had ptosis, four had complex (internal and external) ophthalmoplegia, one had external ophthalmoplegia, and one had unilateral abduction weakness. Five had bilateral and one had unilateral facial weakness. Either two or three had anosmia. Two had high arches and hammer toe deformities (also present in the first-degree relatives of one patient), one had bilateral pes cavus, and one had bilateral transverse above-elbow limb deficiency. Evaluation suggested nonprogressive lower motor neuron abnormalities in two patients, Nonprogressive peripheral neuropathy in two patients, and progressive peripheral neuropathy in two patients. A seventh patient has been reported with ACTH deficiency, slight bilateral abduction and facial weakness, mild appendicular weakness, hammer toes, and peripheral neuropathy.[131]

FIBROSIS SYNDROMES

In 1950, Brown[23] categorized several eye movement disorders with congenital active and passive limitation of globe movement as the "fibrosis syndromes." Because the EOMs felt stiff and tight at surgery and biopsies frequently consisted of fibrous connective tissue, these disorders were felt to result from a primary myopathic process with fibrous changes. Brown[23] included general fibrosis syndrome (clinically affecting three or more of the EOMs), superior oblique tendon sheath syndromes or "Brown syndrome" (affecting inferior and/or superior obliques), horizontal (Duane syndrome) and vertical retraction syndromes, and strabismus fixus (affecting the medial and lateral recti) within this category of disorders. Subsequently, it has been shown that at least some cases of the retraction syndrome are neurogenic, and it is still not known if any of these disorders are truly myopathic.

Congenital Fibrosis of the Extraocular Muscles

General fibrosis syndrome, congenital fibrosis of the extraocular muscles (CFEOMs)[136,184,241] ocular congenital fibrosis syndrome,[173] congenital external ophthalmoplegia,[65,105,114] and congenital external ophthalmoplegia with cocontraction[31,32] have all been used to describe this sporadic or autosomal dominant disorder. Prior to the establishment of linkage of the autosomal dominant families to chromosome 12,[57,58] this disorder was defined clinically.

Individuals with classic CFEOM have bilateral ptosis, bilateral hypotropic strabismus, and severely restricted eye movements with the eyes fixed at 20°–30° below the horizontal. Together with the ptosis, this leads to the patients tilting their head backward with chin elevated in order to see below their eyelids (Fig. 27.6). (Any residual eye movements are typically in the horizontal plane, may vary between the two eyes, and are often notable for aberrant and jerky convergent or divergent movements on attempted vertical gaze.[16,21,28,85,138,206] Affected individuals lack binocular vision, frequently have significant refractive errors with high astigmatism, and can develop amblyopia.[28,36,89,98] Although the neurologic and general physical examinations have usually been reported as

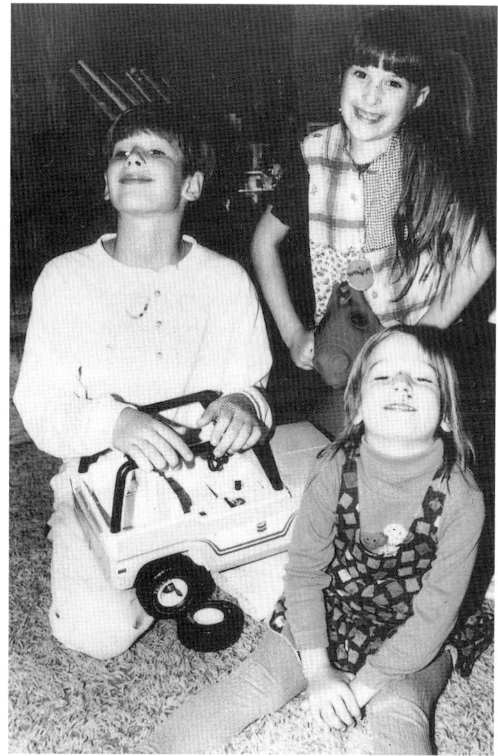

Figure 27.6. Three siblings from a family with chromosome 12-linked congenital fibrosis of the extraocular muscles. The boy on the left and his sister sitting in the foreground are affected. Their sister in the back is unaffected. The two affected children have ptosis and hypotropic strabismus with a compensatory backward tilt to the head. Note also their horizontal smile in comparison with that of their unaffected sister. (From Engle et al.,[57] with permission of The University of Chicago Press).

normal,[102,173] mild facial weakness has been noted in affected individuals and young children may have hypotonia and mild gross motor delay.[56–58]

There have been many attempts to correct this disorder surgically. Typically, the appropriate EOMs are recessed, the position of the globe is adjusted, and the ptosis is corrected.[6,56,89,98,137,146,173] At surgery, forced ductions demonstrate a marked resistance to passive movement.[21,36,56,85,89,98] Movement is most limited in upgaze, somewhat less so in downgaze, and variable in horizontal gaze. The muscles sometimes appear thin and pale. The muscles are taut against the globe, feel stiff, and lack normal stretch and elasticity. In most cases, disinsertion of a muscle frees the globe, although some surgeons have found additional adhesions between muscle, Tenon's capsule, and globe.[6,23,85,173,250] Others have reported anomalous posterior muscle insertions[6,250] or anomalous anatomy with selectively absent muscles and "fragile" conjunctiva.[206]

Occasionally, additional anomalies are reported in association with the fibrosis syndrome. These cases are often sporadic and clinically atypical, or the associations occur in a single member of an otherwise typical pedigree. The anomalies associated with atypical or sporadic CFEOM have been reviewed recently by Kalpakian et al.[116] and by Kishore and Kumar.[130] Ocular anomalies include microphthalmia, corneal opacities, dyscoria, ectopic pupils, choroidal coloboma, congenital cataracts, posterior lentiglobus, optic atrophy, optic disc hypoplasia, and retinitis pigmentosa. Additional neurologic anomalies include mental retardation, Marcus-Gunn phenomenon, internal ophthalmoplegia, syringomyelia, and spina bifida. Systemic anomalies include craniofacial dysmorphism, dental anomalies, Klippel-Feil deformity, cardiac malformations, syndactyly, bilateral inguinal hernias, cryptorchidism, Prader-Willi syndrome, and Joubert syndrome. Chromosomal analyses have been normal.

Pathology and Pathogenesis

It is unclear if CFEOM arises from a primary neurogenic or myopathic process. The congenital and static nature of CFEOM, reports of anomalous insertions on the globe and sparing of the epithelial-derived intrinsic eye muscles, and two atypical cases with associated mesodermal defects[8,130] suggest a primary developmental defect of the mesodermally derived muscle.[62,63,73,215–218] Clinical and EMG features, however, suggest aberrant innervation and a neurogenic etiology. The synergistic convergence or divergence movements on attempted upgaze frequently reported in both autosomal dominant and sporadic cases suggest aberrant innervation, particularly when they occur in combination with the Marcus-Gunn jaw-winking phenomenon.[1,21,190,206,251] EMG interpretation is problematic because abnormal insertions and anatomy can make electrode placement difficult.[28,105,206] Despite this, there is one report of cocontraction of antagonist muscles similar to Duane syndrome, suggesting a neurogenic process.[32] Neuroimaging has not provided much insight into the etiology of CFEOM. CT scans revealed normal brain and EOM in affected members of one pedigree,[105] and a wide variability in size of EOM in several sporadic cases.[108,257] A recent study of an autosomal dominant family found a general reduction in size of the EOM with a particularly marked reduction of the superior recti, and several members had abnormally shaped globes.[74] Some reduction in the relative size of the superior rectus is anticipated, however, given the fixed hypotropic position of the globe and the resultant stretch to this muscle.

Historically, biopsies of the EOMs with sporadic or familial cases of CFEOM contained fibrosis of dense connective tissue and were reported as complete fibrous replacement of the muscle.[23,28,36,89,102,137] Others, however, reported fibrous tissue with "islands of normal muscle,"[6,21] or completely normal muscle.[56,105] Most surgical biopsies have been of sporadic cases and may reflect disorders of varying etiologies. In addition, the presence of fibrosis is not pathognomonic of a myopathic process, and all fibrotic processes are not etiologically related. EOM fibrosis has been reported in primary orbital processes such as tumors and orbital periostitis,[52] as a result of previous muscle surgery, or following muscle entrapment associated with an orbital fracture.[145] In Duane syndrome, fibrosis within the lateral rectus has been shown to result from inadequate innervation secondary to anomalous innervation.[104,165]

It is likely that at least some of the reports of "fibrosis" of the EOMs in CFEOM result from unintentional biopsy of the muscle's long tendonous insertion or its transition zone.[56] The inferior and horizontal recti are typically biopsied as they are recessed to adjust the hypotropic strabismus. The fixed hypotropic position of the globes and tight inelastic muscles severely limit the surgeon's ability to manipulate and expose the muscle, markedly increasing the risk of obtaining a biopsy of the tendon or the transition zone. Some biopsies reported as complete fibrosis may actually be normal tendon and some reported with islands of intermixed muscle may actually be from the normal transition zone.

In 1879, Heuck[97] reported on the postmortem examination of the orbital contents of an affected member of an autosomal dominant pedigree with CFEOM. He described the right levator as "delicate and ill-developed" and could not identify the left. The superior rectus was very thin and almost membranous and the inferior rectus was shortened, thickened, and firm. The superior, lateral, and inferior recti were posteriorly inserted and the superior oblique was anteriorly inserted onto the globe. He felt that the nerves in the orbit appeared normal.

Recently, we had the opportunity to examine the intracranial and orbital pathology of one and the muscle pathology of two other affected members of a family with chromosome 12-linked CFEOM.[56] There was an absence of the superior division of the oculomotor nerve and its corresponding alpha motor neurons, and abnormalities of the levator palpebrae superioris and superior rectus muscles (Fig. 27.7). In addition, the other EOMs contained increased numbers of fibers with internal nuclei and central mitochondrial clumping. The latter

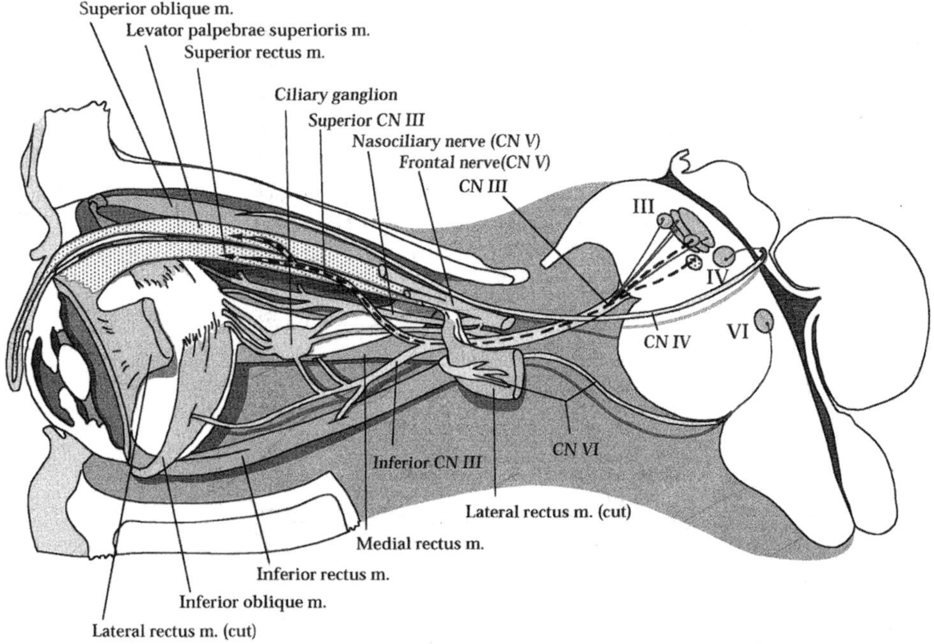

Figure 27.7. Lateral view of the brain stem and orbit showing the pathologic abnormalities in congenital fibrosis of the extraocular muscles. The dotted subnuclei of the oculomotor nucleus and the dotted superior divison of cranial nerve III are absent, the shaded superior rectus is abnormal, and the levator is absent.

changes may reflect lesser susceptibility to the same pathologic process, may be the result of aberrant innervation, or may be secondary changes from lack of normal antagonistic movements during development.

Cloning the gene defective in chromosome 12 CFEOM will lead to the elucidation of the mutated protein and the timing and tissue distribution of its expression. It will result in an understanding of whether the primary etiology has a neurogenic or myopathic basis, and whether it results from aberrant development or early maintenance of the oculomotor system. Given the similarity of the pathologic changes in CFEOM and Duane syndrome, understanding the former may likely lead to a better understanding of the latter.

Genetics

Cases of CFEOM can be sporadic or famlial. CFEOM has been reported in many large families with diverse ethnic backgrounds, and the inheritance pattern is typically autosomal dominant with full penetrance and expressivity. Chromsomal analyses have not assisted in gene localization as they have been normal in all classic CFEOM families,[57] one somewhat atypical family,[168] a sporadic patient with multiple other abnomalities,[8] a sporadic case with associated Prader-Willi syndrome,[116] and a sporadic case with Joubert syndrome and histidinemia.[5]

"Classic CFEOM" with Linkaged to Chromosome 12. When Engle et al.[58] used linkage analysis to screen the human genome, they mapped a gene for autosomal dominant CFEOM to an 8 cM centromeric region of chromosome 12 in two unrelated families.[58] Subsequently, linkage was established to the same region in five additional families (Fig. 27.8).[57] Currently, D12S1584 and D1251668 flank the CFEOM locus, defining a critical region of 3 cM spanning the centromere of chromosome 12. Four internal markers do not recombine with the disease gene and the maximum combined lod scores is 35.7. A physical map of the critical region falls within 12p11.2-q12.[57]

The seven ethnically diverse families with chromosome 12 CFEOM appear to be genetically and clinically homogeneous (Fig. 27.8). The genetic disorder is inherited in an autoso-

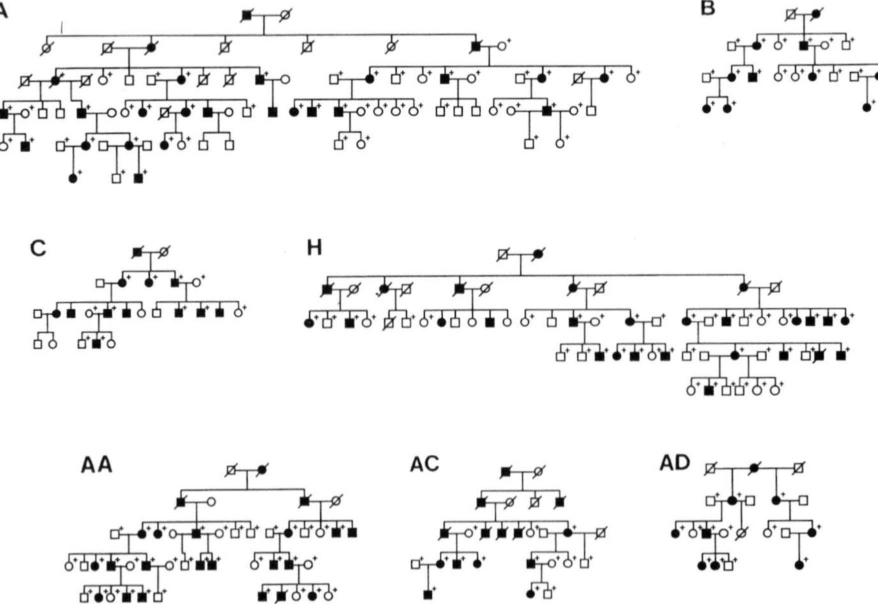

Figure 27.8. Pedigrees of seven families with congenital fibrosis with optic atrophy whose disease gene is linked to chromosome 12. Offspring of unaffected individuals are not shown, as none was clinically affected. (From Engle et al.,[57] with permission of The University of Chicago Press.)

mal dominant fashion with complete penetrance and male to male transmission. Three siblings from a family whose disease gene is linked to chromosome 12 can be seen in Fig. 27.6. Clinically, families are remarkably homogeneous. The involvement is always bilateral with the globe fixed in a hypotropic (and either esotropic or exotropic) position. Within each of the families, the affected members vary in their degree of ptosis, hypotropia, and ophthalmoplegia. Upgaze is completely absent, downgaze is severely limited, and there is variability in the amount of residual horizontal movement. Most affected individuals with any residual horizontal gaze have aberrant fast or slow and sometimes jerky unilateral or bilateral convergent or divergent movements on attempted vertical gaze, and occasionally an affected individual will have aberrant unilateral or bilateral movements on attempted horizontal gaze. Occasionally horizontal or rotary nystagmus is seen in one or both eyes. Movements are not yoked and can vary significantly between the two eyes. Affected individuals seem to have mild facial weakness. Otherwise, there are no associated anomalies and the neurologic examination is normal. Although six of the families were reported to have a congenital static condition, some affected members of one family were said to have progression of their ptosis and eye movement restriction.[173]

Despite their clinical homogeneity, these chromosome 12-linked families had been previously described in the literature under different names, including "congenital familial external ophthalmoplegia with cocontraction,"[31,32] "ocular congenital fibrosis syndrome,"[173] "hereditary congenital external ophthalmoplegia,"[65,105,114] and "congenital fibrosis of the extraocular muscles."[136,184,241]

Linkage analysis now permits us to define CFEOM genetically; we can pool the clinical and laboratory data of these linked families and begin to address the pathologic and pathophysiologic basis of the disorder. In addition, linkage of CFEOM provides the tool to analyze families with the same or slightly different clinical or genetic presentations to determine if these disorders are allelic or separate disease entities. Many published families have not been analyzed but are clinically very similar to the linked families and would be likely to map to the locus on chromosome 12.[19,28,34,36,85,102,138,139,149,153] Most recently, Gillies et al.[74] reported a family with "congenital fibrosis of the vertically acting extraocular muscles" and proposed that this was a new syndrome. This family has fairly good residual horizontal movements and some members have unilateral ptosis. It remains to be determined if this family maps to the chromosome 12 locus.

The elucidation of the mutation and protein product of the CFEOM gene may lead to a better understanding of the development and uniqueness of EOM, as well as provide a framework for examining the genetics of other strabismic disorders. It will be possible to determine if mutations in the same gene cause other "fibrosis" disorders, such as atypical familial "fibrosis syndromes" discussed below, sporadic but clinically typical cases,[6,23,36,89,137] and the related sporadic congenital disorders such as strabismus fixus,[247] vertical retraction syndrome,[125] unilateral fibrosis without ptosis,[183] unilateral fibrosis and ptosis,[54,96,145] and unilateral congenital fibrosis of superior rectus and superior oblique.[195]

Atypical Familial "Fibrosis Syndromes." Families with disorders slightly phenotypically or genotypically variant from CFEOM have been reported. It is now possible to determine if these disorders map to the chromosome 12 locus.

Autosomal dominant congenital external ophthalmoplegia with partial penetrance or variable expressivity: Hiatt and Halle[98] described a three-generation family with six affected members. The four affected members of the first and third generations had ptosis and external ophthalmoplegia clinically indistinguishable from chromosome 12-linked CFEOM. The obligate carrier in the second generation had ptosis but no extraocular muscle impairment, and her brother had EOM impairment but no ptosis. Mollica et al.[168] described a similar family with some affected members who had only ptosis and others who were asymptomatic obligate carriers. Abeloos et al.[1] described a family with some affected members with CFEOM, one with isolated ptosis, three with isolated strabismus, and several with peripheral neuropathies. The author(s) observed several additional pedigrees with variable expressivity including obligate carriers who are clinically normal and families in which some members have only unilateral eye involvement.

X-linked recessive congenital external ophthalmoplegia: There are two reports of an Argentinean family with an X-linked variant of congenital fibrosis.[182,207] Seven affected males had complete bilateral ptosis, external ophthalmoplegia with some slight residual lateral movements, myopia, and eccentric, dyscoric, anisocoric pupils. Affected individuals were strabismic but not consistently hypotropic. Areflexia was found in all of the affected males and both areflexia and goiter in all of the otherwise healthy female obligate carriers.

Unilateral congenital external ophthalmoplegia and ptosis: There is a report of a father and daughter with left-sided ptosis and left eye hypotropia with absence of upgaze.[250] At surgery the daughter's left inferior rectus felt dense, inelastic, and fibrous and there were adhesions between the muscle and the sclera and inferior oblique. In addition, the superior rectus was inserted anomalously and obliquely into the sclera.

Congenital complete (internal and external) ophthalmoplegia and ptosis: Three of five Chinese children of unaffected parents had divergent and slightly hypotropic external ophthalmoplegia with unreactive, miotic pupils.[147] In contrast to CFEOM, at surgery the recti appeared light in color, were flabby, and seemed to lack tone. The results of forced duction testing were not reported. Inheritance could have been autosomal recessive or autosomal dominant with partial penetrance. A second family with a mother and three children affected with hypotropic and exotropic strabismus, ophthalmoplegia, and fixed and slightly dilated pupils has been described.[32]

Brown Syndrome

This motility defect was originally described and classified as one of the "fibrosis syndromes" by Brown.[23] It is manifested by the inability to elevate the adducted eye actively or passively. There is less elevation deficit with the eye in midposition and minimal or no deficit in abduction. There can also be divergence on upgaze, downshoot, or widening of the palpebral fissure on adduction, primary hypotropia, and anomalous head posture.[185,260] Brown syndrome accounts for approximately 2% of strabismus. Ten percent of cases are bilateral, left- and right-sided unilateral cases are equal in frequency, and there is no gender predilection.[260]

Pathology and Pathogenesis

Brown syndrome was originally thought to result from anomalies of the superior oblique tendon sheath and was referred to as the "superior oblique tendon sheath syndrome." It is now believed that the syndrome results from restriction of free movement of the tendon through the trochlea pulley mechanism, due to anomalies of the tendon or the trochlear apparatus.[214,260] The restriction blocks the ability of the superior oblique to stretch with upward movement of the globe in adduction. Similar to the other fibrosis syndromes, the superior oblique can feel inelastic and tight. The restriction can be congenital and has been reported in association with congenital ptosis, Duane syndrome, Marcus-Gunn synkinetic movements, crocodile tears, choroidal coloboma, and congenital heart anomalies.[260] The syndrome can also be acquired, and has been reported in association with trauma and inflammatory disorders.[260] Both congenital and acquired cases can resolve spontaneously or occur intermittently.

Genetics

Most cases of congenital Brown syndrome are sporadic, but familial cases are reported. Twin studies include three reports of concordant monozygotic twins with unilateral mirror image Brown syndrome[64,120,262] and one report of discordant monozyotic twins.[150] Families with affected members in two generations include one family with four individuals unilaterally affected,[81] one with two siblings and a maternal aunt affected,[24] one with a child with the congenital constant form whose mother had an intermittent form,[154] and one in whom both child and father had an intermittent form.[154]

Families with one generation affected include one with two siblings bilaterally affected,[169] one with two siblings unilaterally affected,[81] and one with one sibling bilaterally and one unilaterally affected.[186] It is possible that these familial cases reflect autosomal dominant inheritance with incomplete penetrance.

ISOLATED CRANIAL NERVE PALSIES

Familial Third Nerve Palsy

Complete third nerve palsy results in down-and-out globe deviation, ptosis, and a dilated, unreactive pupil. There is at least one report of familial third nerve palsy with pupillary involvement.[246] Some authors refer to autosomal dominant congenital ptosis with isolated weakness of the superior rectus and levator as a "partial third nerve paralysis." This entity is discussed in detail in Chapter 29, by Sinha and Small.

Familial Fourth Nerve Palsy

Superior oblique muscle weakness and fourth nerve palsy cannot be differentiated clinically. Astle and Rosenbaum[9] reported three pedigrees, each with two members affected. In the first family, a mother had right eye and daughter had left eye involvement, in the second family a brother had left and a sister right eye involvement, and in the third family two brothers had left eye involvement. Four of these six affected individuals did not manifest hypotropia until 7–10 years of age. Harris et al.[91] reported an additional four pedigrees. In two of the families, two generations were affected: a father and daughter with right-sided involvement and a mother and daughter with left-sided involvement. In two of the families a sister and brother were affected. Astle and Rosenbaum[9] also noted left-sided predominance and felt that the inheritance pattern was likely to be autosomal dominant with partial penetrance. No pathologic studies are available, and the authors felt the localization could fall anywhere from the CN IV nucleus and the tendon of the superior oblique. Again, it is unclear if this truly is a fourth nerve palsy or a primary abnormality of the superior oblique muscle.

Familial Sixth Nerve Palsy

Lateral rectus weakness and sixth nerve palsy are not always clinically distinguishable. Lateral rectus weakness without associated retraction syndrome or facial weakness has been reported in multiple family members of several generations and appears to be transmitted as an autosomal dominant trait.[72,136] Lateral rectus palsy should always suggest the possibility of Duane or Möbius syndromes, both of which have been discussed. It is not known if familial isolated lateral rectus palsy and Duane or Möbius are genetically or otherwise etiologically related.

STRABISMUS IN NEUROMUSCULAR DISORDERS

The EOMs are affected or spared quite specifically and predictably in particular inherited neuromuscular disorders. For example, neither ptosis nor strabismus are clinical features of Duchenne/Becker, Emery-Dreifuss, facioscapulohumeral, and limb girdle muscular dystrophies, the spinal muscular atrophies, and most myotonias. The pathophysiologic basis of the sparing of EOMs in these disorders is unknown, although recent work has begun to explore this question in Duchenne muscular dystrophy (DMD). DMD is X-linked and caused by mutations in the dystrophin gene at Xq21. Dystrophin deficiency results clinically in progressive muscular weakness and pathologically in dystrophic changes with progressive fiber size variation, increased central nuclei, fatty changes, and fibrosis of striated muscle. Although the EOMs of boys with DMD lack dystrophin, it has been shown that EOM is spared both the clinical[118] and pathological[126] sequela of this dystrophin absence. Khurana et al.[126] recently proposed that this results from the intrinsic ability of EOM to maintain calcium homeostasis more effectively than other striated muscle. Understanding the basis of this selective sparing may have therapeutic implications for the treatment of DMD and other neuromuscular diseases.

Muscular Dystrophies

Although DMD and other muscular dystrophies spare EOM, several dystrophies specifically target these muscles. Oculopharyngeal muscular dystrophy (OPMD) is selective for extraocular and pharyngeal musculature. The onset of the disorder is variable but typically begins in the fifth or sixth decade with ptosis and dysphagia. As the disease evolves there may be impairment of extraocular movement and rarely complete ophthalmoplegia.[239] Although the pathogenesis of OPMD has not been elucidated and it is not known if it is a primary neurogenic or myopathic process, it is well established that most cases of OPMD are inherited as an autosomal dominant trait with complete penetrance.[239] Brais et al.[20] studied a homogeneous group of OPMD families and demonstrated linkage of their disease locus to markers spanning a 5 cM region of chromosome 14q11.2-q13. Current candidate genes in the region include cardiac beta-myosin heavy chain genes MYH6 and MY7.[20] Of the congenital muscular dystrophies, only children with the most severe form, muscle-eye-brain disease (Santavuori congenital muscular dystrophy), occasonally manifest strabismus.[50] The genetic data are consistent with autosomal recessive inheritance and it is unclear if this disorder results from a myopathic or neurogenic process.

Congenital Myopathies

EOM involvement can assist in the clinical differentiation of the various congenital myopathies. Infants with the early-onset form of centronuclear myopathy (myotubular myopathy) frequently present with ptosis and strabismus, typically in the setting of hypotonia, facial weakness, weak suck and cry, respiratory distress, and dysmorphic features including pectus excavatum and talipes equinovarus.[59] The inheritance pattern of individual cases of centronuclear myopathy can be confusing. There is an early-onset X-linked form and an early- and late-onset autosomal dominant form with partial penetrance. An autosomal recessive form may exist as well. A gene for the severe X-linked form was mapped by several investigators to Xq28[42,141,229,237,238] and, more recently, a female with an interstitial X-chromosome deletion and moderate signs of myotubular myopathy led to refinement of this locus to a 600 kb region of Xq28.[40] In addition, ptosis and ophthalmoplegia are occasionally noted in multicore disease and rarely noted in nemaline myopathy.[59]

Myotonias

Of the myotonias, myotonic dystrophy is the only disorder with abnormalities of the EOM. Myotonic dystrophy is a systemic disorder that can lead not only to weakness and myotonia of skeletal muscle but also dysfunction of smooth and cardiac muscle, peripheral nerve, brain, skin, lungs, and the skeletal and endocrine systems. Eye involvement can include ptosis, strabismus, cataracts, and retinal degeneration.[90] Facial weakness and ptosis are characteristically seen in affected adults and may be present for years before diagnosis.[90] Infants with congenital myotonic dystrohy typically have bilateral facial weakness, hypotonia, and frequently respiratory distress, but they do not usually have ptosis and strabismus until later in the course of the disease. Although myotonic dystrophy has an autosomal dominant pattern of inheritance, investigators have puzzled over the occurrence of remarkable intrafamilial variation in age of onset and degree of severity, by the presence of anticipation, and by the observation that the severe congenital form is transmitted only from an affected mother.[90] The recent discovery that myotonic dystrophy results from the expansion of a trinucleotide repeat has helped to explain some of these atypical genetic features. Myotonic dystrophy was mapped to the proximal arm of chromosome 19 in 1983,[43] and in 1992 the genetic defect was determined to be amplification of a trinucleotide repeat in the 3′ untranslated region of a serine-threonine kinase gene.[22,88] Unaffected individuals have between 5 and 27 repeats, and individuals with myotonic dystrophy have at least 50 and sometimes up to several thousand repeats, with some correlation between the size of the repeat and the severity of the disease.[22]

Neuromuscular Junction Defects

EOMs are specifically targeted in myasthenia gravis, and ptosis with or without ophthalmoplegia may be the only clinical manifestations of this disorder. Adult myasthenia is associated with autoimmunity and the rare familial cases may reflect a general predisposition to autoimmune disorders.[172] The congenital myasthenic syndromes, however, result from nonautoimmune defects of presynaptic and/or postsynaptic transmission at the neuromuscular junction. EOM weakness is seen in the autosomal recessive syndromes of acetylcholinesterase deficiency, postsynaptic acetylcholine receptor deficiency, paucity of postsynaptic folds, and high-conductance fast-channel defect, and in the autosomal dominant postsynaptic slow-channel syndrome.[50,55] Understanding the molecular basis of the congenital myasthenic syndromes may help elucidate the basis of extraocular muscle involvement in these disorders.

Mitochondrial Disorders

Ptosis and external ophthalmoplegia are key components of many of the mitochondrial myopathies, likely because the energy demand of EOM is high and the density of mitochondria is several times greater in extraocular than in limb muscle.[142,170] The extraocular symptoms tend to be progressive and occur in a variety of different mitochondrial disorders including the infant or childhood mitochondrial encephalomyopathy Leigh disease, as well as Kearns–Sayre syndrome (KSS), and progressive external ophthalmoplegia (PEO). Because normal mitochondrial metabolism requires the function of gene products encoded by both nuclear DNA (nDNA) and mitochondrial DNA (mtDNA), mitochondrial myopathies with EOM involvement can have autosomal dominant, autosomal recessive, or maternal inheritance patterns. PEO and Leigh disease show a maternal inheritance pattern when they result from point mutations in mtDNA. Sporadic cases of PE, KSS, and Leigh disease occur with mtDNA large single deletions or tandem duplications. PEO can also be inherited in an autosomal dominant fashion and is proposed to result from nDNA mutation causing secondary multiple deletions of mtDNA ("multiple deletion syndrome").[171]

Spinocerebellar Ataxias

Strabismus can occur with both the autosomal dominant and recessive spinocerebellar ataxias. Typically, the common oculomotor findings are limited gaze (particularly upgaze) with or without primary gaze strabismus, nystagmus, and defective pursuit movements. Of the seven autosomal dominant spinocerebellar ataxias, oculomotor involvement is found in spinocerebellar ataxias (SCA) II, III, and VII. SCA III, or Machado-Joseph disease, results from a trinucleotide expansion of the MJD1 gene located at 14q32.1.[122] Strabismus is also frequent in the autosomal recessive SCA. These include Friedreich ataxia, which was mapped to 9q13-q21.1 in 1990,[220] and ataxia-telangiectasia, which was recently shown to result from mutations in the AT gene on 11q.[210]

Acknowledgments: The author thanks Craig McKeown and Alan Beggs for their critical review of the manuscript. Figures 27.2, 27.4, and 27.7 were adapted with permission from the ciba connection of Medical Illustrations, illustrated by John Craig or Frank Netter, MD. This work was supported by National Eye Institute grant K11-EY00336.

REFERENCES

1. Abeloos M-C, Cordonnier M, Van Nechel C, et al. Fibrose Congenitale des muscles ocularies: Un diagnostic pour plusieurs tableaux. cliniques. *Bull Soc Belge Ophtalmol* 1990;239:61–74.
2. Abid F, Hall R, Hodgson P, et al. Moebius syndrome, peripheral neuropathy and hypogonadotropic hypogonadism. *J Neurol Sci* 1978;35:309–315.
3. Aicardi J. Diseases of the nervous system in children. *Clinics in Developmental Medicine*, Vol. 115/118. London: Mac Keith Press, 1992:1408.
4. Apple, C. Congenital abducens paralysis. *Am J Ophthal Mol* 1939;22:169–173.
5. Appleton RE, Chitayat D, Jan JE, et al. Joubert's syndrome associated with congenital ocular fibrosis and histidinemia. *Arch Neurol* 1989;46:579–582.

6. Apt L, Axelrod, RN. Generalized fibrosis of the extraocular muscles. *AM J Ophthalmol* 1978;85:822–829.
7. Arias S, Penchaszadeh V, Pinto-Cisternos J, et al. The IVIC syndrome: A new autosomal dominant complex pleiotropic syndrome with radial ray hypoplasia, hearing impairment, external ophthalmoplegia, and thrombocytopenia. *Am J Med Genet* 1980;5:25–59.
8. Arruga A, Henriquez AS, Delachaux, AM. Congenital "frozen eyes," with other mesodermal abnormalities. *Adv Ophthalmol* 1978;36:107–117.
9. Astle W, Rosenbaum, A. Familial congenital fourth cranial nerve palsy. *Arch Ophthalmol* 1985;103:532–535.
10. Baraitser M. Genetics of Möbius syndrome. *J Med Genet* 1977;14:415–417.
11. Baraitser M, Reardon W. New case of the Carey-Fineman-Ziter syndrome. *Am J Med Genet* 1994;53:163–164.
12. Barre P, Keith M, Sobel M, et al. Vascular insufficiency in Okihiro's syndrome secondary to hypothenar hammer syndrome. *J Hand Surg* 1987;12A:401–405.
13. Basson C, Cowley G, Solomon SD, et al. The clinical and genetic spectrum on the Holt-Oram syndrome (heart-hand syndrome). *N Engl J Med* 1994;330:885–891.
14. Becker-Christensen F, Lund HT. A family with Möbius syndrome. *J Pediatr* 1974; 84:115–117.
15. Beetz P. Beitrag zur Lehre von den angeborenen beweglichkeitsmusculatur (infantiler kernschwund Moebius). *J Psychiatr Neurol* 1913;20:137–140.
16. Bielschowsky A. Lectures on motor anomalies VIII. Paralysis of individual eye muscles: Abducens-nerve paralysis. *Am J Ophthalmol* 1939;22:357–367.
17. Bouwes-Bavinck J, Weaver D. Subclavian artery supply disruption sequence: Hypothesis of a vascular etiology for Poland, Kippel-Feil and Möbius anomalies. *Am J Med Genet* 1986;23:903–918.
18. Brackett LE, Demers LM, Mamourian AC, et al. Moebius syndrome in association with hypogonadotropic hypogonadism. *J Endocrinol Invest* 1991;14:599–607.
19. Bradburn AA. Herditary ophthalmoplegia in five generations. *Trans Ophthalmol Soc UK* 1912;32:142–153.
20. Brais B, Xie Y-G, Sanson M, et al. The oculopharyngeal muscular dystrophy locus maps to the region of the cardiac alpha and beta myosin heavy chain genes on chromosome 14q11.2-q13. *Hum Mol Genet* 1995; 4:429–434.
21. Brodsky MC, Pollock SC, Buckley EG. Neural misdirection in congenital ocular fibrosis syndrome: Implications and pathogenesis (see comments). *J Pediatr Ophthalmol Strabismus* 1989;26:159–161.
22. Brook J, McCurrach M, Harley HG, et al. Molecular basis of myotonic dystrophy: Expansion of a trinucleotide (CTG) repeat at the 3-prime end of a transcript encoding a protein kinase family member. *Cell* 1992;68:799–808.
23. Brown H. Congenital structural muscle anomalies. In *Strabismus Ophthalmic Symposium.* JH Allen, ed. St. Louis: C. V. Mosby, 1950:205–236.
24. Brown H. True and simulated superior oblique tendon sheath syndromes. *Doc Ophthalmol* 1973;34:123–126.
25. Brueckner J, Itkis O, Porter JD. Spatial and temporal patterns of myosin heavy chain expression in developing rat extraocular muscle. *J Muscle Res Cell Motil* 1996;17(3):297–312.
26. Carey J, Fineman R, Ziter FA. The Robin sequence as a consequence of malformation, dysplasia and neuromuscular syndromes. *J Pediatr* 1982;101:858–864.
27. Carpenter E, Goddard J, Chisaka D, et al. Loss of Hox-A1 (Hox-1.6) function results in the reorganization of the murine hindbrain. *Development* 1993;11:1063–1075.
28. Catford GV. A familial musculo-fascial anomaly. *Trans Ophthalmol Soc UK* 1966; 86:19–36.
29. Chew C, Foster P, Hurst JA, et al. Duane's retraction syndrome associated with chromosome 4q27-31 segment deletion. *Am J Ophthalmol* 1995;119:807–809.
30. Chisolm JJ. Congenital paralysis of the sixth and seventh pairs of cranial nerves in the adult. *Arch Ophthalmol* 1882;11:323.
31. Cibis GW. Congenital familial external ophthalmoplegia with co-contraction. *Ophthalmic Paediatr Genet* 1984;163–168.
32. Cibis GW, Kies R, Lawwill T, et al. Electromyography in congenital familial ophthalmoplegia. In *Strabismus II*, R.D. Reinecke, ed. New York: Grune & Stratton, 1984: 379–390.
33. Collins DL, Schimke RN. Moebius syndrome in a child and extremity defect in her father. *Clin Genet* 1982;22:312–314.

34. Cooper H. A series of cases of congenital ophthalmoplegia external (nuclear paralysis) in the same family. *Br Med J* 1910;1:917.
35. Couly G, Coltey P, LeDouarin NM. The development fate of the cepthalic mesoderm in quail-chick chimeras. *Development* 1910; 114:1–15.
36. Crawford JS. Congenital fibrosis syndrome. *Can J Ophthalmol* 1970;5:331–6.
37. Cullen P, Rodgers C, Callen DF, et al. Association of familial Duane anomaly and urogenital abnormalities with a bisatellited marker derived from chromosome 22. *Am J Med Genet* 1993;47:925–930.
38. Czeizel A, Goblyos P, Kodaj I. IVIC syndrome: Report of a third family. *Am J Med Genet* 1989;32:282–283.
39. D'Cruz OF, Swisher CN, Jaradeh S, et al. Möbius syndrome: Evidence for a vascular etiology. *J Child Neurol* 1993;8:260–265.
40. Dahl N, Hu L, Chevy M, et al. Myotubular myopathy in a girl with a deletion at Xq27-q28 and unbalanced X inactivation assigns the MTM1 gene to a 600-kb region. *Am J Hum Genet* 1995;56:1108–1115.
41. Danis P. Sur les anomalies congenitale de la motilite oculaire d'origine musculaire et en particular sur le sundrome de Stilling-Turk-Duane. *Ann d'Ocul* 1948;1811:148.
42. Darnfors C, Larsson H, Oldfors A, et al. X-linked myotubular myopathy: A linkage study. *Clin Genet* 1990;37:335–340.
43. Davies K, Jackson J, Williamson R, et al. Linkage analysis of myotonic dystrophy and sequences on chromosome 19 using a cloned complement 3 gene probe. *J Med Genet* 1983;20:259–263.
44. Davis A, Witte D, Hsieh-Li HM, et al. Absence of radius and ulna in mice lacking hoxa-11 and hoxd-11. Nature 1995;375:791–795.
45. DeRespinis PA, Caputo AR, Wagner RS, et al. Duane's retraction syndrome. *Surv Ophthalmol* 1993;38:258–288.
46. Dietz HC, Cutting GR, Pyeritz RE, et al. Marfan syndrome caused by a recurrent de novo missense mutation in the fibrillin gene (see comments). *Nature* 1991;352:337–339.
47. Donahue SP, Wenger SL, Steek MW, et al. Broad-spectrum Möbius syndrome associated with a 1;11 chromosome translocation. *Ophthalmic Paediatr Genet* 1993; 14:17–21.
48. Drachman DA, Wetzel N, Wasserman M, et al. Experimental denervation of ocular muscles. A critique of the concept of "ocular myopathy." *Arch Neurol* 1969;21:170–183.
49. Duane A. Congenital deficiency of abduction, associated with impairment of adduction, retraction movements, contraction of the palpebral fissure and oblique movements of the eye. *Arch Ophthalmol* 1905;34: 133–159.
50. Dubowitz V. *Muscle Disorders in Childhood.* London: W.B. Saunders, 1995:540.
51. Dufier J, Briard M, Bonaiti C, et al. Inheritance in the etiology of convergent squint. *Ophthalmologica* 1979;179:225–234.
52. Duke-Elder, S. *Textbook of Ophthalmology.* St. Louis: C. V. Mosby, 1952.
53. Durston JH. Histochemistry of primate extraocular muscles and the changes of denervation. *Br J Ophthalmol* 1974;58:193–216.
54. Effron L, Price RL, Berlin AJ, et al. Congenital unilateral orbital fibrosis with suspected prenatal orbital penetration. *J Pediatr Ophthalmol Strabismus* 1985;22:133–136.
55. Engel, A. Myasthenic syndromes. In *Myology,* vol. 2, A. Engel and C. Franzini-Armstrong, eds. New York: McGraw-Hill, 1995: 1798–1835.
56. Engle E, Goumnerov B, McKeown CA, et al. Oculomotor nerve and muscle abnormalities in congenital fibrosis of the extraocular muscles. *Ann Neurol* 1997;41:314–325.
57. Engle E, Marondel I, Houtman WA, et al. Congenital fibrosis of the extraocular muscles (autosomal dominant congenital external ophthalmoplegia): Genetic homogeneity, linkage refinement, and physical mapping on chromosome 12. *Am J Hum Genet* 1995; 57:1086–1094.
58. Engle EC, Kunkel LM, Specht LA, et al. Mapping a gene for congenital fibrosis of the extraocular muscles to the centromeric region of chromosome. 12. *Nature Genet* 1994;7:69–73.
59. Fardeau M, Tome F. Congenital myopathies. In *Myology,* vol. 2, A. Engel and C. Franzini-Armstrong, eds. New York: McGraw-Hill, 1995:1487–1532.
60. Fenyes I. Zur Frage der Entstehung von angeborenen Beweglichkeitsstorungen im Gehirnnervenbereich: Ein klinisch-anatomischer Beitrag. *Arch Psychiatr Nervenkr* 1937;106:296–311.
61. Ferrell R, Jones, B, Lucas RV. Simultaneous occurrence of the Holt-Oram and the Duane syndromes. *J Pediatr* 1966;69:630–634.
62. Fink WH. The development of the extrinsic

muscles of the eye. *Am J Ophthalmol* 1953;36:10–36.

63. Fink WH. The development of the orbital fascia. *Am J Ophthalmol* 1956;42:269–277.
64. Finlay A, Powell S, Brown's syndrome in identical twins. *Br Orthop J* 1982;39:73–77.
65. Flieringa HJ. Familiare Ptosis congenita kombiniert mit anderen angeborenen Beweglichkeitsdefekten der Bulbusmuskulatur. *Z Augenheilkd* 1924;52:1–14.
66. Frazetto F, Deller M. Jumelles monozygotes et syndrome de Duane. *Bull Soc Fr Ophthalmol* 1971;84:580.
67. Friede R. *Developmental Neuropathology.* Berlin: Springer-Verlag, 1989:577.
68. Fritzsch B, Nichols D, Echelard Y, et al. (1995). Development of midbrain and anterior hindbrain ocular motoneurons in normal and Wnt-1 knockout mice. *J Neurobiol* 1995;27:457–469.
69. Fry FR, Kasak M. Congenital facial paralysis. *Arch Neurol Psychiatry* 1919;2:638–644.
70. Fujita I, Koyanagi T, Kukita J, et al. Moebius syndrome with central hypoventilation and brainstem calcification: A case report. *Eur J Pediatr* 1991;150:582–583.
71. Gedda L, Magistretti S. Paracinesia adduttorio-enoftalmica gemello-familiare e albinismo oculare in altra famiglia. *Acta Genet Med Gemellol* 1956;5:291.
72. Gifford H. Congenital defects of abduction and other ocular movements and their relation to birth injuries. *Am J Ophthalmol* 1926;9:3.
73. Gilbert PW. The origin and development of the human extrinsic ocular muscles. *Contrib Embryol* 1957;36:59–78.
74. Gillies W, Harris A, Brooks AM, et al. Congenital fibrosis of the vertically acting extraocular muscles: A new group of dominantly inherited ocular fibrosis with radiologic findings. *Ophthalmology* 1995;102:607–612.
75. Goldblatt J, Viljoen D. New autosomal dominant radial ray hypoplasia syndrome. *Am J Med Genet* 1987;28:647–654.
76. Goldfarb C, Gannon F. Familial congenital lateral rectus palsy with retraction. *Dis Nerv Syst* 1964;25:17–21.
77. Gonzalez CH, Vargas FR, Perez AB, et al. Limb deficiency with or without Möbius sequence in seven Brazilian children associated with misoprostol use in first trimester of pregnancy. *Am J Med Genet* 1993;47:59–64.
78. Gorlin R, Cohen M, Levin LS. Syndromes of the head and neck. *Oxford Monographs on Medical Genetics No. 19.* New York: Oxford University Press, 1990.
79. Govaert P, Vanhaesebrouck P, DePracter C, et al. Moebius sequence and prenatal brainstem ischemia. *Pediatrics* 1989;84:570–573.
80. Gover M, Yankey J. Physical impairments of members of low-income farm families—11,490 persons. *Public Health Rep* 1944; 59:1163–1184.
81. Gowan M, Levy J. Heredity in the superior oblique tendon sheath syndrome. *Br Orthop* 1968;25:91–93.
82. Gunderson T, Zeavin B. (1956). Observations on the retraction syndrome of Duane. *Arch Ophthalmol* 1956;55:576.
83. Halal F, Homsy M, Perreault G. Acro-renal-ocular syndrome: Autosomal dominant thumb hypoplasia, renal ectopia, and eye defect. *Am J Med Genet* 1984;17:753–762.
84. Hanissian AS, Fuste F, Hayes WT, et al. Möbius syndrome in twins. *Am J Dis Child* 1970;120:472–475.
85. Hansen E. Congenital general fibrosis of the extraocular muscles. *Acta Ophthalmol (Copenh)* 1968;46:469–476.
86. Hanson PA, Rowland LP. Möbius syndrome and fascioscapulo-humeral muscular dystrophy. *Arch Neurol* 1971;24:31–39.
87. Harlan GC. Congenital paralysis of both abducens and both facial nerves. *Trans Am Ophthalmol Soc* 1881;3:216.
88. Harley H, Brook J, Rundle SA, et al. Expansion of an unstable DNA region and phenotypic variation in myotonic dystrophy. *Nature* 1992;355:545–546.
89. Harley RD, Rodrigues MM, Crawford JS. Congenital fibrosis of the extraocular muscles. *J Pediatr Ophthalmol Strabismus* 1978; 15:346–358.
90. Harper P, Rudel R. Myotonic dystrophy. In Myology, vol 2, A. Engel and C. Franzini-Armstrong, eds. New York: McGraw-Hill, 1995:1192–1219.
91. Harris D, Memmen J, Katz NNK, et al. Familial congenital superior oblique palsy. *Ophthalmology* 1986;93:88–90.
92. Hayes A, Costa T, Polomeno RC. The Okihiro syndrome of Duane anomaly, radial ray abnormalities, and deafness. *Am J Med Genet* 1985;22:273–280.
93. Helveston E. 19th Annual Frank Costenbader Lecture—The origins of congenital esotropia. *J Pediatr Ophthalmol Strabismus* 1993;30:215–232.
94. Henderson JL. The congenital facial diplegia

syndrome: Clinical features, pathology, and aetiology. A review of sixty-one cases. *Brain* 1939;62:381–403.

95. Herrman J, Pallister P, Gilbert EF, et al. Studies of malformation syndromes of man. Nosologic studies in the Hanhart and the Möbius syndrome. *Eur J Pediatr* 1976; 122:19–55.
96. Hertle RW, Katowitz JA, Young TL, et al. Congenital unilateral fibrosis, blepharoptosis, and enophthalmos syndrome. *Ophthalmology* 1992;99:347–355.
97. Heuck G. Ueber angeborenen vererbten Beweglichkeits—Defect der Augen. *Klin Monatsbl Augenkeilkd* 1879;17:253–278.
98. Hiatt RL, Halle AA. General fibrosis syndrome. *Ann Ophthalmol* 1983;15:1103–1109.
99. Hicks AM. Congenital paralysis of lateral rotators of eyes with paralysis of muscles of face. *Arch Ophthalmol* 1943;30:38–42.
100. Hofmann R. Monozygotic twins concordant for bilateral Duane's retraction syndrome. *Am J Ophthalmol* 1985;99:563–566.
101. Holm S. Le strabisme concomitant chez les palenegrides au Gabon, Afrique equatoriale francaise. *Acta Ophthalmol (Copenh)* 1939; 17:367.
102. Holmes WJ. Hereditary congenital ophthalmoplegia. *Trans Am Ophthalmol Soc* 1956;41:245–253.
103. Horton RM, Manfredi AA, Conti-Tronconi BM. The "embryonic" gamma subunit of the nicotinic acetylcholine receptor is expressed in adult extraocular muscle. *Neurology* 1993;43:983–986.
104. Hotchkiss MG, Miller NR, Clark AW, et al. Bilateral Duane's retraction syndrome: A clinical-pathological case report. *Arch Ophthalmol* 1980;98:870–874.
105. Houtman WA, vanWeerden TW, Robinson PH, et al. Hereditary congenital external ophthalmoplegia. *Ophthalmologica* 1986; 193:207–218.
106. Huber A. Electrophysiology of the retraction syndrome. *Br J Ophthalmol* 1974;58:293.
107. Huber A. Duane's retraction syndrome: Consideration of pathophysiology and etiology. In *Strabismus II*, R. Reinecke, ed. Orlando, FL: Grune & Stratton, 1984:345–361.
108. Hupp SL, Williams JP, Curran JE. Computerized tomography in the diagnosis of the congenital fibrosis syndrome. *J Clin Neuro-Ophthalmol* 1990;10:135–139.
109. Ing M, Pang S. The racial distribution of strabismus. *Strabismus: Proceedings of the Third Meeting of the International Strabismological Association.* New York: Grune & Stratton, 1978:107–110.
110. Isenberg S, Blechman B. Marcus-Gunn jaw winking and Duane's retraction syndrome. *J Pediatr Ophthalmol Strabismus* 1983;20: 235–237.
111. Isenberg S, Urist M. Clinical observations in 101 consecutive patients with Duane's retraction syndrome. *Am J Ophthalmol* 1974; 84:419–425.
112. Izquierdo N, Traboulsi E, Enger C, et al. Strabismus in the Marfan syndrome. *Am J Ophthalmol* 1994;117:632–635.
113. Jabs E, Li X, Scott AF, et al. Jackson-Weiss and Crouzon syndromes are allelic with mutations in fibroblast growth factor receptor 2. *Nature Genet* 1994;8:275–279.
114. Jonkers GH. Familiaire ptosis congenita, gecombineerd met andere aangeboren defecten in de motiliteit van de bulbusmusculatuur. *Ned Tijdschr Geneesk* 1950;94:1471–1472.
115. Journel H, Roussey M, Le Marec B. MCA/MR syndrome with oligodactyly and Möbius anomaly in first cousins: New sequence or familial facial-limb disruption sequence? *Am J Med Genet* 1989;34:506–510.
116. Kalpakian B, Bateman BJ, Sparkes RS, et al. Congenital ocular fibrosis syndrome associated with the Prader-Willi syndrome. *J Pediatr Ophthalmol Strabismus* 1986;23: 170–173.
117. Kalpakian B, Choy A, Sparkes RS, et al. Duane syndrome associated with features of the cat-eye syndrome and mosaicism for a supernumerary chromosome probably derived from number 22. *J Pediatr Ophthalmol Strabismus* 1988;25:293–297.
118. Kaminski HJ, al Hakim M, Leigh RJ, et al. Extraocular muscles are spared in advanced Duchenne dystrophy. *Ann Neurol* 1992; 32:586–588.
119. Kaminski HJ, Maas E, Spiegel P, Ruff RL. Why are eye muscles frequently involved in myasthenia gravis? *Neurology* 1990;40:1663–1667.
120. Katz N, Whitmore P, Beauchamp GR. Brown's syndrome in twins. *J Pediatr Ophthalmol Strabismus* 1981;18:32–34.
121. Kaur S, Singh G, Stock JL, et al. Dominant mutation of the murine Hox-2.2 gene results in developmental abnormalities. *J Exp Zool* 1992;264:323–336.

122. Kawaguchi Y, Okamoto T, Taniwaki M, et al. CAG expansions in a novel gene for Machado-Joseph disease at chromosome 14q32.1. *Nature Genet* 1994;8:221–228.
123. Kawai M, Momoi T, Fujii T, et al. The syndrome of Möbius sequence, peripheral neuropathy, and hypogonadotropic hypogonadism. *Am J Med Genet* 1990;37:578–582.
124. Keynes R, Lumsden A. Segmentation and the origin of regional diversity in the vertebrate central nervous system. *Neuron* 1990;4:1–9.
125. Khodadoust AA, von Noorden GK. Bilateral vertical retraction syndrome: A family study. *Arch Ophthalmol* 1967;78:606–612.
126. Khurana T, Prendergast R, Alameddine HS, et al. Absence of extraocular muscle pathology in Duchenne's muscular dystrophy: Role for calcium homeostasis in extraocular muscle sparing. *J Exp Med* 1995;182:467–475.
127. Kinney H, Filiano J, Brazy JE, et al. Congenital apnea with medullary and olivary hypoplasia: A pathologic study with computer reconstructions. *Clin Neuropathol* 1989;8: 163–173.
128. Kirkham T. Duane's syndrome and familial perceptive deafness. *Br J Ophthalmol* 1969; 53:335–339.
129. Kirkham T. Inheritance of Duane's syndrome. *Br J Ophthalmol* 1970;54:323–329.
130. Kishore K, Kumar H. Congenital ocular fibrosis with musculoskeletal abnormality: A new association. *J Pediatr Ophthamol Strabismus* 1991;28:283–286.
131. Koide Y, Yamashita N, Kurasa T, et al. Association of isolated adrenocorticotropin deficiency without a variety of neuro-somatic abnormalities in congenital facial diplegia (Moebius) syndrome. *Endocrinol Jpn* 1983; 30:499.
131a. Kremer H, Kuyt L, van den Helm B, et al. Localization of a gene for Möbius syndrome to chromosome 3q by linkage analysis in a Dutch family. *Hum Mol Genet* 1996;5:1367–1371.
132. Krueger KE, Friedrich D. Familiaere kongenitale Motilitaetsstoerungen der Augen. *Klin Mschr. Augenheilkd* 1963; 142:101–117.
133. Kuhn MJ, Clark HB, Morales A, et al. Group III Möbius syndrome: CT and MR findings. *Am J Neurol Res* 1990;11:903–904.
134. Kumar D. Moebius syndrome. *J Med Genet* 1990;27:122–126.
135. Kumar S, Kimberling W, Kenyon WJ, et al. Autosomal dominant branchio-oto-renal syndrome—Localization of a disease gene to chromosome 8q by linkage in a Dutch family. *Hum Mol Genet* 1992;1:491–495.
136. Laughlin R. Hereditary paralysis of the abducens nerve. *Am J Ophthalmol* 1937;20:396.
137. Laughlin RC. Congenital fibrosis of the extraocular muscles; A report of six cases. *Am J Ophthalmol* 1956;41:432–438.
138. Lawford JB. Congenital hereditary defect of ocular movements. *Trans Ophthalmol Soc UK* 1888;8;262–274.
139. Lees F. Congenital static familial ophthalmoplegia. *J Neurol Neurosurg Psychiatry* 1960;23:46–51.
140. Legum C, Godel V, Nemet P. Heterogeneity and pleiotropism in the Moebius syndrome. *Clin Genet* 1981;20:254–259.
141. Lehesjoki A-E, Sankila E-M, Miao J, et al. X-linked neonatal myotubular myopathy: One recombination detected with four polymorphic DNA markers from Xq28. *J Med Genet* 1990;27:288–291.
142. Leigh R, Zee D. The neurology of eye movements. In *Contemporary Neurology Series*, vol. 1, F. Plum, ed. Philadelphia: F. A. Davis Co., 1991:293–377.
143. Lennerstrand G. Motor dysfunction in strabismus. In *Strabismus and Amblyopia*, G. Lennerstrand, G. von Noorden, and E. Campos, eds. New York: Plenum Press, 1988:5–21.
144. Lennon MB. Congenital defects of the muscles of the face and eyes. *Calif State J Med* 1910;8:115–117.
145. Leone, CR, Weinstein GW. Orbital fibrosis with enophthalmos. *Ophthalmic Surg* 1972; 3:71–75.
146. Letson RD. Surgical management of the ocular congenital fibrosis syndrome. *Am Orthop J* 1980;30:97–101.
147. Li TM. Congenital total bilateral ophthalmoplegia. *Am J Ophthalmol* 1923;6:816–821.
148. Lipson AH, Webster WS, Brown-Woodman PDC, et al. Moebius syndrome: Animal model-human correlations and evidence for a brain-stem vascular etiology. *Teratology* 1989;40:339–350.
149. Llouquet JL, Lequoy O, Maurani O. Congenital ophthalmoplegia due to fibrosis of the external ocular muscles. *Orbit* 1985;4: 101–103.
150. Lowe R. Bilateral superior oblique tendon sheath syndrome—Occurrence and sponta-

neous recovery in one of uniovular twins. *Br J Ophthalmol* 1969;53:466.

151. MacDermot K, Winter R. Radial ray defect and Duane anomaly: Report of a family with autosomal dominant transmission. *Am J Med Genet* 1987;27:313–319.
152. MacDermot KD, Winter RM, Taylor D, et al. Oculofacial bulbar palsy in mother and son: Review of 26 reports of familial transmission with the "Möbius spectrum of defects." *J Med Genet* 1990;27:18–26.
153. Mace J, Sponaugle H, Mitsunage RY, et al. Congenital hereditary nonprogressive external ophthalmoplegia. *Am J Dis Child* 1971; 122:261–263.
154. Magli A, Fusco R, Chiosi E, et al. Inheritance of Brown's syndrome. *Ophthalmologica* 1986;192:82–87.
155. Martinez AJ, Biglan AW, Hiles DA. Structural features of extraocular muscles of children with strabismus. *Arch Ophthalmol* 1980;98:533–539.
156. Masaki S. Congenital bilateral facial paralysis. *Arch Otolaryngol* 1971;94:260–263.
157. Mash A, Grutzner P, Hegmann JP, et al. Strabismus. In *Genetic and Metabolic Eye Disease,* M. Goldberg, ed. Boston: Little, Brown, 1974:261–277.
158. Mash A, Spivey B. Genetic aspects of strabismus. *Doc Ophthalmol* 1973;34:285–291.
159. Maumenee I, Alston A, Mets MB, et al. Inheritance of congenital esotropia. *Trans Am Ophthalmol Soc* 1986;34:85–93.
160. McGowan K, Pagon R. Okihiro syndrome. *Am J Med Genet* 1994;51:89.
161. Mehdorn E, Kommerell G. Inherited Duane's syndrome: Mirror-like localization of oculomotor disturbances in monozygotic twins. *J Pediatr Ophthalmol Strabismus* 1979;16:152–154.
162. Merlin S. Strabismus. In *Inherited Eye Diseases. Diagnosis and Clinical Management,* S. Merlin, ed. New York: Marcel Dekker, 1981:401–409.
163. Miller M. Thalidomide embryopathy: A model for the study of congenital incomitant horizontal strabismus. *Trans Am Ophthalmol Soc* 1991;89:623–674.
164. Miller MT, Ray V, Owens P, et al. Möbius and Möbius-like syndromes (TTV-OFM, OMLH). *J Pediatr Ophthalmol Strabismus* 1989;26:176–188.
165. Miller NR, Kiel SM, Green WR, et al. Unilateral Duane's retraction syndrome (type 1). *Arch Ophthalmol* 1982;100:1468–1472.
166. Möbius PJ. Uber infantilen Kernschwund. *Munch Med Wochenschr* 1892;39:17–58.
167. Möbius, PJ. Uber angeborenen doppelseitige Abducens—Facialis—Lahmung. *Munch Med Wochenschr* 1888;35:91–94.
168. Mollica F, Li VS, Incorpora J, et al. Variabilite intrafamiliale de l'ophtalmoplegie exter etude d'une famille sicilienne. *J Genet Hum* 1980;28:23–30.
169. Moore A, Walker J, Taylor D. Familial Brown's syndrome. *J Pediatr Ophthalmol Strabismus* 1988;25:202–204.
170. Moraes C, DiMauro S, Zeviani M, et al. Mitochondrial DNA deletions in progressive external ophthalmoplegia and Kearns-Sayre syndrome. *N Engl J Med* 1989;320:1293–1299.
171. Morgan-Hughes J. Mitochondrial diseases. In *Myology,* vol. 2, A. Engel and C. Franzini-Armstrong, eds. New York: McGraw-Hill, 1994:1610–1660.
172. Namba T, Brunner NG, Brown SB, et al. Familial myasthenia gravis: Report of 27 patients in 12 families and review of 164 patients in 73 families. *Arch Neurol* 1971; 25:49–60.
173. Nemet P, Godel V, Ron S, et al. Ocular congenital fibrosis syndrome. *Metab Pediatr Syst Ophthalmol* 1985;8:172–174.
174. Noden D. Vertebrate craniofacial development: The relation between ontogenetic process and morphological outcome. *Brain Behav Evol* 1991;38:190–225.
175. Noden D. Vertebrate craniofacial development: Novel approaches and new dilemmas. *Curr Opinion Genet Dev* 1992;2:576–581.
176. Nordlow W. Squint: The frequency of onset at different ages and the incidence of associated defects in a Swedish population. *Acta Ophthalmol* 1964;42:1015–1037.
177. O'Malley E, Helveston E, Ellis FD. Duane's retraction syndrome—Plus. *J Pediatr Ophthalmol Strabismus* 1982;19:161–165.
178. Oda K, Shibasaki H. Antigenic difference of acetylcholine receptor between single and multiple form endplates of human extraocular muscle. *Brain Res* 1988;449:337–340.
179. Ohashi H, Wakui K, Nishimoto H, et al. Klippel-Feil syndrome and de novo balanced autosomal translocation [46,XX,t(5,17)(q11.2;q23)]. *Am J Hum Genet* 1992;51 (suppl):A294.
180. Okihiro M, Tasaki T, Nakano KK, et al. Duane syndrome and congenital upper-limb anomalies. *Arch Neurol* 1977;34:174–179.

181. Olson WH, Bardin CW, Walsh GO, et al. Lower motor neuron involvement and hypogonadotropic hypogonadism. *Neurology* 1970;20:1002–1008.
182. Ortiz de Zarate JC. Recessive sex-linked inheritance of congenital external ophthalmoplegia and myopia coincident with other dysplasias; A reappraisal after 15 years. *Br J Ophthalmol* 1966;50:606–607.
183. Paolillo RD, Burch PG, Torchia, RT. Infantile contracture of the inferior rectus muscle with resultant mechanical hypotropia. *Am J Ophthalmol* 1969;68:1057–1060.
184. Parks M. *Ocular Motility and Strabismus, Fibrosis Syndrome.* Hagerstown, MD: Harper & Row, 1975:170–172.
185. Parks M. The superior oblique tendon. *Trans Ophthalmol Soc UK* 1977;97:288–304.
186. Parks M, Eustis H. Simultaneous superior oblique tenectomy and inferior oblique recession in Brown's syndrome. *Ophthalmology* 1987;94:1043–1048.
187. Paul T, Hardage L. The heritability of strabismus. *Ophthalmic Genet* 1994;15:1–18.
188. Pfaffenbach D, Cross H, Kearns TP. Congenital anomalies in Duane's retraction syndrome. *Arch Ophthalmol* 1972;88:635.
189. Pitner SE, Edwards JE, McCormick WF. Observations on the pathology of Moebius syndrome. *J Neurol Neurosurg Psychiatry* 1965;28:362–374.
190. Pollock SC, Brodsky MC, Buckley EG. Congenital fibrosis syndrome (response to letter; comment). *J Pediatr Ophthalmol Strabismus* 1990;27:329.
191. Porter J, Baker R. Muscles of a different "color": The unusual properties of the extraocular muscles may predispose or protect them in neurogenic and myogenic disease. *Neurology* 1996;46:30–37.
192. Porter JD, Baker R, Ragusa RJ, et al. Extraocular muscles: Basic and clinical aspects of structure and function. *Surv Ophthalmol* 1995;39(6):451–484.
193. Porter JD, Burns LA, May PJ. Morphological substrate for eyelid movements: Innervation and structure of primate levator palpebrae superioris and orbicularis oculi muscles. *J Comp Neurol* 1989;287:64–81.
194. Porter JD, Burns LA, McMahon EJ. Denervation of primate extraocular muscle. A unique pattern of structural alterations. *Invest Ophthalmol Vis Sci* 1989;30:1894–1908.
195. Prakash P, Menon V, Ghosh G. Congenital fibrosis of superior rectus and superior oblique: A case report. *Br J Ophthalmol* 1985;69:57–59.
196. Prendergast RA, Khurana TS, Alameddine H, et al. Relative sparing of extraocular muscles in Duchennes muscular dystrophy. *Invest Ophthalmol Vis Sci* (suppl) 1993; 34:1120.
197. Ramsay J, Taylor D. Congenital crocodile tears: A key to the aetiology of Duane's syndrome. *Br J Ophthalmol* 1980;64:518–522.
198. Richards RN. The Möbius syndrome. *J Bone Jt Surg* 1953;35-A:437–444.
199. Richter S. Untersuchungen ueber die Hereditaet des Strabismus concomitans. *Humangenetik* 1967;4:235–243.
200. Ro A, Chernoff G, MacRae D, et al. Auditory function in Duane's retraction syndrome. *Am J Ophthalmol* 1990;109:75–78.
201. Rojas-Martinez A, Garcia-Cruz D, Rodriguez GA, et al. Poland-Moebius syndrome in a boy and Poland syndrome in his mother. *Clin Genet* 1991;40:225–228.
202. Rosenbaum A, Weiss S. Monozygotic twins discordant for Duane's retraction syndrome. *J Pediatr Ophthalmol Strabismus* 1978; 15:359.
203. Rozen S, Rozenman Y, Arnon N, et al. Marfanoid hypermobility syndrome associated with Duane's retraction syndrome. *Ann Ophthalmol* 1983;15:862–864.
204. Rubinstein AE, Lovelace RE, Behrens MM, et al. Moebius syndrome in association with peripheral neuropathy and Kallmann syndrome. *Arch Neurol* 1975;32:480–482.
205. Ruff R, Kaminski H, Mass E, et al. Ocular muscles: Physiology and structure-function correlations. *Bull Soc Belge Ophthalmol* 1989;237:321–352.
206. Rumph M. Fibrose du muscle droit inferieur, anomalies d'insertions et aplasies musculaires, une cause rare de troubles héréditaires non progressifs et congénitaux de la motilité oculaire. *Ann Ocul* 1974;207:829–831.
207. Salleras J, Ortiz De Zarate JC, Recessive sex-linked inheritance of external ophthalmoplegia and myopia coincident with other dysplasias. *Br J Ophthalmol* 1950;34:662–667.
208. Sammito V, Motta D, Capodieci G, et al. IVIC syndrome: Report of a second family. *Am J Med Genet* 1988;29:875–881.
209. Satokata I, Maas R. Msx1 deficient mice exhibited cleft palate and abnormalities of craniofacial and tooth development. *Nature Genet* 1994;6:348–355.

210. Savitsky K, Bar-Shira A, Gilad S, et al. A single ataxia telangiectasia gene with a product similar to P1-3 kinase. *Science* 1995;268:1749–1753.
211. Schimke RN, Collins DL, Hiebert JM. Congenital nonprogressive myopathy with Möbius and Robin sequence—The Carey-Fineman-Ziter syndrome: A confirmatory report. *Am J Med Genet* 1993;46:721–723.
212. Schlossman A, Priestley B. Role of heredity in etiology and treatment of strabismus. *Arch Ophthalmol* 1952;47:1–20.
213. Schneider-Maunoury S, Topilko P, Seitanidou T, et al. Disruption of Krox-20 results in alterations of rhombomeres 3 and 5 in the developing hindbrain. *Cell* 1993;75:1199–1214.
214. Sevel D. Brown's syndrome—A possible etiology explained embryologically. *J Pediatr Ophthalmol Strabismus* 1981;18:26–31.
215. Sevel D. A reappraisal of the origin of human extraocular muscles. *Ophthalmology* 1981; 88:1330–1338.
216. Sevel D. Development of the nerves of the extraocular muscles. In *Strabismus II,* R.D. Reinecke, ed. New York: Grune & Stratton, 1984:645–657.
217. Sevel D. The origins and insertions of the extraocular muscles: Development, histologic features, and clinical significance. *Trans Am Ophthalmol Soc* 1986;84:488–526.
218. Sevel D. Development of the connective tissue of the extraocular muscles and clinical significance. *Graefes Arch Clin Exp Ophthalmol* 1988;226:246–251.
219. Shauly Y, Weissman A, Meyer E. Ocular and systemic characteristics of Duane syndrome. *J Pediatr Ophthalmol Strabismus* 1993; 30:178–183.
220. Shaw J, Lichter P, Driesel AJ, et al. Regional localisation of the Friedreich ataxia locus to human chromosome 9q13-q21.1. *Cytogenet Cell Genet* 1990;53:221–224.
221. Sidman R, Rakic P. Development of the human central nervous system. In *Histology and Histopathology of the Nervous System,* vol. 1, W. Haymaker and R. Adams, eds. Springfield, IL: Charles C Thomas, 1982:1–145.
222. Singh B, Shahwan SA, Singh P, et al. Möbius syndrome with basal ganglia calcification. *Acta Neurol Scand* 1992;85:436–438.
223. Singh P, Patnaik B. Heredity in Duane's syndrome. *Acta Ophthalmol (Copenh)* 1971; 49:103–110.
224. Slee JJ, Smart RD, Viljoen DL. Deletion of chromsome 13 in Moebius syndrome. *J Med Genet* 1991;28:413–414.
225. Spencer R, Porter J. Structural organization of the extraocular muscles. In *Reviews in Oculomotor Research, Neuroanatomy of the Oculomotor System,* vol. 2, J. Buttner-Ennever, ed. New York: Elsevier, 1988:33–79.
226. Sprofkin BE, Hillman JW. Moebius syndrome: Congenital oculofacial paralysis. *Neurology (Minneap)* 1956;6:50–54.
227. St. Charles S, Dimario FJ, Grunnet ML. Möbius sequence: Further in vivo support for the subclavian artery supply disruption sequence. *Am J Med Genet* 1993;47: 289–293.
228. Stabile M, Cavaliere ML, Scarano G, et al. Abnormal B.A.E.P. in a family with Moebius syndrome: Evidence for supranuclear lesion. *Clin Genet* 1984;25:459–463.
229. Starr J, Lamont M, Iselius J, et al. A linkage study of a large pedigree with X-linked centronuclear myopathy. *J Med Genet* 1990;27:2881–2883.
230. Sudarshan A, Goldie WD. The spectrum of congenital facial diplegia (Moebius syndrome). *Pediatr Neurol* 1985;1:180–184.
231. Sugarman GI, Stark HH. Möbius syndrome with Poland's anomaly. *J Med Genet* 1973; 10:192–196.
232. Tabin C. Why we have (only) five fingers per hand: Hox genes and the evolution of paired limbs. *Development* 1992;116:289–296.
233. Temtamy S, Shoukry A, Ghaly I, et al. The Duane/radial dysplasia syndrome: An autosomal dominant disorder. *Birth Defects Orig Art Ser* XI 1975;XI(5):344–345.
234. Temtamy SA, McKusick VA, The genetics of hand malformations. *Birth Defects Orig Art Ser* XIV 1978;3:82–85.
235. Terrett J, Newbury-Ecob R, Cross GS, et al. Holt-Oram syndrome is a genetically heterogeneous disease with one locus mapping to human chromosome 12q. *Nature Genet* 1994;6:401–404.
236. Thakkar N, O'Neil W, Duvally J, et al. Moebius syndrome due to brain stem tegmental necrosis. *Arch Neurol* 1977;34:124–126.
237. Thomas N, Sarfaraze M, Roberts K, et al. X-linked myotubular myopathy (MTM1): Evidence for linkage to Xq28 DNA markers (abstract). *Cytogenet Cell Genet* 1987;46: 704.
238. Thomas N, Williams H, Cole G, et al. X-linked neonatal centronuclear/myotubular myopathy: Evidence for linkage to Xq28

DNA marker loci. *J Med Genet* 1990; 27:284–287.

239. Tome F, Fardeau M. Oculopharyngeal muscular dystrophy. In *Myology*, vol. 2, A. Engel and C. Franzini-Armstrong, eds. New York: McGraw-Hill, 1994:1233–1245.
240. Towfighi J, Marks K, Palmer E, et al. Moebius syndrome. Neuropathologic observations. *Acta Neuropathol (Berl)* 1979;48: 11–17.
241. Traboulsi E, Jaafar M, Kattan HM, et al. Congenital fibrosis of the extraocular muscles: Report of 24 cases illustrating the clinical spectrum and surgical management. *Am Orthop J* 1993;43:45–53.
242. Traboulsi E, Maumenee I. Extraocular muscle aplasia in Moebius syndrome. *J Pediatr Ophthalmol Strabismus* 1986;23:120–122.
243. Turleau C, de Grouchy J, Chavin-Colin F, et al. Two patients with interstitial del (14q), one with features of Holt-Oram syndrome: Exclusion mapping of PI (alpha-1-antitrypsin). *Ann Genet* 1984;27:237–240.
244. Van Allen MW, Blodi FC. Neurologic aspects of the Möbius syndrome. *Neurology* 1960; 10:249–259.
245. Van der Wiel HJ. Hereditary congenital facial paralysis. *Acta Genet Stat Med* 1957;7:348.
246. Victor D. The diagnosis of congenital unilateral third-nerve palsy. *Brain* 1967;99: 711–718.
247. Villaseca A. Strabismus fixus. *Am J Ophthalmol* 1959;48:751–762.
248. Vincent C, Kalatzis V, Compain S, et al. A proposed new contiguous gene syndrome on 8q consists of branchio-oto-renal (BOR) syndrome, Duane syndrome, a dominant form of hydrocephalus and trapeze aplasia: Implications for the mapping of the BOR gene. *Hum Mol Genet* 1994;3:1859–1866.
249. von Graefe A, Saemisch T. *Handbuch der gesamten Augenheilkunde,* vol. 6. Leipzig: Wilhelm Engelmann, 1880.
250. Von Noorden GK. Congenital hereditary ptosis with inferior rectus fibrosis. Report of two cases. *Arch Ophthalmol* 1970;83:378–380.
251. Vossius A. Zwei Falle von angeborener fast vollstandiger Unbeweglichkeit beider Augen und der oberen Augenlider. *Beitr Augenheilkd* 1982;5:1–10.
252. Waardenburg P. Squint and heredity. *Doc Ophthalmol* 1954;7:422.
253. Wahl C, Noden D, Baker R. Developmental relations between sixth nerve motor neurons and their targets in the chick embryo. *Dev Dyn* 1994;201:191–202.
254. Weekers R, Moureau P, Hacourt J. Contribution a l'etiologie du syndrome de retraction oculaire (syndrome de Stilling-Turk-Duane). *Acta Ophthalmol* 1956;34:343.
255. Weleber R, Walknowska J, Peatman D. Cytogenetic investigation of cat-eye syndrome. *Am J Ophthalmol* 1977;84:477–486.
256. Wieczorek DF, Periasamy M, Butler B, et al. Co-expression of multiple myosin heavy chain genes, in addition to a tissue-specific one, in extraocular musculature. *J Cell Biol* 1985;101:618–629.
257. Wilder WM, Williams JP, Happ SL. Computerized tomographic findings in two cases of congenital fibrosis syndrome. *Comput Med Imaging Graph* 1991;15:361–363.
258. Wildervanck L. The cervico-oculo-acusticus syndrome. In *Handbook of Clinical Neurology,* vol. 32, P.J. Vinken, G. Bruyn, and N. Myranthopoulos, eds. Amsterdam: North-Holland, 1978:123–130.
259. Wilson ER, Mirra SS, Schwartz JF. Congenital diencephalic and brain stem damage: Neuropathologic study of three cases. *Acta Neuropathol (Berl)* 1982;57:70–74.
260. Wilson M, Eustis H, Parks MM. Brown's syndrome. *Surv Ophthalmol* 1989;34; 153–172.
261. Wolff J. The occurrence of retraction movements of the eyeball together with congenital defects in the external ocular muscles. *Arch Ophthalmol* 1900;29:297–309.
262. Wortham E, Crawford J. Brown's syndrome in twins. *Am J Ophthalmol* 1988;105:562–563.
263. Wurst W, Auerbach A, Joyner AL. Multiple developmental defects in Engrailed-1 mutant mice: An early mid- and hindbrain deletion and patterning defects in forelimbs and sternum. *Development* 1994;120:2065–2075.
264. Yang S, Sherman S, Derstine JB, et al. Holt-Oram syndrome gene may be on chromosome 20. *Pediatr Res* 1990;27:137A.
265. Ziter FA, Wiser WC, Robinson A. Three-generation pedigree of a Möbius syndrome variant with chromosome translocation. *Arch Neurol* 1977;34:437–442.

28

Congenital Nystagmus

JOHN B. KERRISON
IRENE H. MAUMENEE

Congenital nystagmus is an idiopathic disorder characterized by ocular oscillations typically manifest during infancy. Traditionally, it has been divided into "sensory" and "motor" types.[38] Patients in whom nystagmus is associated with defects in the visual sensory system[85,170,204,231] are thought to have ocular oscillations secondary to the visual deficit. These patients have the sensory form of nystagmus. If no primary visual disturbance is present, the nystagmus is of the motor form.

When nystagmus occurs as part of an ocular genetic syndrome such as achromatopsia, albinism, or Leber's congenital amaurosis, it is considered a feature of that syndrome. The ocular oscillations presumably arise from developmental abnormalities in the visual system, leading to ocular motor instability. When nystagmus occurs without apparent damage to the visual system, it is simply referred to as *congenital motor nystagmus*. Several genetic mutations are responsible as X-linked (MIM31700),[86,114,137,155,163,180,226] autosomal recessive (MIM257400),[67,155,230] and autosomal dominant (MIM164100)[16,64,128,155,169] patterns of inheritance have been described. Often, no family history is present, in which case the congenital motor nystagmus is referred to as *simplex*.

Most cases of congenital motor nystagmus have their onset in the first few months of life rather than immediately at birth.[128,177] Hence several authors prefer to use the term *infantile nystagmus* rather than *congenital nystagmus*.[87,104,124,177] Other synonyms include *manifest congenital nystagmus*[224] and *hereditary congenital nystagmus*.[59]

The traditional nosological division of congenital nystagmus into sensory and motor subtypes does not necessarily represent a difference in developmental pathophysiology. The nystagmus waveforms are similar in both types; nonetheless, it is a clinically useful classification that we will use in this chapter.

EPIDEMIOLOGY

In 1927, based on his examination of military recruits, Hemmes estimated an overall prevalence of hereditary nystagmus in the Netherlands of 1 in 6500 people.[116] Forssman and Ringnér estimated a prevalence among school children in Sweden between 1941 and 1959 of 1/1500 males and 1/1000 females, with an overall frequency of 1/2800 students.[80] Among visually handicapped children, nystagmus is relatively common. In a United Kingdom cohort of 10-year-old children born in 1970, the prevalence of blindness (visual acuity worse than 6/60) was 1 per 2500 to 2941 children while the prevalence of partial sight (visual acuity between 6/24 and 6/60) was 1 per 1149 to 1852 children. The most common cause of partial sight or blindness was congenital cataracts, followed by nystagmus. The overall rate of congenital nystagmus was estimated to be 10.7 per 10,000.[211] This should be viewed as the prevalence of congenitally blinding disorders associated with nystagmus.

The incidence of congenital nystagmus has been crudely estimated. Based on patients who had contacted the Eye Clinic of the Danish Institute for the Blind and Partially Sighted between 1927 and 1963, Norn estimated the incidence of idiopathic nystagmus in the general population to be 1 per 20,000 per year. He noted a male predominance and stressed that his estimate included only those with the poorest vision.[165] Anderson estimated an incidence of 1 new case per 324 patients per year based on 30 years of private practice.[17]

Congenital sensory nystagmus is more common than congenital motor nystagmus. In 1978, Pearce reported that among 40 children registered with the Canadian National Institute for the Blind as having nystagmus, 80% had a sensory defect.[170] The most common visual sensory system disorders associated with nystagmus are ocular or oculocutaneous albinism, optic nerve hypoplasia, or an inherited disturbance of the retina such as Leber's congenital amaurosis. The remaining 10%–20% of patients have congenital motor nystagmus.[85,231]

About 25%–60% of patients with congenital nystagmus have a family history of the disease.[85,231] Although congenital motor nystagmus may be X-linked, autosomal dominant or autosomal recessive, it is not known which form is the most common.

ASSOCIATIONS

Nystagmus at birth or during infancy is a finding that may be associated with metabolic abnormalities,[145,202] teratogens,[151] abnormalities of the brain,[142,143,205] systemic abnormalities as part of a genetic syndrome, or ocular abnormalities alone.

Metabolic abnormalities that are associated with abnormal eye movements include inborn errors of metabolism and endocrinologic abnormalities. Inborn errors of metabolism may lead to corneal opacification, cataracts, retinal degeneration, or optic atrophy with a sensory type congenital nystagmus (Table 28.1). As inborn errors of metabolism are addressed elsewhere in this book, they will not be addressed here with the exception of those of particular neurologic interest. Hyperbilirubinemia may be associated with congenital nystagmus.[175] Endocrinologic abnormalities such as hypothyroidism may be associated with congenital nystagmus.[202]

Teratogenic effects of alcohol and medicines may also lead to congenital nystagmus.[175] Magee and colleagues reported that 1 of 6 children with first trimester exposure to amiodarone, used to treat cardiac arrythmias, developed congenital nystagmus.[151] Although amiodarone may lead to perinatal thyroid dysfunction, the aforementioned patient had normal thyroid function tests. Furthermore, this patient's mother had been taking a beta blocker during pregnancy.

Central nervous system abnormalities that may present with nystagmus include structural defects, inherited metabolic defects, and tumors. *Joubert syndrome* is characterized by neonatal episodes of tachypnea and apnea, hypotonia, ataxia, cerebellar vermis hypoplasia, and nystagmus.[122,125] In some patients, retinal dystrophy and renal cysts are present.[189] *Orofaciodigital syndrome type III* is an autosomal recessive disorder characterized by mental retardation, lingual hamartomas, postaxial polydactyly, malformations of the cerebellar vermis, and characteristic "metronome" eye movements.[205,214] *Dandy-Walker syndrome* is characterized by a dilated fourth ventricle appearing as a posterior fossa cyst with cranial nerve palsies, truncal ataxia, and nystagmus. *Arnold-Chiari malformation* is characterized by extension of a tongue of cerebellar tissue posterior to the medulla and spinal cord into the cervical canal and displacement of the medulla into the cervical canal along with the inferior part of

Table 28.1 Disorders Associated with Nystagmus in Infancy[181,112]

Metabolic Abnormalities

- Albinism
- Inborn errors of metabolism[39]
  - Abetalipoproteinemia
  - Biotin reversible neurodegeneration[145]
  - Gangliosidosis (GM_1 type 1; GM_1 type 2; GM_2 type 1 [Tay-Sachs])
  - Hartnup disease
  - Krabbe disease
  - Metachromatic leukodystrophy
  - Refsum disease
- Hyperbilirubinemia[175]
- Endocrine
  - Hypothyroidism

Teratogens

- Amiodarone
- Alcohol[175]

Brain Abnormalities

- Structural
  - Joubert syndrome
  - Dandy–Walker syndrome
  - Arnold–Chiari malformation
  - Schizencephaly[148]
  - Orofacialdigital syndrome type III
- Degeneration
  - Infantile subacute necrotizing encephalomyopathy (Leigh disease)
  - Pelizaeus–Merzbacher disease
  - Spongy degeneration of infancy (Canavan disease)
- Tumors
  - Astrocytoma
  - Glioma
  - Medulloblastoma
  - Neuroblastoma (associated with opsoclonus)
  - Posterior fossa ependymoma

Syndromes

- Alport syndrome
- Alstrom syndrome
- Cornelia de Lange syndrome[141]
- De Morsier syndrome
- Essential tremor, nystagmus, duodenal ulcer, narcolepsylike episodes
- Familial remitting chorea
- Fanconi syndrome with pancytopenia
- Hallermann-Streiff syndrome
- Jeune syndrome
- Karsch-Neugebauer syndrome
- Klippel-Trenaunay-Weber syndrome
- Lowry-Wood syndrome
- Marinesco-Sjögren syndrome
- Oculocerebrorenal syndrome of Lowe
- Partial deletion of the short arm of chromosome 3 (46,XY,del(3)(p2.53))
- Partial deletion of the long arm of chromosome 18 (18q-)
- trisomy 21 (Down syndrome)
- Turner Syndrome
- Wolfram syndrome (DIDMOAD: diabetes insipidus, diabetes mellitus, optic atrophy, deafness)

Ocular Abnormalities

- Cataracts and anterior segment opacities
  - Peters' anomaly
- Foveal hypoplasia
  - Albinism
  - Aniridia
- Isolated foveal hypoplasia
- Retinal defects
  - Achromatopsia
  - Åland eye disease
  - Congenital stationary night blindness, X-linked and autosomal recessive
  - Leber's congenital amaurosis
  - Retinopathy of prematurity
  - Macular colobomata
  - Norrie disease
  - Retinitis pigmentosa
- Optic nerve atrophy and abnormalities
  - Autosomal recessive optic atrophy
  - Behr optic atrophy
  - Optic nerve hypoplasia
  - Secondary to optic canal compression
    - Apert syndrome
    - Albers-Schonberg syndrome
    - Crouzon disease

the fourth ventricle.[14] Patients may have downbeat nystagmus.

In addition to structural defects, inherited metabolic abnormalities of the central nervous system may lead to nystagmus. *Pelizaeus-Merzbacher disease* is an X-linked disorder with diffuse cerebral sclerosis beginning in infancy and characterized by pendular eye movements, head shaking, hypotonia, choreoathetosis, and pyramidal signs due in some patients to a defect in a gene that encodes lipophilin, a constituent of myelin.[213,220] *Leigh disease* (subacute necrotizing encephalopathy) is an autosomal recessive disorder of thiamine metabolism presenting with loss of head control, hypotonia, vomiting, generalized seizures, myoclonic jerks, and nystagmus. *Canavan disease* (spongy degeneration of infancy) is characterized by psychomotor degeneration, optic atrophy, nystagmus, and spongy degeneration of the deep layers of the cerebral cortex and subcortical white matter.

Some central nervous system tumors may manifest spontaneous ocular movements. These include astrocytoma,[36,219] glioma,[136] medulloblastoma,[68,126] and posterior fossa ependymoma.[150] In addition, neuroblastoma may be associated with the paraneoplastic manifestation of ocular flutter/opsoclonus,[188] probably mediated by an antibody that reacts with the tumor and is sometimes responsive to intravenous immunoglobulin.[74]

Congenital nystagmus has been reported as a feature of several syndromes. *De Morsier syndrome* (septooptic dysplasia) is characterized by optic nerve hypoplasia, absence of the septum pellucidum, short stature, and pituitary endocrinologic abnormalities. Patients may have an associated seesaw nystagmus. *Karsch–Neugebauer syndrome* is characterized by a characteristic split hand/split foot deformity associated with cataracts and nystagmus.[172] *Klippel-Trenaunay-Weber syndrome* is characterized by a triad of cutaneous angiomas, varicosities that appear in childhood, and bony and soft tissue hypertrophy of the involved limb that may be associated with ocular manifestations, including nystagmus and strabismus.[30] Deletion of the long arm of chromosome 18 is associated with psychomotor retardation, microcephaly, prominent chin, optic disc pallor, nystagmus, and tapetoretinal degeneration.[112] Partial deletion of the short arm of chromosome 3 [46,XY, del(3)(p2.53)] results in a syndrome of mental retardation, congenital heart disease, hypertelorism, ptosis, epicanthus, blepharophimosis, strabismus, nystagmus, synophrys, low-set ears, frequent infections, epilepsy, rocker-bottom feet, flat occiput, and muscle hypotonia.[158] *Down syndrome* may be associated with nystagmus in 9%–30% of patients.[198,227] *Wolfram syndrome* (DIDMOAD) is characterized by *d*iabetes *i*nsipidus, *d*iabetes *m*ellitus, *o*ptic *a*trophy, nystagmus, and *d*eafness. *Jeune syndrome* is characterized by thoracic deformities, short limb dwarfism, nephronophthisis, and congenital retinal dystrophy. An autosomal dominant disorder consisting of essential tremor, congenital nystagmus, duodenal ulcers, and narcolepsy-like sleep episodes has been described.[164]

Patients with *Lowry-Wood syndrome* have multiple epiphyseal dysplasia, short stature, microcephaly, mental retardation, and congenital nystagmus, developing features of retinitis pigmentosa after toddler age.[146,147] Yamamoto and colleagues described a $3\frac{1}{2}$-year-old boy with features of Lowry-Wood syndrome, including congenital nystagmus with hypoplasia of the corpus callosum, leukonychia totalis, and a normal visual evoked potential (VEP) and electroretinogram (ERG).[234] Wang et al. observed an early-onset syndrome in siblings of poor weight gain, hypotonia, truncal ataxia, horizontal pendular nystagmus, and poor auditory evoked response attributed to a dysgenetic lesion.[228] Familial remitting chorea has been associated with an infantile monocular horizontal nystagmus and cataracts characterized by peripheral wedge-shaped subcapsular opacities.[232]

Ocular abnormalities may have nystagmus as a manifestation. Usually, these are associated with poor visual acuity. Strabismus and nystagmus are commonly associated with congenital cataracts.[123] *Congenital rubella* may be associated with nystagmus, cataracts, and a salt-and-pepper retinopathy.[17] Nystagmus is present in patients with *Peters' anomaly.* Foveal hypoplasia, as seen in *aniridia* and *albinism,* is associated with nystagmus. However, not all patients with oculocutaneous albinism have nystagmus, even in the same sibship.[34] *Foveal hypoplasia* may also occur as an isolated disorder with no other findings except nystagmus. Hammerstein and Gebauer reported a reciprocal, balanced 5/16 translocation in three patients with foveal hypoplasia and familial nystagmus.[109] More recently, isolated foveal hypoplasia has been associated with mutations in PAX6.[19a] Other retinal diseases associated with nystagmus include: *achromatopsia, Åland eye disease, X-linked and autosomal recessive congenital stationary night blindness, Leber's congenital amaurosis, retinopathy of prematurity, macular colobomata, and retinitis pigmentosa.* Optic nerve abnormalities associated with nystagmus include autosomal recessive optic atrophy, *Behr optic atrophy,*[200] and compression of the optic nerve in the optic canal from *Crouzon syndrome, Apert syndrome* (acrocephaly, syndactyly, exophthalmos, and exotropia) or *Albers-Schonberg syndrome* (osteopetrosis).

CLINICAL FEATURES

Age of Onset

Onset of congenital nystagmus occurs typically during infancy, with oscillations present throughout life. Several authors have reported patients in whom the presence of ocular oscillations was noticed at birth.[128,177,183] The youngest patient to undergo electronystagmography was 2 months old. In infancy (less than 6 months), the most common waveform is triangular (70%), but by 19–24 months, waveforms are jerk or pendular.[177] The large amplitude of triangular waveforms makes the nystagmus readily apparent. As the waveforms assume a pendular or jerk appearance, the nystagmus may appear less noticeable. Patients have also been reported in whom congenital nystagmus waveforms emerged during adolescence or adulthood,[102] and in whom nystagmus disappeared during late childhood only to reappear after minor head trauma.[82] The latter patient had excellent foveation dynamics. His nystagmus was inapparent at times, suggesting that this represented a case of worsening of nystagmus with minor trauma.

Waveforms

Congenital nystagmus is characterized by bilateral conjugate oscillations with onset during infancy. The oscillations are typically horizontal and remain so on upgaze and downgaze. Rarely is the nystagmus vertical or monocular.[64,81,83,117,153] When vertical oscillations are present, they are most evident on upgaze or downgaze and usually coexist with horizontal nystagmus. Congenital motor nystagmus with vertical oscillations is transmitted in an autosomal dominant pattern.[27,64] Vertical nystagmus may also occur with Leber's congenital amaurosis or albinism.[118] Vertical nystagmus may be present without a horizontal component initially only to become horizontally directed with time.[73,118] The cases of intermittent hereditary vertical nystagmus reported by Sogg and Hoyt as congenital nystagmus are questionable because of the presence of oscillopsia.[206]

Two basic congenital nystagmus waveforms may be observed: jerk and pendular (see below). The jerk waveform has a characteristic exponentially increasing velocity slow waveform, followed by a saccade that refoveates the eyes. Jerk, pendular, or both waveforms may be present even in the same individual. Waveforms may vary among affected family members of a single pedigree[45] and even between identical twins with congenital motor nystagmus[5,209] or albinism.[11] Although a single individual may have a variety of waveforms, one waveform may predominate. Once it is established in childhood, the prevailing waveform appears to be stable over time.

The classification and observation of a multitude of waveforms has led to the understanding that no waveform is specific for a particular underlying etiology. These patterns do not help distinguish the sensory form from motor type congenital nystagmus.[6,235] Previous classifications of pendular nystagmus with no apparent fixation as a "sensory nystagmus" and jerk nystagmus with refoveating saccades as a "motor nystagmus" are not valid.

Other waveforms that have been described include a congenital *seesaw nystagmus* that may occur alone[240] or in association with retinitis pigmentosa.[24] An X-linked congenital *peri-*

odic alternating nystagmus has been described.[120] Periodic alternating nystagmus may also occur with albinism.[12,106] A *unilateral-pursuit–induced congenital nystagmus* has been described in which patients showed nystagmus, with waveforms typical of infantile nystagmus, during any task that required visual following toward the left.[127] Achromatopsia may be associated with a horizontal jerk nystagmus with *exponentially decreasing velocity slow phases,* a feature of latent/manifest latent nystagmus.[93,236] A form of congenital *convergence pendular nystagmus* evoked by accommodative vergence has been described.[110,199]

The waveform of the nystagmus in an individual is predominantly affected by the state of attention.[6] The intensity (frequency and amplitude) of nystagmus is accentuated by visual fixation,[45] attention, or anxiety. It is often reported that nystagmus intensity is dampened by lid closure and enhanced by darkness.[45,201,235] These effects are thought to be related to absence of fixation attempt rather than retinal illumination. Waveform and intensity also depend on the position of the eye in the orbit. In contrast, Tusa et al. presented three patients with congenital nystagmus who were able to voluntarily suppress and release their nystagmus by fixating an object in a well-lit room.[218]

"Reversed" or "Inverted" Optokinetic Nystagmus

Another distinctive feature of congenital motor nystagmus is the appearance of "inverted" or "reversed" optokinetic nystagmus (OKN), which is elicited with a optokinetic drum. Instead of quick phases being directed in the opposite direction of drum rotation, they are directed in the same direction as drum rotation.[108]

Null Region

The null region or neutral zone is the eye position or gaze angle at which the intensity of oscillations is dampened.[130] Jerk nystagmus reverses direction on opposite sides of this zone, with slow phases directed toward (centripetal) the zone and quick phases away (centrifugal) from the zone. The null region has a characteristic width and position. It typically measures between 1° and 3° in width and is located off-center and/or in convergence. Not all patients with congenital nystagmus have a gaze or convergence null position. Patients may adapt head tilts or turns in order to place their null point straight ahead.[9] In some patients, poor visual acuity is present without a well-developed null point.

Visual Acuity and Fixation

Visual acuity may vary from 20/20 to 20/400, even within a single pedigree,[129] depending on the foveation dynamics of each patient. It is accepted that the cause of decreased vision is slippage of images across the fovea. Visual acuity correlates with nystagmus intensity (amplitude and frequency at a given gaze position). More specifically, the visual acuity is dependent on the accuracy of target fixation, the duration of target fixation, and the retinal slippage velocity during foveal fixation (see below). The term *foveation dynamics* encompasses these variables.

Thus, patients with better visual acuity are able to adapt strategies that involve *(1)* beat-to-beat foveal fixation with low retinal/target slippage velocity and *(2)* use of the null point, which is the position of the eye in the orbit where oscillations are dampened.

With jerk nystagmus, saccades bring the object of regard onto the fovea, allowing beat-to-beat fixation. As these saccades interrupt the slow movement of eyes away from the target and allow a brief foveal fixation time when the eyes are still, they are referred to as "breaking" saccades. With pendular nystagmus, beat-to-beat foveal fixation occurs during the turnaround of the sinusoidal wave when eye velocity is lowest.

Role of Amblyopia and Astigmatism

Amblyopia may play a role in those patients with strabismus or uncorrected refractive errors. In addition, bilateral amblyopia may contribute to the decreased visual acuity in congenital motor nystagmus.[208] It has also been hypothesized that meridional amblyopia may partially explain decreased visual acuity in patients with astigmatism.[21] Corneal topography and refractions of patients with albinism and congenital nystagmus revealed a greater than normal incidence of high spectacle astigmatism, which was predominantly with-the-rule and corneal in origin.[66] In patients with horizontal nystagmus, the contrast sensitivity and spatial resolution of a sinusoidal grating are greater for horizontally oriented gratings than for vertically oriented gratings in congenital motor[1] and sensory nystagmus.[144] This distinction is present even when the effects of eye movements are eliminated, leading to the conclusion that a meridional amblyopia is present for vertically oriented patterns.[3]

Oscillopsia

Patients with congenital nystagmus do not typically experience oscillopsia (see below). However, as in normal individuals with damage to the vestibuloocular reflex, they cannot suppress the sensation of movement and can develop oscillopsia due to vestibular disease.

Stereopsis

Stereopsis is present in patients with congenital nystagmus unless a sensory abnormality is present. In a study comparing stereopsis in albino patients versus patients with idiopathic infantile nystagmus, 86% of congenital motor nystagmus patients passed the stereofly test, a gross test of stereopsis, in contrast with 5% of albino patients.[104] The authors concluded that this difference reflects asymmetry in decussating retinal ganglion cell axons present in albinism but not in congenital motor nystagmus.

Strabismus

Strabismus is present in 15%–30% of patients. Esotropia is most common.[85,104,128] In nystagmus blockage syndrome, patients with congenital nystagmus present with esotropia.[207] Patients may fixate with either eye, using a head turn when fixing with the esotropic eye and no head turn when fixing with the eye in primary position. As the viewing eye follows a target laterally into abduction, the esotropia decreases and nystagmus increases.[49] It is presumed that adduction represents an effort to dampen the nystagmus and improve vision by dampening a congenital nystagmus waveform[131] or converting to a low-amplitude manifest latent nystagmus.[49] Nystagmus blockage syndrome may be confused with combined esotropia and a manifest latent nystagmus.[49]

Head Posture

A head turn may be present in congenital motor and sensory nystagmus although its overall frequency is not known.[6,75] It is usually adopted between 24 and 52 weeks postnatally.[6] One or multiple postures may be adopted by a patient.[9] Such an adjustment is presumed to be an attempt to position the null region to straight ahead gaze to obtain optimal visual acuity.[9] This torticollis can be cosmetically or physically debilitating and is an indication for surgical intervention. In a series of patients who underwent surgery for a head turn, the average preoperative turn was 41.3°.[162] Head turn may be measured with a orthopedic goniometer. Albino patients do not typically develop abnormal posture.[12]

Head Shaking

Some patients with congenital nystagmus have head shaking that is usually intermittent and may have a frequency similar to that of their nystagmus. Head shaking may be seen in both congenital motor and sensory nystagmus.[94,95] The tremor typically has a frequency of 2–4 Hz and an amplitude of 2°–3°.[98] Patients are usually aware of their head shaking and can voluntarily suppress it.[97] The etiology of the head shaking is unclear, but some patients report improved vision with head shaking (see following.[32,97,99,159]

PHYSIOLOGY

Waveforms of Congenital Nystagmus

Dell'Osso and Daroff have described 12 waveforms that may occur in congenital nystagmus.[46] These waveforms may broadly be divided into pendular, jerk, and dual when pendular and jerk occur simultaneously. They cannot easily be recognized without eye movement recordings, which includes both position and velocity tracings.

Pendular waveforms include *pendular* with a sinusoidal waveform, *asymmetric pendular* with a skewed sinusoidal waveform, and *pendular with foveating saccades* in which small breaking saccades stop the eye movement after bypassing the target, allowing refoveation. The latter pendular waveform may be clinically mistaken for a jerk nystagmus. Eye position and velocity recordings, however, clearly distinguish this waveform as pendular.

Jerk waveforms may be unidirectional or bidirectional. There are four unidirectional forms. In *pure jerk* and *jerk with extended foveation waveforms,* the direction of the fast phase is considered the direction of nystagmus. These fast phases refoveate the eye after the exponentially increasing velocity slow phase take the eyes off target. These fast phases are distinguished as saccades by their amplitude–peak velocity relationship ("main sequence"). The fast phase is in the direction of gaze in the horizontal plane. Thus on right gaze, the patient has a rightward fast phase on right gaze and a leftward fast phase on left gaze. More complex unidirectional jerk waveforms include *pseudocycloid,* in which braking saccades give the impression of a pendular nystagmus, and *pseudojerk,* in which the apparent direction of the fast phase on position recording is opposite the direction of the saccade on velocity tracings. In these two forms, the saccades do not fully refoveate the target. Four bidirectional jerk waveforms include *pseudopendular, pseudopendular with foveating saccades, triangular,* and *bidirectional jerk.* These waveforms occur at gaze angles in the transition or neutral zone in which the direction of jerk nystagmus is reversed and not amenable to good vision.

Dual waveforms consist of the simultaneous admixture of pendular and jerk waveforms. A rapid small amplitude oscillation is superimposed on a larger amplitude jerk nystagmus.

The multitude of waveforms are thought to represent varied expressions of a single underlying developmental ocular motor instability. Most broadly defined, congenital nystagmus represents a single motor deficit that differs only in the magnitude and variation of gaze or convergence angle position and pursuit optokinetic or vestibuloocular velocities.[59]

Fixation in Congenital Nystagmus

Although it has been hypothesized that patients with congenital nystagmus have defective fixation reflexes, this does not appear to be the case, particularly in those individuals with good vision. Parameters used to describe foveal fixation periods include the accuracy of target fixation, the duration of target fixation, and retinal slip velocity, which can be quantified and compared among individuals in terms of standard deviations. In congenital motor nystagmus with relatively good vision, foveal fixation has been shown to be accurate and repeatable, leading to the conclusion that fixation reflexes are normal.[54] In patients with afferent defects, foveal fixation periods are present but not as accurate.[7] In addition, infants with congenital nystagmus do not have well-developed fixation periods.[177] These periods usually improve with age if the afferent system is intact. If they do not, despite an apparently normal visual sensory system, they may be responsible for poor visual acuity. In turn, abnormalities of the visual sensory system with absence of good vision may preclude development of strong fixation reflexes. Overall, patients with congenital nystagmus have accurate fixation reflexes and good vision. Despite the presence of accurate fixation reflexes, the abnormality in congenital nystagmus is associated with the inability to sustain fixation rather than the ability to achieve fixation.

As mentioned previously, the visual acuity of patients depends on accuracy of target fixation, the duration of target fixation, and the retinal slippage velocity during foveal fixation. The mean and standard deviations of these variables can be used to characterize a patient's fixation. The standard deviation for accuracy of target foveation is 0.21°. Retinal slip velocities below 1.67–4°/sec are the upper bounds of normal for good visual acuity.[52] It has been shown that the standard deviation of these quantities is higher in patients with albinism than in patients with congenital motor nystagmus.[20] Compared with congenital motor nystagmus, underlying defects in the visual sensory system preclude development of strong fixations reflexes.[52]

Ocular Motor Control in Congenital Nystagmus: Saccades, Smooth Pursuit, and Vestibuloocular Reflex Saccades

Saccades in patients with congenital nystagmus are normal if assessed in terms of beat-to-beat-fixation. In normal individuals, a saccade is characterized by a burst of neural activity that generates a rapid eye movement followed by continuous tonic activity maintaining the position of the eye. It is thought that a neural network, referred to as the *neural integrator,* exists that mathematically converts the pulse or velocity command into a step or position command as reviewed by Leigh and Zee.[139] A direct relationship exists between the velocity and amplitude of a saccade, and is referred to as the *main sequence.* This relationship is present during the fast phases of congenital nystagmus, identifying them as saccadic in nature.[8] The time interval between quick phases of nystagmus ranges from 100 to 600 msec, averages 240 ms, and has a Gaussian distribution for values less than 300 msec. This was considered the distribution of intersaccadic latencies in normal humans.[29] However, peak velocities are slower than saccades in normal individuals.[8] In most individuals with congenital nystagmus, saccades are accurate and sustained; however, Dell'Osso and colleagues described a family in which individuals had gaze-holding failure as assessed by analysis of foveation windows.[59] This inability to maintain the position signal is referred to as a "leaky" neural integrator.

Pursuit and Optokinetic Response

The ability of an individual to track a target is dependent on the occipitomesencephalic pursuit subsystem and a subcortical optokinetic system.[238] In cortical blindness, optokinetic nystagmus may still be elicited.[222] Patients with congenital motor nystagmus are clearly able to perform tasks and play sports, such as tennis, which require the ability to follow targets.[55]

It has been stated that smooth pursuit was abnormally "reversed" or "inverted" in congenital motor nystagmus.[108,140] This was concluded because of the observed phenomenon that slow phases of optokinetic nystagmus (OKN) move the eyes in the direction opposite to target motion. Although most patients display slow phases directed opposite to an optokinetic stimulus, they may be normally directed in some patients. In patients in whom the optokinetic nystagmus was normally directed, the OKN gain was found to be low and optokinetic afternystagmus (OKAN) was found to be absent.[236] Later investigations of smooth pursuit in congenital motor nystagmus concluded that pursuit gain was normal.[50,133]

Measurements of repeated fixation periods reveal that pursuit gain is normal at a range of target velocities.[55] There is correspondence between target velocity and the beat-to-beat velocity of the foveal fixation. However, the neutral zone was found to shift in the direction opposite the target. The shift is by an amount proportional to the target velocity. Therefore, the waveforms at each angle of gaze during pursuit movements do not correspond to the waveforms measured at fixation of each position. As a result, when the shift is large enough, the slow phase is in the opposite direction of target motion throughout the range of pursuit angles tested, giving the impression of "inverted" OKN.

Optokinetic response has also been evaluated in patients with sensory type congenital nystagmus. In albinism, OKN and OKAN are absent.[62] In achromatopsia, the pursuit gain was found to be decreased. Evaluation of monocular OKN in achromats demonstrated a gradual increase in the velocity of the slow phase of OKN and directional asymmetry, with higher OKN gain during rotation of the OKN drum in a temporal-to-nasal direction compared with rotation in a nasal-to-temporal direction.[237] Similar findings are present in afoveate animals such as the rabbit, but are not present in normal human subjects or in patients with congenital motor nystagmus.[236,238]

Vestibuloocular Reflex

Patients with congenital nystagmus appear to have normal vestibular function. Neurootologically, they have normal righting reactions.[79] The vestibuloocular reflex (VOR) functions to maintain the fovea on target despite head movement. When the VOR is functioning properly, visual acuity is not reduced during passive head oscillation. Furthermore, the ratio of head velocity to eye velocity (gain) is 1, which is normal, when assessed by eye movement recordings during head rotation. Evaluation of the VOR may be difficult because of the superimposition of spontaneous nystagmus.[101]

Some investigators have concluded that the VOR was deficient.[32,62,79,84] In patients with albinism and congenital nystagmus, Demer and Zee were unable to elicit a caloric response. They were only able to observe a normal VOR gain at higher frequencies (1 Hz) of sinusoidal head oscillation.[62] They also concluded that the VOR time constants were shortened for constant velocity head rotations.[62] Decreased VOR time constants were also demonstrated in congenital motor nystagmus patients with bidirectional jerk nystagmus.[101]

Others investigators have concluded that the VOR was not deficient.[50,97,101,133,238] Assessment of target foveation windows in congenital nystagmus has determined that the vestibuloocular gain is approximately 1 and therefore normal.[56] In addition, it was observed that the neutral zone shifted in a direction opposite the target and proportional to target velocity, similar to the shift observed in OKN (see above).[56]

Oscillopsia

In normal individuals in whom retinal image velocity or retinal slip exceeds 4°/sec, visual acuity begins to decline and oscillopsia, an illusory movement of the stationary world, results.[138] Patients with idiopathic nystagmus rarely complain of this sensation; and when they do, it is not considered to be due to the infantile nystagmus. Several reasons for this have been postulated: coexistent afferent visual defects might increase the threshold for oscillopsia, visual information might be suppressed except during fixation, extraretinal signals or efference copy may cancel out the effects on vision due to oscillations, or an elevated central threshold for detection of motion may be present.[13,22,23,57,58,138] Patients may observe visual stimuli at all phases of their nystagmus; therefore information may be processed at times other than fixation.[87,124,229] Insensitivity to motion is not thought to underlie the lack of oscillopsia. Reduced sensitivity to an oscillating target in congenital nystagmus is due primarily to the nystagmus and is reduced in normal individuals by imposing similar oscillations on a target that is itself oscillating[22] It has been shown that an extraretinal signal or efference copy is present in congenital nystagmus, which allows individuals to locate objects presented during various times in the waveform cycle; nonetheless, pointing errors occurred and varied in counterphase with changes in eye position by approximately 25% of the nystagmus amplitude.[22] Thus, efference copy is available but would only represent 75% of the changes in eye position during nystagmus. Furthermore, artificial stabilization of images of stationary objects on the retina in individuals with congenital nystagmus may cause oscillopsia. Repeatable, accurate foveation periods (along with an efference copy) appears to be required to preclude oscillopsia.[57,58] In effect, an internal representation of the motor output cancels out the movement of images across the retina and avoids oscillopsia.

Head Shaking

The intermittent head shaking seen in some individuals with congenital nystagmus may improve vision in some patients. The head shaking may reflect an adaptive strategy to mullify nystagmus in some patients, and is referred to as "nodding," whereas in others it may be an associated abnormal oscillation in the cephalomotor control system, and is referred to as a "tremor."[98] If the vestibuloocular reflex is functioning properly, each head movement would lead to an equal and opposite eye movement with no resultant stabilization of images on the retina and no improvement in visual acuity. This appears to be the more common situation. In these patients, the head shaking may represent an associated pathologic head tremor rather than an adaptive phenomenon.

In those patients with improved visual acuity, the head shaking is adaptive by one of two mechanisms. In one, the vestibuloocular reflex is dampened, and the head shaking is the same frequency as the nystagmus but in appropriate phase to cancel it.[32,98] This allows the stabilization of images on the retina. In the other, spontaneous eye movements are diminished by head shaking through a central inhibitory effect in which the VOR functions with a normal gain.[99] Thus, each head movement results in an equal and opposite eye movement with an associated decrease in spontaneous movements. This has been observed in spasmus nutans.[92,98]

Accommodation and Convergence

In comparison with the static accommodation function in normal individuals, the overall accommodative stimulus to response function is not different in congenital motor nystagmus; however, it is more variable.[166] In addition, congenital motor nystagmus patients have a statistically significant increased depth of focus compared to normal individuals.[166]

During convergence, the amplitude, mean velocity, and frequency of nystagmus is reduced with monocular or binocular viewing.[65] This dampening may be created for distance fixation with base-out prisms. In contrast, von Noorden found that visual acuity improved with near fixation despite a failure to consistently reduce nystagmus intensity.[223] Analysis of slow phase waveforms during convergence does not show increasing velocity exponentials but constant velocity exponentials. Some studies have shown that position variability during foveation windows increases with near viewing, leading to the conclusion that nystagmus worsens with near viewing.[221]

CLINICAL GENETICS

Perhaps, the earliest and most comprehensive report on hereditary forms of congenital nystagmus was by Nettleship in 1911.[163] Investigation of nine pedigrees revealed two hereditary patterns: X-linked recessive and autosomal dominant with incomplete penetrance. He states that "in some stocks the nystagmus affects both sexes and may descend through either parent, whilst in other stocks only males are attacked with descent through the unaffected mother, as in colour-blindness, haemophilia, and some other conditions."[163] In another early work in 1927, Hemmes reported on five pedigrees he examined and an additional six examined by two colleagues. He states that, "the anomaly can be transmitted after two methods. In the first group both sexes are affected, and in the second the men only are affected and the nystagmus is transmitted through women, who themselves are free."[116]

Since these early works, several classic X-linked recessive (MIM31700)[155] pedigrees have been reported with only males affected.[26,86,180,183,226] Of note, the pedigree reported by Lein et al.[137] as X-linked recessive congenital motor nystagmus was later reported by Fialkow and colleagues as ocular albinism.[71a] Irregularly dominant X-linked inheritance (no male-to-male transmission and the presence of affected females) have been described.[105,114,192,230] We have also observed such pedigrees. Autosomal dominant (MIM 164100)[155] pedigrees have also been well characterized.[16,59,64,128,169]

Less well described is autosomal recessive (MIM257400)[155] inheritance.[67,230] In 1908, Dudley described a four-generation family that included 27 affected individuals among 47 members.[67] The high prevalence of nystagmus was attributed to the frequent intermarrying caused by a desire to "keep the money in the family."[67] Waardenburg presented six pedigrees in which nystagmus appeared to be transmitted in an autosomal recessive pattern.[230] The pedigree described by Cox likely represents autosomal recessive inheritance.[41]

Of these various patterns of inheritance, it is not known which one is most common. Waardenburg stated that "the majority of instances concern families which comprise affected males and affected females," in reference to irregularly dominant X-linked inheritance.[230] It appears that various patterns of genetic inheritance cannot be distinguished clinically by waveform or visual acuity.

Unaffected relatives of patients with congenital nystagmus may show eye movement abnormalities on careful observation. Saccadic instabilities may be present in clinically unaffected relatives of patients with congenital motor nystagmus.[59,196] These take the form of square wave jerks, square wave oscillations, and square wave pulses (macro square-wave jerks). These individuals typically are asymptomatic. Although square wave jerks are seen in normal individuals, they typically occur at a frequency of 9–15 per minute with amplitudes of 2–4°. In relatives of patients with congenital motor nystagmus, square wave jerks are more frequent and occur with square wave oscillations or square wave pulses, the presence of all three of which is considered abnormal. Carriers of blue cone monochromatism may have fixation instabilities associated with upbeat or downbeat nystagmus.[93]

CYTOGENETICS AND MOLECULAR GENETICS

At least three genes are responsible for autosomal dominant, autosomal recessive, and X linked heredity patterns. Patton and co-workers described a mother and child with isolated congenital motor nystagmus and a balanced 7 : 15 translocation.[169] Kerrison and co-workers described a large pedigree with autosomal dominant congenital nystagmus in which linkage analysis was performed.[129] Two-point analysis localized six markers linked at $(\theta) = 0$ in the 6p12 region. Haplotype analysis localized the gene to a region spanning 18 cM.

Several X-linked disorders may be associated with nystagmus: Nettleship-Falls ocular albinism p22.3, Forsius-Erickson syndrome p21, complete congenital stationary night blindness p11.3, Pelizaeus-Merzbacher disease q21-22, blue cone monochromatism q27, and adrenoleukodystrophy q28. The X-linked form of hereditary congenital nystagmus has not been localized. In a large X-linked pedigree with congenital motor nystagmus, an affected female was a (46,XX/45,X) mosaic.[25,105]

PATHOLOGY AND ANIMAL MODELS OF CONGENITAL NYSTAGMUS

No postmortem anatomical studies have been performed on patients with congenital motor nystagmus. A study of extraocular muscle tissue obtained at the time of strabismus surgery demonstrated mitochondrial cores and concentric myofibrils. On ultrastructural study, mitochondria contained concentric cristae surrounding a highly electron-dense spherical body and numerous large rods.[156] Although little is known about the etiology of congenital motor nystagmus, the nystagmus in patients with albinism is thought to be related to misrouting of axons in the anterior visual pathways. Ample pathologic and electrophysiologic evidence exists in albino animals and humans that a larger than normal number of fibers cross the chiasm to synapse in the contralateral lateral geniculate body.[19,42,43,103,104,149] Although it was initially thought that a similar abnormality was present in patients with congenital motor nystagmus,[157] several studies using VEPs have failed to demonstrate the asymmetry between voltage amplitudes recorded from opposite sides of the occipital cortex present with monocular stimulation, as observed in albinos.[19,104,197]

Two animal models of congenital nystagmus have been described. In an experimental model, Tusa and colleagues observed nystagmus, amblyopia, and exotropia in macaque monkeys that underwent neonatal reverse eyelid suture.[217] In that study, newborn monkeys had one eye sewn closed for 25 days followed by opening and suturing of the fellow eye for 25 days. Three rhesus monkeys developed a conjugate nystagmus with pendular and jerk waveforms, with slow phases having velocity-increasing profiles.[217] In another model, Dell'Osso and Williams described mutant Belgian sheepdogs born without a chiasm, a trait thought to be transmitted in an autosomal recessive pattern.[61] These achiasmatic mutants developed spontaneous ocular oscillations with waveforms occasionally similar to human congenital nystagmus.[61]

ETIOLOGY

Waardenburg suggested that congenital nystagmus was due to a defect in the "optomotor reflex path."[230] He states that, "it is possible that part of the nucleus of Deiters forms a relay centre between the vestibular and optomotor reflex systems . . . as the seat of this hereditary defect."[230] Evidence of a defect in the brain stem has been presented by Davis and colleagues, who found a delay between the N_{III} and N_V acoustic brainstem electrical response (ABER) in patients with congenital motor nystagmus.[44] Although the etiology of congenital motor nystagmus remains to be discovered, several theories address what is thought to be the underlying ocular motor control deficit. These theories are based on control systems analysis of models of eye movement. Various models have been subjected to computer simulations in order to reproduce eye movements. Optican and Zee introduced a model that included an inappropriate position feedback of eye velocity to the neural integrator from an afferent (such as misdirected afferents from extraocular muscle proprioceptors) or efferent (efferent copy of eye velocity) source.[167] They were able to simulate a variety of congenital nystagmus waveforms based on this model.[167] Expanding on this premise, Tusa and co-workers emphasized two abnormalities: a gaze-holding deficit due to a low-gain, positive position feedback loop and a velocity-increasing slow phase due to an abnormal positive velocity feedback loop.[218] In another model, Harris proposed that excessive gain in the velocity efference copy of the smooth pursuit system combined with a leaky neural integrator could produce congenital nystagmus waveforms.[113] Although computer simulations of these models may reproduce nystagmus waveforms, the anatomic substrates of congenital nystagmus will likely be identified after responsible genes are identified.

DIFFERENTIAL DIAGNOSIS

Congenital nystagmus has several distinct clinical features and must be distinguished from three other forms of ocular oscillations that occur in infancy: spasmus nutans, latent/manifest latent nystagmus, and ocular flutter/opsoclonus. Furthermore, children with congenital nystagmus may present with esotropia as in the nystagmus blockage syndrome.[49] Finally, one must consider acquired forms of nystagmus, particularly in older individuals.[70]

Spamus nutans is characterized by unilateral ocular oscillations, head turn, and head nodding.[92] It is a benign disorder of unknown etiology that in the past has been thought to remit spontaneously. Recently, it has been recognized that although these children have potential for good vision and stereoacuity, pendular movements continue into adolescence.[96] Children with tumors of the anterior visual pathways may present with the same constellation of features.[91]

Latent nystagmus and manifest latent nystagmus occur in patients with horizontal tropias. Latent nystagmus is defined as nystagmus not present under binocular viewing conditions that develop in both eyes during monocular viewing. Manifest latent nystagmus is defined as nystagmus present with both eyes open but when only one eye is being used for vision. Both latent and manifest latent nystagmus are jerk-type nystagmus. The fast phase characteristically beats toward the viewing eye, and the slow phases have an exponentially decreasing velocity waveform. This contrasts with the exponentially increasing velocity waveforms of congenital motor nystagmus.[47,60] Patients with esotropia and manifest latent nystagmus should be differentiated from those with nystagmus blockage syndrome. According to Dell'Osso et al., one can only distinguish the nystagmus blockage syndrome by using eye movement recording to demonstrate the characteristic exponentially increasing velocity waveform of congenital nystagmus recordings, which diminishes with esotropia.[49]

Saccades that occur without an intersaccadic interval are referred to as *ocular flutter* when horizontal and *opsoclonus* when multiplanar and random. These are easily distinguished from congenital nystagmus on clinical exam by their high amplitude and frequency.

Acquired forms of nystagmus must also be considered in the differential diagnosis of congenital nystagmus, particularly when atypical features such as vertical waveforms or dissociation between the eyes are present. Vertical nystagmus makes one think of Arnold-Chiari malformation but may also be present with congenital sensory nystagmus from albinism or Leber's congenital amaurosis.[118] Rarely do congenital motor nystagmus patients have vertical waveforms. In contradistinction, when one evaluates an adult patient with nystagmus and neurologic complaints, one must consider the possibility that the nystagmus is congenital.[100] Sustained nystagmus is not typically seen with cortical visual impairment.[73]

WORK-UP

The work-up of a patient with possible congenital nystagmus will depend on the age of the patient.[72] In infants with spontaneous ocular oscillations, one has to determine whether the patient has congenital nystagmus, ocular flutter/opsoclonus, or an atypical form of nystagmus that may be due to a structural brain lesion. Spasmus nutans and latent/manifest latent nystagmus do not typically present in infancy.

History should include maternal drug ingestion, health of pregnant mother, complications of delivery, prematurity, and developmental history. A history that the infant is feeding well and achieving developmental milestones argues against a structural brain lesion leading to the movements. Important information includes when the parents first noted the movements, the nature of the movements, and ocular alignment. However, the nystagmus blockage syndrome presents with esotropia. Careful family history includes asking about nystagmus in other family members, vision loss, difficulty seeing colors, and night blindness. Examining other family members when available and appropriate may be helpful.

When examining infants, assess fixation and following alignment, spontaneous eye movements and waveform, head shaking, and abnormal head posture. When oscillations are atypical, consider neuroimaging. When ocular flutter/opsoclonus are present the child should be evaluated for neuroblastoma. On hand light exam, look for aniridia or iris transillumination defects as seen in oculocutaneous albinism. On ophthalmoscopy, examine the macula and optic nerve, looking for hypoplasia. If poor vision is apparent, consider neuroimaging, electroretinography, or VEPs. The most likely retinal disorders to have a normally appearing retina with abnormal ERG include Leber's congenital amaurosis, achromatopsia, congenital stationary night blindness, and Joubert syndrome.[111,134] Among 64 children presenting with poor vision and infantile nystagmus, electroretinography established a diagnosis of achromatopsia in 29%.[89] Some authors feel that a diagnosis of congenital nystagmus cannot be made without ERG.[35] Prudent discussion with parents regarding the timing and rationale for these studies is advised and should be done with care and sensitivity. In toddlers, one may be able to better assess vision and ocular alignment. In children presenting with typical features of spasmus nutans, consider neuroimaging.[18] Although strabismus may be seen with all of the above disorders, normal alignment argues against latent/manifest latent nystagmus. There is, however, a need to rule out a microtropia. In an older individual, the clinician must establish whether the nystagmus is congenital or acquired. Patients with acquired forms of nystagmus will typically complain of oscillopsia, which helps to differentiate them from patients with congenital nystagmus.

THERAPY

Goals of Therapy

At this point, no therapy described has alleviated nystagmus, although in infants with congenital cataracts associated with infantile nystagmus, abatement of the eye movements has been reported with removal of cataracts.[123,178,233] The goals of therapy are to improve visual acuity, correct strabismus, and alleviate abnormal head posture. Surgery and prisms rely on exploitation of a gaze or a convergence null zone. Other treatments that have been used include biofeedback, contact lenses, the porthole method, and medications.

Optical: Prisms

Many patients will have dampening of their nystagmus with convergence or in a particular position of gaze. Bilateral base-out prisms (seven prism diopters) may be used in patients with good fusion to stimulate convergence. Minus lenses may also stimulate accommodation and convergence. Furthermore, bilateral prisms may be used to shift the gaze null to the primary position.[160] For example, an individual with nystagmus and a gaze null 2° to the left of center might be fitted with 11Δ base out right eye and 3Δ base out left eye to provide 14Δ of convergence and 4Δ shift of the null point toward the primary position.[45] These optical manipulations may result in dampened nystagmus and better visual acuity.

Optical: Contact Lenses

Contact lenses may be used to correct refractive errors in patients with congenital nystagmus,[88] but they also may improve acuity by dampening nystagmus.[2,15] When contact lenses are removed some patients may show a transient rebound phenomenon with oscillopsia.[184] It is not thought that the effect is due to increased inertia, as it has been shown that scleral search coils have a negligible effect on saccadic dynamics.[179] Dell'Osso and co-workers studied one patient whose visual acuity was improved by contact lenses and had lower intensity when eyes were treated with a topical anesthetic than when no anesthetic was applied.[51] The effect was more pronounced at gaze angles further from the null. Dampening of nystagmus may have resulted from tactile feedback, as nystagmus intensity may be decreased by other forms of stimulation to the ophthalmic division of the trigeminal nerve: acupuncture, touching the upper eyelid, rubbing the forehead lightly, pressing on the forehead, vibration on the forehead at both 30 and 110 Hz, and both supra- and subthreshold electrical stimuli to the forehead.[53]

Biofeedback

Some patients have been described who could voluntarily suppress their nystagmus.[218] In addition, a method has been described in which nystagmus was dampened using acoustic signals generated from eye movements as a form of biofeedback.[4,37,121,161] On average, the nystagmus intensity was decreased by 40%, and foveal fixation periods were prolonged by 190%. After training, all patients reported a subjective improvement in vision when suppressing their nystagmus.[161]

Porthole Method

The porthole method consists of a bilateral peripheral occlusion, which gets its name from the similarity of the glasses to the windows on a sailboat.[190] Treatment with this method in 38 cases of congenital nystagmus over 5 years was reported to have a beneficial effect on nystagmus intensity and torticollis.

Afterimage Treatment and Intermittent Photic Stimulation

Developed initially by Hans Goldmann, the afterimage technique consists of presenting congenital nystagmus patients with a bright electronic flash from an isolated source. This makes the patients aware of their movements, allowing them to adapt a head position where they might be "blocked" and improve visual acuity.[212]

With intermittent photic stimulation, a synoptophore slide with a red background intermittently illuminated at a frequency of 3–4 Hz is presented separately to each eye in a series of treatment sessions.[152] This allows constant refinement of the "fixation reflex" with resultant increase in visual acuity.[152]

Botulinum Injection

Botulinum injection into the extraocular muscles has been used to dampen acquired forms of nystagmus.[176,182,216] This treatment has been performed on some patients with congenital nystagmus with dampening of nystagmus amplitude (M.X. Repka, personal communication). Some of the problems encountered included ptosis, diplopia, and limited duration of effect.

Medical

Congenital periodic alternating nystagmus has responded to baclofen in some patients[33,120] but not in others.[107] Other forms of congenital nystagmus may respond to baclofen[239] or 5-hydroxytryptophan.[135]

Surgery: Anderson and Kestenbaum Procedures

In planning a surgical intervention in patients with congenital nystagmus, patients should be divided into two categories as described by Sandall.[186,187] The surgical intervention differs for the two groups. In the first group, patients with single binocular vision, stereopsis and no tropia, require balanced surgery between eyes, usually to correct an abnormal head posture. Patients in the second group have a constant tropia with abnormal head posture. Careful attention should be paid to the fixation behavior of a patient.[77] Surgery is planned on the fixing eye to correct posture and on the fellow eye to correct the tropia.[194] This may be performed in a two-stage surgery[48,69,185] or in a single operation.[31,191,194]

Three basic surgical interventions were described in the 1950s which in effect resulted in a shift of the null zone to primary position: *Kestenbaum,*[130] *Anderson,*[17] and *Goto.*[90] The goal of each surgery is to eliminate abnormal head posture by rotating the eyes in the direction of the head turn and so bring the null point into primary position. Kestenbaum recommended a two-stage surgery to all four horizontal rectus muscles with equal recession/resection on each eye separately. Anderson reasoned that the slow wave driving the eyes off target was the basic defect and usually in a direction opposite the head turn. He advocated large recession of a single horizontal muscle in each eye that was responsible for the slow dominant phase in order to correct the head turn and reduce the intensity of nystagmus.[215] Goto advocated, based on eye movement recordings, the resection and advancement of the muscles responsible for the quick phases of nystagmus.[90]

Since these descriptions there have been many modifications. The *modified Kestenbaum* involves surgery on all four horizontal rectus muscles but at one operation. The *modified Anderson–Kestenbaum* procedure involves surgery on all four muscles with emphasis on agonist muscles, acting in the slow phase. In most instances, the surgery is performed in a single step, but a two-stage procedure with an Anderson procedure performed initially followed by an Anderson–Kestenbaum procedure has been described.[215] Finally, a *monocular recess/resect procedure* may be performed in patients with an estropia who fixate with the eye in adduction in order to correct both head turn and tropia.[40,194]

How much surgery? Controversy has centered on the amount of surgery required to obtain optimal correction. Several authors feel that the medial rectus should not be recessed more than 3 mm[210] to 5 mm.[40,191] For the *modified Kestenbaum,* the amount of surgery commonly performed was the "classic maximum"[31] using the Parks 5-6-7-8 scheme[71,168] in which for a face turn to the right, the surgery would be right medial rectus recession 5 mm, right lateral rectus resection 8 mm, left lateral rectus recession 7 mm and left medial rectus resection 6 mm. However, this may leave patients undercorrected.[193] As such, the Parks 5-6-7-8 scheme was "augmented" for head turns between 25° and 45° by 10% to 40% and up to 60% for a 50° head turn.[31,194] A 40% augmentation for a right head turn would be 7 mm right medial rectus recession, 11 mm right lateral rectus resection, 10 mm left lateral rectus recession, and 8.5 mm left medial rectus resection. Larger augmentations may result in some gaze limitation.[76] As such, some surgeons advocated only recessing the medial rectus 5 mm while augmenting surgery on the other muscles.[186] D'Esposito and colleagues reported a direct relationship between the degrees of null point shift and the combined millimeters of recession and resection. They suggested that 4 mm of surgery on each eye would result in 10° of shift.[63]

Anderson performed bilateral 5 mm recessions.[17] Taylor and Jesse[215] augmented the *Anderson procedure* such that for a right head turn with left slow phase he performed a 6–7 mm right medial rectus recesssion and a 9–10 mm left lateral rectus recession.

Suggested surgery for a *modified Anderson–Kestenbaum* procedure for a right head turn with a dominant slow phase to the left is as follows: right medial rectus recession 6–7 mm, right lateral rectus resection 6 mm, left lateral rectus recession 10 mm, left medial rectus resection 5 mm. Note that in the Kestenbaum procedure the total amount of resection is greater than recession, whereas in the modified Anderson–Kestenbaum procedure, the total amount of recession is greater than the amount of resection.[215]

The choice of surgical intervention will vary with the severity of abnormal head posture, intensity of nystagmus, and binocular visual acuity. For a large head turn one might choose an augmented Kestenbaum. For a small head turn with high-intensity nystagmus, one might choose the Anderson procedure. For a larger head turn with a high-intensity nystagmus, one might choose the modified Anderson–Kestenbaum procedure. Prior to performing augmented surgery one should discuss with the patient which is more important, abnormal head posture or the possibility of postoperative gaze limitation.

Surgical intervention may also be designed to correct abnormal vertical head posture. For severe chin-down posture, bilateral superior rectus recessions of 5–6 mm may be performed along with bilateral inferior myectomies. For severe chin-up posture, bilateral inferior rectus recessions of 5 mm combined with superior oblique tenotomies may be performed.[171] Torsional head posture is uncommon.[203] Finally, with associated horizontal head turns associated with vertical head turns, vertical transposition of the horizontal recti may be performed up or down in the direction of the vertical head turn.[215]

Eye movement recordings have demonstrated that surgery may benefit abnormal head posture by shifting the null to primary positions, broadening the null position, and decreasing nystagmus intensity.[10,48,76] Increasing the time constant of the slow phase, allowing longer fixation, is another potentially beneficial effect of surgery.[28] In patients with single binocular vision and no constant tropia, surgery for head posture may have a satisfactory result (less than 15°) in 70%–80%[132,162,194,215] and an excellent result (less than 5°) in up to a third of cases.[194] For patients with a abnormal head posture combined with a tropia, the results are more favorable for correction of the tropia than correction of both.[194] Monocular surgery corrected both head posture and esotropia in 57% of patients and tropia alone in 71% of patients.[194] Although the beneficial effect of surgery on head position may last as long as 6 years,[10] several investigators have reported a late failure.[31,162,174,194,210] The factors responsible for late failure and its prevention are not known. In addition to the beneficial effect on torticollis, visual acuity may improve 1.5 to 2.5 Snellen lines[48,72,210,215] in up to 61% of patients.[194] Others have reported no improvement.[119,131]

Surgery: Artificial Divergence Surgery and Recession of All Horizontal Muscles

In patients with good binocular function who have responded to treatment with base-out prisms, an "artificial divergence surgery" has been performed in combination with a classic Kestenbaum procedure, with improvement.[195] Favorable results have also been reported in congenital nystagmus patients who underwent large recessions of four horizontal recti leading to decreased nystagmus amplitude and improved vision.[115,225]

REFERENCES

1. Abadi RV, Sandikciopglu M. Visual resolution in congenital pendular nystagmus. *Am J Optom Physiol Opt* 1975;52:573–581.
2. Abadi RV. Visual performance with contact lenses and congenital idiopathic nystagmus. *Br J Physiol Opt* 1979;33:32–37.
3. Abadi RV, King-Smith PE. Congenital nystagmus modifies orientational detection. *Vision Res* 1979;19(12):1409–1411.
4. Abadi RV, Carden D, Simpson J. A new treatment for congenital nystagmus. *Br J Ophthalmol* 1980;64(1):2–6.
5. Abadi RV, Dickinson CM, Lomas MS, Ackerley R. Congenital idiopathic nystagmus in identical twins. *Br J Ophthalmol* 1983; 67(10):693–695.
6. Abadi RV, Dickinson CM. Waveform characteristics in congenital nystagmus. *Doc Ophthalmol* 1986;64(2):153–167.

7. Abadi RV, Pascal E, Whittle J, Worfolk R. Retinal fixation behavior in human albinos. *Optom Vis Sci* 1989;66:276–280.
8. Abadi RV, Worfolk R. Retinal slip velocities in congenital nystagmus. *Vision Res* 1989;29: 195–205.
9. Abadi RV, Whittle J. Nature of head postures in congenital nystagmus. *Arch Ophthalmol* 1991;109(2):216–220.
10. Abadi RV, Whittle J. Surgery and compensatory head postures in congenital nystagmus. A longitudinal study. *Arch Ophthalmol* 1992; 110:632–635.
11. Abadi RV, Pascal E. Ocular motor behavior of monozygotic twins with tyrosinase negative oculocutaneous albinism. *Br J Ophthalmol* 1994;78:349–352.
12. Abadi RV, Pascal E. Periodic alternating nystagmus in humans with albinism. *Invest Ophthalmol Visual Sci* 1994;35:4080–4086.
13. Abel LA, Williams IW, Levi L. Intermittent oscillopsia in a case of congenital nystagmus: Dependence on waveform. *Invest Ophthalmol Visual Sci* 1990;32:3104–3108.
14. Adams RD, Victor M. *Principles of Neurology*, 4th ed. New York: McGraw-Hill, 1989: 978–980.
15. Allen ED, Davies PD. Role of contact lenses in the management of congenital nystagmus. *Br J Ophthalmol* 1983;67(12):834–836.
16. Allen M. Primary hereditary nystagmus: Case study and genealogy. *J Hered* 1942;33: 454–455.
17. Anderson JR. Causes and treatment of congenital eccentric nystagmus. *Br J Ophthalmol* 1953;37:267–281.
18. Antony JH, Ouvrier RA, Wise G. Spasmus nutans. A mistaken identity. *Arch Neurol* 1980;37:373–375.
19. Apkarian P, Shallo-Hoffmann J. VEP projections in congenital nystagmus; VEP asymmetry in albinism: A comparison study. *Invest Ophthalmol Visual Sci* 1991;32:2653–2661.
19a. Azuma N, Nishina S, Yanagisawa H, Okuyama T, Yamada M. PAX6 missense mutations in isolated foveal hypoplasia. *Nature Genet* 1996; 13:141–142.
20. Bedell HE, White JM, Abplanalp PL. Variability of foveations in congenital nystagmus. *Clin Vision Sci* 1989;4:247–252.
21. Bedell HE, Loshin DS. Interrelations between measures of visual acuity and parameters of eye movement in congenital nystagmus. *Invest Ophthalmol Visual Sci* 1991;32:416–421.
22. Bedell HE. Sensitivity to oscillatory target motion in congenital nystagmus. *Invest Ophthalmol Visual Sci* 1992;33:1811–1821.
23. Bedell HE, Currie DC. Extraretinal signals for congenital nystagmus. *Invest Ophthalmol Visual Sci* 1993;34:2325–2332.
24. Bergin DJ, Halpern J. Congenital see-saw nystagmus associated with retinitis pigmentosa. *Ann Ophthalmol* 1986;18(12):346–349.
25. Berry AC, Docherty Z. X-linked nystagmus and 45,X/46,XX mosaicism [letter; comment]. *Am J Med Genet* 1992;43:896–897.
26. Billings ML. Nystagmus through four generations. *J Hered* 1942;33:457.
27. Bixenman WW. Congenital hereditary downbeat nystagmus. *Can J Ophthalmol* 1983; 18(7):344–348.
28. Bosone G, Reccia R, Roberti G, Russo P. On the variations of the time constant of the slow-phase eye movements produced by surgical therapy of congenital nystagmus: a preliminary report. *Ophthalmic Res* 1989;21:345–351.
29. Bosone G, Reccia R, Roberti G, Russo P. Frequency distribution of the time interval between quick phase nystagmic eye movements. *Ophthalmic Res* 1990;22:178–182.
30. Burke JP, West NF, Strachan IM. Congenital nystagmus anisomyopis, and hemimaglencephaly in the Klippel-Trenaunay-Weber syndrome. *J Pediatr Ophthalmol Strabismus* 1991;28:41–44.
31. Calhoun JH, Harley RD. Surgery for abnormal head position in congenital nystagmus. *Trans Am Ophthalmol Soc* 1973;71:70–87.
32. Carl JR, Optican LM, Chu FC, Zee DS. Head shaking and vestibulo-ocular reflex in congenital nystagmus. *Invest Ophthalmol Visual Sci* 1985;26:1043–1050.
33. Carlow TJ. Medical treatment of nystagmus and other ocular motor disorders. *Int Ophthalmol Clin* 1986;26:251–264.
34. Cheong PY, King RA, Bateman JB. Oculocutaneous albinism: Variable expressivity of nystagmus in a sibship. *J Pediatr Ophthalmol Strabismus* 1992;29:185–188.
35. Cibis GW, Fitzgerald KM. Electroretinography in congenital idiopathic nystagmus. *Pediatr Neurol* 1993;9:369–371.
36. Ciccarelli EC, Huttenlocher PR. Diencephalic tumor. A cause of infantile nystagmus and cachexia. *Arch Ophthalmol* 1967;78(3): 350–353.
37. Ciuffreda KJ, Goldrich SG, Neary C. Use of eye movement auditory feedback in the control

of nystagmus. *Am J Optom Physiol Opt* 1982; 59:396–409.

38. Cogan DG. Congenital nystagmus. *Can J Ophthalmol* 1967;2:4–10.
39. Cogan DG, Chu FC, Reingold D, Barranger J. Ocular motor signs in some metabolic diseases. *Arch Ophthalmol* 1981;99:1802–1808.
40. Cooper EL, Sandall GS. Surgical treatment of congenital nystagmus. *Arch Ophthalmol* 1969; 81:473–480.
41. Cox RA. Congenital head-nodding and nystagmus. *Arch Ophthalmol* 1936;15:1032–1036.
42. Creel D, O'Donnell FE Jr, Witkop C Jr. Visual system anomalies in human ocular albinos. *Science* 1978;201:931–933.
43. Creel DJ. Visual system anomaly associated with albinism in the cat. *Nature* 1971;231: 465–466.
44. Davis AE, Maw AR, Coleman M. Acoustic brainstem electrical responses in congenital nystagmus. *J Laryngol Otol* 1985;99(2): 147–150.
45. Dell'Osso LF, Flynn JT, Daroff RB. Hereditary congenital nystagmus. An intrafamilial study. *Arch Ophthalmol* 1974;92:366–374.
46. Dell'Osso LF, Daroff RB. Congenital nystagmus waveforms and foveation strategy. *Doc Ophthalmol* 1975;39:155–182.
47. Dell'Osso LF, Schmidt D, Daroff RB. Latent, manifest latent, and congenital nystagmus. *Arch Ophthalmol* 1979;97:1877–1885.
48. Dell'Osso LF, Flynn JT. Congenital nystagmus surgery: A quantitative evaluation of the effects. *Arch Ophthalmol* 1979;97:462–469.
49. Dell'Osso LF, Ellenberger C Jr, Abel LA, Flynn JT. The nystagmus blockage syndrome. Congenital nystagmus, manifest latent nystagmus, or both? *Invest Ophthalmol Visual Sci* 1983;24(12):1580–1587.
50. Dell'Osso LF. Evaluation of smooth pursuit in the presence of congenital nystagmus. *Neuro-ophthalmology* 1986;6:383–406.
51. Dell'Osso LF, Traccis S, Abel LA, Erzurum SI. Contact lenses and congenital nystagmus. *Clin Vision Sci* 1988;3:229–232.
52. Dell'Osso LF. Eye movements, visual acuity and spatial constancy. *Acta Neurol Belge* 1991;91:105–113.
53. Dell'Osso LF, Leigh RJ, Daroff RB. Suppression of congenital nystagmus by cutaneous stimulation. *Neuro-ophthalmology* 1991;11: 173–175.
54. Dell'Osso LF, Van der Steen J, Steinman RM, Collewijn H. Foveation dynamics in congenital nystagmus I: Fixation. *Doc Ophthalmol* 1992;79:1–23.
55. Dell'Osso LF, Van der Steen J, Steinman RM, Collewijn H. Foveation dynamics in congenital nystagmus II: Smooth pursuit. *Doc Ophthalmol* 1992;79:25–49.
56. Dell'Osso LF, Van der Steen J, Steinman RM, Collewijn H. Foveation dynamics in congenital nystagmus III: Vestibulo-ocular reflex. *Doc Ophthalmol* 1992;79:51–70.
57. Dell'Osso LF, Leigh RJ. Foveation period stability and oscillopsia suppression in congenital nystagmus. An hypothesis. *Neuro-ophthalmology* 1992;12(3):169–183.
58. Dell'Osso LF, Leigh RJ. Ocular motor stability of foveation periods. Required conditions for suppression of oscillopsia. *Neuro-ophthalmology* 1992;12(5):303–326.
59. Dell'Osso LF, Weissman BM, Leigh RJ, Abel LA, Sheth NV. Hereditary congenital nystagmus and gaze holding failure: The role of the neural integrator. *Neurology* 1993;43:1741–1749.
60. Dell'Osso LF. Congenital and latent/manifest latent nystagmus: Diagnosis, treatment, foveation, oscillopsia, and acuity. *Jpn J Ophthalmol* 1994;38:329–336.
61. Dell'Osso LF, Williams RW. Ocular motor abnormalities in achismatic mutant Belgian sheepdogs. Unyoked eye movements in a mammal. *Vision Res* 1995;35:109–116.
62. Demer JL, Zee DS. Vestibulo-ocular and optokinetic defects in albinos with congenital nystagmus. *Invest Ophthalmol Visual Sci* 1984; 25:739–745.
63. D'Esposito M, Reccia R, Roberti G, Russo P. Amount of surgery in congenital nystagmus. *Ophthalmologica* 1989;198:145–151.
64. Dichgans J, Kornhuber HH. Eine seltene Art des hereditäen Nystagmus mit autosomal-daminantem Erbgang und besonderem Erscheinungsbild: Verikale Nystmuskomponete und Störung des vertikalen und horizontalen optokinetischen Nystagmus. *Acta Genet Stat Med* 1964;14:240–250.
65. Dickinson CM. The elucidation and use of the effect of near fixation in congenital nystagmus. *Ophthalmol Physiol Optom* 1986;6:303–311.
66. Dickinson CM, Abadi RV. Corneal topography of humans with congenital nystagmus. *Ophthalmol Physiol Optom* 1984;4(1):3–13.
67. Dudley WH. Consanguinity. A cause of congenital nystagmus. *Arch Ophthalmol* 1908; 34:565–567.

68. Elliot AJ, Simpson EM, Oakhill A, Decock R. Nystagmus after medulloblastoma. *Dev Med Child Neurol* 1989;31(1):43–46.
69. Estes RL, Sandall GS, Martonyi J. Congenital rotary nystagmus associated with head turning—Successful surgical management. *Ophthalmic Surg* 1981;12:834–837.
70. Evans N. The significance of nystagmus. *Eye* 1989;3:816–835.
71. Fells P, Dulley B. Surgical management of compensatory head posture. *Trans Ophthalmol Soc UK* 1976;96:90–95.
71a. Fialkow PJ, Giblett ER, Motulsky AG. Measurable linkage between ocular albinism and Xg. *Am J Hum Genet* 1967;19:63–69.
72. Fielder AR, Russell-Eggitt IR, Dodd KL, Mellor DH. Delayed visual maturation. *Trans Ophthalmol Soc UK* 1985;104:653–661.
73. Fielder AR, Evans NM. Is the geniculostriate system a prerequisite for nystagmus? *Eye* 1988;2:628–635.
74. Fisher PG, Wechsler DS, Singer HS. Anti-Hu antibody in a neuroblastoma-associated paraneoplastic syndrome. *Pediatr Neurol* 1994; 10(4):309–312.
75. Flanders M, Young D. Atypical sensory nystagmus and its surgical management. *Can J Ophthalmol* 1983;18(7):349–351.
76. Elynn JT, Dell'Osso LF. The effects of congenital nystagmus surgery. *Ophthalmology* 1979;86:1414–1425.
77. Flynn JT, Dell'Osso LF. Surgery of congenital nystagmus. *Trans Ophthalmol Soc UK* 1981; 101:431–433.
78. Forssman B. A study of congenital nystagmus. *Acta Otolaryngol* 1964;57:427–449.
79. Forssman B. Vestibular reactivity in cases of congenital nystagmus and blindness. *Acta Otolaryngol* 1964;57:539–555.
80. Forssman B, Ringnér B. Prevalence and inheritance of congenital nystagmus in a Swedish population. *Ann Hum Genet* 1971;35:139–147.
81. Forsythe WT. Congenital hereditary vertical nystagmus. *J Neurol Neurosurg Psychiatry* 1955;18:196–198.
82. Friedman DI, Dell'Osso LF. "Reappearance" of congenital nystagmus after minor head trauma. *Neurology* 1993;43:2414–2416.
83. Funahashi K, Kuwata T, Yabumoto M, Nakai M, Komai N, Ohmi E. Congenital vertical pendular nystagmus in sisters. *Ophthalmologica* 1988;196(3):137–142.
84. Furman JM, Stoyanoff S, Barbere HO. Head and eye movements in congenital nystagmus. *Otolaryngol Head Neck Surg* 1984;92: 656–661.
85. Gelbart SS, Hoyt CS. Congenital nystagmus: A clinical perspective in infancy. *Graefe's Arch Clin Exp Ophthalmol* 1988;226:178–180.
86. Glover PL. Congenital nystagmus. *Arch Ophthalmol* 1937;17:705–706.
87. Goldstein HP, Gottlob I, Fendick MG. Visual remapping in infantile nystagmus. *Vision Res* 1992;32:1115–1124.
88. Golubovic S, Marjanovic S, Cvetkovic D, Manic S. The application of hard contact lenses in patients with congenital nystagmus. *Fortschr Ophthalmol* 1989;86(5):535–539.
89. Good PA, Searle AE, Campbell S, Crews SJ. Value of the ERG in congenital nystagmus. *Br J Ophthalmol* 1989;73:512–515.
90. Goto N. A study of optic nystagmus by electro-oculogram. *Acta Soc Ophthalmol Jpn* 1954; 58:851–865.
91. Gottlob I, Zubcov A, Catalano RA, Reinecke RD, Koller HP, Calhoun JH, Manley R. Signs distinguishing spasmus nutans (with and without central nervous system lesions) from infantile nystagmus. *Ophthalmology* 1990;97(9): 1166–1175.
92. Gottlob I, Zubcov AA, Wizov SS, Reinecke RD. Head nodding is compensatory in spasmus nutans. *Ophthalmology* 1992;99(7):1024–1031.
93. Gottlob I. Eye movement abnormalities in carriers of blue-cone monochromatism. *Invest Ophthalmol Visual Sci* 1994;35(9):3556–3560.
94. Gottlob I, Reinecke RD. Eye and head movements in patients with achromatopsia. *Graefes Arch Clin Exp Ophthalmol* 1994;232(7): 392–401.
95. Gottlob I, Wizov SS, Reinecke RD. Quantitative eye and head movement recordings of retinal diseases mimicking spasmus nutans. *Am J Ophthalmol* 1995;119(3):374–376.
96. Gottlob I, Wizov SS, Reinecke RD. Spasmus nutans. A long-term follow-up. *Invest Ophthalmol Visual Sci* 1995;36(13):2768–2771.
97. Gresty MA, Halmagyi GM, Leech J. The relationship between head and eye movements in congenital nystagmus with head shaking: objective recordings of a single case. *Br J Ophthalmol* 1978;62:533–535.
98. Gresty MA, Halmagyi GM. Abnormal head movements. *J Neurol Neurosurg Psychiatry* 1979;42:705–714.
99. Gresty MA, Helmagyi GM. Head nodding associated with idiopathic childhood nystagmus. *Ann NY Acad Sci* 1981;374:614–618.
100. Gresty M, Page N, Barratt H. The differential diagnosis of congenital nystagmus. *J Neurol Neurosurg Psychiatry* 1984;47:936–942.

101. Gresty MA, Barratt HJ, Page NGR, Ell JJ. Assessment of vestibulo-ocular reflexes in congenital nystagmus. *Ann Neurol* 1985;17:129–136.
102. Gresty MA, Bronstein AM, Page NG, Rudge P. Congenital-type nystagmus emerging in later life. *Neurology* 1991;41:653–656.
103. Guillery RW, Okore AN, Witkop C Jr. Abnormal visual pathways in the brain of a human albino. *Brain Res* 1975;96:373–377.
104. Guo S, Reinecke RD, Fendick M, Calhoun JH. Visual pathway abnormalities in albinism and infantile nystagmus. VECPs and stereoacuity measurements. *J Pediatr Ophthalmol Strabismus* 1989;26:97–104.
105. Gutmann DH, Brooks ML, Emanuel BS, McDonald-McGinn DM, Zachai EH. Congenital nystagmus in a (46,XX/45,X) mosaic woman from a family with X-linked congenital nystagmus. *Am J Med Genet* 1991;39:167–169.
106. Guyer DR, Lessell S. Periodic alternating nystagmus associated with albinism. *J Clin Neuro-Ophthalmol* 1986;6:82–85.
107. Halmagyi GM, Rudge P, Gresty MA, Leigh RJ, Zee DS. Treatment of periodic alternating nystagmus. *Ann Neurol* 1980;8:609–611.
108. Halmagyi GM, Gresty MA, Leech J. Reversed optokinetic nystagmus (OKN): Mechanism and clinical significance. *Ann Neurol* 1980;7:429–435.
109. Hammerstein W, Gebauer HJ. Familial nystagmus and hypoplasia of the macular in a reciprocal, balanced translocation of 5/16. *Fortschr Ophthalmol* 1989;86:718–721.
110. Hara T, Kawazawa S, Abe Y, Hiyoshi M, Mizuki Y, Yamada M. Conjugate pendular nystagmus evoked by accommodative vergence. *Eur Neurol* 1986;25:369–372.
111. Harcourt B. Hereditary nystagmus in early childhood. *J Med Genet* 1970;7:253–256.
112. Harley RD, ed. *Pediatric Ophthalmology*. Philadelphia: W.B. Saunders, 1975:36–56; 463–467.
113. Harris CM. Problems in modelling congenital nystagmus towards a new model. In *Eye Movements Research. Mechanisms, Processes, and Applications*, J.M. Findlay, R. Walker, R.W. Kentridge, eds. Amsterdam: Elsevier, 1995: 239–253.
114. Hayasaka S. Hereditary congenital nystagmus. A Japanese pedigree. *Ophthalmic Paediatr Genet* 1985;7:73–76.
115. Helveston EM, Ellis FD, Plager DA. Large recession of horizontal recti for treatment of nystagmus. *Ophthalmology* 1991;98:1302–1305.
116. Hemmes GD. Hereditary nystagmus. *Am J Ophthalmol* 1927;10:149–150.
117. Hoyt CS, Aicardi E. Acquired monocular nystagmus in monozygotic twins. *J Pediatr Ophthalmol Strabismus* 1979;16(2):115–118.
118. Hoyt CS, Gelbert SS. Vertical nystagmus in infants with congenital ocular abnormalities. *Ophthalmic Paediatr Genet* 1984;4(3):155–161.
119. Hugonnier R. Notre position actuelle sur les operations dirigees contre le nystagmus. *Ann Inst Barraquer* 1974–75;12:327–340.
120. Huygen PLM, Verhagen WIM, Cruysberg JRM, Koch PAM. Familial congenital periodic alternating nystagmus with presumably X-linked dominant inheritance. *Neuro-ophthalmology* 1995;15:149–155.
121. Ishikawa S, Tanakadate A, Nabatame K, Ishii M. Biofeedback treatment of congenital nystagmus. *Neuro-ophthalmol Jpn* 1985; 2:58–64.
122. Jacobson DM, Johnson R, Frens DB. Joubert's syndrome, ocular fibrosis, and normal histidine levels. *Am J Ophthalmol* 1992;113(6):714–716.
123. Jain IS, Pillay P, Gangwar DN, Dhir SP, Kaul VK. Congenital cataract: Etiology and morphology. *J Pediatr Ophthalmol Strabismus* 1983;20(6):238–242.
124. Jin YH, Goldstein HP, Reinecke RD. Absence of visual sampling in infantile nystagmus. *Korean J Ophthalmol* 1989;3:28–32.
125. Joubert M, Eisenring JJ, Robb JP, Andermann F. Familial agenesis of the cerebellar vermis. A syndrome of episodic hyperpnea, abnormal eye movements, ataxia, and retardation. *Neurology* 1969;19;813–825.
126. Kayama T, Yoshimoto T, Shimizu Y. Neonatal medulloblastoma. *J Neuro-oncol* 1993;15(2): 157–163.
127. Kelly BJ, Rosenberg ML, Zee DS, Optician LM. Unilateral pursuit-induced congenital nystagmus. *Neurology* 1989;39:414–416.
128. Kerrison JB, Koenehoop RK, Zee D, Maumenee IH. Clinical features of autosomal dominant nystagmus linked to chromosome 6p12. *Am J Ophthalmol* 1998;125:64–70.
129. Kerrison JB, Arnould VJ, Barmada MM, Koenekoop RK, Maumenee IH. A gene for autosomal dominant congenital nystagmus localizes to 6p12. *Genomics* 1996;33:523–526.
130. Kestenbaum A. Nouvelle operation de nystagmus. *Bull Soc Ophtalmol Fr* 1953;6:599–602.
131. Kommerell G. Nystagmusoperationen zur korrektur verschied ener kofpzwangshaltungen. *Klin Monatsbl Augenheilkd* 1974;164(2): 172–191.

132. Kraft SP, O'Donoghue EP, Roarty JD. Improvement of compensatory head postures after strabismus surgery. *Ophthalmology* 1992; 99:1301–1308.
133. Kurzan R, Büttner U. Smooth pursuit mechanisms in congenital nystagmus. *Neuro-ophthalmology* 1989;9:313–325.
134. Lambert SR, Taylor D, Kriss A. The infant with nystagmus, normal appearing fundi, but abnormal ERG. *Surv Ophthalmol* 1989;34: 173–186.
135. Larmande P, Pautrizel B. Traitment du nystagmus congenital par le 5-hydroxytryptophane. *Nouv Presse Med* 1981;10:3166.
136. Lavery MA, O'Neill JF, Chu FC, Martyn LJ. Acquired nystagmus in early childhood: A presenting sign of intracranial tumor. *Ophthalmology* 1984;91(5):425–453.
137. Lein JN, Stewart CT, Moll FC. Sex-linked hereditary nystagmus. *Pediatrics* 1956;18:214–217.
138. Leigh RJ, Dell'Osso LF, Yaniglos SS, Thurston SE. Oscillopsia, retinal image stabilization and congenital nystagmus. *Invest Ophthalmol Visual Sci* 1988;29:279–282.
139. Leigh RJ, Zee DS. *The Neurology of Eye Movements*, 2nd ed. Philadelphia: F.A. Davis, 1991.
140. Leliever WC, Barber HO. Observations on optokinetic nystagmus in patients with congenital nystagmus. *Otolaryngol Head Neck Surg* 1981; 89:110–116.
141. Levin AV, Seidman DJ, Nelson LB, Jackson LG. Ophthalmic findings in Cornelia de Lange syndrome. *J Pediatr Ophthalmol Strabismus* 1990;27:94–102.
142. Lo CY. Brain computed tomographic evaluation of noncomitant strabismus and congenital nystagmus. In *ACTA: 24th International Congress of Ophthalmology*, vol. 2, P. Henkind, ed. Philadelphia: Lippincott, 1982:924–928.
143. Lo Cy. Brain lesions in congenital nystagmus as detected by computed tomography. *Jpn J Clin Ophthalmol* 1982;36:871–877.
144. Loshin DS, Browning RA. Contrast sensitivity in albinotic patients. *Am J Optom Physiol Opt* 1983;60:158.
145. Low LB, Stephenson JB, Bartlett K, Seakins JW, Shaikh SA. Biotin-reversible neurodegenerative disease in infancy. *Aust Paediatr J* 1986;22:65–68.
146. Lowry RB, Wood BJ. Syndrome of epiphyseal dysplasia, short stature, microcephaly and nystagmus. *Clin Genet* 1975;8:269–274.
147. Lowry RB, Wood BJ, Cox TA, Hayden MR. Epiphyseal dysplasia, short stature, microcephaly, nystagmus, and retinitis pigmentosa. *Am J Med Genet* 1989;33:341–345.
148. Lu JH, Mielke R, Le TP, Emons D, Kowalski S. Shizenzephalie. *Klin Pediatr* 1990;202: 106–108.
149. Lund RD. Uncrossed visual pathways of hooded and albino rats. *Science* 1965;149:1506.
150. Lyons MK, Kelly PJ. Posterior fossa ependymomas: A report of 30 cases and review of the literature. *Neurosurgery* 1991;28(5):659–664.
151. Magee LA, Downar E, Semar M, Boulton BC, Allen LC, Koren G. Pregnancy outcome after gestational exposure to amiodarone in Canada. *Am J Obstet Gynecol* 1995;172:1307–1311.
152. Mallett RFJ. The treatment of congenital idiopathic nystagmus by intermittent photic stimulation. *Ophthalmol Physiol Optom* 1983;3(3): 341–356.
153. Marmor MF. Hereditary vertical nystagmus. *Arch Ophthalmol* 1973;90:107–111.
154. McCarty JW, Demer JL, Hovis LA, Nuwer MR. Ocular motility anomalies in developmental misdirection of the optic chiasm. *Am J Ophthalmol* 1992;113:86–95.
155. McKusick V. *Mendelian Inheritance in Man: A Catalogue of Human Genes and Genetic Disorders*, 11th ed. Baltimore: Johns Hopkins University Press, 1994:1036, 2082, 2496. World Wide Web URL: http://www3.ncbi.nlm.nih.gov/omim/
156. Mencucci R, Domenici-Lombardo L, Cortesini L, Faussone-Pellegrini MS, Salvi G. Congenital nystagmus: Fine structure of human extraocular muscles. *Ophthalmologica* 1995: 209:1–6.
157. Meienberg O, Hemphill G, Rosenberg M, Hoyt WF. Visual evoked response asymmetries in a family with congenital nystagmus. Possible evidence of abnormal visual projections. *Arch Neurol* 1980;37:697–699.
158. Merrild U, Berggreen S, Hansen L, Mikkelsen M, Henningsen K. Partial deletion of the short arm of chromosome 3. *Eur J Pediatr* 1981; 1365(2):211–216.
159. Metz HS, Jampolsky A, O'Meara DM. Congenital ocular motor nystagmus and nystagmoid head movements. *Am J Ophthalmol* 1972; 74:1131–1133.
160. Metzger EL. Correction of congenital nystagmus. *Am J Ophthalmol* 1950;33:1796–1797.
161. Mezawa M, Ishikawa S, Ukai K. Changes in waveform of congenital nystagmus associated

with biofeedback treatment. *Br J Ophthalmol* 1990;74:472–476.

162. Mitchell PR, Wheeler MB, Parks M. Kestenbaum surgical procedure for torticollis secondary to congenital nystagmus. *J Pediatr Ophthalmol Strabismus* 1987;24:87–93.
163. Nettleship E. On some cases of hereditary nystagmus. *Trans Ophthalmol Soc UK* 1911; 31:159–209.
164. Neuhäuser G, Daly RF, Magnelli NC, Barreras RF, Donaldson RM Jr, Opitz JM. Essential tremor, nystagmus, and duodenal ulcer. A "new" dominantly inherited condition. *Clin Genet* 1976;9:81–91.
165. Norn MS. Congenital nystagmus. Incidence and occupational prognosis. *Acta Ophthalmol* 1964;42:889–896.
166. Ong E, Ciuffreda KJ, Tannen B. Static accommodation in congenital nystagmus. *Invest Ophthalmol Vis Sci* 1993;34:194–204.
167. Optican LM, Zee DS. A hypothetical explanation of congenital nystagmus. *Biol Cybernet* 1984;50(2):119–134.
168. Parks MM. Congenital nystagmus surgery. *Am Othop J* 1973;23:35–39.
169. Patton MA, Jeffery S, Lee N, Hogg C. Congenital nystagmus cosegregating with a balanced 7;15 translocation. *J Med Genet* 1993;30: 526–528.
170. Pearce WG. Congenital nystagmus: Genetic and environmental causes. *Can J Ophthalmol* 1978;13:1–9.
171. Pierse D. Operation on the vertical muscles in cases of nystagmus. *Br J Ophthalmol* 1959; 43:230–233.
172. Pilarski RT, Pauli RM, Bresnick GH, Lebovitz RM. Karsch-Neugebauer syndrome: Split foot/split hand and congenital nystagmus. *Clin Genet* 1985;27(1):97–101.
173. Pratt-Johnson JA. The surgery of congenital nystagmus. *Can J Ophthalmol* 1971;6:268–272.
174. Pratt-Johnson JA. Results of surgery to modify the null-position in congenital nystagmus. *Can J Ophthalmol* 1991;26:219–223.
175. Repka MX. Common pediatric neuro-ophthalmological conditions. *Pediatr Clin N Am* 1993; 40(4):777–788.
176. Repka MX, Savino PJ, Reinecke RD. Treatment of acquired nystagmus with botulinum neurotoxin A. *Arch Ophthalmol* 1994;112: 1320–1324.
177. Reinecke RD, Suqin G, Goldstein HP. Waveform evolution in infantile nystagmus: An Electro-oculographic study of 35 cases. *Binoc Vis* 1988;3:191–202.
178. Robb RM, Petersen RA. Outcome of treatment for bilateral congenital cataracts. *Ophthalmic Surg* 1991;23(10):650–656.
179. Robinson DA. The mechanism of human saccadic eye movement. *J Physiol (Lond)* 1964; 174:245–264.
180. Rosenblum SF, Rosenblum JA. Sex linked hereditary nystagmus. *Metab Pediatr Syst Ophthalmol* 1987;10(4):103–106.
181. Roy FH. *Ocular Differential Diagnosis*, 5th ed. Philadelphia: Lea & Febiger, 1993:173–178.
182. Ruben ST, Lee JP, O'Neil D, Dunlop I, Elston JS. The use of botulinum toxin for treatment of acquired nystagmus and oscillopsia. *Ophthalmology* 1994;101:783–787.
183. Rücker CW. Hereditary nystagmus occurring as a sex-linked character recessive in the female. *Am J Ophthalmol* 1946;29:1534–1541.
184. Safran AB, Gambazzi Y. Congenital nystagmus: Rebound phenomenon following removal of contact lenses. *Br J Ophthalmol* 1992;76: 497–498.
185. Sandall GS, Cooper EL. Surgical treatment of congenital jerk-type nystagmus: Its cause and effect on heterotropia. *Doc Ophthalmol* 1973; 34:361–364.
186. Sandall GS. Surgical treatment of congenital nystagmus in patients with single binocular vision. *Ann Ophthalmol* 1976;8:227–238.
187. Sandall GS. Nystagmus surgery. *Int Ophthalmol Clin* 1976;16:191–196.
188. Sandok BA, Kranz H. Opsoclonus as the initial manifestation of occult neuroblastoma. *Arch Ophthalmol* 1971;86(2):235–236.
189. Saraiva JM, Baraitser M. Joubert syndrome. A review. *Am J Med Genet* 1992;43:726–731.
190. Sasso B. La methode des hublots dans le traitement du nystagmus congenital. *J Fr Ophtalmol* 1986;9(12):848–854.
191. Schlossman A. Nystagmus with strabismus. Surgical management. *Trans Am Acad Ophthalmol Otol* 1972;76:1479–1486.
192. Schneiderman LJ, Bartnof HS, Worthen DM. X-linked congenital nystagmus: A problem in genetic counseling. *Ann Ophthalmol* 1976;8: 444–446.
193. Scott WE, Clarke WN. Surgical treatment of congenital nystagmus. In *Current Concepts in Ophthalmology*, vol. IV. F.C. Blodi, ed. St Louis: C.V. Mosby, 1974:367–370.
194. Scott WE, Kraft SP. Surgical treatment of compensatory head position in congenital nystag-

mus. *J Pediatr Ophthalmol Strabismus* 1984; 21:85–95.

195. Sendler S, Shallo-Hoffmann J, Muhlendyck H. Artificial divergence surgery in congenital nystagmus. *Fortschr Ophthalmol* 1990;87:85–89.
196. Shallo-Hoffmann J, Watermeier D, Petersen J, Mühlendyck H. Electronystagmographic characterization of congenital nystagmus. In *Twenty-Second International Symposium on Strabismus. Congenital Disorders of Ocular Motility,* C de Molina, ed. Barcelona: Editorial JMS, 1989:179–190.
197. Shallo-Hoffmann J, Apkarian P. Visual evoked response asymmetry only in the albino member of a family with congenital nystagmus. *Invest Ophthalmol Visual Sci* 1993;34:682–689.
198. Shapiro MB, France TD. The ocular features of Down's syndrome. *Am J Ophthalmol* 1985; 99(6):659–663.
199. Sharpe JA, Hoyt WF, Rosenberg MA. Convergence-evoked nystagmus. Congenital and acquired forms. *Arch Neurol* 1975;32:191–194.
200. Sheffer RN, Zlotogora J, Elpeleg ON, Paz J, Ben-Ezra D. Behr's syndrome and 3-methylglutaconic acid. *Am J Ophthalmol* 1992;114: 494–497.
201. Shibaski H, Yamashita Y, Motomura S. Suppression of congenital nystagmus. *J Neurol Neurosurg Psychiatry* 1978;41(12):1078–1083.
202. Shulman JD, Crawford JD. Congenital nystagmus and hypothyroidism. *N Engl J Med* 1969;280:708–710.
203. Sigal MB, Diamond GR. Survey of management strategies for nystagmus patients with vertical or torsional head posture. *Ann Ophthalmol* 1990;22;134–138.
204. Simon JW, Kandel GL, Krohel GB, Nelsen PT. Albinotic characteristics in congenital nystagmus. *Am J Ophthalmol* 1984;97:320–327.
205. Smith RA, Gardner-Medwin D. Orofaciodigital syndrome type III in two sibs. *J Med Genet* 1993;30(10):870–872.
206. Sogg RL, Hoyt WF. Intermittent vertical nystagmus in a father and son. *Arch Ophthalmol* 1962;68:515–517.
207. Speilmann A. Blocking convergence, nystagmus blocking syndrome, monocular adduction in infantile esodeviations. In *IInd International Symposium on Strabismus. Congenital Disorders of Ocular Motility,* C. de Molina, ed. Barcelona: Editorial JMS, 1989:195–202.
208. Spierer A. Etiology of reduced visual acuity in congenital nystagmus. *Ann Ophthalmol* 1991; 23:393–397.
209. Spooner SN, Bateman JB, Yee RD. Congenital nystagamus in identical twins: Discordant features. *J Pediatr Ophthalmol Strabismus* 1983; 23(3):115–119.
210. Sternberg-Raab A. Anderson-Kestenbaum operation for assymetric gaze nystagmus. *Br J Ophthalmol* 1963;47:339–345.
211. Stewart-Brown SL, Haslum MN. Partial sight and blindness in children of the 1970 birth cohort at 10 years of age. *J Epidemiol Commun Health* 1988;42:17–23.
212. Stohler T. Afterimage treatment in nystagmus. *Am Orthop J* 1973;23:65–67.
213. Strautnieks S, Rutland P, Winter RM, Baraitser M, Malcolm S. Pelizaeus-Merzbacher disease: Detection of mutations thr181-to-pro and leu223-to-pro in the proteolipid protein gene, and prenatal diagnosis. *Am J Hum Genet* 1992;51:871–878.
214. Sugarman GI, Katakia M, Menkes J. See-saw winking in familial oral-facio digital syndrome. *Clin Genet* 1971;2:248–254.
215. Taylor JN, Jesse K. Surgical management of congenital nystagmus. *Aust NZ J Ophthalmol* 1987;15:25–34.
216. Tomsak RL, Remler BF, Averbuch-Heller L, Chandran M, Leigh RJ. Unsatisfactory treatment of acquired nystagmus with retrobulbar injection of botulinum toxin. *Am J Ophthalmol* 1995;199:489–496.
217. Tusa RJ, Repka MX, Smith CB, Herdman SJ. Early visual deprivation results in persistent strabismus and nystagmus in monkeys. *Invest Ophthalmol Visual Sci* 1991;32(1):134–141.
218. Tusa RJ, Zee DS, Hain TC, Simonsz HJ. Voluntary control of congenital nystagmus. *Clin Vision Sci* 1992;7:195–210.
219. Traccis S, Rosati G, Aiello I, Monaco MF, Loffredo P, Puliga MV, Pirastru MI, Agnetti V. Upbeat nystagmus as an early sign of cerebellar astrocytoma. *J Neurol* 1989;236(6):359–360.
220. Trobe JD, Sharpe JA, Hirsh DK, Gebarski SS. Nystagmus of Pelizaeus-Merzbacher disease. A magnetic search-coil study. *Arch Neurol* 1991;48(1):87–91.
221. Ukwade MT, Bedell HE. Variation of congenital nystagmus with viewing distance. *Optom Vision Sci* 1992;69:976–985.
222. Van Hof-van Duin J, Mohn G. Optokinetic and spontaneous nystagmus in children with neurologic disorders. *Behav Brain Res* 1983; 10(1):163–175.
223. von Noorden GK, La Roche R. Visual acuity and motor characteristics in congenital nystagmus. *Am J Ophthalmol* 1983;95(6):748–751.

224. von Noorden GK, Munoz M, Wong SY. Compensatory mechanisms in congenital nystagmus. *Am J Ophthalmol* 1987;104:387–397.
225. von Noorden GK, Sprunger DT. Large rectus muscle recessions for the treatment of congenital nystagmus. *Arch Ophthalmol* 1991;109: 221–224.
226. Waggoner RW, Boyd D. Sex-linked hereditary nystagmus. *Am J Ophthalmol* 1942;25:177–180.
227. Wagner RS, Caputo AR, Reynolds RD. Nystagmus in Down's syndrome. *Ophthalmology* 1990;97(11):1439–1444.
228. Wang PJ, Chen RL, Shen YZ. Hypotonia, congenital nystagmus, and abnormal auditory brainstem response. *Pediatr Neurol* 1989;5: 381–383.
229. Waugh SJ, Bedell HE. Sensitivity to temporal luminance modulation in congenital nystagmus. *Invest Ophthalmol Visual Sci* 1992;33: 2316–2324.
230. Waardenburg PJ. *Genetics and Opthalmology,* vol. 2. Springfield, IL: Charles C Thomas, 1963:1036–1060.
231. Weiss AH, Biersdorf WR. Visual sensory disorders in congenital nystagmus. *Ophthalmology* 1989;96:517–523.
232. Wheeler PG, Dobyns WB, Plager DA, Ellis FD. Familial remitting chorea, nystagmus, and cataracts. *Am J Med Genet* 1993;47:1215–1217.
233. Yagasaki T, Sato M, Awaya S, Nakamura N. Changes in nystagmus after simultaneous surgery for bilateral congenital cataracts. *Jpn J Ophthalmol* 1993;37:330–338.
234. Yamamoto T, Tohyama J, Koeda T, Maegaki Y, Takahashi Y. Multiple epiphyseal dysplasia with small head congenital nystagmus, hypoplasia of corpus callosum, and leukonychia totalis—A variant of Lowry-Wood syndrome. *Am J Med Genet* 1995;56:6–9.
235. Yee RD, Wong EK, Baloh RW, Honrubia V. A study of congenital nystagmus: Waveforms. *Neurology* 1976;26:326–333.
236. Yee RD, Baloh RW, Honrubia V. A study of congenital nystagmus. Optokinetic nystagmus. *Br J Ophthalmol* 1980;64:926–932.
237. Yee RD, Baloh RW, Honrubia V. Eye movement abnormalities in rod monochromacy. *Ophthalmology* 1981;88(10):1010–1018.
238. Yee RD, Baloh RW, Honrubia V, Kim YS. A study of congenital nystagmus. Vestibular nystagmus. *J Otolaryngol* 1981;10:89–98.
239. Yee RD, Baloh RW, Honrubia V. Effect of baclofen on congenital nystagmus. In *Functional Basis of Ocular Motility Disorders,* G. Lennerstrand, D.S. Zee, E.L. Keller, eds. Oxford: Pergamon Press, 1982:151–158.
240. Zelt RP, Biglan AW. Congenital seesaw nystagmus. *J Pediatr Ophthalmol Strabismus* 1955;22(1):13–16.

29

Blepharoptosis

SUSHANT K. SINHA
KENT W. SMALL

Blepharoptosis refers to drooping of the upper eyelid. The difference in the height of the lid fissures with the eyes in primary position signifies the amount of ptosis. The upper lid normally covers approximately 2 mm of the superior part of the cornea. Unilateral or bilateral ptosis is mild if the eyelid covers up to an additional 2 mm of cornea; it is moderate if the lid covers 3 mm and severe if 6 mm or more of the superior cornea are obscured.[20]

CLASSIFICATION

Ptosis has traditionally been divided into congenital and acquired types. Congenital forms include (*1*) simple isolated ptosis, (*2*) ptosis associated with malformation of the lids, such as the blepharophimosis syndrome (BPES), (*3*) ptosis associated with abnormal extraocular motility, as in congenital fibrosis of the extraocular muscles (CFEOM), (*4*) synkinetic ptosis in the Marcus-Gunn jaw-winking syndrome, and (*5*) ptosis associated with a craniofacial disorder such as Treacher Collins syndrome or fetal alcohol syndrome.

Acquired ptosis can be classified into the following four groups based on etiology: (*1*) traumatic, (*2*) mechanical, (*3*) neurogenic, as in Horner syndrome or myasthenia gravis, and (*4*) myogenic, as in oculopharyngeal muscular dystrophy or the mitochondrial myopathies.[15,52]

In this chapter we review the main genetic disorders that feature ptosis as a major diagnostic criterion, including, in the congenital group, simple isolated ptosis, BPES, Treacher Collins syndrome, fetal alcohol syndrome, and CFEOM, and in the acquired group, the mitochondrial myopathies and oculopharyngeal muscular dystrophy. Some of these diseases are also covered in other chapters.

PERTINENT ANATOMY OF THE UPPER EYELID

The levator palpebrae superioris muscle, supplied by the third cranial nerve, is the primary elevator of the upper lid. Secondary elevators are Müller's muscle, supplied by sympathetic fibers, and frontalis muscle. Embryologically, the levator develops at a later time than the other extraocular muscles from the medial side of the superior rectus, in the third month of gestation. It reaches its final position in the 75 mm stage or fourth fetal month.[124] The levator arises at the orbital apex from the lesser wing of the sphenoid above the annulus of Zinn and runs forward in the orbit dividing into two layers at Whitnall's ligament.

The upper layer, the aponeurosis, passes downward and forward, fanning out to insert into the anterior surface of the tarsus, the adjacent orbicularis muscle, and the overlying skin. This determines the position of the upper eyelid crease. The lower layer, Müller's muscle, inserts into the upper border of the tarsal plate and conjunctiva. The aponeurosis and Müller's muscle are intimately attached. The aponeurosis blends with the orbital septum at varying heights to influence the height of the eyelid crease.[18,109]

CONGENITAL PTOSIS

Simple Isolated Ptosis

Simple isolated ptosis is a subtype of congenital ptosis. Congenital ptosis is usually noted at birth or very early in infancy and may be unilateral or bilateral. There is little change in either the amount of ptosis or the function of the levator muscle with advancing age.[3,161] Patients frequently have amblyopia, anisometropia, astigmatism, strabismus, and abnormalities of eye movement. Ophthalmological examination is therefore indicated in the first year of life,[6,65,112,154,168] and surgery is recommended between the ages of 3.5 and 6 years, unless the drooping of the lid is so severe that the visual axis is occluded and the patient cannot compensate by tilting the head back; in this case, early surgery is indicated.[36,168]

The isolated muscular dystrophy causes inelasticity and fibrosis preventing both elevation and complete relaxation of the muscle, resulting in lid lag and possibly lagophthalmos. The ptosis may be mild, moderate, or severe, and the lid crease may be absent.[72]

The first recorded histological examination of the levator from patients with congenital ptosis was performed in 1987. Light and electron microscopic studies of the levator palpebrae in patients with congenital ptosis show a direct correlation between the number of striated muscle fibers and the degree of ptosis and levator function.[18,72,101] In Berke's[18] report, some normal-appearing striated fibers were found in 100% of patients with congenital ptosis of 2 mm or less, in 54% of patients with ptosis of 3 mm, and in none of those patients with ptosis of 4 mm or more. These findings suggest that congenital ptosis is due to poor development of the levator palpebrae muscle and hence has a myogenic basis.[72]

In most instances, the family history is negative for ptosis.[111] A few large pedigrees of congenital ptosis, however, have been reported where the trait follows an autosomal dominant pattern of inheritance.[23,33] Penetrance is estimated to be 60%.[53] Vestal et al.[169] presented a case of monozygotic twins with concordance for unilateral congenital ptosis, and summarized prior monozygotic and dizygotic twin data. He used Holzinger's formula for the heritability index: $HI = (C(mz) - C(dz))/(100 - C(dz))$, where C is the percent concordance for monozygotic (mz) or dizygotic (dz) twins. HI varies from 0 to 1, with hereditary influence being greater as the value approaches unity. Using all available twin data for unilateral and bilateral congenital ptosis, Vestal et al.[169] obtained a value for C(mz) of 75% and a value for C(dz) of 0. The calculated value for the heritability index, HI, for congenital ptosis was therefore 0.75, suggesting a strong hereditary influence contributing to the development of congenital ptosis. No specific genetic defect has yet been isolated and the precise mechanism remains unknown.

Blepharophimosis Syndrome

Clinical Findings

The three major features of blepharophimosis syndrome (BPES) tend to accentuate one another. Their total effect is to constrict the palpebral fissure by reducing it in both height and width (Fig. 29.1)[96] The three components of the syndrome are (*1*) blepharophimosis, or reduction of the palpebral fissure in the horizontal axis (normal horizontal fissure width in adults is 25–30 mm versus 20–22 mm in this condition),[86] (*2*) ptosis of the upper eyelids that causes a vertical narrowing of the palpebral fissure, and (*3*) epicanthus inversus, which is a fold of skin that arises from the lower lid and extends upward and inward to a point slightly above the inner canthus. In most patients, there is an increased length of the medial canthal ligament resulting in widening of the intercan-

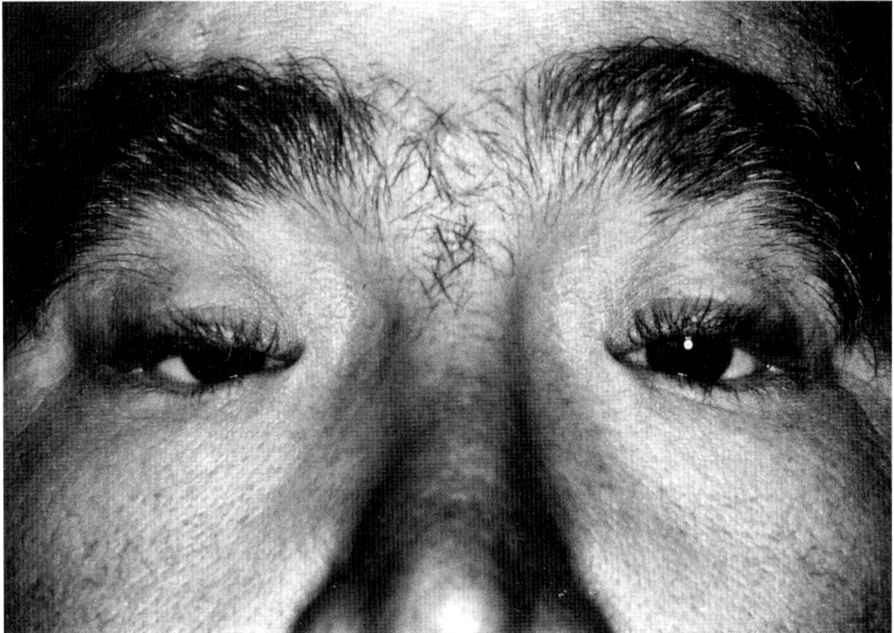

Figure 29.1. Man with the blepharophimosis syndrome. There is bilateral ptosis, horizontal narrowing of the palpebral fissures or blepharophimosis, epicanthus inversus, and telecanthus.

thal distance, or telecanthus. The interpupillary distance remains unchanged. Unlike other types of epicanthus, epicanthus inversus improves very little with age.

To compensate for the ptosis, patients assume a characteristic head posture with chin elevation and furrowing of the eyebrows in order to see under the ptotic lids. Unlike other types of epicanthus, epicanthus inversus improves very little with age. The outer canthal distance is often normal.[87] Only in extreme cases are the medial orbital walls abnormally separated but without true hypertelorism.[85] Eyebrow width is vertically increased and the brows seem to be placed abnormally high on the forehead. This has been attributed to a stretching of the hair-bearing skin from constant contraction of the frontalis muscle to allow vision[128] but may represent a congenital malformation of the brow. The upper eyelid margin is characteristically S shaped while the lower eyelid margin has an abnormal downward concavity, especially laterally, with or without a slight ectropion.[58,85,87,98,133] The eyelids are smooth and inelastic with skin deficiency in both the upper and lower lids.[61,87,104,108,128,167] There is often hypoplasia of the tarsal plates of the upper eyelids.[86,133] Many authors have reported lateral displacement of upper and lower lacrimal puncta, even more than would be expected from the lateral displacement of the medial canthi.[58,76,85,130,167] Other adnexal findings include trichiasis,[78,153] and a hypoplastic appearance of the caruncle and plica semilunaris.[96]

Associated Findings

Additional ophthalmologic, craniofacial, and systemic anomalies are found in both sporadic and familial cases. Occasional ocular findings include microphthalmos,[51,73] anophthalmos,[130] microcornea,[130] cataract,[56] hypermetropia,[87] trabecular dysgenesis,[29] optic disc coloboma,[96] optic nerve hypoplasia,[29] optic atrophy,[4] divergent strabismus and nystagmus,[113,171] superior rectus muscle underaction with limitation of upgaze,[87,108] and poor function of the levator palpebrae superiors and amblyopia.[14]

Patients may have abnormal craniofacial findings such as lop ears (overhanging helix),[87] protruding ears,[96] low-set ears,[4,110] flat, broad nasal bridge,[104,108] bony deficiency of the supraorbital rim and brow with an absent nasoglabellar angle,[104] high arched palate,[78,133] and cleft palate.[110]

Other reported systemic abnormalities include ventricular septal defects,[4,5,16,73,110] polythelia,[178] brachydactyly,[178] muscular hypotonia,[84] cryptorchidism,[32] pectus carinatum,[177] and developmental delay.[32,73] Mental status is usually normal, but some develop secondary psychological problems because of their cosmetic appearance.[86,128]

Surgical correction is usually undertaken between the ages of 3 and 5 years to minimize the psychological problems associated with schooling and to decrease the visual problems associated with blepharophimosis and ptosis. Many surgical techniques have been described that involve initial canthal surgery to improve the blepharophimosis, followed at a later time by ptosis correction.[76,86,153] More recently, one stage operations have been suggested.[92,125]

The association of BPES and female infertility with primary amenorrhea, secondary amenorrhea, or menstrual irregularity[89,119,150,165] led Smith et al.[150] to suggest that BPES may be a contiguous gene disorder resulting from a microdeletion of two or more adjacent or closely linked loci.

Genetics

Several reports of sporadic cases of blepharophimosis and deletions[4,5,54–56,80,84,110,129,177,179] and balanced translocations[21,38,39,57] involving 3q2 have led to the probable localization of the BPES gene to 3q2. Small et al.[149] studied two families with BPES for linkage with 17 polymorphic markers on 3q. Multipoint analysis generated a maximum lod score of 3.23 using the markers RHO, ACPP, and D3S1238. This provided the first noncytogenetic evidence that the gene for the BPES is located on 3q22.[149] Genetic heterogeneity was not observed in this study. At the present time, there are no obvious candidate genes in the BPES region.

Treacher Collins Syndrome

Treacher Collins syndrome (TCOF), also known as mandibulofacial dysostosis (MFD), is a rare autosomal dominant disorder of craniofacial development involving the first and second branchial arches and the first branchial cleft and pouch.[11,141] First described by Thomson[163] in 1846, the syndrome was later named after Treacher Collins, who presented two cases in 1900.[34] Ptosis occurs in 25% (6/24 cases)[67] to 43% (6/14 cases)[174] of patients.

Clinical abnormalities are usually bilateral and symmetrical and include downward slanting of the palpebral fissures, malar and mandibular hypoplasia, hypoplasia or aplasia of the zygomatic arch, malocclusion, hypoplastic supraorbital ridges, temporal lower eyelid coloboma with a paucity of lashes and meibomian glands medially,[66] malformation of the auricle and atresia of the external auditory canals and maldevelopment of the middle ear ossicles, conductive hearing loss, high arched or cleft palate, blind fistula between the angles of the mouth and the ears, flattening of the nasofrontal angle, and projection of scalp hair onto the lateral cheek.[88]

The ocular features of TCOF include blepharoptosis,[67,174] hypoplastic orbicularis oculi muscle, absent lacrimal puncti, absent or hypoplastic tarsal plate,[155] absent or loose and malpositioned lateral canthal tendons,[10,12,175] hyperteloric orbits,[97] ectopia of the pupils, convergent strabismus,[139] and occasional microphthalmia and cataracts.[50]

Other associated features include macrostomia, temporomandibular malarticulation,[78] absence or hypoplasia of the parotid glands, choanal atresia, underdeveloped epiglottis, cardiac anomalies, minor skeletal anomalies, and marked pharyngeal hypoplasia.[139,147]

Reconstructive surgery is aimed at correcting the colobomas, reconstructing the zygomas and the zygomatic arches, reestablishing normal dental occlusion if necessary, harmonizing the profile and the proportional relationship between the different areas of the face, repairing auricular malformations, and correcting the macrostomia.[138]

The incidence of TCOF is approximately 1/50,000 live births,[49] with 50%–60% of cases arising from new mutations.[139] More than 400 cases have been published,[62] with patients reported from all races and nationalities.[139] Penetrance of the trait is almost complete,[151] but the variable expression of the gene[94] makes diagnosis and genetic counseling difficult.

The location of the TCOF locus was first suggested by a case report of a patient with Treacher Collins syndrome and a de novo balanced translocation involving chromosomes 5 and 11, t(5;11)(q11;p11).[13] The gene was later mapped to the distal long arm of chromosome 5 (5q32-33.1) by linkage analysis in informative families.[42,43,81–83] All 43 families studied have supported genetic homogeneity. Multipoint linkage analysis and resolution hybrid mapping have placed the TCOF1 locus in a 2.1 cM interval between d5S519 and SPARC. ANX6, which encodes an intracellular binding protein, lies within the TCOF critical region and is being assessed as a potential candidate for the mutated gene.[41,106] The TCOF critical region has been cloned on yeast artificial chromosomes and a detailed physical map of the region has been created.[41] The candidate gene approach and positional cloning strategies combined with genetic studies should lead to the identification of the disease-causing gene.[45]

The linkage data permit first trimester prenatal DNA diagnosis and enables diagnostic predictions in certain mildly affected and apparently unaffected individuals.[44]

Congenital Fibrosis of the Extraocular Muscles

Congenital fibrosis of the extraocular muscles (CFEOM) is a rare autosomal dominant disorder characterized by bilateral ptosis and external ophthalmoplegia.[35,47,63,68,74,127] The disorder appears to have complete penetrance.[47] CFEOM encompasses a number of different clinical entities that could be classified under the following headings: (*1*) generalized fibrosis syndrome, (*2*) congenital fibrosis of the inferior rectus with blepharoptosis, (*3*) strabismus fixus, (*4*) vertical retraction syndrome, and (*5*) congenital unilateral fibrosis, enophthalmos, and blepharoptosis. Another subtype of congenital fibrosis of the vertically acting extraocular muscles has recently been proposed.[60]

Generalized fibrosis syndrome is the most severe type and is the subject of the remainder of this section. Other names given to this disorder include congenital static ophthalmoplegia, familial musculofascial anomaly, familial ophthalmoplegia with cocontraction, congenital ophthalmoplegia, abiotrophic ophthalmoplegia imperfecta, hereditary congenital ophthalmoplegia, and ophthalmoplegia congenita.[68,74]

Laughlin[100] presented six familial and sporadic cases of this disorder and described the following features: (*1*) fibrosis of all extraocular muscles, (*2*) fibrosis of Tenon's capsule, (*3*) adhesions between muscles, Tenon's capsule, and globe, (*4*) inelasticity and fragility of the conjunctiva, (*5*) no elevation or depression of either eye, (*6*) little or no horizontal movement of the eye, (*7*) both eyes fixed in a downward gaze 20°–30° below the horizontal, (*8*) bilateral blepharoptosis, and (*9*) head tilted backward with the chin elevated.

Additional ophthalmologic abnormalities in familial and sporadic cases include anomalous extraocular muscle insertion on the globe,[9] no levator function,[35] compensatory contraction of the frontalis muscle,[63] no binocular vision,[35] restricted movement of the globes on forced ductions,[9,68] bilateral jerky convergent movements when the patient attempts to look up,[35] intermittent spontaneous convergence,[63] rotary nystagmus,[9,63] strabismus,[35,64,68,74] reduced visual acuity,[35,64,68,74] significant refractive errors,[68] amblyopia,[64,68] and astigmatism.[35,64,74]

Rarely have patients been reported with CFEOM and Marcus-Gunn jaw wink,[24] ventricular septal defect,[63] choroidal coloboma and secondary fibrous bands,[25] bilateral optic disc hypoplasia,[64] bilateral inguinal hernias,[9] cryptorchidism,[9] Prader-Willi syndrome,[90] and Joubert syndrome with histidinemia.[8]

Histopathological studies of extraocular muscles have demonstrated replacement of muscle tissue by fibroblasts[35,63] and parallel bundles of hyalinized collagen enclosed in dense fibrous tissue with no visualization of normal muscle tissue.[100] Apt[9] described multiple dense bands of connective tissue. He observed areas of normal striated muscle in several cases. The muscle tissue was enveloped by a thickened and fibrotic capsule. The intermuscular septum was thickened and fibrotic in all cases. Muscle fibers were present either in tight bundles or in loose ones surrounded by a delicate fibroelastic network. The areas of muscle infiltrated by fibrous tissue lacked the normal fiber orientation and often blended with a fibrotic Tenon's capsule. Apt[9] did not observe any inflammatory infiltrate.

Computed tomography shows asymmetric extraocular muscle atrophy and is helpful in confirming the diagnosis of this condition.[77,176]

Surgery on the ptosis and release of the tight inferior rectus muscles relieve the uncomfortable and fatiguing chin-up head positions.[35] Nemet et al.[127] advised early surgical repair to prevent bilateral amblyopia that may result from severe ptosis and abnormal head posture. Satisfactory results have been obtained with strabismus surgery followed by ptosis surgery.[9]

The pathophysiology of this disorder is unknown, and it is unclear if it is primarily neurogenic[9,24,74] or myopathic[47] etiology. Apt[9] suggested that this disorder results from defective maturation of the extrinsic eye muscles at or before the 20 mm. stage in the seventh week of gestation. Understanding the protein product of the CFEOM gene will give insights into the mechanisms of extraocular muscle development and function.

Using linkage analysis with markers spanning the entire genome, Engle et al.[47] localized the CFEOM gene to the pericentromeric region of chromosome 12, most likely within an 8 cM region flanked by markers D12S87 and D12S85. A marker linked to the Prader-Willi locus on the long arm of chromosome 15 was also investigated because of a report of a sporadic case of one child with both disorders and was found to be unlinked to the CFEOM locus.[90] Engle et al.'s[47] data demonstrates that CFEOM may be a genetically homogeneous disorder. Candidate genes located within this critical region are HOXC, a homeobox gene at 12q12-q13, and COL2A1, a collagen chain gene located at 12q13.[27] (See also section on CFEOM in Chapter 27.)

Fetal Alcohol Syndrome

Fetal alcohol syndrome (FAS), first described in 1968,[102] refers to a constellation of physical abnormalities observed in children born to mothers who have abused alcohol during pregnancy. The three major diagnostic criteria for the FAS are specific craniofacial morphology including short palpebral fissures, elongated midface, a long and flattened philtrum, thin upper vermilion, and flattened maxilla; intrauterine growth retardation; and central nervous system dysfunction.[140,152]

Thirty to forty-five percent of offspring of alcoholic mothers have the complete syndrome.[31] The worldwide incidence of FAS ranges from 0.4 to 3.1 per 1000 live births.[1] There are 1200 children with FAS born each year in the United States.[2]

Ophthalmologic abnormalities are very common in patients with FAS. Characteristic findings include ptosis in 20% of patients,[30,158,159] telecanthus,[115] epicanthus,[159] strabismus,[30,115,159] anterior segment malformations, especially Peters' anomaly,[28,46,158,160,166] myopia,[46,115,157] occasional microphthalmos,[30,159] optic disc anomalies in 48% of patients,[157] and increased tortuosity of the retinal vessel, especially the arteries, in 49% of patients.[158]

The teratogenic effects of alcohol have been established from extensive evidence derived from humans and from experimental animals.[93] The mechanism of the teratogenic action, however, is still unclear.[117] Chromosomes appear normal in children with FAS, implying that chromosomal aberrations are not the cause of the observed pattern of defects.[137] Genetic factors may, however, modulate the expression of the teratogenic effects of alcohol.[156] It is unknown whether the maternal or embryonic genotype is more important in determining susceptibility to alcohol teratogenesis.[59]

ACQUIRED PTOSIS

Mitochondrial Myopathies

The mitochondrial myopathies are a clinically and biochemically heterogenous group of disorders in which defects in mitochondrial metabolism[122] affect multiple systems and organs.[120] Thirty-six percent of patients have a pigmentary retinopathy, which can take the form of "salt-and-pepper" changes or atrophy of the retinal pigment epithelium or may resemble retinitis pigmentosa.[123,136] Some patients have macular degeneration[116]; others have myopia, cataract,[99] optic atrophy,[19] ptosis, diplopia, and restricted eye movements.[136]

Luft[107] introduced the concept of mitochondrial myopathy in 1962 when he described a 35-year-old woman with hypermetabolism without thyrotoxicosis, and mitochondria with poor coupling to oxidative phosphorylation. Since then, over 100 cases of mitochondrial myopathy have been reported in the literature. Disease onset is usually in childhood with a static or progressive disease course.[145]

These disorders are usually defined by morphological abnormalities of mitochondria in skeletal muscle biopsies. The histologic hallmark is the accumulation of abnormal mitochondria at the periphery of muscle fibers, which gives the fibers a "ragged-red" appearance with the modified Gomori trichrome stain.[131] Histologic and electron microscopic studies reveal enlarged mitochondria with altered cristae, characteristic "paracrystalline" inclusions, and excessive accumulation of glycogen particles and triglyceride droplets.[40,105] Sahgal[142] concluded that the mitochondrial changes are a morphological expression of uncoupled but intact mitochondrial respiration.

The mitochondrial myopathies include the following diseases: (*1*) mitochondrial myopathy, encephalopathy, lactic acidosis, and stroke-like episodes (MELAS), (*2*) myoclonic epilepsy and ragged red fiber disease (MERRF), (*3*) chronic progressive external ophthalmoplegia (CPEO), and (*4*) Kearns-Sayre syndrome (KSS).[48]

Mitochondrial myopathies are caused by mutations in the nuclear DNA or mitochondrial DNA, and therefore can be transmitted in a Mendelian or mitochondrial inheritance patterns. The mitochondrial DNA (mtDNA) is a double-stranded, 16,569 base pair-closed circular molecule of DNA located within the mitochondrion.[7] The mtDNA codes for only 13 polypeptides and nuclear DNA controls the synthesis of all mitochondrial proteins. In the formation of the zygote, all the mitochondria are contributed by the ovum. Diseases resulting from mtDNA mutations are transmitted by the mother.[146] Each cell has hundreds to thousands of copies of mtDNA. The phenotypic expression of a mitochondrially encoded gene depends on the relative proportions of mutant and wild-type mtDNA molecules within a cell. The mutation rate of mtDNA is much higher than that of the nuclear DNA.[26] A mutant phenotype is expressed only when the proportion of mutant mtDNA reaches a threshold.[40] Once this threshold is exceeded, the cell phenotype changes abruptly.[146] Mutations result in deficiencies in mitochondrial energy metabolism.[173]

Substantial deletion of a proportion of muscle mtDNA has been demonstrated in 30%–40% of cases of mitochondrial myopathy.[70] Most cases of mitochondrial myopathy and deletions of mtDNA are sporadic.[69,114] Twenty percent of patients with mitochondrial myopathy have similarly affected relatives, and the ratio of maternal to paternal transmission is approximately 9 : 1.[71,75,114] Pedigrees of patients with mitochondrial myopathy have been shown to follow dominant or recessive modes of inheritance.[116] KSS and CPEO are the "ocular mitochondrial myopathies," and are characterized by eyelid ptosis and ophthalmoparesis.[148]

KSS, first described in 1958, is a rare disease characterized by onset before age 20 years, pigmentary degeneration of the retina, progressive external ophthalmoplegia, and at least one of the following abnormalities: heart block, cerebellar ataxia, and cerebrospinal fluid protein greater than 1 g/L. There is often growth retardation, delayed sexual maturation, and mental deterioration.[17,40,95,103,126] The associated bilateral ptosis is due to chronic progressive ocular myopathy.[95] The administration of coenzyme Q has been shown to be of help.[126] Large deletions of mtDNA ranging from 1–8 kb were found in muscle biopsies of patients with KSS.[69,103,118,180] Ota[132] reported finding a mitochondrial gene for KSS between the tRNA Ser gene and the ND5 gene. Most cases with KSS have been sporadic.[40]

CPEO is the most common clinical presentation of mitochondrial myopathy and was present in 45% of a series of 66 patients.[135] CPEO is characterized by progressive weakness of the extraocular muscles and by bilateral ptosis.[48] Early in the course of the disease, patients may have ptosis without ophthalmoplegia.[148] Autosomal dominant, recessive, and maternal patterns of inheritance are described with CPEO.[91] Large deletions of mtDNA can give rise to CPEO.[71,118,180] mtDNA deletions associated with CPEO have been mapped to two sectors of the genome.[172]

Oculopharyngeal Muscular Dystrophy

Oculopharyngeal muscular dystrophy (OPMD) is a recently mapped rare familial disease of late onset characterized by progressive dysphagia and bilateral symmetrical palpebral ptosis.[144,170] First described by Taylor[162] in 1915, the disease has an autosomal dominant mode of inheritance, although both sporadic and familial examples of this disorder have been described.[170] De Braekeleer[37] estimated frequency to be more than 1/7500 in the Saguenay-La-St-Jean region of Quebec, Canada.

Various histological findings from muscle biopsies of affected patients have shown intranuclear filamentary inclusions within muscle fibers,[164] bizarre large mitochondria with abnormal cristae,[134] and replacement of muscle fibers with fatty and fibrous connective tissue.[143] Morgan-Hughes and Mair[121] studied triceps biopsies from four affected patients with oculomusculoskeletal myopathy and showed abnormal muscle fibers ranging from 8%–18%. Electron microscopy showed degenerative muscle fiber changes and ultrastructural changes of the mitochondria including the presence of laminated crystalline inclusions within the crystae.[121]

Brais et al.[22] identified a homogeneous group of OPMD families and studied 166 polymorphic markers to determine that the OPMD locus maps to a 5 cM region of chromosome 14q11.2-q13. A maximum 2-point lod score of 14.73 at theta = 0.03 was obtained in three French-Canadian families for an intronic cardiac beta-myosin heavy chain gene marker. Brais et al.[22] raised the possibility that the cardiac alpha- or beta-myosin heavy chain genes may be the mutated genes in this disorder.

REFERENCES

1. Abel E. *Fetal Alcohol Syndrome and Fetal Alcohol Effects.* New York: Plenum Press, 1984.
2. Abel EL, Sokol RJ. A revised conservative estimate of the incidence of FAS and its economic impact. *Alcoholism Clin Exp Res* 1991;15:514–524.
3. Aberfeld DC. The syndrome of congenital ptosis and development abnormalities of the first visceral arch. *Dev Med Child Neurol* 1968;10:491–496.
4. Al-Awadi SA, Naguib KK, Farag TI, et al. Complex translocation involving chromosomes Y, 1, and 3 resulting in deletion of segment 3q23 to 3q25. *J Med Genet* 1986;23:91–92.
5. Alvarado M, Bocian M, Walker AP. Interstitial deletion of the long arm of chromosome three: Case report, review, and definition of a phenotype. *Am J Med Genet* 1987;27:781–786.
6. Anderson RL, Baumgartner SA. Strabismus in ptosis. *Arch Ophthalmol* 1980;98:1062–1067.
7. Anderson S, Bankier AT, Barrell BG, et al. Sequence and organization of the human mitochondrial genome. *Nature* 1981;290:457–465.
8. Appleton RE, Chitayat D, Jan JE, et al. Joubert's syndrome associated with congenital ocular fibrosis and histidinemia. *Arch Neurol* 1989;46:579–582.
9. Apt L, Axelrod RN. Generalized fibrosis of the extraocular muscles. *Am J Ophthalmol* 1978;85:822–829.
10. Argenta LC, Iacobucci JJ. Treacher Collins syndrome: Present concepts of the disorder and their surgical correction. *World J Surg* 1989;13:401–409.
11. Axelsson A. Dysostosis-mandibulo-facialis. *J Laryngol Otol* 1963;77:575–592.
12. Bachelor EP, Kaplan EN. Absence of the lateral canthal tendon in the Treacher Collins syndrome. *Br J Plast Surg* 1981;34:162–164.
13. Balestrazzi P, Baeteman MA, Mattei MG, Mattei JF. Franceschetti syndrome in a child with a de novo balanced translocation (5;13)(q11;p11) and significant decrease of hexosaminidase B. *Hum Genet* 1983;64:305–308.
14. Beaconsfield M, Walker JW, Collin JR. Visual development in the blepharophimosis syndrome. *Br J Ophthalmol* 1991;75:746–748.
15. Beard C. Ptosis—Current concepts. *Int Ophthalmol Clin* 1978;18:53–73.
16. Beauchamp GR. Blepharophimosis and cardiopathy. *J Pediatr Ophthalmol Strabismus* 1980;17:227–228.
17. Berenberg RA, Pellock JM, DiMauro S, et al. Lumping or splitting? Ophthalmoplegia-plus or Kearns-Sayre syndrome? *Ann Neurol* 1977;1:37–54.

18. Berke RN. Histology of levator muscle in congenital and acquired ptosis. *Arch Ophthalmol* 1955;53:413–428.
19. Berkovic SF, Carpenter S, Evans A, et al. Myoclonus epilepsy and ragged red fibers (MERRF): A clinical, pathological, biochemical, magnetic resonance spectrographic and positron emission tomographic study. *Brain* 1989;112:1231–1260.
20. Beyer-Machule CK. Congenital ptosis and complications of ptosis surgery. *Plast Reconstr Surg* 1988;81:789–799.
21. Boccone L, Meloni A, Falchi AM, Usai V, Cao A. Blepharophimosis, ptosis, epicanthus inversus syndrome, A new case associated with de novo balanced autosomal translocation [46,xy, t(3;7)(q23,q32)]. *Am J Med Genet* 1994;51: 258–259.
22. Brais B, Xie YG, Sanson M, et al. The oculopharyngeal muscular dystrophy locus maps to the region of the cardiac alpha and beta myosin heavy chain genes on chromosome 14q112-q13. *Hum Mol Genet* 1995;4:429–434.
23. Briggs HH. Hereditary congenital ptosis with report of sixty-four cases conforming to the Mendelian rule of dominance. *Am J Ophthalmol* 1919;2:408–417.
24. Brodsky MC, Pollock SC, Buckley EG. Neural misdirection in congenital ocular fibrosis syndrome: Implications and pathogenesis. *J Pediatr Ophthalmol Strabismus* 1989;26:159–161.
25. Brown H. Congenital structural muscle anomalies. In *Strabismus Ophthalmic Symposium*, J. Allen, ed. St. Louis: C. V. Mosby, 1950: 205–236.
26. Brown WM, George M Jr, Wilson AC. Rapid evaluation of animal mitochondrial DNA. *Proc Natl Acad Sci USA* 1979;76:1967–1971.
27. Cannizzaro LA, Croce CM, Griffin CA, et al. Human homeo box-containing genes located at chromosome regions 2q31 to 2q37 and 12q12 to 12q13. *Am J Hum Genet* 1987; 41:1–15.
28. Carones F, Brancato R, Venturi E, et al. Corneal endothelial anomalies in the fetal alcohol syndrome. *Arch Ophthalmol* 1992;110:1128–1131.
29. Chismire KJ, Witkop GS. Optic nerve hypoplasia and angle dysgenesis in a patient with blepharophimosis syndrome. *Am J Ophthalmol* 1994;117:676–677.
30. Clarren SK, Smith DW. The fetal alcohol syndrome. *N Engl J Med* 1978;298:1063–1067.
31. Clarren SK, Smith DW. Recognition of fetal alcohol syndrome. *JAMA* 1981;245:2436–2439.
32. Clayton-Smith J, Krajewska-Walasek M, Fryer A, Donnai D. Ohdo-like blepharophimosis syndrome with distinctive facies, neonatal hypotonia, mental retardation and hypoplastic teeth. *Clin Dysmorphol* 1994;3:115–120.
33. Cohen HB. Congenital ptosis: A new pedigree and classification. *Arch Ophthalmol* 1972;87: 161–163.
34. Collins E. Cases with symmetrical congenital notches in the outer part of each lid and defective development of the malar bones. *Trans Ophthalmol Soc UK* 1900;20:190.
35. Crawford JS. Congenital fibrosis syndrome. *Can J Ophthalmol* 1970;5:331–336.
36. Crawford JS. Repair of ptosis using frontalis muscle and fascia lata: A twenty-year review. *Ophthalmic Surg* 1977;8:31–40.
37. De Braekeleer M. Hereditary disorders in Saguenay-Lac-St-Jean (Quebec, Canada). *Hum Hered* 1991;41:141–146.
38. De Die-Smulders CEM, Engelen JJ, Donk JM, Fryns JP. Further evidence for the location of the BPES gene at 3q2. *J Med Genet* 1991; 28:725.
39. De Almeida JCC, Llerena JC Jr, Goncalves Neto JB, et al. Another example favouring the location of BPES at 3q2. *J Med Genet* 1993; 30:86–88.
40. DiMauro S, Bonilla E, Zeviani M, et al. Mitochondrial myopathies. *Ann Neurol* 1985;17: 521–538.
41. Dixon J, Gladwin AJ, Loftus SK, et al. A YAC contig encompassing the Treacher Collins syndrome critical region at 5q313–32. *Am J Hum Genet* 1994;55:372–378.
42. Dixon MJ, Haan E, Baker E, et al. Association of Treacher Collins syndrome and translocation 6p2131/16p1311: Exclusion of the locus from these candidate regions. *Am J Hum Genet* 1991;48:274–280.
43. Dixon MJ, Dixon J, Raskova D, et al. Genetic and physical mapping of the Treacher Collins syndrome locus: Refinement of the localization to chromosome 5q32-332. *Hum Mol Genet* 1992;1:249–253.
44. Dixon MJ, Dixon J, Houseal T, et al. Narrowing the position of the Treacher Collins syndrome locus to a small interval between three new microsatellite markers at 5q32-331. *Am J Hum Genet* 1993;52:907–914.
45. Edery P, Manach Y, Le Merrer M, et al. Apparent genetic homogeneity of the Treacher Collins-Franceschetti syndrome. *Am J Med Genet* 1994;52:174–177.
46. Edward DP, Li J, Sawaguchi S, et al. Diffuse corneal clouding in siblings with fetal alcohol

syndrome. *Am J Ophthalmol* 1993;115:484–493.
47. Engle EC, Kunkel LM, Specht LA, Beggs AH. Mapping a gene for congenital fibrosis of the extraocular muscles to the centromeric region of chromosome 12. *Nature Genet* 1994;7:69–73.
48. Fang W, Huang CC, Lee CC, et al. Ophthalmic manifestations in MELAS syndrome. *Arch Neurol* 1993;50:977–980.
49. Fazen LE. Mandibulo-facial dysostosis. *Am J Dis Child* 1967;113:405–410.
50. Feingold M. Ocular abnormalities associated with first and second arch syndromes. *Surv Ophthalmol* 1968;14:30–42.
51. Fox SA. Blepharophimosis. *Am J Ophthalmol* 1963;55:469–475.
52. Fox SA. A new ptosis classification. *Arch Ophthal* 1972;88:590–593.
53. Franceschetti A. Un syndrome nouveau: La dysostose mandibulo-faciale. *Bull Schweiz Akad Med Wiss* 1950;1:60.
54. Franceschini P, Cirillo Silengo M, et al. Interstitial deletion of the long arm of chromosome 3 in a patient with mental retardation and congenital anomalies. *Hum Genet* 1983;64:97.
55. Fryns JP, Stromme P, van den Berghe H. Further evidence for the location of the blepharophimosis syndrome (BPES) at 3q223-q23. *Clin Genet* 1993;44:149–151.
56. Fujita H, Meng J, Kawamura M, et al. Boy with a chromosome del (3) (q12q23) and blepharophimosis syndrome. *Am J Med Genet* 1992;44:434–436.
57. Fukushima Y, Wakui K, Nishida T, Ueoka Y. Blepharophimosis sequence and de novo balanced autosomal translocation [46,XY,t(3;4)(q23;p15.2)]: possible assignment of the trait to 3q23. *Am J Med Genet* 1991;40:485–487.
58. Garden JW. Blepharophimosis, ptosis, epicanthus inversus and lacrimal stenosis. *Am J Ophthalmol* 1969;67:153–154.
59. Gilliam DM, Irtenkauf KT. Maternal genetic effects on ethanol teratogenesis and dominance of relative embryonic resistance to malformations. *Alcoholism Clin Exp Res* 1990;14:539–545.
60. Gillies WE, Harris AJ, Brooks AM, Rivers MR, Wolfe RJ. Congenital fibrosis of the vertically acting extraocular muscles: A new group of dominantly inherited ocular fibrosis with radiologic findings. *Ophthalmology* 1995;102:607–612.
61. Girardet P. Epicanthus inversus, ptose palpebrale congenitale et trouble de la motilité oculaire chez un nourrisson de sept mois. *Helv Paediatr Acta* 1951;6:361.
62. Gorlin R. Mandibulofacial dysostosis. In *Syndromes of the Head and Neck.* New York: Oxford University Press, 1990:649–652.
63. Hansen E. Congenital general fibrosis of the extraocular muscles. *Acta Ophthalmol* 1968;46:469–476.
64. Harley RD, Rodrigues MM, Crawford JS. Congenital fibrosis of the extraocular muscles. *J Pediatr Ophthalmol Strabismus* 1978;15:346–358.
65. Harrad RA, Graham CM, Collin JR. Amblyopia and strabismus in congenital ptosis. *Eye* 1988;2:625–627.
66. Harrison S. The Treacher-Collins-Franceschetti syndrome. *J Laryngol Otol* 1957;71:597–604.
67. Hertle RW, Ziylan S, Katowitz JA. Ophthalmic features and visual prognosis in the Treacher Collins syndrome. *Br J Ophthalmol* 1993;77:642–645.
68. Hiatt RL, Halle AA. General fibrosis syndrome. *Ann Ophthalmol* 1983;15:1103–1109.
69. Holt IJ, Harding AE, Morgan-Hughes JA. Deletions of muscle mitochondrial DNA in mitochondrial myopathies: Sequence analysis and possible mechanisms. *Nucleic Acids Res* 1989;17:4465–4469.
70. Holt IJ, Harding AE, Petty RK, Morgan-Hughes JA. A new mitochondrial disease associated with mitochondrial DNA heteroplasmy. *Am J Hum Genet* 1990;46:428–433.
71. Holt IJ, Harding AE, Morgan-Hughes JA. Deletions of mitochondrial DNA in patients with mitochondrial myopathies. *Nature* 1988;331:717–719.
72. Hornblass A, Adachi M, Wolintz A, Smith B. Clinical and ultrasound correlation in congenital and acquired ptosis. *Ophthalmic Surg* 1976;7:69–76.
73. Houlston RS, Ironton R, Temple IK. Association of atrial-ventricular septal defect, blepharophimosis, anal and radial defects in sibs: A new syndrome? *Genet Couns* 1994;5:93–96.
74. Houtman WA, van Weerden TW, Robinson PH, de Vries B, Hoogenraad TU. Hereditary congenital external ophthalmoplegia. *Ophthalmologica* 1986;193:207–218.
75. Hudgson P, Bradley WG, Jenkison M. Familial "mitochondrial" myopathy. A myopathy associated with disordered oxidative metabolism in muscle fibres. 1. Clinical, electrophysiological and pathological findings. *J Neurol Sci* 1972;16:343–370.

76. Hughes WL. Surgical treatment of congenital palpebral phimosis. *Arch Ophthalmol* 1955;54: 586–590.
77. Hupp SL, Williams JP, Curran JE. Computerized tomography in the diagnosis of the congenital fibrosis syndrome. *J Clin Neuro-Ophthalmol* 1990;10:135–139.
78. Hurwitz P. Mandibulofacial dysostosis. *Arch Ophthalmol* 1954;51:69–72.
79. Ionescu A. A surgical solution in the treatment of blepharophimosis. *Rom Med Rev* 1966; 20:62.
80. Ishikiriyama S, Goto M. Blepharophimosis sequence (BPES) and microcephaly in a girl with del (3) (q222q23): A putative gene responsible for microcephaly close to the BPES gene? *Am J Med Genet* 1993;47:487–489.
81. Jabs EW, Coss CA, Hayflick SJ, Whitmore TE, Pauli RM, Kirkpatrick SJ, Meyers DA, Goldberg R, Day DW, Rosenbaum KN. Chromosomal deletion 4p1532 to p14 in a Treacher Collins syndrome patient: Exclusion of the disease locus from and mapping of anonymous DNA sequences to this region. *Genomics* 1991;11:188–192.
82. Jabs EW, Li X, Coss CA, Taylor EW, Meyers DA, Weber JL. Mapping of the Treacher Collins syndrome locus to 5q313 to q333. *Genomics* 1991;11:193–198.
83. Jabs EW. Genetic and physical mapping of the Treacher Collins syndrome locus with respect to loci in the chromosome 5q3 region. *Genomics* 1993;18:7–13.
84. Jewett T, Rao PN, Weaver RG, Stewart W, Thomas IT, Pettenati MJ. Blepharoptosis, ptosis, and epicanthus inversus syndrome (BPES) associated with interstitial deletion of band 3q22: Review and gene assignment to the interface of band 3q223 and 3q23. *Am J Med Genet* 1993;47:1147–1150.
85. Johnson CC. Operations for epicanthus and blepharophimosis: An evaluation and a method for shortening the medial canthal ligament. *Am J Ophthalmol* 1956;41:71–79.
86. Johnson CC. Surgical repair of the syndrome of epicanthus inversus, blepharophimosis and ptosis. *Arch Ophthalmol* 1964;71:510–516.
87. Johnson CC. Epicanthus. *Am J Ophthalmol* 1968;66:939–946.
88. Jones C. *Smith's Recognizable Patterns of Human Malformation*. Philadelphia: W. B. Saunders, 1988:210–211.
89. Jones CA, Collin JR. Blepharophimosis and its association with female infertility. *Br J Ophthalmol* 1984;68:533–534.
90. Kalpakian B, Bateman JB, Sparkes RS, Wood GK. Congenital ocular fibrosis syndrome associated with the Prader-Willi syndrome. *J Pediatr Ophthalmol Strabismus* 1986;23:170–173.
91. Kao K-P, Tsai CP. Mitochondrial disease with chronic progressive external ophthalmoplegia: Clinical analysis of 19 cases. *Chin Med J (Taipei)* 1994;53:95–100.
92. Karacaoglan N, Sahin U, Ercan U, Bozdogan N. One-stage repair of blepharophimosis: A new method. *Plast Reconstr Surg* 1994; 93:1406–1409.
93. Katz LM, Fox DA. Prenatal ethanol exposure alters scotopic and photopic components of adult rat electroretinograms. *Invest Ophthalmol Vis Sci* 1991;32:2861–2872.
94. Kay ED, Kay CN. Dysmorphogenesis of the mandible, zygoma, and middle ear ossicles in hemifacial microsomia and mandibulofacial dysostosis. *Am J Med Genet* 1989;32:27–31.
95. Kearns TP. Retinitis pigmentosa, external ophthalmoplegia and complete heart block. *Arch Ophthalmol* 1958;60:280–289.
96. Kohn R, Romano PE. Blepharoptosis, blepharophimosis, epicanthus inversus, and telecanthus—A syndrome with no name. *Am J Ophthalmol* 1971;72:625–632.
97. Kolar JC, Munro IR, Farkas LG. Anthropometric evaluation of dys-morphology in craniofacial anomalies: Treacher Collins syndrome. *Am J Phys Anthropol* 1987;74:441–451.
98. Komoto J. Ptosis operation. *Klin Monatsbl Augenheilkd* 1921;66:952.
99. Kuchle M, Brenner PM, Engelhardt A, Naumann GO. Augenveranderungen bei melassyndrom. *Klin Monatsbl Augenheilkd* 1990; 197:258–264.
100. Laughlin RC. Congenital fibrosis of the extraocular muscles: A report of six cases. *Am J Ophthalmol* 1956;41:432–438.
101. Lemagne JM, Colonval S, Moens B, Brucher JM. Anatomical modification of the levator muscle of the eyelid in congenital ptosis. *Bull Soc Belge Ophtalmol* 1992;243:23–27.
102. Lemoine P. Les enfants de parents alcooliques: anomalies observees. *Ouest Med* 1968;21: 476–482.
103. Lestienne P, Ponsot G. Kearns-Sayre syndrome with muscle mitochondrial DNA deletion. *Lancet* 1988;i:885.
104. Lewis SR. The congenital eyelid syndrome. *J Plast Reconstr Surg* 1967;39:271.
105. Lindal S, Lund I, Torbergsen T, Aasly J, Mellgren SI, Borud O, Monstad P. Mitochondrial diseases and myopathies: A series of muscle

biopsy specimens with ultrastructural changes in the mitochondria. *Ultrastruct Pathol* 1992; 16:263–275.

106. Loftus SK, Edwards SJ, Scherpbier-Heddema T, Buetow KH, Wasmuth JJ, Dixon MJ. A combined genetic and radiation hybrid map surrounding the Treacher Collins syndrome locus on chromosome 5q. *Hum Mol Genet* 1993; 2:1785–1792.
107. Luft R. A case of severe hypermetabolism of nonthyroid origin with a defect in the maintenance of mitochondrial respiratory control: A correlated clinical, biochemical, and morphological study. *J Clin Invest* 1962;41:1776–1804.
108. Luo TH. Bilateral congenital epicanthus inversus and ptosis: Report of a case. *Chin Med J* 1934;48:814–818.
109. Martin PA, Rogers PA. Congenital aponeurotic ptosis. *Aust NZ J Ophthalmol* 1988;16: 291–294.
110. Martsolf JT, Ray M. Interstitial deletion of the long arm of chromosome three. *Ann Genet* 1983;26:98–99.
111. McCord CD. The evaluation and management of the patient with ptosis. *Clin Plast Surg* 1988;15:169–184.
112. McCulloch DL, Wright KW. Unilateral congenital ptosis: Compensatory head posturing and amblyopia. *Ophthalmic Plast Reconstr Surg* 1993;9:196–200.
113. McIlroy J. Hereditary ptosis with epicanthus: A case with a pedigree extending over four generations. *Proc R Soc Med* 1930;23:285.
114. Mechler F, Fawcett PR, Mastaglia FL, Hudgson P. Mitochondrial myopathy: A study of clinically affected and asymptomatic members of a six-generation family. *J Neurol Sci* 1981; 50:191–200.
115. Miller M, Israel J, Cuttone J. Fetal alcohol syndrome. *J Pediatr Ophthalmol Strabismus* 1981;18:6–15.
116. Modi G, Heckman JM, Saffer D. Vitelliform macular degeneration associated with mitochondrial myopathy. *Br J Ophthalmol* 1992; 76:58–60.
117. Moore GE. Molecular genetic approaches to the study of human craniofacial dysmorphologies. *Int Rev Cytol* 1995;158:215–277.
118. Moraes CT, DiMauro S, Zeviani M, Lombes A, Shanske S, Miranda AF, Nakase H, Bonilla E, Werneck LC, Servidei S, et al. Mitochondrial DNA deletions in progressive external ophthalmoplegia and Kearns-Sayre syndrome. *N. Engl J. Med* 1989;320:1293–1299.
119. Moraine C, Titeca C, Delplace MP, Grenier B, Lenoel Y, Ribadeau-Dumas JL. Familial blepharophimosis and female sterility: pleiotropism or linked genes. *J Genet Hum* 1976;24(Suppl):125–132.
120. Morgan-Hughes J. The mitochondrial myopathies. In *Myology*, A. Engle and B. Banker, eds. New York: McGraw-Hill, 1986:1709–1743.
121. Morgan-Hughes JA, Mair WG. Atypical muscle mitochondria in oculoskeletal myopathy. *Brain* 1973;96:215–224.
122. Morgan-Hughes JA, Hayes DJ, Clark JB, et al. Mitochondrial encephalomyopathies. Biochemical studies in two cases revealing defects in the respiratory chain. *Brain* 1982;105: 553–582.
123. Mullie MA, Harding AE, Petty RK, et al. The retinal manifestations of mitochondrial myopathy: A study of 22 cases. *Arch Ophthalmol* 1985;103:1825–1830.
124. Munn I. *The Development of the Human Eye.* London: Cambridge University Press, 1928.
125. Nakajima T, Yoshimura Y, Onishi K, Sakakibara A. One stage repair of blepharophimosis. *Plas Reconstr Surg* 1991;87:24–31.
126. Nelson I, Degoul F, Obermaier-Kusser B, et al. Mapping of heteroplasmic mitochondrial DNA deletions in Kearns-Sayre syndrome. *Nucleic Acids Res* 1989;17:8117–8124.
127. Nemet P, Godel V, Ron S, Lazar M. Ocular congenital fibrosis syndrome. *Metab Pediatr Syst Ophthalmol* 1985;8:172–174.
128. O'Connor GB. Associated congenital abnormalities of the eyelids and appendages (syndrome). *J Plast Reconstr Surg* 1953;11: 348–352.
129. Okada N, Hasegawa T, Osawa M, Fukuyama Y. A case of de novo interstitial deletion 3q. *J Med Genet* 1987;24:305–308.
130. Oley C, Baraitser M. Blepharophimosis, ptosis, epicanthus inversus syndrome (BPES syndrome). *J Med Genet* 1988;25:47–51.
131. Olson W, Engel WK, Walsh GO, Einaugler R. Oculocraniosomatic neuromuscular disease with "ragged red fibres." *Arch Neurol* 1972; 26:193–211.
132. Ota Y, Miyake Y, Awaya S, et al. Early retinal involvement in mitochondrial myopathy with mitochondrial DNA deletion. *Retina* 1994;14: 270–276.
133. Owens N. Hereditary blepharophimosis, ptosis, and epicanthus inversus. *J Int Coll Surg* 1960;33:558.
134. Pauzner R, Blatt I, Mouallem M, et al. Mitochondrial abnormalities in oculopharyngeal muscular dystrophy. *Muscle Nerve* 1991; 14:947–952.

135. Petty RK, Harding AE, Morgan-Hughes JA. The clinical features of mitochondrial myopathy, (abstract). *J Neurol Neurosurg Psychiatry* 1985;48:604.
136. Petty RK, Harding AE, Morgan-Hughes JA. The clinical features of mitochondrial myopathy. *Brain* 1986;109:915–938.
137. Randall CL, Ekblad U, Anton RF. Perspectives on the pathophysiology of fetal alcohol syndrome. *Alcoholism Clin Exp Res* 1990;14: 807–812.
138. Raulo Y. Treacher Collins syndrome: Analysis and principles of surgery. In *Craniofacial Surgery*. Berlin: Springer-Verlag, 1985:371.
139. Rogers BO. Berry-Treacher Collins syndrome: A review of 200 cases. *Br J Plast Surg* 1964; 17:109–137.
140. Rosett HL. A clinical perspective of the fetal alcohol syndrome. *Alcoholism Clin Exp Res* 1980;4:119–122.
141. Rovin S. Mandibulofacial dysostosis: A familial study of five generations. *J Pediatr* 1964; 65:215–221.
142. Sahgal V, Subramani V, Hughes R, et al. On the pathogenesis of mitochondrial myopathies: An experimental study. *Acta Neuropathol (Berl)* 1979;46:177–183.
143. Schmitt HP, Krause KH. An autopsy study of a familial oculopharyngeal muscular dystrophy (OPMD) with distal spread and neurogenic involvement. *Muscle Nerve* 1981;4:296–305.
144. Schotland DL. Muscular dystrophy. Features of ocular myopathy, distal myopathy, and myotonic dystrophy. *Arch Neurol* 1964;10:433–445.
145. Sengers RC, Stadhouders AM, Trijbels JM. Mitochondrial myopathies: Clinical, morphological and biochemical aspects. *Eur J Pediatr* 1984;141:192–207.
146. Shoffner JM, Lott MT, Wallace DC. MERRF: A model disease for understanding the principles of mitochondrial genetics. *Rev Neurol* 1991;147:431–435.
147. Shprintzen RJ, Croft C, Berkman MD, Rakoff SJ. Pharyngeal hypoplasia in Treacher Collins syndrome. *Arch Otolaryngol* 1979;105:127–131.
148. Siciliano G, Viacava P, Rossi B, et al. Ocular myopathy without ophthalmoplegia can be a form of mitochondrial myopathy. *Clin Neurol Neurosurg* 1992;94:133–141.
149. Small KW, Stalvey M, Fisher L, et al. Blepharophimosis syndrome is linked to chromosome 3q. *Hum Mol Genet* 1995;4:443–448.
150. Smith A, Fraser IS, Shearman RP, Russell P. Blepharophimosis plus ovarian failure: A likely candidate for a contiguous gene syndrome. *J Med Genet* 1989;26:434–438.
151. Smith D. *Recognizable Patterns of Human Malformation: Genetic, Embryologic and Clinical Aspects.* Philadelphia: W. B. Saunders, 1982.
152. Sokol RJ, Clarren SK. Guidelines for use of terminology describing the impact of prenatal alcohol on the offspring. *Alcoholism Clin Exp Res* 1989;13:597–598.
153. Spaeth EB. Further considerations on the surgical correction of blepharophimosis (epicanthus). *Am J Ophthalmol* 1956;41:61–71.
154. Stark N, Walther C. Amblyopie und schieldeviationen bei kongenitaler ptosis. *Klin Monatsbl Augenheilkd* 1984;184:37–39.
155. Stenstrom S. Contribution to the treatment of the eyelid deformities in dysostosis mandibulofacialis. *Plast Reconstr Surg* 1966;38: 567–572.
156. Streissguth AP, Dehaene P. Fetal alcohol syndrome in twins of alcoholic mothers: Concordance of diagnosis and IQ. *Am J Med Genet* 1993;47:857–861.
157. Stromland K. Ocular abnormalities in the fetal alcohol syndrome. *Acta Ophthalmol* 1985 (suppl);171:1–50.
158. Stromland K. Ocular involvement of the fetal alcohol syndrome. *Surv Ophthalmol* 1987;31: 277–284.
159. Stromland K. Contribution of ocular examination to the diagnosis of foetal alcohol syndrome in mentally retarded children. *J Ment Defic Res* 1990;34:429–435.
160. Sulik K. Craniofacial defects from genetic and teratogen-induced deficiencies in presomite embryos. *Brith Defects Orig Art Ser* 1984; 20:79–98.
161. Sutula FC. Histological changes in congenital and acquired blepharoptosis. *Eye* 1988;2: 179–184.
162. Taylor EW. Progressive vagus-glossopharyngeal paralysis with ptosis: Contribution to group of family diseases. *J Nerv Ment Dis* 1915;42:129–139.
163. Thomson A. Notice of several cases of malformation of the external ear, together with experiments on the state of hearing in such persons. *Mon J Med Sci* 1846;7:420.
164. Tome FM, Fardeau M. Nuclear inclusions in oculopharyngeal dystrophy. *Acta Neuropathol* 1980;49:85–87.
165. Townes PL, Muechler EK. Blepharophimosis, ptosis, epicanthus inversus, and primary amenorrhea. *Arch Ophthalmol* 1979;97:1664–1666.
166. Traboulsi EI, Maumenee IH. Peters' anomaly

and associated congenital malformations. *Arch Ophthalmol* 1992;110:1739–1742.

167. Usher C. Epicanthus (Bowman lecture). *Trans Ophthalmol Soc UK* 1935;55:194–232.
168. Van den Bosch WA, Lesnik Oberstein SY. Congenital ptosis of the upper eyelid: Indication for early ophthalmological examination. *Ned Tijdschr Geneeskd* 1995;139:783–788.
169. Vestal KP, Seiff SR, Lahey JM. Congenital ptosis in monozygotic twins. *Ophthalmic Plast Reconst Surg* 1990;6:265–268.
170. Victor M. Oculopharyngeal muscular dystrophy. A familial disease of late life characterized by dysphagia and progressive ptosis of the eyelids. *N Engl J Med* 1962;267:1267–1272.
171. Waardenburg P. Die zuruckfuhrung einer reibe erblich-angeborener familiarer augenmissildungen auf eine fixation normaler fetaler verhaltnisse. *Graefes Arch Ophthalmol* 1930; 124:221.
172. Wallace DC, Lott MT, Shoffner JM, Ballinger S. Mitochondrial DNA mutations in epilepsy and neurological disease. *Epilepsia* 1994;35 (Suppl 1):S43–S50.
173. Wallace DC, Lott MT, Shoffner JM, Brown MD. Diseases resulting from mitochondrial DNA point mutations. *J Inherit Metab Dis* 1992;15:472–479.
174. Wang FM, Millman AL, Sidoti PA, Goldberg RB. Ocular findings in TCS. *Am J Ophthalmol* 1990;110:280–286.
175. Whitaker LA, Katowitz JA, Jacobs WE. Ocular adnexal problems in craniofacial deformities. *J Max-Fac Surg* 1979;7:55–60.
176. Wilder WM, Williams JP, Hupp SL. Computerized tomographic findings in two cases of congenital fibrosis syndrome. *Comput Med Imaging Graph* 1991;15:361–363.
177. Williamson RA. Familial insertional translocation of a portion of 3q into 11q resulting in duplication and deletion of region 3q221 to q24 in different offspring. *Am J Med Genet* 1981;9:105–111.
178. Wittebol-Post D, Hennekam RC. Blepharophimosis, ptosis, polythelia and brachydactyly (BPPB): A new autosomal dominant syndrome? *Clin Dysmorphol* 1993;2:346–350.
179. Wolstenholme J, Brown J, Masters KG, et al. Blepharophimosis sequence and diaphragmatic hernia associated with interstitial deletion of chromosome 3 (46, xy, del(3)(q21q23)). *J Med Genet* 1994;31:647–648.
180. Zeviani M, Moraes CT, DiMauro S, et al. Deletions of mitochondrial DNA in Kearns-Sayre syndrome. *Neurology* 1988;38:1339–1346.

V.

Ocular Manifestations of Inherited Systemic Diseases

30

Ocular Manifestations of Chromosomal Abnormalities

ALEX V. LEVIN
JOANNE SUTHERLAND
ANTHONY G. QUINN

The incidence of congenital ocular malformations is approximately 6/10,000, of which almost 8% are associated with abnormal karyotypes.[172] This chapter is devoted to the description of ocular and systemic anomalies that result from some aberrations of chromosome number or structure. Identification of congenital ocular abnormalities plays an important role in the recognition of chromosomal abnormalities. Likewise, obtaining complete ophthalmologic assessment of children who are known to have chromosomal aberrations is of great value.

The most common chromosomal abnormalities associated with congenital ocular malformations identified at birth are trisomy 13 and trisomy 21.[172] In the presence of an ocular malformation, certain specific systemic malformations appear to be better predictors of an associated chromosomal abnormality: talipes-equinovarus (clubfoot), microcephaly, hydrocephalus, facial dysmorphism, and hypertelorism.[172] Children with congenital ocular malformations tend to be smaller for gestational age and developmentally delayed. They have a higher incidence of consanguineous parents.[172]

Chromosomal aberrations can involve the whole genome, resulting in triploidy, tetraploidy, and polyploidy. They may be numerical (monosomies and trisomies) or structural (translocations, insertions, deletions, or duplications). Because of the size of the chromosomal change, more than one gene is disrupted.

Genetic diseases are usually caused by mutations of a single gene. Detection of these abnormalities requires molecular techniques, because they are not visible by standard cytogenetics. Ocular genetic disorders that are caused by a submicroscopic alteration in a single gene are discussed elsewhere in this book. This chapter deals only with cytogenetically detectable alterations in chromosome structure and number that are compatible with live birth.

The material presented in this chapter will be confined to "pure" chromosomal aberrations. For example, if a deletion of chromosome 1p occurs in association with a partial trisomy of 4q (a 1 : 4 chromosomal translocation), the resulting phenotype may be due to the contribution of the 1p deletion and/or the 4q trisomy. In this chapter, only the phenotypes associated with either the isolated deletion of 1p or iso-

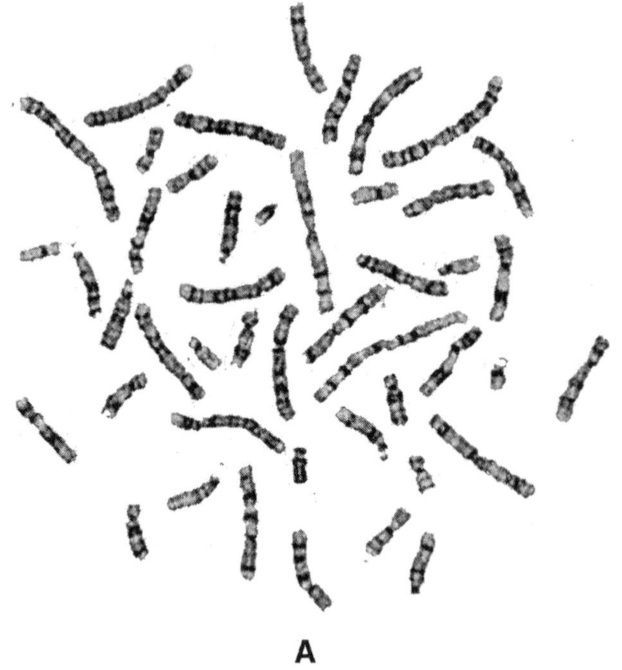

A SPREAD OF CHROMOSOMES
FROM ONE CELL

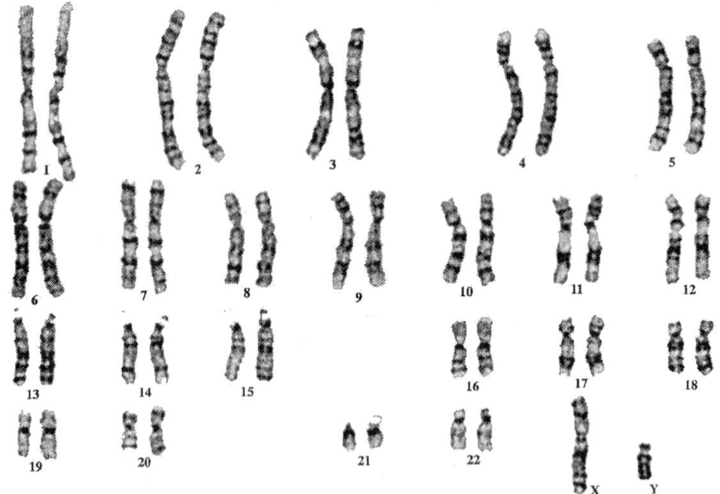

B

A HUMAN MALE KARYOTYPE

Figure 30.1. Cytogenetic photograph of human chromosomes as **A:** spread of chromosomes and **B:** chromosomes sorted into karyotype. (B provided courtesy of the Cytogenetics Laboratory, Hospital for Sick Children, Toronto, Ontario, Canada.)

lated trisomy of 4q will be discussed. It is hoped that the reader will therefore be familar with the phenotypes associated with abnormalities of individual chromosomes so that when more than one chromosome is affected, features of each separate aberration can be considered clinically.

One must be careful in the interpretation of clinical genetic reports in the literature. Sophisticated banding techniques that determine the exact breakpoints in chromosomal anomalies have only been available in relatively recent years. In fact, deletions and ring chromosomes were not even recognized until the late 1950s and early 1960s.[2,71] In addition, many articles in the non-ophthalmologic literature fail to provide adequate ophthalmic information, sometimes precluding the exclusion of ocular malformations.

BASIC CONCEPTS

Every normal cell has two sets of chromosomes. Normal individuals begin life as one diploid cell containing 46 chromosomes formed from the union of one haploid ovum and one haploid sperm. The 46 chromosomes exist as 23 pairs, each pair consisting of one chromosome from the father and one from the mother. Chromosomes 1 to 22 are called "autosomes." The chromosomes that make up pair 23 are called "sex chromosomes"; girls have two X chromosomes in this pair, while boys have one X plus one Y. Chromosomes have a centromere, a short arm (p for "petit") and a long arm (q). One short and one long arm together are known as a single chromatid chromosome.

Figure 30.1*A* shows the 46 chromosomes of one cell as seen under a microscope. The cells have been stained with Giemsa, which causes a striped or banded pattern to appear for each chromosome. Each band may contain hundreds of genes. A trained cytotechnologist can identify each pair of chromosomes based on the size, centromere position, and banding pattern. The chromosomes are cut out of a photograph like the one in Figure 30.1*A* or manipulated as computer images, and placed in a specific order from largest (chromosome 1) to smallest (chromosome 22). The sex chromosomes (XX or XY) are placed in the bottom right corner. This standard picture of chromosomes is called a karyotype (Fig. 30.1*B*).

ABNORMALITIES OF CHROMOSOME NUMBER

Duplications (Trisomies)

Meiotic nondisjunction may result in the presence of two copies of the same chromosome existing in one germ cell (diploid as opposed to haploid). Following conception, the fertilized oocyte would then have three copies of this chromosome and two copies of all of the other chromosomes. Trisomies 13, 18, and 21 are the most common trisomies compatible with life. Mechanisms for creating partial aneuploidy (partial trisomy or monosomy) include rearrangement, duplication, or deletion within a chromosome, or the incomplete formation of a translocation followed by unbalanced segregation.

Duplications can also involve the whole genome, resulting in triploid, tetraploid, and polyploid fetuses that are generally not viable even if the fetus survives to term. Triploid fetuses result from double fertilization (66%), fertilization with a diploid sperm (24%) or the fertilization of a diploid egg (10%). The majority (60%) are XXY and most of the rest are XXX.

Deletions (Monosomies)

The loss of an entire chromosome in human development usually results in spontaneous abortion. One common monosomy that is compatible with life is XO, known as Turner syndrome.

A large piece of DNA can be lost during recombination. Such a deletion can be large enough to result in the loss of part of a gene, all of a gene (loss of heterozygosity) or several genes that are close together. The patient is then monosomic for the deleted segment (partial monosomy). The term *microdeletion syndrome* is used to describe patients who exhibit several diverse phenotypic effects as a result of a missing piece of DNA that is large enough to be detected microscopically by prophase banding or by other methods such as fluorescent in situ hybridization (FISH), but not by standard karyotyping. Two or more genes are usually missing in such patients (contiguous gene deletion syndrome). For example, a microdeletion around Xp21 can result in Duchenne muscular dystrophy (DMD), chronic granulomatous disease (CGD), and several other genetic conditions, including X-linked retinitis pigmentosa. Prader-Willi and Angelman syndromes may be associated with oculocutaneous albinism due to a microdeletion that includes both the PWS/AS locus and the nearby P gene in the region 15q11.2-11.3.

DISORDERS OF CHROMOSOMAL STRUCTURE

Ring chromosomes: Rings can form when the two telomeres of a chromosome fuse or when a chromosome loses the tip of both the p and q arms and the exposed broken ends fuse. The first mechanism is thought to result in no loss of chromosomal material. The second results in a monosomy of part of both the p and the q terminal ends of the involved chromosome.

Intrachromosomal duplications: Throughout the genome there are repeat DNA sequences, some of which occur in tandem. Where these tandem repeats exist, there is a risk of slippage. Segments of DNA within the chromosome can then duplicate by unequal cross over. These duplications tend to occur within the arm of a chromosome (interstitial duplication) as opposed to involving the telomere.

Inversions: When two breaks occur on one chromosome, the intervening segment may invert and reinsert. If that segment includes the centromere, the inversion is denoted as *pericentric* (Fig. 30.2*A*). An inversion that occurs within the long arm or short arm without involving the centromere is denoted as *paracentric* (Fig. 30.2*B*).

Isochromosomes: Isochromosomes only have two short arms or two long arms, separated by the centromere. The centromere appears in the

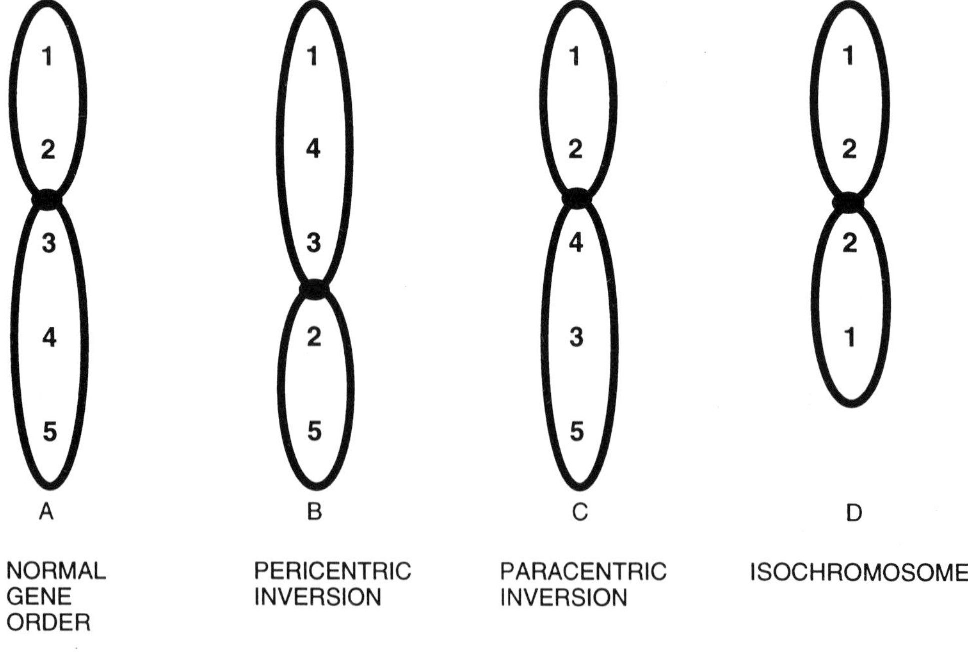

Figure 30.2. Types of inversions. Numbers indicate arbitrary designations of chromosome regions/markers to allow the reader to track their position changes resulting from the indicated inversions. Shaded oval indicates the centromere.

middle of isochromosomes because one arm is deleted and the other duplicated (Fig. 30.2C).

Chromosomal fragments (marker chromosomes): Fragments of chromosomes usually represent trisomic material.

Other more complicated rearrangements are very rare and beyond the scope of this discussion.

TRANSLOCATIONS

Reciprocal Translocation

Most translocations involve only two chromosomes and are referred to as *reciprocal translocations.* Carriers of a balanced translocation are clinically normal because they have no extra or missing chromosomal material: a piece of one chromosome is present but translocated and attached to another chromosome. Some chromosomal rearrangements can pass through cell division unaltered but others are unstable. When the chromosomes involved in the balanced translocation pair at meiosis, there are six segregation products possible (Fig. 30.3). One segregation product involves the normal copy of each chromosome, one involves the balanced translocated chromosomes, and the other four comprise unbalanced segregation products (partial trisomy in two and partial monosomy in two). Individuals with balanced translocations may first be identified when they have recurrent fetal loss or children with malformations caused by unbalanced translocation.

Translocations most commonly occur between autosomes. In autosome/X chromosome translocations, the normal X is usually preferentially inactivated to maintain activation of the complete genomic complement. This can effectively lead to a hemizygosity for a mutated gene resulting in a female affected with a genetic condition usually observed only in males.

Robertsonian Translocation

Five human chromosomes (13, 14, 15, 21, and 22) have very small short arms and are known as *acrocentric chromosomes.* Translocations involving these chromosomes are relatively common (1 in 900 newborns) and usually involve two different chromosomes. The most common Robertsonian translocation involves chromosome 21, resulting in Down syndrome. This translocation should be suspected when there is more than one child in a family with Down syndrome.

Insertional Translocation

A chromosomal segment may be deleted from within a chromosome (donor). Its removal may disrupt a gene at one or both breakpoints on the donor chromosome. When the donor chromosome fragment inserts into another chromosome (recipient), it can disrupt a gene or insert between two genes. If no genes are disrupted, lost, or duplicated on either the donor or recipient chromosome, the result is a balanced translocation.

MOSAIC ABERRATIONS

A mosaic individual has at least two cell lines differing in genotype or karyotype but derived from a single zygote. Mutations or aberrations can arise in a single cell in either prenatal or postnatal life, giving rise to clones of cells genetically different from the original zygote. The effects of mosaicism depend on what stage in development the abnormality occurred.

Somatic Mosaicism

If the aberration occurs in a body cell after conception, the resultant clinical abnormality will involve one or more organs/body parts depending on the embryonic stage of development at which the aberration occured: the later in gestation, the more localized the clinical abnormality. For example, swirling hyperpigmentation following the lines of Blaschko may represent a clone of cells arising from a late-occuring mutation in a surface ectoderm cell. Molecular analyses or karyotypes of the affected tissue is extremely helpful in documenting mosaicism. The karyotype of blood may be normal, but an aberration will be apparent on skin biopsy. Somatic mutations that occur postnatally cause many types of cancer, including 85% of cases of unilateral retinoblastoma.

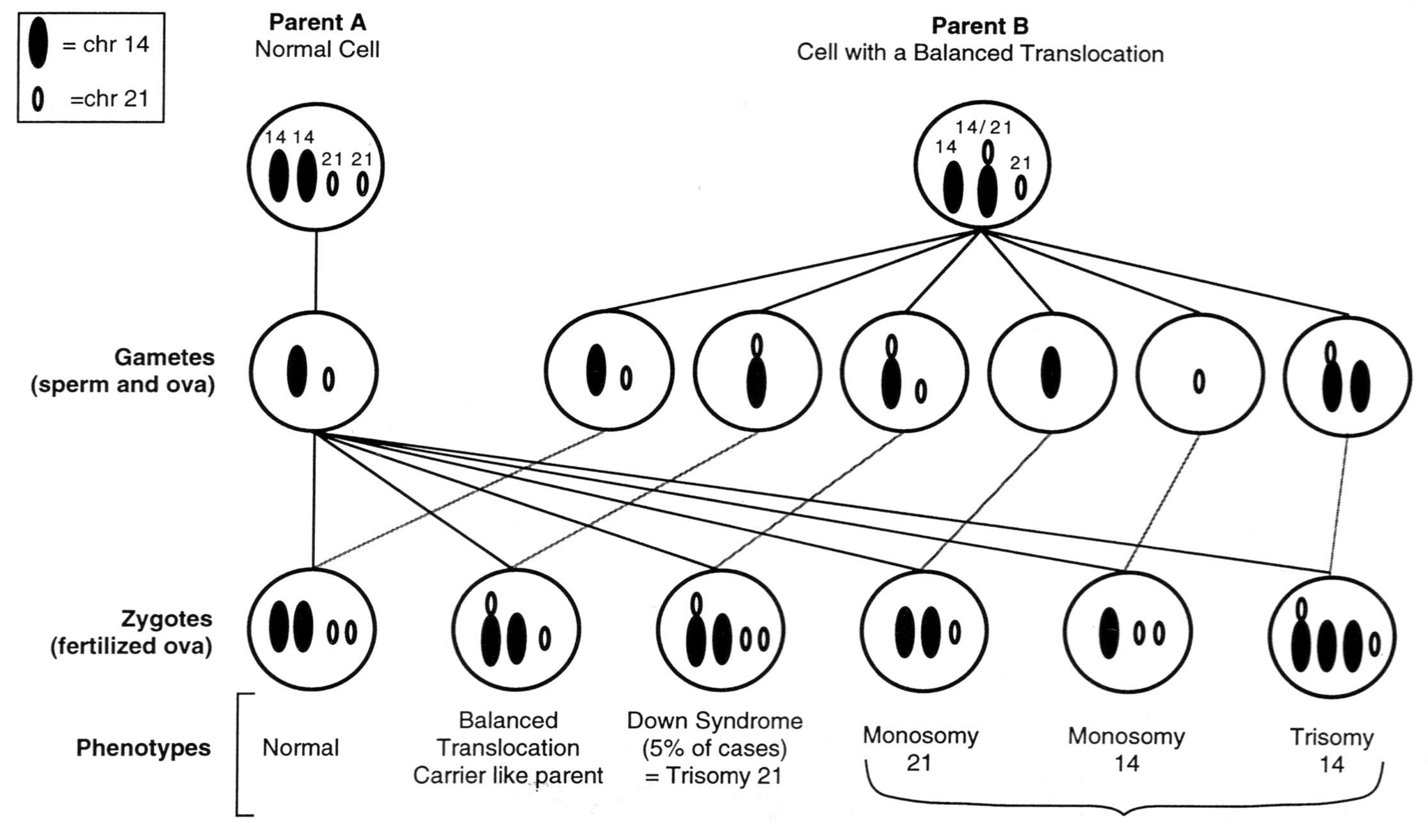

Figure 30.3. Possible products of a mating between a normal individual and a spouse who carries a balanced translocation. The spouse is carrying a common balanced Robertsonian translocation (14/21) wherein all of one chromosome 21 is attached to chromosome 14.

Germline Mosaicism

In females, the germ cells undergo mitotic division about 30 times before meiosis. In males, the germ cells undergo mitotic division several hundred times before meiosis. Mutations thus have many opportunities to occur during germ cell development and may result in germline mosaicism without any somatic abnormalities. Recurrence risks for parents of a child affected with an autosomal dominant or X-linked condition must include a discussion of possible germline mosaicism. If the affected child is the product of an abnormal sperm or egg from a mosaic population of germ cells, then the risk of recurrence is reduced; subsequent pregnancies can result from conception with normal eggs and sperm. The literature is scarce in the estimation of recurrence risk, but it is on the order of 7%–10%, although a risk as high as 22% may be possible.

Placental Mosaicism

Of the cells in the blastocyst, 95% give rise to the placenta and its associated membranes, while only 5% become the embryo. If a mutation or chromosomal aberration takes place in the very early blastocyst stage, the placenta could be mosaic and the embryonic cells could all be normal, or both the placenta and the embryo could carry the aberration and be mosaic.

GENOMIC IMPRINTING

Genomic imprinting is the term used to explain the variation of expression of a disease phenotype depending on which parent the abnormal gene was inherited from. For any given pair of genes, either the maternally or paternally inherited copy may not usually be functional in normal individuals. This can result in two different syndromes depending on which allele is abnormal. For example, when the paternal 15q11-q13 allele is deleted, the phenotype is Prader-Willi syndrome, characterized by obesity, short stature, small hands and feet, and mental retardation. When the maternally inherited chromosome has the deletion, the phenotype is Angelman syndrome, the characteristics of which are dramatically different from Prader-Willi syndrome, with a very happy and social behavior, seizures, and more severe intellectual impairment.

Uniparental disomy occurs when an individual has inherited both copies of all or part of a chromosome from only one parent with no contribution for that chromosome from the other parent. When the whole chromosome from one parent is present in duplicate, the term *isodisomy* is used. *Heterodisomy* refers to situations in which part of a chromosome from one parent is duplicated.

Mosaicism, uniparental disomy, and imprinting should be considered possible causes of genetic disease in the following cases:

- an autosomal recessive disorder found in a patient who has only one identifiable carrier parent in the absence of incorrect paternity
- the syndrome is known but one or more features are uncommon to the disorder; especially if mental retardation or growth deficiency are present
- parent and child have an autosomal recessive condition in the absence of consanguinity or incorrect paternity
- male to male transmission of an X-linked recessive disorder

DETECTION OF CHROMOSOMAL ABERRATIONS

Blood, skin, amniocytes, chorionic villi, and other human tissues can be obtained and cultured for use in cytogenetic analysis. Cells in vivo and in vitro do not divide in a synchronized fashion. To achieve synchronization, colchicine is added to the culture medium, arresting cell division in metaphase. Hypotonic solutions are used to swell the cells and disperse the chromosomes. The cells are dropped onto microscopic slides, causing the cells to burst open resulting in a metaphase spread of chromosomes. Chromosomes can then be stained with different substrates to cause different areas of the chromosome to stain light or dark. Each chromosome has a unique banding pattern.

Giemsa or G-banding: Treating with trypsin followed by Giemsa stain results in a black-and-white banding pattern. This is the most common method of staining (Fig. 30.1A).

Quinacrine or Q-banding: Chromosomes are treated with quinacrine and viewed under UV light.

Centromere or C-banding: This method is useful for examining the Y chromosome or the centromeric regions of chromosomes.

Reverse banding or replication banding: This technique is used to determine whether a particular segment of a chromosome is early or late in the replication cycle. Usually the banding pattern is the negative of the image seen by G-banding.

Silver staining: When marker chromosomes or ribosomal gene regions need to be identified, silver staining is used to blacken the genes that are actively producing rRNA.

Fluorescein in situ hybridization (FISH): Rather than banding, fluoresceinated DNA probes or "paints" can be used to identify segments of DNA or whole chromosomes. This technique is particularly useful in identifying marker chromosomes or microdeletion syndromes. DNA sequences can be recognized if the probe is at least 2000 base pairs (2Kb) in size. Other applications of FISH include:

- rapid detection of aneuploidy in uncultured aminocytes
- detection of deletions, translocations, and other structural abnormalities
- characterization of cell hybrids when human chromosomes are lost or rearranged during culture
- mapping sequences of DNA (resolution of 3 Mb or more)
- resolving the order of probes (resolution of 20 Kb)

OCULAR MANIFESTATIONS OF SPECIFIC CHROMOSOMAL SYNDROMES

Chromosome 1

In a study of 5049 consecutive liveborn children, Friedrich and Neilsen found a balanced translocation rate of 1.39 per 1000 children.[57] Chromosome 1 was involved in 43% of these translocations. Although balanced translocations involving chromosome 1 may be relatively common, the rarity of deletions and trisomies suggests the severity of the respective phenotypes.

Deletion: 1p Minus

Definition. A variety of breakpoints have been described as a result of interstitial deletions, malsegregation of a familial balanced translocation, and de novo translocation with deletion.[86,171] Most terminal deletions have clustered distal to and/or inclusive of 1p34.[86] Interstitial proximal deletions cluster in the 1p22-p31 region.[86,171] The hypervariable repeat region at 1p36.3 may be a "hot spot" for breaks.[17]

History. Aarskog's patient with a large terminal deletion of 1p was the first reported with a 1p− syndrome.[1]

Incidence. Interstitial deletions of chromosome 1p are particularly rare, with fewer than 15 cases reported.[171] Deletions of 1p36 are probably under-recognized because of difficulties in cytogenetic detection of this light distal band.[165] One group has estimated an incidence higher than 1 : 10,000.[165]

Systemic manifestations. As a result of the dissimilar deletion patterns, the reported phenotypes have been quite variable and not clearly related to particular breakpoints.[86] Mental retardation, developmental delay, or psychiatric /behavioral disturbances have been found in all reported cases.[17,86,188] Malformations present in more than 30% of cases include low-set and or posteriorly rotated anomalous ears,[2,86,145,148,171] short neck, bulbous nose, clinodactyly of the fifth finger (as well as several less commonly reported anomalies of the digits, including absent thumb),[2,11,71,86,145,148,171] and congenital heart disease.[86,171] Nonfocal neurologic signs such as mild ataxia or dysarthria, as well as generalized hypotonia[2,188] or seizures,[17] may also occur; yet postmortem brain evaluation has been normal.[2,86] Other anomalies reported in some cases include high arched or cleft palate with or without cleft lip,[2,86,145,171] microcephaly,[145,148] hypertrichosis,[145,148] cryptorchidism,[145,188] dental anomalies,[148] micrognathia,[11,148,188] and preauricular tags.[86] Blennow and co-workers reported a child with a terminal deletion and deafness.[17] The facies has been described as rounded.[11,148]

Stockton and co-workers reported a child with del1p21-22.3 and a particularly severe phenotype in comparison to other similar deletions.[171] The child had severe congenital heart disease, absent thumb, vertebral anomalies, and bilateral cleft lip and palate. The authors speculate that the phenotype could be due to the unmasking of an autosomal recessive mutation on the other allele, or to imprinting.

When deletions are confined to chromosome 1p36, moderate mental retardation and hypotonia are still found in almost all patients.[165] Speech may be particularly impaired.[165] Although usually normal at birth, an obese phenotype is rarely present but feeding problems and poor weight gain are common.[165] The del1p36 phenotype also includes large anterior fontanelle (100%), pointed chin (80%), seizures (72%), flat nasal bridge (65%), clinodactyly and short fifth finger (64%), low-set ears (59%), hearing deficits (56%), and abusive behavior (56%).[105a] Congenital heart disease and cleft lip/palate are less common.[105a]

Survival of 5 months[2] to 30 years[148] has been reported and appears to be unrelated to any particular deletion pattern.[86]

Ophthalmic manifestations. The only oculofacial feature reported in more than 30% of reported cases is small palpebral fissures.[86] However, the exact nature of this defect has not been described. Howard reported an infant with "narrow" palpebral fissures.[86] It is not stated whether this apparent narrowness is in the vertical or horizontal plane. Wenger described a patient with "slightly almond-shaped" eyes.[188] Upslanting of the fissures has been reported in one case,[2] whereas Palova simply described "slanting" of the eyes in an affected child.[145] Two patients had epicanthal folds.[145,188] Hypertelorism and hyperopia were described in one boy.[145] Terminal deletions may be associated with "deep-set" eyes.[17] Both long eyelashes and synophyrs have been reported.[86,148]

Two patients with deletions in the region of 1p22.1-22.2 had bilateral coloboma.[86,148] One woman with bilateral microphthalmia had iris and choroidal coloboma.[148] Gray reported one child with "tiny bilateral central" cataracts, although chromosomal rearrangement may have played a role in generating the clinical characteristics (see below).[71] The patient reported by Stockton and co-workers had no ophthalmic findings despite a deletion of 1p21-22.3 and an otherwise uncharacteristically severe phenotype.[171] Unfortunately, other reports of patients with deletions in this region have not provided adequate ophthalmologic data.[86] Yunis's patient with "scare" [*sic*] eyebrows and enophthalmia but normal ophthalmologic examination is an example.[198]

Blennow's patient with a terminal deletion with a breakpoint in the 1p36.31-36.33 region had optic atrophy with "impaired vision."[17] Although not broken down per patient, the series of patients with del1p36 reported by Shapira and co-workers revealed a wide range of eye/vision problems (75% of patients), including strabismus, 6th cranial nerve palsy, amblyopia, refractive errors, anomalous optic discs, and lacrimal defects.[165] No further details are given.

Diagnosis. FISH has been used to identify small deletions.[17]

Deletion: 1q Minus

Definition. Deletions of 1q can be classified into three groups: del1q21-q25, del1q25-32, and del1q42-qter.[173]

Incidence. The latter group is the most commonly and usually involves 1q42 and/or 1q43.[76] Fewer than 15 cases monosomic for 1q21-q25 have been described.

History. The first patient with a 1q deletion was described in 1972 by Mankinen.[76]

Systemic manifestations. When the deletion is interstitial, involving 1q21-25, features include developmental delay, hypotonia, microbrachycephaly, cleft palate, posteriorly rotated ears, clubfoot, transverse plamar crease, and malformations of the heart, external genitalia, and kidneys.[173] Takano and co-workers reported a patient who also had myelomeningocele with hydrocephalus and anal atresia.[173]

Patients with del1q25-32 show prune belly syndrome and Potter sequence.

The patients with terminal deletions exhibit profound mental retardation, growth deficiency, and microcephaly. Some have abnormalities of the genitals[106] and heart.[63,76] Endocrine abnormalities such as hypothyroidism and growth hormone deficiency have also been reported.[106] As children, patients may also have bursts of spontaneous laughter or unexplained syncope.[76,106] Minor malformations may include a round or broad facies with downturned mouth,[76,106] flat philtrum with thin lips,[76] low-set ears,[63] micrognathia,[63] short broad nose,[76] short or thick neck,[63,106] and clinodactyly.[63,76,106] Halal et al. make the important point that the del1q facies can easily be mistaken for that of Down syndrome, although from the photographs provided, this diagnostic confusion appears to be more prominent in adulthood.[76]

Although approximately one-third of patients die in the first 2 years of life,[76] the two oldest reported survivors are a severely retarded 12-year-old,[76] and a 35-year-old woman.[76]

Ophthalmic manifestations. Epicanthal folds appear to be a constant feature of the distal 1q deletions. Halal et al. have also reported upslanting palpebral fissures.[76] Strabismus (unclassified, exotropia by photograph) was seen in Halal's 35-year-old patient but it is not stated if she had this finding in childhood, and childhood photographs do not allow for adequate assessment.[76] No further ophthalmologic details are given. Garver et al. reported two affected siblings with "protuberant eyes."[63]

Merlob has described a girl with sparse eyebrows and lashes, and bilateral retinal and optic nerve colobomas, as well as absent foveal reflexes as a result of an unbalanced translocation with a partial trisomy of 4q and a terminal deletion of 1q.[84] Although neither dup4q nor del1q has been reported to be associated with these oculofacial abnormalities, a patient with del1q and bilateral iris colobomas has been reported.[41] However, that patient's sibling, with the same 1q deletion, did not have coloboma. Merlob observed that the majority of his patient's systemic defects were more similar to del1q than dup4q. Merlob's patient had hypotelorism, whereas the patient with a pure 1q deletion reported by Koivisto had hypertelorism.[106]

Duplications: 1

Definition. Complete trisomy of chromosome 1 is incompatible with life and results in fetal death.[181] As with many partial trisomies resulting from unbalanced translocations, the duplicated portion of chromosome 1q is found attached to another chromosome from which there will be a small terminal deletion. The "recipient" chromosome reported for the 1q+ has been 2q,[110] 3p,[141] 12p,[181] and 4q.[136] Garver et al. reported an interstitial trisomy of 1q as a result of a rearrangement between 1p and 1q.[63]

Systemic manifestations. Multiple malformations, including congenital heart disease,[136,181] micrognathia,[63,136,141,181] cleft lip and palate,[141] hirsutism,[136,141] cryptorchidism,[141,181] renal dysplasia and hypoplasia[141,181] possibly with calcifications,[136] and absence of the gallbladder[141,181] are part of the 1q+ phenotype. The brain shows microgyria,[141] absent olfactory nerves,[141] and other evidence of cerebral dysgenesis[141] or hydrocephalus.[136]

Infants with trisomy 1 usually die on the first day of life.[141,181] Garver's patient,[63] who had a small interstitial trisomy, lived at least to 4 years of age. This patient had severe physical and mental retardation.

Ophthalmic manifestations. Ocular malformations are not a major part of this syndrome. Minor reported malformations have included "small and wide-set" eyes[63,181] and downslanting of the palpebral fissures.[141] Small eyes were also a feature in Laing's patient with dup1q42.3-qter associated with a monosomy for part of 2q.[110] Verbraak and co-workers reported a child with congenital glaucoma and trisomy 1q41-qter but ascribed the ocular abnormality to the associated monosomy 9p23-pter because of a previous report.[182]

Ring Chromosome 1

Incidence. Fewer than five cases have been reported.

History. Gordon's report of a 5-year-old girl with a mosaic ring 1 was the first published, although it is likely that the patient also had other chromosomal abnormalities.[71] Wolf then reported a girl with ring 1 in all cells but mosaic for an absence of either chromosome 1 or chromosome 3.[193] Kjessler's patient was also mosaic with some cells having a normal karyotype and others having one or more ring 1 chromosomes.[104]

Systemic manifestations. The major systemic features of ring 1 are microcephaly, mental retardation, and short stature.[19,71,193] Wolf has also described an "elfin" facies with upturned mouth.[193] Cleft palate,[104] abnormal ears,[104] congenital hip dislocation,[19] preauricular sinuses,[19] clinodactyly,[19] and ascites[104] may also occur. Affected patients are noted to have a particularly pleasant and lively personality.[11] Reported patients have survived to at least 9 years of age.[71] No autopsies have been reported. Bobrow's patient died of leukemia at 9 years of age.[11]

Ophthalmic manifestations. Gordon and Wolf did not report any ocular abnormalities.[71,193] However, Kjessler's patient had small palpebral fissures, epicanthal folds, and downslanting.[104] Bobrow's patient had a slight upslanting.[11] Retinal examination was normal.

Chromosome 2

Deletion: 2q Minus

Definition. Deletion of 2q33 may be associated with a Seckel syndrome phenotype (bird-headed dwarfism),[37] a syndrome otherwise known to be autosomal recessive.

Incidence. Over 50 patients with interstitial deletion of 2q have been reported.[37] Most often, these deletions are proximal to or up to and including 2q33. Deletion of 2q36 is extremely rare.[129]

Systemic manifestations. The Seckel syndrome phenotype associated with del2q33.3-q34 includes intrauterine and postnatal growth retardation, developmental delay, microcephaly, receding forehead, large beaked nose, micrognathia, radial head dislocation, clinodactyly, and absent earlobes.[37] Hypotonia and hypospadias may also be observed. Deletion of 2q36 has been associated with myelomeningocele, mild congenital heart disease, developmental delay, and minor dysmorphic features, including a long philtrum, hypoplastic nasal bridge, prominent anteverted nasal tip, and mild abnormalities of the fingers.[129]

Ophthalmic manifestations. Downslanting palpebral fissures are seen in the Seckel phenotype. "Small eyes" have been reported in a case of del2q37.1-qter, but this may have been an effect of the concomitant duplication of part of the 1q terminus as discussed previously.[110] Melnyk and Muraskas described "apparent narrowness of the palpebral fissures" in a child with deletion of 2q36, but this is not readily apparent in the accompanying photographs.[129] That child also had hypertelorism. No other ocular abnormalities are described, and the child was noted to have normal visual behavior.

Duplication: 2q Plus

Definition. Most duplications of 2q result from unbalanced translocation, which leads to trisomy for the entire q arm.[9]

Epidemiology. Various interstitial duplications of distal 2q have been reported. Barbicoat and co-workers reported two siblings trisomic for 2q24.3-q32.1 by virtue of an insertion if this material into the long arm of chromosome 5.[9] Their father had a balanced translocation and was clinically normal.

Systemic manifestations. There is evidence that the extent of the trisomic region correlates with phenotypic severity. Features common to virtually all distal trisomies of 2q include developmental delay, prominent forehead, depressed nasal bridge, anteverted nares, and long philtrum with thin upper lip. Ear anomalies include earlobe creases.[9] Other reported findings include inguinal hernia, brachycephaly, clinodactyly, and pectus excavatum.[9]

Ophthalmic manifestations. Hypertelorism has been reported in all cases of distal dup2q. The patients reported by Barnicoat and co-workers also had upslanting palpebral fissures and epicanthal folds.[9] One of the sibling pair had esotropia.

Trisomy 2

Definition. Complete trisomy of chromosome 2 is present in liveborn infants only as mosaicism.

Incidence. This is a very uncommon chromosomal anomaly.

Systemic manifestations. Despite trisomic cells only detected on liver biopsy, Sago and co-workers reported a child with multiple nonhepatic malformations including congenital heart disease, growth failure, hydronephrosis, gastrointestinal dysfunction, brain dysgenesis, hypotonia, microcephaly, and developmental delay.[159] The child had cholestasis and hepatic fibrosis. Perhaps tissues inaccessible to biopsy would also show the trisomy, although it was not found in intestinal mucosa, skin, ascitic fluid, or blood.

Ophthalmic manifestations. The patient reported by Sago and co-workers had "prominent lower canthal folds," although these are not obvious in the photograph provided.[159]

Chromosome 3

Duplication: 3q Plus

Definition. A 3q duplication syndrome has been described in which affected individuals have a phenotypic resemblance to the Brachmann-de Lange syndrome (Cornelia de Lange syndrome, CdLS). These patients are triploid for a region involving all or part of chromosome 3q21-qter.[154]

Systemic manifestations. Patients demonstrating the CdLS phenotype in association with dup3q show hirsutism, anteverted nares, carp shaped mouth with downturned corners, ear malformations, cardiac malformations, and mental, as well as growth retardation. There are some distinctions in that limb reduction anomalies are more often associated with CdLS syndrome without chromosomal aberration, whereas craniosynostosis, urinary malformations, and cleft palate are more often seen in dup3q.[154] Rizzu and co-workers reported a mother and child with dup3q25-q26 who had a mild phenotype.[154] The absence of severe mental retardation as well as some other minor dysmorphic characteristics led the authors to conclude that dup3q25-q26 lies proximal to the critical region for the CdLS phenotype, which as a result of their literature review, they specify as 3q26.3-q27. However, with the exception of craniosynostosis, the majority of features they report are seen in mild forms of CdLS. It may be that CdLS, with its wide spectrum of expression, may be a contiguous gene syndrome with more severe manifestations seen with duplication of more distal genes.

Ophthalmic manifestations. The dup3q CdLS phenotype is associated with hypertelorism, synophrys, and epicanthal folds. Other more compromising ocular abnormalities seen in patients with CdLS but no chromosomal aberration are usually absent. In the more proximal interstitial duplication reported by Rizzu, the patients had only high arched eyebrows and upslanting palpebral fissures.[154]

Chromosome 4

Deletion: 4p Minus (Wolf-Hirschhorn Syndrome [WHS], Pitt-Rogers-Danks Syndrome [PRDS])

Definition. The cardinal features of this condition are related to a deletion of a distal piece of 4p in the region of 4p16.3. The critical region has been narrowed by Reid and co-workers, as well as other laboratories,[62,152] and lies distal to the Huntington disease locus. No patient with both Wolf-Hirschhorn syndrome (WHS) and Huntington disease has been reported, perhaps because of death prior to the usual adult age of onset for Huntington disease. The phenotype remains fairly constant despite significant variations in the deletion size.[50,62,150] Attempts have been made to map clinical features based on comparative deletion analysis.[50,91] Growth retardation and developmental delay cannot be isolated to a particular region, suggesting that more than one locus may be contributing.[50] It appears that WHS represents a contiguous gene deletion syndrome. Some traits, such as strabismus and epicanthus, may also show variable penetrance.[50] Likewise, the association of PRDS with del4p16.3 suggests either variable expression, different deletions in the same gene, or an overlapping contiguous gene syndrome.

Interstitial deletions proximal to the WHS region are usually found within 4p12-p16 and have a somewhat different phenotype.[190]

History. The features of this syndrome were first recognized independently by Wolf and Hirschhorn in two separate 1965 publications, but Hirschhorn may actually have described the first case in 1961.[92] More recently, several authors simultaneously published the association of the PRDS phenotype with del4p16.3.[32,117]

Incidence. The incidence of WPS is 1:50,000 live births.[49] Approximately 90% of cases are the result of a de novo event, while 10%–15% represent the product of a familial balanced translocation. De novo deletions are usually on the paternal chromosome.[49,121,135] Fewer than 20 patients with PRDS have been described.

Systemic manifestations. (Fig. 30.4) The major manifestations of Wolf-Hirschhorn syndrome include developmental delay (100%), growth retardation (90%), cleft lip and/or palate (57%) with or without micrognathism (70%), genital abnormalities (65%), congenital heart disease (50%), and seizures (50%).[49,62,70,91,133,150,152] Microcephaly (90%) along with a prominent glabella (50%) and long nasal root (beaked nose) have led to comparison of the head shape to that of a Greek helmet in profile.[49,51,92,135,150] Minor features include low-set posteriorly rotated ears, with or without preauricular tags and/or hearing loss, short philtrum, bowed or carp-shaped mouth, and scalp defects.[49,62,70,135,150,152] Hypotonia, decreased tendon reflexes and abnormalities of the corpus callosum have been noted in over half of all patients.[70,135,150] Minor skeletal anomalies may include tapered fingers, scoliosis, concave or hyperconvex nails, and clinodactyly.[49,62,150] Other uncommon associations include congenital heart disease, cleft lip and/or palate, and hypospadias.[51,92,135] Fused teeth and hypospadias seem to map distal to the WHS region but may be present in terminal deletions.[50] Most children with WHS die in the first 2 years of life, and those who survive longer have severe mental retardation.[92] The most common causes of death are respiratory and cardiac.[92]

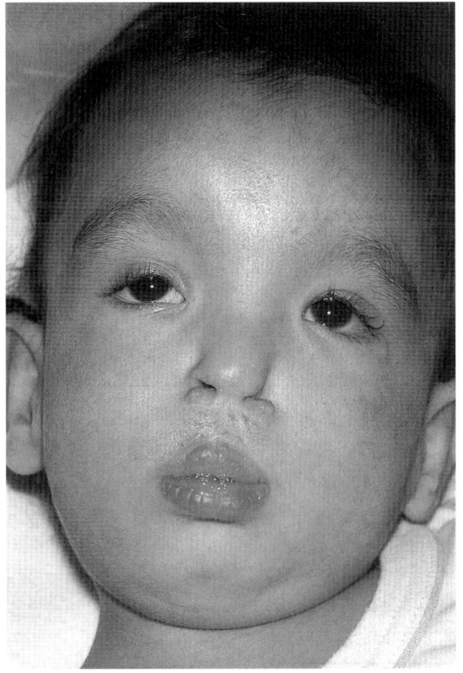

Figure 30.4. Patient with typical facial features of Wolf-Hirschhorn syndrome (del4p). There was mild anterior segment dysgenesis. (Reproduced by permission from Kozma et al. *Am J Ophthalmol* 1986;102:592–597.)

The PRDS and WHS phenotypes share moderate to severe developmental delay, seizures, growth retardation, and hypotonia (often with neonatal feeding difficulties).[32,117] The prominent glabella is not seen and instead midfacial/maxillary hypoplasia with or without micrognathism, exorbitism, a short philturm, wide mouth, prominent (or beaked) nose, and microcephaly are characteristic, giving the lower face the appearance of being vertically compressed.[32,117] Cleft palate is not seen. Patients with PRDS often have abnormal palmar creases and simplified ears.[32] Their life span is significantly longer than that of WHS patients, probably because of the infrequency of heart anomalies, with several patients living into their 50s.[117]

Deletions proximal to the WHS region, involving 4p14-p16, present with variable developmental delay, hypotonia, high arched palate, thick lower lip, micrognathia, and prominent nose. They differ from WHS patients particularly in their tall thin habitus, myopathic facies, and abnormalities of nipple position and number.[190]

Ophthalmic manifestations. Minor oculofacial features may include hypertelorism (65%–75%), arched eyebrows with medial thinning/flare (55%), epicanthus (25%–50%), upslanting or downslanting palpebral fissures (5%), and, less commonly, inferior scleral show, periorbital swelling[150]/proptosis[92]/shallow orbits,[50] or blue sclerae.[49–51,62,70,91,92,135,150] "Brushfield" spots on the iris[121] and iris heterochromia are rare.[150] The spots tend to be atypical and more centrally located than those commonly seen in trisomy 21.[150] Cataracts may occur in up to 25% of children,[135,150] although some authors have found this to be a rare anomaly.[92] Perhaps the most common ocular malformation is coloboma (over 30%) or corectopia, with or without microphthalmia.[92,135] Coloboma may be unilateral[91,92,121] or bilateral. Nasolacrimal duct obstruction, esotropia,[62] exotropia,[92,121] and nystagmus have also been reported.[49,50,150] Strabismus is seen overall in approximately one-third to two-thirds[49,50,92,135] of all patients. Ptosis is seen in about 20%–25%.[49,50,92]

Comparative deletion-phenotype analysis suggests that the loci for strabismus, hypertelorism, epicanthal folds, and abnormalities of the eyebrows occur with deletions that extend proximally, whereas less proximal involvement may still result in ptosis.[50] Only abnormal slanting of the palpebral fissures seems to map to a specific locus: a 150 kb region between D4F26 and D4S90.[50] Nystagmus has been seen in isolated terminal deletions[50] and also with interstitial deletions proximal to the WHS region.[190] The patients from the study that was used to define the 4p16.3 critical region did not have coloboma.[62,152]

The critical region includes the phosphodiesterase β-subunit (PDEβ) gene. Biallelic mutations in this gene may be associated with retinal dystrophy. However, to our knowledge, retinal dystrophy has not been seen in association with WHS.

PRDS patients do not show the range and severity of ocular malformations seen in WHS.[117] They may have epicanthus and hypertelorism although Clemens and co-workers felt that the apparent hypertelorism was not real.[32,117] The exact cause of reported pseudoproptosis/exorbitism is unclear, but in published photographs there often appears to be inferior scleral show associated with ectropion or euryblepharon of the lateral lower lids.[32,117] One patient was reported to have "irregular pigmentation of the retina," but an electroretinogram (ERG) was not done.[117] Myopia has also been described.[117]

Diagnosis. Although some patients have large, cytogenetically visible deletions, molecular techniques, such as FISH, may be required to make the diagnosis of submicroscopic deletions.[51,62,70,91] Preus and co-workers developed a numerical scoring system for phenotypic features, which may be helpful in identifying patients with normal karyotypes on whom further molecular analysis might be indicated.[150]

Deletion: 4q Minus

Definition. Interstitial deletions are more often distal than proximal.

Incidence. Fewer than 15 cases of proximal interstitial deletion have been reported, almost all of which occurred de novo.[167]

Systemic manifestations. Phenotypes of the 4q deletions are often variable. Deletion of 4q27-31 is associated with mild mental retardation, and micrognathia and dental malocclusion but no other systemic abnormalities.[29] Deletion of 4q12-q13.1 also results in mild mental retardation and dental anomalies, along with hypotonia.[167] Major malformations are uncommon but may include renal malformations, congenital heart disease, or seizures. Dysmorphism characteristically involves a high forehead, flat nasal bridge, and receding chin.[167] Minor anomalies of the digits and nipples may also occur. Deafness or cleft palate are uncommon associations. When the deletion involves 4q12, piebaldism may result due to hemizygosity for the *c-kit* gene.[167]

Ophthalmic manifestations. One case of bilateral type II Duane syndrome with ptosis has been reported in a patient with del4q27-31.[29] Bell's phenomenon was reduced. This is one of the few chromosome anomalies reported in patients with Duane syndrome. When 4q12 is involved, manifestations of piebaldism may include hypopigmentation of the eyebrow and anomalies of iris color.[167] In a patient with del4q12-q13.1, esotropia, refractive error, and epicanthus were present.[167] Oblique palpebral fissures and dystopia canthorum have also been reported. Other reported ocular anomalies associated with proximal interstitial deletions include colobomatous microphthalmia, pigmentary retinopathy, and exotropia.

Ring Chromosome 4

The phenotype of a ring chromosome 4 may be identical to the Wolf-Hirschhorn syndrome or may have additional features due to deletion of 4q such as reduction of the radius or absent thumbs.[121]

Chromosome 5

Duplication: 5p Plus

Systemic manifestations: Leichtman and co-workers reported a patient with almost complete (5p12-pter) duplication and inversion of chromosome 5p. The clinical features of the patient were either identical to the Optiz BBBG syndrome or represented a phenocopy.[113] The patient had an asymmetric skull and facies, macrocephaly, low-set posteriorly rotated ears, retrognathia, wide mouth with short philtrum, cleft palate, pectus excavatum, patent ductus arteriosus with aberrant locations of the coronary ostia, cryptorchidism, urinary reflux, hiatal hernia, anteriorly displaced anus, fifth finger clinodactyly, broad thumbs and large toes, hypoplastic nails and hypotonia, with a weak, hoarse cry.[113] The patient also had a dysplastic cleft larynx and hypospadias, which have not previously been associated with BBBG syndrome. The infant had a stormy clinical course and died at 3 months of age.

Ocular manifestations: Leichtman's patient had orbital hypertelorism, telecanthus, and a mild downslanting of the palpebral fissures.[113]

Chromosome 6

Deletion: 6p Minus

Definition. Most deletions of chromosome 6p are terminal deletions. The 6p23 breakpoint is more common than 6p24.

Epidemiology. Fewer than 20 reports of terminal del6p have been reported.

Systemic manifestations. The terminal 6p deletion phenotype, when 6p23 is involved, is characterized in more than 70% of affected children by craniosynostosis (various types, including coronal synostosis, trigonocephaly), with or without microcephaly, and small, pinched nose with flat bridge and anteverted nostrils.[144] Ninety percent have congenital heart disease.[144] It is unclear whether hepatosplenomegaly and thrombocytopenia are related to congenital heart malformations. Hydrocephalus, hypotonia, malar hypoplasia, high/cleft palate, minor ear abnormalities with or without hearing loss, micrognathia, downturned mouth, and webbed/redundant loose neck skin have also been observed.[144,186,199] Hypoplastic nails, minor extremity malformations, and genitourinary abnormalities may occur.[144,199,186] Various abnormalities of nipple anatomy, position, and number have also been reported.[144,199]

Ophthalmic manifestations. Eye abnormalities are seen in over 70% of patients with terminal deletions involving 6p23, although no characteristic pattern is seen. Reported abnormalities include microphthalmia, iris coloboma, Peters' anomaly/corneal opacification, optic atrophy, nystagmus, and epicanthal folds.[144] The eyes have been described as "bulging" with upslanting or downslanting palpebral fissures, mild synophrys, and hypertelorism.[144,199,186] One child had a hemangioma involving the brow.[144] Blepharophimosis, esotropia, high hyperopia, and "Brushfield spots" have also been reported.[144,186,199]

A number of anterior segment disorders such as iris hypoplasia associated with glaucoma map to 6p25.[128] Walsh and co-workers described an unusual anterior segment malformation associated with deletion of 6p24-pter.[186] The child had white corneal endothelial ridges in a quadrangular configuration to which were attached iris processes. In both eyes this finding was associated with posterior embryotoxon and, in one eye, progressive corectopia and ectropion uveae. The patient did not have glaucoma, but there was bilateral optic nerve hypoplasia. Visual evoked potentials (VEPs) and ERG were normal.

Deletion: 6q Minus

Incidence. Approximately 20 cases of del6q have been reported.

Systemic manifestations. Proximal deletions within the region 6cen-q15 have always been associated with umbilical hernia and developmental delay. Most affected children also show palmar creases, hyperextensible skin, joint laxity, microcephaly, and short stature. Of three reported cases involving 6q13-15, all had ectopic kidneys and short necks, while two had congenital heart disease.[66] Other features which have occurred in less than half but more than one of the patients deleted within the 6cen-q15 region, but which are not assignable to a particular subregion, include genitourinary anomalies, joint contractures, syndactyly, clubfoot, micrognathia, and large/low-set ears.

Ophthalmic manifestations. The child reported by Gershoni-Baruch and co-workers with del6q13-15 had hypotelorism, nystagmus, and blue sclerae.[66] The authors also state that the child had small palpebral fissures, downslanting fissures, and mild synophrys, although the photograph does not demonstrate these anomalies. Of seven reported children with proximal deletions (6cen-q15) downslanting fissures occurred in 6 (83%); epicanthal folds in 4 (57%); small palpebral fissures in 3 (43%); and strabismus in 2 (33%), but none of these features seem phenotypically localized to a particular subregion. Macular abnormalities, epicanthal folds, and strabismus have also been reported in association with terminal deletions.[199]

Duplication: 6q Plus

Definition. It has been suggested that duplication of 6q26 is critical for the 6q syndrome phenotype.[79]

Systemic manifestations. The dup6q syndrome is characterized by developmental delay, feeding difficulties, microcephaly, prominent forehead, midfacial hypoplasia micrognathia with carp-shaped mouth, short webbed neck, and flexion deformities such as clubfoot. Abnormal palmar creases may be seen. Henegariu and co-workers described a child with a more proximal duplication involving 6q23.3-25.3.[79] Although microcephalic, she had delayed fontanelle closure (in particular the metopic) and dolicocephaly due to a flattened prominent occiput. She also had congenital cardiac malformations. Like patients with the typical dup6q syndrome, she had flexion contractures, abnormal palmar creases (single), midfacial hypoplasia, and a carp-shaped mouth, but overall was less affected than those patients with dup6q26.

Ophthalmic manifestations. Oculofacial features of dup6q syndrome include downslanting palpebral fissures and epicanthus. The patient reported by Henegariu and co-workers had infraorbital creases, hypertelorism, epicanthus, and "almond-shaped" palpebral fissures without downslanting.[79] This child also had blue "tinted" sclerae.

Ring 6

Ophthalmic manifestations. Ring 6 is frequently associated with eye abnormalities presumably due to concomitant deletion of 6p chromosome. Reported abnormalities include anterior segment malformations (including aniridia, coloboma, ectropion uveae), glaucoma, optic atrophy, and retinal abnormalities.[199]

Chromosome 8

Deletion: 8p Minus

Incidence. Terminal deletions of chromosome 8p have been increasingly recognized through the identification of small deletions, particularly when distal to or involving 8p23.1, in patients previously thought to have normal chromosomes.[31]

Systemic manifestations. Patients with a deletion of the short arm of chromosome 8 are characterized by low birthweight (93%), short stature (80%), and significant developmental delay/mental retardation (100%).[31,125] Marino et al. reported a boy who was unable to sit and had only a few words at 4 years old,[125] whereas others report only mild developmental delays.[31] The degree of retardation may be related to deletion size.[31] Severe behavioral problems may also occur.[31] The most significant systemic abnormality is congenital heart disease, in particular atrioventricular canal.[31,125] The head tends to be dolichocephalic and microcephalic, with a high forehead.[31,125] Microcephaly is more common when the deletion involves 8p22 or 8p21.[31] Other facial features include low-set and/or malformed ears (93%), micrognathia (85%), arched palate (82%), flat nasal bridge (58%), short neck (55%), short nose (50%), and microstomia (43%).[31,81] Patients may also have abnormal genitalia (57%), cryptorchidism, puffy hands and feet, and a broad chest with wide-set nipples.[125,31] Gastrointestinal malrotation has also been observed.[31]

When terminal deletion extends centromeric to 8p23.1, involving up to 8p21, trigonocephaly, dysplastic ears, short neck, hypotonia, elbow dimples, and narrow thorax may also be observed.[31]

Ophthalmic manifestations: Perhaps the most common oculofacial abnormality is epicanthus, which is seen in 91% of children.[125] Hypertelorism is reported in 30% although it was not clarified how this assessment was made.[125] Marino and co-workers[125] reported a child with del8p21.1-23.1 who had long, thin sparse eyebrows and "deep-set" eyes. The authors' photographs do not clearly support the latter assessment. Claeys and co-workers reported hypertrichosis and synophrys in a child with del8p23.1-ter.[31]

One individual with an interstitial 8p23.1 deletion had strabismus, although further details were not available (presented by the Center for Human Genetics, Bar Harbor, Maine, 1994).

Deletion: 8q Minus

Systemic manifestations. Types I and II of the autosomal dominant tricho-rhino-phalangeal syndrome (TRP type I: early baldness, large nose, cone-shaped epiphyses of the middle phalanges; TRP type II [Langer-Giedion syndrome]: type I plus mental retardation, microcephaly, and multiple exostoses) have been attributed to a deletion of 8q24.1.[125] These may represent contiguous gene syndromes.

Ocular manifestations. Bushy eyebrows without synophrys were part of the TRP phenotype in one patient with an 8q24.1 deletion.[125]

Duplication: 8p Plus

Definition. Duplication of 8p can occur either through trisomy (Warkany syndrome) mosaicism, or "tetrasomy" as a result of a supernumerary isochromosome 8p. Phenotype does not correlate well with degree of mosaicism.

Incidence. Fewer than 15 cases of isochromosome 8p have been reported.[192]

Systemic manifestations. Like trisomy for all of chromosome 8, trisomy 8p is characterized by deep hand and foot creases as well as a short wide neck.[192] One child with an inverted terminal duplication of 8p21.2-8p23.2 presented with a triangular facies, growth and developmental delay, large ears, and a café-au-lait spot.[85] The features of supernumerary i(8p) are similar to trisomy 8p, sharing in common agenesis of the corpus callosum, developmental delay, rib anomalies and congenital heart disease (50%), as well as the deep plantar/palmar furrows.[137,155,162,192] The ribs may even be "absent" with a "flail chest" deformity.[155] Isochromosome 8p is also associated with high/cleft palate, enlarged cerebral ventricles with or without gyral anomalies, and veretebral anomalies with or without scoliosis.[108,137,155,162,192] A wide range of development, from normal to moderate delays, has been reported, although motor delays due to hypotonia seem to be a consistent finding.[108,137,155,162,176] Death may occur in the neonatal period, often from the heart disease, or survival may be prolonged into the second decade.[192]

Although dysmorphism may be absent[108] the appearance may be characterized by a high forehead/frontal bossing, sparse temporal hair, and mild ear abnormalities.[137,155,162] A shy behavioral phenotype with obesity has been described.[176] As seen in trisomy 8, abnormal nails,[162] clinodactyly,[137] or gastrointestinal problems such as duodenitis, hamartomata (intestinal, liver, adrenal), and malrotation of the gut rarely occur.[155] Nevus flammeus may be seen.[155] We have cared for a child with mosaic i(8p) diagnosed from biopsy of swirling hyperpigmented skin streaks, who had mild dysmorphism and mild developmental delay. Although rare, children with virtually none of the clinically detectable malformations above have also been reported.[176]

Ophthalmic manifestations. In general, i(8p) is not associated with ophthalmic findings. However, our patient had bilateral severe congenital glaucoma necessitating multiple procedures but with remarkable preservation of some vision despite long periods of intraocular pressure in excess of 40. Schrander-Stumpel reported one child with "left-sided telecanthus and pseudostrabismus" and slightly upslanting palpebral fissures and another child with epicanthus and pseudoesotropia.[162] Epicanthus has been noted by other authors.[137] The eyebrows and eyelashes may be sparse.[155] Duplication of 8p21.2-8p23.2 has been associated with hypertelorism.[85]

Diagnosis. FISH has been useful in characterizing the isochromosomes.[192]

Trisomy 8 (Warkany Syndrome)

Definition. Trisomy 8 is almost always mosaic or the result of translocation. The average peripheral blood mosaicism is 62% and for fibroblasts 72%.[153] However, severity and degree of mosaicism are not correlated. The most common translocation breakpoint is 8q2, with chromosomes 13, 22, and X involved.[153] Other more proximal breakpoints have been described, but the phenotype is then different from Warkany syndrome, suggesting that 8q2 is a critical region.[153]

Incidence. Trisomy 8 has been reported in close to 100 children.

Systemic manifestations. The clinical features of Warkany syndrome have been reviewed in detail by Riccardi.[153] Trisomy 8 is characterized by mental retardation (IQ range 12–80), a dysmorphic facies (prominent anteverted nasal tip, prominent lower jaw, mouth held open), absent or dysplastic patella, joint contractures (in particular limited supination/pronation), vertebral defects, urinary anomalies, a distinctive toe posture (flexed and turned toward the midline of foot, with digits 2 and 3 having equal length), and deep furrows in the palms and soles.[153] Other features seen in 50% or more of affected individuals include cleft or high palate, sacral dimple/spina bifida occulta, congenital heart disease, clinodactyly/long fingers, slender pelvis, abnormal ears, hip dysplasia, everted lower lip, sternum abnormalities, or abnormal nails.[153] Seizures and gastrointestinal anomalies such as anus abnormalities are seen in less than one-third.[153] Birthweight is usually normal.[153] Behavioral phenotype may include temper tantrums. Rib abnormalities and palmar/plantar furrows are the most distinctive features distinguishing between trisomy 8 and translocation.[153]

Siblings with a paternally derived undefined marker chromosome identified by FISH as a chromosome 8 derivative had a duplicated thumb, developmental delay with autistic features, and coarctation of the aorta.[158]

Ophthalmic manifestations. Trisomy 8 is associated with canthal abnormalities and one-third of affected patients show abnormal palpebral slanting.[153] The broad nasal root gives a false appearance of hypertelorism. Strabismus is seen in one-half of all patients.[153] Although the siblings with a marker 8 chromosome had no reported eye abnormalities, their father, who had 10% mosaicism for the marker chromosome, had high myopia.[158]

Chromosome 9

Deletion: 9p Minus

Ophthalmic manifestations. Verbraak and coworkers reported a child with congenital glaucoma and monosomy 9p23-pter associated with trisomy 1q41-qter.[182] They ascribed the ocular abnormality to the 9p trisomy, as deletions of terminal 1q have not previously been associated with this finding.[182]

Duplication: 9q Plus

Systemic manifestations. Microcephaly is associated with duplication of proximal 9q, and vertebral abnormalities with large low-set ears are associated only with duplication of the last band of 9q34.[170] A number of findings have been seen in patients who share the duplication of 9q32: deep-set eyes, beaked nose, micrognathia, long fingers, and stiff joints. Therefore, it appears that dup9q32 may be a critical region.[170] Global developmental delay is also a part of the 9q duplication syndrome.

Ophthalmic manifestations. Strabismus (esotropia[170]) is only seen with duplication of the proximal segment of 9q. Epicanthal folds, narrow palpebral fissures, and deep-set eyes are variably present. Stalker and co-workers reported one child with dup9q12-q33, who had all of these ocular features as well as synophrys.[170]

Trisomy 9

Incidence. Trisomy 9 is rare in liveborn children. In fact, it may be that many liveborn children actually have cryptic mosaicism and that nonmosaic cases succumb prenatally.[23] It has been shown that the manifestations in mosaic versus nonmosaic infants with trisomy 9 are not significantly different.[23] Therefore, the descriptions of malformations reported herein are combined. In either case, this severe chromosomal aberration is not consistent with survival beyond the neonatal period.

Systemic manifestations. Characteristic features in liveborn infants include intrauterine growth retardation, skeletal anomalies (95%), congenital heart disease (86%), congenital kidney disease (59%) and genitourinary malformations (55%).[23] Minor abnormalities such as rocker-bottom feet, joint contractures, overlapping fingers, and hypoplastic nails have been observed. Dysmorphic craniofacial features include malformed low-set (91%) ears with possible absent external canals, cleft/arched palate (83%), micrognathia (77%), bulbous nose (77%), wide fontanelles (71%), and small mouth (11%).[23] Other reported malformations include abnormalities of the palmar crease (65%), low hairline (21%), and, less commonly, anomalies of the gallbladder or diaphragmatic hernia.[23] The brain may be grossly normal despite a 22% incidence of microcephaly.[23]

Ophthalmic manifestations. Microphthalmia is the most common ocular manifestation (61%).[23,100] Although 45%[23] of patients are reported to have "deep-set eyes," it is not clear if this is always due to microphthalmia. Cantu and co-workers reported a liveborn infant with bilateral microphthalmia, cataracts, corneal clouding, "deep-set eyes," and a "depressed right globe."[23] Although not described further, the latter finding may be related to the facial asymmetry seen in approximately one-third of affected babies.

Chromosome 10

Deletion: 10p Minus

Definition. The majority of cases have their breakpoint at 10p13,[119] although a breakpoint at 10p14 is less common.[119]

Incidence. Fewer than 30 cases have been reported.[119]

Systemic manifestations. The facies associated with interstitial del10p13 may be similar to DiGeorge syndrome, and other characteristic malformations may be present, including posterior cleft palate, tracheomalacia, ventricular septal defect, and a small thymus.[119] Finger contractures may also be seen. Deletion of 10p is felt to be second only to del22q11.2 in causing a DiGeorge phenotype.

Deletion: 10q Minus

Definition. The Bannayan-Riley-Ruvalcaba syndrome is an autosomal dominant disorder characterized by macrocephaly, lipomas, and hemangiomas. Ruvalcaba-Myhre syndrome is characterized by macrocephaly, intestinal polyposis, and pigmentary spotting of the penis. Riley-Smith syndrome overlaps with these syndromes and includes pseudopapilledema. Autosomal dominant Cowden disease, also known as multiple hamartoma syndrome, is characterized by macrocephaly, mucocutaneous abnormalities, and hamartomatous neoplasms. All four syndromes appear to be allelic and can result from del10q23.2-q24.1, a region that includes the *PTEN* gene, mutations in which are known to cause these syndromes.[5] The clinical manifestations of all four syndromes may overlap in any individual.[5]

Incidence. Deletions of 10q23.2-q24.1 are rare.

Systemic manifestations. Other associated features may include midfacial hypoplasia, prominent forehead, developmental delay, and hypotonia. Dermatologic lesions particularly characteristic of Cowden disease include facial tricholemmas, as well as acral keratosis and papillomas. Skin lesions, however, usually do not occur until adulthood.[5]

Ophthalmic manifestations. Hypertelorism may be associated with the midfacial hypoplasia seen in del10q23.2-q24.1.[5] Pseudopapilledema is a more "classic" finding. Anisometropia has also been reported.[5]

Duplication: 10p Plus

Definition. Most cases result from translocation with few reported instances of isolated pure trisomy.[33] The most common proximal breakpoint is at 10p11, and the most common mechanism for pure trisomy is translocation to the short arm of an acrocentric chromosome.[33]

Incidence. Over 60 cases have been reported, including those associated with monosomy of another chromosome due to translocation.

Systemic manifestations. Attempts to delineate a common phenotype have been unsuccessful. Only hypotonia, high arched/cleft palate, frontal bossing, clubfoot, and nasal anomalies are reported in more than half of reported cases. Dolicocephaly, delayed suture closure, and mouth abnormalities are seen in less than 50%.[33] Cardiac malformations and cystic dysplasia of the kidney occurred in 28% and 18%, respectively.[33] Agenesis of the gallbladder may also occur.[33] Only hypotonia has a significant association with isolated trisomy of the largest trisomic segment, 10p11-pter.[33] Only high arched/cleft palate and clubfoot are significantly more frequent in pure trisomy as opposed to translocations with concomitant monosomy.

Ophthalmic manifestations. Considering all trisomy 10p patients (including translocations) as a group, approximately one-fifth have ocular anomalies, in particular colobomatous microphthalmia; epicanthus and/or downslanting palpebral fissures are seen in about one-third.[33] One child with an inverted terminal duplication of 10p12.13-pter was diagnosed with pseudotumor cerebri based on the presence of a bulging fontanelle.[85] She was otherwise entirely well. No opthalmic signs were reported.

Duplication: 10q Plus

Definition. Proximal interstitial trisomies have been reported to involve 10q11-q22 or 10q21-q22.[1]

Incidence. Approximately 30 to 40 cases of distal trisomy of 10q have been reported. Fewer than 10 cases of de novo proximal trisomy appear in the literature.

Systemic manifestations. Trisomy involving the 10q11-q22 region usually manifests with growth retardation, microcephaly, mild to moderate developmental delay, prominent forehead, anteverted nares, bow-shaped mouth, micrognathia, flat thick ear helices with or without ear pits and/or hearing loss, and long slender limbs.[1] There is no clear phenotypic variance between duplicated areas of varying size within this region. A child with an inverted terminal duplication of 10q25.1-qter was described as having a flat occiput, flat face, small nose and mouth, congenital hip dislocation, abnormal thumbs, developmental delay, microcephaly, and hypotonia.[85]

Ophthalmic manifestations. Duplication of the 10q11-q22 region is usually characterized by "small" deep-set eyes,[1] although more precise definition regarding micropthalmia has been lacking. In the case reported by Aalfs, this finding is reported yet not demonstrated by the clinical photograph.[1] Vision was normal in this child. Epicanthus is only seen when the trisomy extends from 10q11.2 to q22.3 or 10q21-q22, but not when the trisomy extends more proximally to involve 10q11.2.[1] Conversely, strabismus is seen only when the more proximal region is involved. Downslanting palpebral fissures have been reported in a child with dup10q11.2-22.3.[1] Iris coloboma and retinal dysplasia have been reported in 2 of 7 cases with duplications in this region, one proximal and one distal, thus showing no clear relationship to the involved regions.[1] Blepharophimosis has only been reported with 2 of 3 reported patients with dup11q21-q22, but not when the same region was involved along with more proximal loci.[1] Duplication of 10q25.1-qter is associated with upslanting palpebral fissures and epicanthus but an otherwise normal ocular examination.[85]

Diagnosis. FISH has been used to characterize proximal interstitial trisomy.[1]

Chromosome 11

Deletion: 11p Minus

Definition. The WAGR syndrome, characterized by Wilms' tumor, *a*niridia, genitourinary anomalies, and *r*etardation, is a contiguous gene deletion syndrome involving *PAX6* at 11p11.3 and extending distally into the Wilms' tumor gene, WT1. (See Chapter 6 for more information.)

History. It was Hittner and Francke who first reported heritable transmission of aniridia due to a deletion of 11p.[82]

Incidence. Compared to other chromosomal deletions, del11p in association with aniridia is less common.

Systemic manifestations. Other features are hypotonia, trigonocephaly, hearing deficits, midline brain anomalies, and minor abnormalities of the fingers.

Ophthalmic manifestations. The best recognized ocular manifestation of del11p is aniridia, which is caused by involvement of the *PAX6* gene. The manifestations of aniridia are variable, reflecting the characteristic variable expression of this disorder. Aniridia (see Chapter 6) may occur with any combination of cataracts, macular hypoplasia, glaucoma, keratopathy, and nystagmus. Dry eyes and ptosis have also been reported.[82] It is important to note that other ocular disorders associated with *PAX6* mutations, such as autosomal dominant keratitis and Peters' anomaly, would be expected with del11p.

Deletion: 11q Minus (Jacobsen Syndrome)

Definition. Although Jacobsen's original report described the 11q deletion in the context of a familial 11;21 translocation, over 90% of terminal deletions arise de novo.[142] Whereas 70%–80% of terminal deletions have a breakpoint at 11q23.3, the Jacobsen eponym is often used for any case of terminal 11q deletion with a breakpoint including or distal to 11q23. It has been suggested, however, that deletion of 11q24.1 is critical for the full Jacobsen phenotype.[38,59,60,143] The eponym is not used for interstitial deletions.

The frequency and preponderance of a breakpoint at 11q23.3 has been attributed to the presence of a fragile site (FRA11B) at this locus.[93,184] Molecular techniques have also suggested that cases assumed to be terminal deletions by cytogenetics or FISH may actually have some preservation of telomeric sequences.[93,147] The most frequent translocation also involves a breakpoint at this location and 22q11.2.[87]

History. Jacobsen originally described terminal deletion of 11q23-qter in 1973.[89]

Incidence. Over 50 cases of terminal deletion with breakpoint 11q21-q24 have been reported. The incidence has been estimated at less than 1 in 100,000.[147] Fewer than 10 cases of interstitial deletions of 11q have been described. The phenotype tends to be less severe than terminal deletions.[80]

Systemic manifestations: (Fig. 30.5) Terminal deletions from 11q23 are most often characterized by developmental delay (100%), trigonocephaly (95%), a flat bulbous nose, depressed nasal bridge (62%), ear abnormalities, micrognathia (76%) with or without abnormal palate, a carp-shaped mouth (74%), pre- and postnatal growth retardation (73%), cardiac abnormalities (67%), minor distal limb anomalies or joint contractures (86%), and transient or intermittent thrombocytopenia or pancytopenia (38%). These features are described in detail in references 27, 52, 56, 59, 60, 80, 89, 96, 56, 134, 142, 147, 161, 179, 184. Hertz and co-workers reported a stillborn child with a subterminal deletion with a proximal breakpoint at 11q21.[80] This child had cleft lip and palate and an absent uvula in addition to the other characteristic facial features and growth retardation. Although cleft lip and palate have been seen in interstitial 11q deletions involving 11q21, they are not associated with more terminal deletions involving the same locus, excepting two cases of translocation with a breakpoint of 11q23 in which the effect of a concomitant partial trisomy can't be ruled out.[80]

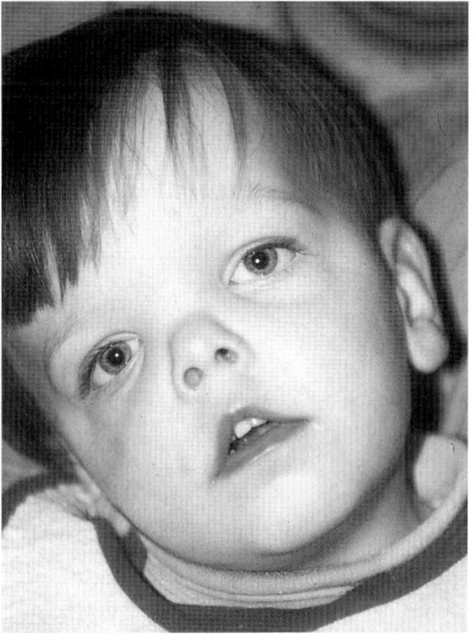

Figure 30.5. Jacobsen syndrome (del11q).

Penny and co-workers used molecular techniques in 17 patients with terminal deletions including or distal to 11q23 to define the following critical regions from centromeric to telomeric: craniosynostosis (11q23.3-11q24.1, between D11S1316 and D11S912), digit anomalies (between D11S933 and D11S912), cardiac defects (distal to D11S933 or D11S912), thrombocytopenia (distal to D11S1351), and facial dysmorphism.[147] However, these findings were not absolute, because in some patients a particular region was involved without the clinical manifestation assigned to that region. The size of the deletion was correlated with the severity of dysmorphism and developmental delay, the latter being most prominent when 11q23 or 11q24.1 are involved. Although they are uncommon, minor structural brain defects are correlated with more proximal deletions,[142,147] as are rare renal or genital anomalies.[89,184] Deafness has been reported in del11q22-qter.[116]

The phenotype for interstitial deletions is more variable. Wakazono and colleagues reported a child with del11q14-q22.[185] The child had transient hypocalcemia, hypotonia, severe growth and developmental retardation, dolichocephaly, anteverted nares, flat nasal bridge, high palate, carp-shaped mouth, and micrognathia. She had repeated respiratory infections despite a normal immunologic evaluation.

The hematologic defect may be associated with recurrent respiratory infections[52,116,134,142] and may be the cause of death. Approximately 25% of affected children will die before 2 years of age, usually because of the cardiac anomaly.[147] Decreased survival in males has been assumed based on the higher incidence in females.[52,56,179] Only one patient is known to be surviving into her late teens.[147] Fryns et al. reported a 21-year-old man with del11q24.2-qter who was also monosomic for part of chromosome 14.[59] Terminal deletions with more proximal breakpoints may be associated with reduced longevity or even lethality. A child with del11q22-qter died at 6 months.[52] Linarelli reported a 12-year-old with del11q22-qter.[116] A 1976 cytogenetic study reported a remarkably mildly affected 4-year-old girl with isolated speech delay despite a del11q23-qter.[48] This is very contrary to all other reports in the literature with similar breakpoints.

Patients with more distal breakpoints show milder phenotypes.[147,164] Schwarz and co-workers reported a 17-year-old-boy with del11q24.2-qter, a breakpoint beyond the presumed "critical region" for Jacobsen syndrome.[164] Although the boy had developmental delay, he enjoyed good health, had no craniosynostosis, hematologic defect, or limb abnormalities, and had only minimal structural brain abnormalities.

Ophthalmic manifestations. The ocular abnormalities most commonly associated with terminal deletions including 11q23 are telecanthus and/or hypertelorism, ptosis, and epicanthal folds. These features are described in references 27, 52, 56, 80, 89, 96, 116, 142, 161. The child reported by Hertz and co-workers with a subterminal deletion had exorbitism in addition to hypertelorism.[80] A patient of Schnizel et al. with a breakpoint of 11q23 had the "impression of a protrusion" of the globes attributed to "hypoplastic orbital roots."[160] Obregon and colleagues also reported hypoplastic roofs.[142] Although hypotelorism is not always reported in this fashion, it is usually hypotelorism rather than hypertelorism that is seen when trigonocephaly of any cause is present, suggesting a more distal, albeit variable, critical region for hypertelorism.[147] Perhaps telecanthus and/or epicanthus has been misinterpreted as hypertelorism in some cases where trigonocephaly is present.[27,160] Hypertelorism can be seen when the deletion starts at the presumed 11q24.1 "critical region,"[143] an observation consistent with Penny's more proximal localization of trigonocephaly.[147]

As described in references 27, 48, 59, 89, 116, 134, 142, 143, 147, 161, 179, epicanthus can be seen with or without a variety of breakpoints, whereas ptosis is usually restricted to deletions involving all or part of 11q23.[27,59,116,142,147,161,179] The ptosis may be mild,[56] unilateral or bilateral, or show absent levator function more consistent with congenital ptosis.[27,160] Upslanting (See references 27, 59, 60, 89, 142, 147, 160, 179 for the former and references 48, 116, 134, and 184 for the latter.) or downslanting of the palpebral fissures has been variably reported. Ectropion has been reported in three cases with del11q23-qter.[147] Lid colobomas with otherwise normal globes were present in a child with del11q22-qter.[52] Short or long eyelashes and eyebrows have been reported with del11q23.

Other reported ocular abnormalities in terminal deletions (breakpoints cited after each anomaly listed as follows) include unilateral or bilateral colobomas of various size and extension with or without microphthalmia with deletion of 11q23,[53,96,116,142,147,160] correctopia (11q23),[27] nuclear cataract (11q23),[53,142] persistent pupillary membrane (11q23),[53] "circular white spots" in the iris stroma (11q23),[160] juvenille glaucoma,[142] and strabismus with breakpoints involving 11q23,[134,147,160] 11q23.3,[179] or 11q24.1.[147]

The retinal examination has not often been commented on. Jacobsen's original description included a normal funduscopy in the first year of life.[89] Schinzel and co-workers also reported a normal fundus in a 1-year-old with del11q23-qter but "poor retinal pigmentation" in a child with a similar breakpoint and other ocular malformations.[160] Felding and Mitelman described a child with del11q22-qter and "progressive pigmentation" of the fundus starting at birth.[52]

Uto and colleagues reported a child (del 11q23.3-qter) born after a full-term gestation with peripheral avascular temporal retina, temporal dragging of retinal vessels, and peripheral vasculopathy.[179] The authors believe that the patient has familial exudative vitreoretinopathy (FEVR). Autosomal dominant FEVR has been mapped to the region 11q13-q23 and was closely linked to marker D11S533, which is proximal to the common breakpoint for terminal deletions.[115]

Although no ocular anomalies were seen, the patient with interstitial del11q14-q22 reported by Wakazono et al. is said to have telecanthus and bilateral ptosis (not confirmed by photographs).[185] Patients with breakpoints distal to 11q24.1 show no ocular abnormalities with the exception of possible hypertelorism, ptosis, esotropia, and in one case, hypertrichosis of the eyebrows.[147,164]

Duplication: 11q Plus

Systemic manifestations. A patient with dup11q22-qter and a phenotype similar to the Pitt-Rogers-Danks syndrome, known to be associated with del4p (*vide supra*) has been reported.[42] This 50-year-old man also had severe kyphoscoliosis, prognathism, severe leg edema, hypertonicity, and spina bifida occulta, features not seen in PRDS.

Ophthalmic manifestations. Unlike patients with PRDS, the adult reported by de Die-Smulders and Engelen, with dup11q22-qter, also had mild ptosis,[42] hypertelorism, and "prominent eyes."

Ring 11

History. The first report of ring 11 was made by Velente and co-workers in 1977.

Systemic manifestations. The patient reported by Cousineau and co-workers had a Jacobsen phenotype, including trigonocephaly, heart defects, micrognathia, and minor ear anomalies, all attributed to del11q24-qter.[38] This is surprising in that some systemic and ocular features were present that are normally associated with a more proximal deletion involving 11q23. This suggests that the early cytogenetic techniques that were used may have failed to detect the full deletion or that the breakpoint at 11p15 is contributing. Similarly, the patient reported by Nikawa and co-workers, with breakpoints at 11p15 and 11q25, shows some features of Jacobsen syndrome (prenatal growth retardation, pancytopenia, minor ear anomaly, micrognathia, arched palate, heart anomaly), several of which are most likely due to the del11p15-pter (genital anomaly, short neck, café-au-lait spots, nail dystrophy).[139] Short neck has also been seen with a single case of del11q23.1-qter.[60] Nikawa's patient was said to have frontal bossing, but there was no mention of trigonocephaly. Both children with ring 11 died in the second year of life.

Ophthalmic manifestations. The patient reported by Cousineau had narrow downslanting palpebral fissures, telecanthus, and epicanthus.[38] Nikawa's patient had hypertelorism, telecanthus, and exotropia.[139]

Chromosome 12

Duplication: 12p Plus

Definition. Pallister-Killian syndrome (PKS) describes the presence of a mosaic supernumerary isochromosome 12p with predilection for the isochromosome to be found in skin but not in lymphocytes.[14,36,16,163] The percentage of mosaicism in peripheral blood does not correlate with severity of the phenotype.[163]

Incidence. Fewer than 100 cases of PKS have been described.[14]

Systemic manifestations. PKS is characterized by coarse facial features, broad high forehead with sparse anterior hair, ear abnormalities, macrostomia, and a short broad nose with anteverted nares and a flat bridge.[36,16,163] Patients have profound developmental delay, seizures, and hypotonia as well as unusual pigmentary abnormalities of the skin.[14,163] Less common features may include anogenital abnormalities, minor finger anomalies, hearing loss, cleft palate, and hemihypertrophy. Bielanska and co-workers review the literature regarding the incidence of these findings.[14] Streaks of hyper/hypopigmentation may be observed due to mosaicism.[36] Early death may occur if multiple organ malformations are present.

Ophthalmic manifestations. Hypertelorism is common (61%).[14,36,16] Approximately half will have epicanthal folds.[14] Other lid anomalies include ptosis, lower lid entropion, and upslanting or downslanting. Patients with PKS often show sparse hair (34%), in particular bitemporal alopecia, as well as sparse eyebrows (24%). Although Bielanska's patient had esotropia,[14] the majority of strabismic patients are exotropic.[16] Other ocular findings include myopia,[14,16] coloboma,[163] "markedly cloudy corneas" (presumably due to anterior segment malformation in a patient with coloboma),[163] and nystagmus (usually horizontal pendular and symmetric).[16] Birch and co-workers have drawn attention to patchy fundus hypopigmentation as a manifestation of the chromosomal mosaicism.[16] The child also had mild iris stromal hypoplasia but no iris transillumination. The laboratory did not have age-matched controls, but the authors report that the electroretinogram was subnormal. As infant electroretinograms have lesser amplitude, this may be a spurious finding. The child also had vertically oval optic nerves and relatively poor visual responses in infancy, which may be due to the nystagmus, retina, or optic nerves.

Diagnosis. FISH may be useful in identifying the isochromosome.[163] Fibroblasts are a more reliable specimen for detection as the isochrome may be absent from lymphocytes.[163]

Chromosome 13

Deletions: 13q Minus

Definition. The q32 region appears to be a particularly important region phenotypically when one considers its relation to the deleted segment. Brown and co-workers have categorized the phenotypes with this in mind.[21]

- Group 1: proximal deletions usually not involving 13q32.
- Group 2: distal deletions involving at least part of 13q32.
- Group 3: more distal deletions involving 13q33-34.

Some of the phenotypic differences may also be due to imprinting.[21]

Systemic manifestations. According to Brown's classification, there appear to be three phenotypic categories based on the relationship of the deletion to 13q32.[21]

- Group 1: mild or moderate mental retardation, growth retardation, hypotonia, and variable minor anomalies, although microcephaly may also occur.
- Group 2: one or more major malformations, in particular microcephaly, brain malformations such as anencephaly or encephalocele, cardiac malformations, distal limb abnormalities, and gastrointestinal tract malformations.
- Group 3: severe mental retardation without major malformations and usually without growth retardation.

Thumb and/or big toe anomalies are associated with deletion of 13q32, and so is Hirschsprung disease. It appears that there may be more than one locus on 13q that affects limb development and colonic innervation. Minor dysmorphic abnormalities such as large ears, beaked nose, facial asymmetry, and protruding upper incisors occur in patients from both groups 2 and 3.[21]

Ocular manifestations. Brown's classification can also be applied to the ophthalmic abnormalities seen in 13q deletions.[21]

Groups 1 and 3:	minor anomalies such as hypertelorism and iris heterochromia with or without retinoblastoma.
Group 2:	minor anomalies including hypertelorism, downslanting of the palpebral fissures and major ocular malformations including "fixed pupils" and the ocular manifestations of severe brain malformations.

Brown and co-workers also reported a child with "partial aniridia," absent corpus callosum, and hypertelorism, although these findings may have been related to the involvement of chromosome 6 in a translocation [46XY, −13, +der(13)t(6 : 13)(q27;q32)].[21]

Trisomy 13 (Patau Syndrome)

Definition. Trisomy 13 as discussed here refers to a complete or near-complete trisomy.

History. Bartholin described what was probably trisomy 13 in 1657, but Patau and coworkers, in 1960, where the first to recognize the relationship of the clinical syndrome to trisomy 13.[146] Trisomy 13 was the second recognized autosomal trisomy in a liveborn child.

Epidemiology. Trisomy 13 is the most common chromosomal abnormality associated with congenital ocular malformations at birth.[172] The reported prevalence varies a great deal, and is likely to change in terms of live births due to increased availability and accuracy of prenatal diagnosis. Three recent studies suggest that the incidence of trisomy 13 in liveborn infants is about 1 in 20,000.[25,69,196] Increased maternal age (mean 30.9 years) is associated with this syndrome. Males and females are affected with equal frequency.

Systemic manifestations. (Fig. 30.6) Partial trisomy for the segment 13 pter-q14 is characterized by a nonspecific pattern of malformations and severe mental deficiency. There is little similarity to the phenotype of patients with full trisomy, and most patients survive. Individuals with partial trisomy for the distal segment of 13q have severe mental deficiency, a characteristic facies including a frontal capillary hemangioma, and a higher death rate, about 25% in the early postnatal period. Trisomy 13 mosaicism is characterized by a less severe phenotype with a wide variation of clinical findings.

Central nervous system anomalies occur in over 50% of patients, with holoprosencephaly being the single most common malformation.[112] Seizures and severe mental deficiency are very common. Moderate microcephaly is common, with a wide sagittal suture and fontanelles. Cardiovascular defects occur in about 80% of patients, cleft lip and/or palate in 60%–80%, and abnormal external ears that may be low-set with/without deafness in over 50%. Capillary hemangiomas, in particular involving the forehead, as well as localized scalp defects in the parieto-occipital area may occur. Other findings seen in more than 50% of affected infants include intrauterine growth retardation, polydactyly, cryptorchidism in males, bicornuate uterus in females, a single umbilical artery, and persistence of embryonic and/or fetal hemoglobin. Polycystic kidneys occur in one-third of patients, along with other less common genitourinary abnormalities. Numerous other abnormalities have been reported. Ninety percent of patients have abnormalities that can be detected on prenatal ultrasound.[112]

Trisomy 13 is usually a lethal condition. One study showed that 28% of surviving newborn infants die in the first week of life, 44% within one month, and 86% in infancy.[123] There are a few long-term survivors. Although there is a very high incidence of congenital heart disease, these lesions are usually not lethal. One study suggested that primary apnea was the most common cause of death.[196] In light of this poor systemic prognosis, ophthalmic treatment has to be carefully considered.

Ophthalmic manifestations. (Fig. 30.6)[18,84,131] Ocular malformations are one of the cardinal signs of trisomy 13. The ocular anomalies are frequently severe and incompatible with vision. Both eyes are affected in nearly all children.

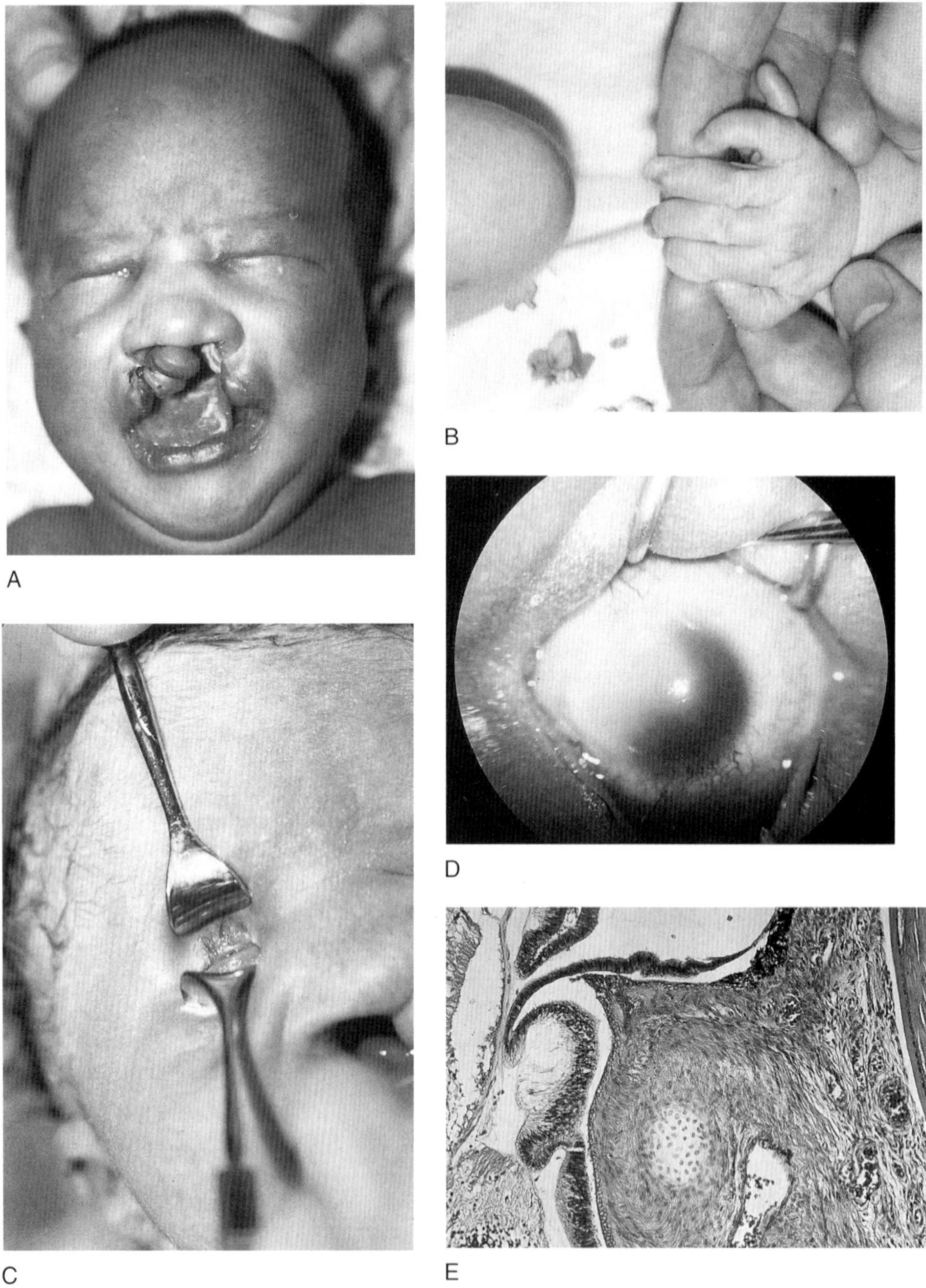

Figure 30.6. Trisomy 13. **A:** facial appearance. **B:** polydactyly. **C:** severe microphthalmia. **D:** partial sclerocornea. **E:** focus of cartilage in ciliary body of an eye from a patient with trisomy 13. (Courtesy of Dr. W. Richard Green.)

In Patau's original report,[146] "apparent anophthalmia" was described although the child more likely had severe microphthalmia as colobomatous microphthalmia is a well-recognized feature of trisomy 13.[68] Trisomy 13 is the most common chromosomal aberration associated with microphthalmia or anophthalmia.[100] Colobomas of the iris and ciliary body are very common and may be associated with cartilage or other choristomatous tissue in the ciliary body.

The retina, choroid, and optic nerve may be involved in the coloboma.

Dysembryogenesis of the anterior segment is common, sometimes phenotypically consistent with Rieger anomaly or, less commonly, Peters' anomaly. The anterior chamber angle is frequently malformed. The cornea may be vascularized and hypercellular with dysgenesis of Descemet's or Bowman's membranes. Cataract is common, with retention of the cell nuclei within the lens nucleus. There may be lens epithelium beneath the posterior half of the lens capsule. Optic nerve hypoplasia may also occur.

Congenital retinal nonattachment or folds due to retinal dysplasia with or without intraocular cartilage may occur. Trisomy 13 is the most common chromosomal aberration found in association with PHPV.[68] Goldberg has suggested that virtually any remnant of the fetal intraocular circulation (e.g., tunica vasculosa lentis) may persist.[68]

Less common ocular findings include shallow supraorbital ridges, slanting palpebral fissures, absent eyebrows, hypertelorism, hypotelorism, synophthalmos, and cyclopia. Congenital unilateral facial paralysis may rarely occur.[166] The child reported by Patau also had "non-elevated simple capillary hemangiomata" involving the upper eyelids as well as other areas typical of newborn nevus flammeus.[146]

Ring 13

Systemic manifestations. Brown and co-workers reported a child with ring 13(p11q13) and major malformations noted at elective abortion which included absent cranial vault, as well as gastrointestinal, genitourinary, limb, and pulmonary malformations.[21] A patient with similar involvement of 13p but less loss of 13q [r(13)(p11q32)] also had a number of major malformations, including microcephaly, absent and hypoplastic thumbs, ambiguous genitalia, anal stenosis, congenital heart disease, probable agenesis of the corpus callosum, multiple skeletal abnormalities, turricephaly with an abnormal ventricular system, and profound developmental delay.[73] Also noted were dysmorphic features, including low-set ears, flat nasal bridge, micrognathia, and arched palate. The authors suggest overlap with the XK syndrome. The child died at the age of 3 years.

Ophthalmic manifestations. Brown's case of ring 13 also had bilateral retinal dysplasia,[21] whereas the child with r(13)(p11q32) had microphthalmia with irido-chorio-retinal coloboma.[73] The latter child also had blepharophimosis with epicanthus, downslanting palpebral fissures, and hypertelorism.

Chromosome 14

Deletions: 14q Minus

Systemic manifestations. Miller and co-workers reported an infant girl with mosaic (64%) deletion of 14q32.3-qter and mental retardation, tracheoesophageal fistula, intestinal malrotation, and coronal synostosis.[132] Other dysmorphic features included low-set ears, midfacial hypoplasia, and maxillary hypoplasia.

Ophthalmic manifestations. Miller's patient with mosaic del14q32.3-ter had a unilateral nuclear cataract, "small orbits," and downslanting palpebral fissures.[132]

Duplication: 14p Plus

Ophthalmic manifestations. Although Fryns and co-workers reported a woman with a visually handicapping tapetoretinal degeneration (no further details given), who had a 14:18 translocation with a breakpoint at 14p11 for which she was trisomic, one cannot rule out the possibility that the ocular finding is due to the coexistent del18q21.[58] Retinal dystrophy has been associated with a deletion at this locus *(vide infra)*. However, the presence of hypotonia, choreoathetosis, sloping forehead, deep-set eyes, upturned nose, and everted upper lid in her affected child all suggest the effect of her dup14p. The patient was severely retarded and small with microcephaly, features known to be associated with del18q21.

Duplication: 14q Plus

Systemic manifestations. North and co-workers reported a child with inverted duplication of 14q22-q24.3 and CHARGE association, including congenital heart disease, choanal stenosis, mental and growth retardation, minor genital abnormalities, and hearing loss.[140] The patient also had clubfoot, pyloric stenosis, gastroesophageal reflux, and recurrent otitis media and sinusitis due to hypogammaglobulinemia. There was a prominent forehead, anteverted nares, bulbous nasal tip, low-set posteriorly rotated ears, micrognathia, and brachydactyly with syndactyly of the second and third toes.

Ophthalmic manifestations. The child reported by North and colleagues had hyperopic astigmatism and bilateral iris colobomas.[140] As with deletions of 14q, one must speculate about the possible role of disruption of the CHX10 gene, which is known to cause ocular malformations in mice although a human phenotype has not yet been identified.

Chromosome 15

Deletions: 15q Minus (Prader-Willi Syndrome, Angelman Syndrome)

Definition. Perhaps the most well-recognized 15q deletion is that involving 15q11-q13. As this is an imprinted region, deletion of the paternal allele will result in Prader-Willi syndrome, whereas deletion of the maternal allele at this region yields the Angelman syndrome phenotype. The syndromes may also result from uniparental disomy in children with normal karyotypes. Approximately 70% of Prader-Willi and Angelman syndromes are due to del15q11-q13. There may be intrachromosomal aberrations in the parental alleles that contribute to creation of a 15q deletion in their offspring.[26] It should be noted that the previous name for Angelman syndrome, "happy puppet syndrome," has been abandoned, as have the pejorative names of many other syndromes (see trisomy 21).

Systemic manifestations. Prader-Willi syndrome is characterized by neonatal hypotonia and feeding difficulties followed later by obesity, developmental delay, and in some children, hyperphagia that may be associated with behavior problems. Other features include small hands and feet, narrow bifrontal skull, and primary hypogonadism with cryptorchidism and small genitals.

Patients with Angelman syndrome have more severe developmental delay and seizures, which may involve inappropriate bouts of laughter and "puppet like" movements of the extremities. They do not demonstrate the obese phenotype seen in Prader-Willi syndrome.

Ophthalmic manifestations. Approximately 1% of patients with either Prader-Willi or Angelman syndrome due to del15q will have oculocutaneous albinism due to contiguous deletion of the P gene (see Chapter 34). In Prader-Willi syndrome the palpebral fissures are often described as "almond shaped."

Trisomy 15

Incidence. Trisomy 15 is generally considered incompatible with live birth, although five cases have been reported.[126] Like most trisomies, this aberration is associated with advanced maternal age, with the trisomic chromosome usually being of maternal origin.

Systemic manifestations. There are no consistent phenotypic features, although multiple congenital anomalies are usually present.

Ophthalmic manifestations. Retinal dysplasia and Bergmeister papilla have been observed.[68]

Chromosome 16

Deletion: 16p Minus

Definition. ATR-16 syndrome is a microdeletion phenotype associated with del16p13.3.

Incidence. Fewer than 10 cases of ATR-16 have been reported.

Systemic manifestations. The hallmark of ATR-16 syndrome is the presence of both alpha thalassemia and developmental delay. Other features may include midfacial hypoplasia, capillary hemangioma, clubfoot, and, less commonly, patent ductus arteriosus, inguinal hernia, hypospadias, cryptorchidism, and speech problems.[18]

Ophthalmic manifestations. Patients with ATR-16 syndrome have a common facial appearance test includes mild hypertelorism, downslanting palpebral fissures, and epicanthal folds. Scant eyebrows with hypoplastic superior orbital ridges and shallow orbits have also been reported.[118] One child is described as having "prominent globes with large-appearing irides" and incomplete closure of the eyes with blinking,[118] although this may all be a relative change due to shallow orbits. This child had del16p13.3-pter. Ophthalmic examination was otherwise normal.

Duplication: 16p Plus

Incidence. Fewer than 20 cases have been reported, mostly secondary to familial balanced translocation.

Systemic manifestations. Reported features of dup16p11.2-p12 have included a distinctive round face with flattened occiput, long philtrum, cleft palate, posteriorly rotated low-set ears, short neck, eczema, truncal hypotonia, hyporeflexia, and moderate developmental delay.[94] A single umbilical artery is seen in 50% of cases.[94]

Ophthalmic manifestations. Juan and coworkers described an infant with dup16p11.2-p12 who had "tremor-like movements and ocular revulsions lasting several seconds without loss of consciousness" that, in the absence of seizure activity on EEG, they attributed to a behavioral disturbance with autistic features.[94] Like other patients with trisomy 16p, this child had sparse eyebrows, hypertelorism, and epicanthus. The patient also had "alternating" strabismus and microphthalmia. Narrow palpebral fissures which give the patient a "sleepy" appearance have been described in more than one report.[94]

Chromosome 17

Deletions: 17p Minus (Smith-Magenis Syndrome)

Definition. The Smith-Magenis syndrome (SMS) phenotype is attributed to a microdeletion of 17p11.2.[54] One of the mechanisms for this contiguous gene deletion syndrome is homologous recombination of flanking repeat gene clusters.[27a]

Systemic manifestations. The Smith-Magenis syndrome is a specific phenotype that includes characteristic physical and behavioral manifestations: developmental delay/mental retardation, self-injurious behavior, and hyperactivity.[54,95] Patients have a flattened midface, brachycephaly, broad nasal bridge, short stature, and brachydactyly.[95]

Yang and co-workers reported a child with a deletion within the 17p11.2 region that did not involve the entire Smith-Magenis region and a phenotype more similar to Smith-Lemli-Opitz syndrome with micropenis and hypogonadism, laryngomalacia, polydactyly, craniofacial dysmorphism (anteriorly displaced parietal hair whorl, abnormal ears, long philtrum with thin upper lip, anteverted nares, small tongue, high palate, and midface hemangioma), and 2–3 toe syndactyly, but normal cholesterol levels.[197] The child died at the age of 2 years. The authors postulate that the phenotypic difference, as compared with Smith-Magenis syndrome, may either be due to position effects caused by the rearrangement (derived from a paternal inversion of 17p) or an unrecognized mutation on the other allele.

Ophthalmic manifestations. Finucane et al. reported a boy with a mosaic 17p11.2 deletion and a phenotype consistent with Smith-Magenis syndrome.[54] He had epicanthal folds, "Brushfield spots," and mild myopia that progressed to −6.00 sphere between the ages of 10 and 14 years. High myopia with retinal detachment has also been observed in nonmosaic patients.[95] Epicanthus may occur.[197] Iris coloboma is a very uncommon finding.

Diagnosis. FISH has been used, particularly in mosaic cases.[95]

Deletion: 17q Minus

Systemic manifestations. Deletions of 17q23.1-24.2 have been associated with the Hunter-McAlpine syndrome phenotype: autosomal dominant craniosynostosis (coronal, lamboidal, metopic) with developmental delay, downturned mouth, short stature, and minor skeletal anomalies.[175] Other features associated with this deletion are polydactyly, clubfoot, genitourinary anomalies, ankyloglossia, seizures, thin upper lip, dental anomalies, and low-set simple ears.

Ophthalmic manifestations. Almond-shaped palpebral features are one of the cardinal phenotypic features of the Hunter-McAlpine phenotype. In the del17q23.1-24.2 reported by Thomas and co-workers, the child had hyperopia, esotropia, and amblyopia with short palpebral fissures.[175]

Chromosome 18

Deletion: 18q Minus (De Grouchy Syndrome)

Definition. Although the eponym de Grouchy syndrome is often used to describe all deletions of the long arm of chromosome 18, the phenotype described by de Grouchy, prior to the days when more accurate banding could be done, seems to be associated with deletions distal to and including 18q21. More proximal deletions are less common and show a different phenotype.

History. The first report of an isolated deletion of 18q was made by de Grouchy et al. in 1964.[43]

Epidemiology. Well over 100 patients have been reported.

Systemic manifestations. (Fig. 30.7) The cardinal features of del18q reported by de Grouchy et al.[43] have been confirmed by other authors who describe patients with deletions usually distal to and including 18q21. The features include severe mental and motor retardation,[102,187,191] failure to thrive, short stature,[102,191] palmar creases,[88,191] and abnormal external ears.[102,187] Postsynaptic hearing loss can be present with or without[187] external ear abnormalities. Some patients with deletions distal to the proximal portion of 18q21.3 have been reported with milder developmental delay.[187] The correlation of severe phenotype with larger deletions has been confirmed using molecular techniques by Kline et al.[105] These authors established a phenotype map with microcephaly and severe mental retardation in the region of 18q21.2-21.3, abnormal brain on MRI at 18q21.2-22.2, and dysmorphic features with extremity abnormalities and hypotonia distal to 18q22.2.

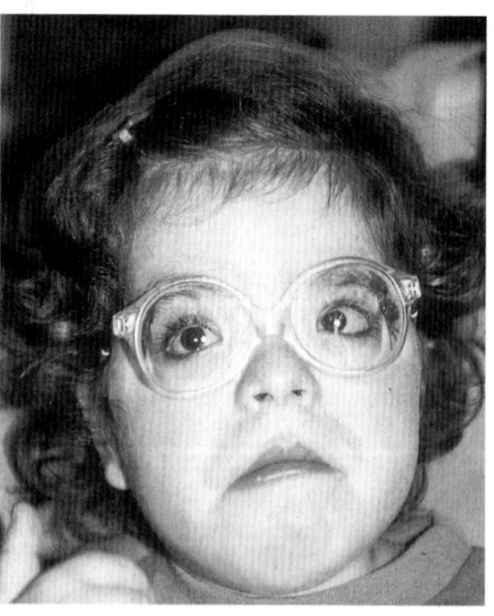

Figure 30.7. Facial features of a girl with de Grouchy syndrome (del18q).

Other features include microcephaly,[187,191] delayed secondary sexual features[187] with or without absent labia minora,[191] cleft lip and palate,[187,191] cutaneous hemangiomas,[187] congenital heart disease,[191] clubfeet,[187] and minor distal skeletal anomalies,[87,191] in particular cutaneous dimples in the fossae overlying the extensor surfaces of joints.[191] A characteristic facies may include mild hypotelorism[187] and a large downturned mouth.[102,187,191]

Although much less common, patients have been reported with deletions proximal to the region associated with the de Grouchy phenotype. Wilson and colleagues reported a patient who had an interstitial deletion extending either from 18q11 to 12.2 or from q12.2 to q21.1.[191] Although this patient had severe developmental delay and a transverse palmar crease, he had numerous features that differed from the de Grouchy phenotype, including, an anteverted nose, protruding upper lip, retrognathism, cryptorchidism, polymicrogyria, an anomalous pectoral muscle, and bronchopulmonary anomalies. Isolated case reports include one girl with del18q21-q32 who had chronic granulomatous disease.[102] The myelin basic protein gene has been mapped to 18q22.3, and patients with deletions involving this region have abnormalities in myelination on MRI[133,156] or at autopsy.[52] IgA deficiency is seen in 26% of del18q− patients.[64]

Ophthalmic manifestations. The first patient reported by de Grouchy et al. was said to have had poor visual responses at 1 year of age, nystagmus, mild optic atrophy, and a possible tapetoretinal degeneration.[43] An electroretinogram was not done. Because high-resolution banding and molecular genetics were not available, the exact location of the deletion breakpoint remains unknown. However, de Grouchy and colleagues were the first to suggest that a locus for a tapetoretinal degeneration may be chromosome 18q. It was 27 years later that Warburg et al. gave further support to de Grouchy's hypothesis in reporting another affected patient who demonstrated hand motion vision, lateral gaze nystagmus, and retinal changes consisting of marked vessel attenuation, optic atrophy, absent foveal reflexes, and "tigroid" retinas without typical pigmentary clumping or "bone spicule" pigmentation.[187] An electroretinogram showed cone–rod dystrophy. Warburg et al. felt that the retinal abnormalities were not attributable to pathologic myopia which might independently alter the electroretinogram. The authors comment that the boy's hearing deficit was postsynaptic and therefore not consistent with Usher syndrome. The patient had del18q21.1-qter. Three other patients presented in the same paper had deletions not involving 18q21.1 but normal retinas.[187] Ishihara color vision testing was normal but electroretinograms were not done on these other patients.

The 18q− Registry and Research Society in San Antonio, Texas, reports nystagmus (35%) and optic atrophy (28%) as common abnormalities.[64] In one literature review, 29% of patients had fundus abnormalities, but cytogenetic correlation and clinical details were not provided.[120] Wolf and co-workers reported a child with "ocular funduscopic anomalies" and strabismus, but the breakpoint was not given.[194] Similarly, Lafourcade reports 14 of 21 patients to have ocular anomalies without correlation to genotype or further detail other than to report that 9 had optic atrophy.[109] Other authors have cited optic atrophy and retinal abnormalities, but some of these reports predate precise cytogenetic breakpoint identification.[44] Some children had no symptoms or signs of a retinal dystrophy despite involvement of the putative critical region, but these children may have been too young to demonstrate evidence of the retinal disorder.[180] Yet, it has become clear that retinal dystrophy is not detected, even well into adulthood, with deletions distal to 18q21.1.[183] However, visual loss may occur as a consequence of abnormalities in visual pathway myelination or gliosis when 18q22 is involved.[52,133,156,183] Either the retinal dystrophy or the visual pathway disorder might be the cause of nystagmus in some patients with breakpoints for deletion in the 18q21 region.[59,161,191]

A patient with a translocation [46XY, t(17;18)(q25;q21)] breakpoint at 18q21 also had retinal abnormalities.[168] At 6 years this patient's eye examination was normal following esotropia surgery. At 10 years of age, he once again showed esotropia, this time in association with a unilateral tractional retinal detachment with tortuous retinal vessels and severe retinal and preretinal fibrosis. The fellow eye had a "misshapen" disc with nasal elevation and, on the provided figure, some abnormalities of the nerve fiber layer and/or internal limiting membrane of the macula are apparent. Photopic and scoptic ERGs were of low amplitude in both eyes, although worse in the eye with the detachment. Although Smith et al. postulate a relationship to del18q21, the breakpoint for the translocation, this child had several other ocular and nonocular features not usually associated with del18q, such as hypertrichosis, high bossed forehead, prominent upper teeth, distichiasis, and multiple iris nevi.[168] Although the presence of an abnormal electroretinogram and the retinal internal limiting membrane changes in the eye without retinal detachment suggest the presence of a retinal dystrophy, traction retinal detachment is not usually associated with del18q. It must also be recognized that Smith and co-workers[168] were unable to demonstrate the deletion cytogenetically, and the ERG testing conditions done at that time may have been suboptimal.

Izquierdo et al. reported a child with esotropia, epicanthus, moderate myopia(−7.00 and −5.00 sphere), microphthalmia (corneal diameters 8 mm and 5 mm), unilateral opacification of the inferior half of the cornea, iris hypoplasia with full-thickness defects and correctopia, peripapillary staphylomas, and straightening of the retinal vessels.[88] This child had a deletion involving 18q21 but was not reported to have signs of a retinal dystrophy. An electroretinogram was not done. Warburg reported a patient who also had microcornea (10 mm) associated with a deletion at 18q23, along with mild nystagmus, mild bilateral ptosis, and an otherwise normal eye examination (refraction not given).[187] Ptosis, strabismus (exotropia), and mild microcornea have also been reported in other patients with deletions involving this region.[187,191] Another child reported by Izquierdo who had a deletion between the 18q21 and 18q23 regions (del18q21.1-22) showed only moderate myopia, epicanthus, and esophoria.[88] However, this patient also had pericentric inversion of chromosome 21. Another child with del18q22.3-qter had microcornea with opaque corneas but an otherwise normal eye at autopsy.[52] In a patient with del18q21.3 there was strabismus but no myopia.[187] Warburg et al.'s patient with del18q21.1-qter also had approximately −10.00 sphere myopia.[187] This patient had a posterior staphyloma demonstrated by ultrasound. Wilson and colleagues reported six children with terminal or subterminal deletions sharing a del18q21.3 with proximal breakpoints varying from 18q21.3 to 18q21.[191] No refractions are cited and electroretinograms were not done. In four of the six patients, who ranged in age from 1 to 13 years, the fundi are described as normal. One child with a normal retina also had nystagmus and strabismus. Another had ptosis with "Brushfield spots." One child had optic atrophy associated with nystagmus. The only child whose deletion extended proximally to involve 18q21.1 was described to have a normal fundus at 1 year of age but poor visual responses. Choroidal coloboma was present in one child with del18q21-qter.[161]

Although the interpretation of many of the foregoing cases may be limited by the accuracy of cytogenetic studies at the time of their publication,[191] it appears reasonable to conclude that there is a critical locus for retinal dystrophy at 18q21.1. More distal deletions may result in strabismus with or without myopia. Microphthalmia with anterior segment anomalies may be the result of deletions proximal to 18q21.1 with a mild degree of microcornea associated with ptosis and nystagmus in the region of 18q23. Yet several anomalies, including microphthalmia, seem not to map consistently to a particular chromosomal region. Perhaps this can be attributed to the influence of the rest of the genetic background or incomplete penetrance of specific traits.

Other reported oculofacial anomalies include epicanthal folds in six of seven of Wilson et al.'s patients who shared a deletion of 18q21.3[191] and in other children with deletions involving the same region.[102] The 18q− Registry found epicanthal folds in 26% and broad nasal bridge in 26%.[64] Epicanthus is reportedly variable with other more distal loci.[133] Wilson et al.'s patient who had an interstitial deletion extending either from 18q11 to 18q12.2 or from 18q12.2 to 18q21.1 had mild exophthalmos, esotropia, ptosis, and epicanthal folds but lacked anterior chamber anomalies and retinal dystrophy (no electroretinogram or fundus exam reported) suggesting that the patient's deletion did not extend to q21.1.[191]

Diagnosis. FISH probes are available for the myelin basic protein locus.[64]

Trisomy 18 (Edwards Syndrome)

History. This chromosomal abnormality was first described in 1960 by Edwards et al.[47]

Epidemiology. Trisomy 18 is the second most common autosomal trisomy. It has a frequency of about 1 in 6000 live births with a female preponderance of 3:1. Like other autosomal trisomies, it is strongly associated with increased maternal age. The great majority of nondisjunction involves the maternal chromosome.[55]

Systemic manifestations. Major and minor anomalies of almost every organ system have been described. It is a severely handicapping disorder from both the mental and physical points of view. Trisomy 18 is usually lethal with a median survival of 4 days. A recent study showed a 9% survival at 6 months and 5% at 1 year, but cited three other recent studies which showed no survival at 1 year.[157]

Anomalies occurring in more than 50% of patients include intrauterine growth retardation, prematurity or postmaturity, and a single umbilical artery. Affected children have an unusual head shape, with prominent occiput, narrow bifrontal diameter, and narrow forehead. The mouth is small, with micrognathia and a narrow palatal arch. The external ears may be low-set and malformed. Congenital heart disease, mainly septal defects and cardiomegaly, occurs in more than 50% of cases. Other common features include inguinal or umbilical hernia, short sternum, small nipples, redundant skin, cryptorchidism, flexion contractures, scoliosis, clenched hands with overlapping of the index finger over the third and fifth finger, and hypoplasia of the nails. Numerous other abnormalities occur in fewer than half of the cases.[10,169]

Ophthalmic manifestations. Ocular malformations can be detected clinically in approximately 50% of cases, but blindness is rare.[67] The most commonly reported periocular abnormalities include hypoplastic supraorbital ridges, ptosis, blepharophimosis, epicanthus, and hypertelorism. Ankyloblepharon may infrequently be seen.[6] Nystagmus, anisocoria, and strabismus are also seen. The most common globe abnormalities are corneal opacities, uveal and optic nerve colobomas, optic nerve hypoplasia or gliosis, cataract, ciliary process abnormalities, microphthalmos, myopia, and retinal folds. Congenital glaucoma is relatively common, and at histology, abnormalities can be seen in the anterior chamber angle structures, such as incomplete cleavage of the anterior chamber angle. Malformations of the iris pigment, stroma, sphincter, and dilator can also occur. Hypopigmentation of the posterior pole retinal pigment epithelium, along with neural retinal immaturity and focal areas of retinal dysplasia can be seen.[61] Other less common abnormalities have been reported, such as thickened or bluish sclera and scleral icterus. Congenital unilateral facial paralysis may rarely occur.[166]

Trisomy 18 is the second most common chromosomal aberration associated with microphthalmia/anophthalmia.[100] Johnson and Cheng reported a child with bilateral microphthalmia with unilateral primary congenital aphakia with a markedly dysplastic anterior segment.[90] The cornea had the microscopic appearance of sclera with no surface epithelium, Bowman's layer, Descemet's membrane, or endothelium. Histopathologic examination revealed a grey nodule of fibrous tissue at the ciliary body with vitreous strands attached, which the authors suggest might represent a form of PHPV. Persistent hyperplastic primary vitreous and persistent hyaloid artery/tunica vasculosa lentis have been reported in other cases.[22] Retinal dysplasia and Bergmeister's papilla have also been observed.[68] Dysplastic retinal rosettes were seen in the aphakic eye reported by Johnson and Cheng.[90] Choroidal and optic nerve coloboma were present in both the aphakic and microphthalmic phakic eyes, the latter having an otherwise normal anterior segment. In both eyes the dysplastic retina at the coloboma protruded into the meningeal sheath/subarachnoid space of the colobomatous optic nerve. There was severe gliosis of the optic nerve in the aphakic eye.

Chromosome 20

Deletion: 20p Minus

Definition. Evidence suggests that Alagille syndrome is a single gene disorder, with the gene located to the 20p11.23-12 region, rather than a contingous gene disorder.[107] The critical region has most recently been narrowed by Krantz and co-workers to 20p12.[107]

Incidence. Approximately 7% of patients with Alagille syndrome will have a demonstrable deletion of 20p11.23-12.[107]

Systemic manifestations. An Alagille syndrome phenotype is associated with del20 p11.23-12. At least three of the following five primary clinical criteria are present: cholestasis, characteristic facies, posterior embryotoxon, "butterfly" vertebrae (hemivertebrae), and cardiac findings (most often pulmonary tree stenosis).[107] When deletions are present, all five findings are usually present. If a family history is present for this otherwise autosomal dominant condition, characterized by penetrance in excess of 90% and variable expression, then only two of the above criteria are required.[107] The characteristic facies includes triangular chin, prominent forehead, long straight nose with flat tip, and flat midface. Notched nasal alae may be seen.[107] Renal and neurodevelopmental abnormalities are less common. Hearing disorders and developmental delay are more common when deletions are present. The main cause of morbidity is the liver disease, which may require surgical intervention.

Ophthalmic manifestations. When the Alagille phenotype is present in association with del20p11.23-12 characteristic features may include posterior embryotoxon, iris adhesions and retinal dystrophy. The facial features include deep-set eyes, hypertelorism, and short palpebral features. It is interesting that a candidate gene in this region, Plcb4, is known to block invertebrate phototransduction leading to retinal degeneration.[107]

Chromosome 21

Deletion: 21q Minus

Definition. Deletion of the proximal segment of 21q has been called 21q1 monosomy, usually resulting from translocations.[174]

Systemic manifestations. Facial dysmorphism in 21q1 monosomy is characterized by beaked nose, high nasal bridge, wide glabella, micrognathia, midline alveolar notching, cupped ears, preauricular tags, and a midline raphe through the philtrum. Congenital heart disease, as well as genitourinary, rib, and vertebral abnormalities may also be seen. Mild abnormalities of the hands, in particular a hypertonic overlapping of the fingers have been reported.[174] This 21q1 monosomy phenotype has been reported to occur with deletion of 21q22 alone, and review of the literature suggests that the critical region may be within 21q22.1-22.2.[174]

Ocular manifestations. Severe microphthalmia is often seen in 21q1 monosomy. Theodoropoulos et al. reported an infant with del21q22 and severe microphthalmia and cloudy corneas.[174] One eye was more affected than the other.

Trisomy 21 (Down Syndrome)

Definition. The term "mongolism," which is no longer used, was originally used to describe patients due to their facial resemblance to individuals of Mongoloid descent and a mistaken notion about a racial etiology.[35] Trisomy of chromosome 21 is the most common cause of Down syndrome (92%–95%) although a similar phenotype is created by either translocation involving chromosome 21 (3%–4%) or mosaicism for trisomy 21 (1%–4%).[8,35] In complete trisomy 21, the origin of the extra chromosome is almost always maternal. Approximately one-half of all translocations resulting in Down syndrome occur as spontaneous events, and the remainder are due to inheritance from a parent who carries a balanced translocation.[35] Although a specific part of chromosome 21 has not been definitively identified as the area that must be included in the trisomy to result in a Down phenotype, trisomy of the region 21q22 is believed to account for most of the manifestations. The specific gene(s) within that region that are involved are not known.

Incidence. Down syndrome affects approximately 1 in 800 live births, rendering it the most common chromosomal cause of mental retardation.[8,35] Trisomy 21 is one of the most common chromsomal abnormalities associated with congenital ocular malformations at birth.[172] The recurrence risk for parents who already have an affected child is empirically estimated to be 1%.[35] Increasing maternal age is associated with an increased risk of having a child with trisomy 21, although this can occur at any maternal age.

History. The disorder was first recognized by J. L. H. Down as a form of "idiocy."

Systemic manifestations. Up to 75% of affected fetuses are aborted spontaneously. Survival rate for liveborns with trisomy 21 at 30 years is 71%.[7] The highest chance of death occurs in the first year of life (9% overall, 24% of those with congenital heart disease).[7] Survival is higher in the absence of congenital heart disease (80% at 30 years) but is still lower than that of other mentally retarded patients.[7] Fewer than half of patients with congenital heart disease will be alive at 30 years. However, if a child with congenital heart disease survives beyond 10 years, the rate of subsequent mortality is not different from those children without heart disease.[7] No significant improvement in survival has occurred between 1952 and 1981.

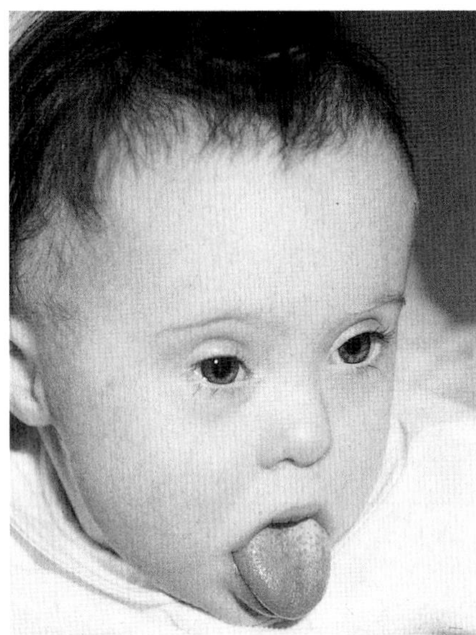

Figure 30.8. Down syndrome (trisomy 21) facial appearance. Note midfacial hypoplasia, upslanted palpebral fissures, macroglossia, and protrusion of the tongue.

The characteristic facies (Fig. 30.8) and variable degree of mental retardation are perhaps the most recognizable features of Down syndrome. Constant features include a flattened facies with a hypoplastic midface and depressed nasal bridge, small ears and mouth, prominent tongue, shortened forehead-to-occiput distance (brachycephaly), flattened occiput, and a narrow palate with prominent ridges. True macroglossia is actually uncommon, although the normal tongue is relatively large compared to the airway in approximately 60% of patients.[35] There may also be redundant skin on the nape of the neck, brachydactyly with fifth finger clinodactyly, a single palmar crease (historically referred to as a simian crease) and abnormal dermatoglyphics.[35] Affected children tend to have short stature, and alternative growth charts are available to allow comparison to other children with the same diagnosis.[35] All children with trisomy 21 have some degree of retardation with an IQ usually less than 70. Language skills tend to lag behind. In addition to mental retardation, other neurologic problems can occur such as seizures (5%–10%) and Tourette syndrome.[35] True psychiatric disorders may occur in adolescence. Affected individuals also have a predisposition to the development of Alzheimer disease in the fourth and fifth decades of life.

Congenital heart disease occurs in 40%–50% of patients and represents the major life-threatening systemic manifestation of trisomy 21, although many children are not symptomatic as neonates.[35,127] Approximately 30%–60% have complete atrioventricular canal and an additional half have isolated atrial septal defects, ventricular septal defects, atrioventricular valvular abnormalities, or combinations of these defects.[35,127] Patent ductus arteriosus, tetralogy of Fallot, and mitral valve prolapse also occur with some frequency.[35] Complications of cardiac disease are the cause of death in one-half of the patients with congenital cardiac abnormalities.[127] Patients who undergo cardiac surgery have a survival rate of 70% at 3 years of age, whereas those with inoperable conditions (either for cardiac or noncardiac) have a much higher mortality rate, such that only 50% are alive at 5 years and 30% at 10 years of age.[127] These findings, however, will need to be updated to keep pace with more recent advances in surgical technique, anesthesia, and medical intervention.

In the first year of life, the most common causes of death are congenital anomalies (63% have congenital heart disease); respiratory infection, particularly pneumonia; and perinatal complications. The rate of perinatal complications, however, does not differ from the rate in the general population.[8] Patients with Down syndrome are at increased risk for infection with subsequent higher risk of complications and morbidity. Even otitis media, which occurs with a higher frequency in these patients, can be life threatening.[8]

For children 1–10 years of age, congenital heart disease and respiratory infection continue to be the leading causes of death.[8] Leukemia, and occasionally lymphoma, begins to appear in this age range, where they have their highest effect on mortality rates. Some children with trisomy 21 may have a spontaneously remitting form of congenital leukemia known as the leukemoid reaction or transient myeloproliferative disorder.[13,35] Although congenital anomalies and respiratory disease are still the leading causes of death during adolescence, other illnesses such as diabetes mellitus, intestinal obstruction, and renal disease may become important sources of morbidity.[8]

Other major systemic problems include obstructive bowel anomalies (12%) such as duodenal atresia, tracheoesophageal fistula, Hirschsprung disease, and imperforate anus. These children have poor muscle tone and may begin life with feeding problems or constipation. Genitourinary problems include obstructive hydronephorsis, renal dysfunction, hypospadias (5%), and undescended testicles (25%–50%).[35] In addition, children with Down syndrome have an increased incidence of autoimmune phenomena, in particular thyroiditis or alopecia areata, which occur in 10%–15% of patients.[35] Congenital hypothyroidism may also occur. Unfortunately, the diagnosis of thyroid dysfunction may be missed when symptoms and signs of this disorder are mistakenly thought to be general characteristics of the developmentally delayed hypotonic child with Down syndrome.

Airway problems such as obstructive sleep apnea and chronic daytime fatigue may occur.[35] The airway, and the spinal cord, may also be endangered by cervical subluxation or dislocation due to ligamentous laxity and hypotonia resulting in atlantoaxial instability. Pulmonary hypertension with or without cardiac disease may be a contributing factor. Dental anomalies such as missing teeth, anomalous teeth, and malocclusion are not uncommon.

Ophthalmic manifestations

Lids and nasolacrimal system. Although Caputo et al. have described epiphora in 15% of patients, only one-third of these had evidence of nasolacrimal duct obstruction.[24] Epiphora in the absence of nasolacrimal duct obstruction has been confirmed by the fluorescein dye disappearance test and may be related to hypotonia (Fig. 30.9).[122] It is essential to rule out the presence of blepharitis, which may cause symptoms and signs that mimic nasolacrimal duct obstruction. Lacrimal sac fistulas have also been reported.

Upward slanting of the palpebral fissures (historically referred to as "mongoloid slant") and epicanthal folds are almost always present.

Chronic xeroderma can occur in up to 90% of children,[35] and we have seen children with dry skin or eczema affecting the periorbital area

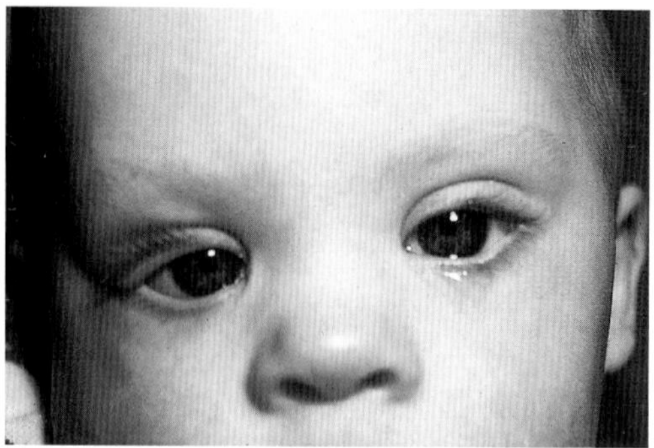

Figure 30.9. Epiphora due to lid hypotonia in child with Down syndrome.

and eyelids. Syringoma, a benign sweat gland tumor, occurs with greater frequency in children with Down syndrome.[35] The tumors are more common in girls and often begin at puberty. They appear as soft yellow or skin-colored papules, 2–3 mm in size, that have a predisposition for the periorbital area, but may occur elsewhere.

Refractive error. Approximately one-fifth of affected children will have greater than 1 diopter (D) of astigmatism, one-fifth will have greater than 1D of myopia, and one-fifth will have greater than 3D of hyperopia.[24] Unfortunately, studies like that of Caputo and coworkers, have not broken down refractive error for different age groups, making it difficult to compare the data in children with Down syndrome with those in the general population.[24] Caputo also found that 2% of patients had high astigmatism (>3D), 8.5% had high myopia (>5D), and 5% had high hyperopia (>5D).[24] Of the children with strabismus, 14% have anisometropia of ≥1.50 diopters spherical equivalent.[81]

Strabismus. Strabismus, has been reported in 33%–57% of patients.[24,81] Approximately 80% of strabismic patients have esotropia and 5%–20% have exotropia.[24,81] Although 35%–50% of esotropic patients may be hyperopic, up to 12% are high myopes, suggesting that accommodative esotropia is not the sole explanation for the strabismus.[24,81] Exotropic patients may be either myopic or hyperopic. A high accommodative convergence to accommodation ratio is present in 5% of strabismic children.[81] Some patients may exhibit irregular spontaneous convergence movements unrelated to true strabismus.[81]

Hypertropia occurs in approximately 5% of patients and may occasionally be due to congenital superior oblique palsy, dissociated vertical deviation, or Brown syndrome. Hamed and co-workers reported one child with idiopathic superior oblique overaction, but there were more patients (3) in the randomly selected control group unaffected with superior oblique dysfunction, suggesting that superior oblique overaction is less common in children with Down syndrome.[77]

One-fourth of esotropic patients will have a hyperdeviation usually in association with an A or V pattern.[81] Although many exotropes with Down syndrome have hypertropia, only 25% will have an A or V pattern.[81] Hiles reported that two of five patients with exotropia and hypertropia out of over 100 children with Down syndrome, had third cranial nerve palsy: one related to myelomeningocele, and one postmeningitis.[81] Caputo described head tilts in 19% of children with Down syndrome; 17% had vertical deviations.[24]

The results of standard medical and surgical strabismus treatment in children with Down syndrome are the same as those with normal children.[81]

Nystagmus. Caputo et al. reported a 29% incidence of nystagmus in an outpatient ophthalmology setting but did not characterize the nystagmus.[24] Hiles and co-workers found that 35% of esotropes and 25% (two of eight) of exotropes had nystagmus that was either horizontal pendular, horizontal jerk, or rotary.[81]

Optic nerve. A characteristic "spoke wheel" disc may be observed in some patients; the vessels radiate out from the disc at multiple clock hours. Optic nerve hypoplasia, pseudopapilledema/crowded disc, and myopic tilted disc may also be seen. Berk and co-workers look for 18 or more vessels crossing the optic nerve margin, which continued to extend at least one disc diameter off the nerve head.[12] This sign was found in 38% of patients suggesting possible diagnostic significance in the neonatal period prior to chromosomal confirmation. However, we would advise the karyotype confirmation be used rather than this sign.

Cornea. Up to 15% of patients with Down syndrome will develop keratoconus, with the lower incidence figures often reflecting younger study populations.[12] We used videophotokeratoscopy to study a population of affected children and found subclinical signs of keratoconus in almost all, perhaps suggesting the presence of a gene on chromosome 21 involved in the development of keratoconus. Yet, linkage studies in families with autosomal dominant keratoconus in the absence of Down syndrome have failed to demonstrate such an association.

Lens. The risk of cataract in children with Down syndrome is about 300 times higher than the general population.[99] The cumulative incidence of all types of lens opacities is approximately 20%,[12] but there is a wide variability in opacity type ranging from visually significant dense total congenital cataract to visually insignificant cortical cataract in adulthood.[12] In a large surveillance study the incidence of cataract at birth was 2.9 per 1000.[99] Caputo et al. found "snowflake" opacities in 10% of their patients and dense cataracts in 2% (Fig. 30.10).[24] Posterior lenticonus has also been reported.[28] Bilateral lens subluxation may occur.[24] Premature development of nuclear sclerosis may occur as part of the overall precocious aging seen in these children.

Iris. Among the ocular hallmarks of Down syndrome are "Brushfield spots" (Fig. 30.11). These are found in approximately one-third of patients, being more prevalent in those with blue or hazel irides.[12] As a result, studies in ethnic groups with more racial pigmentation are more likely to yield a lower incidence of

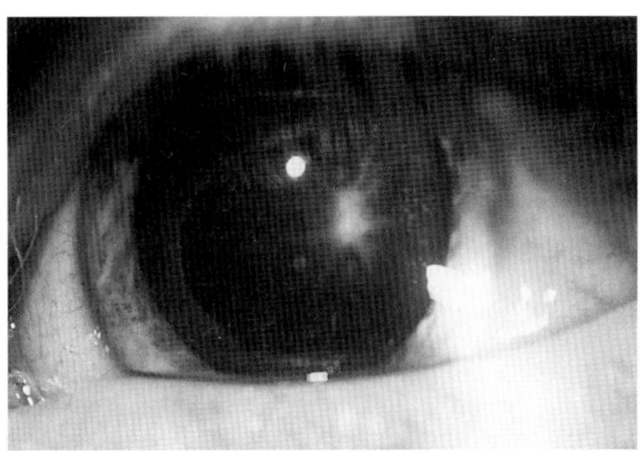

Figure 30.10. Down syndrome cataract consisting of both characteristic "snowflake" cortical opacities and a posterior subcapsular opacity.

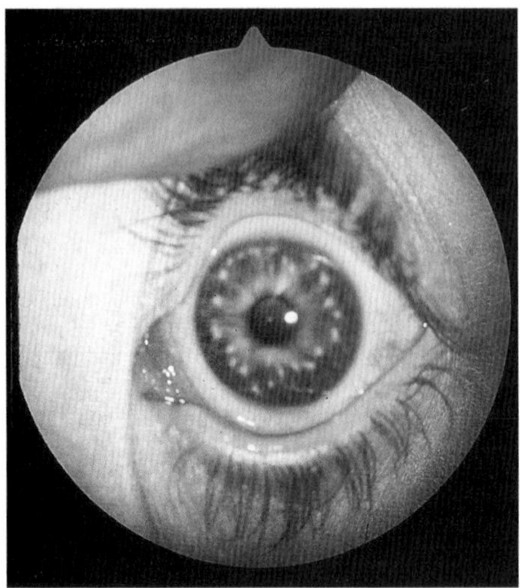

Figure 30.11. "Brushfield spots" appear as circumferentially distributed white spots on iris in Down syndrome.

Brushfield spots. Peripheral circumferential regularly spaced lesions, virtually identical to Brushfield spots, may also be observed commonly in normal individuals. Peripheral iris stromal hypoplasia has also been noted in Down syndrome with or without Brushfield spots.[12]

Retina. There have been isolated reports of retinal detachment (without refraction data) as well as unilateral optic atrophy with accompanying clinical signs of unilateral retinitis pigmentosa.[12] No further details are given to allow analysis.

Visual function. Although visual function is proportional to the degree of ocular abnormality, there is evidence to suggest that, despite their mental retardation, patients with Down syndrome are relatively better at visual tasks as opposed to auditory processing.[35] Therefore, teaching methods that rely on visual rather than auditory stimuli may be more beneficial.[35] Patients may recognize things visually before they are able to vocalize correctly what they are seeing.[35] Due to the high prevalence of ocular abnormalities, we recommend an opthalmologic screening exam twice a year for the first 3 years, and annually thereafter.

Other. Microphthalmia or anophthalmia may occasionally occur.[100]

Diagnosis. In addition to diagnostic chromosome testing of the index case, it is important to note that prenatal testing is available using a combination of ultrasound, maternal serum alpha-fetoprotein levels (low), maternal serum human chorionic gonadotropin levels (high), and maternal serum unconjugated estriol levels (low), particularly for those women at higher risk: those over 35 years of age and/or with a prior history of an affected child.[45,74] The latter three tests are often referred to as the "triple screen." Mothers identified by these means to be at high risk for carrying an affected fetus may elect to undergo amniocentesis or chorionic villus sampling for chromosome analysis of their fetus.[45]

Because of the higher incidence of ocular abnormalities, more frequent screening visits may be indicated.[35]

Treatment. The treatment of ocular problems in patients with Down syndrome is not significantly different from treating those same problems in otherwise normal children, with the exception of the special systemic concerns. The results of standard medical and surgical strabismus treatment in children with Down syndrome are generally the same as with normal children.[81]

One must certainly consider the possibility of complications secondary to underlying systemic abnormalities that may not have been identified. In particular, preoperative assessment should include evaluation of cardiac and respiratory status and complete blood count with differential. Screening for cardiac anomalies on the basis of physical examination is not sufficient, as some children will be asymptomatic and without a heart murmur.[35] Endocarditis prophylaxis may be indicated if cardiac disease is present. If the child has problems with instability of the cervical spine, hyperextension for intubation or positioning at the time of surgery may present additional risks. Although standards have not been firmly established, if preoperative radiologic assessment is desired, an atlanto-dens space in excess of 5 mm may warrant precautions.[35]

Perhaps because of the frequency of this syndrome, many controversial treatments have been proposed, including vitamin and mineral supplementation, thyroid extracts, craniosacral manipulations, patterning, and injection of freeze-dried cells from fetal vertebrate animals. None of these treatments have been shown to result in any demonstrable benefit in well-designed controlled studies.

Cosmetic intervention has generated much controversy and may or may not result in improved appearance, developmental functioning, behavior, or social/family acceptance.[35] The appearance of the eyes affects parental percepton of syndromic status more than any other feature except the relative macroglossia and articulation.[189] Lateral canthoplasty to lower the position of the lateral canthal tendon and thus normalize (or "Westernize") the palpebral fissure slant is usually successful in improving parental perception of appearance, although 50% of the operating surgeons in one study were dissatisfied with the result.[189] In performing reconstructive facial surgery in these patients, one must be aware that the correction of one problem may lead to a heightened parental awareness of other stigmata.[189]

Chromosome 22

Deletion: 22q Minus

Definition. DiGeorge syndrome (DGS) is a developmental field defect that has been recognized following prenatal exposures and other chromosomal aberrations. It may therefore be more appropriate to refer to it as the DiGeorge sequence, although there is some controversy in this regard.[195] The same deleted area, 22q11.2 is known to be associated with a spectrum of phenotypes, including DGS, velocardiofacial syndrome (VCFS), and conotruncal anomalies face syndrome (CTFA). The region is now commonly referred to as the DiGeorge critical region and the phenotypes as either the 22q11.2 syndrome or DiGeorge/velocardiofacial (DG/VCF) syndrome in recognition of the wide variable expression even within the same family.[111,195] There has been no correlation between phenotype and the deletion size.[195] It had been proposed that del22q11.2 be referred to as CATCH 22 (*c*ardiac, *a*bnormal facies, *t*hymus hypoplasia, *c*left palate, *h*ypocalcemia) syndrome, but we agree with other authors[111,195] that to eliminate pejorative terms, this acronym should not be used.

Incidence. Deletion of 22q11.2 is one of the more common chromosomal aberrations in humans, with hundreds of cases described in the literature. It is the second most common chromosomal aberration detected in our cytogenetics laboratory. The majority of children with VCFS and DGS, as well as many patients with congenital conotruncal heart anomalies have del22q11.[138,195]

Systemic manifestations. The DiGeorge sequence includes absent or hypoplastic thymus, hypocalcemia due to hypoparathyroidism, conotruncal heart anomalies, a characteristic facies, and possible developmental delay; VCFS involves velopalatal insufficiency or cleft palate, conotruncal heart anomalies, facial dysmorphism, and learning disability; CTAF describes patients with only conotruncal heart anomalies, facial dysmorphism, and developmental delay. The common facial appearance in these disorders is characterized by mildly dysplastic ears, a laterally built-up nose with bulbous tip, and a small jaw.[111] Phenotypes range from lethal DGS to individuals with only mild developmental delay and subtle facial dysmorphism with other more serious malformations. Long tapered fingers and other minor limb malformations may be seen.[111,149] An arthropathy similar to that of juvenile rheumatoid arthritis (JRA) may be associated as well.[101] Neural tube defects may also be seen, particularly when in association with conotruncal heart defects either in the affected individual or a first-degree relative.[138]

Ophthalmic manifestations. The facial appearance includes "lateral displacement of the outer canthi" (increased outer canthal distance in the absence of hypertelorism).[111] Other ocular abnormalities are uncommon. Although patients may have JRA, there is insufficient data to assess their risk for JRA iritis and other related ocular complications.

Diagnosis. Although deletions are sometimes detectable cytogenetically, most cases require FISH using probes within the DiGeorge critical region for diagnosis. It is recommended that parents of all affected children be tested in recognition of the extremely mild phenotypes that would otherwise be missed.[111]

Trisomy 22

Definition. Complete trisomy of chromosome 22 must first be distinguished from partial trisomies, in particular the cat-eye syndrome, which may have similar ocular findings.[3] Mosaicism may occur in skin fibroblasts with normal blood lymphocyte chromosomes.[40,114] Mosaicism can also be confined to the placenta or amniotic fluid.[114] Pericentric inversion may result in partial trisomy for the distal end of the long arm.[15]

Incidence. Fewer than 15 cases of mosaic trisomy 22 have been reported.

History. Antle and co-workers have presented the most detailed ocular pathology reports to date.[3] Patients reported prior to 1980 have been excluded from this section due to a recognized problem of misdiagnosis prior to that time.[40]

Systemic manifestations. With complete trisomy, the fetus usually exhibits intrauterine growth retardation, and premature birth is not uncommon.[3] Abnormal nonocular facial features characteristically include dysmorphic ears, small ovoid mouth, preauricular pits, and cleft palate. Rocker-bottom feet, ankyloglossia, hypoplastic nails, and single palmar creases have also been reported. Variable cardiac, gastrointestinal, pancreatic, genitourinary, and central nervous system malformations have been reported, although these brain abnormalities are not constant findings despite the usual presence of microcephaly.

Children with mosaicism may also be severely affected. Lessick reported a small-for-gestational-age infant who demonstrated pulmonary stenosis, developmental delay, microcephaly, and dysmorphic features, including preauricular pits, protruding upper lip, and hypoplastic toenails.[114] Unexplained eosinophilia was also present. Biesecker reported a child with duplication of 22q13.2-qter who exhibited hypotonia, retarded growth, cleft lip and palate, hearing loss, seizures, developmental delay and abnormal teeth.[15] MRI showed mild abnormalities.

Trisomy 22 is most often lethal either antepartum or in the immediate postpartum period. Only one of every 1450 fetuses conceived with trisomy 22 is carried beyond 20 weeks of gestation.[3] Congenital cardiac anomalies and related respiratory disease are the most common cause of death, usually in infancy.[41]

Ophthalmic manifestations. In complete trisomy 22, the major reported malformation is retinochoroidal coloboma with or without microphthalmia with cyst.[3] Trisomy 22 is responsible for almost 2% of all chromosome aberrations associated with microphthalmia.[100] The optic nerve is often involved and may be hypoplastic.

Facial. Epicanthal folds, hypertelorism, and proptosis have been described in one infant[3] and are seen in over 40% of mosaic infants as are downslanting or upslanting fissures, synophrys, ptosis, and epicanthal folds.[40] Duplication of 22q13.2-qter may also result in hypertelorism.[15]

Cornea. Although the cornea is usually clear, defects in Bowman's membrane with thin epithelium and stroma may occur.[3] The posterior cornea appears to be normal, although stromal vascularization may be present.[3] Limbal dermoid may also be seen.

Anterior chamber. Although glaucoma has not been a reported complication of trisomy 22, anomalous angle morphology has been noted.[3]

Lens. Cataract is an inconstant feature. There is one report of an inferior lens subluxation, perhaps related to ciliary body hypoplasia.[3]

Uvea. In addition to coloboma, ciliary body and iris hypoplasia are also recognized.[3] The former may account for the absence of glaucoma despite the abnormal anterior chamber angle formation. One child had an unusual bifid iris with the posterior leaflet extending posteriorly into the retinochoroidal colobomatous cyst.[3]

Retina and vitreous. Retinal dysplasia with rosette formation is characteristic. PHPV has been documented histologically.[3] In one of Antle's two cases, the macula was not visualized pathologically.[3] However, the reader is not told if this was due to true macular aplasia or a problem with technique.

Strabismus. Exotropia was present in one child with duplication of q13.2-qter[15] and is observed in over 40% of reported cases with mosaic trisomy 22.[40]

Diagnosis. Given the small size of this acrocentric chromosome, the detection of small deletions or duplications may require FISH studies.[3]

Cat-Eye Syndrome

Definition. The cat-eye syndrome (CES) phenotype is associated with a supernumerary marker chromosome derived from 22 q. The phenotype is particularly associated with having four copies of the region due to an inverted duplication in the marker.[39] Some individuals with a supernumerary 22 can have a normal phenotype, particularly when only trisomic for 22q or when the marker contains only pericentric duplicated material.[39]

History. The first description of the association between anal atresia and coloboma has been attributed to Haab in 1878.[98]

Systemic manifestations. The CES phenotype may include cleft palate, preauricular pits, congenital heart disease (tetralogy of Fallot), sensorineural and conductive hearing impairment, hemivertebrae, cryptorchidism, and failure to thrive.[39,98] Kalapakian et al. reported a child with an inverted duplicated extra chromosome 22 and some features thought to be part of CES.[98] However, this patient did not have anal atresia or coloboma. The patient had blood mosaism (40%) but complete tissue effect (100% of skin fibroblasts). Perhaps this is better considered a case of trisomy 22.

Ophthalmic manifestations. The name of the syndrome reflects the common (but not obligate) association with iris coloboma. The coloboma can involve the posterior segment with or without iris involvement.

Facial features include downslanting palpebral fissures and epicanthal folds.[98] Various forms of Duane syndrome have been reported and suggest the possibility of an important gene on chromosome 22q.[39] One patient had a visual acuity of only 6/18 in each eye, although the reasons are not given.[98] In another patient, who had developmental delay, hypotonia and seizures, the fixation and following was said to be "poor" for age.[39]

X Chromosome

Fragile X (*fra*(X), Martin-Bell Syndrome)

Definition. Four fragile sites are known on the X chromosome: FRAXA, FRAXD, FRAXE, and FRAXF. Only FRAXA and FRAXE are associated with clinical manifestations. Each fragile site is caused by a hypermethylated expansion of either a CCG or CGG repeat, the size of which determines the range from normality, to carrier, to affected. Hypermethylation switches off transcription of the gene.[65,178] The same effect may result from a deletion of the gene or a mutation within the gene.[78,177] The term "folate sensitive" is often applied to the fragile sites, reflecting cytogenetic detection techniques that either limit the availability of folic acid or interfere with thymidylate production necessary for DNA replication.[151] A fragile site at Xq27.2 or lesions at Xq26 may be found in normal individuals and retarded patients under these conditions, but are not diagnostic of the syndrome.[151] Although there appears to be some correlation between frequency of fragile X expression on cytogenetic testing (percent fragility) and clinical degree of retardation,[30] the amount of fragile X expression does not appear to be related to phenotype in females.[75]

In this section the term "fragile X syndrome" will refer to FRAXA unless otherwise specified.

Incidence. Fragile X is the most common cause of hereditary mental retardation.[30] The incidence of fragile X syndrome is between 1 : 1200 and 1 : 4000 depending on the population studied.[178] Since males have only one X chromosome, they are more susceptible to the effects of fragile X. However, approximately 20% of males carry the gene without any apparent deleterious effects.[30]

Females may become heterozygotes for the fragile X by inheriting the abnormal chromosome from either parent. As female heterozygotes also have a normal X chromosome, they are more "protected" from the effects of the fragile X with a higher percentage of unaffected carriers than males.[75] Up to 70% of females have a nonpenetrant fragile site.[30] The expression of the fragile X in females may be in part dependent on Lyonization and/or the parental source of the abnormal X (imprinting).[75]

Systemic manifestations. The syndrome has very variable expressivity. Ten percent of prepubertal boys with fragile X may have IQs in the borderline to low-normal range.[83] However, some children will have intelligence quotients below 20.[30] The mean IQ in fragile X positive females is 80, with 25% functioning in the mentally retarded range.[75] Almost one-third may be functioning as normal or borderline normal.[75] Affected females also tend to have more stable IQs and better outcomes.[75]

Whether there is a global intelligence deficit or specific cognitive deficits in patients with the fragile X syndrome remains an area of debate. Autism or attention deficit disorders may be present in more severely affected individuals. It has been postulated that some boys who have been classified as shy, learning-disabled students may actually have the syndrome. Self-abusive behavior, hyperactivity, and temper tantrums may also be seen.[30,75,83] Language abnormalities may include echolalia, perseveration, and poor auditory memory.[83]

The most characteristic abnormality besides mental retardation is the facial appearance, with large ears, broad nasal bridge, long prominent chin, and narrow face. Dental anomalies (47%) and a flat occiput (61%) are also common.[30] Patients characteristically have joint hypermobility (89%), and males have large testes. Various heights have been observed. In girls, the only physical features that are seen more often in fragile X positive patients are prominent ears and a long face.[75]

FRAXE syndrome is characterized by borderline to mild developmental delay, which may manifest as no more than learning difficulties regardless of whether it is caused by an FMR2 microdeletion or a CCG expansion.[65]

Ophthalmic manifestations. Visual motor integration is delayed.[83] Several authors have reported "gaze avoidance" behaviors with poor eye contact.[30,75] There are no consistent ocular malformations. Strabismus occurs in up to one-third of patients.

XXY (Klinefelter Syndrome)

Incidence. XXY is the most common sex chromosome abnormality in males and one of the more common chromosomal aberrations associated with male developmental delay.

Systemic manifestations. Klinefelter syndrome is characterized by delayed development of secondary sex characteristics due to primary hypogonadism. Patients have mild to moderate developmental delay, learning difficulties, gynecomastia, and in some, a behavioral phenotype characterized by introversion or social immaturity. Major malformations are not usually found. Minor facial dysmorphism may include low-set ears and asymmetric facies.[34] Some individuals have been described with a Marfanoid habitus, including tall stature and mild arachnodactyly.[34]

Ophthalmic manifestations. Eye abnormalities are uncommon. Microphthalmia[100] and coloboma of the iris and choroid have been described, although some authors have questioned whether the latter is a chance occurrence unrelated to the genotype.[4,34] Ectopia lentis may occur, presumably secondary to zonular deficiency in the area of a uveal coloboma.[34]

Other anterior segment abnormalities are occasionally observed. One patient had superior superficial corneal pannus and prominent corneal nerves with an unusual corneal dystrophy consisting of peripheral radial linear double-lined corneal stromal opacities, which originated 2 mm from the limbus but did not involve the visual axis.[34] This patient also had a bilateral deepened anterior chamber overlying an inferior quadrant of iris with anterior stromal hypoplasia, which might perhaps represent a putative coloboma. The iris insertion of this atrophic region was noted to be high. The patient had associated miotic pupils, asymmetric optic discs with situs inversus, and optic disc anomalies consistent with mild colobomas. Chorioretinal changes, including pigmentary alterations, suggested that the discs possibly represent myopic abnormalities. The patient had dyschromatopsia and visual field abnormalities that were also ascribed to myopia. No electrophysiologic studies were performed.

I am aware of one man who had had "left eye strabismus," observed to be an exotropia, since childhood, although he was unable to provide further details (presented by Center for Human Genetics, Bar Harbor, ME, 1994). Collier and Chami reported esotropia with convergence insufficiency.[34] They also make reference to a patient described by Zellweger with strabsimus, myopia, and congenital cataract, although no citation is given. We have cared for an infant with bilateral anterior polar cataracts associated with microphthalmia and an unusual dysgenesis of the iris such that the pupillary axis in each eye was virtually absent. The patient underwent surgical pupilloplasty and cataract extraction complicated by postoperative aphakic glaucoma.

Mild unilateral congenital ptosis, mild proptosis, long palpebral fissures, and forshortened inferior conjunctival fornices have also been observed.[34] X-linked color blindness occurs in 0.4%–7.8% of patients with Klinefelter syndrome.[34]

Triploidy

Definition. Triploidy occurs when there are 3 sets of each chromosome in all or some cells. Therefore, the total number of chromosomes in an affected cell would be 69.

Incidence. Triploidy occurs in 1% of all conceptions and in 15% of all chromosomally abnormal fetuses.[46] Most triploid fetuses abort. Only 1 of 10,000 liveborn infants are triploid.[46]

Systemic manifestations. Two distinct phenotypes are recognized. In type I triploidy, fetal death usually occurs before 8 weeks. The more common type II triploidy results in intrauterine growth retardation and macrocephaly. Type I triploidy usually results from inheritance of an extra haploid set of paternal chromosomes, whereas type II is usually due to maternal inheritance.[46]

Systemic abnormalities may include hydrocephalus, agenesis of the corpus callosum, congenital heart disease, myelomeningocele, adrenal hypoplasia, cryptorchidism, hypogonadism, and intestinal malrotation. Facial dysmorphism may be characterized by malformed low-set ears, large bulbous nose, and micrognathia with or without cleft lip and palate. Minor skeletal abnormalities such as vertebral malformations, clubfoot and syndactyly of the third and fourth fingers may occur.[103]

Ophthalmic manifestations. Coloboma and microphthalmia may occur.[103] Sphenoid wing ossification abnormalities have been observed in stillborn fetuses,[103] but the effect on liveborn orbital development is unknown. Hypotelorism may also occur.

REFERENCES

1. Aalfs CM, Hoovers LMN, Nieste-Otter MA, et al. Further delineation of the proximal trisomy 10q syndrome. *J Med Genet* 1995;32:968–971.
2. Aarskog D. A large deletion of chromosome No. 1 (46,XY,1?−). *J Med Genet* 1968;5:322–325.
3. Antle CM, Pantzar JT, White VA. The ocular pathology of trisomy 22: report of two cases and review. *J Pediatr Ophthalmol Strabismus* 1990;27:310–314.
4. Appelmans M, Michiels J, Guzik A. Colobome bilatéral complet associé au syndrome de Klinefelter, Albright, Reifenstein par erreur chromosomiale XXY. *Bull Soc Belg Ophtal* 1965;140:456–468.
5. Arch EM, Goodman BK, Van Wesep RA, et al. Deletion of PTEN in a patient with Bannayan-Riley-Ruvalcaba syndrome suggests allelism with Cowden disease. *Am J Med Genet* 1997;71:489–493.
6. Bacal DA, Nelson LB, Zackai EH, et al. Ankyloblepharon filiforme adnatum in trisomy 18. *J Pediatr Ophthalmol Strabismus* 1993;30:337–339.
7. Baird PA, Sadovnick AD. Life expectancy in Down syndrome. *J Pediatr* 1987;110:849–854.
8. Baird PA, Sadovnick AD. Causes of death to age 30 in Down syndrome. *Am J Hum Genet* 1988;43:239–248.
9. Barnicoat AJ, Abusaad I, Mackie CM, Robards MF. Two sibs with partial trisomy 2q. *Am J Med Genet* 1997;70:166–170.
10. Baty BJ, Blackburn BL, Carey CC. Natural history of trisomy 18 and trisomy 13: I. Growth, physical assessment, medical histories, survival, and recurrence risk. *Am J Med Genet* 1994;49:175–188.
11. Bene M, Duca-Marinescu D, Loan D, Maximillian C. *De novo* interstitial deletion del(1)(p21p32). *J Med Genet* 1979;16:323–327.
12. Berk AT, Saatci AO, Erçal MD, et al. Ocular findings in 55 patients with Down's syndrome. *Ophthalmic Genet* 1996;17:15–19.
13. Bhatt S, Schreck R, Graham JM, et al. Transient leukemia with trisomy 21: Description of a case and review of the literature. *Am J Med Genet* 1995;58:310–314.
14. Bielanska MM, Khalifa MM, Duncan AM. Pallister-Killian syndrome: a mild case diagnosed by fluorescence in situ hybridization. Review of the literature and expansion of the phenotype. *Am J Med Genet* 1996;65:104–108.
15. Biesecker LG, Rosenberg M, Dziadzio, et al. Detection of a subtle rearrangement of chromosome 22 using molecular techniques. *Am J Med Genet* 1995;58:389–394.

16. Birch M, Patterson A, Fryer A. Hypopigmentation of the fundi associated with Pallister-Killian syndrome. *J Pediatr Ophthalmol Strabismus* 1995;32:128–131.
17. Blennow E, Bui T, Wallin A, Kogner P. Monosomy 1p36.31-33→pter due to a paternal reciprocal translocation: prognostic significance of FISH analysis. *Am J Med Genet* 1996; 65:60–67.
18. Blodi FC. Trisomy 13. Patau's syndrome. In *The Eye in Systemic Disease,* D. Goldstein, T. Weingeist, eds. Philadelphia: J. B. Lippincott, 1990:30–32.
19. Bobrow M, Emerson PM, Spriggs AI, et al. Ring-1 chromosome, microcephalic dwarfism, and acute myeloid leukemia, *Am J Dis Child* 1973;126:257–260.
20. Bowcock AM, Farrer LA, Herbet JM, et al. Eight closely linked loci place Wilson disease locus within 13q14-21. *Am J Hum Genet* 1988;43:664–674.
21. Brown S, Gersen S, Anyane-Yeboa K, Warburton D. Preliminary definition of a "critical region" of chromosome 13 in q32: report of 14 cases with 13q deletions and review of the literature. *Am J Hum Genet* 1993;45:52–59.
22. Calderone JP, Chess J, Borodic G et al. Intraocular pathology of trisomy 18 (Edward's syndrome): Report of a case and review of the literature. *Br J Ophthalmol* 1983;67:162–169.
23. Cantu ES, Eicher DJ, Pai GS, et al. Mosaic vs. nonmosiac trisomy 9: report of a liveborn infant evaluated by fluorescence in situ hybridization and review of the literature. *Am J Med Genet* 1996;62:330–335.
24. Caputo AR, Wagner RS, Reynolds DR, et al. Down syndrome: clinical review of ocular features. *Clin Pediatr* 1989;28:355–358.
25. Carothers AD. A cytogenetic register of trisomies in Scotland: results of the first 2 years (1989, 1990). *Clin Genet* 1994;6:405–409.
26. Carrozzo R, Rossi E, Christian SL, et al. Inter- and intrachromosomal rearrangements are both involved in the origin of 15q11-q13 deletions in the Prader-Willi syndrome. *Am J Hum Genet* 1997;61:228–231.
27. Cassidy SB, Heller RM, Kilroy AW, et al. Trigoncephaly and the 11q− syndrome. *Ann Genet* 1997;20:67–69.
27a. Chen K, Manian P, Koeuth T, et al. Homologous recombination of a flanking repeat gene cluster is a mechanism for a common contiguous gene deletion syndrome. *Nature Genet* 1997;17:154–163.
28. Cheng KP, Hiles DA, Biglan AW, Pettapiece MC. Management of posterior lenticonus. *J Pediatr Ophthalmol Strabismus* 1991;28: 143–149.
29. Chew CK, Foster P, Hurst JA, Salmon JF. Duane's retraction syndrome associated with chromosome 4q27-31 segment deletion. *Am J Ophthalmol* 1995;119:807–809.
30. Cianchetti C, Sannio-Fancello G, Fratta A, et al. Neuropsychological, psychiatric, and physical manifestations in 149 members from 18 fragile X families. *Am J Med Genet* 1991; 40:234–243.
31. Claeys I, Holvoet M, Eyskens B, et al. A recognizable behavioral phenotype associated with terminal deletions of the short arm of chromosome 8. *Am J Med Genet* 1997;74:515–520.
32. Clemens M, Martsolf JT, Rogers JG, et al. Pitt-Rogers-Danks syndrome: the result of a 4p microdeletion. *Am J Med Genet* 1996; 66:95–100.
33. Clement SJ, Leppig KA, Jarvik GP, et al. Trisomy 10p: Report of an unusual mechanism of formation and critical evaluation of the clinical phenotype. *Am J Med Genet* 1996; 65:197–204.
34. Collier M, Chami M. Les manifestations ophthalmologiques dans le syndrome de Klinefelter. *Bull Soc Ophthalmol Fr* 1969;69:1073–1089.
35. Cooley WC, Graham JM. Down syndrome—An update and review for the primary pediatrician. *Clin Pediatr* 1991;30: 233–253.
36. Cormier-Daire V, Le Merrer M, Gigarel N, et al. Prezygotic origin of the isochromosome 12p in Pallister-Killian syndrome. *Am J Med Genet* 1997;69:166–168.
37. Courtens W, Speleman F, Messiaen L, et al. Interstitial deletion 2q33.3-q34 in a boy with a phenotype resembling the Seckel syndrome. *Am J Med Genet* 1997;71:479–485.
38. Cousineau AJ, Higgins JV, Scott-Emuakpor AB, Mody G. Ring-11 chromosome: phenotype–karyotype correlation with deletions of 11q. *Am J Med Genet* 1983;14:29–35.
39. Crolla JA, Howard P, Mitchell C, et al. A molecular and FISH approach to determining karyotype and phenotype correlations in six patients with supernumerary marker(22) chromosomes. *Am J Med Genet* 1997; 72:440–447.
40. Crowe CA, Schwartz S, Black CJ, Jaswaney V. Mosaic trisomy 22: a case presentation and literature review of trisomy 22 phenotypes. *Am J Med Genet* 1997;71:406–413.

41. Cunningham C, Turner S, Sloper P, Knussen C. Is the appearance of children with Down syndrome associated with their development and social functioning? *Dev Med Child Neurol* 1991;33:285–295.
42. de Die-Smulders CE, Engelen JJ. 11q duplication in a patient with Pitt-Rogers-Danks phenotype. *Am J Med Genet* 1996;66: 116–117.
43. de Grouchy J, Royr P, Salmon C, Lamy M. Délétion partielle des bras longs du chromosome 18. *Pathol Biol* 1964;2:579–582.
44. Destiné ML, Punnett HH, Thovichit S, et al. La délétion partielle du bras long du chromosome 18 (syndrome 18q−). Rapport de deux cas. *Ann Genet* 1967;10:65–69.
45. Dick P and the Candian Task Force on the Periodic Health Examination. Periodic health examination, 1996 update: 1. Prenatal screening for diagnosis of Down syndrome. *Can Med Assoc J* 1996;154:465–479.
46. Dietzsch E, Ramsay M, Christianson AL, et al. Maternal origin of extra haploid set of chromosome in third trimester triploid fetuses. *Am J Med Genet* 1995;58:360–364.
47. Edwards JH, et al. A new trisomic syndrome. *Lancet* 1960;1:787–789.
48. Engel E, Hirshberg CS, Cassidy SB, McGee BJ. Chromosome 11 long arm partial deletion: a new syndrome. *Am J Ment Defic* 1976;80: 473–475.
49. Estabrooks LL, Lamb AN, Aylsworth AS, et al. Molecular characterisation of chromosome 4p deletions resulting in Wolf-Hirschhorn syndrome. *J Med Genet* 1994;31:103–107.
50. Estabrooks LL, Rao KW, Driscoll DA, et al. Preliminary phenotypic map of chromosome 4p16 based on 4p deletions. *Am J Med Genet* 1995;57:581–586.
51. Fagan K, Colley P, Partigton M. A practical application of fluorescent in situ hybridization to the Wolf-Hirschhorn syndrome. *Pediatrics* 1994;93:826–827.
52. Felding I, Mitelman F. Deletion of the long arm of chromosome 11. *Acta Paediatr Scand* 1974;68:635–638.
53. Ferry AP, Marchevsky A, Strauss L. Ocular abnormalities in deletion of the long arm of chromosome 11. *Ann Ophthalmol* 1981;13: 1373–1377.
54. Finucane BM, Kurtz MB, Babu VR, Scott CI. Mosaicism for deletion 17p11.2 in a boy with Smith-Magenis syndrome. *Am J Med Genet* 1993;45:447–449.
55. Fisher JM, Harvey JF, Lindenbaum RH, et al. Molecule studies of trisomy 18. *Am J Hum Genet* 1993;52:1139–1144.
56. Frank J, Riccardi VM. The 11q− syndrome. *Hum Genet* 1977;35:241–246.
57. Friedrich U, Nielsen J. Autosomal reciprocal translocations in newborn children and their relatives. *Humangenetik* 1974;21:133–144.
58. Fryns JP, Logghe N, van Eygen M, van den Berghe H. 18q− syndrome in mother and daughter. *Eur J Pediatr* 1979;130:189–192.
59. Fryns JP, Kleczowska A, Buttiens M, et al. Distal 11q monosomy. The typical 11q monosomy syndrome is due to deletion of subband 11q24.1. *Clin Genet* 1986;30:255–260.
60. Fryns JP, Kleczowska A, Smeets E, Van den Berghe H. Distal 11q deletion: a specific clinical entity. *Helv Paediatr Acta* 1987;42: 191–194.
61. Fulton AB, Craft JL, Zokov ZN, et al. Retinal anomalies in trisomy 18. *Graefes Arch Klin Exp Ophthalmol* 1980;213:195–205.
62. Gandelman KY, Gibson L, Meyn MS, Yang-Feng TL. Molecular definition of the smallest region of deletion overlap in the Wolf-Hirshhorn syndrome. *Am J Hum Genet* 1992;51: 571–578.
63. Garver KL, Ciocco AM, Turack NA. Partial monosomy or trisomy resulting from crossing over within a rearranged chromosome 1. *Clin Genet* 1976;10:319–324.
64. Gay CT, Hardies LJ, Rauch RA, et al. Magnetic resonance imaging demonstrates incomplete myelination in 18q− syndrome: Evidence for myelin basic protein haploinsufficiency. *Am J Med Genet (Neuropsych Genet)* 1997;74:422–431.
65. Gecz J, Gedeon AK, Sutherland GR, Mulley JC. Identification of the gene FMR2, associated with FRAXE mental retardation. *Nature Genet* 1996;13:105–108.
66. Gershoni-Baruch R, Mandel H, Bar El H, et al. Interstitial deletion (6)q13q15. *Am J Med Genet* 1996;62:345–347.
67. Ginsberg J, Perrin EV, Sueoka WT. Ocular manifestations of trisomy 18. *Am J Ophthalmol* 1988;66:59–67.
68. Goldberg M. Persistent fetal vasculature (PFV): An integrated interpretation of signs and symptoms associated with persistent hyperplastic primary vitreous (PHPV). LIV Edward Jackson Memorial Lectures. *Am J Ophthalmol* 1997;124:587–626.
69. Goldstein H, Nielsen KG. Rates and survival of individuals with trisomy 13 and 18. *Clin Genet* 1988;34:366–372.

70. Goodship J, Curtis A, Cross I, et al. A submicroscopic translocation, t(4;10), responsible for recurrent Wolf-Hirschhorn syndrome identified by allele loss and fluorescent in situ hybridisation. *J Med Genet* 1992;29:451–454.
71. Gordon RR, Cooke P. Ring-1 chromosome and microcephalic dwarfs. *Lancet* 1964;2: 1212–1213.
72. Gray JE, Syrett JE, Ritchie KM, Elliot WD. An interstitial translocation: chromosome no. 1p to 4q. *Lancet* 1972;2:92–93.
73. Guala A, Dellavecchia C, Mannarino S, et al. Ring chromosome 13 with loss of region D13S317–D13S285: Phenotypic overlap with XK syndrome. *Am J Med Genet* 1997;72: 319–323.
74. Haddow JE, Palomaki GE, Knight GJ, et al. Prenatal screening for Down's syndrome with use of maternal serum markers. *N Engl J Med* 1992;327:588–593.
75. Hagerman RJ, Jackson C, Amiri K, et al. Girls with fragile X syndrome: physical and neurocognitive status and outcome. *Pediatrics* 1992;89:395–400.
76. Halal F, Vekemans M, Kaplan P, Zeesman S. Distal deletion of chromosome 1q in an adult. *Am J Med Genet* 1990;35:379–382.
77. Hamed LM, Fang EN, Fanous MM, et al. The prevalence of neurologic dysfunction in children who have superior oblique overaction. *Ophthalmology* 1993;100:1483–1487.
78. Hammond LS, Macias MM, Tarleton JC, Pai GS. Fragile X syndrome and deletions of FMR1: New case and review of the literature. *Am J Med Genet* 1997;72:430–434.
79. Henegariu O, Heerema NA, Vance GH. Mild "duplication 6q syndrome": A case with partial trisomy (6)(q23.3q25.3). *Am J Med Genet* 1997;68:450–454.
80. Hertz JM, Tommerup N, Sørensen FB, et al. Partial deletion of 11q: report of a case with a large terminal deletion 11q21-qter without loss of telomeric sequences, and review of the literature. *Clin Genet* 1995;47:231–235.
81. Hiles DA, Hoyme SH, McFarlane F. Down's syndrome and strabismus. *Am Orthop J* 1974; 24:63–68.
82. Hittner HM, Francke U. Aniridia caused by a heritable chromosome 11 deletion. *Ophthalmology* 1979;86:1173–1183.
83. Ho HH, Eaves LC, Payne E. Variability of development in three siblings with Fragile X syndrome. *Clin Pediatr* 1991;30:318–321.
84. Hoepner J, Yanoff M. Ocular anomalies in trisomy 13-15. *Am J Ophthalmol* 1972;74: 729–737.
85. Hoo JJ, Chao M, Szego K, et al. Four new cases of inverted terminal duplication: a modified hypothesis of mechanism of origin. *Am J Med Genet* 1995;58:299–304.
86. Howard PJ, Porteus M. Deletion of chromosome 1p: a short review. *Clin Genet* 1990; 37:127–131.
87. Iselius L, Lindsten J, Aurias A, et al. The 11q;22q translocation: a collaborative study of 20 new cases and analysis of 110 families. *Hum Genet* 1983;64:343–355.
88. Izquierdo NJ, Maumenee IH, Traboulsi EI. Anterior segment malformations in 18q− (de Grouchy) syndrome. *Opthalmic Paediatr Genet* 1993;14:91–94.
89. Jacobsen P, Hauge M, Henningsen K, et al. An (11;21) translocation in four generations with chromosome 11 abnormalities in the offspring. *Hum Hered* 1973;23:568–585.
90. Johnson BL, Cheng KP. Congenital aphakia: a clinicopathologic report of three cases. *J Pediatr Ophthalmol Strabismus* 1997;34:35–39.
91. Johnson VP, Altherr MR, Blake JM, Keppen LD. FISH detection of Wolf-Hirschhorn syndrome: exclusion of D4F26 as critical site. *Am J Med Genet* 1994;52:70–74.
92. Johnson VP, Mulder RD, Hosen R. The Wolf-Hirschhorn (4p−) syndrome. *Clin Genet* 1976;10:104–112.
93. Jones C, Slijepcevic P, Marsh S, et al. Physical linkage of the fragile site FRA11B and a Jacobsen syndrome chromosome deletion breakpoint in 11q23.3. *Hum Mol Genet* 1994;3:2123–2130.
94. Juan JL, Cigudosa JC, Gómez AO, et al. De novo trisomy 16p. *Am J Med Genet* 1997; 68:219–221.
95. Juyal RC, Kuwano A, Kondo I, et al. Mosaicism for del(17)(p11.2p11.2) underlying the Smith-Magenis syndrome. *Am J Med Genet* 1996;66:193–196.
96. Kaffe S, Hsu LY, Sachdev RK, et al. Partial deletion of long arm of chromosome 11:del(11)(q23). *Clin Genet* 1977;12:323–328.
97. Kainulainen K, Pulkkinen L, Savolainen A, et al. Location on chromosome 15 of the gene defect causing Marfan syndrome. *N Engl J Med* 1990;14:935–939.
98. Kalapakian B, Choy AE, Sparkes RS, Schreck RR. Duane syndrome associated with features of the cat-eye syndrome and mosaicism for a supernumerary chromosome probably derived from number 22. *J Pediatr Ophthalmol Strabismus* 1988;25:293–297.

99. Källén B, Mastroiacovo P, Robert E. Major congenital malformations in Down syndrome. *Am J Med Genet* 1996;65:160–166.
100. Källén B, Robert E, Harris J. The descriptive epidemiology of anophthalmia and microphthalmia. *Int J Epidemiol* 1996;25:1009–1016.
101. Keenen GF, Sullivan KE, McDonald-McGinn DM, Zackai EH. Arthritis associated with deletion of 22q11.2: more common than previously suspected. *Am J Med Genet* 1997;71:488.
102. Kimpen J, Damme-Lombaerts RV, Van den Berghe G, Proesmans W. Autosomal recessive chronic granulomatous disease associated with 18q− syndrome and end stage renal failure due to Henoch-Schönlein nephritis. *Eur J Pediatr* 1991;150:325–326.
103. Kjær I, Keeling JW, Smith NM, Hansen BF. Pattern of malformations in the axial skeleton in human triploid fetuses. *Am J Med Genet* 1997;72:216–221.
104. Kjessler B, Gustavson KH, Wigertz A. Apparently non-deleted ring-1 chromosome and extreme growth failure in a mentally retarded girl. *Clin Genet* 1978;14:8–15.
105. Kline AD, White ME, Wapner R, et al. Molecular analysis of the 18q− syndrome—and correlation with phenotype. *Am J Hum Genet* 1993;52:895–906.
106. Koivisto M, Akerblom HK, Remes M, De La Chapelle A. Primary hypothyroidism, growth hormone deficiency and congenital malformations in a child with the karyotype 46,XY, del(1)(q25q32). *Acta Paediatr Scand* 1976;65: 513–518.
107. Krantz ID, Rand EB, Gennin A, et al. Deletions of 20p12 in Alagille syndrome: frequency and molecular characterization. *Am J Med Genet* 1997;70:80–86.
108. Kristoffersson U, Lagergren J, Heim S, Mandahl N. Four copies of 8p in a mentally retarded boy in the mosaic karyotype 47,XY,+i(8p)/46,XY. *Clin Genet* 1988;34: 201–203.
109. Lafourcade J, LeJeune J. La déficience du bras long d'un chromosome 18 (18q−). *L'Union Med Can* 1968;97:936–940.
110. Laing IA, Lyall EG, Hendry LM, Ellis PM. "Typus Edinburgensis" explained. *Pediatrics* 1991;88:151–153.
111. Leanna-Cox J, Pangkanon S, Eanet KR, et al. Familial DiGeorge/velocardiofacial syndrome with deletions of chromosome area 22q11.2: report of five familes with a review of the literature. *Am J Med Genet* 1996; 65:309–316.
112. Lehman CD, Nyberg DA, Winter TC, et al. Trisomy 13 syndrome: prenatal ultrasound findings in a review of 33 cases. *Radiology* 1995;194:217–222.
113. Leichtman LG, Werner A, Bass WT, Smith D, Brothman AR. Apparent Opitz BBBG syndrome a partial duplication of 5p. *Am J Med Genet* 1991;40:173–176.
114. Lessick ML, Szego K, Wong PW. Trisomy 22 mosaicism with normal blood chromosomes. *Clin Pediatr* 1988;27:451–454.
115. Li Y, Muller B, Fuhrmann C, et al. The autosomal dominant familial exudative vitreoretinopathy locus maps on 11q and is closely linked to D11S533. *Am J Hum Genet* 1992; 51:749–754.
116. Linarelli LG, Pai KG, Pan SF, Rubin HM. Anomalies associated with partial deletion of long arm of chromosome 11. *J Pediatr* 1975;86:750–752.
117. Lindeman-Kusse MC, Van Haeringen A, Hoorweg-Nijman JJ, Brunner HG. Cytogenetic abnormalities in two new patients with Pitt-Rogers-Danks phenotype. *Am J Med Genet* 1996;66:104–112.
118. Lindor NM, Valdes MG, Wick M, Thibodeau SN, Jalal S. De novo 16p deletion: ATR-16 syndrome. *Am J Med Genet* 1997;72:451–454.
119. Lipson A, Fagan K, Colley A, Colley P, Sholler G, Isaacs D, Oates RK. Velo-cardio-facial and partial DiGeorge phenotype in a child with interstitial deletion at 10p13—implications for cytogenetics and molecular biology. *Am J Med Genet* 1996;65:304–308.
120. Lurie IW, Lazjuk G. Partial monosomies 18: review of cytogenetical and phenotypical variants. *Humangenetik* 1972;15:203–222.
121. Lurie IW, Lazjuk GI, Ussova YI, et al. The Wolf-Hirschhorn syndrome: I. Genetics. *Clin Genet* 1980;17:375–384.
122. MacEwen CJ, Young JD. The fluorescein disappearance test (FDT): an evaluation of its use in infants. *J Pediatr Ophthalmol Strabismus* 1991;28:302–305.
123. Magenis RE, Hecht F, Milham S. Trisomy 13 (D) syndrome: studies on parental age, sex ratio and survival. *J Pediatr* 1968;73:222–228.
124. Marchau FE, Van Roy BC, Parizel PM, et al. Tricho-rhino-phalangeal syndrome type I (TRP I) due to an apparently balanced translocation involving 8q24. *Am J Hum Genet* 1993;45:450–455.
125. Marino B, Reale A, Giannotti A, et al. Nonrandom association of atrioventricular canal and del(8p) syndrome. *Am J Med Genet* 1992;42: 424–427.

126. Markovic VD, Chitayat DA, Ritchie SM, et al. Trisomy 15 mosaic derived from trisomic conceptus: report of a case and a review. *Am J Med Genet* 1996;61:363–370.
127. Mathew P, Moodie D, Sterba R, et al. Long term follow-up of children with Down syndrome with cardiac lesions. *Clin Pediatr* 1990;29;569–574.
128. Mears AJ, Mirzayans F, Gould DB, et al. Autosomal dominant iridogoniodysgenesis anomaly maps to 6p25. *Am J Hum Genet* 1996;59:1321–1327.
129. Melnyk AR, Muraskas J. Interstitial deletion of chromosome 2 region in a malformed infant. *Am J Hum Genet* 1993;45:49–51.
130. Merlob P, Kohn G, Litwin A, et al. New chromosome aberration: duplication of a large part of chromosome 4q and partial deletion of chromosome 1q. *Am J Med Genet* 1989; 32:22–26.
131. Michon JJ, Borges JM, Tso MO. Heterotopic ciliary epithelial differentiation in a patient with trisomy 13. *J Pediatr Ophthalmol Strabismus* 1991;28:23–27.
132. Miller BA, Jaafar MS, Capo H. Chromosome 14-terminal deletion and cataracts. *Arch Ophthalmol* 1992;110:1053.
133. Miller G, Mowrey PN, Hopper KD, et al. Neurologic manifestations in 18q− syndrome. *Am J Med Genet* 1990;37:128–132.
134. Mulcahy MT, Jenkyn J. The 11q− syndrome: another case report. *Hum Genet* 1977; 36:239–242.
135. Murray JC. Deletion of the short arm of chromosome 4: Wolf-Hirschhorn syndrome, 4p− syndrome. In *The Eye in Systemic Disease*, D. Gold, T. Weingeist, eds. Philadelphia: J. B. Lippincott, 1990:16–18.
136. Neu RL, Gardner LI. A partial trisomy of chromosome 1 in a family with a t(1q−;4q+) translocation. *Clin Genet* 1973;4:474–479, 1973.
137. Newton D, Hammond L, Wiley J, Kushnick T. Mosaic tetrasomy 8p, *Am J Med Genet* 1993;46:513–516.
138. Nickel RE, Magenis RE. Neural tube defects and deletions of 22q11. *Am J Med Genet* 1996;66:25–27.
139. Nikawa N, Jinno Y, Tomiyasu T, et al. Ring chromosome 11[46,XX,r(11)(p15-q25)] associated with clinical features of the 11q− syndrome. *Ann Genet* 1981;24:172–175.
140. North KN, Wu BL, Cao BN, et al. CHARGE association in a child with de novo inverted duplication (14)(q22-q24.3). *Am J Med Genet* 1995;57:610–614.
141. Norwood TH, Hoehn H. Trisomy of the long arm of human chromosome 1. *Humangenetik* 1974;25:79–82.
142. Obregon MG, Mingarelli R, Digilio MC, et al. Deletion 11q23-qter (Jacobsen syndrome): report of three new patients. *Ann Genet* 1992;35:208–212.
143. O'Hare AE, Grace E, Edmunds AT. Deletion of the long arm of chromosome 11 [46,XX, del(11)(q24.1-qter)]. *Clin Genet* 1984;25: 373–377.
144. Palmer CG, Bader P, Slovak ML, et al. Partial deletion of chromosome 6p: delineation of the syndrome. *Am J Med Genet* 1991;39:155–160.
145. Palova A, Halasova E, Kamenicka E, Kadasi L. *De novo* deletion 1p(34-pter). *Hum Genet* 1985;69:94.
146. Patau K, Smith DW, Therman E, et al. Multiple congenital anomaly caused by an extra autosome. *Lancet* 1960;1:790–793.
147. Penny LA, Dell'Aquila M, Jones MC, et al. Clinical and molecular characterization of patients with distal 11q deletions. *Am J Hum Genet* 1995;56:676–683.
148. Peterson MB, Warburg M. Interstitial deletion 1p in a 30 year old woman. *J Med Genet* 1987;24:229–231.
149. Prasad C, Quackenbush EJ, Whiteman D, Korf B. Limb anomalies in DiGeorge and CHARGE syndrome. *Am J Med Genet* 1997;68:179–181.
150. Preus M, Aymé S, Kaplan P, Vekemans M. A taxonomic approach to the del(4p) phenotype. *Am J Med Genet* 1985;21:337–345.
151. Ramos FJ, Emanuel BS, Spinner NB. Frequency of the common fragile site at Xq27.2 under conditions of thymidylate stress: implications for cytogenetic diagnosis of the fragile X syndrome. *Am J Med Genet* 1992;42: 835–838.
152. Reid E, Morrison N, Barron L, et al. Familial Wolf-Hirschhorn syndrome resulting from a cryptic translocation: a clinical and molecular study. *J Med Genet* 1996;33:197–202.
153. Riccardi VM. Trisomy 8: an international study of 70 patients. *Birth Defects: Orig Art Ser* 1977;13:171–184.
154. Rizzu P, Haddad BR, Vallcorba I, et al. Delineation of a duplication map of chromosome 3q: a new case confirms the exclusion of 3q25-q26.2 from the duplication 3q syndrome critical region. *Am J Med Genet* 1997;68:428–432.
155. Robinow M, Haney N, Chen H, et al. Secondary trisomy or mosaic "tetrasomy" 8p. *Am J Med Genet* 1989;32:320–324.

156. Rodichok L, Miller G. A study of evoked potentials in the 18q− syndrome which includes the absence of the gene locus for myelin basic protein. *Neuropediatrics* 1992;23:218–220.
157. Root S, Carey JC. Survival in trisomy 18. *Am J Med Genet* 1994;49:170–174.
158. Rothenmund H, Chudley AE, Dawson AJ. Familial transmission of a small supernumerary marker chromosome 8 identified by FISH: an update. *Am J Med Genet* 1997;72:339–342.
159. Sago H, Chen E, Conte WJ, et al. True trisomy 2 mosaicism in amniocytes and newborn liver with multiple systemic abnormalities. *Am J Med Genet* 1997;72:343–346.
160. Schinzel A, auf der Maur P, Moser H. Partial deletion of long arm of chromosome 11[del (11)(q23)]: Jacobsen syndrome. *J Med Genet* 1977;14:438–444.
161. Schinzel A, Hayashi K, Schmid W. Structural aberrations of chromosome 18. II. The 18q− syndrome. Report of three cases. *Humangenetik* 1975;26:123–132.
162. Schrander-Stumpel CT, Govaerts LC, Engelen JJ, et al. Mosaic tetrasomy 8p in two patients: clinical data and review of the literature. *Am J Med Genet* 1994;50:377–380.
163. Schubert R, Viersbach R, Eggerman T, et al. Report of two new cases of Pallister-Killian syndrome confirmed by FISH: tissue-specific mosaicism and loss of i(12p) by in vitro selection. *Am J Med Genet* 1997;72:106–110.
164. Schwarz C, Mpofu C, Wraith JE. A terminal deletion of 11q. *J Med Genet* 1992;29: 511–512.
165. Shapira M, Dar H, Bar-el H, et al. Inherited inverted duplication of X chromosome in a male: report of a patient and review of the literature. *Am J Med Genet* 1997;72:409–414.
166. Shapiro NL, Cunningham MJ, Parikj SR, et al. Congenital unilateral facial paralysis. *Pediatrics* 1996:261–265.
167. Slavotinek A, Kingston H. Interstitial deletion of bands 4q12-q13.1: case report and review of proximal 4q deletions. *J Med Genet* 1997;34:862–865.
168. Smith A, Caradus V, Henry JG. Translocation 46XY,t(17;18)(q25;q21) in a mentally retarded boy with progressive eye abnormalities. *Clin Genet* 1979;16:156–162.
169. Smith DW. The 18 trisomy and the 13 trisomy syndromes. *Birth Defects: Orig Art Ser* 1969; 5:67.
170. Stalker HJ, Aymé S, Delneste D, et al. Duplication of 9q12-q33: a case report and implications for the dup(9q) syndrome. *Am J Hum Genet* 1993;45:456–459.
171. Stockton DW, Ross HL, Bacino CA, et al. Severe clinical phenotype due to an interstitial deletion of the short arm of chromosome 1: a brief review. *Am J Med Genet* 1997;71: 189–193.
172. Stoll C, Alembik Y, Dott B, Roth MP. Epidemiology of congenital eye malformations in 131,760 consecutive births. *Ophthalmic Paediatr Genet* 1992;13:179–186.
173. Takano T, Yamanouchi Y, Mori Y, et al: Interstitial deletion of chromosome 1q [del(1) (q24q25.30)] identified by fluorescence in situ hybridization and gene dosage analysis of apolipoprotein A-II, coagulation factor V, and antithrombin III. *Am J Med Genet* 1997;68: 207–210.
174. Theodoropoulos DS, Cowan JM, Elias ER, Cole C. Physical findings in 21q22 deletion suggest critical region for 21q− phenotype in q22. *Am J Med Genet* 1995;59:161–163.
175. Thomas JA, Manchester DK, Prescott KE, et al. Hunter-McAlpine craniosynostosis phenotype associated with skeletal anomalies and interstitial deletion of chromosome 17q. *Am J Med Genet* 1996;62:372–375.
176. Tilstra DJ, Grove M, Spencer AC, et al. Mosaic isochromosome 8p. *Am J Med Genet* 1993;46:517–519.
177. Tonsgard JH, Yelavarthi KK, Cushner S, et al. Do NF1 gene deletions result in a characteristic phenotype? *Am J Med Genet* 1997; 73:80–86.
178. Turner G, Webb T, Wake S, Robinson H. Prevalence of fragile X syndrome. *Am J Med Genet* 1996;64:196–197.
179. Uto H, Shigeto M, Tanaka H, et al. A case of 11q− syndrome associated with abnormalities of the retinal vessels. *Ophthalmologica* 1994; 208:233–236.
180. Valtuena MM, Garcia-Sagredo JM, Villa AM, et al. 18q− syndrome and extraskeletal Ewing's sarcoma *J Med Genet* 1986;23:426–441.
181. van den Berghe H, van Eygen M, Fryns JP, et al. Partial trisomy 1, karyotype 46,XY,12, t(1q,12p)+. *Humangenetik* 1973;18:225–230.
182. Verbraak FD, Pogany K, Pilon J, et al. Congenital glaucoma in a child with partial 1q duplication and 9p deletion. *Ophthalmic Paediatr Genet* 1992;13:165–170.
183. Vogel H, Urich H, Horoupian DS, Wertelecki W. The brain in the 18q− syndrome. *Dev Med Child Neurol* 1990;32:725–742.
184. Voullaire LE, Webb GC, Leversha MA. Chromosome deletion at 11q23 in an abnormal child from a family with inherited fragility at 11q23. *Hum Genet* 1987;76:202–204.

185. Wakazono A, Masumo M, Yamaguchi S, et al. Interstitial deletion of the long arm of chromosome 11: report of a case and review of the literature. *Jpn J Hum Genet* 1992;37;229–234.
186. Walsh LM, Lynch SA, Clarke MP. Ocular abnormalities in a patient with partial deletion of chromosome 6p: a case report. *Ophthalmic Genet* 1997;18:151–156.
187. Warburg M, Sjo O, Tranebjaerg L, Fledelius HC. Deletion mapping of a retinal cone-rod dystrophy: assignment to 18q211. *Am J Med Genet* 1991;39:288–293.
188. Wenger SL, Steele MW, Becker DJ. Clinical consequences of deletion 1p35. *J Med Genet* 1988;25:263.
189. Wexler M, Peled IJ, Rand Y, et al. Rehabilitation of the face in patients with Down's syndrome. *Plast Reconstr Surg* 1986;7:383–391.
190. White DM, Pillers DM, Reiss JA, et al. Interstitial deletions of the short arm of chromosome 4 in patients with a similar combination of multiple minor anomalies and mental retardation. *Am J Med Genet* 1995;57:588–597.
191. Wilson MG, Towner JW, Forsman I, Siris E. Syndromes associated with deletion of the long arm of chromosome 18[del(18q)]. *Am J Med Genet* 1979;3:155–174.
192. Winters J, Markello T, Nance W, Jackson-Cook C. Mosaic "tetrasomy" 8p: case report and review of the literature. *Clin Genet* 1995;48:195–198.
193. Wolf CB, Peterson JA, LoGrippo GA, Weiss L. Ring 1 chromosome and dwarfism—a possible syndrome. *J Pediatr* 1967;71:719–722.
194. Wolf U, Reinwein H, Gorman LZ, Künzer W. Deletion on long arm of a chromosome 18 (46XX, 18q−). *Humangenetik* 1967;5:70–71.
195. Wulfsberg EA, Leanna-Cox J, Neri G. What's in a name? Chromosome 22q abnormalities and the DiGeorge, velocardiofacial, and conotruncal anomalies face syndromes. *Am J Med Genet* 1996;65:317–319.
196. Wyllie JP, Wright MJ, Burn J, Hunter S. Natural hisory of trisomy 13. *Arch Dis Child* 1994;7:343–345.
197. Yang SP, Bidichandani SI, Figuera LE, et al. Molecular analysis of deletion (17)(p11.2 p11.2) in a family segregating a 17p paracentric inversion: implications for carriers of paracentric inversions. *Am J Hum Genet* 1997; 60:1184–1193.
198. Yunis E, Quintero L, Leibovici M. Monosomy 1pter. *Hum Genet* 1981;56:279–282.
199. Zurcher VL, Golden WL, Zinn AB. Distal deletion of the short arm of chromosome 6. *Am J Med Genet* 1990;35:261–265.

31

Subluxation of the Crystalline Lens and Associated Systemic Disease

ELIAS I. TRABOULSI
IRENE H. MAUMENEE

The crystalline lens collects light rays and images and keeps them in focus on the retina by changing its refractive power through the complex process of accommodation. The zonular fibers connect the ciliary processes to the equatorial region of the lens and suspend the latter in a centered position behind the pupil. Zonular fibers are rich in fibrillin and in cysteine and are hence disrupted in diseases of sulfur metabolism such as homocystinuria and sulfite oxidase deficiency, and in the Marfan syndrome. Loss of normal zonular support leads to displacement of the lens from its normal position and to changes in its curvature and refractive power.

PATTERNS OF LENS SUBLUXATION AND DISLOCATION: ECTOPIA LENTIS

Ectopia lentis refers to the displacement of the crystalline lens away from its position in the center of the visual axis. When the lens is displaced but remains attached to the ciliary processes by some zonules, it is said to be *subluxated.* The term *dislocation* is reserved to situations where there is complete disruption of all zonular attachments and free movement of the lens in the eye. When zonular fibers stretch or break in one sector of the lens circumference, the latter moves in the opposite direction, and the equatorial zone, which is no longer under tension by intact zonules, loses its rounded appearance. Notching of the equatorial area of the lens secondary to loss of some zonular fibers has been referred to as a *coloboma* of the lens. Such irregularities of lens contour develop because the lens substance is soft and relaxation of the pull exerted by the zonular fibers leads to the recoil of the capsule in that area. A true coloboma of the lens is a rare developmental abnormality that results from faulty embryonic formation of a sector of ciliary processes. Persistence of a portion of the anterior fetal vasculature in the area of the coloboma is believed to be responsible for the defective ciliary processes and for the coloboma.

Changes in the distribution of the zonular traction forces that are exerted by the zonules on the deformable lens lead to a modification of its contour and shape, and hence to a change in its refractive power. When all the zonules are disrupted, as in untreated homocystinuria, the lens becomes globular, its diameter is reduced, and high myopia develops. This is called *microspherophakia.* Microspherophakia may also be present in Marfan syndrome, Weill-Marchesani syndrome, or in ectopia lentis et pupillae. In Marfan syndrome, astigmatism may result from irregularities in the contour of the lens in different meridians.

The direction of lens subluxation or dislocation and the appearance of the zonules can provide a clue to the systemic diagnosis. In Marfan syndrome, the lens most often moves superotemporally, and stretched zonules may be visible before or after pupillary dilation (Fig. 31.1*A–C*). In normal individuals, zonules may only be seen occasionally after maximal dilation of the pupil. When a patient is evaluated for the presence of lens subluxation to rule out Marfan syndrome, he or she is asked to look down while positioned at the slit lamp. Using retroillumination, the examiner looks for evidence of posterior and superior displacement of the lens by observing the inferior portion of the lens behind the iris. If the lens is in its physiologic position, there is no separation between the pupillary margin and the lens, and the equator of the lens is not visible. If the equatorial region is seen, the lens is considered to be subluxated. The mere visualization of zonules on downgaze is not sufficient to diagnose lens subluxation. A proposed grading scheme for subluxation of the lens (assuming that the pupil dilates to at least 7 mm) is given in Table 31.1 and shown in Figure 31.1*A–C*.

In untreated homocystinuria the lenses become dislocated after the patient reaches 4 or 5 years of age; the lenses move initially in an inferior direction behind the iris but may later occlude the pupil or dislocate into the anterior chamber. Dislocation of the crystalline lens into the anterior chamber is almost pathognomonic of homocystinuria.

Another differentiating clinical finding is the appearance of the zonules that are nearly absent in homocystinuria (the equatorial area of the lens only has a fuzz of zonular remnants), as opposed to the elongated and sometimes rarefied zonules of patients with Marfan syndrome.

Iridodonesis, or movement of the iris with ocular movements, results from loss of the pos-

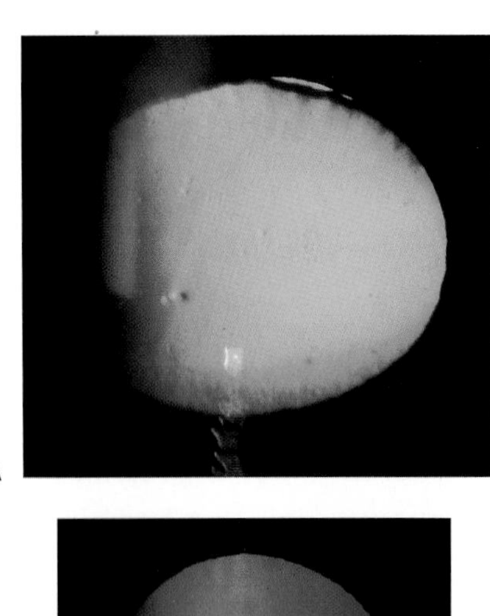

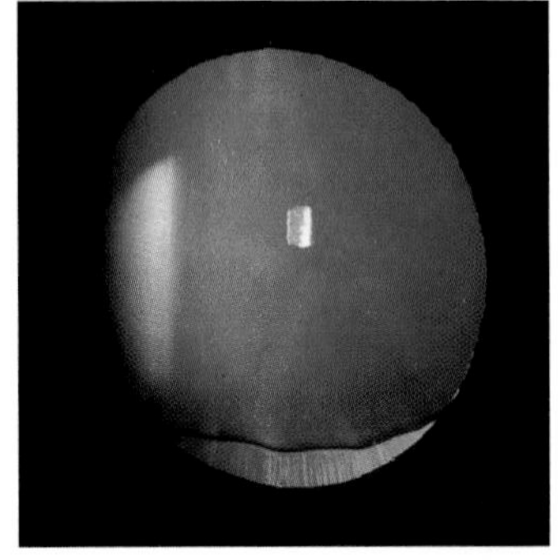

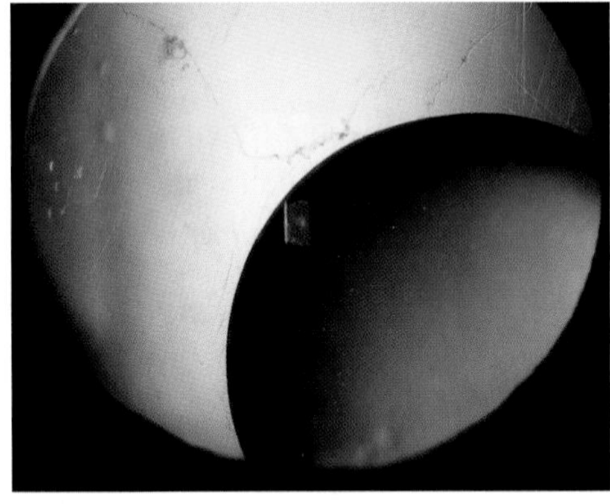

Figure 31.1. **A:** Retroillumination in this slit-lamp photograph reveals a characteristic inferior equatorial notch in a patient with Marfan syndrome and very mild subluxation of the lens. **B:** Superior subluxation of the lens in another patient with Marfan syndrome. The equatorial contour is crenated because of uneven zonular support. The zonular fibers are elongated and clearly visible. **C:** The lens in this patient with Marfan syndrome is almost completely dislocated and was causing significant visual dysfunction from intermittent movements into and out of the visual axis, depending on head position. The few remaining zonular fibers are markedly stretched.

Table 31.1. Clinical Grading of Ectopia Lentis

Grading of Subluxation	Findings
Minimal subluxation	The equator of the lens is seen only in downgaze.
Mild subluxation	The equatorial edge of the lens is visible in primary gaze, but only through a dilated pupil.
Moderate subluxation	The equatorial portion of the lens is visible through the undilated pupil.
Dislocation	The lens has lost all zonular attachments and moves freely behind or in front of the iris.

terior support that the lens and zonules provide to the iris diaphragm. Iridodonesis is more evident with increasing degrees of lenticular displacement.

CLASSIFICATION OF DISEASES MARKED BY ECTOPIA LENTIS

In the absence of trauma and a history of syphilis, ectopia lentis may be an isolated ocular abnormality, a component of a developmental malformation syndrome affecting the eye, or a manifestation of a metabolic disorder, a disease of connective tissue, or other rare inherited syndromes (Table 31.2). The following sections give an overview of some of the conditions that are associated with subluxation of the crystalline lens.

SIMPLE ECTOPIA LENTIS

This is an autosomal dominant condition in which the characteristics of lens subluxation are indistinguishable from those of patients with Marfan syndrome (vide infra) (Fig. 31.2*A*,*B*). The gene for simple ectopia lentis was mapped to chromosome 15 and linked to FBN1, the gene coding for fibrillin, which is also responsible for Marfan syndrome. It is most likely that families with simple ectopia lentis represent an extreme of the variable expressivity of FBN1 mutations, some mutations would result in simple ectopia lentis, while others would cause the full-blown Marfan phenotype. Tsipouras et al.[107] found a linkage between FBN1 and simple ectopia lentis in two families.[107] Kainulainen et al.[47] reported a mutation in FBN1 in a family with what these authors diagnosed as "simple ectopia lentis," despite the presence of skeletal abnormalities compatible with Marfan syndrome in some family members. Edwards et al.[30] also found linkage to the FBN1 region in

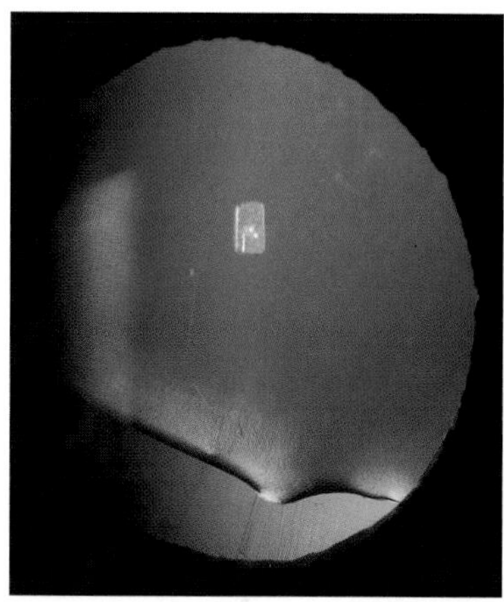
A

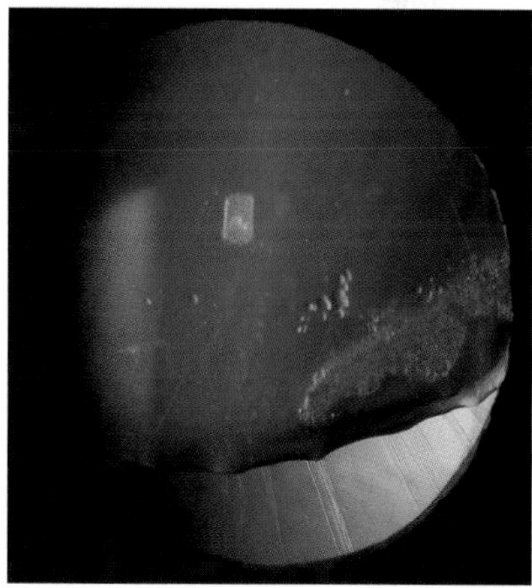
B

Figure 31.2. Slit-lamp photographs of subluxated left (**A**) and right (**B**) lenses of a 4-year-old boy with simple ectopia lentis. A small cataract is present on the right. His older brother was similarly affected. Both parents were of normal stature and had no lens subluxation. This may be an example of autosomal recessive ectopia lentis et pupillae, without a visible displacement of the pupil. Simple ectopia lentis is generally inherited in an autosomal dominant fashion.

Table 31.2. Classification of Diseases Marked by Ectopia Lentis

Disease	Defect	Inheritance	Gene Map	MIM	Prevalence of Ectopia lentis
Disorders of Collagen Metabolism					
Stickler syndrome	Collagen type 2A	AD		108300	Rare
Kniest dysplasia	Collagen type 2A	AD		156550	15%
Spondyloepiphyseal dysplasia congenita	Collagen type 2A	AD	12q13.11 − q13.2	183900	Rare
Osteogenesis imperfecta congenita	Collagen type 1A1 and collagen 1A2	AR/AD			Rare
Disorder of Fibrillin Formation					
Marfan syndrome	Fibrillin 1	AD	15q21.1	154700	60%–70%
Simple ectopia lentis	Fibrillin 1	AD	15q21.1	129600	>90%
Weill-Marchesani syndrome	Fibrillin 1 ?	AR	15q21.1	277600	>90%
Shprintzen-Goldberg syndrome	Fibrillin 1	AD	15q21.1	182212	
Developmental Disorders					
Aniridia	PAX6	AD	11p13		10%–20%
Congenital glaucoma		AR	2p21 1p36.2 − p36.1		Rare
Other Connective Tissue Diseases					
Blepharoptosis, myopia, and ectopia lentis		AD		110150	All
Kniest-like dysplasia with pursed lips and ectopia lentis		AD		245160	All
Craniofacial dysmorphism with ocular coloboma, absent corpus callosum, and aortic dilatation (Temtamy syndrome)		AD			
Craniofacial dysostosis with ectopia lentis and anterior segment dysgenesis		AD vs AR		601552	All
Spondyloepimetaphyseal dysplasia with joint laxity (SEMDJL)		AD			Rare
Metabolic Disorders					
Homocystinuria	Cystathionine-beta-synthase deficiency	AR	21q22.3	236200	All untreated

(continued)

Table 31.2. Classification of Diseases Marked by Ectopia Lentis—Continued

Disease	Defect	Inheritance	Gene Map	MIM	Prevalence of Ectopia lentis
Hyperlysinemia	Lysine : alpha-ketoglutarate reductase deficiency		238700		
Sulfocysteinuria	Sulfite oxidase deficiency		272300		
Molybdenum cofactor deficiency types a and B	Combined deficiency of sulfite oxidase, xanthine dehydrogenase, and aldehyde oxidase	AR		252150 252160	
Miscellaneous Disorders					
Ectopia lentis et pupillae		AR		225200	95%
Late subluxation of the lenses		AD		185450	All
Iridoschisis		Sporadic/ AD		147610	Rare
Megalocornea		XR			Rare
Blepharoptosis, myopia, and ectopia lentis		AD		110150	All

AD = autosomal dominant; AR = autosomal recessive; MIM = Mendelian Inheritance in Man (World Wide Web URL :http://www.ncbi.nlm.nih.gov/Omim/).

a four-generation family with simple ectopia lentis. Some members of this family were tall, but none had echocardiographic evidence of abnormalities diagnostic of Marfan syndrome.

A recessive form of simple ectopia lentis is listed in McKusick's *Mendelian Inheritance in Man* (MIM225100; World Wide Web URL: http://www.ncbi.nlm.nih.gov/omim/). This entity is not well established, and autosomal recessive inheritance of subluxated lenses should suggest the diagnosis of ectopia lentis et pupillae, homocystinuria, the Weill-Marchesani syndrome, or the entity of craniofacial dysostosis, dislocation of the lens, and anterior segment dysgenesis (vide infra).

ECTOPIA LENTIS ET PUPILLAE

Ectopia lentis et pupillae is an autosomal recessive, purely ocular disease characterized by the presence of congenital, and sometimes progressive, subluxation of the crystalline lens.[15,35] The pupil is frequently eccentric, miotic, and sometimes difficult to dilate (Fig. 31.3). The lens and pupil are usually displaced in opposite directions. There may be remnants of the pupillary membrane and subtle signs of anterior segment dysgenesis.

In ectopia lentis et pupillae, the lenses can

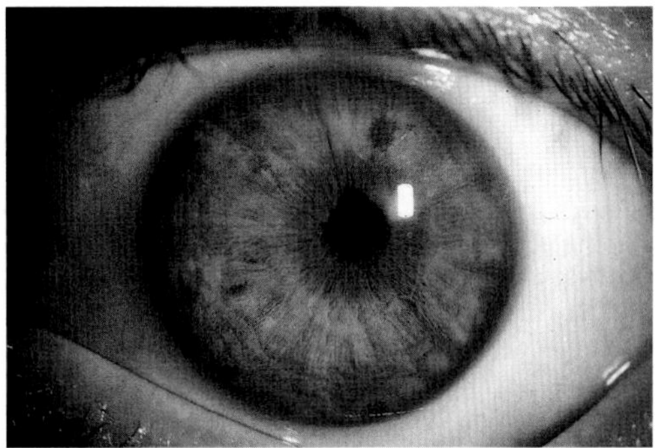

Figure 31.3. Miotic and nasally displaced pupil in a patient with ectopia lentis et pupillae. The lens was displaced temporally.

be displaced in any direction, and zonules are generally stretched but may be disrupted. The lenses may become totally loose with age and may cause pupillary block. Open-angle glaucoma and retinal detachment are not uncommon and can occur spontaneously or following lens extraction.[35]

Table 31.3 summarizes the ocular findings in a series of 16 patients with ectopia lentis et pupillae reported by Goldberg.[35] Forty percent of eyes had visual acuity better than or equal to 20/40, and 90% had vision better than or equal to 20/400. Two eyes had very poor vision from failed retinal reattachment surgery, and one eye had very poor vision from amblyopia. Perimetry could not document glaucomatous damage in any eye.

Patients are refracted through the phakic or aphakic part of the pupil if the edge of the lens is visible in the pupillary area, and the glasses or contact lenses are prescribed accordingly. If optical correction is difficult, most often from constant movement of the lens in and out of the visual axis, lens extraction may become necessary. Frequent measurements of the intraocular pressure are necessary because of the increased prevalence of glaucoma. Periodic ultrasonographic examination of the eye or visual field testing is indicated in the occasional patient with severely miotic and nondilating pupils. Laser and surgical iridoplasties have been used to visualize the fundus and to permit retinoscopy.

Table 31.3. Ocular Findings in 16 Patients with Ectopia Lentis et Pupillae

Ocular Finding	Frequency (%)
Ectopia lentis	94
Persistent pupillary membrane	87.5
Prominent iris processes in the angle	80
Axial elongation of the globe	78
Poor pupillary dilatation	60
Ectopia pupillae	59
Enlarged corneal diameter	44
Cataract	34
Iridohyaloid adhesions	29
Elevated intraocular pressure	15
Retinal detachment	9

Lenses are extracted if they move into and out of the visual axis, or if there is recurrent pupillary block glaucoma. If lens extraction is planned, automated suction/cutting lensectomy is preferred and may be performed through the limbus or the pars plana, depending on the surgeon's preference. The vitreous is well formed and the lens does not sink back toward the retina (personal observations).

MARFAN SYNDROME

A disease named for the French pediatrician Antoine Marfan[61] was first reported by him in a 5.5-year-old girl whom he described as having dolichostenomelia, or long, thin limbs. The occurrence of dislocated lenses in patients with this condition was noted by Boerger,[7] and the eponym Marfan syndrome is attributed to Carrau.[13] McKusick[69] suggested that the defect in Marfan syndrome lies in a constituent common to the suspensory ligament of the lens and the media of the aorta. He[70] was proved right when the disease was discovered to be due to an abnormality in fibrillin, a major component of the lens zonule and of all connective tissue.

Clinical Manifestations and Diagnostic Criteria

The three systems that are most prominently involved in Marfan syndrome are the skeleton, the heart, and the eye. Common and major manifestations of the disease include subluxation of the crystalline lens; dilatation of the aortic root and aneurysm of the ascending aorta; and skeletal abnormalities such as kyphoscoliosis, an upper segment/lower segment ratio 2 standard deviations below the mean for age, and pectus excavatum.[4,82,104] Auxiliary signs such as myopia, mitral valve prolapse, arachnodactyly, joint laxity,[59] tall stature, pes planus, striae atrophicae, pneumothorax, obstructive sleep apnea,[14] and dural ectasia may also be present.[84]

The 1986 Berlin diagnostic criteria for Marfan syndrome were as follows: *(1)* in the absence of an unequivocally affected first-degree relative, an individual is diagnosed with the syndrome if he or she has involvement of the skeleton and at least two other systems, with a minimum of one major manifestation (ectopia lentis, aortic dilation/dissection, dural ectasia); or *(2)* in the presence of an unequivocally affected first-degree relative, the diagnosis is made if only two systems are involved.[4] The criteria were revised in 1996 when it became evident that overdiagnosis was being made in relatives of unequivocally affected individuals. The new diagnostic criteria are summarized in Table 31.4.[21]

The clinical diagnosis of Marfan syndrome is relatively easy in patients with the full-blown clinical phenotype and in those with a positive family history of the disease, but it may be difficult in patients with mild or absent skeletal, ocular, or cardiac abnormalities. Because of the variable manifestations of the disease and the wide spectrum in the severity of clinical abnormalities in patients with connective tissue abnormalities simulating Marfan syndrome, detailed ophthalmologic, cardiac, and skeletal evaluations should be performed in patients in whom the diagnosis is suspected.[82,83] About one-third of patients may have mitral valve prolapse and/or aortic root enlargement that can be detected on echocardiography in the absence of auscultatory signs.[10,82]

In addition to connective tissue disorders of unclear etiology and Ehlers-Danlos syndrome, the differential diagnosis of Marfan syndrome includes the mosaic trisomy 8 syndrome[44,79] and multiple endocrine neoplasia type 2B. Patients with the latter two conditions have a body habitus similar to that of patients with Marfan syndrome but none of the ocular or cardiac features. Patients with homocystinuria may also have a body habitus indistinguishable from that of patients with Marfan syndrome, which when added to the presence of subluxated lenses makes the differentiation between the two diseases difficult unless biochemical screening for homocystinuria is performed. The exclusion of homocystinuria using biochemical testing is a criterion for the diagnosis of Marfan syndrome.[21]

Although mortality from cardiac disease at an early age was very high in patients with Marfan syndrome,[78] advances in the medical and surgical diagnosis and management of these patients have resulted in an approximate 25% increase in survival.[36,38,62,75,77,87,99]

Genetics

Marfan syndrome is inherited in an autosomal dominant fashion. About 25% of cases arise as new mutations. Virtually all are believed to be due to FBN1 mutations. Kainulainen et al.,[47] however, could identify mutations in FBN1 in only 25% of patients. The family with skeletal and cardiac abnormalities, but no ocular abnormalities, initially reported by Boileau et al.[8,9] did not map to 15q, and was later linked to markers on 3p25-p24.2.[16]

Fibrillin and Marfan Syndrome

Following the mapping of the genes for one of the two types of fibrillin[56,58] and for Marfan syndrome to chromosome 15,[26,48,107,108] the disease and the molecule were matched. The structure of fibrillin had been determined,[92] the cDNA was sequenced,[17,63] and mutations were soon identified in FBN1, the fibrillin gene, in numerous patients with Marfan syndrome.[23,24,25,27,40,47,72]

Fibrillin is a 350 kDa glycoprotein. It is the principal structural component of a class of connective tissue microfibrils found in virtually all extracellular matrices. It contains approximately 14% cysteine, of which one-third is in the free sulfhydryl form.[51,92,93,113] Ultrastructural analysis shows the microfibrils to exhibit a beaded morphology, with a fiber diameter of 10–12 nm, and an average periodicity of 55 nm. Fibrillin structures serve as a scaffold for the deposition of elastin in elastic tissues.[71,92]

The fibrillin polypeptide chain contains several types of repetitive sequences, including EGF-like motifs, seven 8-cysteine motifs, other unique regions, and hybrid motifs.[17] Dietz and co-workers[27] found clustering of FBN1 mutations in Marfan syndrome at cysteine residues in EGF-like domains. Normal calcium-binding EGF-like domains in the fibrillin molecule appear to allow fibrillin monomers to aggregate into microfibrils.[28] Fibrillin molecules that are missing an EGF-like domain are secreted normally and participate in the formation of microfibrils, but they are associated with the Marfan phenotype, and thus demonstrate a dominant negative effect.[57]

Monoclonal antibodies to fibrillin have been developed and the distribution of fibrillin in

Table 31.4. Current Diagnostic Criteria[a] for the Diagnosis of Marfan Syndrome[21]

System	Criteria
Family/Genetic History	***Major***
	One parent who meets diagnostic criteria independently FBN1 mutation known to cause Marfan syndrome inherited by descent FBN1 haplotype inherited by descent and known to be associated with Marfan syndrome
Skeletal	***Major—At Least Four of the Following:***
For the skeletal system to be involved, at least two of the components of the major criterion or one of the components of the major criterion plus two of the minor criteria must be present	Pectus excavatum requiring surgery *or* pectus carinatum
	Reduced upper-to-lower segment ratio *or* arm span-to-height ratio >1.05
	Positive wrist *and* thumb signs
	Scoliosis >2°
	Reduced extension of the elbows to <170°
	Medial displacement of the malleolus *and* pes planus
	Protrusio acetabulae of any degree as detected by radiographic studies
	Minor
	Pectus excavatum of moderate severity
	Joint hypermobility
	Highly arched palate with dental crowding
	Typical facies (dolichocephaly, malar hypoplasia, enophthalmos, retrognathia, downslanting palpebral fissures)
Ocular	***Major***
For the ocular system to be affected, at least two of the minor criteria must be present	Ectopia lentis
	Minor
	Flat cornea (as measured by keratometry)
	Increased axial length of the globe (as measured by A-scan ultrasonography)
	Miosis and hypoplastic ciliary muscle
Cardiovascular	***Major***
For the cardiovascular system to be involved, only one of the minor criteria must be present	Aortic root dilatation with or without aortic regurgitation and involving at least the sinuses of Valsalva
	Aortic dissection
	Minor
	Mitral valve prolapse with or without mitral valve regurgitation
	Dilatation of the proximal main pulmonary artery (in the absence of peripheral pulmonic stenosis or other cause) before the age of 40
	Calcification of the mitral annulus before age 40
	Dilatation of the abdominal or descending thoracic aorta before age 50

Table 31.4. Continued

System	Criteria
Pulmonary	***Major***
For the pulmonary system to be involved, one of the minor criteria must be present	None
	Minor
	Spontaneous pneumothorax Apical blebs on chest radiography
Dura	***Major***
	Lumbosacral dural ectasia by CT or MRI
	Minor
	None
Skin and Integument	***Major***
For the skin and integument system to be involved, one of the minor criteria must be present	None
	Minor
	Striae atrophicae in the absence of marked weight changes, pregnancy, or repetitive stress Recurrent *or* incisional hernia

[a] The requirements for diagnosis are *(1)* for the index case. At least two major criteria in different systems *and* involvement of a third system and exclusion of homocystinuria by plasma amino acid analysis. *(2)* For a family member: major criterion in family history *and* one major criterion in one system *and* involvement of a second system and exclusion of homocystinuria by plasma amino acid analysis.

skin and fibroblasts of individuals with Marfan syndrome and other diseases of connective tissue has been determined.[41,73,85] In a study of the synthesis, secretion, and incorporation of fibrillin in the extracellular matrix of 26 probands with Marfan syndrome, Milewicz et al.[73] found four groups of patients: *(1)* those whose cells synthesized and secreted normally half the normal amount of fibrillin, *(2)* those whose cells synthesized normal amounts of fibrillin, but failed to secrete it efficiently, *(3)* those whose cells synthesized and secreted normal amounts of fibrillin, but who failed to incorporate the fibrillin normally into the extracellular matrix, and *(4)* those who had apparently normal synthesis, secretion, and incorporation of fibrillin. The abnormalities were consistent within families and were absent in nonaffected family members.[73]

Wheatley and co-workers[116] studied the distribution of fibrillin in normal ocular tissues and found the glycoprotein to be ubiquitous in the cornea, sclera, anterior chamber angle, uvea, zonules, lens capsule, and optic nerve septae. These authors concluded that ocular abnormalities in Marfan syndrome could be correlated to the pattern of distribution fibrillin in the eye.[116] Further studies by Mir et al.[74] sought to determine the localization, distribution, and structure of fibrillin microfibrils in the lens capsule of normal individuals and of subjects with Marfan syndrome, in order to gain a better understanding of the pathogenesis of ectopia lentis and of myopia in this condition. We examined sections and/or flat mounts of lens capsules from normal autopsy eyes and surgical capsulotomy specimens from patients with senile cataracts and from patients with Marfan syndrome. Based on fibrillin staining patterns, we identified three distinct and adjacent zones in the equatorial and periequatorial regions of the normal lens capsule (Fig. 31.4). Zone I was a 0.75 mm-wide peripheral ring of the anterior capsule that contained radial bundles of fibrillin fibers that appeared to suspend the central part of the capsule (Fig. 31.5). Zone II was a 1 mm-wide meshwork of fibrillin-rich fibers that encircled the equator and

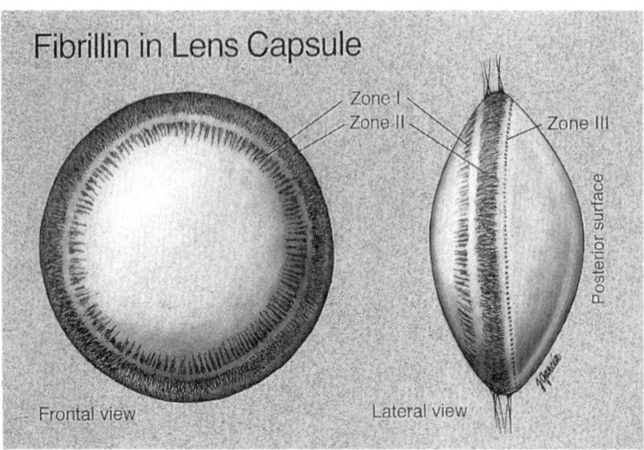

Figure 31.4. Artist's rendering of the three zones of fibrillin staining in the equatorial region of the lens capsule. The sketches are drawn to scale assuming a lens diameter of 11 mm. Frontal and lateral views are shown. (Reproduced with permission from Mir et al.[74])

served as an insertion platform for zonular fibers. Zone III was composed of radial, 0.1 mm-wide bands arranged in a periodic fashion in the most peripheral part of the posterior capsule (Fig. 31.6). Fibrillin fibers were abnormal and disrupted in all three zones in patients with

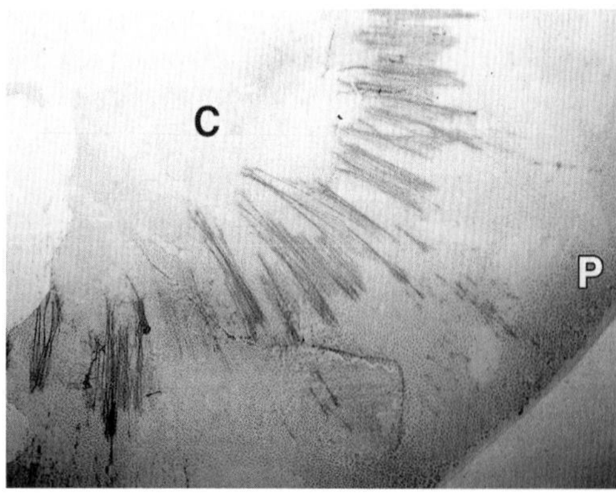

Figure 31.5. Immunohistochemical detection of fibrillin distribution in normal human lens capsule. This is a low-power view of a flat-mounted capsulotomy specimen obtained during routine cataract surgery. The capsule was stained by ABC immunoperoxidase methods for fibrillin (red reaction product is seen as black). Fiber bundles are organized in a radial configuration peripheral to the central anterior region. Smaller fiber bundles or individual microfibrils are located more peripherally. C = central anterior capsule; P = peripheral anterior capsule. Original magnification 10×. (Reproduced with permission from Mir et al.[74])

Marfan syndrome. From these observations, we concluded that fibrillin is a major constituent of the peripheral and equatorial areas of the lens capsule, that it may play a role in the ability of the lens to change its configuration during accommodation, and that the observed qualitative and quantitative abnormalities in fibrillin expression in the lens capsule of patients with Marfan syndrome support a causal relationship to lens abnormalities in these patients.

Kielty and co-workers[50] found abnormal fibrillin microfibrils in tissues and cell cultures from two cousins with Marfan syndrome who had ectopia lentis and skeletal involvement, but no cardiovascular defects. Ultrastructural analysis of ciliary zonules showed abundant loose and disorganized microfibril bundles. Microfibrils from ciliary zonules and vitreous were highly fragmented when examined by rotary shadowing electron microscopy. Microfibrils elaborated by patient dermal fibroblasts showed remarkable variations in periodicity and packing. The synthesis and secretion of fibrillin by these cells were confirmed electrophoretically with the identification of metabolically labeled immunoprecipitated fibrillin in medium and cell layer compartments. It was concluded that fibrillin expression was normal but that assembled microfibrils were abnormal both morphologically and functionally.

Genotype-Phenotype Correlation

Most Marfan syndrome families have unique FBN1 mutations at residues with putative importance for calcium binding to EGF-like domains; these mutations generally result in moderate to severe disease.[27] Mutations that result in premature termination of translation of mRNA and reduced mutant allele transcript may be associated with a clinically mild phenotype, supporting the view that a dominant negative mechanism plays an important role in the pathogenesis of this disorder.[24] Liu and co-workers[57] identified exon-skipping mutations in six probands with severe Marfan syndrome and concluded that this type of mutation is associated with a severe phenotype.

In patients with severe neonatal Marfan syndrome, where the diagnosis is made in the first 3 months of life, there is severe cardiac involve-

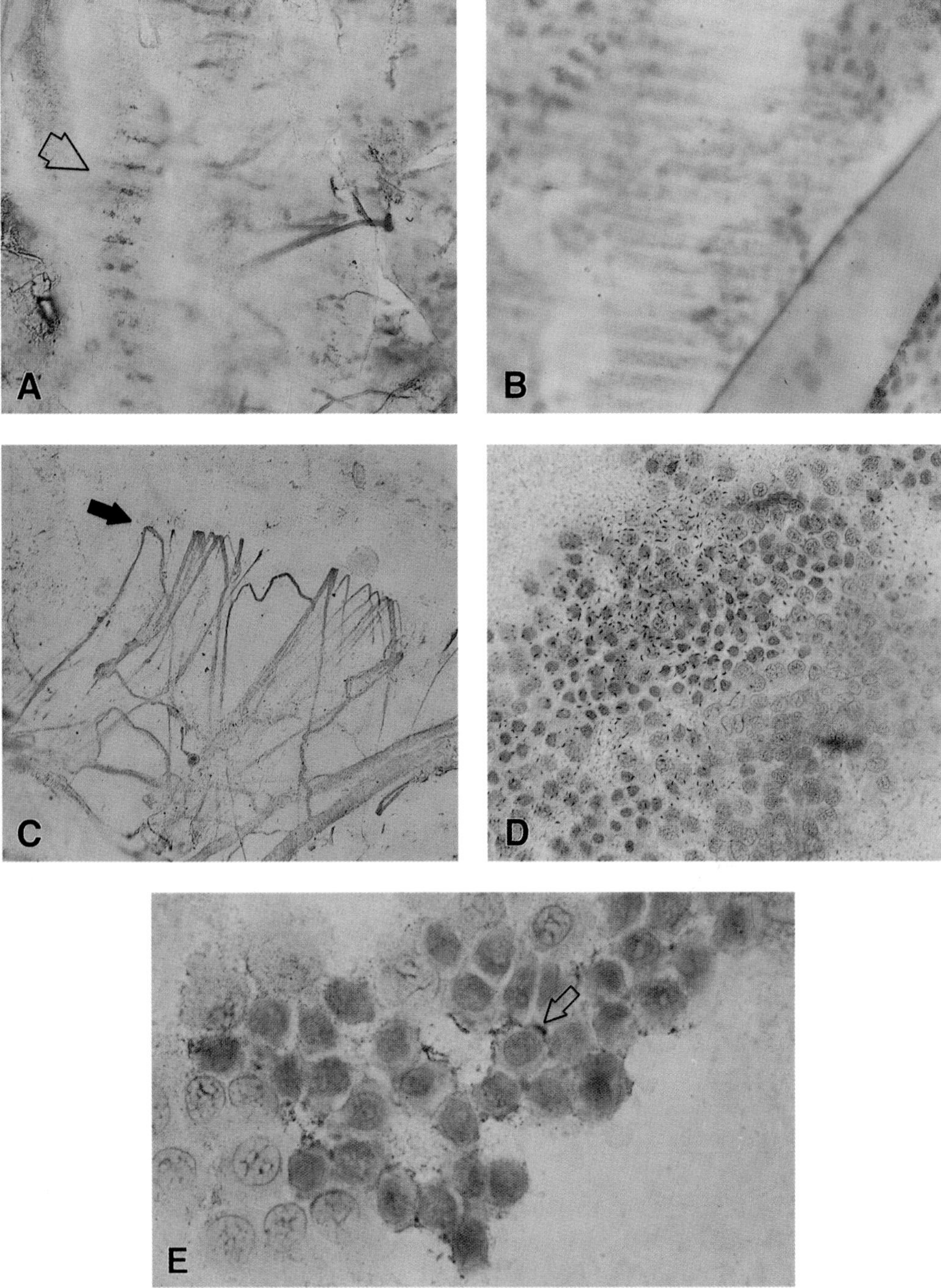

Figure 31.6. Fibrillin abnormalities in lens capsules of Marfan syndrome patients. Flat-mounted capsule specimens were stained by ABC immunoperoxidase for fibrillin. **A:** Irregular periodic segments in the retro-equatorial (zone III) region of capsule (arrowhead). Portions of ragged-appearing zonular attachments are seen to the right in the figure. Original magnification, 100×. **B:** Normal capsule exhibits more intense, regular, and larger periodic segments. These contrasting distributions are supported by the serial-sectioned samples shown in Figure 7**A–D**. Original magnification, 100×. **C:** Zonular fibers are elongated and floppy. Some have a striking hairpin shape. No staining was observed in the area corresponding to zone II. Original magnification, 100×. **D:** Large bundles normally present in zone I were absent in the Marfan capsule. Instead, a bed of granular fibrillin-positive material was present over the epithelial cell layer. Original magnification, 100×. **E:** Some epithelial cell membranes appeared to be immunoreactive for fibrillin (arrows). Immunoreactive fibrillin (red); counterstain, Harris's hematoxylin (blue). Original magnification, 250×. (Reproduced with permission from Mir et al.[74])

ment and congenital joint contractures.[75] A cluster of mutations leading to the severe neonatal form of Marfan syndrome may be located at the beginning of the longest stretch of EGF-like motifs in the fibrillin molecule and between exons 24 and 32.[47,57a,94,114] Some of these patients, such as the ones reported by Schollin et al.[94] and by Karttunen et al.,[49] may be homozygous or compound heterozygous for mutations in FBN1.

Associated Shprintzen-Goldberg Syndrome

Dietz and co-workers[22] found a de novo G-to-A mutation at nucleotide 3668 in a 7-year-old girl with typical ocular, skeletal, and cardiovascular features of Marfan syndrome and additional clinical abnormalities consistent with Shprintzen-Goldberg syndrome[98] (hypotonia, scaphocephaly, craniosynostosis, low-set anomalous ears, hyperelastic skin, diastasis recti, vertical talus, and mental retardation). Sood and co-workers found another mutation, this time at nucleotide 1148, associated with the Shprintzen-Goldberg phenotype.[102] This last mutation, however, was also detected in patients with classic Marfan syndrome or with isolated aortic aneurysm. This led Sood et al.[102] to suggest that this mutation produces a fibrillin allele that is subject to extreme modification by epistatic, stochastic, and/or environmental factors.

Ocular Complications

Subluxation of the crystalline lens is the diagnostic ocular abnormality in this disease. It is present in 65%–70% of patients and varies from a mild superior and posterior displacement of the lens, which is only evident on maximal pupillary dilation, to significant subluxation that places the equator of the lens in the pupillary axis (Fig. 31.7). Rarely is the lens totally dislocated into the vitreous cavity or into the anterior chamber. Although superior and temporal displacement of the lens is most common, inferior, nasal, or lateral subluxation can also occur. The zonular fibers are stretched and may be reduced in number. Subluxation of the lens is slowly progressive in the first two decades of life.[64] Further displacement may take place at a later age but is uncommon. Total dislocation into the vitreous cavity occurs rarely in older patients and may be complicated by phacolytic uveitis and glaucoma, necessitating lens extraction and vitrectomy.[42] Anterior dislocation of the lens into the pupil or anterior chamber is characteristic of untreated homocystinuria, and is rare, but not unheard of, in Marfan syndrome.

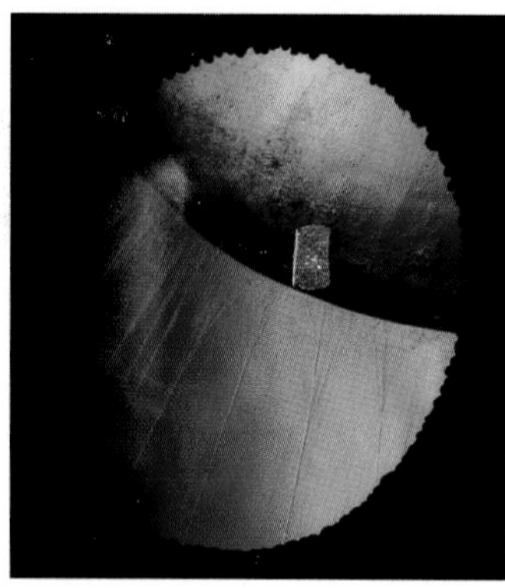

Figure 31.7. Significant superotemporal displacement of the lens in a patient with Marfan syndrome. There is a fair complement of extremely stretched zonules.

Other lenticular abnormalities include microspherophakia, which was diagnosed in only 2 of 160 patients examined by Maumenee.[64] In this condition, the lens has a smaller diameter than normal, assumes a globular configuration, and results in high myopia. Microspherophakia is presumed to be due to the defective fibrillin in the lens capsule and zonule.[74]

Cataracts develop 10–20 years earlier in patients with Marfan syndrome than in the general population. The typical Marfan cataract is of the nuclear sclerotic type. The indications for, and techniques of, clear subluxated lens removal in patients with Marfan syndrome continue to be controversial subjects. A cataractous lens that obscures the visual axis obviously needs to be removed; this can be achieved using intracapsular, endocapsular, or extracapsular techniques.[1,91] Removing clear subluxated lenses that bisect the visual axis or that render refraction very difficult can be avoided by diligent efforts at refracting the patient through the phakic or aphakic portions of the pupil. Sufficient time, in the order of several months, should be allowed for the patient to adapt to a new corrective refractive method before a decision to perform a lensectomy is taken. Some clinicians maintain that limbal or pars plana lensectomy can be performed safely in patients with Marfan syndrome and that these procedures result in a clear pupillary axis that allows a stable refraction and excellent vision. Halpert and BenEzra[39] reported the results of lens extraction in 59 eyes of 37 patients with ectopia lentis of genetic origin. In all, there were 65 patients with this category of ocular problems in these authors' practice. Twenty-seven eyes were in patients with Marfan syndrome, 23 eyes had simple ectopia lentis, and 9 eyes were in patients with homocystinuria, aniridia, microphthalmia, or Weill-Marchesani syndrome. The indications for surgery were best-corrected visual acuity of less than 20/70, luxation of the lens into the anterior chamber, monocular diplopia, or rapidly progressing posterior subluxation of the lens. Fifty-four eyes with subluxation of the crystalline lens behind the iris underwent pars plana lensectomy combined with anterior vitrectomy. The lenses were removed through a limbal approach in 5 eyes with dislocation of the lens in the anterior chamber. After a postoperative follow-up ranging from 12 to 144 months (average, 55 months), 52 eyes (88% of the entire group) improved two lines or more on the Snellen chart in best-corrected visual acuity. Seven eyes (12%) retained the same visual acuity as before the surgery. Retinal detachment was detected in one eye 2 years after surgery and was the only major postoperative complication. The authors concluded that lensectomy of subluxated lenses, combined with anterior vitrectomy using a closed-system technique, is a beneficial and relatively safe procedure.[39]

Patients with an increased axial length are probably at higher risk of retinal detachment following lens extraction,[64] although no extensive statistics are available that address this specific issue.

The corneal curvature is flatter than normal in most patients with Marfan syndrome. The average keratometric values are 41.38 ± 2.04D compared to 43.44 ± 0.19D for normal males and 44.00 ± 0.19D for normal females. Corneal thickness is not reduced.[64]

The anterior chamber is very deep with prominent iris processes to Schwalbe's line in some patients. The iris is often thin and velvety, with absent crypts and convolutions. The pupil may be difficult to dilate, especially in the more severely affected patients.

Izquierdo and co-workers[43] studied 573 patients with Marfan syndrome for the presence of ocular misalignment, refractive errors, and amblyopia. A total of 110 patients (19.2%) had strabismus. Exotropia occurred in 67 (11.7%), esotropia in 12 (2.1%), vertical deviations in 8 (1.4%), and primary inferior oblique muscle overaction in 3 patients (0.5%). Of the 67 patients with exotropia, 18 had anisometropia and 39 had amblyopia. Of the 12 patients with esotropia, 4 had amblyopia and none had anisometropia. Exotropia and esotropia were more common in patients with Marfan syndrome than in the general population of the United States ($p < 0.001$ for exotropia and $0.05 < p < 0.10$ for esotropia).[43] Amblyopia in patients with Marfan syndrome responds surprisingly well to optical correction and visual penalization, sometimes despite years of uncorrected high errors of refraction.

The vitreous is well formed in patients with Marfan syndrome. The retinal appearance is generally normal; no posterior staphylomas were detected in a large number of patients examined by Maumenee.[64] Peripheral areas of white without pressure may be present, and retinal breaks may be visualized. Retinal detachment may occur spontaneously in eyes with axial myopia, or may follow lens extraction, especially in eyes with increased axial length. Greco and Ambrosino[37] reported on the surgical repair of six eyes with retinal detachment and ectopia lentis; they achieved a good surgical outcome in five of the six eyes.

In a retrospective review of more than 500 patients with Marfan syndrome, Izquierdo and co-workers[42] found that open-angle glaucoma was significantly more common in all age groups compared to the general population. Pupillary block glaucoma is rare in Marfan syndrome, but cases have been documented (and personal observation). Two older patients in the series by Izquierdo et al.[42] had phacolytic glaucoma from mature totally dislocated lenses; both patients needed vitreoretinal surgery to extract the hard cataractous lenses. It is conceivable that glaucoma in Marfan syndrome results, at least in part, from abnormalities in the connective tissue components of the anterior chamber angle and from mechanical factors at the level of the optic nerve head and the lamina cribrosa.

Ocular Histopathology

A number of ocular histopathological studies in Marfan syndrome have been published.[11,29,32,87,111] The most prominent findings consist of increased axial length of the globe; stretching or ectasia of the cornea in the limbal area, absence of pigment in the iris pigment epithelium, hypopigmentation, and thinning of the iris stroma, especially in the periphery; hypoplasia of the dilator muscles of the iris; hypoplasia of the circular component of the ciliary muscle; and attenuation of the zonular fibers as they attach to the lens capsule, with lack of separation into a fan of filaments. Farnsworth et al.[32] presented an electron microscopic study of the zonules and lens capsule in a 19-year-old patient with Marfan syndrome. Compared to normal zonules, the ones in Marfan syndrome were few and malformed; they were composed of irregular aggregates of their subunits, which in the normal zonule were arranged in a parallel fashion. The posterior capsular epithelial cells in the Marfan specimen lacked the normal meridional row alignment, had irregular borders, and contained numerous abnormally large granules.[32]

Now that fibrillin has been identified as the defective protein in Marfan syndrome and as a major constituent of the zonular suspensory fibers of the crystalline lens,[105,116] the findings of Farnsworth et al.[32] and of Mir et al.[74] (vide supra) can be interpreted: abnormal fibrillin molecules cannot aggregate appropriately into parallel microfibrils to form the normal zonules and allow them to attach properly to the lens capsule. The abnormal protein aggregates accumulate in or around the epithelial cells, where they appear as granular inclusions or extracellular aggregates.

The same defect in fibrillin probably leads to abnormal scleral structure and tensile strength, with subsequent elongation of the globe and axial myopia. Other ocular abnormalities in Marfan syndrome such as increased depth of the anterior chamber, flat cornea, abnormalities of iris structure, presenile cataracts, and a predisposition for retinal detachment may all represent changes resulting from a defective backbone of fibrillin in the connective tissue matrix.[116]

Treatment

Orthopedic and Cardiac Considerations. Infants and children with Marfan syndrome can be severely affected and present major therapeutic orthopedic and cardiovascular challenges.[38,75] Recent advances in the medical and surgical management of these problems have allowed longer survival than existed two decades ago.[36,62,77] Mitral valve disease in childhood and dissecting aortic aneurysm in adults remain the most frequent causes of death. The mainstay in the treatment relies on the prevention of cardiac complications using beta-blocking agents. Shores et al.[97] showed a significantly lower rate of dilatation of the aortic root, and improvement of survival of patients treated with propranolol over 10 years, compared to patients who were not given the medication. Surgical repair of the ascending aorta using a composite aortic valve–ascending aortic conduit (Bentall operation) is performed on patients with moderate aortic regurgitation or dilation of the aortic root to more than 5.5 cm.[67]

Ophthalmologic Considerations. Careful and repeated phakic or aphakic refraction is necessary to achieve the best possible vision. Patients with subluxated lenses that are bisecting the pupillary aperture should try both aphakic and phakic corrections and see which one they prefer. Lens extraction should be avoided unless absolutely necessary because of the high risk of retinal detachment, especially in elongated globes. Large argon laser burns may be applied on the iris over areas of elongated zonules in the hope that the dissipated heat may result in further subluxation of the lens, allowing aphakic correction. Visual prognosis is good if amblyopia is treated and appropriate optical correction is instituted early. Retinal detachment remains the leading cause of severe visual loss. Early detection of glaucoma is essential.

Prenatal Diagnosis

Prenatal diagnosis of Marfan syndrome is possible using ultrasonography if the fetus is severely affected. In families where linkage to chromosome 15q markers is possible, or where a specific mutation in the fibrillin gene is present, linkage analysis or direct gene sequencing may allow prenatal diagnosis.[34]

WEILL-MARCHESANI SYNDROME

Clinical Findings and Genetics

Weill-Marchesani syndrome is a rare autosomal recessive disease characterized by congenital short stature, brachycephaly, short stubby spadelike hands and feet, microspherophakia, and subluxated lenses.[60,65,89,115] The disease occurs in 1 : 100,000 individuals. Patients are of normal intelligence. Although the disease is recessive, parents may be comparatively short, with or without stubby hands and no ocular abnormalities. Family members in previous generations may be identified as carriers of the mutated gene based on stature.[52,81]

Wirtz et al.[118a] studied two families with affected members in three generations. There was possible linkage to 15q21.1 where the genes for fibrillin 1 and microfibril-associated protein 1 are located. There was reduced fibrillin staining in skin sections from one family compared to normal controls.[118a]

Ocular Findings

Ocular abnormalities occur only in homozygotes.[45] The microspherophakic lens tends to move into the pupillary area causing pupillary block and glaucoma.[117] Total dislocation into the anterior chamber is uncommon but may occur. Myopia results from spherophakia but may be axial. The lens diameter may be as small as 6.75 mm, and the lens may be increased by 25% in thickness.[68] The anterior chamber is usually shallow, predisposing to angle-closure glaucoma.

Treatment

A peripheral iridectomy should be performed to prevent or relieve pupillary block. Lens extraction may be necessary to control intraocular pressure elevation in some patients. Although mydriatics are preferred over miotics for the relief of pupillary block, cycloplegics have been reported to induce pupillary block in patients with Weill-Marchesani syndrome.[119] Trabeculectomy may be necessary in patients with chronic glaucoma. The anterior chamber may remain shallow for a prolonged period following surgery, but if the fistula is open, there is adequate control of the intraocular pressure (personal observation).

HOMOCYSTINURIA

Clinical Findings and Genetics

Untreated patients with this autosomal recessive disease have mental retardation, coarse fair hair, a Marfanoid body habitus, and a thromboembolic diathesis. These patients are frequently misdiagnosed with Marfan syndrome because of their slender body and the presence of lens dislocation. Accumulation of homocysteine may be responsible for the arteriosclerosis, the abnormal platelet adhesiveness, and frequent cerebral thromboses. It has also been proposed that the accumulated homocysteine interferes with collagen and elastin crosslinking, hence leading to the observed connective tissue defects and ectopia lentis.

Two major categories of homocystinuria are recognized. Cystathionine-β-synthase deficiency is responsible for the more common variety of the disease. This enzyme catalyzes the transsulfuration of homocysteine to cystathionine in the presence of vitamin B6. Fifty percent of patients with cystathionine-β-synthase deficiency respond to vitamin B6 supplementation with clearing of their urine of homocysteine. Mental retardation occurs mostly in vitamin B6 nonresponders. The gene for cystathionine-β-synthase has been mapped to 21q22.3[55] and the sequence of its cDNA has been determined.[54] A less common variety of homocystinuria results from reduced activity of 5-methyltetrahydrofolate-homocysteine methyltransferase.

Ocular Findings

All untreated patients with homocystinuria develop dislocation of both lenses, about 40% of them by the age of 5 years. The lenses dislocate completely in an inferior or inferonasal direction (Fig. 31.8).[19] Anterior movement of the unrestrained lenses leads to pupillary block and to glaucoma (Fig. 31.9). Patients may initially present with a red eye and cloudy cornea. In contradistinction to the elongated but intact zonules in Marfan syndrome, a fringe of ragged zonular remnants is present in the equatorial zone of the lenses in patients with homocystinuria.[86,88] The appearance of the zonular remnants may help differentiate patients with homocystinuria from those with Marfan syndrome (Figs. 31.3, 31.4). A characteristic thick periodic acid–Schiff-positive layer of short filaments of zonular origin is demonstrated histopathologically over the ciliary epithelium.

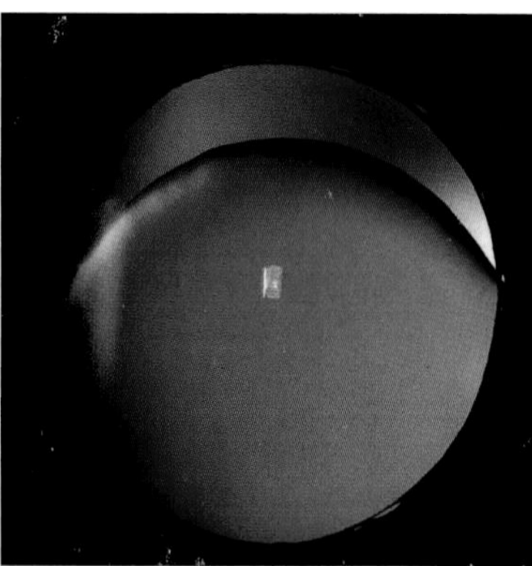

Figure 31.8. Inferior displacement of the lens in a 10-year-old boy with homocystinuria. Note the absence of zonules. This patient was initially misdiagnosed with Marfan syndrome because of his thin body habitus, the absence of mental retardation, and the presence of subluxated lenses. Biochemical studies confirmed a diagnosis of homocystinuria. The boy has a similarly affected older brother.

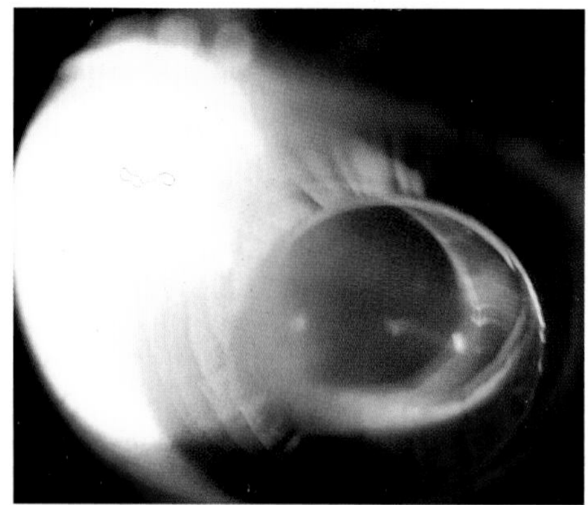

Figure 31.9. The lens is in the anterior chamber in a young girl with homocystinuria. The pupillary space is blocked, and the lens is touching the corneal endothelium.

High myopia is the result of microspherophakia. Cystic and pigmentary changes of unclear significance have been noted in the retinal periphery of some patients with the disease.

Treatment

Medical Management

All patients with dislocated lenses without a clear history of trauma should undergo quantitation of urine and serum amino acids to rule out homocystinuria.[103] Conversely, an episode of dislocation of the crystalline lens into the anterior chamber in a patient with presumed Marfan syndrome should suggest the diagnosis of homocystinuria.

Supplementation with 50–1000 mg/day of oral vitamin B6 clears the urine from methionine in the subgroup of vitamin B6 responders. Nonresponders do not receive further vitamin supplementation and are started on a diet low in methionine. They are also given cystine supplements. Betaine supplementation facilitates the conversion of serum homocysteine to methionine and significantly reduces the symptoms of homocystinuria.

Recent studies have demonstrated that neonatal screening, detection of the disease at birth, and appropriate therapy prevent the development of mental retardation, myopia, and lens subluxation. Platelet antiaggregation agents such as dipyridamole and acetylsalicylic acid are given to prevent vasocclusive or thromboembolic events. A normal life span is expected in vitamin B6 responders. Patients with other types of homocystinuria have shortened survival depending on the type of mutation, severity of the disease at diagnosis, and time of institution of therapy.

Management of the Dislocated Lens

If the crystalline lens dislocates into the anterior chamber, the pupil is dilated and the patient is placed in a supine position to reposition the lens behind the pupil. Digital pressure on the cornea may be a helpful maneuver. Miotics are then prescribed, and a peripheral laser iridotomy is performed. In some patients, and with the passage of time, the pupillary sphincter infarcts, the pupil dilates, and miotics become ineffective in keeping the lens behind the iris. Lens extraction may then become necessary. Because of the increased risk of thromboembolic phenomena with general anesthesia, local anesthesia is preferred if surgery is inevitable. Intravenous hydration is instituted prior to surgery to reduce the risk of thrombosis.

MOLYBDENUM COFACTOR DEFECTS AND SULFITE OXIDASE DEFICIENCY

Lens dislocation is probably not present at birth but develops in the first year or two of life in this group of metabolic diseases characterized by severe neurologic abnormalities.[31,100] Some cases are due to isolated sulfite oxidase deficiency, but more patients have a molybdenum-containing cofactor deficiency that results in deficient activities of the three enzymes that require this cofactor: sulfite oxidase, xanthine dehydrogenase, and aldehyde oxidase.[112] Urinary excretion of sulfite, thiosulfate, S-sulfocysteine, taurine, hypoxanthine, and xanthine is increased, whereas sulfate and urate excretion is markedly reduced. Urinary urothione is nondetectable.[90] The diagnosis may be made by assaying for urinary sulfite.[112] In addition to dislocated lenses, patients have convulsions, feeding difficulties, and mental retardation. In the form due to the cofactor defect, abnormal muscle tone, myoclonic spasms, and dysmorphic facies have been reported.[46]

Mudd et al.[76] reported an infant with a fatal neurologic disease, ectopia lentis, and increased levels of sulfite in the urine, with markedly decreased inorganic sulfate excretion. The authors postulated a defect in sulfite oxidase, an enzyme that catalyzes the conversion of sulfite to sulfate. It is postulated that the accumulated sulfite combines to aldehyde groups in the zonules and leads to their dissolution, as is the case with homocysteine in homocystinuria. Another child with this disorder was reported by Shih et al.[96]; the child had acute infantile hemiplegia and ectopia lentis. A low-sulfur amino acid diet resulted in an improvement of the biochemical profile.[96] Other cases of sulfite oxidase deficiency have been reported by Vianey-Liaud et al.,[110] van der Klei-van Moorsel et al.,[109] and Barbot et al.[2] Not all patients had dislocated lenses.

HYPERLYSINEMIA

There is only one patient with hyperlysinemia who was reported to have dislocated lenses,[101] and the association has been considered fortuitous by some authors.[20] The features of this autosomal recessive condition are mental retardation, impaired sexual development, lax ligaments and muscles, convulsions in early life, and mild anemia. The patient reported by Smith et al.[101] may have had a second recessive disorder responsible for lax ligaments and ectopia lentis. Lysine levels are elevated in blood and in spinal fluid. There is reduced activity of two successive enzymes in the major pathway of lysine degradation: lysine ketoglutarate reductase and saccharopine dehydrogenase.[18] The two enzymes are coded for by a single gene and are components of a homotetrameric bifunctional enzyme called aminoadipic semialdehyde synthase, which has both lysine ketoglutarate reductase and saccharopine dehydrogenase activity. In hyperlysinemia, both enzymatic functions of the bifunctional enzyme are defective, whereas in saccharopinemia, some of the first enzymatic function is retained.[18]

CRANIOFACIAL DYSOSTOSIS WITH ECTOPIA LENTIS, ANTERIOR SEGMENT DYSGENESIS, AND GLAUCOMA

Shawaf and co-workers[95] reported a family with a presumed autosomal recessive syndrome characterized by craniofacial dysmorphism and severe ocular anomalies that included totally dislocated lenses, anterior segment dysgenesis, severe glaucoma, and progressive spontaneous thinning and perforation of the perilimbal sclera (Fig. 31.10). There were no cardiac or skeletal abnormalities compatible with Marfan syndrome. Patients were of normal stature and intelligence. Facial features consisted of downslanting of the palpebral fissures, a beaked nose, and crowding of the teeth. Another unrelated Lebanese Druze family had the same syndrome in several members of one generation with normal parents (Traboulsi, personal observation).

KNIEST DYSPLASIA (METATROPIC DWARFISM II)

This is an autosomal dominant disorder that results from a defect in type II procollagen.[80,118]

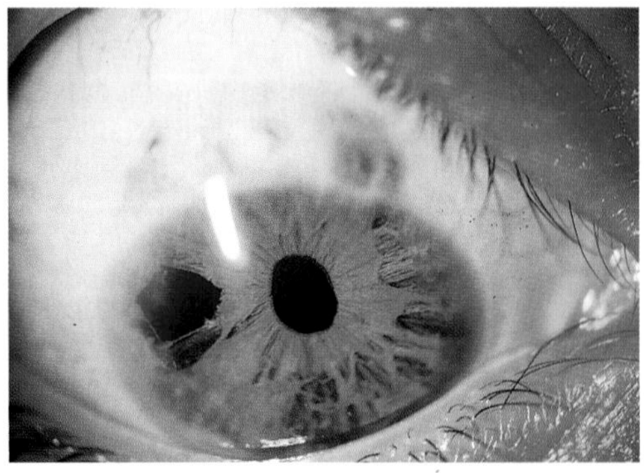

Figure 31.10. Right eye of a 15-year-old girl with ectopia lentis, anterior segment dysgenesis, and spontaneous filtering blebs. The sclera is extremely thin superiorly. There is true polycoria and the anterior leaflet of the iris is poorly developed. The dislocated lens was extracted.

Patients have a flat face, wide and stiff joints, short stature, kyphoscoliosis, and severe ocular abnormalities.[53] In a series of seven patients, Maumenee and Traboulsi[66] found congenital and severe myopia and vitreoretinal degeneration in all patients, rhegmatogenous retinal detachment in four, cataracts in two, and subluxated lenses in one patient.

KNIEST-LIKE DYSPLASIA WITH PURSED LIPS AND ECTOPIA LENTIS

This rare autosomal recessive syndrome has been described in only one family. A brother and sister had clinical and radiologic features similar to those of Kniest dysplasia but did not have the characteristic "Swiss cheese" appearance of the cartilage on histopathology; there were rather scattered thick collagen fibers in the cartilage matrix. In addition to Kniest-like features, both patients had pursed lips such as those seen in the whistling-face syndrome, and bilateral inferior subluxation of their lenses.[12]

SPONDYLOEPIMETAPHYSEAL DYSPLASIA WITH JOINT LAXITY (SEMDJL)

This condition was described by Beighton and Kozlowski.[6] Patients have a distinctive form of skeletal dysplasia with characteristic facial appearance, joint laxity, and severe scoliosis. The face is oval with prominent eyes, a long philtrum, and a small mandible. Most patients die in the first decades of life from spinal compression.[3] Cleft palate is common. Subluxated lenses have been reported in one patient.[5] Most patients have blue sclerae.

CRANIOFACIAL DYSMORPHISM WITH OCULAR COLOBOMA, ABSENT CORPUS CALLOSUM, AND AORTIC DILATATION (TEMTAMY SYNDROME)

Temtamy et al.[106] described three siblings with craniofacial dysmorphism, absent corpus callosum, and chorioretinal coloboma. The lenses were subluxated superiorly. Facial features consisted of macrodolichocephaly, arched eyebrows, antimongoloid slanting of the palpebral fissures, low-set simple lop ears, a beaked nose, long philtrum, short upper lip, and micrognathia. Two of the three children had aortic dilatation with aortic regurgitation. One child was moderately retarded. There were abnormalities of the intercellular space and of collagen fibrils on gingival biopsies.

BLEPHAROPTOSIS, MYOPIA, AND ECTOPIA LENTIS

This condition has also been described in only one family.[33] A woman and her two daughters had bilateral congenital ptosis, high myopia, and subluxated lenses. An abnormality of connective tissue was presumed to cause all three components of the syndrome.

REFERENCES

1. Adank AM, Hennekes R. Phacoemulsification of the subluxated or atopic lens. *Bull Soc Belge Ophtalmol* 1993;249:33–39.
2. Barbot C, Martins E, Vilarinho L, Dorche C, Cardoso M. A mild form of infantile isolated sulphite oxidase deficiency. *Neuropediatrics* 1995;26:322–324.
3. Beighton P. Spondyloepimetaphyseal dysplasia with joint laxity (SEMDJL). *J Med Genet* 1994;31:136–140.
4. Beighton P, de Paepe A, Danks D, et al. International nosology of heritable disorders of connective tissue, Berlin 1986. *Am J Med Genet* 1988;29:581–594.
5. Beighton P, Gericke G, Kozlowski K, Grobler L. The manifestations and natural history of spondylo-epi-metaphyseal dysplasia with joint laxity. *Clin Genet* 1984;26:308–317.
6. Beighton P, Kozlowski K. Spondylo-epi-metaphyseal dysplasia with joint laxity and severe, progressive kyphoscoliosis. *Skeletal Radiol* 1980;5:205–212.
7. Boerger F. Ueber zwei Falle von Arachnodaktylie. *Z Kinderheilkd* 1914;12:161–184.
8. Boileau C, Coulon M, Junien C. [Marfan syndrome. Current molecular data]. *Arch Fr Pediatr* 1992;49(10):941–943.
9. Boileau C, Jondeau G, Babron MC, Coulon M, Alexandre JA, Sakai L, et al. Autosomal dominant Marfan-like connective-tissue disorder with aortic dilation and skeletal anomalies not linked to the fibrillin genes [see comments]. *Am J Hum Genet* 1993;53(1):46–54.
10. Brown O, DeMots H, Kloster F, Roberts A, Menashe V, Beals R. Aortic root dilatation and mitral valve prolapse in Marfan's syndrome: An echocardiographic study. *Circulation* 1975; 53:651–657.
11. Burian A, Allen L. Histologic study of patients with Marfan's syndrome. *Arch Ophthalmol* 1961;65:323–333.
12. Burton B, Sumner T, Langer L, Rimoin D, Adomian GE, Lachman R, et al. A new skeletal dysplasia: Clinical, radiologic, and pathologic findings. *J Pediatr* 1986;109:642–648.
13. Carrau A. Sur la dolichosténomélie: Maladie de Marfan. *Le Nourrisson* 1929;17:82–92.
14. Cistulli P, Sullivan C. Sleep apnea in Marfan's syndrome: Increased upper airway collapsibility during sleep. *Chest* 1995;108:631–635.
15. Colley A, Lloyd I, Ridgway A, Donnai D. Ectopia lentis et pupillae: The genetic aspects and differential diagnosis. *J Med Genet* 1991;28:791–794.
16. Collod G, Babron MC, Jondeau G, Coulon M, Weissenbach J, Dubourg, et al. A second locus for Marfan syndrome maps to chromosome 3p24.2-p25 [see comments]. *Nature Genet* 1994;8:264–268.
17. Corson GM, Chalberg SC, Dietz HC, Charbonneau NL, Sakai LY. Fibrillin binds calcium and is coded by cDNAs that reveal a multidomain structure and alternatively spliced exons at the 5′ end. *Genomics* 1993;17(2):476–484.
18. Cox R, Markovitz PJ, Chuang D. Familial hyperlysinemias—Multiple enzyme deficiencies associated with the bifunctional aminoadipic semialdehyde synthase. *Trans Am Clin Climatol Assoc* 1985;97:69–81.
19. Cross H, Jensen A. Ocular manifestations in the Marfan syndrome and homocystinuria. *Am J Ophthalmol* 1973;75:405–420.
20. Dancis J, Hutzler J, Ampola M, Shih V, van Gelderen H, Kirby L, et al. The prognosis of hyperlysinemia: An interim report. *Am J Hum Genet* 1983;35:438–442.
21. De Paepe A, Devereux RB, Dietz HC, Hennekam RC, Pyeritz RE. Revised diagnostic criteria for the Marfan syndrome. *Am J Med Genet* 1996;62:417–426.
22. Dietz H, Sood I, McIntosh I. The phenotypic continuum associated with FBN1 mutations

includes the Shprintzen-Goldberg syndrome. *Am J Hum Genet* 1995;57:(abstract) A211.

23. Dietz HC, Cutting GR, Pyeritz RE, Maslen CL, Sakai LY, Corson GM, et al. Marfan syndrome caused by a recurrent de novo missense mutation in the fibrillin gene [see comments]. *Nature* 1991;352:337–339.
24. Dietz HC, McIntosh I, Sakai LY, Corson GM, Chalberg SC, Pyeritz RE, et al. Four novel FBN1 mutations: Significance for mutant transcript level and EGF-like domain calcium binding in the pathogenesis of Marfan syndrome. *Genomics* 1993;17:468–475.
25. Dietz HC, Pyeritz RE. Mutations in the human gene for fibrillin-1 (FBN1) in the Marfan syndrome and related disorders. *Hum Mol Genet* 1995;4(spec. no.):1799–1809.
26. Dietz HC, Pyeritz RE, Hall BD, Cadle RG, Hamosh A, Schwartz J, et al. The Marfan syndrome locus: Confirmation of assignment to chromosome 15 and identification of tightly linked markers at 15q15-q21.3. *Genomics* 1991;9:355–361.
27. Dietz HC, Saraiva JM, Pyeritz RE, Cutting GR, Francomano CA. Clustering of fibrillin (FBN1) missense mutations in Marfan syndrome patients at cysteine residues in EGF-like domains. *Hum Mutat* 1992;1:366–374.
28. Downing AK, Knott V, Werner JM, Cardy CM, Campbell ID, Handford PA. Solution structure of a pair of calcium-binding epidermal growth factor-like domains: Implications for the Marfan syndrome and other genetic disorders. *Cell* 1996;85:597–605.
29. Dvorak-Theobald G. Histologic eye findings in arachnodactyly. *Am J Ophthalmol* 1941;24: 1132–1137.
30. Edwards MJ, Challinor CJ, Colley PW, Roberts J, Partington MW, Hollway GE, et al. Clinical and linkage study of a large family with simple ectopia lentis linked to FBN1. *Am J Med Genet* 1994;53:65–71.
31. Endres W, Shin Y, Gunther R, Ibel H, Duran M, Wadman S. Report on a new patient with combined deficiencies of sulphite oxidase and xanthine dehydrogenase due to molybdenum cofactor deficiency. *Eur J Pediatr* 1988;148: 246–249.
32. Farnsworth P, Burke P, Dotto M, et al. Ultrastructural abnormalities in Marfan's syndrome lens. *Arch Ophthalmol* 1977;95:1601–1606.
33. Gillum W, Anderson R. Dominantly inherited blepharoptosis, high myopia, and ectopia lentis. *Arch Ophthalmol* 1982;100:282–284.
34. Godfrey M, Vandemark N, Wang M, Velinov M, Wargowski D, Tsipouras P, et al. Prenatal diagnosis and a donor splice site mutation in fibrillin in a family with Marfan syndrome. *Am J Hum Genet* 1993;53(2):472–480.
35. Goldberg M. Clinical manifestations of ectopia lentis et pupillae in 16 patients. *Ophthalmology* 1988;95:1080–1087.
36. Gott V, Pyeritz R, Magovern GJ, et al. Surgical treatment of aneurysm of the ascending aorta in the Marfan syndrome: Results of composite-graft repair in 50 patients. *N Engl J Med* 1986;314:1070–1074.
37. Greco GM, Ambrosino L. Treatment of retinal detachment in Marfan syndrome. *Ann Ophthalmol* 1993;25:72–76.
38. Gruber M, Graham TJ, Engel E. Marfan syndrome with contractural arachnodactyly and severe mitral regurgitation in a premature infant. *J Pediatr* 1978;93:80–82.
39. Halpert M, BenEzra D. Surgery of the hereditary subluxated lens in children. *Ophthalmology* 1996;103:681–686.
40. Hewett DR, Lynch JR, Smith R, Sykes BC. A novel fibrillin mutation in the Marfan syndrome which could disrupt calcium binding of the epidermal growth factor-like module. *Hum Mol Genet* 1993;2:475–477.
41. Hollister DW, Godfrey M, Sakai LY, Pyeritz RE. Immunohistologic abnormalities of the microfibrillar-fiber system in the Marfan syndrome. *N Engl J Med* 1990;323:152–159.
42. Izquierdo NJ, Traboulsi EI, Enger C, Maumenee IH. Glaucoma in the Marfan syndrome. *Trans Am Ophthalmol Soc* 1992;90:111–117; discussion 118–122.
43. Izquierdo NJ, Traboulsi EI, Enger C, Maumenee IH. Strabismus in the Marfan syndrome. *Am J Ophthalmol* 1994;117:632–635.
44. James R, Jacobs P. Molecular studies of the aetiology of trisomy 8 in spontaneous abortions and the liveborn population. *Hum Genet* 1996;97:283–286.
45. Jensen A, Cross H. Ocular complications in the Weill-Marchesani syndrome. *Am J Ophthalmol* 1974;77:261–269.
46. Johnson J, Waud W, Rajagopalan K, Duran M, Beemer F, Wadman S. Inborn errors of molybdenum metabolism: Combined deficiencies of sulfite oxidase and xanthine dehydrogenase in a patient lacking the molybdenum cofactor. *Proc Natl Acad Sci USA* 1980;77: 3715–3719.
47. Kainulainen K, Karttunen L, Puhakka L, Sakai L, Peltonen L. Mutations in the fibrillin gene responsible for dominant ectopia lentis and neonatal Marfan syndrome. *Nature Genet* 1994;6:64–69.

48. Kainulainen K, Pulkkinen L, Savolainen A, Kaitila I, Peltonen L. Location on chromosome 15 of the gene defect causing Marfan syndrome [see comments]. *N Engl J Med* 1990;323: 935–939.
49. Karttunen L, Raghunath M, Lonnqvist L, Peltonen L. A compound-heterozygous Marfan patient: Two defective fibrillin alleles result in a lethal phenotype. *Am J Hum Genet* 1994;55:1083–1091.
50. Kielty CM, Davies SJ, Phillips JE, Jones CJ, Shuttleworth CA, Charles SJ. Marfan syndrome: Fibrillin expression and microfibrillar abnormalities in a family with predominant ocular defects. *J Med Genet* 1995;32:1–6.
51. Kielty CM, Shuttleworth CA. Fibrillin-containing microfibrils: structure and function in health and disease. *Int J Biochem Cell Biol* 1995;27:747–760.
52. Kloepfer H, Rosenthal J. Possible genetic carriers in the spherophakia-brachymorphia syndrome. *Am J Hum Genet* 1955;7:398–419.
53. Kniest W. Zur Abgrengzung der Dysostosis enchondralis von der Chondrodystrophie. *Z Kinderheilkd* 1952;43:633–640.
54. Kraus J, Le K, Swaroop M, et al. Human cystathionine beta-synthase: Sequence, alternative splicing and expression in cultured cells. *Hum Mol Genet* 1993;2:1633–1638.
55. Kraus J, Williamson C, Firgaira F, et al. Cloning and screening of nanogram amounts of immunopurified mRNAs: cDNA cloning and chromosomal mapping of cystathionine-beta-synthase and the beta subunit of propionyl-CoA carboxylase. *Proc Natl Acad Sci USA* 1986;83:2047–2051.
56. Lee B, Godfrey M, Vitale E, Hori H, Mattei MG, Sarfarazi M, et al. Linkage of Marfan syndrome and a phenotypically related disorder to two different fibrillin genes [see comments]. *Nature* 1991;352:330–334.
57. Liu W, Qian C, Comeau K, Brenn T, Furthmayr H, Francke U. Mutant fibrillin-1 monomers lacking EGF-like domains disrupt microfibril assembly and cause severe Marfan syndrome. *Hum Mol Genet* 1996;5:1581–1587.
57a. Lonnqvist L, Karttunen L, Rantamaki T, et al. A point mutation creating an extra N-glycosylation site in fibrillin-1 results in neonatal Marfan syndrome. *Genomics* 1996;3:468–475.
58. Magenis RE, Maslen CL, Smith L, Allen L, Sakai LY. Localization of the fibrillin (FBN) gene to chromosome 15, band q21.1. *Genomics* 1991;11:346–351.
59. Magid D, Pyeritz RE, Fishman EK. Musculoskeletal manifestations of the Marfan syndrome: Radiologic features. *Am J Roentgenol* 1990;155:99–104.
60. Marchesani O. Brachydaktylie und angeborene Kugelinse als Systemerk-rankung. *Klin Monatsbl Augenheilkd* 1939;103:392–406.
61. Marfan A. Un cas de deformation congenitale des quatres membres, plus prononcee aux extremites, characterisee par l'allongement des os, avec un certain degre d'amaincissement. *Bull Mem Soc Med Hop (Paris)* 1896;13: 220–226.
62. Marsalese D, Moodie D, Vacante M, et al. Marfan's syndrome: Natural history and long-term follow-up of cardiovascular involvement. *J Am Coll Cardiol* 1989;14:422–428.
63. Maslen CL, Corson GM, Maddox BK, Glanville RW, Sakai LY. Partial sequence of a candidate gene for the Marfan syndrome [see comments]. *Nature* 1991;352:334–337.
64. Maumenee I. The eye in the Marfan syndrome. *Trans Am Ophthalmol Soc* 1981;79:696–733.
65. Maumenee I. The Weill-Marchesani syndrome. In *Heritable Disorders of Connective Tissue*. P. Beighton, ed. St. Louis: C.V. Mosby, 1993, pp. 179–187.
66. Maumenee I, Traboulsi E. The ocular findings in Kniest dysplasia. *Am J Ophthalmol* 1985;100:155–160.
67. McDonald G, Schaff H, Pyeritz R, McKusick V, Goh V. Surgical management of patients with the Marfan syndrome and dilatation of the ascending aorta. *J Thorac Cardiovasc Surg* 1981;81:180–186.
68. McGavic J. Weill-Marchesani syndrome. *Am J Ophthalmol* 1966;62:820–823.
69. McKusick V. *Heritable Disorders of Connective Tissue*. St. Louis: C.V. Mosby, 1956.
70. McKusick V. The defect in the Marfan syndrome. *Nature* 1991;352:279–281.
71. Mecham RP, Broekelmann T, Davis EC, Gibson MA, Brown-Augsburger P. Elastic fibre assembly: macromolecular interactions. *Ciba Found Symp* 1995;192:172–181.
72. Milewicz DM, Duvic M. Severe neonatal Marfan syndrome resulting from a de novo 3-bp insertion into the fibrillin gene on chromosome 15. *Am J Hum Genet* 1994;54(3):447–453.
73. Milewicz DM, Pyeritz RE, Crawford ES, Byers PH. Marfan syndrome: Defective synthesis, secretion, and extracellular matrix formation of fibrillin by cultured dermal fibroblasts. *J Clin Invest* 1992;89:79–86.
74. Mir S, Whittum-Hudson J, Wheatley H, Hussels I, Traboulsi E. A comparative histological study of the fibrillin microfibrillar system in the lens capsule of normal and Marfan syndrome

subjects. *Invest Ophthalmol Visual Sci* 1998;39:84–93.

75. Morse RP, Rockenmacher S, Pyeritz RE, Sanders SP, Bieber FR, Lin A, et al. Diagnosis and management of infantile Marfan syndrome. *Pediatrics* 1990;86:888–895.
76. Mudd S, Irreverre F, Laster L. Sulfite oxidase deficiency in man: Demonstration of the enzymatic defect. *Science* 1967;156:1599–1602.
77. Murdoch J, Walker B, Halpern B, et al. Life expectancy and causes of death in the Marfan syndrome. *N Engl J Med* 1972;286:804–808.
78. Murdoch J, Walker B, Halpern B, Kuzma J, McKusick V. Life expectancy and causes of death in the Marfan syndrome. *N Engl J Med* 1972;286:804–808.
79. Pai G, Thomas G, Leonard C, Ward J, Valle D, Pyeritz R. Syndromes due to chromosomal abnormalities: Partial trisomy 22, interstitial deletion of the long arm of 13, and trisomy 8. *Johns Hopkins Med J* 1979;145:162–169.
80. Poole A, Pidoux I, Reiner A, Rosenberg L, Hollister D, Murray L, et al. Kniest dysplasia is characterized by an apparent abnormal processing of the C-propeptide of type II cartilage collagen resulting in imperfect fibril assembly. *J Clin Invest* 1988;81:579–589.
81. Probert L. Spherophakia with brachydactyly: Comparison with Marfan's syndrome. *Am J Ophthalmol* 1953;36:1571–1574.
82. Pyeritz R, McKusick V. The Marfan syndrome: Diagnosis and management. *N Engl J Med* 1979;300:772–777.
83. Pyeritz RE. Marfan syndrome [editorial; comment]. *N Engl J Med* 1990;323:987–989.
84. Pyeritz RE, Fishman EK, Bernhardt BA, Siegelman SS. Dural ectasia is a common feature of the Marfan syndrome. *Am J Hum Genet* 1988;43(5):726–732.
85. Raghunath M, Superti-Furga A, Godfrey M, Steinmann B. Decreased extracellular deposition of fibrillin and decorin in neonatal Marfan syndrome fibroblasts. *Hum Genet* 1993;90:511–515.
86. Ramsey M, Dickson D. Lens fringe in homocystinuria. *Br J Ophthalmol* 1975;59:338–342.
87. Ramsey M, Fine B, Shields J, et al. The Marfan syndrome. *Am J Ophthalmol* 1973;76:102–116.
88. Ramsey M, Yanoff M, Fine B. The ocular histopathology of homocystinuria. A light and electronmicroscopic study. *Am J Ophthalmol* 1972;74:377–385.
89. Rennert O. The Marchesani syndrome. A brief review. *Am J Dis Child* 1969;117:703–705.
90. Roesel R, Bowyer F, Blankenship P, Hommes F. Combined xanthine and sulphite oxidase defect due to a deficiency of molybdenum cofactor. *J Inherit Metab Dis* 1986;9:343–347.
91. Roussat B, Chiou AG, Quesnot S, Hamard H, Godde-Jolly D. Surgery of ectopia lentis in Marfan disease in children and young adults. *J Fr Ophtalmol* 1995;18(3):170–177.
92. Sakai L, Keene D, Engvall E. Fibrillin, a new 350-kD glycoprotein, is a component of extracellular microfibrils. *J Cell Biol* 1986;103:2499–2509.
93. Sakai L, Keene D, Glanville R, Bachinger H. Purification and partial characterization of fibrillin, a cysteine-rich structural component of connective tissue microfibrils. *J Biol Chem* 1992;266:14,763–14,770.
94. Schollin J, Bjarke B, Gustavson KH. Probable homozygotic form of the Marfan syndrome in a newborn child. *Acta Paediatr Scand* 1988;77:452–456.
95. Shawaf S, Noureddin B, Khouri A, Traboulsi E. A family with a syndrome of ectopia lentis, spontaneous filtering blebs, and craniofacial dysmorphism. *Ophthalmic Genet* 1995;1995:163–169.
96. Shih V, Abrams I, Johnson J, Carney M, Mandell R, Robb R, et al. Sulfite oxidase deficiency: Biochemical and clinical investigations of a hereditary metabolic disorder in sulfur metabolism. *N Engl J Med* 1977;297:1022–1028.
97. Shores J, Berger K, Murphy E, Pyeritz R. Progression of aortic dilatation and the benefit of long-term beta-adrenergic blockade in Marfan's syndrome. *N Engl J Med* 1994;330:1335–1341.
98. Shprintzen R, Goldberg R. Dysmorphic facies, omphalocele, laryngeal and pharyngeal hypoplasia, spinal anomalies, and learning disabilities in a new dominant malformation syndrome. *Birth Defects Orig Art Ser* 1979;XV(5B):347–353.
99. Silverman D, Burton K, Gray J, Bosner M, Kouchokos N, Roman M, et al. Life expectancy in the Marfan syndrome. *Am J Cardiol* 1995;75:157–160.
100. Slot H, Overweg-Plandsoen W, Bakker H, Abeling N, Tamminga P, Barth P, et al. Molybdenum-cofactor deficiency: An easily missed cause of neonatal convulsions. *Neuropediatrics* 1993;24:139–142.
101. Smith T, Holland M, Woody N. Ocular manifestations of familial hyperlysinemia. *Trans Am Acad Ophthalmol Otolaryngol* 1971;75:355–360.
102. Sood S, Eldadah ZA, Krause WL, McIntosh

I, Dietz HC. Mutation in fibrillin-1 and the Marfanoid-craniosynostosis (Shprintzen-Goldberg) syndrome. *Nature Genet* 1996;12: 209–211.

103. Spaeth G, Barber G. Prevalence of homocystinuria among the mentally retarded: Evaluation of a specific screening test. *Pediatrics* 1967;40:586–589.
104. Sponseller P, Hobbs W, Riley L, Pyeritz R. The thoracolumbar spine in Marfan syndrome. *J Bone Joint Surg* 1995;77-A:867–876.
105. Streeten B, Licari P, Marucci A, Dougherty R. Immunohistochemical comparison of ocular zonules and the microfibrils of elastic tissue. *Invest Ophthalmol Visual Sci* 1981;21: 130–135.
106. Temtamy S, Salam M, Aboul-Ezz E, Hussein H, Helmy S, Shalash B. New autosomal recessive multiple congenital abnormalities/mental retardation syndrome with craniofacial dysmorphism, absent corpus callosum, iris colobomas and connective tissue dysplasia. *Clin Dysmorphol* 1996;5:231–240.
107. Tsipouras P, Del Mastro R, Sarfarazi M, Lee B, Vitale E, Child AH, et al. Genetic linkage of the Marfan syndrome, ectopia lentis, and congenital contractural arachnodactyly to the fibrillin genes on chromosomes 15 and 5. The International Marfan Syndrome Collaborative Study. *N Engl J Med* 1992; 326:905–909.
108. Tsipouras P, Sarfarazi M, Devi A, Weiffenbach B, Boxer M. Marfan syndrome is closely linked to a marker on chromosome 15q1.5-q2.1. *Proc Natl Acad Sci USA* 1991;88:4486–4488.
109. van der Klei-van Moorsel J, Smit L, Brockstedt M, Jakobs C, Dorche C, Duran M. Infantile isolated sulphite oxidase deficiency: Report of a case with negative sulphite test and normal sulphate excretion. *Eur J Pediatr* 1991;150: 196–197.
110. Vianey-Liaud C, Desjacques P, Gaulme J, Dorche C, Vanliefringhe P, Dechelotte P, et al. A new case of isolated sulphite oxidase deficiency with rapid fatal outcome. *J Inherit Metab Dis* 1988;11:425–426.
111. Wachtel J. The ocular pathology of Marfan's syndrome. *Arch Ophthalmol* 1966;76: 512–522.
112. Wadman S, Cats B, de Bree P. Sulfite oxidase deficiency and the detection of urinary sulfite (letter). *Eur J Pediatr* 1983;141:62–63.
113. Wallace R, Streeten B, Hanna R. Rotary shadowing of elastic system microfibrils in the ocular zonule, vitreous, and ligamentum nuchae. *Curr Eye Res* 1991;10:99–109.
114. Wang M, Price C, Han J, Cisler J, Imaizumi K, Van Thienen MN, et al. Recurrent missplicing of fibrillin exon 32 in two patients with neonatal Marfan syndrome. *Hum Mol Genet* 1995;4:607–613.
115. Weill G. Ectopie des crystallines et malformations generales. *Ann Ocul* 1932:169:21–44.
116. Wheatley HM, Traboulsi EI, Flowers BE, Maumenee IH, Azar D, Pyeritz RE, et al. Immunohistochemical localization of fibrillin in human ocular tissues. Relevance to the Marfan syndrome. *Arch Ophthalmol* 1995;113: 103–109.
117. Willi M, Kut L, Cotlier E. Pupillary block glaucoma in the Marchesani syndrome. *Arch Ophthalmol* 1973;90:504–508.
118. Winterpacht A, Superti-Furga A, Schwarze U, Stoss H, Steinmann B, Spranger J, et al. The deletion of six amino acids at the C-terminus of the alpha 1(II) chain causes overmodification of type II and type XI collagen: Further evidence for the association between small deletions in COL2A1 and Kniest dysplasia. *J Med Genet* 1996;33:649–654.

118a. Wirtz MK, Samples JR, Kramer PL, et al. Weill-Marchesani syndrome—Possible linkage of the autosomal dominant form to 15q21.1. *Am J Med Genet* 1996;65:68–75.

119. Wright K, Chrousos G. Weill-Marchesani syndrome with bilateral angle closure glaucoma. *J Pediatr Ophthalmol Strabismus* 1985;22: 129–132.

32

Pigmentary Retinopathy and Systemic Disease

ELIAS I. TRABOULSI
ARLENE V. DRACK
HESHAM SALAMA

Pigmentary retinopathy refers to the migration and proliferation of retinal pigment epithelial cells into the retina of patients with degenerative, infectious, or systemic diseases. Pigmentary retinopathy mimics retinitis pigmentosa because of the presence of retinal dystrophic and pigmentary changes and the frequent occurrence of night blindness, reduction of visual acuity, constriction of visual fields, and abnormal electroretinographic findings. Hence, pigmentary retinopathy is the final common outcome of many retinal and chorioretinal disorders and one manifestation of numerous metabolic and neurodegenerative diseases.

The evaluation of patients with a pigmentary retinopathy is a special challenge. The same fundus picture may represent a primary ocular process, a harbinger of neurologic degeneration, a remote effect of cancer, or just one feature in a constellation of signs comprising a genetic syndrome. The work-up of the patient with a pigmentary retinopathy should include the meticulous extraction of the history of onset and course of ocular symptoms, as well as a complete review of systems with special emphasis on signs and symptoms that may indicate disease processes known to be associated with retinal degeneration. A detailed family history of blinding conditions is essential to rule out primary retinal degenerations such as retinitis pigmentosa, choroideremia, or juvenile macular degeneration. A general physical examination should be performed by a pediatrician, internist, or clinical geneticist in search of physical findings that would clinch a systemic diagnosis. The electroretinogram (ERG) may detect retinal dysfunction before the occurrence of pigmentary alterations in the retina, but is rarely diagnostic. Biochemical, metabolic and DNA tests, neurologic imaging, and referral to the appropriate specialists must be obtained as needed.

The etiology of retinitis pigmentosa (RP) is being unraveled through the discovery of mutations in genes coding for molecules involved in the phototransduction cascade and other retinal cellular functions. Retinitis pigmentosa and the primary retinal dystrophies are discussed elsewhere in this text (see chapters 17–25). In secondary pigmentary retinopathies where an underlying systemic abnormality is known, we have the unique opportunity to study the effect of various metabolic defects on the retina.

Table 32.1. Systemic Syndromes Associated with Pigmentary Retinopathy

Disorders of Amino Acid, Protein, and Lipoprotein Metabolism	Friedreich ataxia
Gyrate atrophy of the choroid and retina	Retinitis pigmentosa with pallidal degeneration
Cystinosis	Saldino-Mainzer syndrome
Cobalamin-C defects (methylmalonic aciduria with homocystinuria)	Charcot-Marie-Tooth disease
Abetalipoproteinemia (Bassen-Kornzweig syndrome)	Marinesco-Sjögren syndrome
Hypobetalipoproteinemia	Joubert syndrome
Lysosomal Storage Diseases	***Dermatologic Disorders***
Mucopolysaccharidoses I-H (Hurler); I-S (Scheie); I-HS (Hurler-Scheie compound); III A and B (Sanfilippo)	Darier disease
Peroxisomal Disorders	Incontinentia pigmenti (Bloch-Sulzberger disease)
Cerebro-hepato-renal syndrome (Zellweger syndrome)	Rud syndrome
Neonatal adrenoleukodystrophy	Sjögren-Larsson syndrome (fatty alcohol oxidoreductase deficiency)
Infantile Refsum disease	***Renal Disease***
Acylcoenzyme oxidase deficiency	Renal-retinal dysplasia (Senior-Loken syndrome)
Peroxisomal thiolase deficiency	Hereditary hemorrhagic nephritis (Alport syndrome)
Primary hyperoxaluria	***Skeletal Anomalies/Dwarfism***
Neurologic Disorders	Asphyxiating thoracic dystrophy (Jeune syndrome)
Neuronal ceroid lipofuscinoses	Cockayne syndrome
Olivopontocerebellar atrophy with retinal degeneration (spinocerebellar ataxia type II)	Osteopetrosis
Kearns-Sayre syndrome	***Other Multisystem Disorders***
Myotonic dystrophy	Bardet-Biedl syndrome
Hallervorden-Spatz syndrome	Cohen syndrome
	Retinitis Pigmentosa and Deafness
	Usher syndrome
	Flynn-Aird syndrome
	Alstrom syndrome

This chapter covers some of the diseases that are associated with a pigmentary retinopathy (Table 32.1); others are discussed elsewhere in this text.

GYRATE ATROPHY OF THE CHOROID AND RETINA

Gyrate atrophy is an autosomal recessive disease caused by a deficiency of the enzyme ornithine aminotransferase (OAT). This defect results in hyperornithinemia.[101,169] The gene was mapped to 10q and was later cloned.[135] A number of mutations and deletions have been described.[83,134,188]

Patients with hyperornithinemia and gyrate atrophy present in the first decade of life with progressive myopia, night blindness, enlarging and coalescing chorioretinal atrophic lesions, and peripheral visual field loss.[96] Blindness ensues by age 40 to 50 years in most untreated patients.[179] There are no systemic abnormalities except for mild proximal muscle weakness and

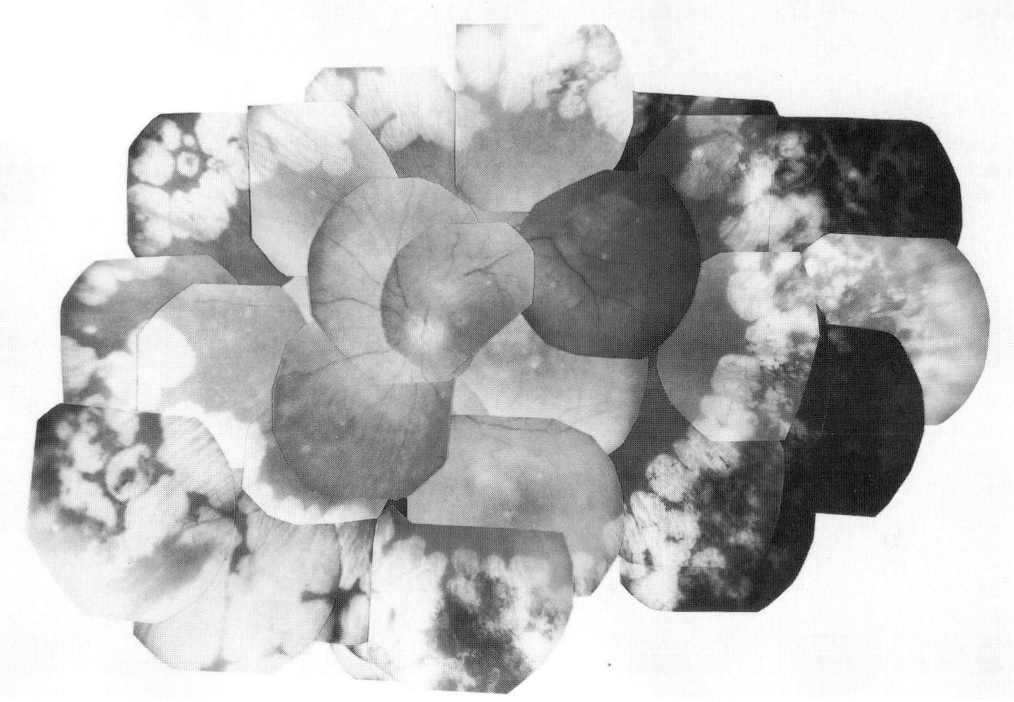

Figure 32.1. Collage of fundus photograph shows peripheral scalloped lesions characteristic of gyrate atrophy. (Courtesy of Drs. Irene Maumenee and Linn Murphree.)

fine sparse hair in a minority of patients.[94] Abnormalities in mitochondria and type 2 muscle fibers are present in biopsies from most patients.[170] About one-third of patients have slow waves on electroencephalography.[178]

The fundus appearance of gyrate atrophy is characteristic (Fig. 32.1). Small, geographic, round or oval areas of choroidal and retinal atrophy appear in the peripheral fundus around the age of 5 years; these areas enlarge and coalesce, giving the fundus an appearance similar to cerebral gyri, hence the descriptive name (Fig. 32.2). Peripapillary lesions may be present, but the optic disc remains pink and healthy. The atrophic areas may be separated from adjacent normal appearing retina by hyperpigmentation, and crystals have been reported at the margins of the atrophic areas.[94] Posterior subcapsular cataracts appear by the second or third decade of life and require surgery.[95] The electroretinogram (ERG) is decreased late in the course of the disease but before the atrophy becomes complete. Fluorescein angiography shows hyperfluorescence in atrophic areas with staining at the edges of normal-appearing retina. Wilson and co-workers described the ocular histopathologic findings in a 98-year-old patient with vitamin B6–responsive mild disease.[202] There were areas of atrophy of the retina that were adjacent to areas of normal retina. There were also focal areas of photoreceptor

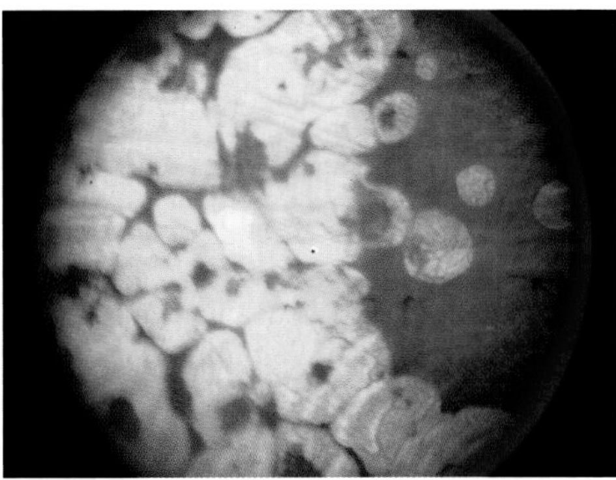

Figure 32.2. Peripheral fundus in a 10-year-old patient with gyrate atrophy. Round lesions enlarge and become confluent, forming gyrate pattern.

atrophy. Photoreceptor mitochondria were swollen. Mitochondrial abnormalities were also present in corneal epithelium and nonpigmented ciliary epithelium.

A diet restricted in arginine (a precursor of ornithine) has been shown to reduce plasma ornithine levels into the normal range[189] and may halt the progression of the retinopathy in some cases.[92] Proline supplementation has also been postulated to slow the retinopathy.[176] Plasma levels of ornithine can be reduced by about 50% in some patients with gyrate atrophy when they are treated with pharmacological (500–1000 mg/day) doses of pyridoxine.[196] This reduction, however, does not significantly slow the progression of the retinopathy.

Gyrate atrophy should be differentiated from pathologic high myopia in which very high myopia(usually greater than 10 diopters) is present from infancy or very early childhood, ERG is normal or mildly depressed, and atrophic round or oval areas appear in the posterior pole only. This disorder is usually autosomal recessive.

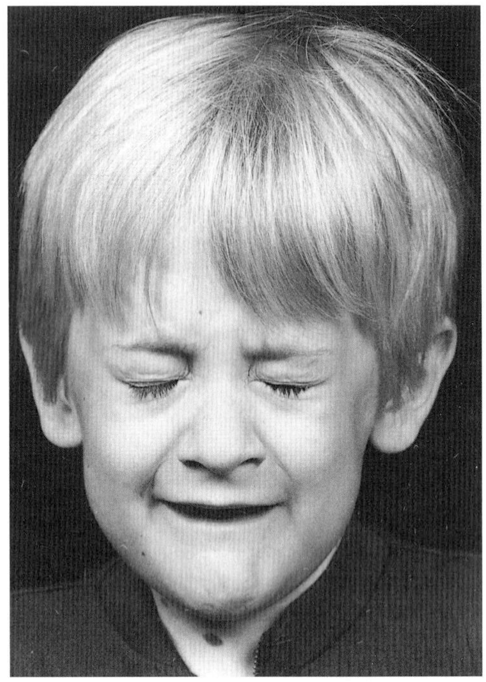

Figure 32.3. Nine-year-old boy with cystinosis. He is short and markedly photophobic. He does not have rickets but is hypothyroidic. (Courtesy of Drs. Irene Maumenee and Linn Murphree.)

CYSTINOSIS

There are three clinical forms of cystinosis: *(1)* the most common, an early infantile nephronopathic form in which patients present at 8 to 12 months of age with polydypsia, polyuria, recurrent fever, acidosis, and rickets. Renal failure occurs in the first decade of life and frequently necessitates kidney transplantation; *(2)* a less common, late-onset form where renal failure does not occur until the second or third decade; and *(3)* a benign form in which retinopathy and renal failure do not occur.[124] The infantile and juvenile forms are allelic and map to 17p.[88,130] Cystinosis occurs in about 1/100,000 to 1/200,000 individuals except in Brittany, France, where its incidence is 1/26,000.[17]

The infantile nephronopathic type of cystinosis is an autosomal recessive lysosomal storage disease characterized by progressive renal failure, retinopathy, growth retardation (Fig. 32.3), and deposition of cystine crystals in body tissues leading to organ failure.[60] Endocrine gland dysfunction leads to hypothyroidism and diabetes mellitus. Dysphagia and neurologic changes have also been reported. A lysosomal defect probably prevents the transport of cystine from lysosomes into the cytosol and crystals form inside these organelles.[203] Plasma levels of cystine are below saturation, indicating a cellular defect of cystine transport. Cystinosis is diagnosed by the presence of crystals in biopsy material and by an 80–100-fold increase in free cystine in peripheral leukocytes or cultured skin fibroblasts.

Cystine crystals deposit in the cornea and other ocular tissues. The corneal crystals are best detected by slit-lamp examination (Fig. 32.4). Patients are very photophobic (Fig. 32.3),[104] and some develop recurrent corneal erosions. Retinal pigmentary changes initially appear in the periphery of the fundus and progress to involve the macula.[204] There are mottled areas of depigmentation and pigment clumping with or without yellowish macular

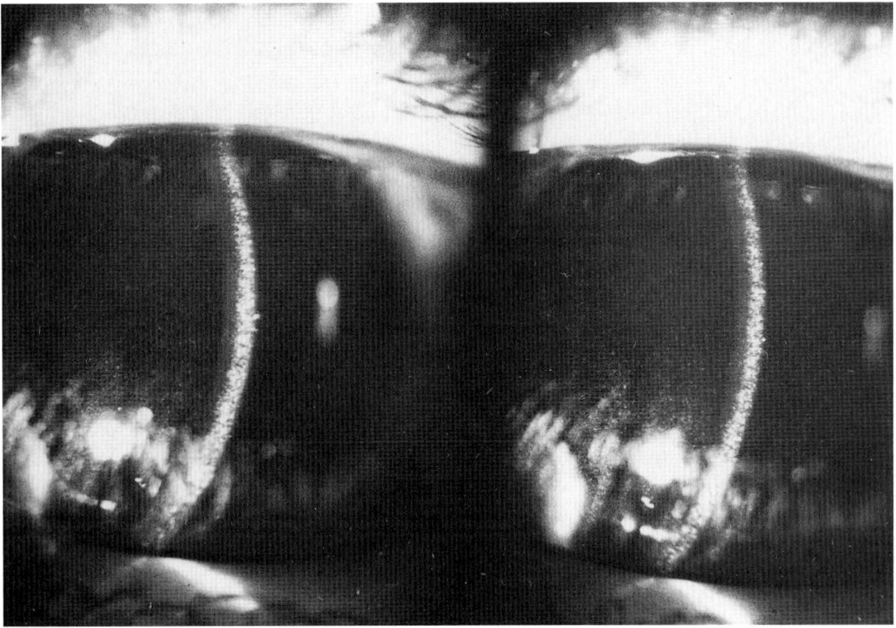

Figure 32.4. Views of the cornea under wide and narrow slit beam. These are advanced cases of cystinosis and the corneal crystals are present in the full thickness of the cornea centrally and peripherally. (Courtesy of Drs. Irene Maumenee and Linn Murphree.)

changes. Retinal changes may precede the appearance of corneal crystals. The retinopathy is more common in the infantile nephronopathic form and was present in all patients with the infantile form by age 7 years in one long-term study.[46] Tests of visual function are generally normal. The ERG may, however, decrease in amplitude with time.[46]

The secondary metabolic and hormonal abnormalities in cystinosis are treated as necessary.[58,199] Renal transplantation is usually required in the nephronopathic varieties. The systemic administration of cysteamine has been beneficial in a large number of patients.[59] In a series of 76 children with cystinosis treated with cysteamine at the National Institutes of Health, Markello and co-workers found that patients who were treated early and adequately have renal function that increases during the first 5 years of life and then declines at a normal rate.[129] These authors further showed that patients who do not comply with the treatment regimen and those who are treated at a later age have poor outcomes. Cysteamine has also been used topically on the cornea of two patients with reduction in the number of corneal crystals and improvement of corneal clarity after several months of therapy.[93]

METHYLMALONIC ACIDURIA WITH HOMOCYSTINURIA

Methylmalonic aciduria with homocystinuria results from at least three autosomal recessive disorders of cobalamin transport and metabolism.[54] Patients usually present in the first few months of life with failure to thrive, developmental delay, seizures, and megaloblastic anemia. Others are diagnosed later in childhood following the appearance of fatigue and neurologic symptoms.

Methylmalonic aciduria with homocystinuria is due to an abnormality of cobalamin metabolism (possibly a defect of cytosolic cobalamin reductase) that leads to deficient activity of L-methylmalonyl CoA mutase and *N*-methyltetrahydrofolate : homocysteine methyltrans-

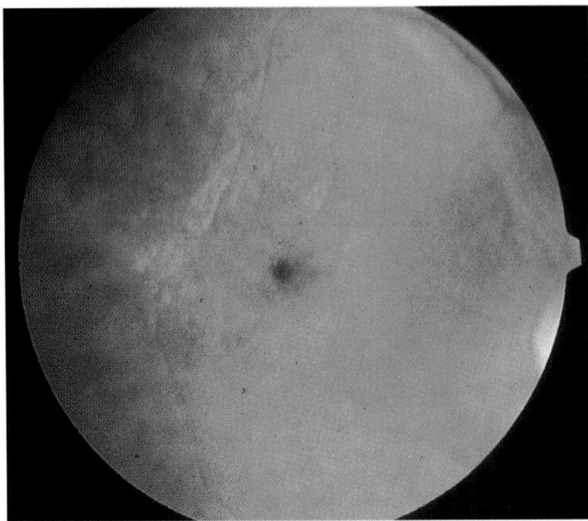

Figure 32.5. Macular pigmentary changes in a patient with methylmalonic aciduria with homocystinuria. (Courtesy of Dr. Irene Maumenee.)

ferase. This results in elevated levels of homocysteine and methylmalonic acid in the urine, and in reduced levels of methionine in serum.

Patients develop fine pigmentary changes in the retinal periphery and/or a granular or bull's-eye maculopathy (Fig. 32.5).[27,152] Nystagmus, optic nerve pallor, attenuated retinal vessels, and strabismus can occur. The ERG is attenuated early in the course of the disease and there is retinal degeneration (Fig. 32.6).[183]

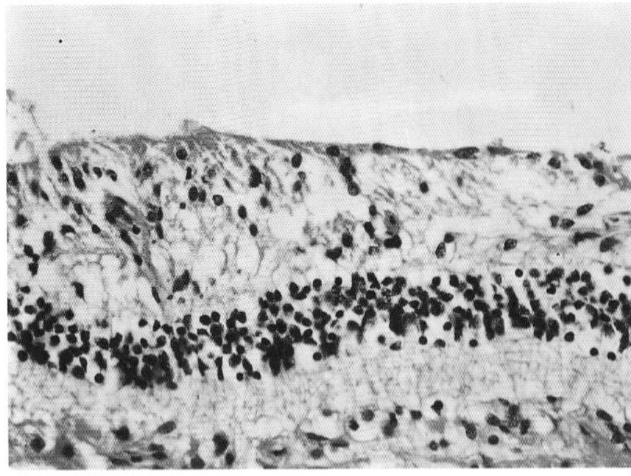

Figure 32.6. Retinal degeneration in a patient with methylmalonic aciduria and homocystinuria. The photoreceptor outer segments are atrophic and there is disorganization and paucity of inner segments. (H&E; original magnification ×100.) (Courtesy of Dr. W. R. Green.)

Early treatment with very large doses (up to 1 mg IM daily) of hydroxycobalamin with or without betaine improves the biochemical profiles and possibly the outcome of some patients.[10] There is evidence that metronidazole may be helpful in reducing gut flora that produce propionic acid, which in turn is metabolized to methylmalonic acid.[8]

ABETALIPOPROTEINEMIA (BASSEN-KORNZWEIG DISEASE)

Abetalipoproteinemia is a rare autosomal recessive disorder[11] that was initially described in Ashkenazi Jews. Subsequent cases have been reported in other ethnic groups as well.[65] The disease results from a defect in microsomal triglyceride transfer protein.[166,197]

Patients have a characteristic "burr-cell" malformation of the red blood cells called *acanthocytosis*. They also develop a celiac syndrome of mild fat malabsorption and steatorrhea, progressive ataxic neuropathy, and abnormal levels of plasma lipids with total absence of beta lipoproteins and chylomicra and very low cholesterol. All major plasma lipids are reduced to less than 50% of normal levels. The deficiency in chylomicra prevents the absorption of fat-soluble vitamins from the intestine leading to low serum levels of vitamins A and E.[155,159]

The main ocular manifestation of abetalipoproteinemia is an atypical pigmentary retinopathy that usually develops in the early teens but that may present at any age. Patients are night blind and have fundus changes similar to retinitis pigmentosa (RP) in some and to retinitis punctata albescens in others.[66,111] Rod and cone dysfunction is evident on electroretinography and dark adaptation thresholds may be elevated before the appearance of ophthalmoscopic changes.[113] The macula may or may not be affected. The low serum levels of the fat-soluble vitamins A and E may account for the pigmentary retinopathy.[111,155] Vitamin A supplementation has been reported to have beneficial retinal effects[66] and there is evidence that oral vitamin E therapy improves the neuropathy and slows down or prevents the retinopathy.[137,159]

THE MUCOPOLYSACCHARIDOSES

Six main types and 16 subtypes of mucopolysaccharidosis have been described. Facial and bony changes, variable mental retardation, mucopolysaccharides in the urine, corneal clouding, and retinal degeneration are features. Pigmentary retinopathy and retinal degeneration only occur in mucopolysaccharidoses where there is storage of heparan sulfate. These types are discussed in detail in this chapter. The salient systemic and ocular characteristics of the other types of MPS are presented in Table 32.2.

The nomenclature can be confusing; Roman

Table 32.2. Ocular and Systemic Findings in the Mucopolysaccharidoses

Disease	Systemic Findings	Glaucoma	Corneal Clouding	Retinal Degeneration	Optic Nerve Swelling	Optic Atrophy	Enzyme Defect
MPS IH Hurler	AR Severe dysostosis multiplex; coarse facies; cardiac disease; psychomotor delay; early death	+	+++ By 6 months	+++	+	+++	α-L-Iduronidase
MPS IS Scheie	AR, allelic with MPS I-H; mild systemic findings; normal life span	+	+++ By 1 to 2 years	++ Late finding	+		α-L-Iduronidase
MPS IH/S Hurler-Scheie compound	AR; compound heterozygote for MPS I-H and MPS I-S; systemic findings of intermediate severity	+	+++ By 1 to 2 years	+++	+		α-L-Iduronidase
MPS II Hunter	XR, one mild and one severe form; Variable severity of systemic features depending on subtype; skin pebbling	+	−	+/−	++	++	Iduronate sulfatase
MPS III Sanfilippo	AR; four types A–D; hyperactivity in preschool years; deterioration of psychomotor functions; mild coarse dysmorphic features	−	+ Mild	++	+/−	+/−	A: Heparan sulfate sulfatase B: *N*-acetyl-α-D-glucosaminidase C: Acetyl coenzyme A: α-glucosaminide *N*-acetyltransferase D: *N*-acetylglucosamine 6-sulfatase

(continued)

Table 32.2. Ocular and Systemic Findings in the Mucopolysaccharidoses—Continued

Disease	Systemic Findings	Glaucoma	Corneal Clouding	Retinal Degeneration	Optic Nerve Swelling	Optic Atrophy	Enzyme Defect
MPS IV Morquio	AR; severe type A and milder type B; short trunk dwarfism; kyphoscoliosis with vertebral defects; and spinal compression	−	+++ By age 10 years	−	−	−	A: Galactose 6-sulfatase B: β-Galactosidase
MPS VI Maroteaux-Lamy	AR; one mild and one severe form; systemic features similar to MPS IH; normal intelligence	++	+++ After age 5 years with peripheral vascularization	−	++	++	Arylsulfatase B
MPS VII Sly	AR; severe, mild and intermediate forms; Hurler-like findings in severe form	−	++ In severe form	−	+	−	β-Glucuronidase

AR = autosomal recessive; MPS = mucopolysaccharidoses; XR = X-linked recessive; −, +/−, +, ++, and +++ indicate increasing degrees of frequency of the individual clinical findings ranging from absent (−) to uniform (+++).

numerals after the initials MPS divide the groups into I (iduronase deficient), II (iduronase sulfate sulfatase deficient), III (subdivided into A–D, depending on enzyme deficiency), IV (galactosamine-6-sulfatase deficient in subtype A; β-galactosidase, in B), VI (*N*-acetylgalactosamine-4-sulfatase deficient), and VII (β-glucuronidase deficient). There is no group V. The group I disorders are further subdivided by adding the letters H, S, or H/S, referring to the historical eponyms. Disorders that include retinal degeneration are MPS-IH, MPS-IS, MPS-II, MPS-III, and MPS-VI. MPS-IV patients have cloudy corneas but no retinal degeneration and normal intelligence. MPS-II and III patients rarely have cloudy corneas.

Hurler Syndrome

Hurler syndrome is the prototype of the mucopolysaccharidoses. This autosomal recessive disorder occurs in about 1 : 100,000 individuals. Approximately 30 new patients are born annually in the United States. The carrier frequency is 1 in 160 persons. The disease results from absence of the activity of the lysosomal enzyme alpha-L-iduronidase. This renders cells incapable of cleaving iduronic acid residues in polysaccharide chains. Both heparan sulfate and dermatan sulfate contain the residue and cannot be degraded. As a result, heparan and dermatan sulfate are excreted in the urine and stored in tissues.

The clinical manifestations start in infancy, but patients appear normal at birth. Development is normal in the first few months of life, but progressive mental and physical deterioration follow. Photophobia, corneal clouding, a coarse facial appearance, stiff joints, chest deformity, rhinitis, or visceromegaly prompt the initial medical consultation. Short stature and typical skeletal changes become apparent by 2

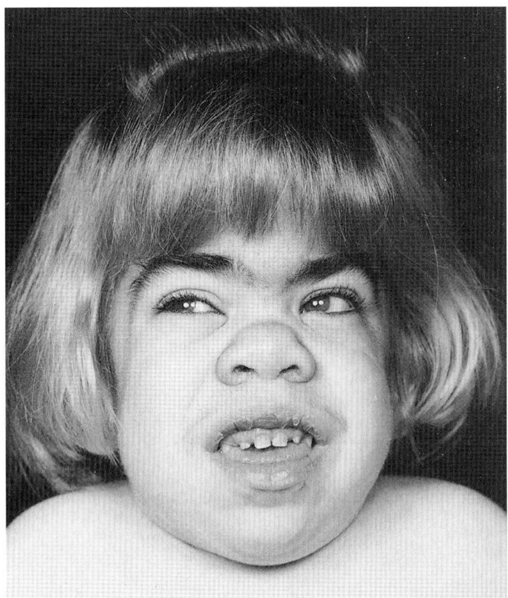

Figure 32.7. Four-year-old girl with Hurler's syndrome (MPS-IH). She is short with coarse features, limitation of joint mobility, umbilical hernias, hepatosplenomegaly, and corneal clouding. She died 6 months later from cardiopulmonary failure. MPS = mucopolysaccharidosis. (Courtesy of Drs. Irene Maumenee and Linn Murphree.)

to 3 years of age (Fig. 32.7). The liver and spleen enlarge, increasing abdominal girth. Death usually occurs before the age of 10 years from pulmonary infections or cardiac failure secondary to mucopolysaccharide deposition in the aortic or mitral valves, the intima of the coronary arteries, or the myocardium. Mental deterioration is evident after 1 year of age and hydrocephalus is a frequent finding. Other clinical features include deafness, a short neck, and wide-spaced teeth with hypertrophy of the gums. The reduced range of joint motion is especially striking in the fingers, resulting in a claw-hand deformity.

Corneal opacification appears early in life and is slowly progressive (Fig. 32.8). The accumulation of cytoplasmic and extracellular mucopolysaccharide is the cause of the ground-glass clouding of the cornea.[31,103] Numerous massively swollen histiocytes give the cornea the appearance of hypercellularity on light microscopy. Intralysosomal inclusions in the form of single-membrane–bound vacuoles are detected using electron microscopy. The ERG is abolished by age 5 or 6 years.[120] Papilledema and/or optic atrophy may be present along with a pigmentary retinopathy.[36] Chan et al. showed storage of mucopolysaccharides in all parts of the eye[31]; these authors postulated that the optic atrophy is due to both descending degeneration from hydrocephalus and to accumulation of storage material in the ganglion cells.[31] An alternative mechanism was proposed by Collins and co-workers, who attributed the papilledema, at least in part, to the compression of the optic nerve fibers at their exit from the globe by a thickened posterior sclera (Fig. 32.9).[36] These authors also showed that optic atrophy may follow papilledema and may hence be partially due to chronic optic nerve compression. The orbits of patients with Hurler syndrome are shallow as a result of premature closure of cranial sutures; proptosis may ensue. Glaucoma may occur and is presumed to result from accumulation of mucopolysaccharides in the trabecular meshwork.

The diagnosis of Hurler syndrome is based on the presence of the clinical signs, mucopolysacchariduria (heparan sulfate and dermatan sulfate), and on demonstration of deficient alpha-L-iduronidase in leukocytes or cultured fibroblasts.

MPS-I (Hurler syndrome) should be differentiated from mucolipidosis-II (I-cell disease—*vide infra*), in which patients, although clinically similar to those affected with MPS-I, have abnormalities at birth, whereas the clinical

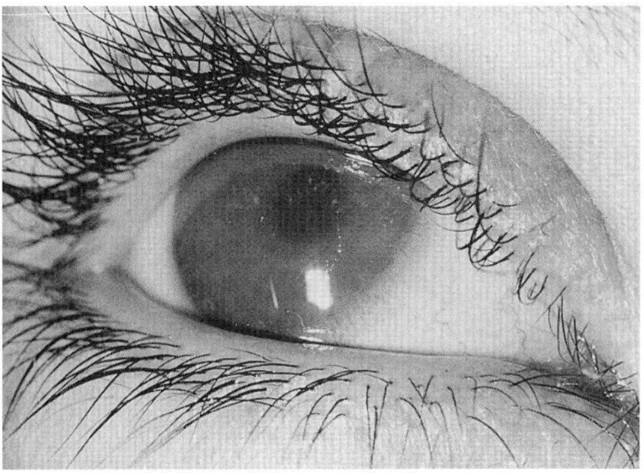

Figure 32.8. Corneal clouding in patient with MPS-IH shown in figure. MPS = mucopolysaccharidosis. (Courtesy of Drs. Irene Maumenee and Linn Murphree.)

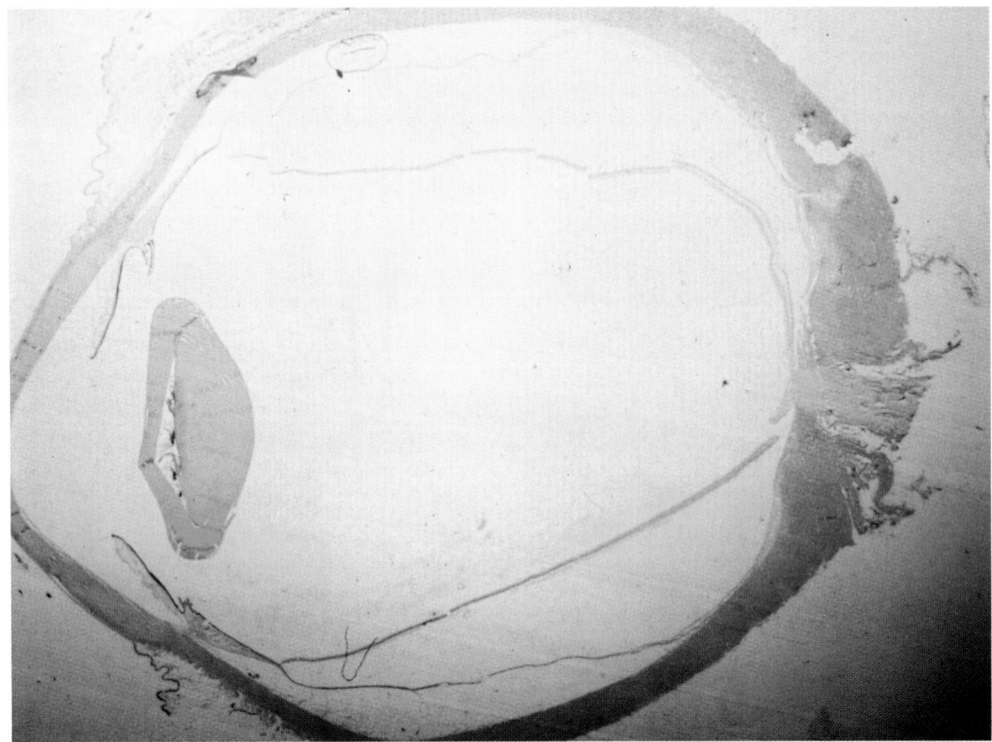

Figure 32.9. Histologic section of the eye of a patient with mucopolysaccharidosis reveals thickening of the sclera because of accumulation of mucopolysaccharides. The process is most marked posteriorly and presumably leads to compression of the optic nerve axons, papilledema, and optic atrophy (Used with permission from K. R. Kenyon, Ocular pathology of the Maroteaux-Lamy syndrome [systemic mucopolysaccharidosis type VI] *Am J Ophthalmol* 73:718–741, 1972.)

features of Hurler syndrome develop concurrently with progressive accumulation of storage material, and the child with MPS-I appears normal at birth. Hurler syndrome is also differentiated from MPS-II (Hunter syndrome) by the absence of corneal clouding in the latter disorder. Patients with mucolipidosis III (pseudo-Hurler polydystrophy) are less severely affected, with mild corneal clouding and pigmentary retinopathy. Mannisodosis, multiple sulfatase deficiency, fucosidosis, asparthylglycosaminuria, and the GM1 (monosialoganglioside) gangliosidosis must all be considered in the differential diagnosis of Hurler syndrome because of clinical similarities.

Bone marrow transplantation can improve the somatic features of MPS-IH. Following transplantation, serum and leukocyte levels of alpha-L-iduronidase and urinary excretion of glycosaminoglycans are normalized, and hepatomegaly is decreased. The skeletal abnormalities are not reversed but long bone growth continues. Facial dysmorphism is improved and hydrocephalus does not develop. Hearing, vision, joint motility, and cardiac and respiratory functions are all improved.[138] Corneal transplantation is not recommended because of limited life span, concurrent retinal degeneration, the difficulty in maintaining a clear graft in a child, and the potentially serious anesthesia problems that patients with MPS-IH may develop due to upper airway obstruction and excessive secretions.

MPS-IS (Scheie Syndrome)

MPS-IS (Scheie syndrome) laboratory findings are identical to those of MPS-IH. The difference between the two diseases is severity: hepatosplenomegaly, mental retardation, and dwarfism do not occur in MPS-IS. Facial features are less dysmorphic. Deafness, genu valgaum, and joint stiffness develop with increasing age, and aortic regurgitation and psychosis are occasional findings.[138] Corneal clouding and retinal dystrophy are present. Diagnostic techniques are the same as in MPS-IH; however, supportive treatment may be more successsful since patients often live to adulthood.

MPS-II (Hunter Syndrome)

Allelic mild and severe forms of Hunter syndrome result from mutations at the X-chromosomal locus for the enzyme iduronate sulfate sulfatase. Patients with the severe phenotype die prior to age 20 years. They share a lot of the clinical features with Hurler syndrome, but corneal clouding is absent and skeletal and mental changes are milder in Hunter syndrome. Patients with the mild form may survive beyond age 50; intelligence is normal and the skeletal involvement only moderate. Pebbling of the skin over the scapula, neck, chest, or thigh is a characteristic clinical finding in Hunter syndrome.[144]

Patients with Hunter syndrome have clear corneas. Pigmentary retinopathy with an extinguished ERG may lead to severe visual impairment in the severe phenotype or be more benign in the mild phenotype. Elevated and blurred disc margins have led to the diagnosis of chronic papilledema.[36] Long-standing papilledema may result in secondary optic atrophy and loss of vision, even in the mild phenotype. Retinal pigmentary degeneration has been documented histologically.[64]

The diagnosis of Hunter syndrome is based on the demonstration of deficient activity of alpha-L-sulfoiduronate sulfatase. Dermatan and heparan sulfate are present in the urine. Prognosis depends on the clinical type.

MSP-III (Sanfilippo Syndrome)

Four enzyme defects result in the single phenotype of Sanfilippo syndrome.[138] There is urinary excretion of heparitin sulfate. The accumulation of mucopolysaccharides is generalized, and although the somatic stigmata are mild, the central nervous system consequences are devastating. Patients are normal in appearance and development in infancy. Motor delay, intellectual deterioration, and behavioral problems become apparent by school age. There is rapid clinical deterioration, and if patients live to adulthood, they are bedridden and may have abnormal mentation. Deafness may also develop.

Corneal clouding does not occur in MPS-III, but there is a pigmentary retinopathy similar to that of Hurler and Scheie syndromes. Ocular histopathology in type IIIA has been reported by Del Monte et al.[43] and includes intracellular accumulation of fibrogranular and membraneous lamellar vacuoles in all ocular structures. Marked photoreceptor loss was noted.

MUCOLIPIDOSES

The mucolipidoses (ML) cause disease that resembles mucopolysaccharidoses and neurolipidoses, but without mucopolysaccharide excretion in urine. There are four types. Type I patients have corneal clouding and cherry red spot. Type II have retinal degeneration and resemble MPS-IH (Hurler syndrome). Type III have stiff joints, a more chronic course, and wrinkled or hazy retinas, which may be seen despite normal ERG. Mucolipidosis IV is the most important to ophthalmologists. It is an autosomal recessive disease that was originally described by Merin and co-workers in four Ashkenazi children of Southern Polish ancestry.[131] It has also been reported in non-Jewish families.[67] Patients with ML-IV develop normally in the first few months of life, but hypotonia, psychomotor retardation, corneal clouding, retinal degeneration, athetosis, and progressive motor and mental disability set in during infancy and early childhood (Fig. 32.10). There are no skeletal or visceral abnormalities and there is no cellular metachromasia or mucopolysacchariduria.[3] Progressive corneal epithelial clouding prevents visualization of the fundus (Fig. 32.11). Optic atrophy and retinal degeneration are present. Diagnosis is based on clinical findings and on the demonstration of two characteristic types of intracellular inclusions in conjunctival biopsies[102]: *(1)* single-membrane–bound cytoplasmic vacuoles con-

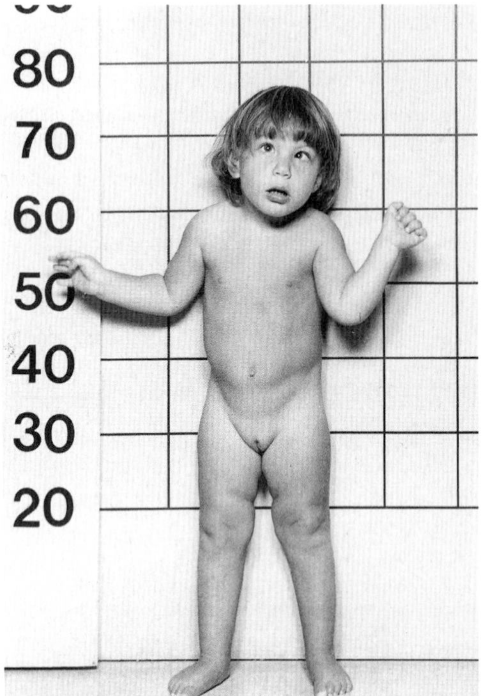

Figure 32.10. Two-year-old patient with a clinical diagnosis of mucolipidosis IV, confirmed by conjunctival biopsy (strabismus is not usually a feature of this disorder). (Courtesy of Drs. Irene Maumenee and Linn Murphree.)

taining fibrillogranular material and membranous lamellae and *(2)* lamellar and concentric bodies. Amir et al.[3] reviewed the clinical findings and natural history of the disease in 20 patients ranging in age from 2 to 17 years. The age at onset and severity of corneal opacification were variable. One patient had retinal degeneration but no corneal opacification at the age of 5 years while 11 patients had congenital corneal opacification.

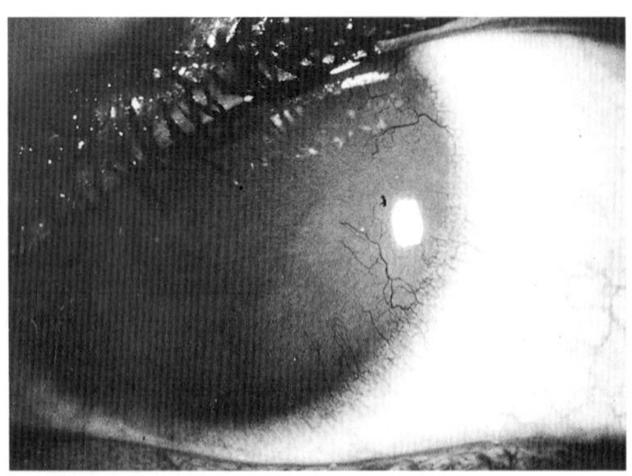

Figure 32.11. Superficial corneal opacification in an 18-year-old patient with mucolipidosis IV. (Courtesy of Drs. Irene Maumenee and Linn Murphree.)

The ocular histopathology was studied by Riedel et al. who found retinal degeneration and widespread intracellular inclusions.[151] Deficiency of ganglioside sialidase in ML-IV[7] has been refuted.[123] Folkerth and colleagues[56] found that the storage material in neurons differed from that in nonneural cells. The material in neural cells contained nonpolar lipids, whereas nonneural cells contained carbohydrates with vicinal glycol structures. Hepatocytes, kidney cells, and myocytes contained polar lipids. Because of the variability in storage materials, Folkerth and colleagues[56] suggested that ML-IV was not due to a single enzyme defect but rather to a defect in intracellular packaging or transport.

Corneal clarity can be achieved temporarily by removal of the corneal epithelium and by limbal conjunctival transplantation using donor tissue from unaffected siblings.[41] Patients may survive into early adulthood but may be profoundly retarded.[2]

Conjunctival biopsy is often helpful in diagnosis of the mucolipidoses.

PEROXISOMAL DISORDERS

Peroxisomal disorders are discussed in great detail by Weleber in Chapter 33.

THE NEURONAL CEROID LIPOFUSCINOSES

The term *neuronal ceroid lipofuscinoses* (NCL) was coined by Zeman and Dyken in 1969 to describe the storage of ceroid and lipofuscin in neuronal cells.[205] These autosomal recessive, progressively disabling, and uniformly fatal and blinding neurodegenerative diseases were previously grouped under the familial amaurotic idiocies (which include Tay-Sachs disease). These diseases have an overall incidence of 1 to 5 in 100,000 live births indicating carrier frequency of 1 in 150.[79,150] Juvenile NCL is probably the most common neurodegenerative disease of children, with an incidence of about 1 in 25,000 live births.

Six major clinical types of human NCL have been described, as well as variants thereof.[47] The six types differ in age of onset, clinical course, and neuropathologic findings (Table 32.3). Five types have their onset in infancy and childhood.[24,63] *(1)* Congenital NCL presents at birth[61,141]; *(2)* infantile NCL (INCL, Santavuori-Haltia disease) presents between 8 and 18 months with myoclonus, delayed development, and vision loss; *(3)* late infantile NCL (LINCL, Jansky-Bielchowsky disease) presents from 2 to 4 years of age with seizures, mental deterioration, and vision loss; *(4)* LINCL variant; and *(5)* juvenile NCL (JNCL, Batten disease, Spielmeyer-Vogt disease), which presents between 4 and 10 years of age with vision loss followed by neurologic disease. Adult NCL (Kufs disease)[14,39] will not be discussed in this chapter because of the absence of clinical ocular abnormalities. There are also atypical rare clinical forms of NCL that are difficult to classify.[147]

The NCLs are characterized by the accumulation of intracellular autofluorescent lipopigments in a number of cell types. Ultrastructurally, the characteristic intracellular granules have a curvilinear or fingerprint-like profile (Fig. 32.12). Electron-dense and lucent round granules are also present. Loss of cerebral neurons and of photoreceptor cells leads to severe neurologic and visual defects.[22,23,147] The storage material has been identified as subunit c of mitochondrial adenosine triphosphate (ATP) synthase in late infantile NCL (LINCL) and in juvenile NCL (JNCL).[109,142] Tyynela and coworkers[185] found the sphingolipid activator proteins saponins A and D to constitute a major

Table 32.3. Characteristics of Six Clinical Types of Neuronal Ceroid Lipofuscinosis (NCL)

Characteristic	Congenital NCL (CNCL)	Infantile NCL (Santavuori-Haltia) (INCL)	Late Infantile NCL (Jansky-Bielschowsky) (LINCL)	Variant of LINCL	Juvenile NCL (Spielmeyer-Vogt) (Batten) (JNCL)	Adult NCL (Kufs Disease)
Age of onset	Immediately after birth	First 2 years of life	2–4 yr	4–7 yr	4–10 yr	3rd, 4th decade
Visual loss	—	Relatively early	Late	Late	Early presenting symptom	None
Ataxia	—	Moderate	Marked	Marked	Marked, late finding	With type B (mild)
Seizures	Fulminant generalized convulsions	Constant	Constant	Constant	Mild	With type A (mild)
Gene locus	—	1p	Not allelic with INCL or JNCL	13q31-32	16p	—
Ultrastructure of storage material	Membrane-bound globular aggregates with amorphous internal structure	Granular amorphic profiles	Curvilinear profiles	Curvilinear or fingerprint or mixture of both	Fingerprint profiles	Curvilinear and/or multilaminated profiles
Age at death	24 h–7 wk	8–14 years	6–15 yr	Live longer than INCL	13–40 yr	Delayed

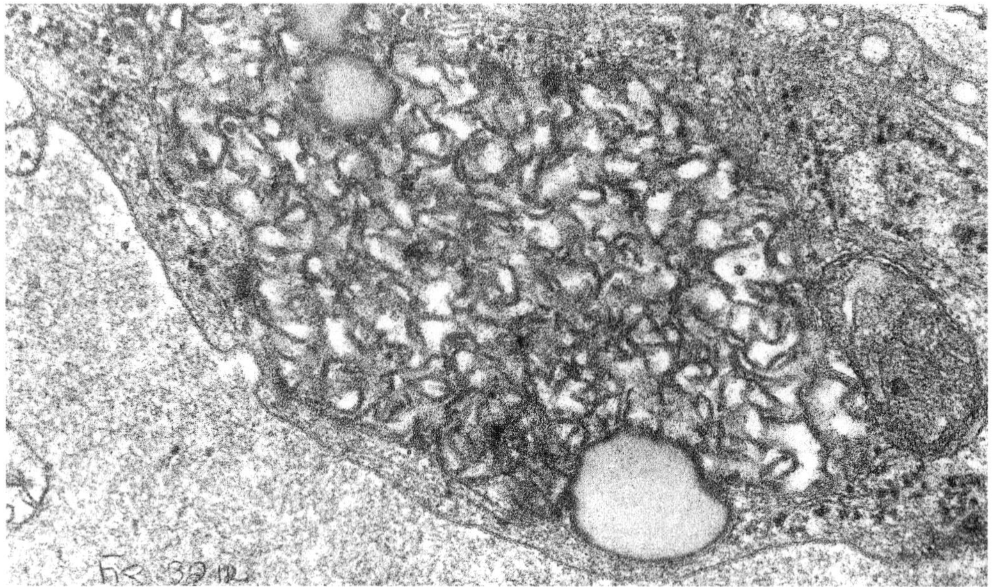

Figure 32.12. Electron micrograph of a conjunctival fibroblast from a patient with juvenile neuronal ceroid lipofuscinosis (Batten's disease) shows characteristic curvilinear profiles in a large inclusion body that also contains a few lipid granules. (Courtesy of Dr. W. R. Green.)

component of the proteins stored in infantile NCL (INCL).

In the infantile and late infantile forms of NCL, neurologic symptoms usually precede retinopathy and visual loss. Patients with juvenile NCL (Batten disease) present first to the ophthalmologist with complaints of decreased vision (Fig. 32.13). It may be difficult for the neurologist to differentiate the infantile form of NCL from Rett syndrome if patients have the hand stereotypies of the latter; the ophthalmologist may be able to make the correct diagnosis of INCL if retinal degeneration is present.[72] The clinical classification of the NCLs, which is based on the age at onset, clinical signs and symptoms, and type of intracellular inclusions, appears simple but raises problems with so-called variant forms.[161] The most important clinical differentiating criterion for classifying patients into specific subgroups of NCL is the pattern of the evolution of the disease and the magnitude of seizure activity, with the age of onset of the disease and the fine structure of the storage material being less important. A more accurate classification is based on chromosomal localization and analysis of responsible mutant genes, or one based on specific biochemical abnormalities. Animal models of NCL have been identified in the dog,[110] sheep,[89,90] cattle, and most recently in the mouse.[26,32,143]

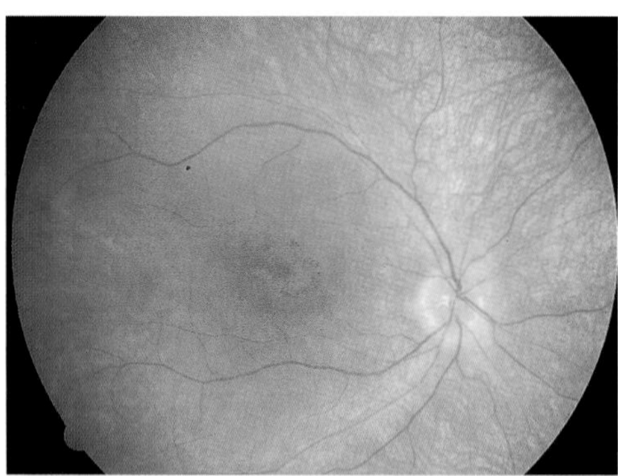

Figure 32.13. Retinal dystrophy with macular bull's-eye lesion in a child with juvenile neuronal ceroid lipofuscinosis. The patient presented with visual loss and was misdiagnosed with retinitis pigmentosa.

The ocular manifestations of the NCLs include night blindness, progressive loss of acuity and field of vision, retinal degeneration, and a reduced or unrecordable electroretinogram.[182] Patients with infantile NCL have optic atrophy, pigmentary changes in the macula and retinal periphery, and a reduced or absent ERG and VER[46]; cataracts have also been reported.[12] In the late infantile form there is a bull's-eye maculopathy, pigment mottling and granularity, optic atrophy, and attenuation of retinal blood vessels. Patients with the juvenile form have an absent macular reflex and occasionally a bull's-eye macular lesion (Fig. 32.14); peripheral retinal signs of degeneration are also present.[182]

We found that it takes an average of 3 years for JNCL patients who present with visual loss to develop neurologic symptoms (Salama, Naidu, Maumenee, and Traboulsi, unpublished data); it takes an average of 1 year for patients with LINCL and the variant form of LINCL to develop visual loss following the onset of neurologic symptoms. By 8 years, most patients with any type of NCL have lost vision completely and have developed neurologic signs and symptoms.

In the course of our examination of three patients with JNCL who have survived into their early twenties, we discovered two presumably late ocular manifestations of the disease. All three patients had cataracts (total cataracts in one, and cortical cataracts in two; Fig. 32.15); and one had corneal epithelial opacification in the form of cornea verticillata that progressed to diffuse epithelial involvement (Fig. 32.16). We presume that this is due to the storage of lipopigment in the corneal epithelium.

The diagnosis of NCL should be suspected in children with dementia, behavioral changes, psychomotor deterioration, ataxia, and seizures and, in the case of JNCL, in those who may present with visual loss from a retinal dystrophy before the onset of neurologic deterioration. A recent onset of nightmares combined with loss of scholastic skills or behavioral changes in a child with a retinal dystrophy should prompt an investigation for JNCL. Other metabolic disorders and post-infectious disorders such as subacute sclerosing panencephalitis should be ruled out, using the appropriate tests as deemed necessary based on clinical findings and differential diagnosis. Ophthalmoscopy

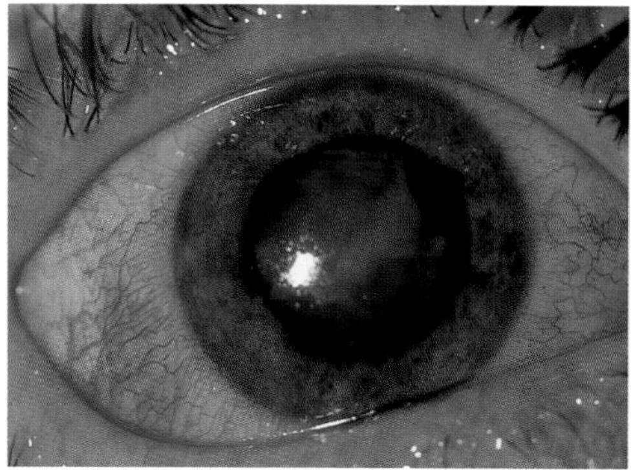

Figure 32.15. Cataract in an adult with juvenile neuronal ceroid lipofuscinosis.

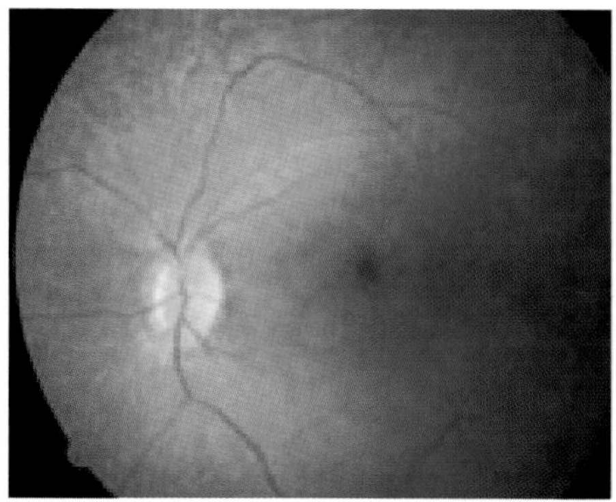

Figure 32.14. Retinal dystrophy in a child with neuronal ceroid lipofuscinosis. The optic nerve is pale, retinal vessels are attenuated, and there are fine pigmentary changes in the macula.

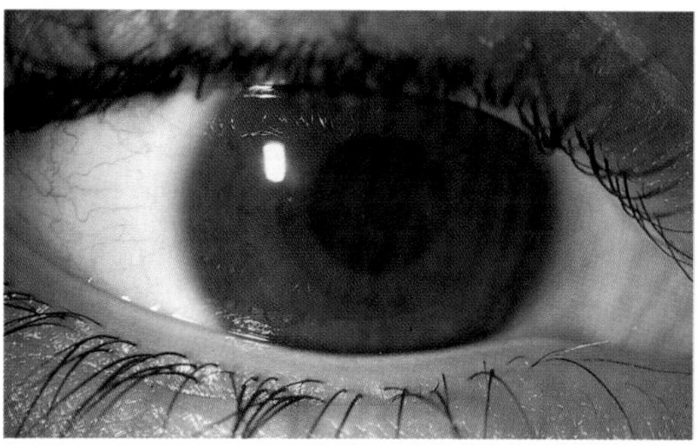

Figure 32.16. Corneal epithelial opacification in an adult with juvenile neuronal ceroid lipofuscinosis.

and electrophysiological testing are important to establish the presence of retinal degeneration. Neuroradiological imaging studies may show atrophic changes that appear early and progress rapidly and simultaneously in all areas of the central nervous system. The presence of white matter hypodense lesions in patients with advanced INCL is used to differentiate INCL from other clinical subtypes of NCL.[145] The diagnostic step in the investigation of patients with suspected NCL is the demonstration on electron microscopy of intracellular storage of lipopigments in biopsy specimens.[122] The presence of vacuolated lymphocytes in peripheral blood is a highly suggestive finding.[25] Lymphocytes may also be examined electron microscopically for the characteristic cytosomes found in all types of NCL. The most commonly biopsied sites are skin, conjunctiva, and rectal mucosa.[122] The conjunctiva is easily accessible and biopsies are obtained under topical anesthesia. Skin specimens offer the advantage of containing several types of tissues such as sweat glands, blood vessels, smooth muscle, and myelinated and nonmyelinated nerves with Schwann cells and fibrocytes. We have biopsied conjunctiva, skin, or rectal mucosa in our patients, and we find that all three tissues yield adequate diagnostic information if appropriately processed and interpreted by an experienced pathologist.

Eiberg et al.[48] presented initial evidence of linkage of JNCL to the haptoglobin locus on chromosome 16. This was confirmed by the studies of Callen and co-workers,[29] who mapped the gene to 16p12. The International Batten Disease Consortium reported the isolation of a candidate novel gene from the Batten disease region bound by markers D16S299 and D16S298.[38] The gene was disrupted by a 1 kb genomic deletion in all patients carrying the so-called 56 chromosome haplotype; two additional deletions and a point mutation were identified in three unrelated families. In studies of 15 Finnish families, Jarvela et al.[86] reported that INCL is not linked to chromosome 16 markers but maps to chromosome 1p. Using positional candidate gene methods, Vesa et al. identified defects in the palmitoyl protein thioesterase gene in all of their 42 Finnish patients and in several non-Finnish patients.[192] Locus heterogeneity between late infantile NCL and infantile and juvenile NCL has been demonstrated, providing evidence that classical LINCL is not an allelic form of the juvenile or infantile subtypes.[198] The locus of the variant form of LINCL was assigned to chromosome 13q31-23, demonstrating that at least four genetic loci are involved in the pathogenesis of human NCL.[163]

Prenatal diagnosis of NCL using electron microscopic search for the characteristic intracellular inclusions in chorionic villus samples has been performed successfully.[37,148] There is, however, a risk of sampling error involved in this technically very demanding analysis. Prenatal diagnosis can also be performed using linkage analysis of INCL and JNCL to several informative DNA markers.[85,187] With the current markers, the risk of error due to recombination is still 3%–5%, a rate acceptable to most families. A combination of DNA testing and electron microscope analysis of choroinic villus biopsy specimens is currently used in Finland.[78]

OLIVOPONTOCEREBELLAR ATROPHY WITH RETINAL DEGENERATION OR AUTOSOMAL DOMINANT CEREBELLAR ATAXIA TYPE II (OPCA TYPE III; ADCAII/SCAII)

Olivopontocerebellar atrophy (OPCA) is present in a heterogeneous group of neurodegenerative disorders.[75] One subtype, OPCA type III in the classification of Koenigsmark and Weiner,[108] is associated with retinal degeneration and is inherited in an autosomal dominant fashion with a significant degree of variability in severity of neurologic and ocular symptomatology and age of onset within and among families.[4,184] There is evidence of anticipation and higher rates of paternal transmission of the disorder. The gene for this disease, now referred to as spinocerebellar ataxia type II was mapped to 3p12-p21.1.[13,68]

When OPCA presents in infancy, there is developmental delay, ataxia, and poor vision. Seizures are uncommon and head circumference is normal. There is poor vision with diffuse pigmentary mottling of the retina and reduced

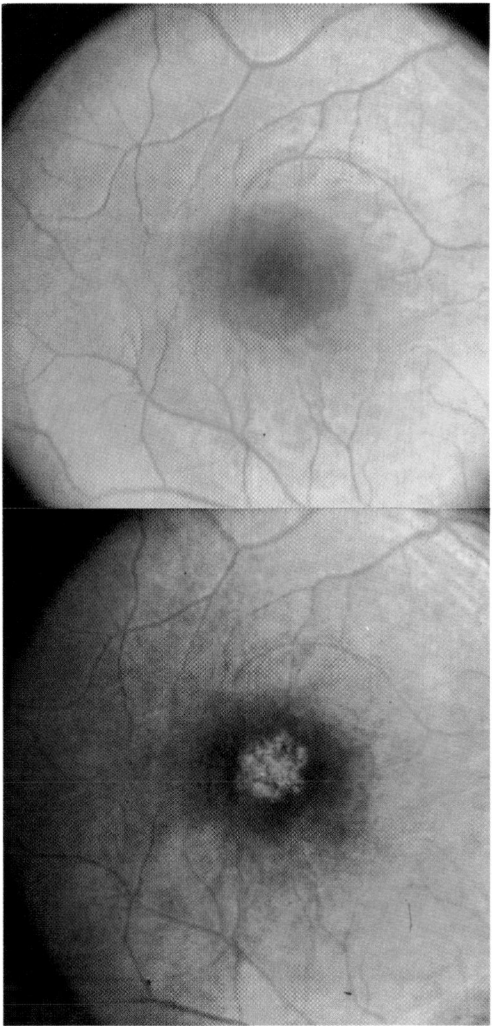

Figure 32.17. Progression of retinal degenerative changes in an adult with olivopontocerebellar atrophy type III or spino-cerebellar atrophy type II. Top and bottom photographs were taken 10 years apart. (From ref. 45, used with permission.)

or nonrecordable ERG. Patients may have strabismus. Death occurs in the first few years of life. If patients become symptomatic in childhood or adolescence, there is progressive cerebellar ataxia, dysarthria, external ophthalmoplegia, and blindness. Patients become wheelchair-bound or bedridden and need substantial supportive care. Adult-onset disease has a very insidious and slowly progressive course with gradually increasing ataxia and decreasing vision. Visual loss with predominant macular involvement may be the presenting findings in older patients, and may be misdiagnosed as age-related macular degeneration. Diffuse pigmentary retinopathy and peripheral punched-out chorioretinal lesions resembling gyrate atrophy may be present in young adults (Figs. 32.17 and 32.18),[45] and are accompanied by progressive severe loss of vision.[42,157,184] Subtle cerebellar signs should be looked for. Traboulsi et al.[184] found photoreceptor degeneration with sparing of the ganglion cells and optic nerve in the eyes of twin boys who

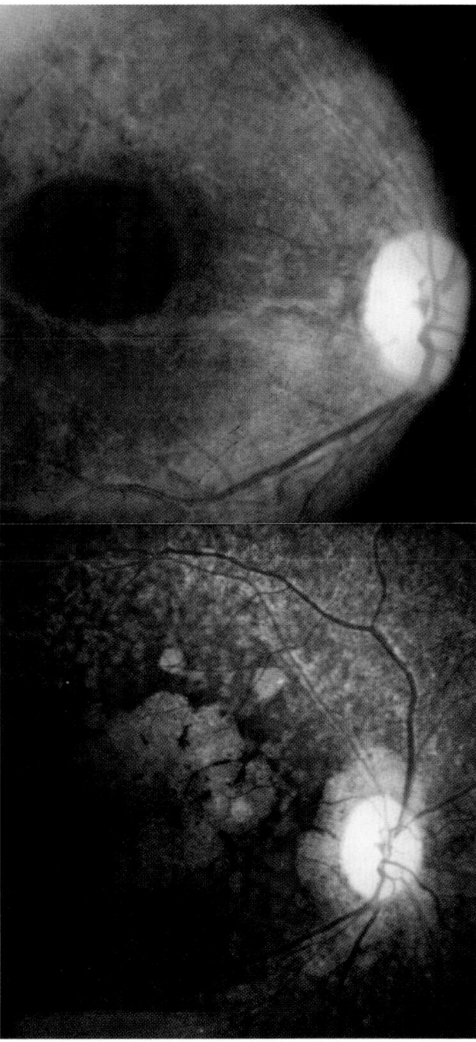

Figure 32.18. Eye of daughter of patient whose fundus is shown in Figure 32.17. Top and bottom photographs were taken several years apart. (From ref. 45, used with permission.)

died from complications of early onset disease. Ryan and co-workers found similar histologic changes in adults.[156]

The diagnosis of olivopontocerebellar atrophy with retinal degeneration is based on clinical and neuroradiologic findings. Neuroimaging reveals pontine and cerebellar atrophy. The disease should be suspected in infants presenting with a neurodegenerative disease and retinal dystrophy. The differential diagnosis includes infantile phytanic acid storage disease, abetalipoproteinemia, recessive neonatal adrenoleukodystrophy, and the infantile form of NCL. One parent is frequently mildly affected and may not be diagnosed at the time the child presents with severe neurologic and retinal signs and symptoms. The dominant mode of inheritance and the presence of ataxia are the best differential diagnostic clues.

KEARNS-SAYRE SYNDROME

This disease is discussed in Chapters 27 and 35.

HALLERVORDEN-SPATZ DISEASE

Hallervorden and Spatz[73] first reported five sisters in a sibship of 12 with progressive dysarthria and dementia. All five died before the age of 25 years. Autopsy findings consisted of brown discoloration of the globus pallidus and substantia nigra. Patients with this disease develóp progressive rigidity of the lower then upper extremities, extrapyramidal motor signs, dysarthria, chorioathetoid movements, difficulties in chewing and swallowing, dementia, and ultimately die. Because early symptoms are insidious and unusual, psychological disorders may be suspected. Some patients may be depressed. The hallmark of this condition is the deposition of iron, most notably in the globus pallidus and the substantia nigra. Diagnosis is hence made on clinical and neuroradiologic grounds.[165] Another distinctive feature of this disease is neuroaxonal degeneration with formation of spheroid bodies or inclusions, which are also present in Schindler's disease, Seitelberger disease and neuroaxonal dystrophy. Almost 25% of patients with Hallervorden-Spatz disease have retinal degeneration. Such individuals are usually young and have a rapidly progressive disease. There is a fleck type of retinopathy with a bulls-eye maculopathy. Typical RP-like changes and optic atrophy develop later in the course of the disease. The ocular histopathology has been reported by Roth et al.[154] and by Luckenback et al.[127]

DARIER DISEASE

Patients with Darier disease, a rare autosomal dominant disorder, have a follicular keratosis with papules, scaly crusty lesions, and papillomatous masses. The nails are dystrophic and there may be pitting of the palms. Itin et al.[84] reported two brothers with typical RP-like retinal changes, cataracts at an early age, and characteristic skin changes. The ERG was nonrecordable at the ages of 48 and 52 years. Deficient dark adaptation without pigmentary retinopathy has also been described.[50] Vitamin A therapy improves the skin lesions but not the retinopathy of this disease.

SENIOR-LOKEN SYNDROME (NEPHRONOPHTHISIS-RETINOPATHY SYNDROME)

The renal disease in the recessively inherited Senior-Loken syndrome[126] is histologically similar to juvenile nephronophthisis and to medullary cystic disease.[164] Patients develop renal failure in the first decade of life. There are two patterns of ocular disease associated with this syndrome. In the first type, children present in the first year of life with blindness and a clinical picture identical to Leber's congenital amaurosis. There is nystagmus, a nonrecordable ERG, and the retina may appear normal or show areas of hypo- and hyperpigmentation with arteriolar narrowing. In the second type, the retinal dystrophy may not become apparent until later in life. Families of patients with a diagnosis of Leber's congenital amaurosis should be warned that the Senior-Loken syndrome is one of the possible systemic diseases associated with the retinal dystrophy. There are also reports of congenital hepatic fibrosis associated with nephronophthisis and retinal degeneration.[44] The relationship between the Senior-Loken syndrome and the Saldino-Mainzer syndrome,[128] and the syndrome of nephronophthisis, deafness, and retinal dystrophy reported by Clarke et al.[33] is not clear. Senior-Loken syndrome does not map to the chromosome 2 region where one gene for isolated juvenile nephronophthisis resides.[6]

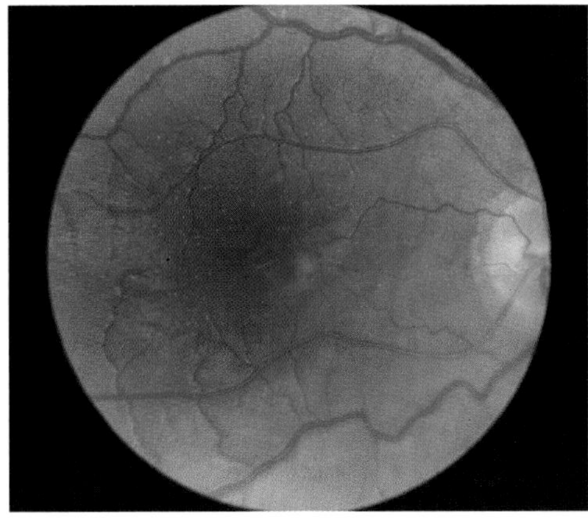

Figure 32.19. Fine yellow flecks at the level of Bruchs' membrane in a child with Alport syndrome.

HEREDITARY HEMORRHAGIC NEPHRITIS (ALPORT SYNDROME)

Hereditary hemorrhagic nephritis is characterized by progressive nephritis with hematuria and proteinuria, and by sensorineural deafness. It is inherited in an X-linked fasion in 85% of cases and results from mutations in the COL4A5 gene that codes for the α-5-polypeptide of type IV collagen.[9,149] This gene is located at Xq22. The autosomal recessive forms may be caused by mutations in the autosomal genes coding for other chains of type IV collagen.

Clinical manifestations occur earlier and are more severe in males than in females of the same family. Patients may come to medical attention in childhood or in adulthood, although hematuria may be present at birth. Renal biopsy may be required for the diagnosis. Patients may need renal transplantation and supportive therapy.

There is a characteristic thinning and splitting of the renal glomerular basement membrane. The lens capsule and Bruchs' membrane are also affected, leading to ocular findings of cataracts and flecked retinopathy in about 15% of patients. The retinopathy is characterized by the presence of pale yellow flecks at the level of the retinal pigment epithelium (RPE) (Fig. 32.19). The flecks are most prominent in the macula and at the posterior pole. Cataracts are most characteristically of the anterior lenticonus type (Fig. 32.20), but nuclear, cortical, and posterior subcapsular opacities may be present. In 41 of 58 patients who were examined for ocular abnormalities, 10 boys had anterior lenticonus and macular changes, but 8 patients had macular changes only. Of the 18 patients with macular changes, 13 had fine yellow-white drusenlike lesions around the fovea. Fluorescein angiography shows patchy hyperfluorescence. The electroretinogram and electrooculogram may be abnormal.

ASPHYXIATING THORACIC DYSTROPHY (JEUNE SYNDROME)

Asphyxiating thoracic dystrophy is an autosomal recessive disorder characterized by short-limbed dwarfism, thoracic dysplasia with a narrow rib cage and respiratory insufficiency, brachydactyly and rarely polydactyly, and progressive renal failure from chronic nephritis. Jeune syndrome should be differentiated from Ellis-van Creveld syndrome in which patients

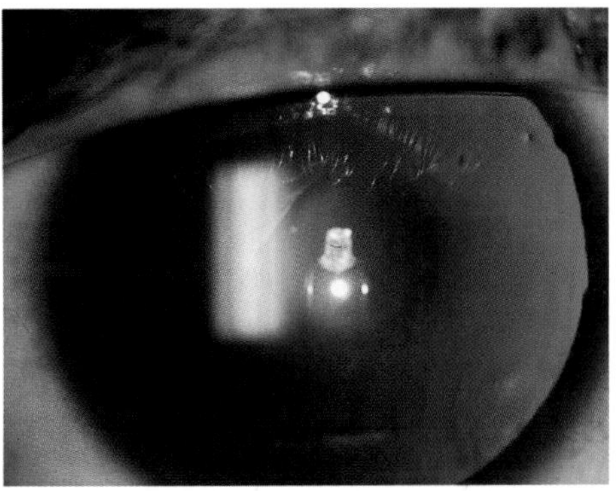

Figure 32.20. Anterior lenticonus in a teenaged girl with Alport syndrome.

have similar changes in the pelvis and limbs but also have nail dysplasia and a peculiar upper lip; furthermore, polydactyly is a constant feature of the Ellis-van Creveld syndrome and patients with the latter syndrome have cardiac defects rather than renal disease. The underlying genetic or metabolic defect in Jeune syndrome is not known. Respiratory insufficiency frequently results in death in infancy, but some patients survive to adulthood. Ocular findings consist of midperipheral and at times macular retinal pigment epithelial atrophic and hypertrophic changes. Visual acuity may be reduced, and myopia, photophobia, nystagmus, and strabismus have been described. Electroretinographic and visual field defects are progressive. Histopathologic study of the retina of one patient showed mild changes of the RPE, marked loss of photoreceptor cells with relative sparing of cones, and moderate loss of peripheral ganglion cells.[201]

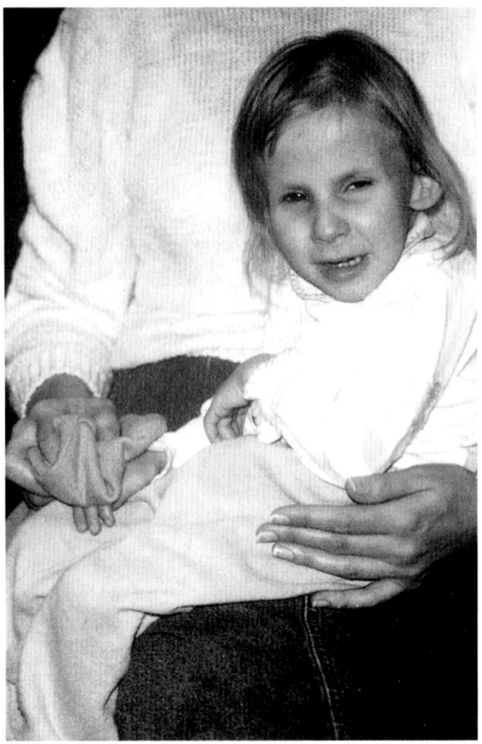

Figure 32.21. Young girl with Cockayne syndrome. There is growth retardation, facial features of premature aging, and enophthalmos.

COCKAYNE SYNDROME (CS)

A rare group of autosomal recessive disorders, Cockayne syndrome is characterized by dwarfism, progeria (Fig. 32.21), deafness, mental retardation, skin photosensitivity, and retinal degeneration. Development may be normal in the first year of life with deterioration thereafter. Death usually occurs before the teenage years with occasional survival into the third decade.[190] There is a variability in the severity of clinical findings that may depend on the genetic subtype. There is a defect in the ability of cells to repair ultraviolet-induced DNA damage[191] while repair of total genomic DNA is normal. The increased rate of repair of active genes in repair-proficient cells is absent in CS cells. There is delayed recovery of DNA and RNA synthesis following UV radiation. This property is used as a basis for prenatal diagnosis.[118] Three complementation groups are differentiated on the basis of rate of recovery of DNA and RNA repair, suggesting genetic heterogeneity.[117]

Enophthalmos (sunken eyes) is universal and results from loss of subcutaneous and orbital fat. There is poor pupillary dilation due to hypoplasia of the dilator muscle with iris transillumination. Cataracts are present in some patients as early as the first year of life (Fig. 32.22), but may develop later in others.[139] There is an atypical pigmentary retinopathy characterized

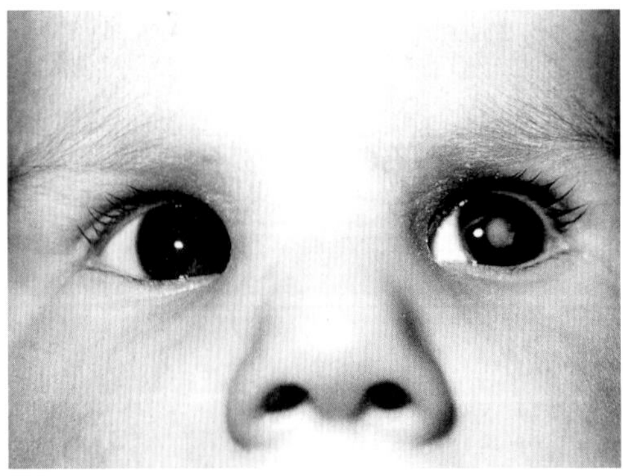

Figure 32.22. Cataract in the left eye of a patient with Cockayne syndrome.

by fine granular pigment spots, attenuated retinal vessels, and optic atrophy. Heavy scattered black pigmentation may be pronounced in the posterior pole. The ERG is decreased or extinguished. High hyperopic and astigmatic refractive errors are universal. Corneal dystrophic changes and recurrent erosions have been described in several patients and usually involve the lower half of the cornea. Photophobia may be extreme. Surprisingly, visual acuity may be relatively well preserved despite marked retinal dystrophic changes and a nonrecordable ERG.[180]

Diagnosis may be aided by magnetic resonance imaging of the brain, which demonstrates hypomyelination, cerebellar atrophy, and calcification of the basal ganglia. Ultraviolet irradiation of cultured fibroblasts results in abnormal DNA repair. The differential diagnosis of Cockayne syndrome includes Bloom syndrome, Rothmund-Thompson syndrome, xeroderma pigmentosum, and progeria.

BARDET-BIEDL SYNDROME

The cardinal features of the autosomal recessive Bardet-Biedl syndrome are obesity (Fig. 32.23), postaxial polydactyly (Fig. 32.24), hypogenitalism (Fig. 32.23), hypogonadism, mental retardation, and renal anomalies that lead to renal insufficiency and hypertension. Diabetes mellitus or glucose intolerance occurs in about one-third of patients.[52,70] Echocardiographic abnormalities are found in one third to one-half of patients and include valvular malformations and thickening of the interventricular septum.[49] Although structural genital anomalies are more prominent in males, females may have vaginal atresia or other external or internal genital abnormalities.[175] Harnett and co-workers reported on 32 Canadian patients and found retinal dystrophy in all, but typical retinitis pigmentosa in only two; 18 patients had polydactyly, but all patients had syndactyly, brachydactyly, or both; obesity was present in all except one patient; 12 of 32 patients were severely retarded; 7 of 8 men had hypogenitalism not due to hypogonadotropism; all 12 women in the study had menstrual irregularities; 9 of 20 patients had diabetes mellitus; all 21 patients studied had renal disease, including 3 with end-stage renal failure.[76]

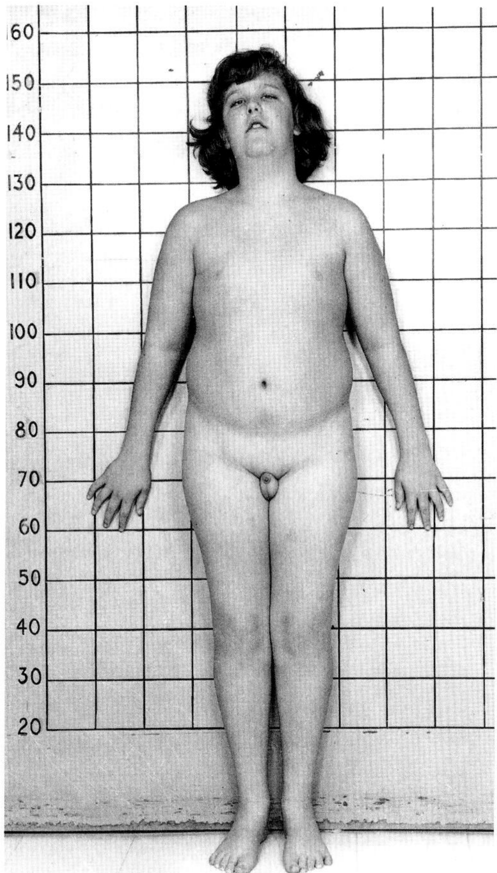

Figure 32.23. Prepubescent boy with Bardet-Biedl syndrome. Note obesity and hypogenitalism. (Courtesy of Drs. Irene Maumenee and Linn Murphree.)

The disease has a frequency of 1 in 100,000 worldwide but is more common in certain geographically isolated populations in Switzerland, Newfoundland in Canada, the Negev region of Israel, and among the Bedouins in Kuwait, where the prevalence is about 1 in 13,500.[53]

The first genetic locus for the Bardet-Biedl phenotype (BBS1) was mapped to chromosome 11q.[119] Three additional genes were mapped in three unrelated Arab-Bedouin families in the Negev region of Israel.[30,112,167] BBS2 maps to chromosome 16q21,[112] BBS3 to chromosome 3,[167] and BBS4 to chromosome

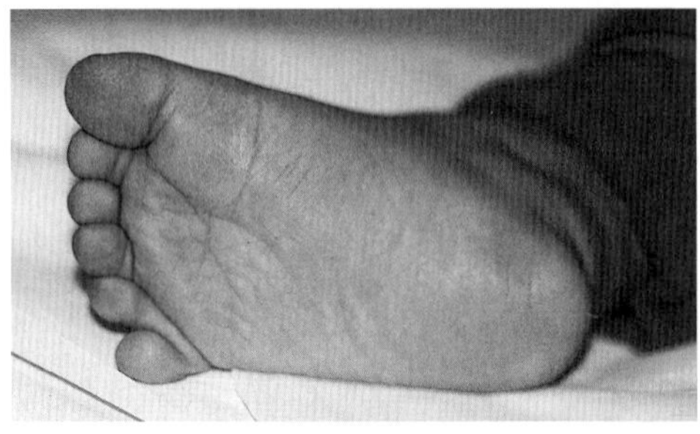

A

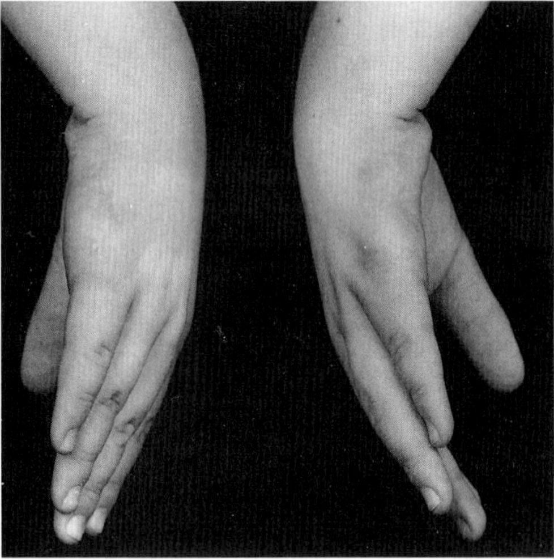

B

Figure 32.24. **A:** Polydactyly in a patient with Bardet-Biedl syndrome. **B:** Scars on hypothenar area of both hands of a patient with Bardet-Biedl syndrome. The sixth digits had been amputated. (Courtesy of Drs. Irene Maumenee and Linn Murphree.)

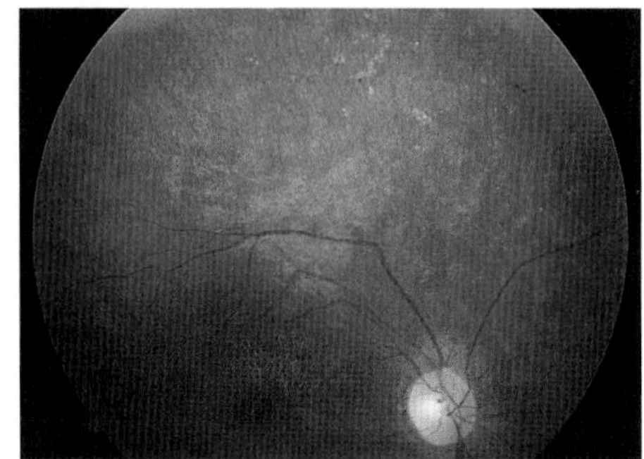

Figure 32.25. Retinal dystrophic changes with attenuated blood vessels and atrophic macular changes in a teenager with Bardet-Biedl syndrome.

15q22.3-q23.[30] Patients with BBS2 appear to be the leanest, while those with BBS4 have early-onset morbid obesity.[30] Patients with BBS3 tend to have polydactyly of all four limbs, while those with BBS4 have polydactyly of the hands.[30] The BBS gene may predispose male heterozygote carriers to obesity, and male and female carriers of the gene are significantly taller than the average population.[40]

The Laurence-Moon syndrome is differentiated from Bardet-Biedl syndrome by the presence of spastic paraplegia and the absence of polydactyly and obesity.[5] The two conditions may indeed be distinct, with the Laurence-Moon syndrome being much less common than the Bardet-Biedl phenotype. Alstrom syndrome *(vide infra)* has clinical features that overlap with those of Bardet-Biedl syndrome (Table 32.4) but appears to be genetically distinct. Biemond syndrome differs from the BBS by the presence of colobomas of the iris.[15,16,69]

A progressive retinal dystrophy begins in childhood in patients with BBS and progresses moderately rapidly to severe visual loss and constriction of visual fields. Ophthalmoscopic changes include macular atrophic and pigmentary changes, sometimes in a bull's-eye configuration; optic nerve pallor and arteriolar narrowing occur, but peripheral pigmentary changes may be modest (Fig. 32.25). The ERG is nonrecordable in early childhood. The retinal dystrophy of Bardet-Biedl syn-

Table 32.4. Genetic Types of Bardet-Biedl Syndrome (BBS)

Type	Chromosomal Locus	Polydactyly	Obesity	Retinal Dystrophy
BBS 1	11q13	Present	Present	Present
BBS 2	16q21	All four limbs	Leanest	Present
BBS 3	3p13-p12	All four limbs	Present	Present
BBS 4	15q22.3-q23	Hands	Early onset, morbid	Present

drome may be best characterized as a cone-rod dystrophy.

COHEN SYNDROME

The main clinical features of Cohen syndrome, an autosomal recessive condition, include nonprogressive mental retardation, microcephaly, short stature, hypotonia, and hypermobility of the joints, long and narrow hands, and truncal obesity. Patients have a characteristic facial appearance with a prominent bridge of the nose and upper central incisors.[35] There may be a mild, intermittent, and clinically insignificant neutropenia. Ophthalmologic findings include myopia, decreased visual acuity, night blindness, pigmentary retinopathy, and a nonrecordable ERG.[140,193]

The gene for Cohen syndrome is more common in Finland[140] and in Israel than in other parts of the world, with about 20 patients diagnosed in the former country[177] and 39 in the latter.[158] Tahvanainen and co-workers mapped the gene for Cohen syndrome to chromosome 8q22 in the Finnish families.[177] The differential diagnosis of the Cohen syndrome is identical to that of Bardet-Biedl syndrome, and it may be identical to Mirhosseini-Holmes-Walton syndrome.[174]

THE USHER SYNDROMES

The Usher syndromes, a group of genetically and clinically distinct autosomal recessive conditions named for Charles Usher,[186] are characterized by sensorineural hearing loss accompanied by a retinal dystrophy indistinguishable from retinitis pigmentosa. Hallgren reported on 177 patients from 102 families.[74] Most patients developed cataracts by the age of 40; about one-fourth had mental retardation or psychosis and a majority had gait disturbances that were attributed to labyrinthine dysfunction. Hallgren estimated the frequency of Usher syndrome to be 3.0 per 100,000 in Scandinavia. The prevalence in the United States is estimated to be about 4.4 per 100,000.[21] The Usher syndromes constitute about 2.5% of families with retinitis pigmentosa[87] and 24%–54% of deaf-blind persons registered at the Helen Keller National Center for Deaf-Blind Youths and Adults have Usher syndrome.[21] Thirty percent of deaf French-Acadians in Louisiana have Usher syndrome, now identified as type IC.[107] From his studies of 133 Finnish Usher syndrome patients, Forsius concluded that there were two distinct forms of the disease: a common severe congenital form (USH1) and a less common milder form (USH2). The criteria for the clinical diagnosis of Usher syndrome that were adopted by the Usher Syndrome Consortium are given by Smith and co-workers,[171] who stressed the importance of excluding intrauterine infections and perinatal problems that may cause profound hearing loss and retinal damage before making a diagnosis of Usher syndrome. At present there are at least four distinct genetic USH1 loci—two USH2 loci and one USH3 locus (Table 32.5).

Night blindness starts in childhood or early teens in type 1, and later in type 2. Central visual acuity is often decreased late in the course of type 1, whereas it may remain at acceptable levels for a longer period in type 2. Ophthalmoscopy reveals findings of typical retinitis pigmentosa. Diagnosis is made on the basis of combined otologic and ophthalmologic testing after other causes of syndromic deafness have been ruled out.

Type I (USH1)

In type I patients, a severe hearing deficit is present from birth and speech rarely develops. Vestibular responses are abnormal. Visual symptoms are apparent by age 10 years and the ERG is markedly diminished or absent. Ataxia, psychosis, and mental retardation may develop. One gene for USH1 was mapped to 14q32.[97] There is genetic heterogeneity for USH1 in France.[114] The gene in the families originating from the Poitou-Charentes region in western France (USH1A) maps to 14q32.[114] The Acadian variety of Usher syndrome in Louisiana (USH1C) maps to 11p15.1[100,172] and the non-Acadian, non 14q variety (USH1B) maps to 11q13.5.[20,105,172] There is an abnormality of the axoneme (a component of ciliated cells such as photoreceptors, auditory hair cells, and vestibular cells) structure in patients with

Table 32.5. Types of Usher Syndrome (USH)

Type	Night Blindness	Hearing Loss	Vestibular Function	Neurologic Signs	Gene Map/ Defective Gene
USH IA	By age 10 yr	Congenital and severe	Abnormal	May develop	14q32
USH IB	By age 10 yr	Congenital and severe	Abnormal	May develop	11q13.5 Myosin VIIA
USH IC	By age 10 yr	Congenital and severe	Abnormal	May develop	11p15.1
USH I non-A,B,C	By age 10 yr	Congenital and severe	Abnormal	May develop	Unknown
USH IIA	Adulthood	Congenital, milder	Normal	None	1q41
USH IIB	Adulthood	Congenital, milder	Normal	None	Unknown
USH III	Adulthood	Progressive	Abnormal	None	3q21-q25

Usher syndrome.[19,82,168] Weil and co-workers demonstrated mutations in the gene coding for myosin VIIA, a gene that maps to 11q13.5, in 75% of patients with type I Usher syndrome, suggesting that 75% of type I Usher syndrome are USH1B.[194]

Gerber and colleagues[62] suggested the existence of a fourth locus for Usher syndrome type I since the loci for types IA, IB, and IC were excluded by linkage studies in two families of Moroccan and Pakistani ancestry.

Type II (USHII)

In type II patients, congenital hearing loss is less severe than in type 1 and speech may develop. Vestibular and neurologic functions are normal. Visual symptoms start in the late teens. The ERG is usually decreased, but a wave is recordable. The locus for the USH2A gene has been mapped to chromosome 1q41.[106,121]

Type III (USHIII)

There is a third, apparently distinct form of the syndrome that is characterized by progressive hearing loss and vestibular hypoactivity.[98] USH3 comprises 2% of all Usher syndrome cases, except in Finland, where it accounts for 42% of patients. The USH3 locus was assigned to 3q21-q25 by Sankila et al.[160]

FLYNN-AIRD SYNDROME

Flynn-Aird syndrome is a rare autosomal dominant condition that combines deafness, neurologic degeneration, atypical seizures, and skin and bone defects. Deafness is usually the presenting sign in early adulthood. Ataxia, neuritic pain, atrophic skin lesions, and joint stiffness follow. The underlying defect is unknown. Ocular findings include high myopia, cataracts, and a retinitis pigmentosalike appearance of the ocular fundus.[55]

ALSTROM SYNDROME

Alstrom syndrome seems to be most prevalent among the French Acadians of Yarmouth County in Nova Scotia and those living in Louisiana. In this autosomal recessive disease obesity, sensorineural deafness and cone-rod dystrophy are diagnosed in the first decade of life.[2] The phenotype resembles that of the Bardet-Biedl syndrome, but there is no polydactyly, mental retardation, or hypogonadism. Although intellect is generally believed to be normal, some patients have been found to have learning disabilities.[132] Males have hypogonadotropic hypogonadism with normal virilization. Most patients do not reproduce, although the patients reported by Cohen and Kisch were fertile.[34] Chronic nephritis and diabetes caused by insulin resistance develop in the second and third decades of life. Even in childhood, systemic steroids may cause severe hyperglycemia necessitating insulin; cessation of steroids reverses the hyperglycemia (Drack, unpublished data). Dilated cardiomyopathy is an underrecognized feature of the disease in infancy and early childhood.[132] Patients suspected of having this syndrome should have a thorough cardiac evaluation.

Nystagmus and photophobia are noted in the first year of life. Salt-and-pepper retinal pigmentary changes are present along with areas of atrophy and retinal pigment epithelium (RPE) clumping. Electroretinographic studies in very young patients reveal that the cones are affected first, followed by the rods. Optic atrophy and arteriolar attenuation are present and functional blindness by adolescence is usual.[133]

ALAGILLE SYNDROME (ARTERIOHEPATIC DYSPLASIA)

Patients with Alagille syndrome have hepatic cholestasis because of congenital hypoplasia of the interlobular bile ducts.[1,136] System abnormalities include dysmorphic facies, congenital heart disease, pulmonary stenosis, and vertebral and renal anomalies. Jaundice and failure to thrive are noted in infancy or in childhood. Some patients have skin photosensitivity with blistering and scarring similar to those of porphyria. Long-term prognosis for liver function is fairly good, although some patients require liver transplants. Hepatocarcinoma has been reported.[99] The inheritance is autosomal dominant with variable penetrance. Family studies reveal that some parents may have subclinical evidence of the disease.[51]

The gene for Alagille syndrome has been localized to chromosome 20p11.2 because of a number of patients who had deletions[28,173] and by linkage analysis.[80]

Mild anterior segment dysgenesis (posterior embryotoxon) and/or a pigmentary retinopathy are inconsistent ocular findings.[51,153] When retinal changes are present, the ERG findings are consistent with a rod–cone dystrophy; this may be secondary to low levels of the fat soluble vitamins. The diagnosis is made on the basis of clinical, laboratory, and or liver biopsy findings. Oral supplementation of vitamins A and E and triglycerides should be considered.[1]

JOUBERT SYNDROME

This autosomal recessive condition is named after Joubert,[91] who described four French-Canadian sibs with partial or total absence of the cerebellar vermis, episodic hyperpnea, abnormal eye movements, and psychomotor retardation; one of the four had an occipital meningomyelocele. Bolthauser and Isler suggested the designation of Joubert syndrome and reported two sibs and an isolated case.[18] The neuropathologic findings of one of these three cases were reported by Friede and Bolthauser.[57] Saraiva and Baraitser reviewed the clinical findings in 94 patients who fulfilled a number of diagnostic criteria that these authors set forth and concluded that there were two major categories of patients: those with and those without a retinal dystrophy.[162] All patients with renal cysts had retinal degeneration. When the retinopathy is present, the ERG is abnormal. An ocular motility disorder similar to oculomotor apraxia, and nystagmus may be present. Some patients with a clinical diagnosis of Joubert syndrome have uveal or optic nerve colobomas.[115,125] It is unclear whether these patients have the same, or a related condition.

BIETTI'S CRYSTALLINE RETINOPATHY

Bietti's crystalline retinopathy is a progressive chorioretinal degeneration characterized by the deposition of crystalline material in the retina of all patients and in the peripheral cornea of some.[195] The disease may be relatively common in China.[81] Symptoms of night blindness, decreased vision, and restricted visual fields become evident in the late teens or early twenties. Patients are otherwise healthy, although abnormalities of serum lipids have been described in some. In a study of three patients, Wilson et al. described inclusions resembling cholesterol or cholesterol esters in corneal and

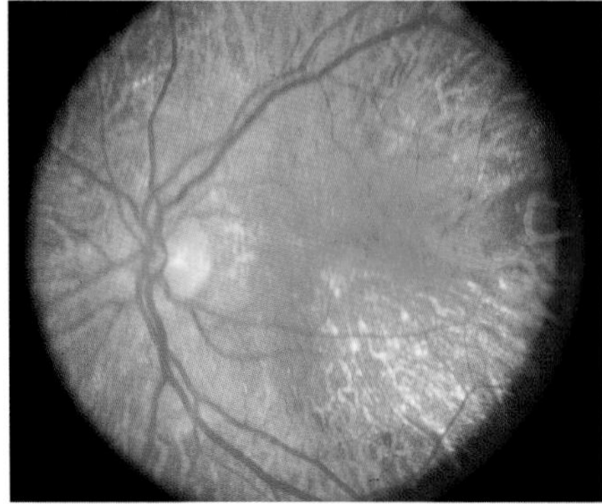

A

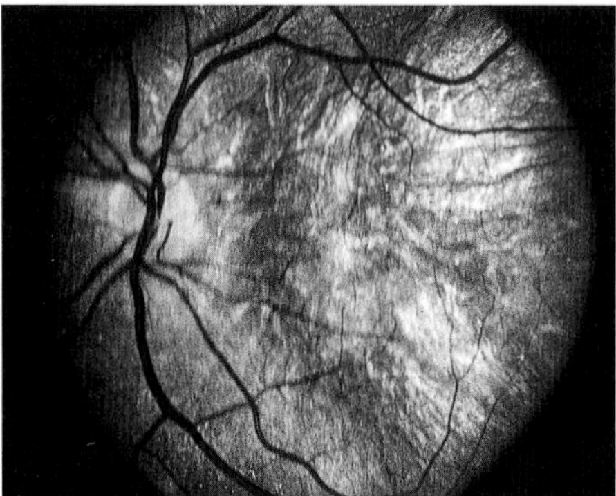

B

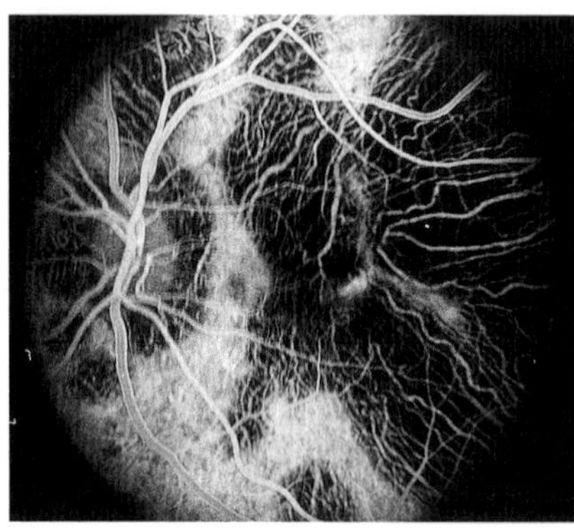

C

Figure 32.26. A: Fundus of patient with Bietti's crystalline retinopathy. Many of the crystals have disappeared and there is atrophy in the macular area. **B:** Red-free photograph demonstrates retinal crystals in the same patient. **C:** Angiogram shows characteristic geographic areas of retinal pigment epithelium and choriocapillaris atrophy.

conjunctival cells.[200] Similar inclusions were present in lymphocytes, suggesting that the disease may be one of lipid metabolism.[200] The disease is inherited in an autosomal recessive fashion.[81]

Fluorescein angiographic findings are characteristic: there are progressively enlarging geographic areas of choriocapillaris atrophy in the posterior pole (Fig. 32.26*C*).[71,181] The retinal crystals can be observed in the superficial and deep retinal layers (Fig. 32.26*B*) and tend to disappear as the disease advances and the chorioretinal layers atrophy in the posterior pole (Fig. 32.26*A*). The optic nerve head and retinal vessels are normal. Corneal crystals may be more common in occidental than oriental patients.[77,181]

The differential diagnosis of crystalline retinopathy includes fundus albipunctatus, retinitis punctata albescens, drusen, oxalosis, cystinosis, Sjögren-Larsson syndrome, and tamoxifen retinopathy.

REFERENCES

1. Alagille D, Odievre M, Gautier M, Dommergues J. Hepatic ductular hypoplasia associated with characteristic facies, vertebral malformations, retarded physical, mental and sexual development, and cardiac murmur. *J Pediatr* 1975;86:63–71.
2. Alstrom C, Hallgren B, Nilsson L, Asander H. Retinal degeneration combined with obesity; diabetes mellitus and neurogenous deafness: A specific syndrome (not hitherto described) distinct from the Laurence-Moon-Bardet-Biedl syndrome. *Acta Psychiatry Neurol Scand* 1959;129(suppl):1–35.
3. Amir N, Zlotogora J, Bach G. Mucolipidosis type IV; Clinical spectrum and natural history. *Pediatrics* 1987;79:953–959.
4. Amit R, Granit G, Shapira Y. Familial ataxia with extreme difference in age of clinical onset. *Neuropediatrics* 1986;17:165–167.
5. Ammann F. Investigations cliniques et génétiques sur le syndrome de Bardet-Biedl en Suisse. *J Genet Hum* 1970;18(suppl):1–310.
6. Antignac C, Arduy C, Beckmann J et al. A gene for familial juvenile nephronophthisis (recessive medullary cystic kidney disease) maps to chromosome 2 p. *Nature Genet* 1993;3:342–345.
7. Bach G, Zeigler M, Schaap T et al. Mucolipidosis type IV: Ganglioside sialidase deficiency. *Biochem Biophys Res Commun* 1979;90:1341–1347.
8. Bain M, Jones M, Borriello S et al. Contribution of gut bacterial metabolism to human metabolic disease. *Lancet* 1988;1:1078–1079.

9. Barker D, Hostikka S, Zhou J, Chow L, Oliphant A, Gerben S et al. Identification of mutations in the COL4A5 collagen gene in Alport syndrome. *Science* 1990;248:1224–1227.
10. Bartholomew DW, Batshaw ML, Allen RH, Roe CR, Rosenblatt D, Valle DL et al. Therapeutic approaches to cobalamin-C methylmalonic acidemia and homocystinuria. *J Pediatr* 1988;112(1):32–39.
11. Bassen F, Kornzweig A. Malformation of the erythrocytes in a case of atypical retinitis pigmentosa. *Blood* 1950;5:381.
12. Bateman B, Philippart M. Ocular features of the Hagberg-Santavuori syndrome. *Am J Ophthalmol* 1986;102:262–271.
13. Benomar A, Krols L, Stevanin G et al. The gene for autosomal dominant cerebellar ataxia with pigmentary macular dystrophy maps to chromosome 3p12-p21.1. *Nature Genet* 1995; 7:84–88.
14. Berkovic S, Carpenter S, Andermann F, Andermann E, Wolfe L. Kufs' disease: A critical reappraisal. *Brain* 1988;111:27–62.
15. Biemond A. Het syndroom van aurence-Biedl en een aanverwaant; nieuw syndroom. *Ned Tijdschr Geneeskd* 1934;78:1801–1814.
16. Blumel J, Kniker W. Laurence-Moon-Berdet-Biedl syndrome: Review of the literature and a report of five cases including a family group with three affected males. *Texas Rep Biol Med* 1959;17:391–410.
17. Bois E, Feingold J, Frenay P, Briard M-L. Infantile cystinosis in France: Genetics; incidence; geographic distribution. *J Med Genet* 1976;13:434–438.
18. Bolthauser E, Isler W. Joubert syndrome: Episodic hyperpnea, abnormal eye movements, retardation and ataxia, associated with dysplasia of the cerebellar vermis. *Neuropaediatrie* 1977;8:57–66.
19. Bonneau D, Raymond F, Kremer C, Klossek J-M, Kaplan J, Patte F. Usher syndrome type I associated with bronchiectasis and immobile nasal cilia in two brothers. *J Med Genet* 1993;30:253–254.
20. Bonne-Tamir B, Korostishevsky M, Kalinsky H, Seroussi E, Beker R, Weiss S et al. Genetic mapping of the gene for Usher syndrome: Linkage analysis in a large Samaritan kindred. *Genomics* 1994;20:36–42.
21. Boughman J, Vernon M, Shaver K. Usher syndrome: Definition and estimate of prevalence from two high-risk populations. *J Chronic Dis* 1983;36:596–603.
22. Boustany R, Kolodny E. Neurological progress. The neuronal ceroid lipofuscinoses: A review. *Rev Neurol (Paris)* 1989;145(2):105–110.
23. Boustany R-M. Neurology of the neuronal ceroid lipofuscinoses: Late infantile and juvenile types. *Am J Med Genet* 1992;42:533–535.
24. Boustany R-M, Alory J, Kolodny E. Clinical classification of neuronal ceroid lipofuscinosis subtypes. *Am J Med Genet* 1988(suppl);5: 47–58.
25. Brod R, Packer A, Van Dyk H. Diagnosis of neuronal ceroid lipofuscinosis by ultrastructural examination of peripheral blood lymphocytes. *Arch Ophthalmol* 1987;105:1388–1393.
26. Bronson R, Lake B, Cook S, Taylor S, Davisson M. Motor neuron degeneration of mice is a model of neuronal ceroid lipofuscinosis (Batten's disease). *Ann Neurol* 1993;33:381–385.
27. Brown R, Maumenee I. Methymalonic aciduria and homocystinuria—A disorder of intracellular vitamin B12 metabolism. *Invest Ophthalmol Visual Sci* 1989(suppl);30:307.
28. Byrne J, Harrod M, Friedman J et al. Del (20p) with manifestations of arteriohepatic dysplasia. *Am J Med Genet* 1986;24:673–678.
29. Callen DF, Baker E, Lane S, Nancarrow J, Thompson A, Whitmore SA et al. Regional mapping of the Batten disease locus (CLN3) to human chromosome 16p12. *Am J Hum Genet* 1991;49(6):1372–1377.
30. Carmi R, Rokhlina T, Kwitek-Black A, Elbedour K, Nishimura D, Stone E et al. Use of a DNA pooling strategy to identify a human obesity syndrome on chromosome 15. *Hum Mol Genet* 1995;4:9–13.
31. Chan C, Green W, Maumenee I et al. Ocular ultrastructural studies of two cases of the Hurler syndrome (systemic mucopolysaccharidosis I-H). *Ophthalmic Paediatr Genet* 1983; 2:3–19.
32. Chang B, Bronson R, Hawes N et al. Retinal degeneration in motor neuron degeneration: a mouse model of ceroid lipofuscinoses. *Invest Ophthalmol Visual Sci* 1994;335:1071–1076.
33. Clarke M, Sullivan T, Francis C, Baumal R, Fenton T, Pearce W. Senior-Loken syndrome: Case report and association with sensorineural deafness. *Br J Ophthalmol* 1992;76:171–172.
34. Cohen J, Kisch E. Alstrom syndrome: A new variant? *Israel J Med Sci* 1994;30:234–236.
35. Cohen M, Hall B, Smith D, Graham C, Lambert K. A new syndrome with hypotonia, obesity, mental deficiency, and facial, oral, ocular and limb anomalies. *J Pediatr* 1973;83: 280–284.

36. Collins M, Traboulsi E, Maumenee I. Optic nerve head swelling and optic atrophy in the mucopolysaccharidoses. *Ophthalmology* 1990;97:1445–1449.
37. Conradi N, Uvebrant P, Hokegard K, Wahlstrom J. First-trimester diagnosis of juvenile neuronal ceroid lipofuscinosis by demonstration of fingerprint inclusions in chorionic villi. *Prenat Diagn* 1989;9:283–287.
38. Consortium International Batten Disease. Isolation of a novel gene underlying Batten disease. *Cell* 1995;82:949–957.
39. Constantinidis J, Wisniewski K, Wisniewski T. The adult and a new late adult forms of neuronal ceroid lipofuscinosis. *Acta Neuropathol* 1992;83:461–468.
40. Croft J, Morrell D, Chase C, Swift M. Obesity in heterozygous carriers of the gene for the Bardet-Biedl syndrome. *Am J Med Genet* 1995;55:12–15.
41. Dangel M, Bremer D, Rogers G. Treatment of corneal opacification in mucolipidosis IV with conjunctival transplantation. *Am J Ophthalmol* 1985;99:137–141.
42. de Jong P, de Jong J, de Jong-Ten Doeschate J et al. Olivopontocerebellar atrophy with visual disturbances. An ophthalmologic investigation into four generations. *Ophthalmology* 1980; 87:793–804.
43. Del Monte M, Maumenee I, Green W et al. Clinical and ocular histopathologic studies of mucopolysaccharidosis type III-A: The Sanfilipo syndrome. *Arch Ophthalmol* 1983;101: 1255–1262.
44. Delaney V, Mullaney J, Bourke E. Juvenile nephronophthisis: Congenital hepatic fibrosis and retinal hypoplasia in twins. *Q J Med* 1978;186:281–296.
45. Drack A, Traboulsi E, Maumenee I. Progression of fundus findings in olivopontocerebellar atrophy with retinal degeneration. *Arch Ophthalmol* 1992;110:712–713.
46. Dufier J, Dhermy P, Gubler M et al. Ocular changes in long-term evaluation of infantile cystinosis. *Ophthalmic Pediatr Genet* 1987; 8:131–137.
47. Dyken P. Reconsideration of the classification of the neuronal ceroid lipofuscinosis. *Am J Med Genet* 1988(Suppl);5:69–84.
48. Eiberg M, Gardiner R, Mohr J. Batten disease (Spielmeyer-Sjögren disease) and haptoglobin (HP): Indication of linkage and assignment to chromosome 16. *Clin Genet* 1989;36:217–218.
49. Elbedour K, Zucker N, Zalzstein E, Barki Y, Carmi R. Cardiac abnormalities in the Bardet-Biedl syndrome: Echocardiographic studies of 22 patients. *Am J Med Genet* 1994;52:164–169.
50. Elliott S, Buxman M, Weleber R. Abnormal dark adaptation in Darier's disease. *J Invest Dermatol* 1979;72:207.
51. Elmslie F, Vivian A, Gardiner H, Hall C, Wowat A, Winter R. Alagille syndrome: Family studies. *J Med Genet* 1995;32:264–268.
52. Escallon F, Traboulsi E, Infante R. A family with the Bardet-Biedl syndrome and diabetes mellitus. *Arch Ophthalmol* 1989;107:855–857.
53. Farag T, Teebi A. High incidence of Bardet-Biedl syndrome among the Bedouin. *Clin Genet* 1989;36:463–465.
54. Fenton W, Rosenberg L. Inherited disorders of cobalamin transport and metabolism. In *The Metabolic Basis of Inherited Disease.* C. Scriber, A. Beaudetn, W. Sly, D. Valle, eds. New York: McGraw-Hill, 1989:2065–2082.
55. Flynn A, Aird R. A neuroectodermal syndrome of dominant inheritance. *J Neurol Sci* 1965;2: 161–182.
56. Folkerth R, Alroy J, Lomakina I, Skutelsky E, Raghavan S, Kolodny E et al. Morphology and histochemistry of an autopsy case. *J Neuropathol Exp Neurol* 1995;54:154–164.
57. Friede R, Bolthauser E. Uncommon syndromes of cerebellar vermis aplasia I: Joubert syndrome. *Dev Med Child Neurol* 1978;20: 758–763.
58. Gahl W, Bernardini I, Dalakas M et al. Oral carnitine therapy in children with cystinosis and Fanconi syndrome. *J Clin Invest* 1988; 81:549–560.
59. Gahl W, Reed G, Thoene J et al. Cysteamine therapy for children with nephropathic cystinosis. *N Engl J Med* 1987;316:971–977.
60. Gahl W, Schneider J, Aula P. Lysosomal transport disorders: Cystinosis and sialic acid storage disorders. In *The Metabolic and Molecular Bases of Inherited Disease,* C. R. Scriver, A. Bardet, W. S. Sly, D. Valle, eds. New York: McGraw-Hill, 1995:3763–3797.
61. Garborg I, Torvik A, Hals J, Tangsrud S, Lindemann R. Congenital neuronal ceroid lipofuscinosis. A case report. *Acta Pathol Microbiol Immunol* 1987;95:119–125.
62. Gerber S, Larget-Piet D, Rozet J-M et al. Evidence for a fourth locus in Usher syndrome type I. *J Med Genet* 1996;33:77–79.
63. Goebel H. Neuronal ceroid lipofuscinoses: The current status. *Brain Dev* 1992;14:203–211.
64. Goldberg M, Duke J. Ocular histopathology in Hunter's syndrome. *Arch Ophthalmol* 1967; 77:503–512.

65. Goodman R. *Genetic Disorders of the Jewish People.* Baltimore: Johns Hopkins University Press. 1979:69, 71.
66. Gouras P, Carr R, Gunkel R. Retinitis pigmentosa in abetalipoproteinemia: Effects of vitamin A, *Invest Ophthalmol* 1971;10:784.
67. Goutieres F, Arsenio-Nunes M-L, Aicardi J. Mucolipidosis IV. *Neuropaediatrie* 1979;10: 321–330.
68. Gouw L, Kaplan C, Haines J, Digre K, Rutledge S, Matilla A et al. Retinal degeneration characterizes a spinocerebellar ataxia mapping to chromosome 3p. *Nature Genet* 1995;7: 89–93.
69. Grebe H. Contribution au diagnostic differentiel du syndrome de Bardet-Biedl. *J Genet Hum* 1953;2:127–144.
70. Green J, Parfrey P, Harnett J, Farid N, Cramer B, Johnson G et al. The cardinal manifestations of Bardet-Biedl syndrome; A forme of Laurence-Moon-Biedl syndrome. *N Engl J Med* 1989;321:1002–1009.
71. Grizzard W, Deutman A, Nijhuis F et al. Crystalline retinopathy. *Am J Ophthalmol* 1978; 86:81–88.
72. Hagberg B, Witt-Engerstrom I. Early stages of Rett syndrome and infantile neuronal ceroid lipofuscinosis—A difficult differential diagnosis. *Brain Dev* 1990;12:20–22.
73. Hallervorden J, Spatz H. Eigenartige Erkrankung im extrapyramidalen System mit besonderer Beteiligung des Globus pallidus und der Substantia nigra: Ein Beitrag zu den Beziehungen zwischen diesen beiden Zentren. *Z Gesamte Neurol Psychiatry* 1922;79:254–302.
74. Hallgren B. Retinitis pigmentosa combined with congenital deafness, with vestibulocerebellar ataxia and mental abnormality in a proportion of cases. A clinical and geneticostatistical study. *Acta Psych Scand* 1959 (suppl);138:5–101.
75. Harding A. Classification of the hereditary ataxias and paraplegias. *Lancet* 1983;1:1151–1154.
76. Harnett J, Green J, Cramer B, Johnson G, Chafe L, McManamon P et al. The spectrum of renal disease in Laurence-Moon-Biedl syndrome. *N Engl J Med* 1988;319:615–618.
77. Hayasaka S, Okuyama S. Crystalline retinopathy. *Retina* 1984;4:177–181.
78. Hellsten E, Vesa J, Jarvela I et al. Refined assignment of the infantile neuronal ceroid lipofuscinosis (INCL) locus at 1p32 and the current status of prenatal and carrier diagnosis. *J Inherit Metab Dis* 1993;16:335–338.
79. Hofman I. *The Batten-Spielmeyer-Vogt Disease.* Doorn, The Netherlands: Bartimeus Foundation, 1990.
80. Hol F, Hamel B, Geurds M, Hansmann I, Nabben F, Daniels O et al. Localization of Alagille syndrome to 20p112-p12 by linkage analysis of a three-generation family. *Hum Genet* 1995;95:687–690.
81. Hu D-N. Ophthalmic genetics in China. *Ophthalmic Paediatr Genet* 1983;2:39–45.
82. Hunter D, Fishman G, Mehta R, Kretzer F. Abnormal sperm and photoreceptor axonemes in Usher's syndrome. *Arch Ophthalmol* 1986; 104:385–389.
83. Inana G, Chambers C, Hatta Y et al. Point mutation affecting processing of the ornithine aminotransferase precursor protein in gyrate atrophy. *J Biol Chem* 1989;264:17,432–17,436.
84. Itin P, Buchner S, Gloor B. Darier's disease and retinitis pigmentosa; Is there a pathogenetic relationship? *Br J Dermatol* 1988; 119:397–402.
85. Jarvela I, Santavuori P, Puhakka L, Haltia M, Peltonen L. Linkage map of the chromosome region surrounding the infantile neuronal ceroid lipofuscinosis on 1p. *Am J Med Genet* 1992;42:546–548.
86. Jarvela I, Scheulker J, Haltia M et al. Infantile form of neuronal ceroid lipofuscinosis (CLN) maps to the short arm of chromosome 1. *Genomics* 1991;9:170–173.
87. Jay M. Figures and fantasies: The frequencies of the different genetic forms of retinitis pigmentosa. *Birth Defects Orig Art Ser* 1982; 18(6):167–183.
88. Jean G, Fuchshuber A, Town M, Gribouval O, Schneider J, Broyer M et al. High resolution mapping of the gene for cystinosis: Using combined biochemical and linkage analysis. *Am J Hum Genet* 1996;58:535–543.
89. Jolly R, Martinus R, Palmer D. Sheep and other animals with ceroid-lipofuscinoses: Their relevance to Batten disease. *Am J Med Genet* 1992;42:609–614.
90. Jolly R, West D, Janmaat A, Morrison I. Ovine ceroid lipofuscinoses: A model of Batten's disease. *Neuropathol Appl Neurobiol* 1980;6: 195–209.
91. Joubert M, Eisenring J, Robb J, Andermann F. Familial agenesis of the cerebellar vermis. A syndrome of episodic hyperpnea, abnormal eye movements, ataxia, and retardation. *Neurology* 1969;19:813–825.
92. Kaiser-Kupfer M, Caruso R, Valle D. Gyrate

atrophy of the choroid and retina: Chronic reduction of ornithine slows retinal degeneration. *Arch Ophthalmol* 1991;109:1539.

93. Kaiser-Kupfer M, Gazzo M, Datiles M et al. A randomized placebo-controlled trial of cysteamine eyedrops in nephropathic cystinosis. *Arch Ophthalmol* 1990;108:689–693.
94. Kaiser-Kupfer M, Kuwabara T, Askanas V, Brody L, Takki K, Dvoretzky I et al. Systemic manifestations of gyrate atrophy of the choroid and retina. *Ophthalmology* 1981;88:302–306.
95. Kaiser-Kupfer M, Kuwabara T, Uga S et al. Cataracts in gyrate atrophy: Clinical and morphologic studies. *Invest Ophthalmol Visual Sci* 1983;24:432.
96. Kaiser-Kupfer M, Ludwig I, DeMonasteris F et al. Gyrate atrophy of the choroid and retina: Early findings. *Ophthalmology* 1985;92:394.
97. Kaplan J, Gerber S, Bonneau D, Rozet J, Delrieu O, Briard M et al. A gene for Usher syndrome type I (USH1A) maps to chromosome 14q. *Genomics* 1992;14:979–987.
98. Karjalainen S, Vartiainen E, Terasvirta M, Karja J, Kaariainen H. An unusual otological manifestation of Usher's syndrome in 4 siblings. *Adv Audiol* 1985;3:32–40.
99. Kaufman S, Wood R, Shaw B Jr, Markin R, Gridelli B, Vanderhoff J. Hepatocarcinoma in a child with the Alagille syndrome. *Am J Dis Child* 1987;141:698–700.
100. Keats B, Nouri N, Pelias M, Deininger P, Litt M. Tightly linked flanking microsatellite markers for the Usher syndrome type I locus on the short arm of chromosome 11. *Am J Hum Genet* 1994;54:681–686.
101. Kennaway N, Weleber R, Buist N. Gyrate atrophy of the choroid and retina. Deficient activity of ornithine ketoacid aminotransferase in cultured skin fibroblasts. *N Engl J Med* 1977; 297:1180.
102. Kenyon KR, Maumenee I, Green W et al. Mucolipidosis IV. Histopathology of conjunctive, cornea, and skin. *Arch Ophthalmol* 1979;97: 1106–1111.
103. Kenyon KR, Quigley H, Hussels I, Wyllie R. The systemic mucopolysaccharidoses. Ultrastructural and histochemical studies of conjunctiva and skin. *Am J Ophthalmol* 1972;73: 811–833.
104. Ketz B, Melles R, Schneider J. Glare disability in nephropathic cystinosis. *Arch Ophthalmol* 1987;105:1670–1671.
105. Kimberling W, Moller C, Davenport S et al. Linkage of Usher syndrome type I gene (USH1B) to the long arm of chromosome 11. *Genomics* 1992;14:988–994.
106. Kimberling W, Weston M, Moller C et al. Localization of Usher syndrome type II to chromosome 1q. *Genomics* 1990;7:245–249.
107. Kloepfer H, Laguaite J, McLaurin J. The hereditary syndrome of congenital deafness and retinitis pigmentosa: (Usher's syndrome). *Laryngoscope* 1966;76:850–862.
108. Koenignsmark BW, Weiner LP. The olivopontocerebellar atrophies: a review. *Medicine* 1970;49:227–242.
109. Kominami E, Ezaki J, Muno D et al. Specific storage of subunit c of mitochondrial ATP synthase in lysosomes of neuronal ceroid lipofuscinosis (Batten's disease). *J Biochem* 1992; 111:278–282.
110. Koppang N. The English Setter with ceroid lipofuscinosis: A suitable model for the juvenile type of ceroid lipofuscinosis in humans. *Am J Med Genet* 1988(suppl);5:117–125.
111. Kornzweig A, Bassen F. Retinitis pigmentosa, acanthocystosis, and heredodegenerative neuromuscular disease. *Arch Ophthalmol* 1957; 58:183.
112. Kwitek-Black A, Carmi R, Duyk G, Buetow K, Elbedour K, Parvari R et al. Linkage of Bardet-Biedl syndrome to chromosome 16q and evidence for non-allelic geneticheterogenetity. *Nature Genet* 1993;5:392–396.
113. Lamy M, Frezal J, Polonovski J, Rey J. L'absence congenitale des beta-lipoproteines. *Presse Med* 1961;69:1511.
114. Larget-Piet D, Gerber S, Bonneau D, Rozet J-M, Marc S, Ghazi I et al. Genetic heterogeneity of Usher syndrome type 1 in French families. *Genomics* 1994;21:138–143.
115. Laverda A, Saia O, Drigo P, Dnieli E, Clementi M, Tenconi R. Chorioretinal coloboma and Joubert syndrome: A nonrandom association. *J Pediatr* 1984;105:282–284.
116. Lavery M, Green W, Jabs E et al. Ocular histopathology and ultrastructure of Sanfilipo's syndrome; Type III-B. *Arch Ophthalmol* 1983; 101:1263–1274.
117. Lehmann A. Three complementation groups in Cockayne syndrome. *Mutat Res* 1982;106:347.
118. Lehmann A, Francis A, Giannelli F. Prenatal diagnosis of Cockayne syndrome. *Lancet* 1985; 1:486.
119. Leppert M, Baird L, Anderson K, Otterud B, Lupski J, Lewis R. Bardet-Biedl syndrome is linked to DNA markers on chromosome 11q and is genetically heterogeneous. *Nature Genet* 1994;7:108–112.

120. Leug L-S, Weinstein G, Hobson R. Further electroretinographic studies of patients with mucopolysaccharidoses. *Birth Defects Orig Art Ser* 1971;VII(3):32–40.
121. Lewis R, Otterund B, Stouffer D, Lalouel J-M, Leppert M. Mapping recessive ophthalmic diseases: Linkage of the locus for Usher syndrome type II to a DNA marker on chromosome 1q. *Genomics* 1990;7:250–256.
122. Libert J. Diagnosis of lysosomal storage disorders by the ultrastructural study of conjunctival biopsies. In *Pathology Annual,* S. Sommers, P. Rosen, eds. New York: Appleton-Century-Crofts, 1980:37–66.
123. Lieser M, Harms E, Kern H et al. Ganglioside GM3 sialidase activity in fibroblasts of normal individuals and of patients with sialisosis and mucolipidosis IV. Subcellular distribution and some properties. *Biochem J* 1989;260:69–74.
124. Lietman P, Frazier P, Wong V et al. Adult cystinosis: A benign disorder. *Am J Med* 1966; 40:511–517.
125. Lindhout D, Barth P, Valk J, Boen-Tan T. The Joubert syndrome associated with bilateral chorioretinal coloboma. *Eur J Pediatr* 1980; 134:173–176.
126. Loken A, Hanssen O, Halvorsen S, Jolster N. Hereditary renal dysplasia and blindness. *Acta Paediatr (Copenh)* 1961;50:177–184.
127. Luckenback M, Green W, Miller N et al. Ocular clinicopathologic correlation of Hallervorden-Spatz syndrome with acanthocytosis and pigmentary retinopathy. *Am J Ophthalmol* 1983;95:369–382.
128. Mainzer F, Saldino R, Ozonoff M, Minagi H. Familial nephropathy associated with retinitis pigmentosa, cerebellar ataxia and skeletal abnormalities. *Am J Med* 1970;49:556–562.
129. Markello T, Bernardini I, Gahl W. Improved renal function in children with cystinosis treated with cysteamine. *N Engl J Med* 1993; 328:1157.
130. McDowell G, Gahl W, Stephenson L, Schneider J, Weissenbach J, Polymeropoulos M et al. Linkage of the gene for cystinosis to markers on the short arm of chromosome 17. *Nature Genet* 1995;10:246–248.
131. Merin S, Livni N, Berman E, Yatziv S. Mucolipidosis IV: Ocular systemic, and ultrastructural findings. *Invest Ophthalmol* 1975;14: 437–448.
132. Michaud J, Héon E, Guilbert F et al. Natural history of Alström syndrome in early childhood: Onset with dilated cardiomyopathy. *J Pediatr* 1996;128:225–229.
133. Millay R, Weleber R, Heckenlively J. Ophthalmologic and systemic manifestations of Alstrom's disease. *Am J Ophthalmol* 1986;102: 482–490.
134. Mitchell G, Brody L, Looney J et al. An initiator cordon mutation in ornithine-delta-aminotransferase causing gyrate atrophy. *J Clin Invest* 1988;81:630.
135. Mitchell G, Looney D, Brody L et al. Human ornithine-delta-aminotransferase: CDNA cloning and analysis of the structural gene. *J Biol Chem* 1988;263:14288.
136. Mueller R, Pagon R, Pepin M, Haas J, Kawabori I, Stevenson J et al. Arteriohepatic dysplasia: Phenotypic features and family studies. *Clin Genet* 1984;25:323–331.
137. Muller D, Lloyd J, Bird A. Long term management of abetalipoproteinemia. Possible role for vitamin E. *Arch Dis Child* 1977;52:209.
138. Neufeld E, Muenzer J. The mucopolysaccharidoses. In *The Metabolic and Molecular Bases of Inherited Disease,* C. Scriver, A. Beaudet, W. Sly, D. Valle, eds. New York: McGraw-Hill, 1995:2465–2494.
139. Newsome D, Quinn T, Hess A et al. Cellular immune status in retinitis pigmentosa. *Ophthalmology* 1988;95:1696–1703.
140. Norio R, Raitta C, Lindahl E. Further delineation of the Cohen syndrome: Report on chorioretinal dystrophy, leukopenia and consanguinity. *Clin Genet* 1984;25:1–14.
141. Norman R, Wood N. Congenital form of amaurotic family idiocy. *J Neurol Psychiatry* 1941; 4:175–190.
142. Palmer D, Fearnley I, Walker J et al. Mitochondrial ATP synthase subunit c storage in the ceroid lipofuscinoses (Batten disease). *Am J Med Genet* 1992;42:561–567.
143. Pardo C, Rabin B, Palmer D, Price D. Accumulation of the adenosine triphosphate synthase subunit c in the mnd mutant mouse. A model for neuronal ceroid lipofuscinosis. *Am J Pathol* 1994;144:829–835.
144. Prystowsky S, Maumenee I, Freeman R, Herndon J Jr, Harrod M. A cutaneous marker in the Hunter Syndrome. *Arch Dermatol* 1977; 113:602–605.
145. Raininko R, Santavuori P, Heiskala H, Sainio K, Palo J. CT findings in neuronal ceroid lipofuscinosis. *Neuropediatrics* 1990;21:95–101.
146. Raitta C, Santavuori P. Ophthalmological findings in the infantile type of so-called neuronal ceroid-lipofuscinosis. *Acta Ophthalmol (Copenh)* 1973;51:755–763.
147. Rapola J. Neuronal ceroid lipofuscinosis in

childhood. In *Genetic Metabolic Diseases*, B. Landing, M. Haust, J. Bernstein, H. Rosenberg, eds. Basel: Karger, 1993:7–44.

148. Rapola J, Salonen R, Ammala P, Santavuori P. Prenatal diagnosis of the infantile type of neuronal ceroid lipofuscinosis by electron microscopic investigations of human chorionic villi. *Prenat Diagn* 1990;10:553–559.
149. Renieri A, Bruttini M, Galli L et al. X-linked Alport syndrome: An SSCP-based mutation survey over all 51 exons of the COL4A5 gene. *Am J Hum Genet* 1996;58:1192–1204.
150. Rider J, Rider D. Batten disease: Past; present and future. *Am J Med Genet* 1988 (suppl);5:21–26.
151. Riedel K, Zwaan J, Kenyon K, Kolodny E, Hanninen L, Albert D. Ocular abnormalities in mucolipridosis IV. *Am J Ophthalmol* 1985; 99:125–136.
152. Robb R, Dowton S, Fulton A et al. Retinal degeneration in vitamin B12 disorder associated with methylmalonic aciduria and sulfur amino acid abnormalities. *Am J Ophthalmol* 1984;97:691–696.
153. Romanchuk K, Judisch G, LaBrecque D. Ocular findings in arteriohepatic dysplasia (Alagille's syndrome). *Can J Ophthalmol* 1981; 16:94–99.
154. Roth A, Helper R, Mukoyama M et al. Pigmentary retinal dystrophy in Hallervoden-Spatz disease: Clinicopathological report of a case. *Surv Ophthalmol* 1971;16:24–35.
155. Runge P, Muller D, McAllister J et al. Oral vitamin E supplements can prevent the retinopathy of abetalipoproteinemia. *Br J Ophthalmol* 1986;70:166–173.
156. Ryan S, Knox D, Green W, Konigsmark B. Olivopontocerebellar degeneration. Clinicopathologic correlation of the associated retinopathy. *Arch Ophthalmol* 1975;93:169–172.
157. Ryan S, Smith R. Retinopathy associated with hereditary olivopontocerebellar degeneration. *Am J Ophthalmol* 1971;71:838–843.
158. Sack J, Friedman E. The Cohen syndrome in Israel. *Israel J Med Sci* 1986;22:766–770.
159. Salt H, Wolff O, Lloyd J et al. On having no beta-lipoprotein: A syndrome comprising abetalipoproteinemia; acanthocytosis; and steatorrhea. *Lancet* 1960;2:325–329.
160. Sankila E-M, Pakarinen L, Kaariainen H. Assignment of an Usher syndrome type III (USH3) gene to chromosome 3q. *Hum Mol Genet* 1995;4:93–98.
161. Santavuori P, Vanhanen S-L, Sainio K et al. New aspects in the diagnosis of NCL. *Brain Dysfun* 1991;4:211–216.
162. Saraiva J, Baraitser M. Joubert syndrome: A review. *Am J Med Genet* 1992;43:726–731.
163. Savukoski M, Kestila M, Williams R et al. Defined chromosomal assignment of CLN5 demonstrates that at least four genetic loci are involved in the pathogenesis of human ceroid lipofuscinoses. *Am J Hum Genet* 1994;55: 695–701.
164. Schimke R. Hereditary renal-retinal dysplasia. *Ann Intern Med* 1969;70:735–744.
165. Sethi K, Adams R, Loring D, El Gammal T. Hallervorden-Spatz syndrome: Clinical and magnetic resonance imaging correlations. *Ann Neurol* 1988;24:692–694.
166. Sharp D, Blinderman L, Combs K, Kienzle B, Ricci B, Wager-Smith K et al. Cloning and gene defects in microsomal triglyceride transfer protein associated with abetalipoproteinemia. *Nature* 1993;365:65–69.
167. Sheffield V, Carmi R, Kwitek-Black A, Rokhlina T, Nishimura D, Duyk G et al. Identification of a Bardet-Biedl syndrome locus on chromosome 3 and evaluation of an efficient approach to homozygosity mapping. *Hum Mol Genet* 1994;3:1331–1335.
168. Shinkawa H, Nadol J Jr. Histopathology of the inner ear in Usher's syndrome as observed by light and electron microscopy. *Ann Otol Rhinol Laryngol* 1986;95:313–318.
169. Simell O, Takki K. Raised plasma ornithine and gyrate atrophy of the choroid and retina. *Lancet* 1973;1:1031–1033.
170. Sipila I, Simell O, Rapola J et al. Gyrate atrophy of the choroid and retina with hyperornithinemia tubular aggregates and type 2 fiber atrophy in muscle. *Neurology* 1979;29:996–1005.
171. Smith R, Berlin C, Hejmancik J, Keats B, Kimberling W, Lewis R et al. Clinical diagnosis of the Usher syndromes. *Am J Med Genet* 1994;50:32–38.
172. Smith R, Lee E, Kimberling W, Daiger S et al. Localization of two genes for Usher syndrome type I to chromosome 11. *Genomics* 1992;14: 995–1002.
173. Spinner N, Rand E, Fortina P, Genin A, Taub R, Semeraro A et al. Cytologically balanced t(2;20) in a two-generation family with Alagille syndrome: Cytogenetic and molecular studies. *Am J Hum Genet* 1994;55:238–243.
174. Steinlein O, Tariverdian G, Boll H, Vogel F. Taperoretinal degeneration in brothers with apparent Cohen syndrome: Nosology with

Mirhosseini-Holmes-Walton syndrome. *Am J Med Genet* 1991;41:196–200.

175. Stoler J, Herrin J, Holmes L. Genital abnormalities in females with Bardet-Biedl syndrome. *Am J Med Genet* 1995;55:276–278.
176. Tada K, Saito T, Hayasaka S et al. Hyperonithinemia with gyrate atrophy: pathophysiology and treatment. *J Inherit Metab Dis* 1983; 6:105–106.
177. Tahvanainen E, Norio R, Karila E, Ranta S, Weissenbach J, Sistonen P et al. Cohen syndrome gene assigned to the long arm of chromosome 8 by linkage analysis. *Nature Genet* 1994;7:201–204.
178. Takki K. Gyrate atrophy of the choroid and retina associated with hyperornithinaemia. *Br J Ophthalmol* 1974;58:3–23.
179. Takki K, Milton R. The natural history of gyrate atrophy of the choroid and retina. *Ophthalmology* 1981;88:292.
180. Traboulsi E, DeBecker I, Maumenee I. Ocular findings in Cockayne syndrome. *Am J Ophthalmol* 1992;114:579–583.
181. Traboulsi E, Faris B. Crystalline retinopathy. *Ann Ophthalmol* 1987;19:156–158.
182. Traboulsi E, Green W, de la Cruz Z et al. The neuronal ceroid lipofuscinoses. Ocular histopathologic studies in the late infantile, juvenile and adult forms. *Graefes Arch Clin Exp Ophthalmol* 1987;225:391–402.
183. Traboulsi E, Maumenee I, Geraghty M, Valle D, Silva J, Green W. Ocular histopathology in the cobalamin C type of vitamin B12 defect with methylmalonic aciduria and homocystinuria. *Am J Ophthalmol* 1992;113:268–290.
184. Traboulsi E, Maumenee I, Green W et al. Olivopontocerebellar atrophy with retinal degeneration. A clinical and ocular histopathologic study. *Arch Ophthalmol* 1988;106:801–806.
185. Tyynela J, Palmer D, Baumann M, Haltia M. Storage of saposins A and D in infantile neuronal ceroid lipofuscinosis. *FEBS Lett* 1993; 330:8–12.
186. Usher C. Bowman's lecture: On a few hereditary eye affections. *Trans Ophthalmol Soc UK* 1935;55:164–245.
187. Uvebrant P, Bjork E, Conradi N et al. Successful DNA-based prenatal exclusion of juvenile neuronal ceroid lipofuscinosis. *Prenat Diagn* 1993;13:651–657.
188. Valle D, Simell O. The hyperonithinemias. In *The Metabolic and Molecular Bases of Inherited Diseases,* C. Scriver, A. Beaudet, W. Sly, D. Valle, eds. New York: McGraw-Hill, 1995: 1147–1185.
189. Valle D, Walser M, Brusilow S, Kaiser-Kupfer M. Gyrate atrophy of the choroid and retina. Amino acid metabolism and correction of hyperonithinemia with an arginine-deficient diet. *J Clin Invest* 1980;65:371–378.
190. van der Pol B, Planten J. A non-metastatic remote effect of lung carcinoma. *Doc Ophthalmol* 1987;67:89–94.
191. Venema J, Mullenders L, Natarajan A, Van Zeeland A, Mayne L. The genetic defect in Cockayne syndrome is associated with a defect in repair of UV-induced DNA damage in transcriptionally active DNA. *Proc Natl Acad Sci USA* 1990;87:4707.
192. Vesa J, Hallsten E, Verkruyse L et al. Mutations in the palmitoyl protein thioesterase gene causing infantile neuronal ceroid lipofuscinosis. *Nature* 1995;376:584–588.
193. Warburg M, Pedersen S, Hertwyk H. The Cohen syndrome: Retinal lesions and granulocytopenia. *Ophthalmic Paediatr Genet* 1990; 11:7–13.
194. Weil D, Blanchard S, Kaplan J et al. Defective myosin VIIA gene responsible for Usher syndrome type 1B. *Nature* 1995;374:60–61.
195. Welch R. Bietti's tapetoretinal degeneration with marginal corneal dystrophy: Crystalline retinopathy. *Trans Am Ophthalmol Soc* 1977; 75:164–175.
196. Weleber R, Kennaway N, Buist N. Vitamin B6 in the management of gyrate atrophy of the choroid and retina. *Lancet* 1978;2:1213.
197. Wetterau J, Aggerbeck L, Bouma M-E, Eisenberg C, Munck A, Hermier M et al. Absence of microsomal triglyceride transfer protein in individuals with abetalipoproteinemia. *Science* 1992;258:999–1001.
198. Willams R, Vesa J, Jarvela I et al. Genetic heterogeneity in neuronal ceroid lipofuscinosis (NCL): Evidence that the late-infantile subtype (Jansky-Bielchowsky disease; CLN2) is not an alleic form of the juvenile or infantile subtypes. *Am J Hum Genet* 1993;53: 931–935.
199. Wilson D, Jelley D, Stratton R et al. Nephropathic cystinosis: improved linear growth after treatment with recombinant human growth hormone. *J Pediatr* 1989;115:758–761.
200. Wilson D, Weleber RG, Klein M, Welch R, Green W. Bietti's crystalline dystrophy: A clinicopathologic correlative study. *Arch Ophthalmol* 1989;107:213–221.
201. Wilson D, Weleber R, Beals R. Retinal dystrophy in Jeune's syndrome. *Arch Ophthalmol* 1987;105:651–657.

202. Wilson D, Weleber R, Green W. Ocular clinicopathologic study of gyrate atrophy. *Am J Ophthalmol* 1991;111:24–33.
203. Wong V, Kuwabara T, Brubaker R et al. Intralysosomal cystine crystal in cystinosis. *Invest Ophthalmol Visual Sci* 1970;9:83–88.
204. Wong V, Lietman P, Seegmiller J. Alterations of pigment epithelium in cystinosis. *Arch Ophthalmol* 1967;77:369.
205. Zeman W, Dyken P. Neuronal ceroid lipofuscinosis (Batten's disease): Relationship to amaurotic family idiocy? *Pediatrics* 1969;44: 570–583.

33

Peroxisomal Disorders

RICHARD G. WELEBER

Peroxisomes are subcellular single-membrane-bound organelles (measuring 0.1–1.0 μm in diameter) that are present in almost all eukaryotic cells. They were first described in mouse kidney cells by Rhodin[110] in 1954 as small organelles filled with a homogeneous, moderately electron-dense matrix. Because of their nondescript appearance, they were first called microbodies. Peroxisomes were characterized biochemically in 1960 by de Duve et al.,[29] who found them to contain catalase, hydrolases, and oxidases. de Duve and Baudhuin[28] were the first to propose the name peroxisome because the reactions within these microbodies consumed and produced hydrogen peroxide. Peroxisomes, thus, appeared to be specialized organelles for oxidative reactions that use molecular oxygen.[28]

BIOGENESIS OF PEROXISOMES

The half-life of peroxisomes has been estimated to be 1.5–2.0 days. Peroxisomal proteins are synthesized in free polysomes and are imported into preexisting peroxisomes, which then bud or divide.

The proteins are targeted for import into peroxisomes by *cis*-acting peroxisomal targeting signals (PTSs).[48,92,131,134] PTS1, a tripeptide of the sequence Ser-Lys/His-Leu (the so-called SKL motif), is located at the carboxy-terminus and is involved in the import of a number of peroxisomal enzymes, including catalase, hydratase:dehydrogenase, D-amino acid oxidase, and acylcoenzyme A (acyl-CoA) oxidase.[48] Defects in the PTS1 receptor gene *PXR1* have been reported in two patients with a neonatal adrenoleukodystrophy (NALD) phenotype. PTS1 defects define complementation group 2 of peroxisome biogenesis disorders.[31,125] PTS2 is a string of about 11 amino acids at or near the amino-terminal end of the peptide in a presequence that is eventually proteolytically cleaved after the peptide enters the peroxisomes.[131,134] PTS2 directs the import of 3-ketoacyl CoA thiolase, alkyl-dihydroxyacetonephosphate synthase, and phytanoyl-CoA α-hydroxylase into peroxisomes.[29a,79b,134] Loss of PTS2 import is the cause of the most common form of rhizomelic chondrodysplasia punctata.[92a,125]

From an evolutionary perspective, peroxisomes are considered to be endosymbiants similar to mitochondria and chloroplasts. This may account for the primitive nature of many of the peroxisomal biochemical reactions.

FUNCTIONS OF PEROXISOMES

Close to 50 biochemical reactions have been identified that take place in whole or in part within peroxisomes.[131,142] The catabolic reactions do not generate ATP but produce heat and may play a role in thermogenesis. Disorders of peroxisomal biogenesis usually result in severe deficiency of many of these reactions.

Anabolic Reactions

Biosynthesis of Bile Acids

Di- and trihydroxycoprostanoic acid are converted within peroxisomes to cholic acid. Hence, peroxisomal disorders are often associated with elevation of serum bile acids.

Biosynthesis of Ether-Phospholipids (Plasmalogens and Alkyl-Glycerides)

Plasmalogens, which are unsaturated long-chain alcohols in vinyl ether linkage to the glycerol backbone of a phospholipid (Fig. 33.1), account for 5%–20% of phospholipids in most mammalian cell membranes and constitute about one-third of phospholipids in the brain. Certain classes of phospholipids contain high proportions of plasmalogens. Plasmalogens constitute 80%–90% of the ethanolamine class of phospholipids in myelin. Platelet-activating factor also represents an ether lipid, but it is unknown whether deficiency of this factor plays a role in the bleeding tendency that has been reported in some disorders of peroxisomal biogenesis. The first two steps of plasmalogen synthesis from dihydroxyacetonephosphate occur exclusively in peroxisomes. The rest of the reactions occur in the endoplasmic reticulum.

The major peroxisomal enzymes involved in synthesis of ether-phospholipids are dihydroxyacetonephosphate acyltransferase (DHAP-AT) and alkyl-dihydroxyacetonephosphate synthase (alkyl-DHAP synthase). Plasmalogens are deficient in plasma and tissues of virtually all patients with disorders of peroxisomal biogenesis, particularly those with rhizomelic chondrodysplasia punctata.

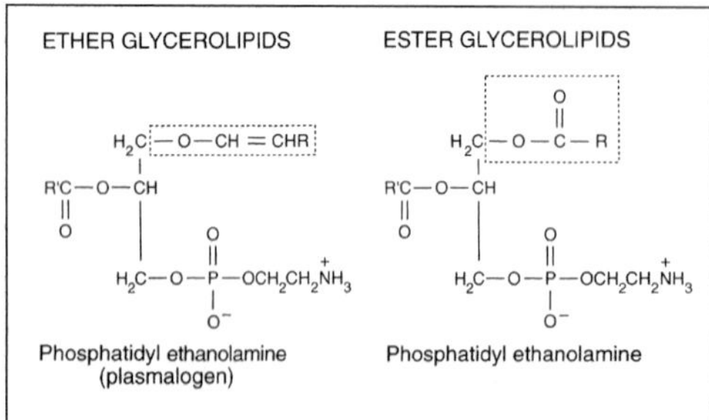

Figure 33.1. Structure of ether-linked glycerolipids (plasmalogens) and the more common ester-linked glycerolipids. (Modified from Moser,[83] with permission.)

Biosynthesis of Cholesterol

Peroxisomes contain several enzymes involved in cholesterol synthesis and may be required for maintenance of normal cholesterol levels.[7,57,67] Hydroxymethylglutaryl-CoA reductase, the primary enzyme involved in cholesterol biosynthesis, is located in the endoplasmic reticulum and can also be induced in peroxisomes by cholestyramine. Peroxisomes can convert mevalonic acid to cholesterol.[67] Mevalonate kinase is localized to peroxisomes and is deficient in disorders of peroxisomal biogenesis.[7] Mevalonic aciduria, manifested clinically by failure to thrive, anemia, gastroenteropathy, hepatosplenomegaly, psychomotor retardation, hypotonia, ataxia, cataract, and dysmorphic features, may be classified as a disorder of a single peroxisomal function—that of mevalonate kinase.[7]

Biosynthesis of Docosahexaenoic Acid

The levels of docosahexaenoic acid (DHA) are reduced in multiple tissues of patients with disorders of peroxisomal biogenesis.[75,76] Although suggested to be the result of a deficiency of Δ_4 desaturase,[75] there is evidence that the decreased DHA levels are due to deficient β-oxidation of a 24-carbon intermediate[146] or possibly to coexistent liver disease.[69] The significance of decreased levels of DHA and the biochemical origin of the defect in these patients remain unknown.

Catabolic Reactions

Hydrogen Peroxide (H_2O_2)-Based Cellular Respiration

Peroxisomes contain enzymes that consume molecular oxygen and produce hydrogen peroxide. Peroxisomal oxidases can have as their substrates D- and L-amino acids, L-α-hydroxy acids, glutaryl-CoA, oxalate, CoA derivatives, and polyamines. The hydrogen peroxide that is produced can be converted to oxygen and water by catalase or by peroxidation to form water. Many compounds, including ethanol, methanol, nitrites, quinones, and formate, can be substrates for peroxisomal-based peroxidation. Peroxisomal respiration accounts for approximately 20% of oxygen consumption by the liver.[28] Thus, one very important function of peroxisomes is to compartmentalize H_2O_2-generating reactions within the organelle and thus protect cells against oxidative damage.

Peroxisomal β-Oxidation, Including Catabolism of Very-Long-Chain Fatty Acids

One of the most important reactions that takes place within peroxisomes is the β-oxidation of fatty acids, particularly very-long-chain fatty acids (VLCFAs) (Fig. 33.2). Peroxisomal β-oxidation is not merely a duplication of mitochondrial β-oxidation. Peroxisomal β-oxidation occurs in all animals, in plants, and in unicellular eukaryotes, whereas mitochondrial β-oxidation appears to take place only in animals. The substrates for peroxisomal β-oxidation include VLCFAs, long-chain fatty acids (LCFAs), polyunsaturated fatty acids, dicarboxylic fatty acids, prostaglandins, and the side chain of cholesterol. A carnitine acyl transferase carrier system is needed for entry of fatty acids into mitochondria in preparation for mitochondrial β-oxidation, whereas peroxisomes do not require carnitine for entry of fatty acids but utilize carnitine to facilitate the exit of shortened reaction products. Mitochondrial β-oxidation is capable of handling fatty acids up to only 18 carbons long (C18) and can generate adenosine triphosphate (ATP). Peroxisomes have essentially no activity below C8 but are the only organelles that can oxidize VLCFAs of C24 to C26.

The fatty acid activation that is required for initiation of β-oxidation in peroxisomes occurs through the action of two membrane-bound acyl-CoA ligases or synthetases, one for chain lengths of 12 carbons or more, and another exclusively for 24 carbons or more (as will be explained later, it is the latter enzyme that is deficient in X-linked adrenoleukodystrophy).

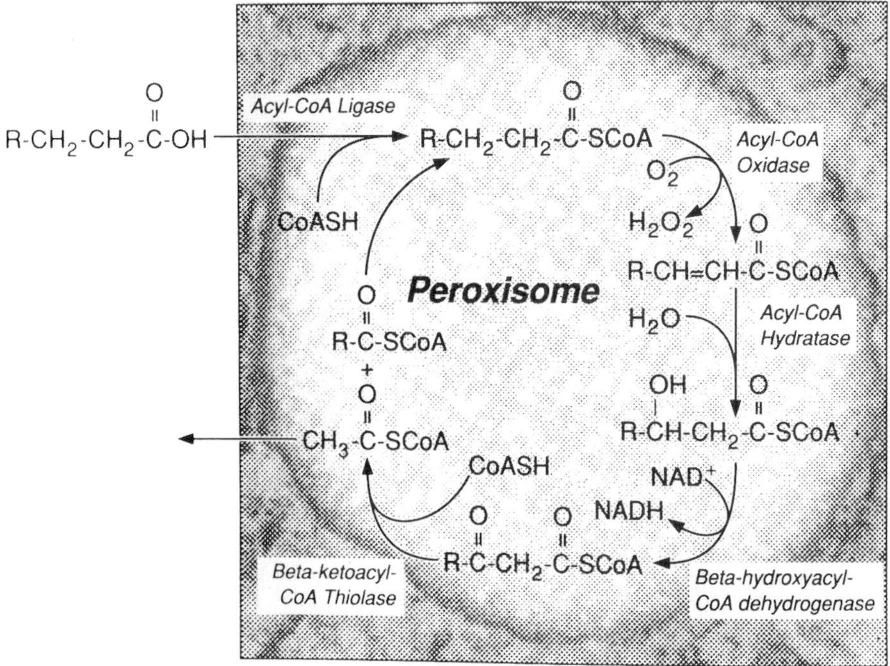

Figure 33.2. β-Oxidation pathways within peroxisomes. The acylcoenzyme A (acyl-CoA) hydratase and β-hydroxyacyl-CoA dehydrogenase steps are catalyzed by different domains of the peroxisomal bifunctional protein. (From Folz and Trobe,[38] with permission.)

Rather than using acyl-CoA dehydrogenase, as is the case for mitochondria, the first stage of β-oxidation in peroxisomes takes place by two acyl-CoA oxidases: one a branched-chain oxidase for activated pristanic acid and di- and trihydroxycholestanoic acid, and the other is a separate oxidase for activated LCFAs and VLCFAs.

By a series of successive steps of dehydrogenation, hydration, dehydrogenation, and thiolytic cleavage, peroxisomal β-oxidation shortens the fatty acid chains by two carbon fragments in the form of acetyl-CoA until the carbon chain is suitable for further β-oxidation within mitochondria and eventual entry into the tricarboxylic acid cycle for generation of ATP. Whereas in mitochondria separate enzymes are used for the hydration and dehydrogenation steps, these reactions in peroxisomes are catalyzed by a single enzyme, known as peroxisomal bifunctional protein (this protein, which is sometimes called trifunctional protein, also has a third enzymatic role, that of 3/2-enoyl CoA isomerase, which is needed for oxidation of unsaturated fatty acids).

Peroxisomal β-oxidation may also play an important role in the regulation of oxidation of LCFAs. Mitochondrial β-oxidation is capable of being induced to, at most, only a twofold increase in activity. Peroxisomal β-oxidation, on the other hand, is capable of increasing up to 15- to 20-fold in activity in response to a fatty diet, starvation, cold, increases in intracellular ATP concentrations, and certain chemicals. There is no electron transport chain, no citric acid cycle, and no phosphorylation within peroxisomes. Peroxisomal β-oxidation, thus, may be of importance in the supply of acetyl CoA for anabolic reactions during times when energy stores are high. Plasma VLCFAs are elevated in all disorders of peroxisomal biogenesis and also in X-linked adrenoleukodystrophy but not in rhizomelic chondrodysplasia punctata.

Catabolism of Pipecolic Acid

Pipecolic acid is an intermediate in the degradation of L-lysine and is oxidized further to α-aminoadipic acid. This pathway may be extremely important for the catabolism of lysine in the brain.[19,20] L-pipecolate oxidase is absent in Zellweger syndrome. Blood levels of pipecolic acid are usually elevated in disorders of peroxisomal biogenesis. Measurements of serum levels of pipecolic acid were often used as an initial test for these diseases. The greater availability and decreasing cost of the determination of plasma levels of VLCFAs have led clinicians to order this more specific screening test.

Catabolism of Prostaglandins

Prostaglandins (notably leukotrienes) are degraded within peroxisomes by a process of β-oxidation from the ω-end.[61] In disorders of peroxisomal biogenesis, leukotrienes persist within tissues and may contribute to the promotion of inflammation.[79] Such inflammation may produce edema, vascular leakage, mucus secretion, and muscular contraction.

Catabolism of Dicarboxylic Acids (Omega-Oxidation Products)

Certain medium and long-chain dicarboxylic acids (especially C8 and C10) are preferentially catabolized by ω-oxidation within microsomes, followed by β-oxidation within peroxisomes. Patients with Zellweger syndrome and NALD have elevated urinary concentrations of medium-chain-length dicarboxylic acids. This aciduria is of limited diagnostic value and of little clinical significance.

Catabolism of Phytanic Acid

Phytanic acid is a fully saturated, branched-chain, 20-carbon fatty acid that is normally present in trace amounts in blood and tissues. Phytanic acid is not synthesized in the body and is ingested in the diet in animal fats and dairy products or as its precursor phytol, which can be readily converted to phytanic acid. Plant phytol (principally as chlorophyll) is poorly absorbed and is not a significant dietary source of free or unbound phytol.[130]

Because of the presence of a methyl group at the third carbon position, phytanic acid cannot undergo β-oxidation. Instead, phytanic acid is broken down exclusively by α-oxidation to pristanic acid, followed by subsequent steps of β-oxidation. The α-oxidation of phytanic acid occurs in two stages: (*1*) hydroxylation at the α position followed by (*2*) decarboxylation to yield the $n - 1$ carbon pristanic acid. The first stage, that of formation of α-hydroxyphytanic acid, is deficient in Refsum disease,[130] and the second stage, that of decarboxylation of α-hydroxyphytanic acid to pristanic acid, appears to be deficient in one form of rhizomelic chondrodysplasia punctata (RCDP).[136] Cells from patients with RCDP and Refsum disease will complement one another for the defects in α-oxidation of phytanic acid that are present separately in each.[100]

Serum levels of phytanic acid are often mildly elevated in disorders of peroxisomal biogenesis leading to the use of plasma phytanic acid levels as a screening test for these disorders. However, because its elevation is age dependent, and because it is usually normal in the neonatal period, measurement of phytanic acid levels is not a good screening test for peroxisomal disorders. Phytanic acid α-oxidation is impaired equally in disorders of peroxisomal biogenesis and in adult Refsum disease. At one time, phytanic acid was incorrectly thought to be metabolized in humans only within mitochondria, as it is in rat liver.[154] Because pristanic acid is markedly elevated in disorders of peroxisomal biogenesis, the elevation of phytanic acid in peroxisome deficiency syndromes was suggested to be from a block in the peroxisomal β-oxidation of pristanic acid, the $n - 1$ product of phytanic acid α-oxidation, by deficient pristanoyl-CoA oxidase activity.[104,149] However, Singh and co-workers[123] have shown that differences exist between human and lower species, with 20 times greater peroxisomal than mitochondrial oxidation of phytanic acid in humans. Thus, in humans, phytanic acid α-oxidation to pristanic acid as well as subsequent β-oxidation of pristanic acid, takes place predominantly in peroxisomes. The enzyme that is deficient in Refsum's disease has been shown to be phytanoyl-CoA α-hydroxylase.[60a] This enzyme uses the PST2 signal peptide sequence for transport into peroxisomes.[79b] Mutations within the gene *PAHX*, which encodes the enzyme phytanoyl-CoA α-hydroxylase, have been detected in patients with classic Refsum's disease.[60b,79b]

Catabolism of Polyamines

Spermine and spermidine are catabolized within peroxisomes by polyamine oxidase, producing putrescine, 3-aminopropionaldehyde, and hydrogen peroxide.[58]

Glycolate and Glyoxylate Metabolism

In plants, the enzymes of the glyoxylate cycle are contained within a subclass of peroxisomes called glyoxisomes. Leaf microbodies or peroxisomes have additional enzyme systems involving glycolate and glycerate. These systems are part of the oxidative photosynthetic carbon cycle of photorespiration in plants.[26,55] Many of the enzymes localized to plant peroxisomes have not been detected in mammals. Oxalate appears to serve no useful purpose in mammals and, in general, is regarded as a toxic product of metabolism of sugars and amino acids, particularly glycine. Glycine and glycolate are the immediate precursors of glyoxylate, which is also highly reactive and toxic to animals. Glycine is converted by oxidative deamination to glyoxylate by peroxisomal D-amino acid oxidase, whereas glycolate is oxidized to glyoxylate (and can be further oxidized to oxalate) by peroxisomal L-2-hydroxy acid oxidase A, with both reactions producing H_2O_2 as a byproduct.

The major enzyme that catalyzes a reaction for the detoxification of glyoxylate appears to be hepatic peroxisomal alanine:glyoxylate aminotransferase (AGT), which, in converting glyoxylate back to glycine, changes alanine to pyruvate. AGT has pyridoxal phosphate as its cofactor and is deficient in primary hyperoxaluria type 1. The exact source of the glycolate and glyoxylate that accumulate in tissues of patients with type 1 hyperoxaluria and that would have been converted to glycine by AGT is currently unclear.

PEROXISOMAL DISORDERS

The unraveling of the molecular genetics of peroxisomal disorders has been extremely valuable in the formation of a classification system based on the defective genes. This will allow unambiguous carrier detection, prenatal diagnosis, more precise definition of the natural history of the various diseases, and will form the cornerstone for the early identification of patients for treatment trials by metabolic intervention or gene therapy.

The molecular answers to the cause of certain peroxisomal disease phenotypes are already creating results that may have been anticipated by complementation studies but that are quite remarkable all the same. For example, one form of Zellweger syndrome and one form of NALD can each be caused by separate mutations of the same gene, *PXR1,* which codes for the first of a series of peroxisomal targeting signal receptor proteins (PTS1).[31] This phenomenon of disparate phenotypes being caused by separate mutations within the same gene has been noted with other genetic disorders. Mutations within the rhodopsin gene can cause autosomal dominant retinitis pigmentosa, autosomal recessive retinitis pigmentosa, and autosomal recessive congenital stationary night blindness (for review see Daiger et al.[23]). Mutations of the peripherin/*RDS* gene can cause several different ocular phenotypes, including peripheral retinal degeneration identical to retinitis pigmentosa, cone-rod retinal degeneration, retinitis punctata albescens, Stargardt disease or fundus flavimaculatus, either central or diffuse choroidal atrophy, several variations on pattern macular dystrophy, and even aging macular degeneration.[36,37,47,60,64,66,96,156,160] Different phenotypes have even been reported within the same family.[47,156] Some of the differences in phenotypes may relate to the way the gene mutations influence specific domains or functions of the gene product or to the way the initial mutated gene (or its product) interacts with other genes (or their products). In one instance, digenic inheritance of mutations of both peripherin/*RDS* and *ROM1* genes has been associated with phenotypic expression of retinitis pigmentosa.[63]

Despite these advances in the understanding of the molecular biology of peroxisomal disorders, recognition and identification of the various clinical phenotypes or syndromes remain the cornerstone for the correct use of the information already collected on the biochemical diagnosis, natural history, and subsequent morbidity for these diseases. Accordingly, the following is a classification of peroxisomal diseases based to a large part on clinical and biochemical findings, but including information on complementation studies and peroxisomal import protein defects.[40,81] Eventually, classification systems will evolve and will take into account specific genetic defects.

Peroxisomal disorders can be divided into disorders of peroxisomal assembly or biogenesis and disorders of single peroxisomal proteins. Table 33.1 lists the known peroxisomal disorders by these two categories.

Table 33.1. Classification of Peroxisomal Disorders*

Disorder	Enzyme Defect
Deficiencies of Peroxisomal Assembly	
Zellweger syndrome	Generalized
Neonatal adrenoleukodystrophy	Generalized
Infantile Refsum disease	Generalized
Zellweger-like syndrome	VLCFA oxidation, THCA oxidation, DHAP-AT, phytanic acid oxidation
Rhizomelic chondrodysplasia punctata (classical and atypical phenotypes)	DHAP-AT, alkyl-DHAP synthase, phytanic acid oxidase, unprocessed peroxisomal thiolase
Deficiencies of Single Peroxisomal Enzymes	
Rhizomelic chondrodysplasia punctata†	Isolated DHAP-AT or alkyl-DHAP synthase
X-linked adrenoleukodystrophy	VLCFA-CoA synthetase transport
Pseudo-neonatal adrenoleukodystrophy†	Acyl-CoA oxidase
Bifunctional enzyme deficiency†	Bi(tri)functional enzyme
Pseudo-Zellweger syndrome†	Peroxisomal thiolase
Classical Refsum disease	Phytanic acid oxidase
Hyperoxaluria type 1	Alanine:glyoxylate aminotransferase
Acatalasemia	Catalase

* DHAP = dihydroxyacetonephosphate; DHAP-AT = dihydroxyacetonephosphate acyltransferase; VLCFA = very-long-chain fatty acids; THCA = trihydroxylcholestanoyl. (After Fournier et al.[40] and Moser et al.[81])

† Disorders in which clinical manifestations resemble those of the group with deficiencies of peroxisome assembly.

Disorders of Peroxisomal Biogenesis

In 1964, Bowen et al.[10] described a malformation syndrome in two pairs of sibs that was characterized by severe hypotonia, prominent high forehead, large anterior fontanelle, hypoplasia of the midface, glaucoma, cloudy corneas, cataracts, multiple joint contractures, hepatomegaly, chondrodysplasia punctata, and cysts of the kidneys. Smith et al.[127] in 1965 reported two siblings who probably had the same syndrome. Passarge and McAdams[99] in 1967 reported five additional cases and introduced the term cerebro-hepato-renal syndrome. Opitz et al.[98] reviewed the syndrome in 1969 and proposed the name Zellweger syndrome (ZS) in honor of Hans Zellweger, who had played a major role in the early recognition of the disorder.

In 1973, Goldfischer et al.[46] found peroxisomes to be lacking in the liver and kidneys of patients with ZS. Versmold et al.[145] in 1977 reported that peroxisomes were absent in ZS patients. The first demonstration of a biochemical abnormality in ZS was the finding of an excess of pipecolic acid by Danks et al.[24] The finding in ZS patients of defective bile acid synthesis by Hanson et al.[52] in 1979, the demonstration of excess of VLCFAs by Brown et al.[13] in 1982 and Moser et al.[82] in 1984, and the recognition of the deficiency of the first two steps of plasmalogen synthesis by Heymans et al.,[54] Datta et al.,[27] and Schutgens et al.[114] in 1983–1984 strengthened the appreciation that ZS was a metabolic disorder. Finally, between 1984 and 1987, degradation of VLCFAs was found to be deficient in patients with ZS, defining one of the hallmark biochemical findings in this class of disorders.[121,122]

Opitz[97] emphasized the importance of the reassignment of ZS from a static nonmetabolic malformation syndrome to the metabolic dysplasia-malformation category. Rather than a simple semantic change, the very name "Zellweger syndrome" became equated with a whole new class of genetic disease—the disorders of peroxisome biogenesis.[68]

Additional disorders have been found to be associated with a deficiency of multiple peroxisomal functions in association with absent peroxisomes. These include NALD,[65] infantile Refsum disease (IRD),[102] hyperpipecolic acidemia,[44] and one type of complicated Leber's congenital amaurosis.[33] RCDP is a disease in which patients are deficient in more than one peroxisomal function and has recently been shown also to be a disorder of peroxisomal biogenesis.[92,106,125]

The three characteristics of disorders of peroxisomal assembly or biogenesis are (*1*) decreased size or number of peroxisomes in cells, (*2*) catalase activity detected within the cytosol rather than within peroxisomes where it normally resides, and (*3*) deficient activity of multiple peroxisomal enzyme systems leading to decreased levels of plasmalogens and increased levels of bile acid precursors, phytanic acid, pipecolic acid, and VLCFAs. Even when peroxisomes appear absent or deficient, ghost peroxisomes lacking in imported proteins are present in many people with these disorders.

Table 33.2 summarizes the major clinical findings of 173 patients with the clinical and biochemical manifestations of disorders of peroxisomal biogenesis and compares their occurrence in these and other selected peroxisomal diseases.[81] The great majority of patients had the phenotypes of ZS, NALD, IRD, or RCDP. However, 10 of the 173 had unusually mild clinical manifestations with survival into the fifth decade or had congenital cataracts as the only abnormality.

Except for patients with the RCDP phenotype and possibly those with isolated thiolase deficiency, all children with disorders of peroxisomal assembly who survive long enough, develop a retinal degeneration. Without a normal electroretinogram (ERG), the absence of ophthalmoscopic abnormalities in infancy cannot exclude significant retinal dysfunction that, with time, would be associated with a pigmentary retinopathy.

Cerebro-Hepato-Renal (Zellweger) Syndrome (MIM 214100)

The major features of this disease include a characteristic facial appearance (Fig. 33.3), deformations of the extremities and joints, abnormal cartilage calcification, hypotonia, seizures, profound psychomotor retardation, hepato-

Table 33.2. Clinical Features of Disorders of Peroxisome Assembly and Their Occurrence in Selected Peroxisomal Disorders*

Feature	ZS	NALD	IRD	Oxidase Deficiency	Bifunctional Enzyme Deficiency	Thiolase Deficiency	RCDP	DHAP Synthase Deficiency	DHAP-AT Deficiency
Average age at death or last follow-up (years)	0.76	2.2	6.4	4.0	0.75	0.9	1.0	0.5	?
Facial dysmorphism	++	+	+	0	73%	+	++	++	++
Cataract	80%	45%	7%	0	±	0	72%	+	+
Retinopathy	71%	82%	100%	2+	2+	0†	0	0†	0†
Impaired hearing	100%	100%	93%	2+	?	?	71%	33%	100%
Psychomotor delay	4+	3–4+	3+	2+	4+	4+	4+	4+	?
Hypotonia	99%	82%	52%	+	4+	+	±	±	?
Neonatal seizures	80%	82%	20%	50%	93%	+	±	?	?
Large liver	100%	79%	83%	0	+	+	0	?	
Renal cysts	93%	0	0	0	0	+	0	0	0
Rhizomelia	3%	0	0	0	0	0	93%	+	+
Chondrodysplasia punctata	69%	0	0	0	0	0	100%	+	+
Neuronal migration defect	67%	20%	±	?	88%	+	±	?	?
Coronal vertebral cleft	0	0	0	0	0	0	+	+	+
Demyelination	22%	50%	0	60%	75%	±	0	0	0

* Data are from patients tested at the Kennedy Krieger Institute, Baltimore, MD, as reported by Moser et al.[81] ZS = Zellweger syndrome; NALD = neonatal adrenoleukodystrophy; IRD = infantile Refsum disease; RCDP = rhizomelic chondrodysplasia punctata; DHAP = dihydroxyacetonephosphate; DHAP-AT = dihydroxyacetonephosphate alkyltransferase; % = percentage of patients in whom the feature is present; 0 = feature absent; ± to 4+ = degree to which a feature is present; † = electroretinography not reported.

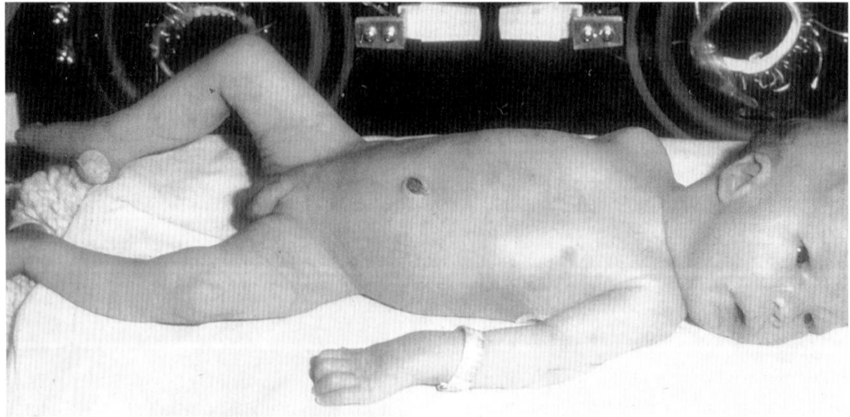

Figure 33.3. *A*: Infant with Zellweger syndrome. Note generalized hypotonia. (Figure continued on facing page.)

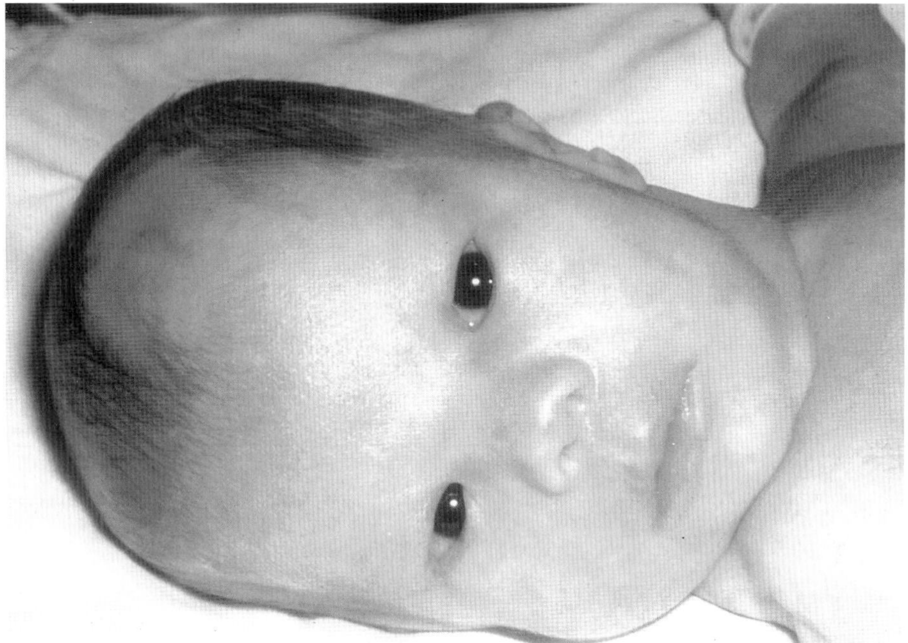

Figure 33.3. *B*: Characteristic facial appearance with large high forehead of Zellweger syndrome.

megaly, hepatic fibrosis, and renal cortical cysts. Histologic examination of the brain shows abnormal neuronal migration and cerebral dysgenesis. The major findings that tend to support the diagnosis of ZS over other disorders of peroxisomal biogenesis are cartilage calcification, the severity of dysmorphic features, congenital deformations of joints from intrauterine hypotonia, and renal cysts. Most patients die within months of birth. Seventy-nine of 90 patients in one survery died at an average age of 12.5 weeks.[161]

Ocular findings include upslanting palpebral fissures, epicanthal folds, cataracts (Fig. 33.4), glaucoma, corneal clouding, retinal degeneration, nonrecordable ERG, and optic atrophy.[41,56] Peroxisomes are absent in liver cells and decreased in fibroblasts. Serum levels of VLCFAs, pipecolic acid, phytanic acid, pristanic acid, and bile acid precursors are elevated. Plasmalogen levels are severely reduced. Abnormalities in plasma levels of phytanic acid and plasmalogens are age dependent and these compounds may be absent in older infants.[69] Urinary excretion of metabolites of leukotrienes are more than tenfold elevated in ZS patients than in normals.[79] Defective catabolism of these mediators of inflammation may play an important role in the pathogenesis of ZS and related syndromes.

At least one form of ZS results from a defect in the import of matrix proteins into peroxisomes. Mutations of the PTS1 receptor gene (PXR1) define this complementation group 2 of disorders of peroxisomal biogenesis, which includes one form of ZS and one form of NALD.[31]

Other cases of ZS are due to defects in other genes. One form, ZWS3 (MIM 170993), is associated with a defect of peroxisomal membrane protein 35K, also called PMP35, PXMP3, peroxisomal assembly factor-1, or PAF1.[119] Cataracts and pigmentary retinopathy are features of this type of ZS.

Neonatal Adrenoleukodystrophy (MIM 202370)

This autosomal recessive disorder was described by Ulrich et al.[141] in 1978 and by Benke et al.[4] in 1981. Kelley et al.[65] reported eight cases and compared the findings to ZS. Chil-

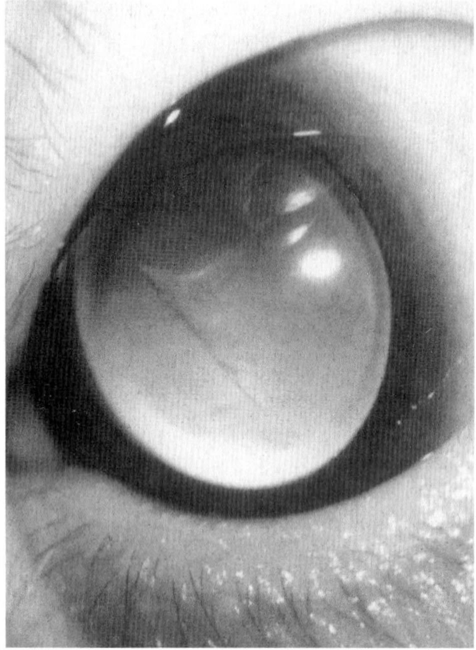

A

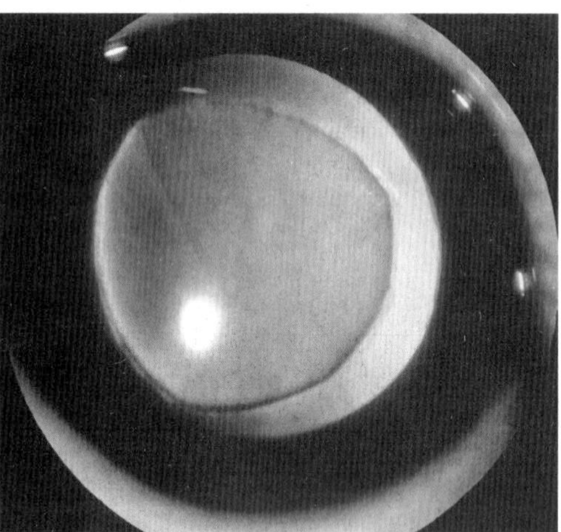

B

Figure 33.4. Typical stellate cataract (*A*), and more extensive cataract (*B*), in two patients with Zellweger syndrome. (Courtesy of Dr. Andrew Q. McCormick, Children's Hospital, Vancouver, BC.)

dren with NALD are less dysmorpic than those with ZS. They have severe hypotonia, profound retardation, progressive neurodevelopmental deterioration, seizures, demyelination of the brain, abnormal neuronal migration, polymicrogyria, and adrenal atrophy. The major findings that help distinguish NALD from ZS are the extent of central nervous system demyelination and the absence of chondrodysplasia punctata and renal cysts. Patients with NALD live longer than those with ZS (in the Kennedy Institute series, the mean age at death was 15 ± 31 months, $n = 16$ for NALD versus 5.7 ± 6.8 months, $n = 50$ for ZS).[68]

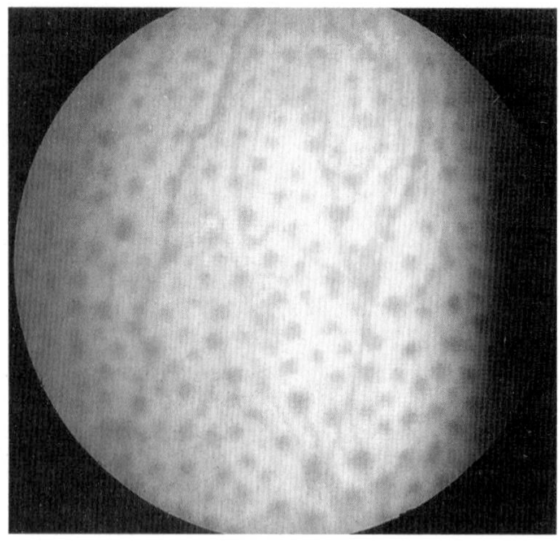

Figure 33.5. Fundus appearance of a child with neonatal adrenoleukodystrophy showing the "leopard spot" pigmentary retinopathy that can be seen in the first year or two of life in patients with generalized disorders of peroxisomal biogenesis. This same appearance also has been seen in infants with infantile Refsum disease. (Courtesy of Dr. Andrew Q. McCormick, Children's Hospital, Vancouver, BC.)

Ocular findings in NALD include esotropia, epicanthal folds, abnormal retinal pigmentation, cataracts, and optic atrophy.[22] Patches of whitish retina in the mid-peripheral retina called "leopard spots" can occur during the first year or two of life but later fade (Fig. 33.5). This flecked retinal appearance can also be seen in IRD (unpublished observations) and in peroxisomal bifunctional enzyme complex deficiency.[1,34] The ERG in NALD is nonrecordable.[38]

Peroxisomes are decreased in size and number. Plasmalogen levels are severely decreased and the peroxisomal enzymes of plasmalogen synthesis are deficient. VLCFAs, phytanic acid, pipecolic acid, and bile precursors are elevated in blood.

At least one form of NALD as well as one form of ZS are caused by mutation of the PTS1 receptor gene (*PXR1*).[31]

Infantile Refsum Disease (Infantile Phytanic Acid Storage Disease) (MIM 266510)

This autosomal recessive disorder was characterized by Scotto and co-workers[115] in 1982. Mild elevation of phytanic acid led earlier investigators to call the disorder infantile phytanic acid storage disease, but the current preferred name is infantile Refsum disease (IRD).[103,105] Craniofacial and systemic malformations (epicanthal folds, low-set ears, and single palmar creases) are present (Fig. 33.6) but are less severe than those in patients with the ZS.[15] Other features include severe hypotonia, profound psychomotor retardation, hepatomegaly, liver dysfunction, anosmia, and severe progressive neurosensory deafness that usually

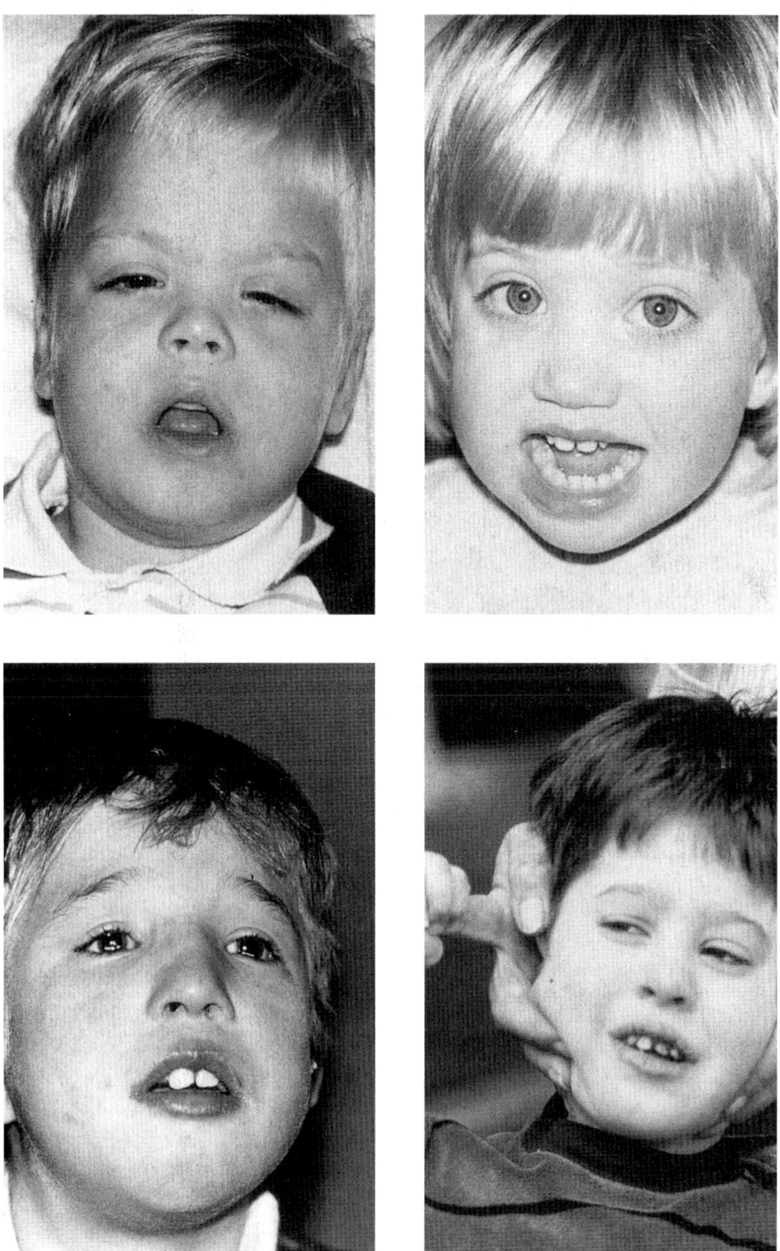

Figure 33.6. Facial appearance of four children with infantile Refsum disease. (From Budden et al.,[15] with permission.)

starts at about 6 months of age. Neonatal bleeding episodes, including intracranial hemorrhage, have been associated with low serum levels of vitamin K.[15] Bilamellar sheetlike structures (Fig. 33.7), presumably representing abnormal storage of phytols or lipid material, have been detected on electron microscopy of biopsied liver and other tissues, including lymph nodes, macrophages, and astrocytes.[15,138] These inclusions are not specific for IRD and have also been found in NALD and uncommonly in ZS.[21,65] Chondrodysplasia punctata and renal cysts have not been reported in IRD.

Patients with IRD may present with severe visual impairment in infancy, hence simulating Leber's congenital amaurosis, or may mistakenly be diagnosed with Usher syndrome because of the deafness.[138,159] The clinical findings in IRD are the mildest of all the disorders of peroxisomal biogenesis. In a subset of patients

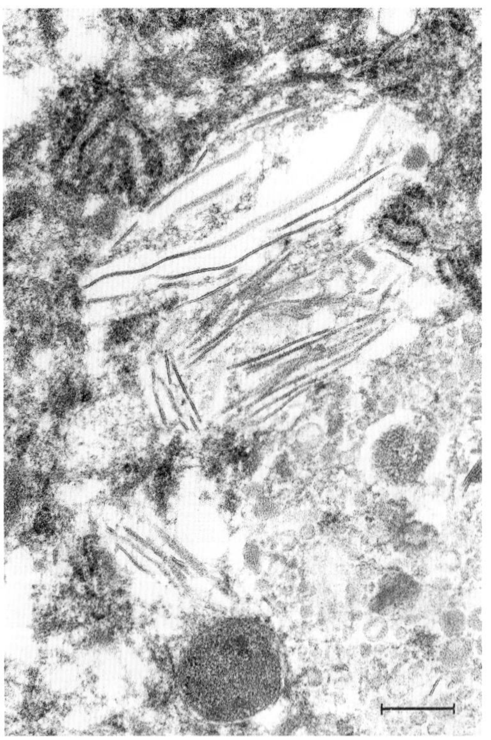

Figure 33.7. Bilamellar sheetlike structures seen on electron microscopy of liver biopsy of a 3.5-year-old girl with infantile Refsum disease. Calibration bar, 300 nm. (From Budden et al.,[15] with permission.)

with IRD, serum levels of phytanic acid and VLCFAs actually become lower with advancing age. Patients usually die late in the second to third decades of life. A single histopathologic report of a child who died at age 12 years has been published.[138] The liver showed micronodular cirrhosis. Reductions of axons and myelin were present in various areas of the central nervous system, including the optic nerve. There was neuronal loss in all layers of the retina. This case was different from NALD and ZS in that the autopsy failed to disclose active central nervous system demyelination, degenerative changes of the adrenals, skeletal changes, or renal cortical cysts.

The ocular features in IRD are nystagmus, strabismus, retinal degeneration, optic atrophy, and cataracts.[15,157,159] The retinal degeneration is prominent in the macular area (Fig. 33.8) relatively early in the course of the disease. In the first year or two of life, the fundus may show characteristic multiple whitish flecks scattered in the midperipheral retina. These lesions are known as leopard spots (Fig. 33.5). They fade with time and are replaced with mottled atrophic retinal pigment epithelium (Fig. 33.9). Prominent pigment clumping in the macula and in the peripheral retina, as well as optic atrophy, are present in late stages of the disease (Figs. 33.10, 33.11). Patients with severe retinal degeneration have lived into the second to third decades of life (unpublished observations). The ERG is profoundly abnormal early in the course of the disease and has an electronegative configuration (Fig. 33.12).[159]

Pipecolic acid, trihydroxycoprostanoic acid, and VLCFAs are elevated in IRD. Peroxisomes are absent in fibroblasts and in liver cells. There is defective plasmalogen synthesis. Patients with IRD have relatively low levels of cholesterol.[15,73,102] The significance of this finding is unclear, but hypocholesterolemia may be the result of an absence of normal peroxisomal reactions involved in cholesterol synthesis.[57,67] DHA (C22:6ω3) levels have been reported to be low in patients with ZS and other disorders of peroxisomal biogenesis and supplementation of DHA in the diet has been proposed as a rational treatment for these disorders.[75–78] No conclusive beneficial effect has been shown yet and IRD remains untreatable.

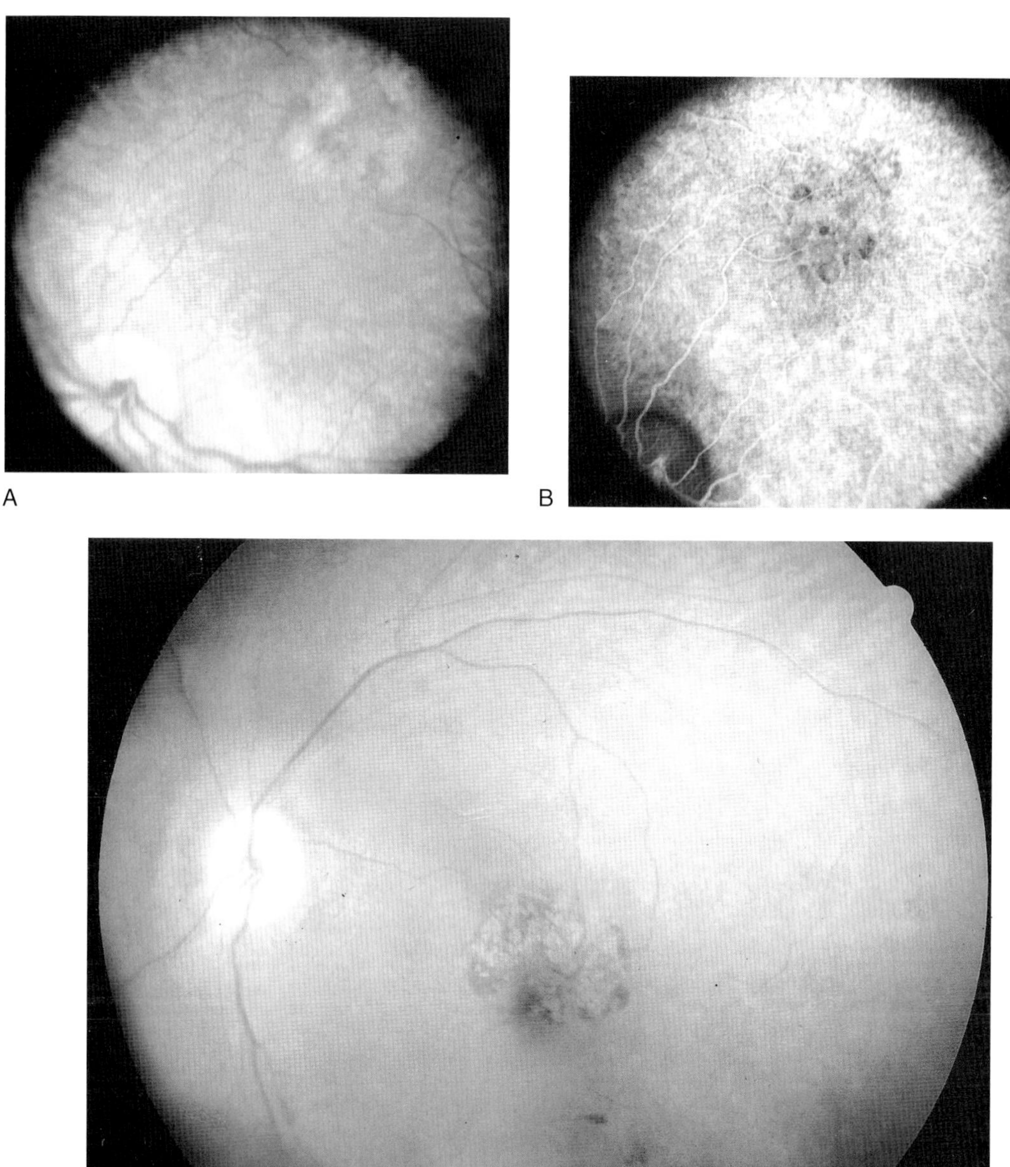

Figure 33.8. Fundus (*A*) and fluorescein angiogram (*B*) of left eye of a 3.6-year-old boy with infantile Refsum disease, showing prominent macular degeneration and atrophy of retinal pigment epithelium and choriocapillaris. *C*: Left eye at age 14 years, showing evolution of maculopathy and further retinal vessel attenuation. (From Weleber et al.,[159] with permission.)

Hyperpipecolic Acidemia (MIM 239400)

Hyperpipecolic acidemia was described by Gatfield et al.[44] in 1968 as a distinct disease but is currently considered to be a variant of ZS or NALD. Gatfield et al.[44] reported mild craniofacial dysmorphism and severe hypotonia and psychomotor retardation. Other features included seizures, hepatomegaly, hepatic fibrosis, retinal degeneration, optic atrophy, impaired hearing, elevated VLCFAs and pipecolic acid, and decreased plasmalogens and DHAP-AT activity.

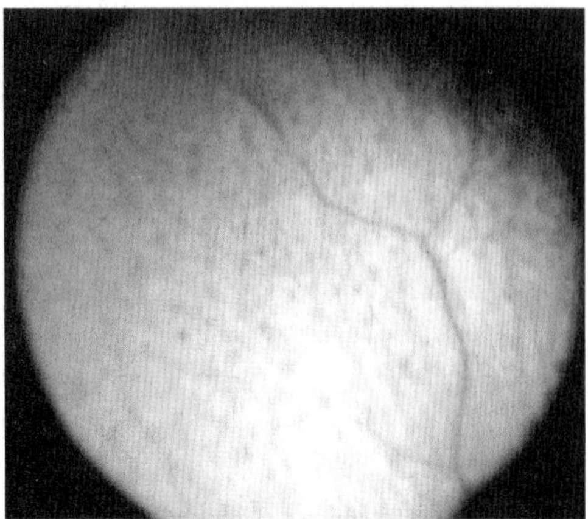

Figure 33.9. Fundus appearance of left eye of a 16-month-old girl with infantile Refsum disease showing pigment mottling, replacing a region that previously displayed the "leopard spot" appearance.

Leber's Congenital Amaurosis

In 1986, Ek and co-workers[33] reported a 7-month-old child with a clinical diagnosis of Leber's congenital amaurosis. The patient was retarded, hypotonic, and had hepatomegaly but was not dysmorphic. Chondrodysplasia punctata was not present, but peroxisomes were absent on liver biopsy and many of the biochemical features of a generalized peroxisomal disorder were demonstrated. Whether this patient has a distinct disease or an unusual presentation of one of the other diseases is unknown. Several children with IRD have ocular findings suggestive of Leber's congenital amaurosis.[138,159] No patients with uncomplicated forms of Leber's congenital amaurosis have been reported to have either deficient peroxisomes or defects of known peroxisomal functions.

Rhizomelic Chondrodysplasia Punctata (MIM 215100)

The rhizomelic form of chondrodysplasia punctata (RCDP) is an autosomal recessive disorder first described by Spranger et al.[128] in 1971. The major features are craniofacial dysmorphism (Fig. 33.13), disproportionate dwarfism (Fig. 33.14), mental retardation, and stippling of epiphyses. There is no demonstrated defect of neuronal migration. Congenital cataracts are

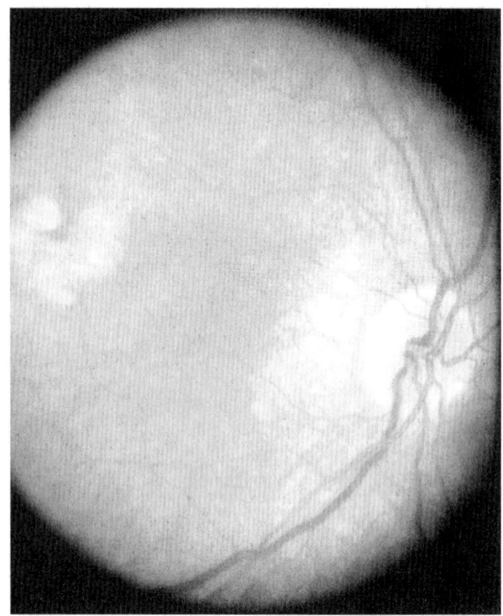

A

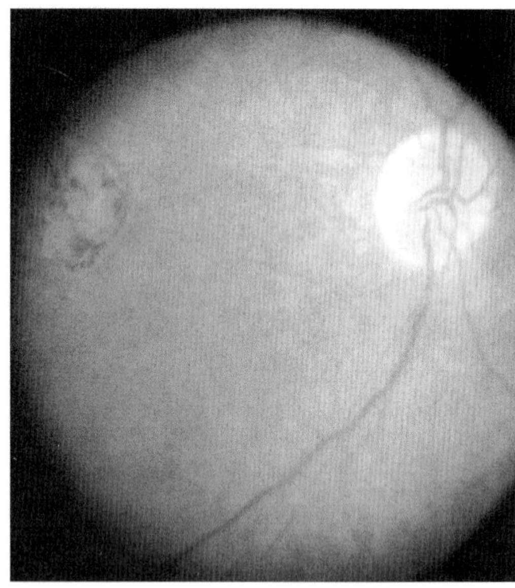

B

Figure 33.10. Fundus appearance of posterior pole of right eye of a boy with infantile Refsum disease at age 4 years 2 months (*A*) and 7 years 6 months (*B*), demonstrating progressive mottling of pigment epithelium in the macula, attenuation of retinal vessels, and optic atrophy. Note the peripapillary halo of pallor, the so-called "golden-ring sign," which is typical for optic nerve head appearance in retinal degenerations.[155] This is the same patient as shown in Figure 33.8.

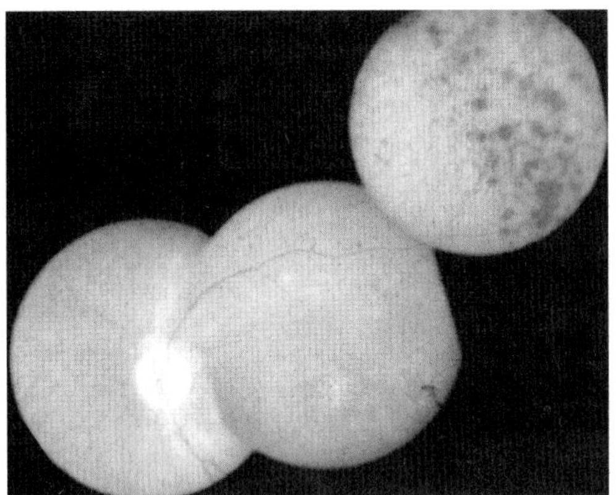

Figure 33.11. Fundus appearance of left eye of a child with infantile Refsum disease at age 10 years 8 months, demonstrating severe optic atrophy, degeneration of the macula, and pigment accumulation in the periphery. Note that the pigment deposition is in the form of clumping rather than the bone-spicule formation that is typical for many forms of retinitis pigmentosa.

present in 72% of cases but retinal degeneration has not been reported. The ERG has been reported to be either normal[38] or abnormal.[49,152] In the case reported by Wardinsky et al.,[152] the ERG was incorrectly reported as abnormal; histopathologic study of the retina at autopsy was normal for this subject (Wilson and Weleber, unpublished observations). Gray et al.[49] did not provide tracings of, or details of the technique for, recording the ERG in their patient.

Peroxisomes are present in fibroblasts of patients with RCDP but may be either deficient or enlarged in the liver.[111] Three biochemical characteristics are typical of classical RCDP. First, phytanic acid levels are variably elevated but pristanic acid levels, VLCFA levels, and peroxisomal β-oxidation are normal. Phytanic acid oxidation is as severely deficient as in patients with ZS and those with adult Refsum disease. Deficient decarboxylation of α-hydroxy-

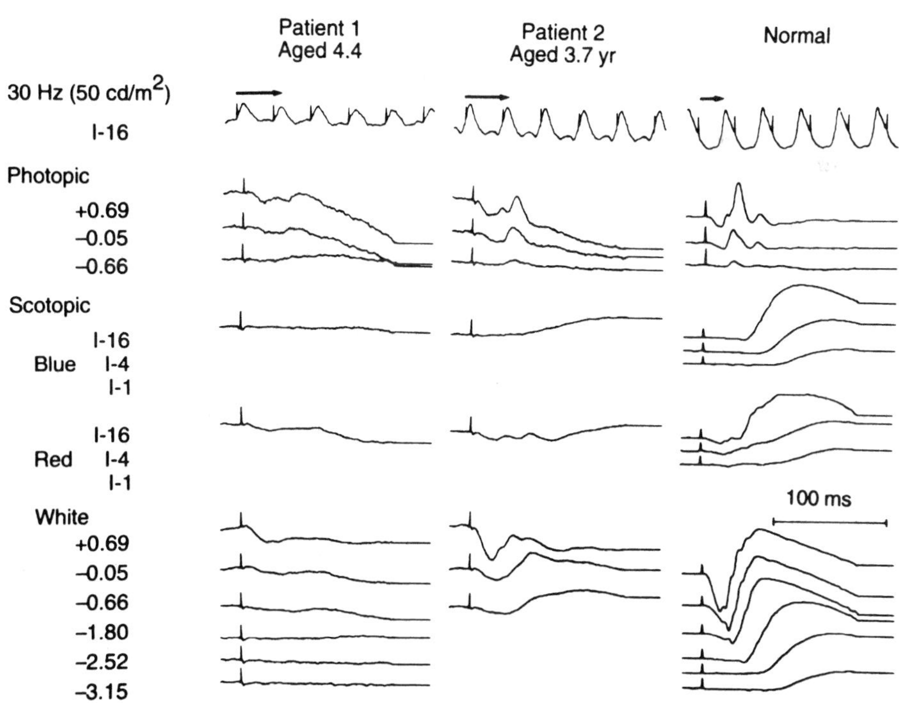

Figure 33.12. Electroretinogram (ERG) of two patients with infantile Refsum disease demonstrating severely subnormal, prolonged responses. Patient 1 is the same one as shown in Figures 33.8 and 33.10. From top to bottom, for the 30 Hz flicker, photopic, and scotopic responses, the stimulus spikes have been set at 5, 5, and 10 μV for patients 1 and 2 and 75, 75, and 100 μV for the normal ERG. The numbers to the left of the photopic and scotopic responses to white light represent the integrated light intensity of the stimulus in log cd-s/m^2. (Modified from Weleber et al.,[159] with permission.)

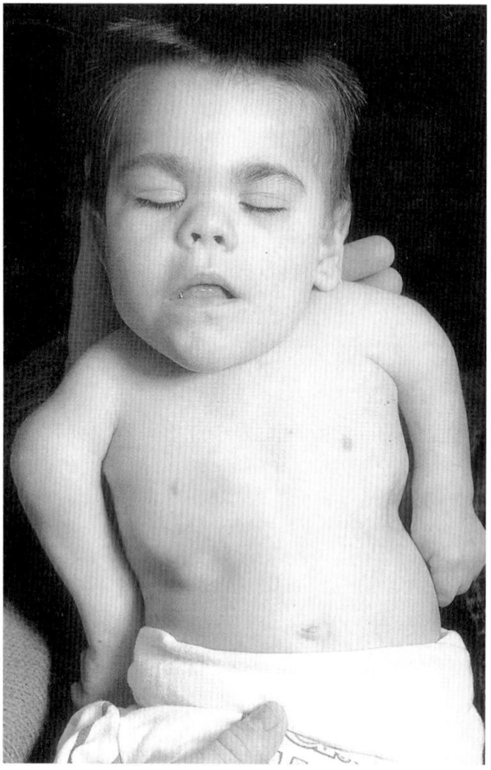

Figure 33.13. Male infant with the rhizomelic form of chondrodysplasia punctata at 4.5 years of age. This child had cataract surgery in each eye at age 2 months. An electroretinogram performed when the child was 4.5 years old was incorrectly reported in a previous paper as abnormal,[152] but the study was, in fact, relatively normal considering the bound-down, extremely miotic pupils secondary to surgery. The child died at age 5 years. The eyes were studied histopathologically and no evidence of retinopathy was found (Wilson and Weleber, unpublished data, 1989).

phytanic acid is believed to be the cause of the block in α-oxidation of phytanic acid in RCDP.[136] Second, plasmalogen levels are lower in RCDP than in disorders of peroxisomal biogenesis, and the enzymes of synthesis, DHAP-AT and alkyl-DHAP synthase, are more deficient in RCDP than in ZS. The third characteristic biochemical defect of RCDP is a failure to process peroxisomal 3-oxoacyl-CoA thiolase in the liver. Recent studies by Motley et al.[92] and by Slawecki et al.[125] provided evidence that the basic defect in the classic form of RCDP involves the receptor for peroxisomal targeting signal 2 (PTS2). *PEX7*, one of over 17 genes encoding for peroxins (proteins involved in peroxisomal import, biogenesis, pro-

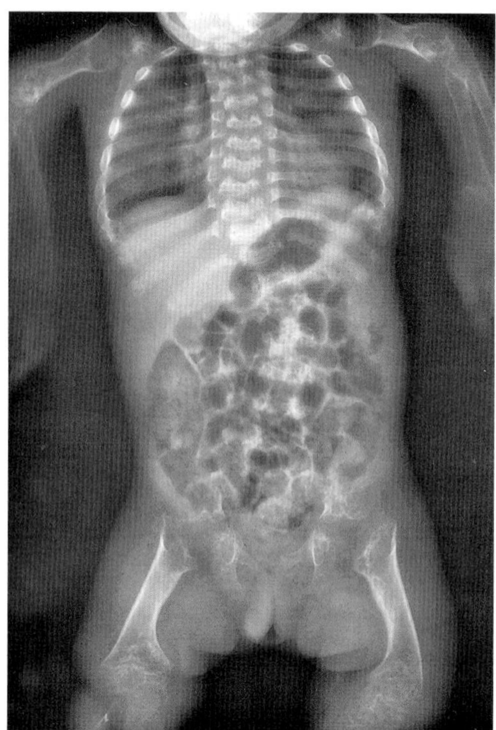

A

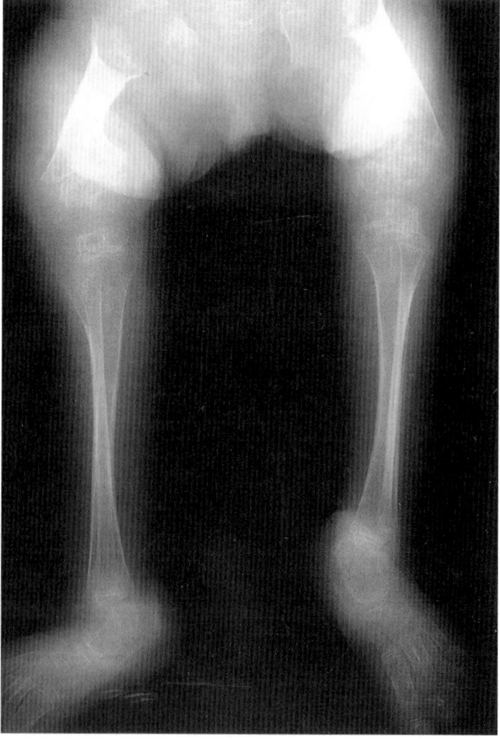

B

Figure 33.14. **A**, **B**: Radiographs demonstrating disproportionate dwarfism of a male child with chondrodysplasia punctata at 4.5 years of age. This is the same patient as shown in Figure 33.13.

liferation, and inheritance), was determined to be the gene that encodes the PTS2 receptor and was found to be mutated in patients with RCDP.[12a,92a,107a] Thus, the most common form of RCDP appears to be a disorder of defective import of proteins into peroxisomes.

Wanders et al.[148] reported a child with clinical and biochemical features suggestive of RCDP with unique, isolated deficiency of DHAP-AT activity in cultured skin fibroblasts. Alkyl-DHAP synthase activity was normal. The plasmalogen level was elevated but the phytanic acid level was normal. Cataracts were present. This condition was called pseudo-RCDP. Subsequent to this report, another child with the RCDP phenotype was described who had isolated deficiency of alkyl-DHAP synthase activity.[147]

Combined Peroxisomal β-Oxidation Enzyme Deficiency with "Zellweger-Like Syndrome"

This syndrome was described in only one child who died at 5 months of age. The patient presented with features similar to those of the ZS and deficiency of all three β-oxidation enzyme proteins by immunoblotting.[132] Peroxisomes were present on electron microscopy. The eye findings were not reported.

Complementation Studies of Disorders of Peroxisomal Assembly or Biogenesis

Information has been gleaned from complementation studies that involve fusion of somatic cells from patients with different clinical diagnoses.[14,69,81,112,118] Cells derived from patients with disorders caused by a different genetic defect would be expected in such a system to complement the deficient peroxisomal function in cells from another patient. These studies allow the distinction among patients with different complementation groups. Complementation has been seen between cells from some patients (but not others) with ZS, NALD, or IRD and cells from patients with hyperpipecolic acidemia, indicating that those patients whose cells showed complementation had disorders of different genes. No complementation was observed among cells from patients with hyperpipecolic acidemia and those from patients with IRD, NALD, or ZS, supporting the concept that these disorders are allelic. Cell complementation can distinguish at least 16 different groups, each presumably corresponding to a different gene involved in peroxisome biogenesis.[81] In general, all three phenotypes (ZS, NALD, IRD) are represented in the largest complementation groups. ZS is represented in nearly all complementation groups, and there appears to be no obvious correlation between complementation group and phenotype.[69,81]

Chromosomal Assignments and Molecular Defects of Disorders of Peroxisomal Assembly or Biogenesis

Recently, gene localization and molecular studies have provided additional information on the causes of defective peroxisomal biogenesis. In virtually all cases where the molecular defect has been identified, the abnormality has involved the failure of importation of matrix or membrane proteins into peroxisomes.

One form of ZS (termed ZWS1, MIM 214100), which complements with NALD and IRD, has been mapped to chromosome 7q11.23 by the finding of two cases of chromosomal rearrangement.[94,95]

A second form of ZS (ZWS2, MIM 170995) has been found to be caused by a defect of peroxisomal membrane protein-70, also called PMP70 or PXMP1.[43] This gene, which is a candidate for transport functions, is located at chromosome 1p22-p21.[42] Cataracts and pigmentary retinopathy are listed as features of this form of ZS. A third form of ZS (ZWS3, MIM 170993) is associated with a defect of peroxisomal membrane protein 35K, also called PMP35, PXMP3, peroxisomal assembly factor-1, or PAF1.[119] This gene is located on chromosome 8q21.1 and defines complementation group 10 using the Kennedy Krieger Classification.[117,118] Cataracts and pigmentary retinopathy were listed as features of this form of ZS.

PTS1 and PTS2 are two *cis*-acting peroxisomal targeting signals that are needed for post-translational import of peroxisomal enzymes into preexisting peroxisomes.[48,92,131,134] Both PTS1 and PTS2 imported proteins are absent or reduced in the vast majority of patients with

ZS, NALD, and IRD. Moreover, no ZS patient has yet been found with the ability to import PTS2 proteins but not PTS1 proteins.[125] Mutations in the PTS1 receptor gene *PXR1* have been reported as the only defect in two NALD patients and in 1 ZS patient who also was defective for PTS2 protein import; these three patients appear to define complementation group 2 of the disorders of peroxisome biogenesis.[31,125]

Disorders of Single Peroxisomal Proteins

Certain disorders result from a defect of a single peroxisomal protein with structurally normal peroxisomes. The recognition that a given disease was due to a defect of a single protein involved in peroxisomal function in nearly all instances came long after the clinical recognition of the disease and, in many cases, even after its biochemical characterization. X-linked adrenoleukodystrophy was known clinically for over one-half century before it was discovered to be a metabolic disorder of singular peroxisomal function.[85,89] Often the determination that a given biochemical reaction or metabolic pathway is localized to the peroxisomes is the first indication that the disorder represents a defect of a single peroxisomal protein. Classic Refsum disease was, until recently, incorrectly classified as a disorder of mitochondrial rather than peroxisomal function.[124,129,154] Other disorders that result from a single peroxisomal protein defect appeared clinically similar to disorders of more generalized peroxisomal dysfunction or disorders of peroxisomal biogenesis but were found on further study not to be deficient in size or number of peroxisomes. The disorders associated with deficiency of one of the three peroxisomal enzymes involved in β-oxidation (acyl-CoA oxidase, bifunctional enzyme, or 3-oxoacyl CoA thiolase) all present with clinical features indistinguishable from disorders of peroxisomal biogenesis, and differentiation among these two groups of diseases can only be achieved by the demonstration of intact peroxisomes in disorders of single enzymatic origin, and on biochemical enzyme testing. At present, virtually all individual enzymes or proteins involved in peroxisomal biochemical functions have a representative genetic disorder associated with a defect of the gene controlling the individual enzymatic reaction.

Adult-Type Refsum Disease (MIM 266500)

Refsum disease was first described in 1946 as an autosomal recessive, progressive neurologic disorder associated with retinitis pigmentosa, peripheral neuropathy, cerebellar ataxia, and elevated cerebrospinal protein levels (without pleocytosis). Less consistent clinical findings include nerve deafness, anosmia, skeletal abnormalities (including epiphyseal dysplasia), ichthyosis, and nonspecific abnormalities of the electrocardiogram.[108] Other reported systemic features are syndactyly, short fourth metatarsal, hammer toe, pes cavus, and osteochondritis dissecans. Cardiac conduction defects can lead to life-threatening arrhythmias. Patients may have cataracts, pupillary abnormalities (miosis and poor pupillary dilation), a degenerative maculopathy relatively early in the course of the disease, and optic atrophy.[129,130,158]

Although most patients begin to experience symptoms in the first two decades of life, neurologic and cardiac dysfunction may be delayed in some patients into the fifth decade. Cerebellar abnormalities lead to an unsteady gait, a positive Romberg sign, intention tremor, and nystagmus that are out of proportion to the peripheral neuropathy that presents as symmetric motor and sensory losses with absent or decreased deep tendon reflexes. Weakness in the extremities, ataxia and night blindness are the most common early symptoms. The electroretinogram is abnormal or nonrecordable in virtually all patients.[6,109]

Blood and tissue levels of phytanic acid are high in Refsum disease. Phytanic acid may account for 5%–30% of fatty acids in serum and up to 50% of fatty acids in tissues such as the liver.

The disease is caused by a deficiency of phytanic acid α-oxidation, which was previously considered to be an exclusively mitochondrial function, and Refsum disease was for many years not classified as a peroxisomal disorder.[129,154] The elevation of phytanic acid (and pristanic acid) concentrations in peroxisome deficiency syndromes was thought to result from a block in the peroxisomal β-oxidation of pristanic acid, the $n - 1$ product of phytanic acid α-oxidation, from deficient pristanoyl-CoA oxidase activity.[104,149] However, pristanic acid levels are not elevated in patients with Refsum disease, a finding consistent with a defect at an earlier step of the biochemical pathway.

Oxidation of phytanic acid in humans proceeds at a rate 20 times greater in peroxisomes than in mitochondria. Studies of oxidation of phytanic acid in normal human fibroblasts and in fibroblasts from patients with Refsum disease demonstrated that, although the mitochondrial activity was normal, peroxisomal oxidation of phytanic acid was virtually absent in cells from patients with Refsum disease.[124] Steinberg[130] has shown that the defect in Refsum disease was the first stage of phytanic α-oxidation: the step that involves hydroxylation of phytanic acid to α-hydroxyphytanic acid by peroxisomal phytanic acid α-hydroxlylase.

The mechanism of retinal degeneration and other features of Refsum disease is unknown but has been the topic of much speculation.[130] One theory is that the rigid, fully saturated phytanic acid molecule is incorporated into brain, nerve, heart, and retinal membranes, interfering with their normal function or stability. Certainly, membranes with phytanic acid substituted for unsaturated straight-chain fatty acids would be expected to have highly different fluidity characteristics. This theory is supported by the fact that dietary restriction of phytanic acid can prevent progression, and can even result in improvement, of some of the features of the disease. Another theory is that, because of the similarity of phytanic acid to the isoprenoid side chains of certain fat-soluble vitamins, its accumulation interferes with the function of certain vitamins. A correlate of this theory is that normal prenylation of proteins may be disrupted by the accumulation of phytanic acid, thereby interfering with the cycling of proteins from cytosol to membranes, or with the interactions of some proteins with others.[18,74] Choroideremia is another degenerative disorder of the choroid and retina that results from a defect of a form of prenylation called geranylgeranylation. The gene product that is deficient in choroideremia is Rab escort protein, REP-1, which is required for the prenylation of a specific subset of Rab proteins essential for the retina.[1a,116] Other possible pathogenetic mechanisms include interference by phytanic acid with the function of coenzyme Q and the possibility that a more widespread, generalized defect in α-oxidation exists, with effects on currently unknown pathways.

The pathophysiology of the ichthyosiform skin lesions may relate to reduction of available free cholesterol because of the conversion of phytanic acid in skin to its ester cholesterol phytanate and/or induced reduction of linoleate, since ichthyosis is also present in essential fatty acid deficiency.

Although Refsum disease shares an elevation of serum and plasma phytanic acid with disorders of peroxisomal biogenesis, the degree of elevation of plasma and tissue phytanic acid is much greater in Refsum disease than in any of the disorders of peroxisomal biogenesis. Dietary restriction of phytanic acid in patients with Refsum disease can lower phytanic acid levels to normal values and can arrest or improve the ichthyosis, peripheral neuropathy, and cardiac conduction defects. Reduction diets may mobilize fatty stores of phytanic acid, and plasmapheresis is sometimes needed to prevent death from cardiac arrhythmias. Studies of individual patients on low phytanic acid diets have shown long-term arrest of progression of the disease, but no improvement in visual and auditory impairment.[30,50,51]

Adrenoleukodystrophy; Adrenomyeloneuropathy (MIM 300100)

X-linked adrenoleukodystrophy (ALD) is the most common of the disorders that are associated with a loss of a single peroxisomal function, in this instance, that of peroxisomal β-oxidation.[83,85,89] First described in 1923 by Siemerling and Creutzfeldt[120] under the term "bronzed sclerosing encephalomyelitis," the name "adrenoleukodystrophy" was first given to this disorder in 1970 by Blaw.[8] The observations that the adrenals of these patients contained lipid inclusions,[62,107] later shown to result from accumulation of VLCFAs,[59] helped in the appreciation that ALD is a metabolic disorder and led to the discovery of elevated VLCFAs in blood and other cells by Moser and co-workers.[86,87]

The incidence of ALD in Caucasians has been estimated to be as high as 1 in 15,000 to 20,000.[90] Because of the defect in peroxisomal β-oxidation, unbranched saturated VLCFAs, particularly hexacosanoate (C26:0), accumulate in blood and virtually all tissues, most strikingly in the white matter of the brain and in the adrenal cortex.[122] The enzyme deficient in X-linked ALD was originally reported to be lignoceroyl-CoA ligase, an enzyme needed for activation of VLCFAs for entry into β-oxidation.[53,70,151] This enzyme is also referred to as very-long-chain acyl-CoA synthetase. However, recently, the gene for ALD, which is called *ALDP,* has been identified as belonging to a superfamily of ATP-binding cassette (ABC) transmembrane transporter genes.[35,90,91] This recent discovery suggests that the deficiency of VLCFA CoA synthetase is secondary to a defect in import of the enzyme into peroxisomal membranes.

The phenotype of individuals who carry the ALD gene mutations is highly variable, suggesting that other genetic or environmental factors influence the expression or effect of the mutant gene.[72,83] Moser and colleagues[88,89] proposed that six different phenotypes can be recognized: childhood cerebral, adolescent cerebral, adult cerebral, adrenomyeloneuropathy (AMN), adrenal insufficiency only, and asymptomatic. The childhood form of the disorder, which accounted for 48% of 1475 cases at the Kennedy Krieger Institute in Baltimore, MD, has its onset in the first decade of life (mean age of onset of 7.7 ± 1.7 years with a mean interval to a vegetative state of 1.9 ± 2 years). Visual impairment is an early sign and strabismus is common. In later stages all vision is lost and the optic nerve heads become severely atrophic.

White matter demyelination results in cerebral blindness, decline of school performance, behavioral disturbance, emotional liability, attention deficit, cognitive decline, hearing loss, seizures, and progessive neurologic deterioration, leading eventually to a vegetative state and death.[85] Although the accumulation of VLCFAs in tissues is believed to lead to demyelination, inflammatory factors appear to play a definite role in the pathogenesis.[89] There is a characteristic appearance on computed tomographic (CT) or magnetic resonance imaging (MRI) scanning of marked loss of periventricular white matter with prominent uptake of contrast media or gadolinium agents (Fig. 33.15) in active areas of disease. Adrenal cortical hypofunction from atrophy usually occurs and darkening of the skin can be a prominent early finding.

The vision may be noted to fluctuate dramatically from one moment to the next during the early phases of the disease. At one point the child may appear to see well, while minutes to hours later he might appear severely visually disoriented. The disturbed visual function and spatial disorientation are presumed to result from demyelination of the periventricular optic radiations. During the early stages of the disease the optic nerve usually appears normal but may rarely demonstrate the typical findings of neuroretinitis (Fig. 33.16). Other reported findings include exotropia, esotropia, disturbance of motility suggesting ocular motor apraxia, macular pigmentation, normal ERG, borderline to abnormal visual evoked response (VER), and, invariably in late stages of the disease, optic atrophy.[140] The ERG and electrooculogram (EOG) are normal in ALD, but the VER is abnormal.[38,140]

The second most common form of the disease, AMN, occurred in about 25% of cases at the Kennedy Krieger Institute in Baltimore, MD, and usually started as a spastic paraparesis in the third decade of life (mean age of onset 27.6 ± 8.7 years).[89] Patients with AMN have a 50% chance to have abnormalities on MRI scans with cognitive decline, but they almost always have abnormal somatosensory and brain stem auditory evoked cortical potentials. Visually evoked cortical potentials are often increased in latency in the presence of cerebral disease (70% of cases) but are less frequent among patients with AMN (17% of cases).

In about 5% of cases, ALD presents in adolescence with an age of onset from 10 to 21 years with symptoms and features similar to those of the childhood form. Addison disease without neurologic involvement occurs in 10% of cases. In 3% of cases, the disorder presents in adulthood with cerebral disease. Ten percent of males with the biochemical defect are initially asymptomatic, but with time many, if not all, convert to other phenotypes.[89]

Different ALD phenotypes commonly occur within the same family and immunologic differences have been suggested to play a role in the neurologic expression of the disease. Moser et al.[88] found Mendelian segregation of clinical

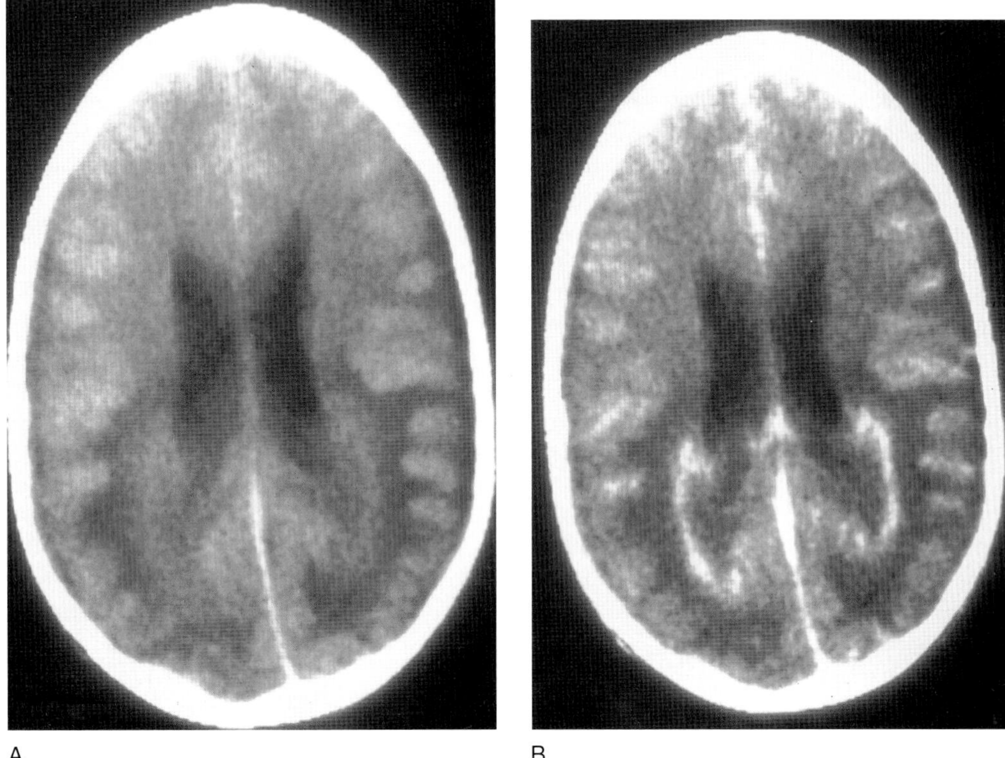

Figure 33.15. Computerized tomographic imaging study of a 7-year-old boy with X-linked adrenoleukodystrophy demonstrating severe loss of myelinated fibers (including optic radiations) in the posterior periventricular region (*A*) and with enhancement after intravenous administration of contrast material (*B*). (Courtesy of Dr. William T. Shults.)

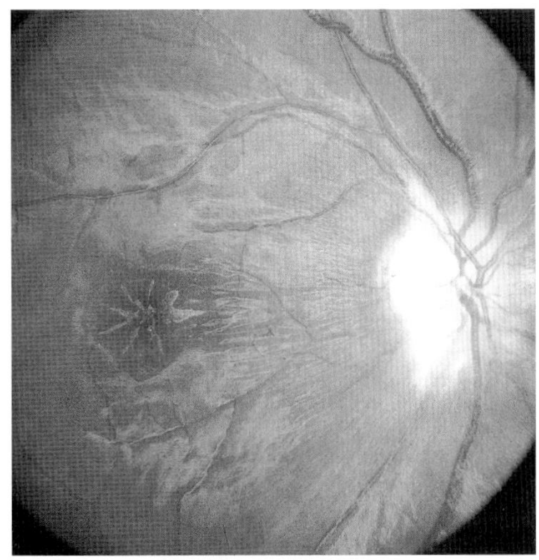

Figure 33.16. Neuroretinitis with stellate maculopathy in right eye of a 7-year-old boy with X-linked adrenoleukodystrophy. This is the same patient as shown in Figure 33.15. (Courtesy of Dr. William T. Shults.)

phenotypes within families, suggesting that modifier genes rather than environmental factors may be the principal determinants of expression differences. Approximately 15% of carrier women develop features similar to, but generally milder than, AMN. In these women, symptoms start at a later age.[85]

The gene for ALD, *ALDP,* codes for a product that demonstrates about 75% homology to another ATP-binding cassette protein, a 70 kD peroxisomal membrane protein (PMP70). The ALDP protein has been hypothesized to be involved in the import of the VLCFA acyl-CoA synthetase within the peroxisomal membrane.[91] Mutations within the *ALDP* gene have been described in patients with ALD.[5,12,17,71,84]

There is no evidence to date to suggest that differences in phenotype, e.g., between childhood cerebral ALD and AMN, relate to the location where the mutation resides in the gene or how the mutation specifically affects the gene product.[12] Indeed, Fanen et al.[35] reported all three phenotypes—ALD, AMN, and Addison disease only—in a family with a splice-site mutation in intron 6. Berger et al.[5] reported five different phenotypes in six affected members of a family with Pro484Arg mutation of the ALD gene. Such families suggest that other genetic (or environmental) influences may prevail in determining the expression of different clinical phenotypes.

Unfortunately, except for the adrenal insufficiency, which readily responds to steroid replacement therapy, the treatment of ALD remains controversial and unproven.[89] Bone marrow transplantation from a fraternal twin reversed the early neuroradiologic and neurologic findings in one case, and although this patient was still normal 3 years after bone marrow transplantation, the long-term clinical course of this child has not been reported.[3] Immunosuppression with cyclophosphamide[93] and intravenous high doses of immunoglobulin therapy[16] have failed to slow the course of deterioration in affected individuals. Dietary treatment with oleic acid/erucic acid ("Lorenzo's oil") can reduce plasma VLCFAs in all phenotypes of ALD. Lorenzo's oil appears to be of no value for symptomatic patients. Earlier hope that Lorenzo's oil would be able to arrest disease progression in patients with AMN has unfortunately not been verified.[2] Whether similar treatment can truly prevent the development of disease or slow the deterioration in asymptomatic patients is yet to be determined, and early findings are encouraging.[84,89]

Pseudo-Zellweger Syndrome-Acetyl-CoA Acyltransferase Deficiency: ACAA Deficiency; 3-Oxoacyl-CoA Thiolase Deficiency (MIM 261510)

Goldfischer et al.[45] in 1986 and Schram et al.[113] in 1987 described an 11-month-old girl with otherwise typical clinical features of ZS who had deficient peroxisomal β-oxidation, elevated VLCFAs and bile acid intermediates, but normal levels of pipecolic and phytanic acids. Plasmalogen levels and the enzymes of plasmalogen synthesis were normal. Peroxisomes were normal in liver cells, and peroxisomal 3-oxoacyl-CoA thiolase was the only enzyme of peroxisomal β-oxidation that was found to be deficient.

Although retinopathy was not visible, the visually evoked cortical potential was reported as abnormal. ERG was not done. The gene for this enzyme resides at 3p23-p22.[9]

Pseudoneonatal Adrenoleukodystrophy (Acyl-CoA Oxidase Deficiency; ACOX) (MIM 264470)

Poll-Thé et al.[101] in 1988 described two children who were not dysmorphic but who had features otherwise similar to NALD (hypotonia, seizures, and severe psychomotor retardation). VLCFAs were elevated, indicating deficient peroxisomal β-oxidation, but plasmalogen levels and enzymes were normal. Peroxisomes that were normal in number and enlarged in size were present in the liver. Bile acid intermediates, pipecolic acid, and phytanic acid levels were normal. Cataracts were not described but retinopathy was present. The ERG was nonrecordable and the flash VER was almost entirely absent. Optic atrophy developed in the late stage of the disease.

The only enzyme deficiency found was that of acyl-CoA oxidase, which is the first enzyme of the peroxisomal β-oxidation pathway, catalyzing acyl-CoA to 2-trans-enoyl-CoA. This enzyme is located at 17q25.[144] In 1994, Fournier et al.[39] reported a large deletion within the ACOX gene in DNA from the patients reported by Poll-Thé et al.[101] Suzuki et al.[133] described two cases (one with retinal degeneration) of acyl-CoA oxidase deficiency with detectable enzyme protein where the diagnosis was established by complementation analysis.

PseudoNeonatal Adrenoleukodystrophy (Peroxisomal Bifunctional Protein Deficiency) (MIM 261515)

Watkins et al.[153] in 1989 reported a male infant with elevated VLCFAs and features suggestive of NALD. There were, however, biochemical findings that distinguished this disorder from NALD. Phytanic acid, pipecolic acid, and plasmalogen levels were normal. Retinopathy was absent (although an ERG was not done). Peroxisomes were present. The deficient β-oxidation was attributed to the absence of the bifunctional protein (with enoyl-CoA-hydratase and 3-hydroxyacyl-CoA dehydrogenase activity).

Suzuki et al.[133] described two additional cases with bifunctional enzyme deficiency identified by complementation analysis. Retinopathy was not reported in either of these patients. Wanders et al.[150] also described a case of bifunctional deficiency with cataracts and abnormal retinal pigmentation; this patient had an inactive form of the enzyme. No ERGs were reported for any of these cases.

Eustis and co-workers[34] in 1995 reported two second cousin girls with a fleck retinopathy similar to the leopard spots that occur in NALD and IRD. These children had elevated VLCFAs and low plasma carnitine. Complementation studies performed at the Kennedy-Krieger Institute revealed a peroxisomal bifunctional enzyme deficiency.[34] The first of these girls had a nondetectable scotopic and photopic ERG at age 10 months: she died at age 12 months. The second child, who also had early cataract in the right eye, died at age 8 months without having had an ERG. Al-Hazzaa and Ozand[1] in 1997 reported another patient with peroxisomal bifunctional enzyme deficiency associated with the leopard spot flecked retina appearance.

Pseudorhizomelic Chondrodysplasia Punctata (Deficiency of Dihydroxyacetonephosphate Actyltransferase, DHAP-AT`Deficiency; Pseudo-RCDP) (MIM 222765)

Wanders and colleagues[148] described a child with typical features of RCDP with isolated deficiency of dihydroxyacetonephosphate acyltransferase (DHAP-AT). The patient was extremely hypotonic and had cataracts. Plasma levels of phytanic acid and phytanic acid α-oxidation were normal. The patient died at the age of 6 months.

Pseudorhizomelic Chondrodysplasia Punctata (Deficiency of Alkyl DHAP Synthase; Pseudo-RCDP)

Wanders and co-workers[147] also reported a child with features of RCDP with an isolated deficiency of alkyl DHAP synthase. The clinical features of this patient were essentially the same as those seen in classical RCDP. Cataracts were present, but there was no retinopathy.

Oxalosis I; Primary Hyperoxaluria Type 1; Glycolic Aciduria; Peroxisomal Alanine: Glyoxylate Aminotransferase Deficiency; Hepatic AGT Deficiency; AGXT (MIM 259900)

Primary hyperoxaluria is the term used to describe two autosomal recessive disorders, primary hyperoxaluria type 1 (PH1) and primary hyperoxaluria type 2 (PH2).[26] PH1 is a disorder of glyoxylate metabolism that results in widespread accumulation of calcium oxalate crystals in tissues, including kidney, bone, myocardium, brain, skin, and peripheral vessels.[26,55] Renal failure, hydrocephalus, osteodystrophy, livedo reticularis, and gangrene can occur. Abnormal urine levels of organic acids (oxalic, glycolic, and glyoxylic acids) assist in the diagnosis. Ocular findings are optic atrophy, unusual-appearing black ringlets (Fig. 33.17) of retinal hyperpigmentation, and retinal fibrosis (Fig. 33.18).[55,126,139] PH2 is a milder disorder with the only clinical feature of urolithiasis.

PH1 results from a deficiency of hepatic peroxisomal AGT, which has pyridoxal phosphate as its cofactor. The gene that encodes this enzyme is located at 2q36-37. Peroxisomes are normal in number and appearance. Although for the great majority of instances the disease results from the lack of a functional gene product, in a few cases it is caused by a misrouting of the enzyme to mitochondria rather than to peroxisomes because of a defect in the targeting signal.[25,135] These cases are examples of a defect in normal protein sorting to peroxisomes. PH2 is due to deficiency of cytosolic *D*-glycerate dehydrogenase/glyoxylate reductase. Supplementation with high doses of pyridoxine decreases oxalate excretion, at least in mild cases, and may slow the deposition of crystals in tissues.[80] However, virtually all patients eventually develop renal failure and require renal transplant. The disease, however, recurs with time in the transplanted kidney. Combined hepatorenal transplantation appears to offer hope for a long-term control of this metabolic disorder.[26]

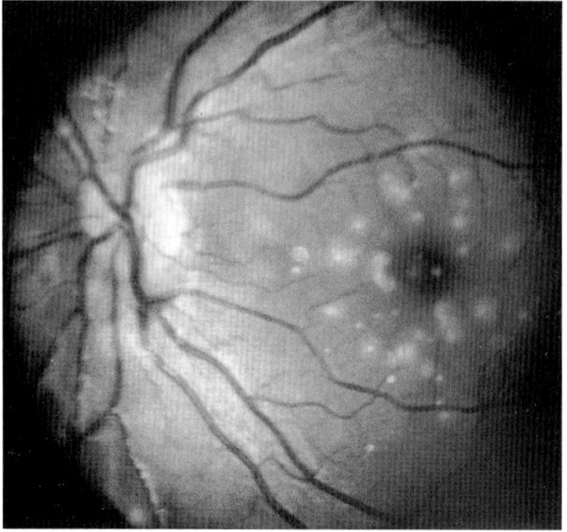

A

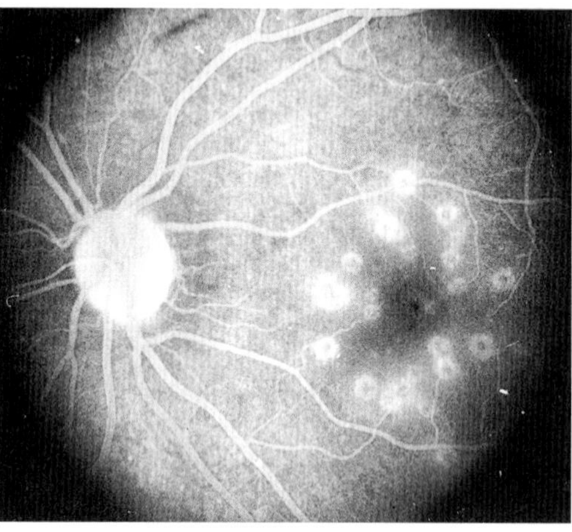

B

Figure 33.17. *A*, *B*: Fundus appearance of a 7-year-old boy with hyperoxaluria type 1. Crystalline deposits are surrounded by ringlets of atrophy (*A*) that hyperfluoresce on angiography (*B*). (From Traboulsi et al.,[139] with permission.)

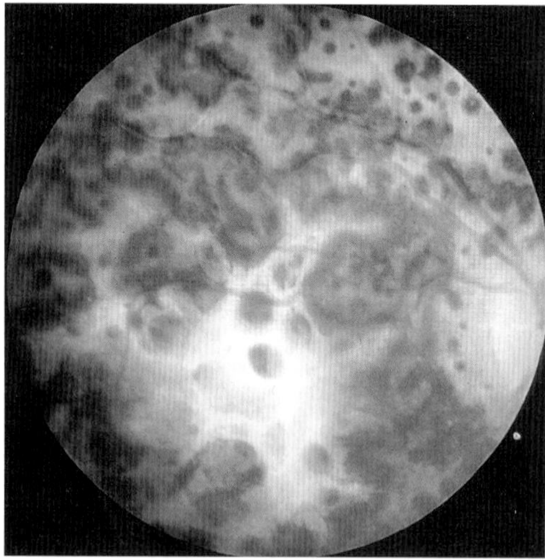

Figure 33.18. Fundus appearance of a 3-year-old girl with hyperoxaluria type 1, showing retinal fibrosis. (From Small et al.,[126] with permission. Copyright 1990, American Medical Association.)

Acatalasemia (MIM 115500)

Acatalasemia is an autosomal recessive disorder that results from the near total deficiency of the enzyme catalase. The disease was mapped to chromosome 11p13.[32] Acatalasemia is not associated with ocular pathology, although it has been associated with ulcerative oral lesions in Japanese patients, where the disorder is known as Takahara disease. Patients are homozygous for the mutant gene, but decreased activity of catalase is present in heterozygotes, who are otherwise normal. This had led McKusick[79a] to classify acatalasemia as an autosomal dominant trait.

The aniridia-Wilms' tumor syndrome is a contiguous deletion syndrome caused by deletion of chromosomal material at chromosome 11p13. Patients with this syndrome who have deletions that are visible on light microscopy will usually have hypocatalasemia from absence of the gene, where as patients without a visible deletion will have normal catalase activity. This had led some investigators to suggest that assay of catalase activity may have diagnostic value in sporadic aniridia. However, one case of aniridia/Wilms' tumor syndrome and five with sporadic aniridia (one with a visible deletion) have been reported with normal catalase activity.[11] Moreover, the gene for catalase appears to reside several thousand base pairs proximal to the loci for aniridia and Wilms' tumor.[143]

SUMMARY AND CONCLUSIONS

Peroxisomes are essential organelles for normal cellular function and are responsible for performing over 50 metabolic reactions, most of which consume or generate molecular oxygen.

They are highly versatile with both anabolic and catabolic functions, many of which are induced only under appropriate conditions. Many reactions, such as β-oxidation of VLCFAs, take place exclusively within peroxisomes. Other reactions, such as β-oxidation of LCFAs, occur in other compartments within the cell but the peroxisomal pathway is highly inducible and allows for fine tuning of the metabolic environment. For many pathways, such as the first steps in plasmalogen synthesis, essential portions of the reactions take place within peroxisomes and intermediates are shunted to other cellular organelles for additional processing.

Much of what has been learned about peroxisomes stems from the search to understand diseases where one or more peroxisomal functions are deficient. Peroxisomal diseases were hence divided into (*1*) disorders of peroxisomal assembly or biogenesis, where peroxisomes are characteristically deficient in size and number (although "ghost" organelles may be present), and (*2*) disorders where only single enzymatic functions of peroxisomes are defective.

Peroxisomal membrane and matrix proteins are synthesized on free ribosomes and transported into existing peroxisomes that bud and divide to form new peroxisomes. The mechanisms of peroxisomal biogenesis involve specific targeting of proteins by PTSs within the amino acid sequence that direct the importation of the protein into the peroxisomes. These PTSs occur at either the carboxy-terminal end of the peptide (PTS1) or within the presequence at the amino-terminus (PTS2). Defects of some of the receptors for these targeting signals have been identified in patients with ZS, NALD, and RCDP. Three ATP-binding cassette (ABC) transporters have been identified in the human peroxisome membrane: ALDP, ALDR, and PMP70. A fourth transporter has been cloned (P70R). All are half ABC transporters that must heterodimerize to form complete, functional transporters.[116a] Much is yet to be discovered about the transportation into peroxisomes of proteins and substrates for metabolic reactions.

The clinician should suspect a disorder of peroxisomal biogenesis, such as ZS, NALD, or IRD, in patients who present early in life with features that are characteristic for these disorders (Table 33.3). The most widely used laboratory test for the diagnosis of children suspected of having a disorder of peroxisomal biogenesis is the measurement of levels of VLCFAs in plasma. However, VLCFA levels are not elevated in RCDP. Other assays that help in the detection and classification of these disorders include measurement of plasma levels of phytanic acid, pristanic acid, pipecolic acid, plasmalogens, and bile acid intermediates. Phytanic acid and plasmalogen levels are age dependent and may not be abnormal in older children with ZS, NALD, and IRD. Disorders where peroxisomes are intact but multiple or single enzyme deficiencies are present, e.g., pseudo-ZS and pseudo-NALD, can present with a variety of phenotypes, some of which are similar to those of disorders of peroxisomal biogenesis. Most of these disorders have ocular or visual system findings, including cataract, glaucoma, retinal degeneration, optic atrophy, and leukodystrophy leading to cortical blindness. Retinopathy cannot be presumed to be absent in infancy without a normal ERG. The ophthalmologist must consider the possibility of a peroxisomal disease whenever findings suggestive of this class of disorders are encountered.

Table 33.3. Features Suggestive of a Generalized Peroxisomal Disorder*

Dysmorphic features (including low or broad nasal bridge, large fontanels, shallow orbital ridges, epicanthus, and anteverted nostrils)[137]
Early hypotonia
Early seizures
Hepatomegaly with impaired function
Psychomotor retardation
Pigmentary retinal degeneration
Impaired hearing
Renal cysts
Aberrant bone calcifications
Adrenal insufficiency (rare)

* Modified from Moser.[81]

This work was supported in part by an unrestricted grant from Research to Prevent Blindness, Inc., New York, NY, and a Center Grant from The Foundation Fighting Blindness, Baltimore, MD.

REFERENCES

1. Al-Hazzaa SAF, Ozand PT. Peroxisomal bifunctional enzyme deficiency with associated retinal findings. *Ophthalmic Genet* 1997;18: 93–99.

1a. Andres DA, Seabra MC, Brown MS, Armstrong SA, Smeland TE, Cremers FPM, Goldstein JL. cDNA cloning of component A of Rab geranylgeranyl transferase and demonstration of its role as a Rab escort protein. *Cell* 1993;73:1091–1099.

2. Aubourg P, Adamsbaum C, Lavallard-Rousseau M-C, Rocchiccioli F, Cartier N, Jambaqu JI, Jakobezak C, Lemaitre A, Boureau F, Wolf C, Bougneres P-F. A two-year trial of oleic and erucic acids ("Lorenzo's oil") as treatment for adrenomyeloneuropathy. *N Engl J Med* 1993;329:745–752.

3. Aubourg P, Blanche S, Jambaque I, Rocchiccioli F, Kalifa G, Naud-Saudreau C, Rolland M-O, Debre M, Chaussain J-L, Griscelli C, Fischer A, Bougneres P-F. Reversal of early neurologic and neuroradiologic manifestations of X-linked adenoleukodystrophy by bone marrow transplantation. *N Engl J Med* 1990;322:1860–1866.

4. Benke PJ, Reyes PF, Parker JC, Jr. New form of adrenoleukodystrophy. *Hum Genet* 1981; 58:204–208.

5. Berger J, Molzer B, Faé I, Bernheimer H. X-linked adrenoleukodystrophy (ALD): A novel mutation of the ALD gene in 6 members of a family presenting with 5 different phenotypes. *Biochem Biophys Res Commun* 1994;205: 1638–1643.

6. Berson EL. Retinitis pigmentosa and allied disease: Applications of electroretinographic testing. *Int Ophthalmol* 1981;4:7–22.

7. Biardi L, Sreedhar A, Zokaei A, Vartak NB, Bozeat RL, Shackelford JE, Kellers G-A, Krisans SL, Mevalonate kinase is predominantly localized in peroxisomes and is defective in patients with peroxisome deficiency disorders. *J Biol Chem* 1994;269:1197–1205.

8. Blaw ME. Melanodermic type leukodystrophy (adreno-leukodystrophy). In *Handbook of Clinical Neurology,* vol. 10, P.J. Vinken and G.W. Bruyn, eds. Amsterdam: North-Holland, 1970:128–133.

9. Bout A, Hoovers JMN, Bakker E, Mannens MMAM, Geurts van Kessel A, Westerveld A, Tager JM, Benne R. Assignment of the gene coding for human peroxisomal 3-oxoacyl-CoA thiolase (ACAA) to chromosome region 3p22-p23. *Cytogenet Cell Genet* 1989;52:147–150.

10. Bowen P, Lee CSN, Zellweger H, Lindenberg R. A familiar syndrome of multiple congenital defects. *Bull Johns Hopkins Hosp* 1964;114; 402–414.

11. Boyd P, van Heyningen V, Seawright A, Fekete G, Hastie N. Use of catalase polymorphisms in the study of sporadic aniridia. *Hum Genet* 1986;73:171–174.

12. Braun A, Ambach H, Kammerer S, Rolinski B, Stöckler S, Rabl W, Gärtner J, Zierz S, Roscher AA. Mutations in the gene for X-linked adrenoleukodystrophy in patients with different clinical phenotypes. *Am J Hum Genet* 1995;56:854–861.

12a. Braverman N, Steel G, Obie C, Moser A, Moser H, Gould S, Valle D. Human *PEX7* encodes the peroxisomal PTS2 receptor and is responsible for rhizomelic chondrodysplasia punctata. *Nature Genet* 1997;15:369–376.

13. Brown FR III, McAdams AJ, Cummins JW, Konkol R, Singh I, Moser AB, Moser HW. Cerebro-hepato-renal (Zellweger) syndrome and neonatal adrenoleukodystrophy: Similarities in phenotype and accumulation of very long chain fatty acids. *Johns Hopkins Med J* 1982;151:344–361.

14. Brul S, Westerveld A, Strijland A, Wanders RJA, Schram AW, Heymans HSA, Schutgens RBH, van den Bosch H, Tager JM. Genetic heterogeneity in the cerebrohepatorenal (Zellweger) syndrome and other inherited disorders with a generalized impairment of peroxisomal functions: A study using complementation analysis. *J Clin Invest* 1988;81: 1710–1715.

15. Budden SS, Kennaway NG, Buist NRM, Poulos A, Weleber RG. Dysmorphic syndrome with phytanic acid oxidase deficiency, abnormal very long chain fatty acids, and pipecolic acidemia: Studies in four children. *J Pediatr* 1986;108:33–39.

16. Cappa M, Bertini E, del Balzo P, Cambiaso P, Di Biase A, Salvati S. High dose immunoglobulin IV treatment in adrenoleukodystrophy. *J Neurol Neurosurg Psychiatry* 1994; 57(suppl):69–70.

17. Cartier N, Sarde C-O, Douar A-M, Mosser J, Mandel J-L, Aubourg P. Abnormal messenger

RNA expression and a missense mutation in patients with X-linked adrenoleukodystrophy. *Hum Mol Genet* 1993;2:1949–1951.
18. Casey PJ. Protein lipidation in cell signaling. *Science* 1995;268:221–225.
19. Chang Y-F. Pipecolic acid pathway: The major lysine metabolic route in the rat brain. *Biochem Biophys Res Commun* 1976;69:174–180.
20. Chang Y-F. Lysine metabolism in the rat brain: Blood-brain barrier transport, formation of pipecolic acid and human hyperpipecolatemia. *J Neurochem* 1978;30:355–360.
21. Cohen SMZ, Brown FR III, Martyn L, Moser HW, Chen W, Kistenmacher M, Punnett H, Grover W, de la Cruz ZC, Chan NR, Green WR. Ocular histopathologic and biochemical studies of the cerebrohepatorenal syndrome (Zellweger's syndrome) and its relationship to neonatal adrenoleukodystrophy. *Am J Ophthalmol* 1983;96:488–501.
22. Cohen SMZ, Green WR, de la Cruz ZC, Brown FR, Moser HW, Luckenbach MW. Ocular histopathologic studies of neonatal and childhood adrenoleukodystrophy. *Am J Ophthalmol* 1983;95:82–96.
23. Daiger SP, Sullivan AS, Rodriguez JA. Correlation of phenotype with genotype in inherited retinal degeneration. *Behav Brain Sci* 1995; 18:452–467.
24. Danks DM, Tippett P, Adams C, Campbell P. Cerebro-hepato-renal syndrome of Zellweger. *J Pediatr* 1975;86:382–387.
25. Danpure CJ, Cooper PJ, Wise PJ, Jennings PR. An enzyme trafficking defect in two patients with primary hyperoxaluria type 1: Peroxisomal alanine/glyoxylate aminotransferase rerouted to mitochondria. *J Cell Biol* 1989; 108:1345–1351.
26. Danpure CJ, Purdue PE. Primary hyperoxaluria. In *The Metabolic and Molecular Bases of Inherited Disease,* 7th ed., vol. 2, C.R. Scriver, A. L. Beaudet, W.S. Sly, and D. Valle, eds. New York: McGraw-Hill, 1995:2385–2424.
27. Datta NS, Wilson GN, Hajra AK. Deficiency of enzymes catalyzing the biosynthesis of glycerol-ether lipids in Zellweger syndrome: A new category of metabolic disease involving the absence of peroxisomes. *N Engl J Med* 1984;311:1080–1083.
28. de Duve C, Baudhuin P. Peroxisomes (microbodies and related particles). *Physiol Rev* 1966; 46:323–357.
29. de Duve C, Beaufay H, Jacques P, Rahman-Li Y, Sellinger OZ, Wattiaux R, de Coninck S. Intracellular localization of catalase and of some oxidases in rat liver. *Biochim Biophys Acta* 1960;40:186–187.
29a. de Vet EC, Zomer AW, Lahaut GJ, van den Bosch H. Polymerase chain reaction-based cloning of alkyl-dihydroxyacetonephosphate synthase complementary DNA from guinea pig liver. *J Biol Chem* 1997;262:8151–8158.
30. Djupesland G, Flottorp G, Refsum S. Phytanic acid storage disease: Hearing maintained after 15 years of dietary treatment. *Neurology* 1983;33:237–240.
31. Dodt G, Braverman N, Wong C, Moser A, Moser HW, Watkins P, Valle D, Gould SJ. Mutations in the PTS1 receptor gene, *PXR1,* define complementation group 2 of the peroxisome biogenesis disorders. *Nature Genet* 1995;9:115–125.
32. Eaton JW, Ma M. Acatalasemia. In *The Metabolic and Molecular Bases of Inherited Disease.* 7 ed., vol. II, C.R. Scriver, A.L. Beaudet, W.S. Sly, and D. Valle, eds. New York: McGraw-Hill, 1995:2371–2383.
33. Ek J, Kase BF, Reith A, Bjòrkhem I, Pedersen JI. Peroxisomal dysfunction in a boy with neurological symptoms and amaurosis (Leber disease): Clinical and biochemical findings similar to those observed in Zellweger syndrome. *J Pediatr* 1986:108:19–24.
34. Eustis HS, Curry T, Superneau DW. Peroxisomal bifunctional enzyme complex deficiency with associated retinal findings. *J Pediatr Ophthalmol Strabismus* 1995;32:125–127.
35. Fanen P, Guidoux S, Sarde C-O, Mandel J-L, Goossens M, Aubourg P. Identification of mutations in the putative ATP-binding domain of the adrenoleukodystrophy gene. *J Clin Invest* 1994;94:516–520.
36. Farrar GJ, Kenna PF, Jordan S, Kumar-Singh K, Humphries MM, Sharp EM, Sheils D, Humphries P. Autosomal dominant retinitis pigmentosa: Identification of mutations in the rhodopsin and peripherin/RDS gene in the original families used to map adRP loci to 3q and 6p. *Am J Hum Genet* 1992;51(4):A94 (abstract 363).
37. Fishman GA, Stone E, Gilbert LD, Vandenburgh K, Sheffield VC, Heckenlively JR. Clinical features of a previously undescribed codon 216 (proline to serine) mutation in the peripherin/retinal degeneration slow gene in autosomal dominant retinitis pigmentosa. *Ophthalmology* 1994;101:1409–1421.

38. Folz SJ, Trobe JD. The peroxisome and the eye. *Surv Ophthalmol* 1991;35:353–368.
39. Fournier B, Saudubray J-M, Benichou B, Lyonnet S, Munnich A, Clevers H, Poll-Thé BT. Large deletion of the peroxisomal acyl-CoA oxidase gene in pseudoneonatal adrenoleukodystrophy. *J Clin Invest* 1994;94:526–531.
40. Fournier B, Smeitink JAM, Dorland L, Berger R, Saudubray JM, Poll-Thé BT. Peroxisomal disorders: A review. *J Inherit Metab Dis* 1994;17:470–486.
41. Garner A, Fielder AR, Primavesi R, Stevens A. Tapetoretinal degeneration in the cerebro-hepato-renal (Zellweger's) syndrome. *Br J Ophthalmol* 1982;66:422–431.
42. Gärtner J, Kearns W, Rosenberg C, Pearson P, Copeland NG, Gilbert DJ, Jenkins NA, Valle D. Localization of the 70-kDa peroxisomal membrane protein to human 1p21-p22 and mouse 3. *Genomics* 1993;15:412–414.
43. Gärtner J, Moser H, Valle D. Mutations in the 70 K peroxisomal membrane protein in Zellweger syndrome. *Nature Genet* 1992; 1:16–23.
44. Gatfield PD, Taller E, Hinton GG, Wallace AC, Abdelnour GM, Haust MD. Hyperpipecolatemia: A new metabolic disorder associated with neuropathy and hepatomegaly: A case study. *Can Med Assoc J* 1968;99:1215–1233.
45. Goldfischer S, Collins J, Rapin I, Newmann P, Neglia W, Spiro AJ, Ishii T, Roels F, Vamecq J, van Hoof F. Pseudo-Zellweger syndrome: Deficiencies in several peroxisomal oxidative activities. *J Pediatr* 1986; 108:25–32.
46. Goldfischer S, Moore CL, Johnson AB, Spiro AJ, Valsamis MP, Wisniewski HK, Ritch RH, Norton WT, Rapin I, Gartner LM. Peroxisomal and mitochondrial defects in the cerebro-hepato-renal syndrome. *Science* 1973;182:62–64.
47. Gorin MB, Jackson KE, Ferrell RE, Sheffield VC, Jacobson SG, Gass JDM, Mitchell E, Stone EM. A peripherin/retinal degeneration slow mutation (Pro-210-Arg) associated with macular and peripheral retinal degeneration. *Ophthalmology* 1995;102:246–255.
48. Gould SJ, Keller G-A, Subramani S. Identification of peroxisomal targeting signals located at the carboxy terminus of four peroxisomal proteins. *J Cell Biol* 1988;107:897–905.
49. Gray RGF, Green A, Chapman S, McKeown C, Schutgens RBH, Wanders RJA. Rhizomelic chondrodysplasia punctata—A new clinical variant. *J Inherit Metab Dis* 1992; 15:931–932.
50. Hansen E, Bachen NK, Flage T. Refsum's disease: Eye manifestations in a patient treated with low phytol low phytanic acid diet. *Acta Ophthalmol (Copenh)* 1979;57:899–913.
51. Hansen E, Refsum S. Heredopathia atactica polyneuritiformis. Phytanic acid storage disease (Refsum's disease). A biochemically well defined disease with a specific dietary treatment. In *Neurogenetics and Neuro-Ophthalmology. Development in Neurology,* vol. 5, A. Huber and D. Klein, eds. New York: Elsevier, 1981:333–339.
52. Hanson RF, Szczepanik-vanLeeuwan P, Williams GC, Grabowski G, Sharp HL. Defects of the bile acid synthesis in Zellweger's syndrome. *Science* 1979;203:1107–1108.
53. Hashmi M, Stanley W, Singh I. Lignoceroyl-CoASH ligase: Enzyme defect in fatty acid β-oxidation system in X-linked childhood adrenoleukodystrophy. *FEBS Lett* 1986;196:247–250.
54. Heymans HSA, Schutgens RBH, Tan R, van den Bosch H, Borst P. Severe plasmalogen deficiency tissues of infants without peroxisomes (Zellweger syndrome). *Nature* 1983; 306:69–70.
55. Hillman RE. Primary hyperoxalurias. In *The Metabolic Basis of Inherited Disease,* 6th ed., vol. 1, C.R. Scriver, A.L. Beaudet, W.S. Sly, and D. Valle, eds. New York: McGraw-Hill, 1989:933–944.
56. Hittner HM, Kretzer FL, Mehta RS. Zellweger syndrome: Lenticular opacities indicating carrier status and lens abnormalities characteristic of heterozygotes. *Arch Ophthalmol* 1981;99:1977–1982.
57. Hodge VJ, Gould SJ, Subramani S, Moser HW, Krisans SK. Normal cholesterol synthesis in human cells requires functional peroxisomes. *Biochem Biophys Res Commun* 1991; 181:537–541.
58. Holtta E. Oxidation of spermidine and spermine in rat liver: Purification and properties of polyamine oxidase. *Biochemistry* 1977;16: 91–100.
59. Igarashi M, Schaumburg HH, Powers J, Kishimoto Y, Kolodny E, Suzuki K. Fatty acid abnormality in adrenoleukodystrophy. *J Neurochem* 1976;26:851–860.
60. Jacobson SG, Kemp CM, Cideciyan AV, Sun XK, Vandenburgh K, Sheffield VC, Stone EM. Spectrum of functional phenotypes in RDS gene mutations. *Invest Ophthalmol Vis Sci* 1994;35(4):1479.

60a. Jansen GA, Wanders RJA, Watkins PA, Milhalik SJ. Phytanoyl-coenzymes A hydoxylase deficiency—The enzyme defect in Refsum's disease. *N Engl J Med* 1997;337: 133–134.

60b. Jansen GA, Ofman R, Ferdinandusse S, Ijlst L, Muijsers AO, Skjeldal OH, Stokke O, Jakobs C, Besley GTN, Wraith JE, Wanders RJA. Refsum disease is caused by mutations in the phytanoyl-CoA hydroxylase gene. *Nature Genet* 1997;17:190–193.

61. Jedlitschky G, Huber M, Völkl A, Müller M, Leier I, Müller J, Lehmann W-D, Fahimi HD, Keppler D. Peroxisomal degradation of leukotrienes by β-oxidation from the ω-end. *J Biol. Chem.* 1991;266:24763–24772.

62. Johnson AB, Schaumburg HH, Powers JM. Histochemical characteristics of the striated inclusions of adrenoleukodystrophy. *J Histochem Cytochem* 1976;24:725–730.

63. Kajiwara K, Berson EL, Dryja TP. Digenic retinitis pigmentosa due to mutations at the unlinked peripherin/*RDS* and *ROM1* loci. *Science* 1994;264:1604–1608.

64. Kajiwara K, Sandberg MA, Berson EL, Dryja TP. A *null* mutation in the human peripherin/RDS gene in a family with autosomal dominant retinitis punctata albescens. *Nature Genet* 1993;3:208–212.

65. Kelley RI, Datta NS, Dobyns WB, Hajra AK, Moser AB, Noetzel MJ, Zackai EH, Moser HW. Neonatal adrenoleukodystrophy: New cases, biochemical studies, and differentiation from Zellweger and related peroxisomal polydystrophy syndromes. *Am J Med Genet* 1986;23:869–901.

66. Kemp CM, Jacobson SG, Cideciyan AV, Kimura AE, Sheffield VC, Stone EM. RDS gene mutations causing retinitis pigmentosa or macular degeneration lead to the same abnormality in photoreceptor function. *Invest Ophthalmol Vis Sci* 1994;35:3154–3162.

67. Krisans SL. The role of peroxisomes in cholesterol metabolism. *Am J Respir Cell Mol Biol* 1992;7:358–364.

68. Lazarow PB, Moser HW. Disorders of peroxisome biogenesis. In *The Metabolic Basis of Inherited Disease,* 6th ed., vol. 2, C. R. Scriver, A. L. Beaudet, W.S. Sly, and D. Valle, eds. New York: McGraw-Hill, 1989:1479–1509.

69. Lazarow PB, Moser HW. Disorders of peroxisome biogenesis. In *The Metabolic and Molecular Bases of Inherited Disease,* 7th ed., vol. 2, C.R. Scriver, A.L. Beaudet, W.S. Sly, and D. Valle, eds. New York: McGraw-Hill, 1995:2287–2324.

70. Lazo O, Contreras C, Hashmi M, Stanley W, Irazu C, Singh I. Peroxisomal lignoceryl-CoA ligase deficiency in childhood adrenoleukodystrophy and adrenomyeloneuropathy. *Proc Natl Acad Sci USA* 1988;85:7647–7651.

71. Ligtenberg MJL, Kemp S, Sarde C-O, van Geel BM, Kleijer WJ, Barth PG, Mandel J-L, van Oost BA, Bolhius PA. Spectrum of mutations in the gene encoding the adrenoleukodystrophy protein. *Am J Hum Genet* 1995;56:44–50.

72. Maestri NE, Beaty TH. Predictions of a 2-locus model for disease heterogeneity: Application to adrenoleukodystrophy. *Am J Hum Genet* 1992;44:576–582.

73. Mandel H, Berant M, Meiron D, Aizin A, Oiknine J, Brook JG, Aviram M. Plasma lipoproteins and monocyte-macrophages in a peroxisome-deficient system: Study of a patient with infantile Refsum disease. *J Inherit Metab Dis* 1992;15:774–784.

74. Marshall CJ. Protein prenylation: A mediator of protein-protein interactions. *Science* 1993; 259:1865–1866.

75. Martinez M. Severe deficiency of docosahexaenoic acid in peroxisomal disorders: A defect of Δ_4 desaturation? *Neurology* 1990;40:1292–1298.

76. Martinez M. Abnormal profiles of polyunsaturated fatty acids in the brain, liver, kidney and retina of patients with peroxisomal disorders. *Brain Res* 1992;583:171–182.

77. Martinez M. Severe changes in polyunsaturated fatty acids in the brain, liver, kidney, and retina in patients with peroxisomal disorders. In *Neurobiology of Essential Fatty Acids,* N.G. Bazan, M. G. Murphy, and G. Toffano, eds. New York: Plenum, 1992: 347–359.

78. Martinez M. Treatment with docosahexaenoic acid favorably modifies the fatty acid composition of erythrocytes in peroxisomal patients. In *New Developments in Fatty Acid Oxidation: Proceedings of the Second International Symposium on Clinical, Biochemical, and Molecular Aspects of Fatty Acid Oxidation,* P.M. Coates and K. Tanaka, eds., New York: Wiley-Liss, 1992:389–397.

79. Mayatepek E, Lehmann W-D, Fauler J, Tsikas D, Frölich JC, Schutgens RBH, Wanders RJA, Keppler D. Impaired degradation of leukotrienes in patients with peroxisome

deficiency disorders. *J Clin Invest* 1993;91: 881–888.

79a. McKusick VA. Catalase [CAT; ACATALASEMIA, INCLUDED; ACATALASIA, INCLUDED; CATALASE DEFICIENCY, INCLUDED]. In *Mendelian Inheritance in Man: A Catalog of Human Genes and Genetic Disorders,* 11th ed., vol. 1, V.A. McKusick, ed., with the assistance of C.A. Francomano, S.E. Antonarakis, and P.L. Pearson. Baltimore: Johns Hopkins University Press 1994:259–261.

79b. Mihalik SJ, Morrell JC, Kim D, Sacksteder KA, Watkins PA, Gould SJ. Identification of *PAHX,* a Refsum disease gene. *Nature Genet* 1997;17:185–189.

80. Milliner DS, Eickholt JT, Bergstralh EJ, Wilson DM, Smith LH. Results of long-term treatment with orthophosphate and pyridoxine in patients with primary hyperoxaluria. *N Engl J Med* 1994;331:1533–1558.

81. Moser AB, Rasmussen M, Naidu S, Watkins PA, McGuinness M, Hajra AK, Chen G, Raymond G, Liu A, Gordon D, Garnaas K, Walton DS, Skjeldal OH, Guggenheim MA, Jackson LG, Elias ER, Moser HW. Phenotype of patients with peroxisomal disorders subdivided into sixteen complementation groups. *J Pediatr* 1995;127:13–22.

82. Moser AE, Singh I, Brown FR III. Solish GI, Kelley RI, Benke PJ, Moser HW. The cerebrohepatorenal (Zellweger) syndrome: Increased levels and impaired degradation of very-long-chain fatty acids and their use in prenatal diagnosis. *N Engl J Med* 1984; 310:1141–1146.

83. Moser HW. The peroxisome: Nervous system role of a previously underrated organelle. *Neurology* 1988;38:1617–1627.

84. Moser HW, Kok F, Neumann S, Borel J, Bergin A, Mostafa SD, Panoscha R, Davoli CT, Shankroff J, Smith KD. Adrenoleukodystrophy update: Genetics and effect of Lorenzo's oil therapy in asymptomatic patients. *Int Pediatr* 1994;9(3):196–204.

85. Moser HW, Moser AB. (1989) Adrenoleukodystrophy (X-linked). In *The Metabolic Basis of Inherited Disease,* 6th ed., vol. 2, C.R. Scriver, A.L. Beaudet, W.S. Sly, and D. Valle, eds. New York: McGraw-Hill, 1989:1511–1532.

86. Moser HW, Moser AB, Frayer KK, Chen W, Schulman JD, O'Neill BP, Kishimoto Y. Adrenoleukodystrophy: Increased plasma content of saturated very long chain fatty acids. *Neurology* 1981;31:1241–1249.

87. Moser HW, Moser AB, Kawamura N, Murphy J, Milunsky A, Suzuki K, Schaumburg H, Kishimoto Y. Adrenoleukodystrophy: Elevated C-26 fatty acid in cultured skin fibroblasts. *Ann Neurol* 1980;7:542–549.

88. Moser HW, Moser AB, Naidu S, Bergin A. Clinical aspects of adrenoleukodystrophy and adrenomyeloneuropathy. *Dev Neurosci* 1991; 13;254–261.

89. Moser HW, Smith KD, Moser AB. X-linked adrenoleukodystrophy. In *The Metabolic and Molecular Bases of Inherited Disease,* 7th ed., vol. 2, C.R. Scriver, A. L. Beaudet, W.S. Sly, and D. Valle, eds. New York: McGraw-Hill, 1995:2325–2349.

90. Mosser J, Douar A-M, Sarde C-O, Kioschis P, Feil R, Moser H, Poustka A-M, Mandel J-L, Aubourg P. Putative X-linked adrenoleukodystrophy gene shares unexpected homology with ABC transporters. *Nature* 1993;361: 726–730.

91. Mosser J, Lutz Y, Stoeckel ME, Sarde CO, Kretz C, Douar AM, Lopez J, Aubourg P, Mandell JL. The gene responsible for adrenoleukodystrophy encodes a peroxisomal membrane protein. *Hum Mol Genet* 1994;3: 265–271.

92. Motley A, Hettema E, Distel B, Tabak H. Differential protein import deficiencies in human peroxisome assembly disorders. *J Cell Biol* 1994;125:755–767.

92a. Motley AM, Hettema EH, Hogenhout EM, Brites P, ten Asbroek ALMA, Wijburg FA, et al. Rhizomelic chondrodysplasia punctata is a peroxisomal protein targeting disease caused by a non-functional PTS2 receptor. *Nature Genet* 1997;15:377–380.

93. Naidu S, Bresnan MJ, Griffin D, O'Toole S, Moser HW. Childhood adrenoleukodystrophy: Failure of intensive immunosuppression to arrest neurologic progression. *Arch Neurol* 1988;45:846–848.

94. Naritomi K, Hyakuna N, Suzuki Y, Orii T, Hirayama K. Zellweger syndrome and a microdeletion of the proximal long arm of chromosome 7. *Hum Genet* 1988;80:201–202.

95. Naritomi K, Izumikawa Y, Ohshiro S, Yoshida K, Shimozawa N, Suzuki Y, Orii T, Hirayama K. Gene assignment of Zellweger syndrome to 7q11.23: Report of the second case associated with a pericentric inversion of chromosome 7. *Hum Genet* 1989;84:79–80.

96. Nichols BE, Sheffield VC, Vandenburgh K, Drack AV, Kimura AE, Stone EM. Butterfly-shaped pigment dystrophy of the fovea caused by a point mutation in codon 167 of the RDS gene. *Nature Genet* 1993;3:202–207.
97. Opitz JM. The Zellweger syndrome: Book review and bibliography. *Am J Med Genet* 1985;22:419.
98. Opitz JM, ZuRhein GM, Vitale L, Shahida NT, Howe JJ, Chou SM, Shanklin DR, Sybers HD, Dood AR, Gerritsen T. The Zellweger syndrome (cerebro-hepato-renal syndrome). *Birth Defects Orig Art Ser* 1969;V(2): 144–160.
99. Passarge E, McAdams AJ. Cerebro-hepato-renal syndrome: A newly recognized hereditary disorder of multiple congenital defects including sudanophilic leukodystrophy, cirrhosis of the liver, and polycystic kidneys. *J Pediatr* 1967;71:691–702.
100. Poll-Thé BT, Skjeldal OH, Stokke O, Poulos A, Demaugre F, Saudubray J-M. Phytanic acid alpha-oxidation and complementation analysis of classical Refsum and peroxisomal disorders. *Hum Genet* 1989;81:175–181.
101. Poll-Thé BT, Roels F, Ogier H, Scotto J, Vamecq J, Schutgens RBH, van Roermund CWT, van Wijland MJA, Schram AW, Tager JM, Saudubray JM. A new peroxisomal disorder with enlarged peroxisomes and a specific deficiency of acyl-CoA oxidase (pseudo-neonatal adrenoleukodystrophy). *Am J Hum Genet* 1988;42:422–434.
102. Poll-Thé BT, Saudubray JM, Ogier H, Schutgens RBH, Wanders RJA, Schrakamp G, van den Bosch H, Trijbels JMF, Poulos A, Moser HW, van Eldere J, Eyssen HJ. Infantile Refsum's disease: Biochemical findings suggesting multiple peroxisomal dysfunction. *J Inherit Metab Dis* 1986;9:169–174.
103. Poll-Thé BT, Saudubray JM, Ogier HAM, Odievre M, Scotto JM, Monnens L, Govaerts LCP, Roels F, Cornelis A, Schutgens RBH, Wanders RJA, Schram AW, Tager JM. Infantile Refsum disease: An inherited peroxisomal disorder—Comparison with Zellweger syndrome and neonatal adrenoleukodystrophy. *Eur J Pediatr* 1987;146:477–483.
104. Poulos A, Sharp P, Fellenberg AJ, Johnson DW. Accumulation of pristanic acid (2,6,10, 14 tetramethylpentadecanoic acid) in the plasma of patients with generalized peroxisomal dysfunction. *Eur J Pediatr* 1988;147: 143–147.
105. Poulos A, Sharp P, Whiting M. Infantile Refsum's disease (phytanic acid storage disease): A variant of Zellweger's syndrome? *Clin Genet* 1984;26:579–586.
106. Poulos A, Sheffield L, Sharp P, Sherwood G, Johnson D, Beckman K, Fellenberg AJ, Wraith JE, Chow CW, Usher S, Singh H. Rhizomelic chondrodysplasia punctata: Clinical, pathologic, and biochemical findings in two patients. *J Pediatr* 1988;113:685–690.
107. Powers JM, Schaumburg HH. Adreno-leukodystrophy: Similar ultrastructural changes in adrenal cortical and Schwann cells. *Arch Neurol* 1974;30:406–408.
107a. Purdue PE, Zhang JW, Skoneczyn M, Lazarow PB. Rhizomelic chondrodysplasia punctata is caused by deficiency of human PEX7, a homologue of the yeast PTS2 receptor. *Nature Genet* 1997;15:381–384.
108. Refsum S. Heredopathia atactica polyneuritiformis: A familial syndrome not hitherto described. *Acta Psychiatr Scand Suppl* 1946; 38:1–303.
109. Refsum S. Heredopathia atactica polyneuritiformis: Phytanic acid storage disease (Refsum's disease) with particular reference to ophthalmological disturbances. *Metab Ophthalmol* 1977;1:73–79.
110. Rhodin J. *Correlation of Ultrastructural Organization and Function in Normal and Experimentally Changed Proximal Convoluted Tubule Cells of the Mouse Kidney*. Stockholm: Aktiebolaget Godvil, 1954. Dissertation.
111. Roels F, Espeel M, De Craemer D. Liver pathology and immunocytochemistry in congenital peroxisomal diseases: A review. *J Inherit Metab Dis* 1991;14:853–875.
112. Roscher AA, Hoefler S, Hoefler G, Paschke E, Paltauf F, Moser A, Moser H. Genetic and phenotypic heterogeneity in disorders of peroxisome biogenesis—A complementation study involving cell lines from 19 patients. *Pediatr Res* 1989;26:67–72.
113. Schram AW, Goldfischer S, van Roermund CWT, Brouwer-Kelder EM, Collins J, Hashimoto T, Heymans HSA, van den Bosch H, Schutgens RBH, Tager JM, Wanders RJA. Human peroxisomal 3-oxoacyl-coenzyme. A thiolase deficiency. *Proc Natl Acad Sci USA* 1987;84;2494–2496.
114. Schutgens RBH, Romeyn GJ, Wanders RJA, van den Bosch H, Schrakamp G, Heymans HSA. Deficiency of acyl-CoA: Dihydroxylacetone phosphate acyltransferase in patients

with Zellweger (cerebro-hepato-renal) syndrome. *Biochem Biophys Res Comm* 1984; 120;179–184.

115. Scotto JM, Hadchouel M, Odievre M, Laudat MH, Saudubray JM, Dulac O, Beucler I, Beaune P. Infantile phytanic acid storage disease, a possible variant of Refsum's disease: Three cases, including ultrastructural studies of the liver. *J Inherit Metab Dis* 1982;8:83–90.
116. Seabra MC, Brown MS, Goldstein JL. Retinal degeneration in choroideremia: Deficiency of Rab geranylgeranyl transferase. *Science* 1993; 259:377–381.
116a. Shani M, Steel G, Dean M, Valle D. Four half ABC transporters may heterodimerize in the peroxisome membrane. *Am J Hum Genet* 1996;59:A42 (abstract 208).
117. Shimozawa N, Masuno M, Suzuki Y, Orii T, Imaizumi K, Kuroki Y, Tsukamoto T, Osumi T, Fujiki Y. A human gene of Zellweger syndrome is mapped to chromosome 8q21.1. *Am J Hum Genet* 1993;53:A947.
118. Shimozawa N, Suzuki Y, Orii T, Moser A, Moser H, Wanders RJA. Standardization of complementation grouping of peroxisome-deficient disorders and the second Zellweger patient with peroxisomal assembly factor-1 (PAF-1) defect. *Am J Hum Genet* 1993; 52:843–844.
119. Shimozawa N, Tsukamoto T, Suzuki Y, Orii T, Shirayoshi Y, Mori T, Fujiki Y. A human gene responsible for Zellweger syndrome that affects peroxisome assembly. *Science* 1992; 255:1132–1134.
120. Siemerling E, Creutzfeldt HG. Bronzekrankheit und sklerosierende Encephalomyelitis (diffuse Skerose). *Arch Psychiatr Nervenkr* 1923;68:217–244.
121. Singh H, Derwas N, Poulos A. Very long chain fatty acid beta-oxidation by rat liver mitochondria and peroxisomes. *Arch Biochem Biophys* 1987;259:382–390.
122. Singh I, Moser AE, Goldfischer S, Moser HW. Lignoceric acid is oxidized in the peroxisomes: Implications for the Zellweger cerebro-hepato-renal syndrome and adrenoleukodystrophy. *Proc Natl Acad Sci USA* 1984; 81:4203–4207.
123. Singh I, Pahan K, Dhaunsi GS, Lazo O, Ozand P. Phytanic acid α-oxidation: Differential subcellular localization in rat and human tissue and its inhibition by Nycodenz. *J Biol Chem* 1993;268:9972–9979.
124. Singh I, Pahan K, Singh AK, Barbosa E. Refsum disease: A defect in the α-oxidation of phytanic acid in peroxisomes. *J Lipid Res* 1993;34:1755–1764.
125. Slawecki ML, Dodt G, Moser AB, Moser HW, Gould SJ. Identification of three distinct peroxisomal protein import defects in patients with peroxisome biogenesis disorders. *J Cell Sci* 1995;108:1817–1829.
126. Small KW, Letson R, Scheinman J. Ocular findings in primary oxalosis. *Arch Ophthalmol* 1990;108:89–93.
127. Smith DW, Opitz JM, Inhorn SL. A syndrome of multiple developmental defects including polycystic kidneys and intrahepatic biliary dysgenesis in 2 siblings. *J Pediatr* 1965; 67:617–624.
128. Spranger JW, Opitz JM, Bidder. Heterogeneity of chondrodysplasia punctata. *Humangenetik* 1971;11:190–212.
129. Steinberg D. Refsum disease. In *The Metabolic Basis of Inherited Disease,* vol. 2, C.R. Scriver, A.L. Beaudet, W.S, Sly and D. Valle eds. New York: McGraw-Hill, 1989:1533–1550.
130. Steinberg D. Refsum disease. In *The Metabolic and Molecular Bases of Inherited Disease,* 7th ed., vol 2, C. R. Scriver A. L. Beaudet W.S, Sly and D. Valle, eds. New York: McGraw-Hill, 1995:2351–2369.
131. Subramani S. Protein import into peroxisomes and biogenesis of the organelle. *Annu Rev Cell Biol* 1993;9:445–478.
132. Suzuki Y, Shimozawa N, Orii T, Igarashi N, Kono N, Hashimoto T. Molecular analysis of peroxisomal β-oxidation enzymes in infants with Zellweger syndrome and Zellweger-like syndrome: Further heterogeneity of the peroxisomal disorders. *Clin Chim Acta* 1988; 172:65–76.
133. Suzuki Y, Shimozawa N, Yajima S, Tomatsu S, Kondo N, Nakada Y, Akaboshi S, Iai M, Tanabe Y, Hashimoto T, Wanders RJA, Schutgens RBH, Moser HW, Orii T. Novel subtype of peroxisomal acyl-CoA oxidase deficiency and bifunctional enzyme deficiency with detectable enzyme protein: Identification by means of complementation analysis, *Am J Hum Genet* 1994;54:36–43.
134. Swinkels BW, Gould SJ, Bodnar AG, Rachubinski RA, Subramani S. A novel, cleavable peroxisomal targeting signal at the aminoterminus of the rat 3-ketoacyl-CoA thiolase. *EMBO J* 1991;10:3255–3262.
135. Takada Y, Kaneko N, Esumi H, Purdue PE, Danpure CJ. Human proxisomal L-ala-

nine:glyoxylate aminotransferase. Evolutionary loss of a mitochondrial targeting signal by point mutation of the initiation codon. *Biochem J* 1990;208:517–520.

136. ten Brink HJ, Schor DSM, Kok RM, Stellaard F, Kneer J, Poll-The BT, Saudubray J-M, Jakobs C. *In vivo* study of phytanic acid α-oxidation in classic Refsum's disease and chondrodysplasia punctata. *Pediatr Res* 1992; 32:566–570.
137. Theil AC, Schutgens RBH, Wanders RJA, Heymans HSA. Clinical recognition of patients affected by a peroxisomal disorder: A retrospective study in 40 patients. *Eur J Pediatr* 1992;151:117–120.
138. Torvik A, Torp, S, Kase BF, Ek J, Skjeldal O, Stokke O. Infantile Refsum's disease: A generalized peroxisomal disorder. Case report with postmortem examination. *J Neurol Sci* 1988;85:39–53.
139. Traboulsi EI, El-Baba F, Barakat AY, Faris BM. The retinopathy of primary hyperoxaluria. *Retina* 1985;5:151–153.
140. Traboulsi EI, Maumenee IH. Ophthalmologic manifestations of X-linked childhood adrenoleukodystrophy. *Ophthalmology* 1987; 94:47–51.
141. Ulrich J, Herschkowitz N, Heitz P, Sigrist T, Baerlocher P. Adrenoleukodystrophy: Preliminary report of a connatal case: Light- and electron microscopical, immunohistochemical and biochemical findings. *Acta Neuropathol (Berlin)* 1978;43:77–83.
142. van den Bosch H, Schutgens RBH, Wanders RJA, Tager JM. Biochemistry of peroxisomes. *Annu Rev Biochem* 1992;61:157–197.
143. van Heyningen V, Boyd PA, Seawright A, Fletcher JM, Fantes JA, Buckton KE, Spowart G, Porteous DJ, Hill RE, Newton MS, Hastie ND. Molecular analysis of chromosome 11 deletions in aniridia-Wilms' tumor syndrome. *Proc Natl Acad Sci USA* 1985; 82:8592–8596.
144. Varanasi U, Chu R, Chu S, Espinosa R, LeBeau MM, Reddy JK. Isolation of the human peroxisomal acyl-CoA oxidase gene: Organization, promoter analysis, and chromosomal localization. *Proc Natl Acad Sci USA* 1994;91:3107–3111.
145. Versmold HT, Bremer HJ, Herzog V, Siegel G, Bassewitz DB, Irle U, Voss H, Lombeck I, Brauser B. A metabolic disorder similar to Zellweger syndrome with hepatic actalasia and absence of peroxisomes, altered content and redox state of cytochromes, and infantile cirrhosis with hemosiderosis. *Eur J Pediatr* 1977;124:261–275.
146. Voss A, Reinhart M, Sankarappa S, Sprecher H. The metabolism of 7,10,13,16,19-docosapentaenoic acid to 4,7,10,13,16,19-docosahexaenoic acid in rat liver is independent of 4-desaturase. *J Biol Chem* 1991;266:19995–20000.
147. Wanders RJA, Dekker C, Hovarth VAP, Schutgens RBH, Tager JM, van Laer P, Lecoutere D. Human alkyldihydroxyacetonephosphate synthase deficiency: A new peroxisomal disorder. *J Inherit Metab Dis* 1994; 17:315–318.
148. Wanders RJA, Schumacher H, Heikoop J, Schutgens RBH, Tager JM. Human dihydroxyacetonephosphate acyltransferase deficiency: A new peroxisomal disorder. *J Inherit Metab Dis* 1992;15:389–391.
149. Wanders RJA, ten Brink HJ, van Roermund CWT, Schutgens RBH, Tager JM, Jakobs C. Identification of pristanoyl-CoA oxidase activity in human liver and its deficiency in the Zellweger syndrome. *Biochem Biophys Res Commun* 1990;172:490–495.
150. Wanders RJA, van Roermund CWT, Brul S, Schutgens RBH, Tager JM. Bifunctional enzyme deficiency: Identification of a new type of peroxisomal disorder in a patient with an impairment in peroxisomal β-oxidation of unknown aetiology by means of complementation analysis. *J Inherit Metab Dis* 1992; 15:385–388.
151. Wanders RJA, van Roermund CWT, van Wijland MJA, Schutgens RBH, van den Bosch H, Tager JM. Direct demonstration that the deficient oxidation of very long chain fatty acids in X-linked adrenoleukodystrophy is due to an impaired ability of peroxisomes to activate very long chain fatty acids. *Biochem Biophys Res Commun* 1988;153:618–624.
152. Wardinsky TD, Pagon RA, Powell BR, McGillivray B, Stephan M, Zonana J, Moser A. Rhizomelic chondrodysplasia punctata and survival beyond one year: A review of the literature and five case reports. *Clin Genet* 1990;38:84–93.
153. Watkins P, Chen WW, Harris CJ, Hoefler G, Hoefler S, Blake DC Jr, Balfe A, Kelly RI, Moser AB, Beard ME, Moser HW. Peroxisomal bifunctional enzyme deficiency. *J Clin Invest* 1989;83:771–777.
154. Watkins PA, Mihalik SJ, Skjedal OH. Mitochondrial oxidation of phytanic acid in human and monkey liver: Implication that Refsum's

disease is not a peroxisomal disorder. *Biochem Biophys Res Commun* 1990;167:580–586.

155. Weleber RG. Retinitis pigmentosa and allied disorders. In *Retina: Basic Science and Inherited Retinal Disease,* 2nd ed., vol. 1, S.J. Ryan, ed., with the assistance of T.E. Ogden. St. Louis: C. V. Mosby, 1994:335–466.
156. Weleber RG, Carr RE, Murphey WH, Sheffield VC, Stone EM. Phenotypic variation including retinitis pigmentosa, pattern dystrophy, and fundus flavimaculatus in a single family with a deletion of codon 153 or 154 of the peripherin/*RDS* gene. *Arch Ophthalmol* 1993;111:1531–1542.
157. Weleber RG, Kennaway NG. Infantile Refsum's disease. In *The Eye in Systemic Disease,* D.H. Gold and T.A. Weingeist, eds. Philadelphia: J. B. Lippincott, 1990:409–411.
158. Weleber RG, Kennaway NG. Refsum's disease. In *The Eye in Systemic Disease,* D.H. Gold and T.A. Weingeist, eds. Philadelphia: J. B. Lippincott, 1990:407–408.
159. Weleber RG, Tongue AT, Kennaway NG, Budden SS, Buist NRM. Ophthalmic manifestations of infantile phytanic acid storage disease. *Arch Ophthalmol* 1984;102:1317–1321.
160. Wells J, Wroblewski J, Keen J, Inglehearn C, Jubb C, Eckstein A, Jay M, Arden G, Bhattacharya S, Fitzke F, Bird A. Mutations in the human retinal degeneration slow (*RDS*) gene can cause either retinitis pigmentosa or macular dystrophy. *Nature Genet* 1993;3:213–218.
161. Wilson GN, Holmes RG, Custer J, Lipkowitz JL, Stover J, Datta N, Hajra A. Zellweger syndrome: Diagnostic assays, syndrome delineation, and potential therapy. *Am J Med Genet* 1986;24:69–82.

34

Albinism

LISA S. ABRAMS
ELIAS I. TRABOULSI

Albinism comprises a heterogeneous group of inherited disorders characterized by the reduction or total absence of pigment from the eye, hair, and skin. All the current known types of albinism are inherited in an autosomal recessive fashion with the exception of Nettleship-Falls ocular albinism, which is X-linked recessive. Albinism has been classified as to type by the degree and the distribution of hypopigmentation as *total versus partial*, and *ocular versus oculocutaneous*. As the molecular genetic understanding of disorders of pigmentation has improved,[72,123] it has become possible to classify albinism more accurately with regard to the specific genetic defect in each clinical subtype (Table 34.1).

The ophthalmologic findings in all forms of albinism are consistent, although variable in severity. Signs include nystagmus, hypopigmentation of the uveal tract and retinal pigment epithelium, iris transillumination, foveal hypoplasia, and abnormal decussation of optic nerve fibers at the chiasm. Strabismus and high refractive errors are common. Symptoms include decreased visual acuity, reduced or absent stereoacuity, and photophobia.

Albinoidism refers to the reduction of ocular and cutaneous pigmentation without visual system abnormalities. *Albinism* results from the defective production of melanin from tyrosine through a complex pathway of metabolic reactions that were worked out partially by Raper[108] early in the twentieth century. Melanogenesis is a complicated pathway involving enzymes and proteins coded for by genes on a number of chromosomes.

HISTORICAL REFERENCES

Sorsby[119] has provided evidence that Noah (builder of the Ark in Hebrew Scripture) was an albino. Another famous albino was William Spooner, a twentieth century British classicist and Warden of New College at Oxford University, whose amusing tendency to errors of speech came to be known as "spoonerism." The aberration of speech was said to be related to his nystagmus, which caused a jumbling of information from the printed page. Other famous albinos include Edward the Confessor, Saxon king from 1042 to 1066, and Tamerlane, the fourteenth century Central Asian conqueror.

EPIDEMIOLOGY

The prevalence of albinism varies with the racial makeup of a particular geographic area.

Table 34.1. Classification of Human Abinism

Clinical Type	Defective Gene	Gene Map
Tyrosinase-negative oculocutaneous albinism	Tyrosinase (TYR)	11q14-q21
Yellow mutant type of oculocutaneous albinism	Tyrosinase (TYR)	11q14-q21
Temperature-sensitive oculocutaneous albinism	Tyrosinase (TYR)	11q14-q21
Rufous albinism (xanthism)	Unknown	
Brown albinism (albinism with only moderate reduction in pigment)	Tyrosinase-related protein (TYRP)	9p
Tyrosinase-positive oculocutaneous albinism	Some cases due to mutations in tyrosinase, others to mutations in P gene	15q11.2-q12 11q14-q21
Nettleship-Falls ocular albinism, X-linked ocular albinism		Xp22.3
Forsius-Eriksson disease (Åland island eye disease)	Unknown	Xp11.4-p11.2
Autosomal recessive ocular albinism	Some cases due to mutations in tyrosinase, others to mutations in P gene	11q14-q21 15q11.2-q12
X-linked albinism with late-onset deafness	Unknown	Xp22.3
Hermansky-Pudlak syndrome	Transmembrane component of cytoplasmic organelles	10q23.1-23.3
Chediak-Higashi syndrome	Important in lysosomal and granular cell compartmentalization	1q43

The frequency of albinism is 1/18,000 among U.S. whites, 1/10,000 among U.S. blacks, and approximately 1/20,000 in the United States overall.[67] The carrier frequency for the type I oculocutaneous albinism (OCA) (tyrosinase-negative) gene is 1 in 99 Caucasians and 1 in 84 African Americans. Witkop found that 9% of partially sighted individuals attending institutions in the United States had some form of OCA.[146] Type II OCA (previously known as "tyrosinase-positive OCA") is the most common type overall, with an incidence of 1 in 36,000 among Caucasians in the United States and 1 in 10,000 among U.S. blacks.[67] Type I OCA (formerly known as "tyrosinase-negative") is slightly less common in whites (1 in 39,000) and much less common in blacks (1 in 28,000).[67] In British Columbia, however, McLeod and Lowry[92] found the incidence of type I OCA to be 1 in 67,800 live births and that of type II OCA to be 1 in 35,700 live births. Type IB OCA (formerly known as "yellow mutant") was first described in, and is most prevalent among the Amish. Type IV ("brown") oculocutaneous albinism occurs in up to 1 in 1100 Nigerians.[105] The Hermansky-Pudlak syndrome is most common among Puerto Ricans but has been reported in other ethnic groups. Among Puerto Ricans it has a prevalence of 1/1800 and a carrier rate of 1/21 persons.[147] Chediak-Higashi syndrome is relatively less common and has been described in an isolated cluster of Venezuelan patients. X-linked Nettleship-Falls ocular albinism affects approximately 1 person in 150,000.[116,134]

MELANOCYTE DEVELOPMENT AND THE SYNTHESIS OF MELANIN

Melanin is synthesized and deposited within specialized intracellular organelles called *melanosomes*. Melanin acts as a barrier against ionizing radiation, participates in the cellular developmental process, and acts as a scavenger of cytotoxic free radicals.

Melanosomes are formed from rough and smooth endoplasmic reticulum in conjunction with vesiculoglobular bodies in the cytoplasm. The process of melanogenesis is identical within neural crest–derived melanocytes of the skin, hair, and uvea, and within the ocular pigment epithelia, which are derived from the optic vesicle neuroectoderm.[95,150] Melanogenesis occurs in four stages and the melanosomes in the four stages are numbered accordingly. Stage I and II melanosomes contain no melanin; they originate from the smooth endoplasmic reticulum as cytoplasmic membrane-bound vesicles (stage I). Tyrosinase is synthesized on the ribosomes and transported from rough endoplasmic reticulum to the Golgi apparatus; it is then glycosylated and secreted into coated vesicles, which are transferred to premelanosomes. The premelanosomes then elongate and become oval, and are filled with parallel filaments (stage II). In stage III, the filaments gradually become completely filled with melanin and thicken to form rodlets; melanin is deposited focally along these filaments. When the rodlets are compacted to form a homogeneously dense structure, and there is no tyrosinase activity remaining, the vesicle is considered a mature (stage IV) melanosome.[95]

The time course in development and morphology of the melanosomes differs between cutaneous and ocular tissues. Whereas skin and hair melanocytes produce melanized melanosomes for exportation to adjacent cells, uveal melanocytes and ocular pigment epithelial cells do not normally release their melanosomes. Thus, melanogenesis is a lifelong activity of skin and hair melanocytes, but it is a transient activity of ocular pigment epithelial cells. Retinal pigment epithelial (neuroectoderm-derived) melanogenesis begins by the third or fourth week of gestation[150] and is thought to be completed shortly after birth. Uveal melanocytes (neural crest cell–derived) appear much later at about 20 weeks of gestation and may continue to produce pigment for several years, thus accounting for darkening of the iris stroma and choroid in childhood. The pigment content of the ocular pigment epithelium is relatively constant and perhaps independent of constitutive pigmentation. Experience with X-linked ocular albinism in blacks suggests that pigment content of the pigment epithelium is partly dependent on constitutive pigmentation, but to a lesser degree than uveal pigmentation. Retinal pigment epithelial (RPE) cells are very reactive to a number of stimuli but do not seem to be able to resume melanogenesis. Cryotherapy, diathermy, and photocoagulation produce hyperpigmented areas of the fundus, but this ophthalmoscopic sign represents pigment clumping rather than renewed or increased melanogenesis.

Melanosomes within the skin, hair, and uvea are typically ellipsoidal, and they measure on the average 0.7 mm × 0.3 mm, with a maximum dimension of about 1.3 mm. On average, pigment epithelial melanosomes are larger than melanocytic melanosomes. Melanosomes of the ocular pigmented epithelia vary in shape from spherical to ellipsoidal. The spherical melanosomes have a maximum diameter of 0.85 mm and the ellipsoidal melanosomes have a maximum axis of 1.45 mm. The iris pigment epithelium has mainly spherical melanosomes, whereas the retinal pigment epithelium mainly has ellipsoidal melanosomes.

Within the melanosomes the copper-containing enzyme tyrosinase catalyzes three of the steps of a series of reactions leading to the formation of melanin from its precursor tyrosine, including the initial, rate-limiting step (Fig. 34.1). Tyrosine is hydroxylated to L-3,4-dihydroxyphenylalanine (DOPA) and then oxidized to dopaquinone; both steps are catalyzed by tyrosinase. Dopaquinone spontaneously rearranges to form leucodopachrome, then dopachrome; however, in the presence of glutathione and/or cysteine, dopaquinone is diverted to the pheomelanin pathway (see below). Dopachrome is decarboxylated to 5,6-dihydroxyindole, which is oxidized to indole-5,6-quinone; this reaction is also catalyzed by tyrosinase.[55] The indole–quinone is converted to melachrome (by tyrosinase or peroxidase), which polymerizes to form eumelanin, a high molecular weight compound that is black-brown. Alternatively, dopachrome may be diverted to 5,6-dihydroxyindole-2-carboxylic acid (DHICA)

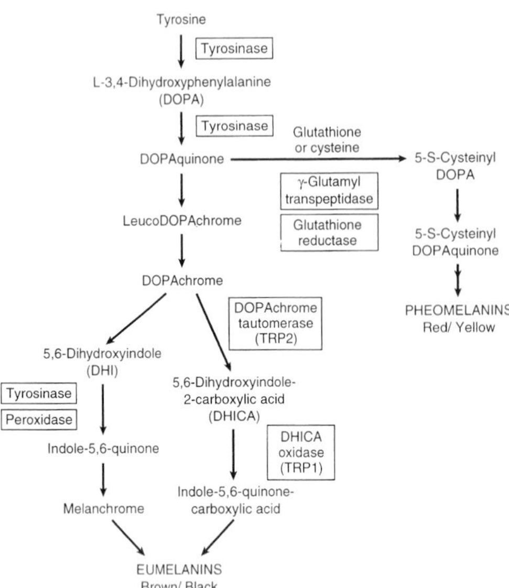

Figure 34.1. Metabolic pathway for the formation of the melanins.

in the presence of dopachrome tautomerase (tyrosinase-related protein-2) or divalent cations. DHICA will be oxidized to indole–quinone carboxylic acid by tyrosinase-related protein-1 and then converted to eumelanin.

Two alternative pathways are available for the processing of dopaquinone. In the presence of high concentrations of cysteine, dopaquinone will form cysteinyl DOPA, which is then oxidized to form pheomelanin (a pigment that has a yellow or reddish-brown color). Alternatively, or concomitantly, DOPA will react with glutathione to form pheomelanin. Trichrome, a third pigmented polymer that is yellow to red in color, is a lower molecular compound than pheomelanin and is produced when oxidized tyrosine reacts with cysteine. Additional proteins involved in melanogenesis include an indole-blocking factor, an indole-converting factor, and a quinone-converting factor.

Ultrastructurally normal melanosomes are present in all subtypes of oculocutaneous albinism, but they are incompletely melanized.[148] Therefore, pigmentary dilution in all subtypes of OCA is due to inadequate amounts of melanin within apparently normal numbers of melanosomes. In contrast, X-linked recessive ocular albinism results from fewer than the normal number of melanosomes, but those that are present are fully melanized.

CLINICAL CHARACTERISTICS AND CLASSIFICATION

In 1904 Durham[35] discovered that albino animals lacked tyrosinase activity. Kugelman and Van Scott[79] demonstrated that some albinos had evidence of tyrosinase activity using the hair bulb tyrosine assay. This led to the classification of oculocutaneous albinism into tyrosinase-negative and tyrosinase-positive categories (Table 34.2). King, Olds, and Witkop[70] demonstrated that the tyrosinase present in the hair bulbs of tyrosinase-positive (type II) albinos was kinetically normal; thus the metabolic defect must be elsewhere in the melanin pathway. As understanding of the molecular genetic basis of albinism has expanded, the older classification of albinism based on tyrosinase activity has given way to one that is based on specific genetic defects. For example, type I OCA results from mutations in the tyrosinase gene (chromosome 11p14-21).[8,102,122] There are two subtypes that are allelic: type Ia with an abolished tyrosinase activity and type Ib with a markedly decreased tyrosinase activity. Type II is due to mutations in the "P" gene (chromosome 15), which corresponds to the pink-eyed dilution mutation (*p*) in mouse and codes for a protein that is an integral component of the cellular membrane and may function in the transport of tyrosine into the melanosome. The range of phenotypes in type II OCA may relate to the extent of P gene function.[111] The gene for type IV OCA has not yet been identified. In mice, the gene encodes a tyrosinase-related protein that is involved in a distal step of eumelanin synthesis. The analogous gene in humans is on chromosome 9p22-23.[68] The X-linked recessive ocular albinism gene was recently cloned and is located on the distal short arm of the X chromosome.[9] Diagnosis relies on the pattern of family history and the identification of female carriers.

Many patients with presumed tyrosinase-positive albinism have actually been found to carry tyrosinase gene mutations with a less severe phenotype than tyrosinase-negative albi-

Table 34.2. Major Features of Disorders of Melanogenesis*

Type	Ia	Ib	II	IV
Name	Tyrosinase negative	Yellow albinism	Tyrosinase positive	Brown albinism
Characteristics	No pigment	Little to no pigment at birth; increases with age	Little pigment at birth; increases with age	Moderate hypopigmentation
	VA around 20/200	Phenotypic variability	VA 20/40–20/400	VA 20/60–20/200
	Nystagmus	—	—	—
	Foveal hypoplasia		—	—
	Strabismus			
Defective gene	Tyrosinase (tyr)	Tyrosinase	P (pink-eyed dilution)	Tyrosinase-related protein 1
Chromosome	11p14-21	11p14-21 (allelic with Ia)	15q11.2-q12	9p22-23
Inheritance	AR	AR	AR	AR
Pathophysiology	Normal number of melanosomes with no melanin	Incomplete and decreased melanization—stage I, II, III premelanosomes	?Abnormal transport of tyrosine across melanosome membrane—stage II and III premelanosomes	Defect in enzyme in melanin biosynthesis—stage II and III premelanosomes with few stage IV melanosomes
Hair-bulb melanosomes	Stage I and II premelanosomes	—	—	—
Diagnostic tests	Hair-bulb test—negative carriers: decreased tyrosinase activity	Hair-bulb test—negative or weakly positive (positive with l-cysteine)	Hair-bulb test—positive Visual evoked potential	Hair-bulb test—positive

Type	XLOA	Hermansky-Pudlak	Chediak-Higashi
Name	Nettleship-Falls	—	—
Characteristics	Mild skin, iris, retinal hypopigmentation; iris transillumination defects	Lightly pigmented skin and iris; normal or decreased VA; bleeding diathesis; pulmonary fibrosis	Variable pigmentation; VA normal to moderately decreased; immune deficiency; decreased life span
Gene function	Unknown	Organelle structural membrane protein defect	Intracellular protein transport defect
Chromosome	Xp22.3	12q12-13	1q43
Inheritance	XR	AR	AR
Pathophysiology	Decreased numbers of melanosomes with normal melanin	Pheomelanosomes; unevenly melanized melanosomes	Giant melanosomes; decreased numbers of melanosomes
Hair-bulb melanosomes	Type IV melanosomes; macromelanosomes	Stage I, II, III premelanosomes	Stage II and III premelanosomes; stage IV melanosomes; macromelanosomes
Diagnostic tests	Hair-bulb test—positive; macromelanosomes; carriers—tigroid fundus	Hair-bulb test—positive; prolonged bleeding time; ceroid accumulation	Hair-bulb test—positive; giant lysosomal granules; decreased natural killer cell activity

* AR = autosomal recessive; VA = visual acuity; XR = X-linked recessive; xLOA = X-linked ocular albinism.

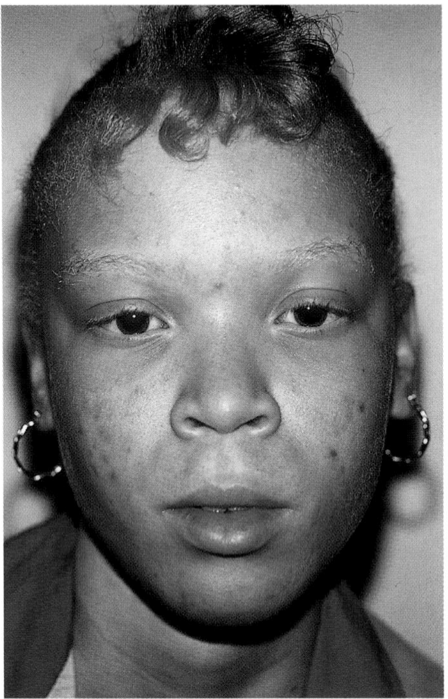

Figure 34.2. Young black girl with type II oculocutaneous albinism.

nos. Recent studies have demonstrated that some patients with so-called autosomal recessive ocular albinism have mutations in the P gene or in the tyrosinase gene, allowing their correct classification into the group of tyrosinase-positive OCA.[123] It has then become evident that autosomal recessive ocular albinism is a clinical variant of oculocutaneous albinism where skin and hair hypopigmentation may be extremely subtle, especially in older children and adults.

Clinically, the severity of the pigmentary dilution in OCA depends on the genetic subtype, the constitutive (racial) pigmentation, and age. For example, a black adult with type II OCA is more darkly pigmented than a white infant with type II OCA. Hair color in OCA ranges from white to dark brown (Fig. 34.2), and iris color ranges from very light blue to light hazel or even brown. The skin may be without pigment or it may have some pigment, especially in nevi and freckles. Van Dorp[134] observed that some patients with OCA may have normal cutaneous pigmentation, that patients with X-linked ocular albinism may be hypopigmented, and that patients with the Hermansky-Pudlak syndrome may have a dark complexion. Obligate carriers of OCA generally have normal pigmentation and ocular examinations. Some white carriers of tyrosinase-negative OCA, however, have a partial transillumination of the iris in a punctate pattern.[136]

The ocular consequences of the pigmentary dilution are identical in all types of albinism. Nystagmus is detected in the first few months of life. Visual acuity ranges from 20/80–20/400 in most patients, but may be as good as 20/30 or 20/40 in some patients with type II OCA. Patients are generally photophobic, and there is a high incidence of strabismus and astigmatic errors of refraction. Color vision is generally normal. The amplitudes of the scotopic electroretinographic responses may be more than normal,[78] and a high electrooculographic Arden ratio[110] may be recorded. These findings have been postulated to result from the increased amount of stimulating light entering the eye through a hypopigmented anterior segment.[138]

On physical examination, a pink reflex is sometimes seen through the undilated iris. Using retroillumination, the iris and the globe diffusely transilluminate and the outline of the lens can be seen (Fig. 34.3). There is prominence of the choroidal vasculature because of the lack or paucity of pigment in the overlying

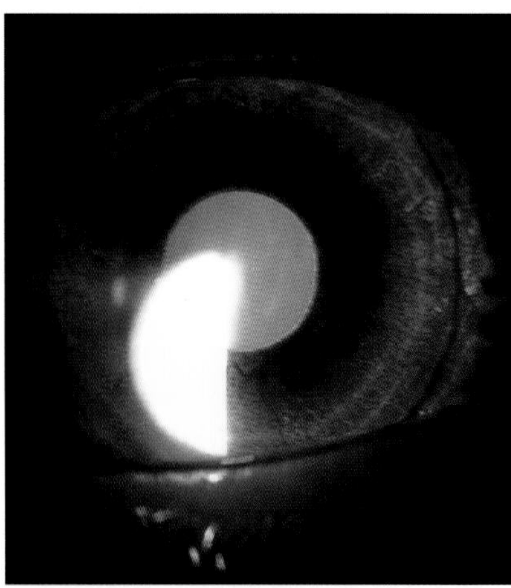

Figure 34.3. Transillumination in this brown-colored iris of a moderately pigmented Middle Eastern boy with type II oculocutaneous albinism.

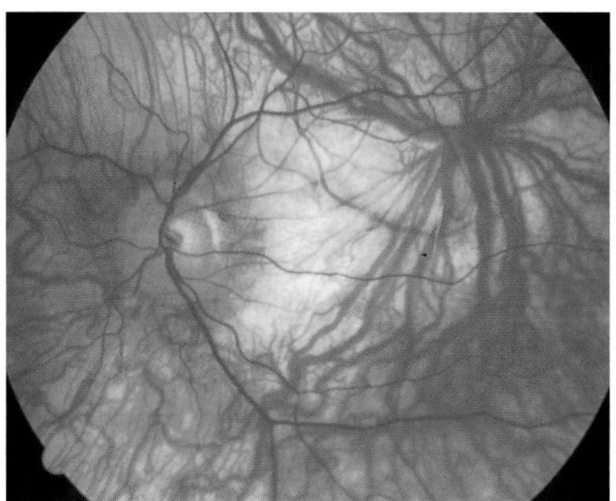

Figure 34.4. Fundus of the patient in Figure 34.2. There is foveal hypoplasia and apparent absence of retinal pigment epithelium and choroidal pigmentation with prominence of choroidal vasculature.

RPE and surrounding choroidal stroma (Fig. 34.4). Some pigment may be present in the presumed macular area, obscuring a view of the submacular choroidal vasculature. The macula is always hypoplastic and the foveal pit is absent. The retinal vessels fail to wreathe the fovea.

There have been a few reports of the association of albinism with anterior segment dysgenesis and glaucoma (personal observations).[22,83,132] Although a possible link between the two conditions may exist, the association may have been fortuitous.

PATHOPHYSIOLOGY OF THE VISUAL IMPAIRMENT IN ALBINISM

Abnormal Decussation of Optic Nerve Fibers at the Chiasm

In a wide variety of animals, albinism is associated with misrouting of the optic nerve fibers.[52] Carroll et al.[19] presented evidence that the human albino has the same pattern of misrouting of the retinogeniculate projections as albinos of other species. It may be that melanin determines neuronal target specificity in the brain. When pigmentation is incomplete, the developing optic tracts take on a near-completely crossed pattern at the chiasm, such as is the case in more primitive panoramic systems. In normal humans, 45% of axons remain uncrossed as they pass through the chiasm and project to the ipsilateral lateral geniculate nucleus, and the greatest number of these fibers subserve the central 20° of the temporal retina. In albinos, however, most of these fibers decussate at the chiasm and synapse in the contralateral lateral geniculate nucleus, leaving only 10%–20% of fibers uncrossed. This leads to a loss of the normal laminar organization of the lateral geniculate nucleus and a predominantly monocular representation of the central visual field in each occipital cortex. Albinos lack the central nervous system substrate for the development of stereopsis. Monocular visual evoked potential (VEP) responses lead to markedly asymmetrical responses from the two hemispheres.[4,29] Such abnormalities in the VEP are not seen in other disorders of pigmentation such as albinoidism, or in other ocular conditions such as congenital motor nystagmus, achromatopsia, and congenital strabismus.[30]

All conditions with oculocutaneous or ocular albinism in humans and animals have shown either electrophysiologic or anatomic evidence of a decussation defect in the optic tracts.[149] Evidence that anomalous decussation exists in the auditory system was presented by Creel et al.[28] The amount of pigment in the inner ear correlates directly with the amount in the iris, and otic pigment is lacking in albinos. Leventhal et al.[85] studied cats who were obligatory heterozygotes for a c-locus tyrosinase-negative allele and were not genetically related to "deaf white cats." In these normally pigmented animals, abnormalities of the retino-geniculo-cortical pathways were found to be similar to those in homozygous albinos. By unilateral injection of horseradish peroxidase into the dorsal lateral geniculate nucleus, Leventhal and co-workers[85] were able to map the labeled retinal ganglion cells. Compared to homozygous normal controls, heterozygotes showed labeling of an abnormally large number of cells, especially large alpha cells, in the contralateral temporal retina. The authors pointed out that 1%–2% of the human population may be heterozygous for albinism and that the above described abnormality may have an adverse effect on binocular depth perception. Castle et al., however, reported that the VEP was normal in African-American carriers of type II OCA.[21]

Wack and co-workers[138] showed that electroretinogram (ERG) recordings in albinos were in the normal range for amplitude and implicit times. At high flash luminance, the amplitudes were at or above normal, and implicit times were shorter than normal. These authors postulate that responses of the anterior retina to trans-scleral illumination lead to the supernormal ERG recording in some patients with tyrosinase-negative albinism. Creel, Conlee, and King[31] reported that patients with tyrosinase-positive and tyrosinase-negative albinism had normal dark adaptation and rod function. Scotopic and flicker ERGs showed slightly decreased amplitude, which Creel and co-workers attributed to photophobia.[31]

Light Scattering

Light scattering within the eye may play a minimal role in the pathophysiology of visual impairment in albinism. This factor may not be very important, because patients with albinoidism who have translucent irides and an albinotic fundus also have normal visual acuity.[34] Some complain of photophobia, which may be a consequence of light scattering. Tinted lenses can be of some help. Corneal contact lenses with an opaque iris portion have not significantly improved visual acuity in albinos.[41]

Light-Induced Retinal Damage

Light-induced retinal damage does not seem to play an appreciable role in the visual impairment of albinos. Extremely intense light can produce nonthermal retinal damage even in normally pigmented animals.[83] Albino animals have a lower threshold for such damage; this has been attributed to an inefficient shielding of light by the iris diaphragm, since normally pigmented animals show somewhat compatible thresholds with pupillary dilatation. There are no data suggesting that visual function in human albinos deteriorates with age. Nevertheless, it seems reasonable to limit exposure to unnatural, moderately intense light sources. It has been hypothesized that light-generated free radicals are responsible for nonthermal light damage. Feeney and Berman[39] have suggested that melanin normally plays a protective role by reducing such free radicals.

Congenital Nystagmus

The congenital nystagmus (onset in the first 3 months of postnatal life) that is invariably present in albinism may contribute to visual impairment. Patients with albinism and some degree of skin pigmentation, especially blacks,[100] are often misdiagnosed as having congenital motor nystagmus[114] or a retinal dystrophy. Waveform analysis of the nystagmus does not show consistent differences between the nystagmus that is secondary to sensorial causes and that resulting from albinism or primary motor defect nystagmus.[152] Both pendular and jerk-type patterns can be found in each group, depending on test conditions. Also, in both groups the nystagmus consists of horizontal and rotary excursions, although a rare vertical form of hereditary motor nystagmus also exists.[91] The nystagmus present in albinism is presumed to be due to foveal hypoplasia or to central nervous system maldevelopment.[149]

Patients without recognizable ophthalmoscopic or sensory defects who have congenital hereditary nystagmus (so-called motor-defect type or congenital motor nystagmus) typically have a visual acuity of 20/40 to 20/60.[26] Thus, it is often assumed that foveal hypoplasia is a greater detriment to visual acuity than nystagmus; however, patients with foveal hypoplasia without manifest nystagmus may have near-normal visual acuity.

In congenital motor-defect type nystagmus, some patients assume a compensatory head position in order to shift their so-called null point (direction of gaze with least nystagmus and best visual acuity), to the straight-ahead position. Kestenbaum,[65] Anderson,[3] and others have advocated muscle surgery on such patients to shift the null point to the primary position of gaze. Although albinos typically do not assume such head positions, we have observed a number of patients to do so. An occasional patient with albinism may require eye muscle surgery to correct the torticollis. An improvement in visual acuity is not to be expected because of the sensorial defect. Davis et al., however, observed two or more Snellen lines of visual improvement in 7 of 12 albinos who underwent retroequatorial horizontal rectus muscle recession.[32a] There was subjective improvement of vision and reduction of the nystagmus.

Macular Hypoplasia

The most significant factor reducing visual acuity in albinos is macular hypoplasia. Clinically, a presumed "hypoplasia" has been posited X for a long time (Fig. 34.5), but earlier histopathologic studies of albino eyes were difficult to interpret. There seems to be a consensus that the macula lutea pigment is absent. Postmortem histopathological studies of serial sections through the presumed maculae of the eyes of oculocutaneous albinos,[44,93,99] and of an ocular albino,[101] have been studied. In each case, no foveal pit or umbo was found, but normally thick central ganglion and nuclear cell layers were present. Rods and parafoveal-type cones were present in the macula of albinos[44]; the outer segments of these cones were tapered (as is normally found in cones in the parafoveal area), as opposed to the normal macular slender and cylindrical configuration. Mietz and coworkers examined the eyes of an 99-year-old tyrosinase-negative albino woman.[93] These authors found a posterior embryotoxon, absence of melanin in all ocular structures, and absence of a foveal pit. In the normal anatomic position of the foveola, the retina was of normal thickness with 5–7 ganglion cell layers (Fig. 34.9). The etiology of foveal hypoplasia in albinism is not understood but may be related to the reduced amount of melanin in the RPE.

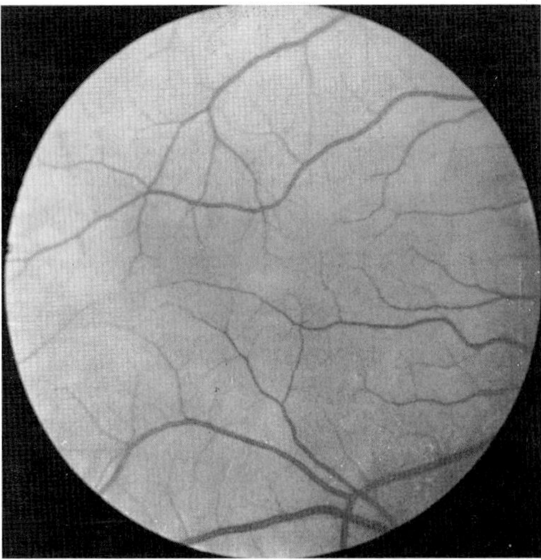

Figure 34.5. Foveal hypoplasia in a patient with X-linked ocular albinism. There is no foveal pit. A retinal vessel courses over the center of the macula.

Although it was originally reported by Ichikara[61] that the retinal vessels fail to wreathe the fovea in patients with albinism, one fluorescein angiographic study of patients with type II OCA demonstrated multiple window defects of the RPE with a normal foveal avascular zone.[49]

Abadi et al.[1] studied the retinal fixation behavior of 17 albino patients and found that in 8 patients, there was consistent fixation with a location compatible with the anatomic fovea. Patients with tyrosinase-positive OCA were more likely to demonstrate foveation than those with tyrosinase-negative disease.

OCULOCUTANEOUS ALBINISM

Oculocutaneous Albinism Type II (Tyrosinase-Positive)

The type II form is the most common type of albinism and is clinically differentiated from tyrosinase-negative or type IA OCA by the presence of some pigment in the hair, skin, and eyes of older patients. Infants with tyrosinase-positive oculocutaneous albinism may be clinically indistinguishable from infants with tyrosinase-negative oculocutaneous albinism, but acquire pigmentation with age. Hair color tends to be yellow at birth, the skin is creamy-white, and the iris is lightly pigmented. Visual acuity is often less severely decreased than in OCA type I and is in the range of 20/40 to 20/200; acuity may improve with age as pigmentation increases. Pigmented nevi and freckles develop at around age 5 to 6 years. There is susceptibility to basal cell and squamous cell carcinoma of the skin, and cutaneous and choroidal malignant melanomas have been reported in a few instances.[20,117] Electron microscopy reveals normal numbers of lightly melanized melanosomes (stages I–III) in the skin and hair of older patients. Kugelman and Van Scott's method[79] of in vitro incubation of hair bulbs in L-tyrosine or L-dopa differentiates this form of OCA from type I in infants. In type II OCA the hair bulbs darken appreciably because of the presence of tyrosinase, and electron microscopy of incubated hair bulbs reveals further melanization of melanosomes. The recent identification of mutations in the P gene in patients with tyrosinase-positive OCA suggests that, at least in some patients, albinism is due to decreased availability of tyrosine in the melanocytes; the P protein is thought to be important in the transport of tyrosine.[111] Ramsay et al.[107] demonstrated linkage of tyrosinase-positive OCA to 15q11.2-q12, the human locus homologous to the *p* gene in the mouse; these authors hence postulated that the genes for tyrosinase-positive OCA and the pink-eyed dilution are homologous. Gardner et al.[45] and Lee et al.[84] demonstrated that the human homologue of the mouse *p* mutation is a gene located on 15q11.2-q12, a region associated with the Prader-Willi and Angelman syndromes, both of which are characterized by hypopigmentation among other clinical abnormalities. Rinchik et al.[111] found a mutation in both copies of the human *P* gene in a patient with tyrosinase-positive OCA. Spritz[123] has shown that *P* gene mutations are more common among African Americans with type II OCA than among Caucasians; he found a *P* gene mutation in 7 of 7 African-American patients, 15 of 16 African patients, and only 6 of 14 Caucasians.

Oculocutaneous Albinism Type IA (Tyrosinase-Negative)

Type IA OCA is the second most common type of oculocutaneous albinism. Patients with this disease do not have any clinically or histopathologically discernible pigmentation as a result of total deficiency of tyrosinase activity. Pigmented nevi and freckles do not occur. Electron microscopy of skin and hair reveals normal numbers of melanosomes but no melanization (stages I-II melanosomes). In vitro hair-bulb incubation in L-tyrosine does not produce melanin. Carriers of this type of oculocutaneous albinism can be identified by King's microassay[76] as they have less than half the normal tyrosinase activity in hair bulbs.[75] Since the mapping of the tyrosinase gene to chromosome 11q and the cloning of the tyrosinase gene, numerous mutations have been identified in a number of patient populations. Kwon et al.[80] showed that human tyrosinase is composed of 548 amino acids and had a molecular weight of 62,610. The cDNA clone isolated by Kwon was mapped to chromosome 7 in the mouse near or at the *c*-albino locus, which codes for tyrosinase. Barton et al. mapped the human tyrosinase gene to 11q14-q21.[8] Giebel et al.[47] demonstrated that the tyrosinase gene contained five exons and spanned more than 50 kb of DNA. Spritz has identified two common polymorphisms among Caucasians (codons 192 and 402), resulting in four slightly different isoforms.[122] Based on analysis of 16 missense mutations, King et al.[69] found that mutations clustered in four areas of the gene; however, deletions in the gene are rare.[123] In a study of tyrosinase gene mutations, Tripathi et al.[131] concluded that in Caucasians, OCA1 results from a great variety of uncommon alleles. About 90% of patients had a total of 29 mutations. Eighty percent of missense substitutions clustered in two relatively small regions of the tyrosinase polypeptide, either near the amino terminus or near the center of the polypeptide. In Tripathi's study, 6 of 17 patients initially classified as having tyrosinase-positive oculocutaneous albinism had mutations in the tyrosinase gene.[131] Other mutations in the tyrosinase gene are reviewed by Oetting and King[102,103] and by Oetting et al.[104]

Oculocutaneous Albinism Type IB (Yellow Albinism)

Type IB albinism is allelic to type IA. There is marked reduction in tyrosinase activity with little pigment at birth, but some increase with age. This type was first described as "yellow mutant OCA" among the Amish.[98] There is a broad range of phenotypes. Caucasian infants may be indistinguishable from type IA infants. African-American patients with this form of OCA will have dark, cream-colored skin and light-red hair. The in vitro hair-bulb test is negative, but with the addition of excess L-cysteine, pheomelanin is produced.[75] Yellow albinism has been shown to be allelic to tyrosinase-negative OCA.[59] In addition, Spritz et al.[121] identified a proline to leucine substitution at codon 406 in a patient with yellow oculocutaneous albinism; this mutation may result in abnormal folding of the tyrosinase polypeptide. To date, this mutation has been identified only in the Amish.

Temperature-Sensitive Albinism

The temperature-sensitive variant of tyrosinase-related oculocutaneous albinism described by King et al.,[73,74] is characterized by the development of some pigmentation in hairs of cooler or exposed parts of the body. Axillary hair is white, but pubic hair and leg hair are darker. There is an absence of ocular pigment. Giebel et al.[46] found an arginine-to-glycine substitution at codon 422 in one family with this condition. In vitro introduction of the codon 422 mutation resulted in thermosensitivity of tyrosinase with 28% activity at 31°C and only 1.4% activity at 37°C.

Oculocutaneous Albinism Type IV (Brown Albinism)

Black individuals with the clinical type IV form of albinism have light-brown skin, light-brown hair, and blue to brown irides with transillumination defects. These patients are often more lightly pigmented than their unaffected relatives but more darkly pigmented than patients with type II OCA. There is little accumulation or change of pigment in the eyes or skin with age. The hair-bulb test is positive.[66] This disorder was first described in Enulu Nigerians, and further characterized in African Americans.[66,68,71] Brown albinism is the human homologue of *brown (b)* mutant mice with a brown rather than black coat color.[87,118] The cDNA of the *b* gene was found to be different from that coding for tyrosinase.[62] However, because of similarities to tyrosinase, the protein, 5,6-dihydroxyindole-2-carboxylic acid (DHICA), was named *tyrosinase-related protein* and the gene was called *TYRP*. This protein catalyzes a distal step in the eumelanin biosynthetic pathway. Human TYRP was mapped to 9p22-p23.[26,97,155] Zhao et al.[154] have shown that TYRP has some tyrosine hydroxylase activity but no DOPA oxidase activity, and they propose that TYRP modulates tyrosinase activity by making available DOPA as a cofactor for melanogenesis. No mutations in the human TYRP gene have yet been identified. There are two reported patients with a deletion of 9p and hypopigmentation,[139] and one patient with Brown albinism has been found to have no immunologically detectable TYRP protein or mRNA.[16]

Rufous Oculocutaneous Albinism (Xanthism)

Walsh described rufous oculocutaneous albinism in New Guinea indigens in 1971.[141] The skin of affected children appears red and becomes reddish-brown with age. The hair is auburn-red and the eyes are brown; mild iris transillumination defects are present. Some of the patients described by Walsh were photophobic and had nystagmus, but he did not provide details of their ocular examination.

Hermansky-Pudlak Syndrome (Albinism-Hemorrhagic Diathesis)

Hermansky-Pudlak syndrome (HPS) consists of the triad of albinism, hemorrhagic diathesis, and the accumulation of ceroidlike material in the reticuloendothelial system and other tissues. Although the original patients described with this condition were from Czechoslovakia,[57] most cases in the United States are from the Arecibo region of Puerto Rico.[147] Clusters of pedigrees have been reported in southern Holland and in Switzerland. There is marked phenotypic variability in hypopigmentation that seems somewhat dependent on age and racial background. Some patients are extremely hypopigmented and are misdiagnosed as having tyrosinase-negative oculocutaneous albinism; others have nearly normal skin color. Hair color ranges from yellow-white to brown, and eye color from blue to hazel. Even when there is little cutaneous pigmentation, pigmented nevi and lentigines are present. The ophthalmologic findings of patients with the Hermansky-Pudlak syndrome have been reviewed by Summers and co-workers,[124] and are practically indistinguishable from those of other types of albinism. Iris transillumination defects, nystagmus, and photophobia are present and visual acuity is in the range of 20/100–20/300. Electron microscopy of skin and hair-bulb melanocytes reveals unevenly melanized melanosomes as well as some giant melanosomes.

HPS results from defective assembly, maturation, and structure of various cytoplasmic organelles such as melanosomes, platelet-dense granules, and lysosomes. Following the mapping of the HPS to 10q23.1-23.3, Oh and colleagues used positional cloning to identify the gene for the HPS.[104a] They found frameshift mutations in Puerto Rican, Swiss, Irish, and Japanese patients. They discovered that the HPS polypeptide is a transmembrane protein that is likely to be a component of multiple cytoplasmic organelles, and that is crucial to their development and function. The HPS gene consists of 20 exons that span 30.5 kb in chromosome region 10q23.1-q23.3.[5a] The gene contains an "AT-AC" intron defined by highly atypical 5′ and 3′ splice site and branch site consensus sequences that provide novel targets for pathologic gene mutations.[5a]

Patients with Hermansky-Pudlak syndrome usually have a history of easy bruisability, epistaxis, or hemoptysis.[57] Prolonged bleeding may occur following dental extractions and childbirth. Some patients have dyspnea because of pulmonary interstitial infiltrates. Respiratory symptoms start between the third and fourth decades of life and are due to the deposition of ceroid-like material in the lungs; these deposits lead to interstitial fibrosis and restrictive lung disease. The catechol-like storage material accumulates in the urine, bone marrow, peripheral leukocytes, and reticuloendothelial cells. It can be identified by yellow fluorescence under ultraviolet light and histochemically in urine. The same ceroid-like material deposits in bone marrow, leukocytes, oral mucosa, and gastrointestinal system, sometimes producing an inflammatory bowel disease–like illness with fever, abdominal pain, and diarrhea. This illness occurs in the second and third decades and may require resection of the affected intestinal segment. Occasionally, the material may deposit in other organs and cause kidney disease and cardiomyopathy.

The hemostatic defect in patients with Hermansky-Pudlak syndrome is the result of platelet dysfunction. Although routine tests of coagulation do not reveal any abnormalities, bleeding time is usually prolonged. A careful history of hemostatic defects is the best screening method. Platelet aggregation studies show poor platelet aggregation, particularly with collagen. Electron microscopy of platelets in plasma shows greatly reduced numbers of "dense bodies."[147] These dense bodies contain serotonin, adenine nucleotides, and calcium, which are necessary factors in normal platelet aggregation. Platelets from patients with Hermansky-Pudlak syndrome show less than 10% of the normal levels of serotonin and adenosine diphosphate. Because aspirin and indomethacin are potent inhibitors of release of these substances from dense bodies, patients with this syndrome must be explicitly advised to avoid all aspirin-containing drugs, indomethacin, and other drugs blocking prostaglandin synthetase because these medications can precipitate life-threatening gastrointestinal hemorrhages. Cryoprecipitate is useful in decreasing the bleeding time before elective surgery. Bleeding emergencies may require platelet transfusions.

Because of the variable clinical appearance of patients with Hermansky-Pudlak syndrome, all patients with oculocutaneous albinism should be asked about a hemorrhagic diathesis; patients with a suspicious history should be referred for hematological consultation. Known patients with this syndrome who are planning to undergo elective ophthalmic surgery should be asked about use of aspirin-containing drugs and indomethacin, and their use should be discontinued permanently, and well in advance of the planned surgery. Consultation with the hematologist should be obtained because platelet transfusions may be indicated. The addition of only a 10% portion of normal platelets to platelet-rich Hermansky-Pudlak plasma restores the in vitro platelet aggregation to normal.

Chediak-Higashi Syndrome

The Chediak-Higashi syndrome (CHS) is characterized by variable oculocutaneous pigmentary dilution, susceptibility to pyogenic infections in childhood (usually gram-positive bacteria) from severe immunologic deficiency with neutropenia and lack of natural killer cells, and a predisposition to develop a lymphoma-like condition in adolescence.[15] The patient's life span is markedly reduced. This condition was first described by BeguezCesar in 1943.[11] Most reported patients have been Caucasians, although Japanese[126] and black[33] patients have been reported. Ocular features are identical to those in other types of albinism. Some patients with CHS have severe generalized pigmentary dilution and resemble oculocutaneous albinos. However, many patients resemble ocular albinos with mild cutaneous pigmentary dilution. Hair color is usually fair to light-brown and the skin is creamy-white. There is often a blue-gray sheen to the scalp hair, and patients have patches of slate gray cutaneous discoloration. A minority of patients lack all stigmata of albinism. The hair-bulb test is positive. Histopathologically, the number of melanosomes within pigment epithelia is reduced,[10,64,120,143] and abnormally large melanosomes are present in the pigment epithelia, skin, and hair.[143,153] When examined by light microscopy, these giant pigment granules are typically nonspherical. On electron microscopy, they appear as large ellipsoidal structures with a normal lamellar substructure, in contrast to the round melanosomes of Nettleship-Falls X-linked ocular albinism.

Chediak-Higashi syndrome appears to represent a generalized abnormality of membrane-bound organelles.[143] Giant, peroxidase-positive lysosomal granules are found within leukocytes, Schwann cells, gastrointestinal mucosa, kidneys, bone marrow, pancreas, and conjunctiva.[15] Abnormal fusion of immature organelles leads to a reduction in the number of mature organelles, such as melanosomes and leukocyte granules and leads to their giant counterparts. In a recent study of cultured melanocytes from a patient with the Chediak-Higashi syndrome, Zhao et al.[153] found giant melanosomes, tyrosinase-containing vesicles that were widely distributed throughout the cytoplasm, and perinuclear melanocyte-specific proteins. The media that were conditioned by Chediak-Higashi melanocytes exhibited significant tyrosine hydroxylase activity. The melanocytes produced a novel DOPA-positive, tyrosinase immunoreactive 100-kd protein that is secreted into the growth medium. This study provided evidence for a functional disorder of protein transport in CHS.

The gene for CHS was identified because of its homology to its murine counterpart the *beige* mouse gene.[18a,99a] The human gene is located on 1q43. The protein coded for by this gene has a modular architecture that is very similar to the yeast vacuolar-sorting protein, VPS15, explaining the defective vesicular transport to and from the lysosome and late endosome, and the aberrant compartmentalization of lysosomal and granular enzymes in cells of patients with this disease.[18a] Nagle and co-workers identified mutations in the CHS gene in three patients with this condition.[99a]

The large leukocytic inclusions are 2–4 mm in diameter and are accompanied by reduced numbers of normal-sized leukocyte granules.[109] These giant granules are associated with inadequate chemotactic and bactericidal activity of leukocytes and delayed fusion with phagocytic vacuoles; they may also affect natural killer cell activity. These deficiencies account for the predisposition to infection, especially with *Staphylococcus aureus*, including recurrent orbital cellulitis.[120] During adolescence, patients with CHS develop lymphohistiocytic infiltration of the liver, bone marrow, and peripheral nervous system. This leads to hepatomegaly, pancytopenia, weakness, paresthesias, muscle atrophy, and decreased deep tendon reflexes. Splenomegaly results from sequestration of platelets. Some patients have signs and symptoms of central nervous system dysfunction. A peripheral neuropathy often develops in childhood.

Albinos of uncertain subtype with a history of recurrent infections should be referred for evaluation to rule out CHS. Examination of hair-bulb and skin-biopsy specimens by light microscopy for giant melanosomes can be used. Because patients with Nettleship-Falls X-linked ocular albinism also have macromelanosomes, electron microscopy of macromelanosomes may be necessary.

Inspection of buffy coats for abnormal leukocyte inclusions in CHS can be utilized. Ascorbate (vitamin C) therapy improves the leukocyte function and may, perhaps, reduce the morbidity and mortality[17] but appears to have no effect on the pigmentary dilution. Combination chemotherapy with vincristine and steroids has been used with some success to treat the pancytopenia. The life expectancy of patients with CHS averages 4.1 years, and the oldest surviving patient in one series was 25 years old.[15]

Cross Syndrome

In 1967, Cross et al. described three siblings in an Amish family with an autosomal recessive syndrome characterized by mental retardation, athetosis, spastic diplegia, cutaneous hypopigmentation, gingival fibromatosis, nystagmus, and microphthalmia with corneal opacification.[32] The tyrosinase test was weakly positive. It is not known for certain whether this syndrome affects the eye in the same fashion as other types of albinism.

Ocular Albinism

X-Linked Recessive Ocular Albinism (Nettleship-Falls)

X-linked ocular albinism occurs with a frequency of about 1 : 150,000 live male births.[123] Cutaneous pigmentation typically falls within the normal range. The hair-bulb incubation test is positive for tyrosinase. The ophthalmologic manifestations of ocular albinism are almost identical to those of the different types of oculocutaneous albinism, except that in ocular albinism, the pigmentary dilution of the eye may be subtle. Nystagmus, decreased visual acuity, and sometimes photophobia are all present. Ocular pigmentation depends on constitutive pigmentation, age, and the presence or absence of axial myopia. In whites, the iris color may be brown, but the iris almost always transilluminates because of a hypopigmented iris pigment epithelium. In blacks, the iris often does not transilluminate, and ophthalmoscopic examination often shows a moderately pigmented, nonalbinotic fundus.[100] Even in darkly pigmented patients, however, there is ophthalmoscopic evidence of foveal hypoplasia (Fig. 34.5). Recognizing foveal hypoplasia alerts the examiner to the possibility of ocular albinism. Infants are easier to detect than adults because the uveal tract is less pigmented. In nonalbinotic patients, axial myopia causes a pigmentary dilution that is presumably due to stretching and thinning of the tissues. In ocular albinism the myopia aggravates the pigmentary dilution and thereby facilitates recognition of the albinism.

X-linked ocular albinos may have relatively good visual acuity, but most often vision is as poor as 20/300. Visual acuity does not improve with age. Color vision is normal. As in oculocutaneous albinism, there is sometimes a supranormal ERG scotopic b wave and an elevated EOG Arden ratio.

Carriers of Nettleship-Falls X-linked ocular albinism have diagnostic ocular findings,[38,48,81,101] although they are generally asymptomatic. There is one report of a white carrier female who had congenital nystagmus and subnormal visual acuity with ocular findings identical to those found in affected males, although she was presumably heterozygous for the trait.[106] White carrier females often, but not always, have a partial translucency of the iris. In contrast, black carriers almost never show iris transillumination[100] but may show a striking pattern of alternating spoke-like pigmentation of the iris stroma that has been attributed to lyonization.[89] In a recent study by Charles and coworkers,[23] 74% of obligate carriers were found to have iris transillumination defects versus 20% of controls; 87%–92% of obligate carriers showed a "mud-splattered" fundus appearance: in the midperiphery of the fundus. Carrier females of X-linked ocular albinism have patches and streaks of hypopigmentation of the retinal pigment epithelium adjacent to areas of normal or even increased pigmentation (Fig. 34.6). This quilt-work disturbance of the retinal pigment epithelium is most noticeable in the midperiphery of the retina, but it affects the entire retinal pigment epithelium, giving a mottled appearance to the macular area and a more streaked appearance to the midperipheral fundus. The findings in the carrier females of Nettleship-Falls X-linked ocular albinism have been attributed by Falls to lyonization of the X chromosome[38,88] (i.e., random inactivation of one X chromosome within a progenitor cell leading to a random pattern of pigmented and

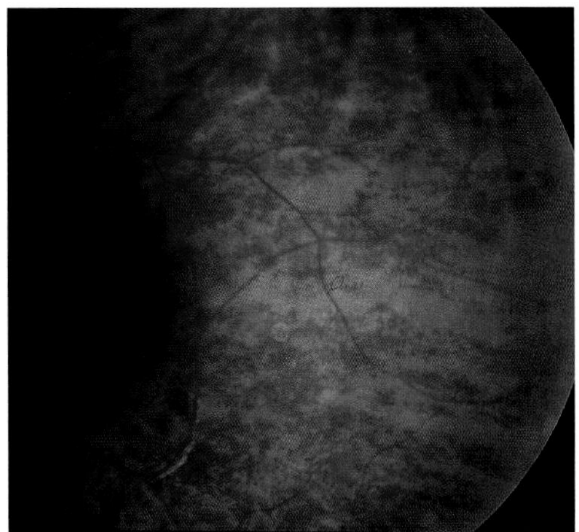

Figure 34.6. Midperiphery of the retinal grounds of a female carrier of X-linked ocular albinism reveals pigmented streaks alternating with depigmented ones, illustrating lyonization.

hypopigmented RPE cells. The relative value of skin biopsy, iris transillumination, and ophthalmoscopy in the diagnosis of patients and female carriers of X-linked albinism has been reviewed by Cortin and co-workers.[27] In female carriers of X-linked ocular albinism, serial sections of biopsied clinically normal skin show macromelanosomes in some melanocytes and keratinocytes.[27,125] This may be useful when the family history is vague or ophthalmologic findings equivocal.

In contrast to oculocutaneous albinism, in which pigmentary dilution is due to inadequate melanization of melanosomes, pigmentary dilution in X-linked ocular albinism appears to be the result of abnormalities in melanosome synthesis resulting in fewer than normal numbers of melanosomes. Some authors, however, suggest that it is probably a disorder of pigment distribution and/or transfer rather than a primary disorder of production.[116] Once melanosomes are produced, they can become fully melanized and are dopa oxidase and tyrosinase positive. Although there is ample clinical and some histopathologic evidence of cutaneous pigmentary dilution in the X-linked form of ocular albinism, the cutaneous manifestations are relatively mild. It is possible that the eye, especially the pigment epithelium, is more severely affected than the skin in ocular albinism because embryonic melanogenesis within the ocular pigment epithelium occurs only for a limited period of time.[18,95] The number of melanosomes of any size in ocular pigment epithelia is reduced in X-linked ocular albinism.[101,151]

Clinically, patients with X-linked ocular albinism are distinguished from those with other forms of albinism by the presence of congenitally hypopigmented cutaneous patches and macules in some patients, especially blacks.[100,101] The pathogenesis of these patches is unknown. One white male was noted to have areas of slate gray discoloration of the skin, similar to those described more commonly in CHS. These patches appear to be due to excessive amounts of pigment within macrophages in the dermis.[101]

Histopathologic examination of the clinically normal skin (Fig. 34.7) in affected males and carrier females[100,101] and ocular pigment epithelia (Fig. 34.8) of two male patients[101,151] with X-linked ocular albinism revealed the presence of abnormally large melanosomes in addition to normal-sized melanosomes. In a study by Charles et al.,[23] all affected males and 84% of obligatory carriers had macromelanosomes. Families where patients and carriers lack macromelanosomes have also been reported.[116]

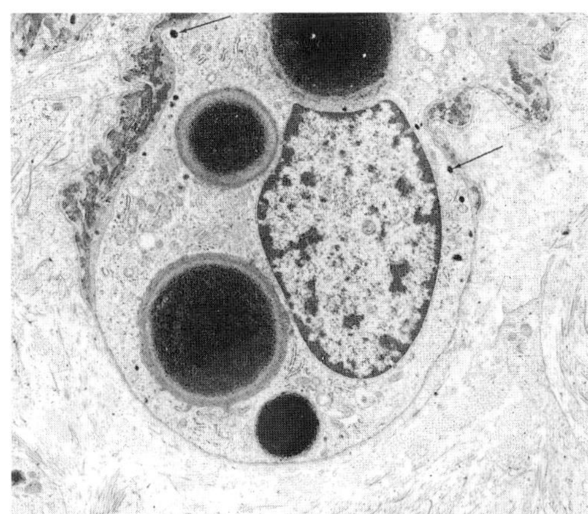

Figure 34.7. Electron micrograph of an epidermal melanocyte from a patient with X-linked ocular albinism. There are several giant melanosomes and a reduced number of normal melanosomes (arrows). (Reproduced with permission from F. E. O'Donnell et al., ref. 101.)

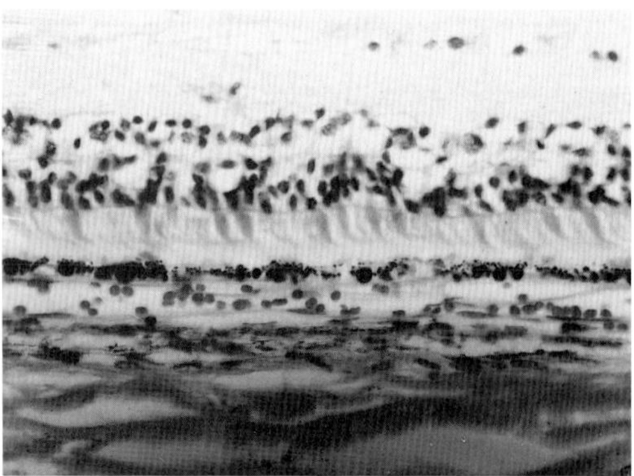

Figure 34.8. Retinal pigment epithelium of a patient with X-linked ocular albinism contains large melanosomes and fewer numbers of normal size melanosomes (arrows). (Courtesy of Dr. W. Richard Green.)

Electron microscopy of skin, hair bulbs, and fetal pigment epithelia has shown ultrastructurally normal melanosomes as well as abnormal melanosomes. The latter have a granular substructure and are spherical. They become fully melanized and can be very large.[150] The cutaneous macromelanosomes are not pathognomonic of X-linked ocular albinism because they also occur in the clinically normal skin of patients with neurofibromatosis[12,63] and xeroderma pigmentosum.[51] Macromelanosomes or melanin macroglobules are thought to represent autophagolysosomes that contain varying numbers of melanosomes.[97] They are present in fetal pigment epithelia as early as 22 weeks.[151]

The genetic locus for X-linked ocular albinism is in the Xp22.3 region[115] and closely linked to the locus for the XgA blood group.[101] Linkage analysis studies include those by Charles et al.[23] and by Bergen et al.[13] A study of 11 families from North America and Australia mapped OA1 between markers DXS85 and DXS143.[116] The gene for XLOA has recently been cloned and found to encode a 424 amino acid protein. This gene is expressed at high levels in the retina and RPE.[9] Schiaffino and co-workers found mutations in 21 of 60 patients with this disorder.[113a] They postulated that mutations in regulatory gene elements or in other gene(s) in the same region account for the disease in the remaining patients.[113a]

Åland Island Disease (Forsius–Eriksson Syndrome)

In 1964, Forsius and Eriksson described an X-linked ocular disorder in 7 male patients from a six-generation family from the Åland Islands, off the coast of Denmark.[42] The disorder is characterized by congenital nystagmus, axial myopia, reduced visual acuity, atypical protanomalous color defect, fundus hypopigmentation, and macular hypoplasia in affected males. Most patients in the original report lacked iris transillumination. Carrier females did not have ocular signs, except for some who had a form of latent nystagmus. Defective dark adaptation and reduced photopic flicker and scotopic b-wave amplitude were also noted. Van Dorp et al.[133] found no evidence of misrouting of the optic pathways in these patients. Thus, some features suggest a variant of X-linked ocular albinism, whereas other findings are atypical and suggest an incomplete form of congenital stationary night blindness[141] as defined by Miyake.[93a] Linkage studies indicated possibly close linkage with the XgA blood group locus, as in X-linked ocular albinism.

X-Linked Ocular Albinism with Late-Onset Sensorineural Deafness

This appears to be a distinct disease in which patients with X-linked ocular albinism develop progressive sensorineural deafness in the fourth and fifth decades.[143a] Patients have normal cutaneous pigmentation and macromelanosomes. Linkage analysis of this disease in a large South African family mapped this disorder to Xp22.3, suggesting that this disorder and X-linked ocular albinism are allelic variants or that they are due to contiguous gene defects.[144]

Syndrome of Ocular Albinism, Congenital Sensorineural Hearing Loss, and Cutaneous Lentigines

Lewis[86] described a syndrome of ocular albinism, congenital sensorineural hearing loss, and cutaneous lentigines inherited as an autosomal dominant trait in three generations of a single white kindred. Histopathologic study of the lentigines revealed macromelanosomes. Clinically normal skin lacked macromelanosomes. This condition appears to be a distinct type of albinism, although it shows some features in common with the Waardenburg-like syndrome described by Bard *(vide infra)*.[7]

ABCD Syndrome and BADS Syndrome

Albinism, black hair lock, cell migration disorder of the neurocytes of the gut, and deafness (ABCD) syndrome and black lock, albinism, and deafness syndrome (BADS) may be the same recessive disorder described initially by Witkop.[146] ABCD syndrome was described in a Kurdish girl who died from complications of aganglionosis of the large intestine; in addition to her intestinal dysfunction she had albinism with depigmentation of her fundus and bilateral deafness.[50a]

ALBINOIDISM

Albinoidism is a form of hypopigmentation that can be differentiated from oculocutaneous and ocular albinism by the lack of significant visual impairment. As in ocular albinism, cutaneous pigmentation falls within the normal range; but, when compared with unaffected siblings, these patients have a lighter complexion. Patients sunburn easily, but they may tan. Unlike patients with albinism, visual acuity is good and there is no nystagmus. Ocular findings that suggest abnormal pigmentary dilution are iris transillumination, hypopigmentation of the fundus, and, sometimes, a dull foveal reflex.

Albinoidism can be an isolated finding, inherited as an autosomal dominant trait (autosomal dominant oculocutaneous albinoidism[35] and punctate oculocutaneous albinoidism[14]), or it may be an inconstant feature of autosomal dominant disorders such as Apert syndrome.[90]

Piebaldism

Piebaldism is a heritable, stable, patterned hypomelanosis lacking extracutaneous manifestations.[95] The hypomelanosis usually involves the central frontal lock of hair in 80%–90% of patients, and the ventral part of the trunk and extremities. The hypomelanotic skin macules are usually stable in size but have occasionally been observed to enlarge; hair growing within these patches is also nonpigmented. Melanocytes in the skin of such patients have unmelanized premelanosomes[53]; however, within the hypomelanotic patches, melanocytes are absent. Associated syndromes that have been previously described as being distinct are autosomal recessive piebaldism and deafness[112]; autosomal dominant piebald trait, ataxia, and deafness[130]; and vitiligo, muscle wasting, achalasia, and deafness.[112] Piebaldism results from defects in the *kit* gene, which encodes a transmembrane cellular receptor for stem cell growth factor.[47a,140a]

Waardenburg Syndromes Types I and II

In 1951 Waardenburg[137] described a syndrome featuring heterochromia or isohypochromia irides, deafness, albinoidism with a white forelock in some patients, and dystopia canthorum in most patients. The affected structures are all derived from neural crest.[127] This autosomal dominant disorder has since been divided into three types. In type I there is lateral displacement of the medial canthi (dystopia canthorum) and lacrimal puncti with normal interpupillary distance (Fig. 34.9); sensorineural deafness is also present. Patients with Waardenburg type II do not have dystopia canthorum[5] but are otherwise clinically similar to those with type I. Other rare associated malformations include Hirschsprung disease and clefting of the lip and/or palate. Patients with Waardenburg syndrome type III, as those with type II, lack dystopia canthorum but have unilateral ptosis and skeletal abnormalities. The gene for Waardenburg syndrome type I was mapped to chromosome 2q35.[44] Tassabehji et al.[127,128] and Baldwin et al.[6] identified mutations in the paired box-containing developmental gene *PAX3* in families with Waardenburg syndrome type I and type III.[58] Six mutations have been identified that are of three different types: alteration of the paired domain of the protein, elimination of a conserved octapeptide and homeobox domain, or complete elimination of

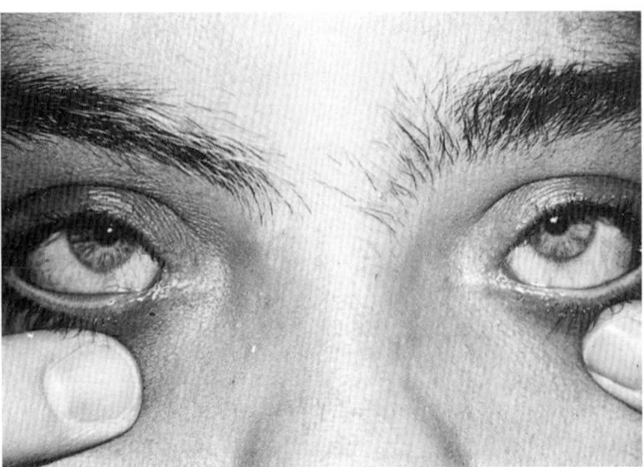

Figure 34.9. Young black patient with Waardenburg syndrome type I. There is a synophris and numerous white hairs in the medial aspect of the eyebrows. The inner canthi are displaced temporally. The distance between the inner canthi and the inferior punctum measures 8 mm. The irides are bright blue. (Courtesy of Drs. F. Char and M. F. Goldberg.)

protein function. Waardenburg syndrome type II was mapped to chromosome 3p14.1-p12.3 near the presumed locus for the human homologue of the murine microphthalmia gene.[60] Subsequently, Tassabehji et al. detected splice site mutations in the human microphthalmia (MITF) gene in two families with Waardenburg syndrome type II.[129]

Patients with Waardenburg syndrome types I and II can have hypopigmentation of the fundus and bright-blue irides or heterochromia irides. Iris transillumination may also be present. Vision is generally unimpaired and there is no nystagmus.

Waardenburg-like Syndrome of Bard

Like patients with Waardenburg syndrome, some patients with the Waardenburg-like syndrome of Bard have congenital sensorineural deafness, broad nasal root, white forelock, light complexion, premature graying of the scalp hair, segmental iris heterochromia, and fundus heterochromia.[7] Unlike patients with Waardenburg syndrome type I, however, they always lack dystopia of the inner canthi. They also often, but not invariably, have two features not associated with classic Waardenburg syndrome: *(1)* hyperopia with esotropia and amblyopia and *(2)* iris transillumination and severe fundus hypopigmentation with an abnormal foveal appearance. Fluorescein angiography reveals no increased transmission at the macula. Visual acuity is 20/30 to 20/40 in the preferred eye, and the hypopigmented fovea has a hypoplastic appearance on ophthalmoscopy; nystagmus is absent. The phenotype appears to be the result of digenic inheritance of a mutation in the MITF gene and homozygosity or heterozygosity for the R402Q polymorphism of the tyrosinase gene.[93b]

Griscelli Syndrome

Griscelli syndrome consists of partial albinism with immunodeficiency and was first described in 1976.[51] Klein et al.[77] refined the characterization of this condition. Patients have silvery-gray hair without ocular or cutaneous hypopigmentation. They have no ophthalmologic abnormalities. There is an abundance of mature melanosomes, but there is failure of their transfer to keratinocytes.[105a,114] Patients are predisposed to acute viral and bacterial infections that lead to lymphohistiocytic infiltration of multiple organs and to pancytopenia. Impaired T helper cell function and natural killer cell function are responsible for the immunologic incompetence. On light microscopy there were no intracellular granules similar to those characteristic of Chediak-Higashi syndrome. The disease is fatal, with a life expectancy of approximately 5 years. Bone marrow transplantation is indicated and may result in a clinical cure. Pastural et al. mapped the disease locus to 15q21 and found the disorder to result from mutations in the myosin-Va gene.[105a]

MANAGEMENT OF PATIENTS WITH ALBINISM

Diagnosing patients with tyrosinase-negative oculocutaneous albinism is not difficult and is made on clinical grounds.[145] If they are examined late in childhood, patients with tyrosinase-positive oculocutaneous albinism are sometimes more difficult to detect because of nystagmus and poor vision. Iris transillumination, foveal hypoplasia, and a history of light cutaneous pigmentation at birth and increased pigmentation thereafter clinch the diagnosis. The hair-bulb incubation assay for tyrosinase activity is not required for the diagnosis of most patients but may prove of help in very unusual cases. X-linked ocular albinism should be suspected in boys who present with nystagmus. Examination of the fundus and iris of carrier mothers is helpful in those patients, especially blacks, who have variable amounts of ocular pigment (ocular albinism *cum pigmento*). Puerto Rican albinos should be screened for a bleeding diathesis and Hermansky-Pudlak syndrome. Albinos with recurrent infections should be suspected of having the Chediak-Higashi-syndrome, and appropriate tests should be undertaken. Haynes and Robertson[54] found that at 16 weeks of gestation, fetal scalp biopsy can diagnose types I and II albinism. Eady et al.[36,37] were able to diagnose albinism prenatally by fetal skin biopsy at 20 weeks gestation, although they were unable to define the level of tyrosinase activity.

Albinism may be a cause of psychological problems because of the patient's unusual appearance, the presence of nystagmus, and because of the handicap resulting from reduced visual acuity. Furthermore, albinism predisposes to actinic-induced cutaneous malignancies. Patients are thus instructed to avoid outdoor occupations, use sunscreens, and have regular examinations for cutaneous neoplasms in sun-exposed areas. Tinted glasses are helpful in patients with excessive photophobia. Optimal correction of refractive errors may improve acuity or sharpness of images; near-vision aids such as magnifiers are also useful. Some studies have suggested that contact lenses may improve visual acuity in patients with congenital motor nystagmus, possibly by stimulation of additional vergence and accommodation.[2] Telescopes may be of help to school children for viewing the blackboard.[40,41] Children with albinism often attend regular school and are seated in the front of the classroom. They should not be discouraged from holding their reading material very close to their faces.

Patients with esotropia or exotropia, both of which are common in albinos, may require patching and/or surgery. Kestenbaum procedures can be helpful in patients with a face turn. Von Noorden and Sprunger[135] and later Helveston et al.[56] proposed large rectus muscle recessions for the treatment of idiopathic and other forms of congenital motor nystagmus, including that associated with albinism; however, this procedure remains controversial. Finally, Zubcov et al.[155] compared the improvement of visual acuity in patients with congenital motor nystagmus after the Anderson-Kestenbaum procedure, an artificial divergence procedure, or both, and they found that the artificial divergence and combined operations gave better results than the Anderson-Kestenbaum procedure.

REFERENCES

1. Abadi RV, Pascal E, Whittle J, Worfolk R. Retinal fixation behavior in human albinos. *Optom Visual Sci* 1989;66:276–280.
2. Allen ED, Davies PD. Role of contact lenses in the management of congenital nystagmus. *Br J Ophthalmol* 1983;67:834–836.
3. Anderson JR. Causes and treatment of congenital eccentric nystagmus. *Br J Ophthalmol* 1953;37:267–281.
4. Apkarian P, Reits D, Spekreijse H, Van Dorp D. A decisive electrophysiological test for human albinism. *Electroencephalogr Clin Neurophysiol* 1983;55:513–531.
5. Arias S. Genetic heterogeneity in the Waardenburg syndrome. *Birth Defects Orig Art Ser* 1971;7:87–101.

5a. Bailin T, Oh J, Feng GH, et al. Organization and nucleotide sequence of the human Hermansky-Pudlak syndrome. *J Invest Dermatol* 1997;108:923–927.

6. Baldwin CT, Hoth CF, Amos JA, da-Silva EO, Milunsky A. An exonic mutation in HuP2 paired domain gene causes Waardenburg's syndrome. *Nature* 1993;355:637–638.
7. Bard LA. Heterogeneity in Waardenburg's syndrome. *Arch Ophthalmol* 1978;96:1193–1198.
8. Barton DE, Kwon BS, Francke U. Human tyrosinase gene, mapped to chromosome 11 (q14-q21), defines second region of homology with mouse chromosome 7. *Genomics* 1988; 3:17–24.
9. Bassi MT, Schiaffino MV, Renieri A, De

Nigris F, Galli L, Bruttini M, Gebbia M, Bergen AAB, Lewis RA, Ballabio AB. Cloning of the gene for ocular albinism type 1 from the distal short arm of the X chromosome. *Nature Genet* 1995;10:13–19.

10. Bedoya V, Grimley PM, Duque O. Chediak-Higashi syndrome. *Arch Pathol* 1969;88: 340–349.
11. Beguez Cesar A. Neutropenia cronica maligna familar con granulaciones atipicas de los leucocitos. *Biol Soc Cubana Pediatr* 1943; 15:900–922.
12. Benedict PH, Szabo G, Fitzpatrick TB, Sinesi J. Melanotic macules in Albright's syndrome and in neurofibromatosis. *JAMA* 1968;205: 618–626.
13. Bergen AAB, Zijp P, Schuurman EJM, Bleeker-Wagemakers EM, Apkarian P, van Ommen G-JB. Refinement of the localization of the X-linked ocular albinism gene. *Genomics* 1993;16:272–273.
14. Bergsma DR, Kaiser-Kupfer M. A new form of albinism. *Am J Ophthalmol* 1974;77: 837–844.
15. Blume RS, Wolff SM. The Chediak-Higashi syndrome: Studies in four patients and a review of the literature. *Medicine* 1972; 51:247–280.
16. Boissy RE, Zhao H, Austin LM, Nordlund JJ, King RA. Melanocytes from an individual with brown oculocutaneous albinism lack expression of TRP-1, the product of human homologue of the murine brown locus. *Am J Hum Genet* 1993;53(suppl):Abstract #160.
17. Boxer LA, Watanabe AM, Rister M, Besch HR, Allen J, Baehner RL. Correction of leukocyte function in Chediak-Higashi syndrome by ascorbate. *N Engl J Med* 1976;295:1041–1045.
18. Breathnach AS, Wyllie L. Ultrastructure of retinal pigment epithelium of the human fetus. *J Ultrastruct Res* 1966;16:584–597.

18a. Burkhardt JK, Wiebel FA, Hester S, Argon Y. The giant organelles in *Beige* and Chediak-Higashi fibroblasts are derived from late endosomes and mature lysosomes. *J Exp Med* 1993;178:1845–1856.

19. Carroll WM, Jay BS, McDonald WI, Halliday AM. Two distinct patterns of visual evoked response asymmetry in human albinism. *Nature* 1980;286:604–606.
20. Casswell AG, McCartney ACE, Hungerford JL. Choroidal malignant melanoma in an albino. *Br J Ophthalmol* 1989;73:840–845.
21. Castle D, Kromberg J, Kowalsky R et al. Visual evoked potentials in Negro carriers of the gene for tyrosinase positive oculocutaneous albinism. *J Med Genet* 1988;25:835–837.
22. Catalano RA, Nelson LB, Schaffer DB. Oculocutaneous albinism associated with congenital glaucoma. *Ophthalmic Paediatr Genet* 1988;9:5–6.
23. Charles SJ, Green JS, Moore AT, Barton DE, Yates JRW. Genetic mapping of X-linked ocular albinism: Linkage analysis in a large Newfoundland kindred. *Genomics* 1993; 16:259–261.
24. Charles SJ, Moore AT, Grant JW, Yates JRW. Genetic counseling in X-linked ocular albinism: clinical features of the carrier state. *Eye* 1992;6:75–79.
25. Chintamaneni CD, Ramsay M, Colman MA, Fox MF, Pickard RT, Kwon BS. Mapping the human CAS2 gene, the homologue of the mouse brown (b) locus to human chromosome 9p22-pter. *Biochem Biophys Res Commun* 1991;178:227–235.
26. Cogan DG. Congenital nystagmus. *Can J Ophthalmol* 1967;2:4–10.
27. Cortin P, Tremblay M, Lemagne JM. X-linked ocular albinism: relative value of skin biopsy, iris transillumination and funduscopy in identifying males and carriers. *Can J Ophthalmol* 1981;16:121–123.
28. Creel D, Garber SR, King RA, Witkop CJ Jr. Auditory brainstem anomalies in human albinos. *Science* 1980;209:1253–1255.
29. Creel D, O'Donnell FE Jr, Witkop CJ Jr. Visual system anomalies in human ocular albinos. *Science* 1978;201:931–933.
30. Creel D, Spekreijse H, Reits D. Evoked potential in albinos: Efficacy of pattern stimuli in detecting misrouted optic fibers. *Electroencephalogr Clin Neurophysiol* 1981;53: 595–603.
31. Creel DJ, Conlee JW, King RA. Dark adaptation in human albinos. *Clin Vision Sci* 1990;5:81–85.
32. Cross HE, McKusick VA, Breen W. A new oculocerebral syndrome with pigmentation. *J Pediatr* 1967;70:398–406.

32a. Davis PL, Bakers RS, Piccione RJ. Large recession nystagmus surgery in albinos: effect on acuity. *J Pediatr Ophthalmol Strabismus* 1997;34:279–283.

33. De Beer HA, Anderson R, Findlay GH. Chediak-Higashi syndrome in a "black" child: Clinical features, immunological studies, and optics of the hair and skin. *S Afr Med J* 1981;60:108–112.

34. Donaldson DD. Transillumination of the iris. *Trans Am Ophthalmol Soc* 1974;72:89.
35. Durham FM. On the presence of tyrosinase in the skin of some pigmented vertebrates. *Proc R Soc Lond* 1904;74:31–313.
36. Eady RAJ, Gunner DB, Garner A, Rodeck CH. Prenatal diagnosis of oculocutaneous albinism by electron microscopy of fetal skin. *J Invest Dermatol* 1983;80:210–212.
37. Eady RAJ. Prenatal diagnosis of oculocutaneous albinism: Implication for other hereditary disorders of pigmentation. *Semin Dermatol* 1984;3:241–246.
38. Falls HF. Sex-linked ocular albinism displaying typical fundus changes in the female heterozygote. *Am J Ophthalmol* 1951;34: 41–50.
39. Feeney L, Berman ER. Oxygen toxicity: Membrane damage by free radicals. *Invest Ophthalmol* 1976;15:789–792.
40. Fonda G, Thomas H, Gore GV. Educational and vocational placement, and low-vision corrections in albinism. *Sight Saving Rev* 1975; 41:29–36.
41. Fonda G. Characteristics and low-vision correction in albinism. *Arch Ophthalmol* 1962; 68:754–761.
42. Forsius H, Eriksson AW. Ein neues augensyndrom mit X-chromosomaler transmission: Eine sippe mit fundusalbinismus, foveahypoplasie, nystagmus, myopie, asstigmatismus und dyschromatopsie. *Klin Monatsbl Augenheilkd* 1964;144:447–457.
43. Foy C, Newton VE, Wellesley D, Harris R, Read AP. Assignment of WS1 locus to human 2q37 and possible homology between Waardenburg syndrome and the Splotch mouse. *Am J Hum Genet* 1990;46:1017–1023.
44. Fulton AB, Albert DM, Craft JL. Human albinism: Light and electron microscopy study. *Arch Ophthalmol* 1978;96:305–310.
45. Gardner JM, Nakatsu Y, Gondo Y, Lee S, Lyon MF, King RA, Brilliant MH. The mouse pink-eyed dilution gene: Association with human Prader-Willi and Angelman syndromes. *Science* 1992;257:1121–1124.
46. Giebel LB, Musarella MA, Spritz RA. A nonsense mutation in the tyrosinase gene Afghan patients with tyrosinase negative (type IA) oculocutaneous albinism. *J Med Genet* 1991;28:464–467.
47. Giebel LB, Strunk KM, Spritz RA. Organization and nucleotide sequences of the human tyrosinase gene and a truncated tyrosinase-related segment. *Genomics* 1991;9:435–445.
47a. Giebel LB, Spritz RA. Mutation of the KIT (mast/stem cell growth factor receptor) protooncogene in human piebaldism. *Proc Natl Acad Sci USA* 1991;88:8696–8699.
48. Gillespie FD, Covelli B. Carriers of ocular albinism with and without ocular changes. *Arch Ophthalmol* 1963;70:209–213.
49. Gregor Z. The perifoveal vasculature in albinism. *Br J Ophthalmol* 1978;62:554–557.
50. Griscelli C, Durandy A, Guy-grand D, Daguillard F, Herzog C, Prunieras M. A syndrome associating partial albinism and immunodeficiency. *Am J Med* 1976;65:691–702.
50a. Gross A, Kunze J, Maier RF, et al. Autosomal recessive neural crest syndrome with albinism, black lock, cell migration disorder of the neurocytes of the gut and deafness: ABCD syndrome. *Am J Med Genet* 1995;56:322–326.
51. Guerrier CJ, Lutzner MA, Devico V. An electronmicroscopical study of the skin in 18 cases of xeroderma pigmentosum. *Dermatologica* 1973;146:211–221.
52. Guillery RW. Visual pathways in albinos. *Sci Am* 1974;230:44–54.
53. Hayashibe K, Mishima Y. Tyrosinase-positive melanocyte distribution and induction of pigmentation in human piebald skin. *Arch Dermatol* 1988;124:381–386.
54. Haynes ME, Robertson E. Can oculocutaneous albinism be diagnosed prenatally? *Prenat Diagn* 1981;1:85–89.
55. Hearing VJ. Invited editorial: Unraveling the melanocyte. *Am J Hum Genet* 1993;52:1–7.
56. Helveston EM, Ellis FD, Plager DA. Large recession of the horizontal recti for treatment of nystagmus. *Ophthalmology* 1991;98:1302–1305.
57. Hermansky F, Pudlak P. Albinism associated with hemorrhagic diathesis and unusual pigmented reticular cells in the bone marrow: Report of two cases with histochemical studies. *Blood* 1959;14:162–169.
58. Hoth CF, Milunsky A, Lipsky N, Sheffer R, Clarren SK, Baldwin OT. Mutations in the paired domain of the human PAX3 gene cause Klein-Waardenburg syndrome (WS-III) as well as Waardenburg syndrome type 1 (WS-1). *Am J Hum Genet* 1993;52:455–462.
59. Hu F, Hanifin JM, Prescott GH, Tongue AC. Yellow mutant albinism: Cytochemical, ultrastructural, and genetic characterization suggesting multiple allelism. *Am J Hum Genet* 1980;32:387–395.
60. Hughes AE, Newton VE, Liu XZ, Read AP. A gene for Waardenburg syndrome type 2

maps close to the human homologue of the microphthalmia gene at chromosome 3p12-p14.1. *Nature Genet* 1994;7:509–512.
61. Ichikawa K. Uber den ophthalmoscopischen befund der area centralis des albinotischen augen. *Klin Monatsbl Augenheilkd* 1913; 51:9–15.
62. Jackson IJ. A cDNA encoding tyrosinase-related protein maps to the brown locus in mouse. *Proc Natl Acad Sci USA* 1988;85: 4392–4396. [Erratum in *Proc Natl Acad Sci USA* 1989;86:997.]
63. Jimbow K, Szabo G, Fitzpatrick TB. Ultrastructure of giant pigment granules (macromelanosomes) in the cutaneous pigmented macules of neurofibromatosis. *J Invest Dermatol* 1973;61:300–309.
64. Johnson DL, Jacobson LW, Toyama R, Monahan RH. Histopathology of eyes in Chediak-Higashi syndrome. *Arch Ophthalmol* 1966; 75:84–88.
65. Kestenbaum A. A nystagmus operation. In *Acta XVII Concilium Ophthalmologicum*, vol. II:1954:1071–1078.
66. King RA, Creel D, Cervenka J, Okoro AN, Witkop CJ. Albinism in Nigeria with delineation of a new recessive oculocutaneous type. *Clin Genet* 1980;17:259–270.
67. King RA, Hearing VJ, Creel DJ, Oetting WS. Albinism. In *The Metabolic and Molecular Basis of Disease*, C. R. Scriver, A. L. Beardet, W. S. Sly, D. Valle, eds. New York: McGraw-Hill, 1995.
68. King RA, Lewis RA, Townsend D, Zelickson A, Olds DP, Brumbaugh J. Brown oculocutaneous albinism. Clinical, ophthalmological, and biochemical characterization. *Ophthalmology* 1985;92:1496–1505.
69. King RA, Mentink MM, Oetting WS. Nonrandom distribution of missense mutations within the human tyrosinase gène in type I (tyrosinase-related) oculocutaneous albinism. *Mol Biol Med* 1991;8:19–29.
70. King RA, Olds DP, Witkop CJ. Characterization of human hairbulb tyrosinase: Properties of normal and albinos enzyme. *J Invest Dermatol* 1978;71:136–139.
71. King RA, Rich SS. Segregation analysis of brown oculocutaneous albinism. *Clin Genet* 1986;29:496–501.
72. King RA, Summers CG, Creel D, Weleber R, Fryer JP, Oetting WS. Mutations of the tyrosinase gene produce autosomal recessive ocular albinism. *Am J Hum Genet* 1994; 55(suppl):A226.
73. King RA, Townsend D, Oetting W, Summers CG, Olds DP, White JG, Spritz RA. Temperature-sensitive tyrosinase associated with peripheral pigmentation in oculocutaneous albinism. *J Clin Invest* 1991;87:1046–1053.
74. King RA, Townsend D, Oetting WS, Spritz RA. An unusual pigment pattern in type I oculocutaneous albinism (OCA) resulting from a temperature-sensitive enzyme (Abstract). *Am J Hum Genet* 1989;45(suppl):A8.
75. King RA, Witkop CJ. Detection of heterozygotes for tyrosinase-negative oculocutaneous albinism by hair-bulb tyrosinase assay. *Am J Hum Genet* 1977;29:164–168.
76. King RA, Witkop CJ. Hairbulb tyrosinase activity in oculocutaneous albinism. *Nature* 1976;263:69–71.
77. Klein C, Philippe N, LeDeist F et al. Partial albinism with immunodeficiency (Griscelli syndrome). *J Pediatr* 1994;125:886–895.
78. Krill AE, Lee GB. The electroretinogram in albinos and carriers of the ocular albino trait. *Arch Opthalmol* 1963;69:32–38.
79. Kugelman TP, Van Scott EJ. Tyrosinase activity in melanocytes of human albinos. *J Invest Dermatol* 1961;37:73–76.
80. Kwon BS, Haq AK, Pomerantz SH, Halaban R. Isolation and sequence of a cDNA clone for human tyrosinase that maps at the mouse c-albino locus. *Proc Natl Acad Sci USA* 1987;84:473–7477.
81. Lang GE, Rott H-D, Pfeiffer RA. X-linked ocular albinism: Characteristic pattern of affection in female carriers. *Ophthalmic Paediatr Genet* 1990;11:265–271.
82. Lanum J. The damaging effects of light on the retina: empirical findings, theoretical and practical implications. *Surv Opthalmol* 1978; 22:221–249.
83. Larkin DFP, O'Donoghue HN. Developmental glaucoma in oculocutaneous albinism. *Ophthalmic Paediatr Genet* 1988;9:1–4.
84. Lee S-T, Nicholls RD, Bundey S et al. Mutations of the P gene in oculocutaneous albinism, ocular albinism and Prader-Willi syndrome plus albinism. *N Engl J Med* 1994; 330:529–534.
85. Leventhal AG, Vitek DJ, Creel DJ. Abnormal visual pathways in normally pigmented cats that are heterozygous for albinism. *Science* 1985;229:1395–1397.
86. Lewis RA. Ocular albinism and deafness (Abstract). *Am J Hum Genet* 1978;30(suppl):57.
87. Lyon M, Searle AG. Genetic Variants and Strains of the Laboratory Mouse. New York: Oxford University Press, 1989.
88. Lyon MF. Sex chromatin and gene action in

the mammalian X-chromosome. *Am J Med Genet* 1962;14:135–148.

89. Maguire AM, Maumenee IH. Iris pigment mosaicism in carriers of X-linked ocular albinism cum pigmento. *Am J Ophthalmol* 1989; 107:298–299.

90. Margolis S, Siegel IM, Choy A, Breinin GM. Depigmentation of hair, skin, and eyes associated with the Apert syndrome. *Birth Defects Orig Art Ser* 1978;14:341–360.

91. Marmor MF. Hereditary vertical nystagmus. *Arch Ophthalmol* 1973;90:107–111.

92. McLeod R, Lowry RB. Incidence of albinism in British Columbia: Separation by hairbulb test. *Clin Genet* 1976;9:77–80.

93. Mietz H, Green WR, Wolff SM, Abundo GP. Foveal hypoplasia in complete oculocutaneous albinism. *Retina* 1992;12:254–260.

93a. Miyake Y, Yagasaki K, Horiguchi M, et al. Congenital stationary night blindness with negative electroretinogram. A new classification. *Arch Ophthalmol* 1986;104:1013–1020.

93b. Morell R, Spritz RA, Ho L, et al. Apparent digenic inheritance of Waardenburg syndrome type 2 (WS2) and autosomal recessive ocular albinism (AROA). *Hum Mol Genet* 1997;6:659–664.

94. Mosher DB, Fitzpatrick TB. Piebaldism. *Arch Dermatol* 1988;124:364–365.

95. Mund ML, Rodrigues MM, Fine BS. Light and electronmicroscopic observations on the pigmented layers of the developing human eye. *Am J Ophthalmol* 1972;73:167–182.

96. Murty VVVS, Bouchard B, Mathew S, Vijayasaradhi S, Houghton AN. Assignment of the human TYRP (brown) locus to chromosome region 9p23 by nonradioactive in situ hybridization. *Genomics* 1992;13:227–229.

97. Nakagawa H, Hori Y, Sato S, Fitzpatrick TB, Martuza RL. The nature and origin of the melanin macroglobule. *J Invest Dermatol* 1984;83:134–139.

98. Nance WE, Jackson CE, Witkop CJ Jr. Amish albinism: A distinctive autosomal recessive phenotype. *Am J Hum Genet* 1970;22: 579–586.

99. Naumann GOH, Lerche W, Schroeder W. Foveola-Aplasie bei tyrosinase-positivem oculocutanen albinismus. *Graefes Clin Exp Arch Ophthalmol* 1976;200:39–50.

99a. Nagle DL, Karim MA, Woolf EA et al. Identification and mutation analysis of the complete gene for Chediak-Higashi syndrome. *Nature Genet* 1996;14:307–312.

100. O'Donnell FE Jr, Green WR, Fleischman JA, Hambrick GW. X-linked ocular albinism in blacks: Ocular albinism cum pigmento. *Arch Ophthalmol* 1978;96:1189–1192.

101. O'Donnell FE Jr, Hambrick GW, Green WR et al. X-linked ocular albinism: An oculocutaneous macromelanosomal disorder. *Arch Ophthalmol* 1976;94:1883–1892.

102. Oetting WS, King RA. Molecular analysis of type I-A (tyrosine negative) oculocutaneous albinism. *Hum Genet* 1992;90:258–262.

103. Oetting WS, King RA. Molecular basis of type I-A (tyrosinase-related) oculocutaneous albinism: Mutations and polymorphisms of the human tyrosinase gene. *Hum Mutat* 1993; 2:1–6.

104. Oetting WS, Mentink MM, Summers CG, et al. Three different frameshift mutations of the tyrosinase gene in type I-A oculocutaneous albinism. *Am J Hum Genet* 1991; 49:199–206.

104a. Oh J, Bailin T, Fukai K, et al. Positional cloning of a gene for Hermansky-Pudlak syndrome, a disorder of cytoplasmic organelles. *Nature Genet* 1996;14:300–306.

105. Okoro AN. Albinism in Nigeria: A clinical and social study. *Br J Dermatol* 1975;92:485–492.

105a. Pastural E, Barrat FJ, Dufourcq-Lagelouse R, et al. Griseelli disease maps to chromosome 15q21 and is associated with mutations in the myosin-Va gene. *Nature Genet* 1997;16: 289–292.

106. Pearce WG, Johnson GL, Gillan JG. Nystagmus in a female carrier of ocular albinism. *J Med Genet* 1972;9:126–128.

107. Ramsay M, Coleman M-A, Stevens G, et al. The tyrosinase-positive oculocutaneous albinism locus maps to chromosome 15q11.2-q12. *Am J Hum Genet* 1992;51:879–884.

108. Raper HS. XIV. The tyrosinase-tyrosine reaction. *Biochem J* 1927;21:89–96.

109. Rausch PDG, Pryzwansky KB, Spitznagel JK. Immunohistochemical identification of azurophilic and specific granule markers in the granules of Chediak-Higashi neutrophils. *N Engl J Med* 1978;298:693–698.

110. Reeser F, Weinstein GW, Feiock KB. Electrooculography as a test of retinal function. *Am J Ophthalmol* 1970;70:505–514.

111. Rinchik EM, Bultman SJ, Horsthemke B, et al. A gene for the mouse pink-eyed dilution locus and for human type II oculocutaneous albinism. *Nature* 1993;361:72–76.

112. Rozycki DL, Ruben RJ, Rapen I, Spiro AJ. Autosomal recessive deafness associated with short stature, vitiligo, muscle wasting and achalasia. *Arch Otolaryngol* 1971;93: 194–197.

113. Saral O, Kucukali T, Esroy F, et al. Griscelli's syndrome: Clinical features of 3 siblings. *Turk J Pediatr* 1993;35:115–119.
113a. Schiaffino MV, Bassi MT, Galli L, et al. Analysis of the OA1 gene reveals mutations in only one-third of patients with X-linked ocular albinism. *Hum Mol Genet* 1995;4:2319–2325.
114. Schneiderman LJ, Bartnof HS, Worthen DM. X-linked congenital nystagmus: A problem in genetic counseling. *Ann Ophthalmol* 1976; 8:444–446.
115. Schnur RE, Trask BJ, van den Engh, et al. An Xp22 microdeletion associated with ocular albinism and icthyosis: Approximation of breakpoints and estimation of deletion size by using cloned DNA probes and flow cytometry. *Am J Hum Genet* 1989;45:706–720.
116. Schnur RE, Wick PA, Bailey C, et al. Phenotypic variability in X-linked ocular albinism: Relationship to linkage genotypes. *Am J Hum Genet* 1994;55:484–496.
117. Scott MJ Jr, Giacobetti R, Zugerman C. Malignant melanoma with oculocutaneous albinism. *J Am Acad Dermatol* 1982;7:684–685.
118. Silvers WK. *The Coat Colors of Mice.* New York: Springer-Verlag, 1979.
119. Sorsby A. Noah—An albino. *Br Med J* 1958;2:1587–1589.
120. Spencer WH, Hogan MJ. Ocular manifestations of Chediak-Higashi syndrome. *Am J Ophthalmol* 1962;50:1197–1960.
121. Spritz RA, Strunk K, King RA. Molecular analyses of the tyrosinase gene in patients with tyrosinase-deficient oculocutaneous albinism (Abstract). *Am J Hum Genet* 1989; 45(suppl):A221.
122. Spritz RA, Strunk KM, Giebel LB, King RA. Detection of mutations in the tyrosinase gene in a patient with type I-A oculocutaneous albinism. *N Engl J Med* 1990;322:1724–1728.
123. Spritz RA. Molecular genetics of oculocutaneous albinism. *Hum Mol Genet* 1994;3: 1469–1475.
124. Summers CG, Knobloch WH, Witkop CJ Jr, King RA. Hermansky-Pudlak syndrome: Ophthalmic findings. *Ophthalmology* 1988; 95:545–554.
125. Szmanski KA, Boughman JA, Nance WE, Olansky DC, Weinberg RS. Genetic studies of ocular albinism in a large Virginia kindred. *Ann Ophthalmol* 1984;16:183–195.
126. Tanaka T. Chediak-Higashi syndrome: Abnormal lysosomal enzyme levels in granulocytes of patients and family members. *Pediatr Res* 1980;14:901–904.
127. Tassabehji M, Read AP, Newton VE, Patton M, Gross P, Harris R, Strachan T. Mutations in the PAX3 gene causing Waardenburg syndrome type 1 and type 2. *Nature Genet* 1993;3:26–30.
128. Tassabehji M, Read AP, Newton VE, et al. Waardenburg syndrome patients have mutations in the human homologue of the Pax-3 paired box gene. *Nature* 1992;355:635–636.
129. Tassabehji M, Newton VE, Read AP. Waardenburg syndrome type 2 caused by mutations in the human microphthalmia (MITF) gene. *Nature Genet* 1994;8:251–255.
130. Telfer MA, Sugar M, Jaeger EA, Mulcahy J. Dominant piebald trait (white forelock and leukoderma) with neurological impairment. *Am J Hum Genet* 1971;23:383–389.
131. Tripathi RK, Strunk KM, Giebel LB, et al. Tyrosinase gene mutations in type I (tyrosinase-deficient) oculocutaneous albinism define two clusters of missense substitutions. *Am J Med Genet* 1992;43:865–871.
132. van Dorp DB, Delleman JW, Loewer-Sieger DH. Oculocutaneous albinism and anterior chamber cleavage malformations. *Clin Genet* 1984;26:440–444.
133. van Dorp DB, Eriksson AW, Delleman JW, et al. Åland eye disease: No albino misrouting. *Clin Genet* 1985;28:526–531.
134. van Dorp DB. Albinism, or the NOACH syndrome. *Clin Genet* 1987;31:228–242.
135. Von Noorden GK, Sprunger DT. Large rectus muscle recessions for the treatment congenital nystagmus. *Arch Ophthalmol* 1991;109: 221–224.
136. Waardenburg PJ. Herkenbaarheid van letente overdragers van albinismus universalis et albinismus oculi. *Ned Tijdschr Geneeskd* 1947; 91:1863–1866.
137. Waardenburg PJ. New syndrome combining developmental anomalies of the eyelids, eyebrows, and nose root with pigmentary defects of iris and head hair and with congenital deafness. *Am J Hum Genet* 1951;3:195–253.
138. Wack MA, Peachy NS, Fishman GA. Electroretinographic findings in human oculocutaneous albinism. *Ophthalmology* 1989;96: 1778–1785.
139. Wagstaff J. A translocation-associated deletion defines a critical region for the $9p^-$ syndrome (Abstract). *Am J Hum Genet* 1993; 53(suppl):A619.
140. Walsh RJ. A distinctive pigment of skin in New Guinea indigines. *Ann Hum Genet* 1971;34:379–388.

140a. Ward KA, Moss C, Sanders DS. Human piebaldism: Relationship between phenotype and site of KIT gene mutation. *Br J Dermatol* 1995;132:929–935.
141. Weleber RG, Pillers DM, Powell BR, et al. Åland Island disease (Forsius-Eriksson syndrome) associated with contiguous gene syndrome at Xp21: Similarity to incomplete congenital stationary night blindness. *Arch Ophthalmol* 1989;107:1170–1179.
142. Windhorst DB, Zelickson AS, Good RA. A human pigmentary dilution based on heritable subcellular structural defect: The Chediak-Higashi syndrome. *J Invest Dermatol* 1966;50:9–18.
143. Windhorst DB, Zelickson AS, Good RA. Chediak-Higashi syndrome: Hereditary gigantism of cytoplasmic organelles. *Science* 1966;151:81–83.
143a. Winship I, Gericke G, Beighton P. X-linked inheritance of ocular albinism with late-onset sensorineural deafness. *Am J Med Genet* 1984;19:797–803.
144. Winship IM, Babaya M, Ramesar RS. X-linked ocular albinism and sensorineural deafness: Linkage to Xp22.3. *Genomics* 1993;18: 444–445.
145. Witkop CJ Jr. Albinism. *Clin Dermatol* 1989;7:80–91.
146. Witkop CJ Jr. Depigmentations of the general and oral tissues and their genetic foundations. *Ala J Med Sci* 1979;16:330–333.
147. Witkop CJ, Almodavar C, Pineiro B, Babcock MN. Hermansky-Pudlak syndrome (HPA). An epidemiologic study. *Ophthalmic Paediatr Genet* 1990;11:245–250.
148. Witkop CJ, Hill CW, Desnick S, et al. Ophthalmologic, biochemical, platelet and ultrastructural defects in the various types of oculocutaneous albinism. *J Invest Dermatol* 1973;60:443–456.
149. Witkop CJ, Jay B, Creel D, Guillery RW. Optic and otic neurologic abnormalities oculocutaneous and ocular albinism. *Birth Defects Orig Art Ser* 1982;18:299–318.
150. Wolff E. *Anatomy of the Eye and Orbit*, 7th ed, Philadelphia: W. B. Saunders, 1976:434.
151. Wong L, O'Donnell FE Jr, Green WR. Giant pigment granules in the retinal pigment epithelium of a fetus with X-linked ocular albinism. *Ophthalmic Paediatr Genet* 1983;2: 47–66.
152. Yee RD, Wong EK, Baloh RW, Honrubia V. A study of congenital nystagmus: Waveforms. *Neurology* 1976;26:326–333.
153. Zhao H, Boissy YL, Abdel-Malek Z, et al. On the analysis of the pathophysiology of Chediak-Higashi syndrome. Defects expressed by cultured melanocytes. *Lab Invest* 1994;71:25–35.
154. Zhao H, Zhao Y, Nordlund JJ, Boissy RE. Human TRP-1 has tyrosine hydroxylase but no DOPA oxidase activity. *Pigment Cell Res* 1994;7:131–140.
155. Zubcov AA, Stark N, Weber A, et al. Improvement of visual acuity after surgery for nystagmus. *Ophthalmology* 1993;100:1488–1497.

35

Mitochondrial Diseases

DAVID MACKEY

Mitochondria are the small organelles inside cells that are responsible for the production of energy via adenosine triphosphate (ATP). They are unusual because they contain several copies of a very small circular DNA that encodes some of the subunits of the respiratory chain proteins required for production of the oxidative phosphorylation pathway and also codes for their transfer and ribosomal RNAs. Each cell contains multiple mitochondria, each with multiple copies of mitochondrial DNA (mtDNA); thus a cell may contain several different types of mtDNA, including some that have pathogenic mutations. In this condition, known as *heteroplasmy*, the mtDNA mutations may consist of deletions, duplications, or point mutations. If a mitochondrion has a deletion or pathological point mutation in one of its mtDNA copies it is still able to produce some of the normal protein from its normal mtDNA copies. If, however, the mitochondrion contains a large number of mutant mtDNA then it no longer can produce normal proteins and the mitochondrion will cease to function properly. If a cell contains a large number of dysfunctional mitochondria it will not be able to utilize enough energy (a particular problem for the highly respiratory-dependent neural tissues) and will die. Thus the phenotype of a disease will not only depend on which mutation is present, but on which cells of the body contain a large percentage of mutant mitochondria.[10] The mtDNA mutations (see Table 35.1) may consist of *(1)* deletions—usually of large portions of the mtDNA loop, with particular areas common as breakpoints (Kearn-Sayre syndrome [KSS] and chronic progressive external ophthalmoplegia [CPEO]), or they may be *(2)* point mutations in the transfer RNA (myoclonus epilepsy, ragged, red, fibers [MERRF], mitochondrial myopathy, lactic acidosis, and strokelike episodes [MELAS]), resulting in abnormalities of the mtDNA coded proteins, or *(3)* point mutations in the coded respiratory chain subunits (Leber's hereditary optic neuropathy [LHON] and neuropathy, ataxia, and retinitis pigmentosa [NARP]). Nuclear-encoded genes involved in the mitochondrial respiratory chain can also result in disease (Leigh syndrome, subacute necrotizing encephalopathy).

Mitochondria and their mtDNA are transmitted almost exclusively from the mother in the ovum, with the sperm contributing very few, if any, mitochondria. Thus diseases of mitochondrial DNA are transmitted by women. The small number of mitochondria from the ovum will populate all the cells of the embryo. If the original mitochondria in the ovum are identical, then every cell will have the same mitochondrial DNA until new mutations arise. If the ovum has two or more different versions of the mtDNA, than these will be distributed

Table 35.1. Ophthalmic Diseases Associated with Mitochondrial Abnormalities

Point Mutation Diseases
Leber's hereditary optic neuropathy (LHON)
Neuropathy ataxia, and retinitis pigmentosa (NARP)
Mitochondrial myopathy, lactic acidosis, and strokelike episodes (MELAS)
Deletion Diseases
Kearn-Sayre syndrome (KSS)/chronic progressive external ophthalmoplegia
Aging
Diseases of the Nuclear DNA that Affect Mitochondria
Leigh syndrome

in a random manner, and thus some cells may have more mutant mtDNA and other cells more normal mtDNA, a condition known as mtDNA heteroplasmy. Thus a mtDNA disease may vary depending on the proportion of mutant and normal mtDNA. Similarly, new mutations may arise in the mtDNA of the embryo and be distributed to the cells descendant from the mtDNA carrying the new mutation. The high level of free radicals in mitochondria—because of the oxidative phosphorylation, the absence of the nuclear DNA repair mechanisms, and the protective effect of histones—means that mtDNA is far more likely to undergo mutation.[9]

Mutations in mtDNA occur as part of aging.[55] Numerous reports have associated particular mtDNA mutations with aging, and many mtDNA mutations have been identified in tissues affected by age-related diseases. It is not clear, however, whether these mutations are pathogenic or just general markers of aging. It may be that any of the mtDNA mutations that decrease the mitochondrial function can cause age-related diseases. However, the alternative possibility—that age-related diseases cause a hostile environment for the mtDNA, resulting in more mutations—has not been ruled out.

Mitochondrial DNA has been used to establish the relatedness of individuals through the female line and is now a powerful tool in forensic pathology. The mtDNA sequence of the Duke of Edinburgh (a direct female-line-descendant of Queen Victoria) was used to identify the bones of the Tsar of Russia's family (also direct female-line-descendants of Queen Victoria).[14] The same mtDNA sequence was used to establish that Anna Anderson Manahan, who had claimed to be the Tsar's daughter, Anastasia, was, in fact, not related.[15] The estimated rate of mtDNA mutation and the diversity of mtDNA sequences have been used to identify human population subgroups and to estimate the time that all the races were descended from a common female ancestor, the mitochondrial Eve hypothesis.[8]

LEBER'S HEREDITARY OPTIC NEUROPATHY (LHON)

Leber's hereditary optic neuropathy (LHON; MIM #535000 with numerous other MIM numbers for established and proposed point mutations) is synonymous with Leber's optic atrophy, Leber's hereditary optic neuroretinopathy, Leber disease, and several permutations of these. LHON should not be confused with three other diseases described by Theodore Leber. Leber's congenital amaurosis (also called Leber disease; see Chapter 21) is a congenital form of retinal dystrophy. Leber's stellate neuroretinitis is a postviral disorder characterized by swelling of the disc and edema residues, giving a stellate maculopathy. Leber's miliary aneurysms are the abnormal retinal vessels, which may leak and result in the exudative retinal detachment of Coat's disease.

Although the first description of LHON is attributed to Beer (1817),[3] it was not until the development of the ophthalmoscope by Helmholtz in 1851[12] that the clinical assessment of optic atrophy was possible. Von Graefe[53] described families with LHON, but it was Leber (also in Berlin at the time), with his two works[27,28] who defined much of the disorder that now bears his name. Numerous other authors described cases and pedigrees, with the first major review by Bell,[4] where she gave details on over 600 patients. In retrospect, some of these patients were probably not LHON, but her work gives us similar data on age of onset sex ratio of those affected, and the clinical features, which still apply today. The inheritance of LHON was initially thought to be X linked, however, the possibility of cytoplasmic inheritance was raised as early as 1936.[22] Subsequent work showed that the mitochondria, which contain a small amount of DNA, were also cytoplasmically inherited. Although the full DNA sequence of the mitochondrial DNA was published in 1980,[1] it was a further 7 years before the most commonly found point mutation at position 11778 was associated with LHON.[54] LHON is an uncommon disorder, although most ophthalmologists will probably see a patient with LHON at some stage. In Australia it accounts for 2% of patients who are legally blind under the age of 65 years.[30] Most data are on populations of Northern European origin, where rates would appear to be similar. However, it is rarely described in other populations, with the exception of Japan.[32]

LHON is characterized by a subacute visual loss, affecting both eyes simultaneously or sequentially. The central vision is lost almost completely, while the peripheral field is spared to varying degrees, resulting in a dense centrocecal scotoma.[51] Patients may notice a small area of visual disturbance that may settle for a period of time, but usually there is a rapid progression of visual loss, with enlargement of the scotoma. The vision may be lost as dramatically as over 1 day, or it may take as much as several months to reach its nadir. The two eyes may be noted to lose vision together; however, many patients may not notice the onset of visual loss in the first eye. All references to the time interval between the two eyes must be interpreted with this in mind, especially as patients will often change the time interval when requestioned and very few patients have been regularly examined prior to the visual loss, allowing exact time intervals to be measured. The color vision is profoundly affected mainly in the red–green axis (Figs. 35.1 and 35.2). Dominant optic atrophy usually causes greater visual loss in the blue–yellow axis, however, when severely affected, color vision may not be useful in distinguishing between the two. The age of onset is usually in early adult life, although it may occur at any age. The youngest known patient to be affected is 4 years and the oldest 86. The median age of visual loss is around 23–26 years, while the 25%–75% range is 18–32 years.[30,36] There is a slightly older age of onset in women. The number of men affected compared to women is around 5 : 1, this varies slightly with different mutations causing LHON. The higher percentage of affected individuals in Japan being women, noted by Kawakami[25] and publicized by Bell,[4] may not be a real phenomenon and may have included cases of dominant optic atrophy. The rate of loss of vision in an eye varies considerably, deteriorating from normal to counting fingers in one day, to a gradual loss over months. The loss has been described as stepwise by some patients and gradual by others. The vast majority of patients only report one episode of visual loss. Once the vision has stabilized, further changes seem rare. Partial recovery of vision usually does not start until 6 months (sometimes years) later, if it occurs at all. This contrasts with optic neuritis or multiple sclerosis, in which visual recovery occurs within weeks after the initial loss.[42] The form of recovery may be in the fenestration of the scotoma, an uncommon event, usually associated with the 11778 mutation.[50] Recovery, which is sometimes dramatic, in the form of constriction of the scotoma, is frequently associated with the 14484 and 3460 mutation.[33]

The funduscopic appearance in the acute stage of LHON is diagnostic but may not easily be seen. Subtle disc elevation, which involves elevation of the disc and surrounding ganglion cells, peripapillary telangiectasia (Figs. 35.3 and 35.4*A*), and absence of leakage of fluorescein angiography.[49] There are patients who present without these features (possibly having them prior to the onset of visual loss). Within a few months the peripapillary telangiectasia disappear, resulting in nonspecific optic atrophy.[32] The late optic atrophy may be localized to temporal pallor (and thus be difficult to distinguish from dominant optic atrophy), but in most cases there is generalized atrophy resulting in a very pale disc (Fig. 35.4*B*). Associated abnormalities with LHON include abnormal electrocardiograph (EKG) findings. Initially described by Rose et al.,[48] and further

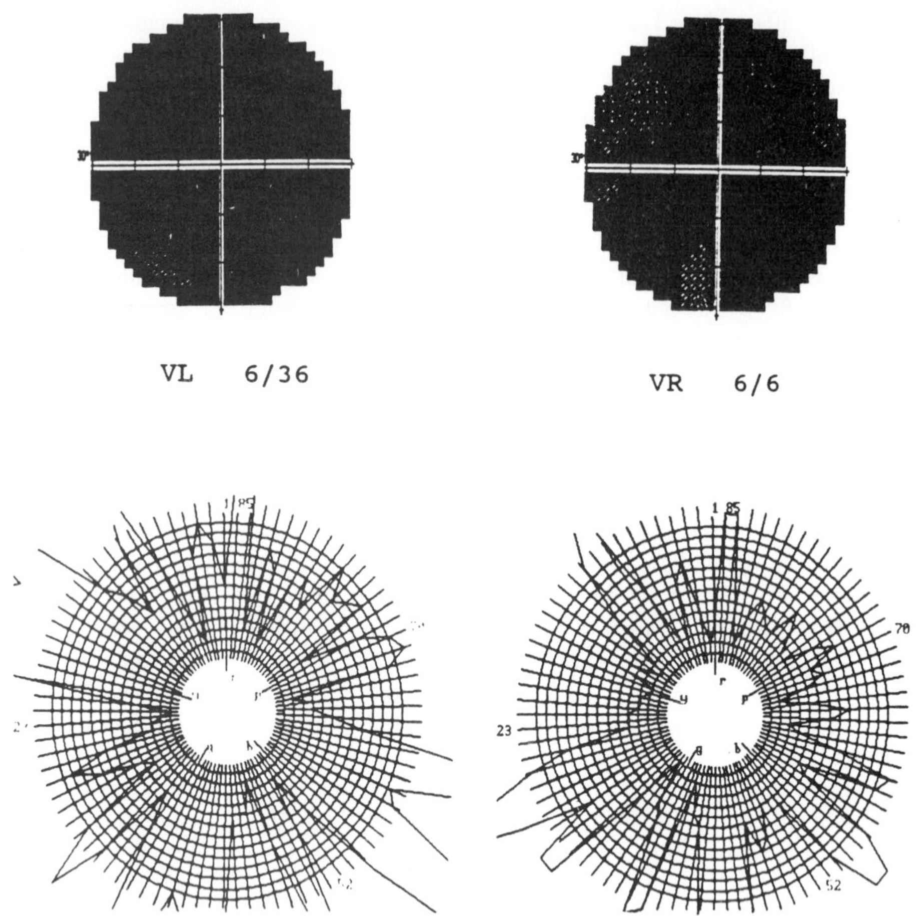

Figure 35.1. Left: Humphrey 30-2 visual fields of a 26-year-old patient with Leber's hereditary optic neuropathy with the 11778 mutation. Visual recovery (VR) in the right eye occurred 1 year after loss of vision. Left visual acuity is 6/36 and right is 6/6. The fenestration of the scotoma is too small to detect on the Humphrey or Goldmann field. **Right:** Farnsworth-Munsell 100 hue showing generalized poor color discrimination, which is slightly better in the right eye.

expanded by Nikoskelainen et al.,[38] there appears to be an increased association with EKG abnormalities such as a prolonged PR interval and Wolff–Parkinson–White (WPW) conduction abnormality. These seem to be concentrated in particular families. Interestingly, Bower et al.[6] reviewed the EKG abnormalities in the large Tasmanian 11778 and 14484 pedigrees and found no difference compared to controls. However, they found a sister of a visually affected 3460 patient, who died suddenly at the age of 20 years. Other neurological abnormalities have been described with LHON. These may be a real association or just be a normal overlap with other neurological findings. The Australian family "NSW1" with the 11778 mutation initially described as having Charcot-Marie-Tooth disease[35] actually appears to be the coincidental overlap of two disease pedigrees. Although LHON was often misdiagnosed as multiple sclerosis (MS) in women, recent work has identified an association between LHON and MS, the "LHON MS-like illness."[18] Again, it is not clear whether this is just the overlap of these two disorders or whether there is a common underlying etiol-

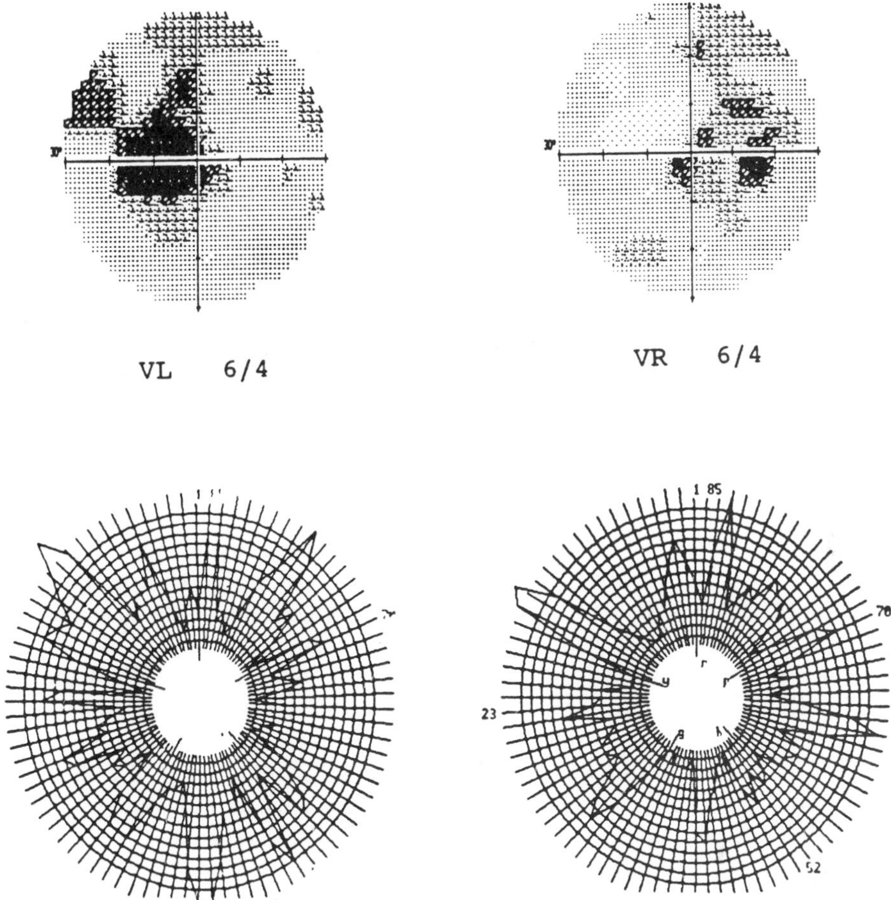

Figure 35.2. Left: Humphrey 30-2 visual fields of a 20-year-old woman with Leber's hereditary optic neuropathy with the 14484 mutation. She lost vision to less than 6/60 at the age of 12 years and noted recovery starting 6 months after the initial loss. Visual fields show the enlarged blind spot of the constricted scotoma. **Right:** Farnsworth-Munsell 100 hue showing generalized, poor color discrimination.

ogy. There are, however, rare specific families in which there are frequent associated neurological abnormalities. The Qld1 family 14484+4160 seems to be unique. There is a high penetrance of optic atrophy, dysarthria, peripheral sensory loss, spasticity, and the often fatal juvenile encephalopathy.[33] Families with dystonia have been described in the United States[39] and the Netherlands.[7] The Hispanic family from the United States has been found to carry a heteroplasmic mutation at position 14595.[23]

The genetics of LHON are fairly well documented for most of the large pedigrees.[33a] The 11778 mutation in ND4 has been found in almost all population groups and accounts for approximately 65% of LHON. The 14484 mutation in ND6 seems to have some geographic origins, being common in the Netherlands, England, and countries with their emigrants. Mutation 14484 accounts for around 25% of LHON. The 3460 mutation in ND1 occurs in somewhat smaller families and accounts for approximately 10% of LHON. The pathogenicity of other mutations remains to be proven,[20] in particular, the 15257 mutation, which seems to be common in controls and has not been found in multiple large LHON pedigrees like the

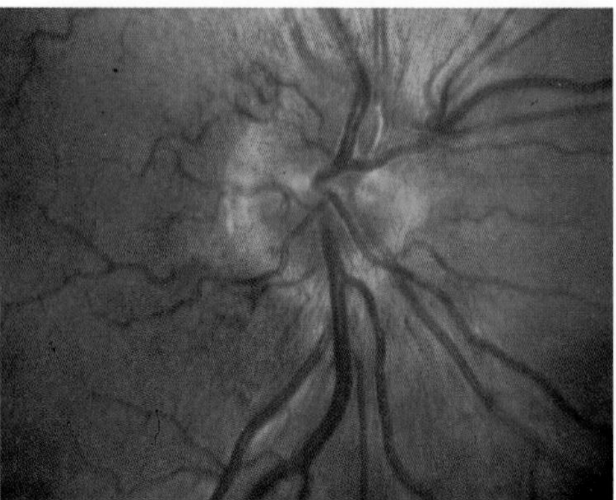

Figure 35.3. Fundus photograph of the acute stage of Leber's hereditary optic neuropathy in a patient with the 11778 mutation, showing subtle disc swelling and peripapillary telangiectasia.

other mutations. The other, so-called secondary, mutations are possibly related to the development of LHON, but this has never been proven. The most difficult thing to understand in LHON is why the vast majority of women and the majority of men carrying the mtDNA mutation never lose vision. Whether there are other factors involved is confusing. An initial study identifying a second X-linked factor,[52] was later refuted.[24] The proposal that a single second X-linked factor (MIM #308905) was involved (or even an autosomal second factor) was refuted by the finding of the low number of blind offspring in women who themselves were blinded by LHON.[31] The relationship of heteroplasmy to the development of LHON is not fully explained. Most pedigrees with heteroplasmy are small, where the mutation seems to have arisen a few generations before the index case. Many large multigeneration pedigrees seem to be homoplasmic for the mutation in every individual tested, affected or unaffected. The mtDNA status of the peripheral blood and other tissues may not reflect the status of the optic nerve. For reasons yet to be explained the risk of losing vision in large LHON pedigrees living in Australia has fallen over the last 150 years.[30] This lower risk contrasts with the United Kingdom, where the risk of losing vision is still high.

Management of LHON in the acute phase can be difficult. Often the diagnosis of LHON is not obvious, particularly if the relevant family history is not known or not disclosed. The most important aspect of the investigation is to exclude other treatable causes of visual loss. At least one neuroimaging test should be performed in most individuals to exclude a space-occupying lesion. The need for other investigations depends on how typical or atypical the patient's presentation was. There is probably no need for DNA testing an individual in a family where there has already been a mtDNA LHON mutation found. Nevertheless, in dis-

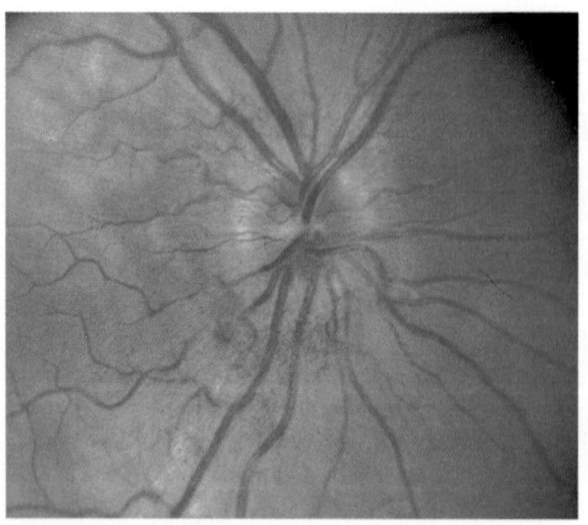

A

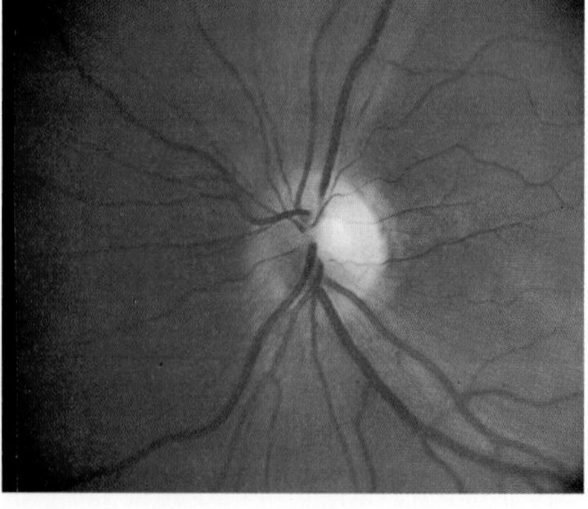

B

Figure 35.4. Sequential fundus photographs taken 4 months apart of a patient with Leber's hereditary optic neuropathy. **A:** Subtle disc swelling and peripapillary telangiectasia. **B:** Temporal pallor of the disc, loss of the maculopapular nerve fibers, and regression of the telangiectatic vessels.

tant relatives in unaffected branches of the family it is worthwhile testing concerned individuals as it may be possible that they do not carry the mutation. DNA testing of family members where there are multiple individuals affected almost always shows 100% mutant mtDNA. Even if relatives carry the mutation, most do not lose vision. The presence of one of the three undisputed mutations—3460, 11778, or 14484—combined with a normal neuroimaging scan makes the diagnosis of LHON almost certain.

There is no proven treatment for the acute phase of LHON. Numerous drugs such as steroids, hydroxycobalamin, coenzyme Q-10, and idebenone[34] have all been tried, but none show any dramatic effect. The most important aspect in management is assessing the psychosocial aspects of the patients. Preventing suicide and family breakdown are very important. LHON patient support groups are invaluable, but are not available in many places. In general, patients who have previously lost vision are usually quite well adjusted. Appropriate rehabilitation is essential. Most patients have profoundly affected central vision, which requires training in magnification, low-vision aids, and closed-circuit television. Eccentric fixation training is also of great value. As the peripheral vision in most LHON patients is retained, the need for guide dogs and canes is uncommon. Mobility training utilizing peripheral vision is helpful. Counseling is of particular importance in LHON, not only for the affected patient but also for the parents and other children at risk. Denial, anger, and despair are common problems. Affected individuals are usually devastated during the initial stages of the disease, but almost all seem to adjust fairly well to their disability. Some even appear to be relieved, because they no longer need to worry whether they might lose vision or not. Previously affected individuals are a good source of support for newly diagnosed patients. Unaffected family members often ask to have DNA testing to tell if they are at risk. In well-established LHON families this is of little practical value. Most will have 100% mutant mtDNA, and as we do not know the associated precipitating factors—environmental or genetic—we can just say they are at risk. The majority of men and the vast majority of women who are homoplasmic (100% mutant) in their peripheral blood never lose vision. In smaller families, usually where there is only one affected member, it is of value to test the relatives. In particular this should be done if anyone exhibits heteroplasmy, as this suggests that the mutations has only arisen recently and may be at low levels in some members. It is not possible to give accurate figures on whether there is a threshold level or a proportional reduction in risk, but it would appear that heteroplasmic individuals are at lower risk of losing vision. Heteroplasmic levels can fluctuate widely from generation to generation in some families, so it is difficult to give the level of risk for their proposed offspring, as the child may well have high levels of mutant DNA. Age-adjusted risk counseling is possible for homoplasmic 100% mutant individuals. This ideally would use the overall risk for their family or the overall risk in their population. In Europe, the risk of visual loss appears to be 40% for males and 10% for females, while in Australia (and probably the United States) the risk is lower, being 20% for males and 4% for females. The median age of visual loss is 24–26 years, with standard deviations around 11–13 years. Thus we can estimate the age-adjusted risk as shown in Table 35.2.

Table 35.2. Risk of Visual Loss from LHON with Age (%) Depending on Overall Risk for Family and Gender

	Remaining Lifetime Risk at Age				
Birth	14 yr	26 yr	37 yr	50 yr	61 yr
50	42	25	8	1	0.07 (e.g., European male)
20	17	10	3	0.4	0.02 (e.g., Australian male)
4	3.3	2	0.7	0.1	0.01 (e.g., Australian female)

NEUROPATHY, ATAXIA, AND RETINITIS PIGMENTOSA (NARP)

Neuropathy, ataxia, and retinitis pigmentosa (NARP; MIM #551500) is a mitochondrial disorder with retinal abnormalities ranging from a mild salt-and-pepper retinopathy to more severe retinitis pigmentosa.[43] Migraine headache, seizures, proximal neurogenic muscle weakness, sensory neuropathy, and developmental delay may all be seen.[19] Mutation of the ATPase 6 gene at position 8993 has been identified in multiple pedigrees.

MITOCHONDRIAL ENCEPHALOPATHY, LACTIC ACIDOSIS, AND STROKELIKE EPISODES (MELAS)

Mitochondrial myopathy, lactic acidosis, and strokelike episodes (MELAS; MIM #590050) presents with episodes of vomiting, headache, seizures, and recurrent strokelike episodes, which may result in hemiparesis, hemianopsia, or cortical blindness.[44] Eighty percent of patients are aged 5 to 15 years.[17] A mtDNA point mutation has been identified in the transfer RNA for mitochondrial leucine, tRNA(leu) (UUR), gene at position 3243.[16]

KEARNS-SAYRE SYNDROME (KSS)/ CHRONIC PROGRESSIVE EXTERNAL OPHTHALMOPLEGIA (CPEO)

Kearns-Sayre syndrome (KSS; MIM #530000) is a mitochondrial cytopathy that is part of a spectrum from mild chronic progressive external ophthalmoplegia (CPEO) through the CPEO plus disorders to KSS.[11] KSS is characterized by the presence of ophthalmoplegia, pigmentary degeneration of the retina, and cardiomyopathy.[26] Lesser features include pharyngeal and facial weakness, skeletal muscle weakness, deafness, small stature and electroencephalographic changes, and markedly raised cerebrospinal fluid protein. Electrocardiographic abnormalities include complete heart block,[48] thus EKGs must be performed on all patients suspected of having KSS. Computed tomography may reveal diffuse leukencephalopathy[5] or cerebellar and brain stem atrophy with calcification of the basal ganglia.[47] Biochemical studies show abnormal pyruvate and lactate metabolism. Biopsy of skeletal muscle shows aggregates of abnormal mitochondria or "ragged red fibers."[2] KSS usually occurs as an isolated case, although occasionally siblings are affected.[21] Egger and Wilson[13] felt that in most pedigrees, KSS was transmitted by the mother and this was consistent with mitochondrial inheritance. Lestienne and Ponsot[29] described a 5 kb deletion in the mtDNA of muscle mitochondria, but not in the mtDNA of lymphocytes or fibroblasts. Holt et al.[19] found 9 of 25 patients that they studied harbored a heteroplasmic mtDNA deletion. Poulton et al.[45] described a patient with KSS and an asymptomatic mother and maternal aunt, all of whom carried the same mtDNA deletion, supporting the possibility for maternal transmission. It is, however, likely that the most severely affected ova are nonviable; thus extensive pedigrees of KSS are not seen. The deletion may be preceded by a mtDNA duplication.[46] The exact site and size of the deletion varies from patient to patient, as well as the proportion of normal and abnormal mitochondria in the cells. This explains the variable clinical presentation. Identical deletions are reported with KSS, CPEO, and Pearson syndrome. In KSS, mutant mitochondria are localized to muscle and central nervous system, whereas in CPEO they are localized to muscle and in Pearson syndrome they are localized to blood. Pearson syndrome may evolve to KSS. Treatment of KSS with coenzyme Q(10) has been promising in some cases.[40,41] Improvement in the first-degree atrioventricular block, improved eye movements, and lessened fatigue are seen with doses of 50 mg three times daily for 3 months.

FRIEDREICH'S ATAXIA

For a comprehensive discussion of Friedreich's ataxia, see Chapter 26.

REFERENCES

1. Anderson S, Bankier AT, Barrell BG et al. Sequence and organization of the human mitochondrial genome. *Nature* 1981;290:457–465.
2. Bastiaenser LAK, Joosten EMG, De Rooij et al. Ophthalmoplegia plus, a real nosological entity. *Acta Neurol Scand* 1978;58:9–34.
3. Beer GJ. Lehre von den Augenkrankheiten 1817;2.
4. Bell J. Hereditary optic atrophy (Leber's disease). In *The Treasury of Human Inheritance,* K. Pearson, ed. Cambridge, England: Cambridge University Press, 1931:325–423.
5. Bertorini T, Engel WK, Di Chiro G, Dalakas M. Leukancephalopathy in oculocraniosomatic neuromuscular disease with ragged red fibres: Mitochondrial abnormalities detected by computerised tomography. *Arch Neurol* 1978;35: 643–647.
6. Bower SPC, Hawley I, Mackey DA. Cardiac arrhythmia and Leber's hereditary optic neuropathy. *Lancet* 1992;339:1427–1428.
7. Bruyn GW, Went LN. A sex-linked heredodegenerative neurological disorder, associated with Leber's optic atrophy. Part 1: clinical studies. *J Neurol Sci* 1964;1:59–80.
8. Cann RL, Stoneking M, Wilson AC. Mitochondrial DNA and human evolution. *Nature* 1987; 325:31–36.
9. Corral-Debrinski M, Stepian G, Shoffner JM, Lott MT, Kanter K, Wallace DC. Hypoxemia is associated with mitochondrial DNA damage and gene induction, implications for cardiac disease. *JAMA* 1992;226:1812–1816.
10. De Vivo DC. The expanding clinical spectrum of mitochondrial diseases. *Brain Dev* 1993;15: 1–22.
11. Drachman DA. Ophthalmoplegia plus. The neurodegenerative disorders associated with progressive external ophthalmoplegia. *Arch Neurol* 1968;18:654–674.
12. Duke-Elder SS. Ophthalmoscopy. In *System of Ophthalmology,* S. S. Duke-Elder, ed. St. Louis: C.V. Mosby, 1962:290.
13. Egger J, Wilson I. Mitochondrial inheritance in a mitochondrially mediated disease. *N Engl J Med* 1983;309:142–146.
14. Gill P, Ivanov PL, Kimpton C et al. Identification of the remains of the Romanov family by DNA analysis. *Nature Genet* 1994;6: 130–135.
15. Gill P, Kimpton C, Aliston-Greiner R et al. Establishing the identity of Anna Anderson Manahan. *Nature Genet* 1995;9:9–10.
16. Goto Y, Nonaka I, Horai S. A mutation in the tRNA(Leu)(UUR) gene associated with the MELAS subgroup of mitochondrial encephalomyopathies. *Nature* 1990;348:651–653.
17. Goto Y, Yonada I, Horai S. A new mtDNA mutation associated with mitochondrial myopathy, encephalopathy, lactic acidosis and stroke-like episodes (MELAS). *Biochem Biophys Acta* 1991;1097:238–240.
18. Harding AE, Sweeney MG, Miller DH et al. Occurrence of a multiple sclerosis-like illness in women who have a Leber's hereditary optic neuropathy mitochondrial DNA mutation. *Brain* 1992;115:979–989.
19. Holt IJ, Harding AE, Petty RK, Morgan Hughes JA. A new mitochondrial disease associated with mitochondrial DNA heteroplasmy. *Am J Hum Genetics* 1990;46:428–433.
20. Howell N. Mitochondrial gene mutations and human diseases: A prolegomenon (editorial). *Am J Hum Genet* 1994;55:219–224.
21. Hurwitz LJ, Carson NAJ, Allen IV, Chopra JS. Congenital ophthalmoplegia, floppy baby syndrome, myopathy and aminoaciduria: Report of a family. *J Neurol Neurosurg Psychiatry* 1969;32:495–508.
22. Imai Y, Moriwaki D. A probable case of cytoplasmic inheritance in man: A critique of Leber's Disease. *J Genet* 1936;33:163–167.
23. Jun AS, Brown MD, Wallace DC. A mitochondrial DNA mutation at nucleotide pair 14459 of the NADH dehydrogenase subunit 6 gene associated with maternally inherited Leber hereditary optic neuropathy and dystonia. *Proc Natl Acad Sci USA* 1994;91:6206–6210.
24. Juvonen V, Vilkki J, Aula P, Nikoskelainen E, Savontaus ML. Reevaluation of the linkage of an optic atrophy susceptibility gene to X-chromosomal markers in Finnish families with Leber hereditary optic neuropathy (LHON). *Am J Hum Genet* 1993;53:289–292.
25. Kawakami R. Beiträge zur Vererbung der familiären Sehnervenatrophie. *Grafe's Arch Ophthalmol* 1926;66:568–595.
26. Kearns TP. External ophthalmoplagia, pigmentary degeneration of the retina and cardiomyopathy: Newly recognised syndrome. *Trans Ophthalmol Soc UK* 1965;63:559–625.
27. Leber T. Ueber hereditare und congenital-angelegte Sehnervenleiden. *Graefe's Arch Ophthalmol* 1871;2:249–291.
28. Leber T. Die Neuritis optica in Folge von Hereditat und congenitaler Anlage. *Graefe-Saemisch Handbuch* 1877;5:824.

29. Lestienne P, Ponsot G. Kearns-Sayre syndrome with muscle mitochondrial DNA deletion. *Lancet* 1988;8590(1):885.
30. Mackey DA, Buttery RG. Leber hereditary optic neuropathy in Australia. *Aust N Z J Ophthalmol* 1992;20:177–184.
31. Mackey DA. Blindness in offspring of women blinded by Leber hereditary optic neuropathy. *Lancet* 1993;341:1020–1021.
32. Mackey DA. Leber's hereditary optic neuropathy, is it a disease of Northern Europe and Asia? (editorial) *Ophthalmic Paediatr Genet* 1993;14:105–107.
33. Mackey DA. Three subgroups of patients with Leber hereditary optic neuropathy from the UK. *Eye* 1994;8:431–436.
33a. Mackey DA, Oostra R-J, Rosenberg T, Nikoskelainen E, Bronte-Stewart J, Poulton J, Harding AE, Govan G, Bolhuis PA, Norby S, Bleeker-Wagemakers EM, Savontaus M-L, Chan C, Howell N. MtDNA mutations in pedigrees of Leber's hereditary optic neuropathy: The 15257 mutation does not have a primary pathogenic role. *Am J Hum Genet* 1996;59: 481–485.
34. Mashima Y, Hiida Y, Oguchi Y. Remission of Leber's hereditary optic neuropathy with idebenone. *Lancet* 1992;340:368–369.
35. McLeod JG, Low PA, Morgan Hughes JA. Charcot-Marie-Tooth disease with Leber optic atrophy. *Neurology* 1978;28:179–184.
36. Newman NJ, Lott MT, Wallace DC. The clinical characteristics of pedigrees of Leber's hereditary optic neuropathy with the 11778 mutation. *Am J Ophthalmol* 1991;111:750–762.
37. Nikoskelainen E, Hoyt WF, Nummelin KU. Ophthalmoscopic findings in Leber's hereditary optic neuropathy. II. The fundus findings in the affected family members. *Arch Ophthalmol* 1983;101:1059–1068.
38. Nikoskelainen E, Wanne O, Dahl M. Pre-excitation syndrome and Leber's hereditary optic neuroretinopathy letter. *Lancet* 1985;1:696.
39. Novotny EJ Jr, Singh G, Wallace DC et al. Leber's disease and dystonia: A mitochondrial disease. *Neurology* 1986;36:1053–1060.
40. Ogasahara S, Engel AG, Frens D, Mack D. Muscle co-enzyme Q deficiency in familial mitochondrial encephalomyopathy. *Proc Natl Acad Sci USA* 1989;86:2379–2382.
41. Ogasahara S, Yorifuji S, Nishikawa Y et al. Improvement of abnormal pyruvate metabolism and cardiac conduction with co-enzyme Q(10) in Kearns-Sayre syndrome. *Neurology* 1985; 35:372–377.
42. Optic Neuritis Study Group. The clinical profile of optic neuritis: Experience of the optic neuritis treatment trial. *Arch Ophthalmol* 1991;109:1673–1678.
43. Ortiz RG, Newman NJ, Shoffner JM, Kaufman AE, Koontz DA, Wallace DC. Variable retinal and neurologic manifestations in patients harboring the mitochondrial DNA 8993 mutation. *Arch Ophthalmol* 1993;111:1525–1530.
44. Pavlakis SG, Phillips PC, DiMauro S et al. Mitochondrial myopathy, encephalopathy, lactic acidosis, and stroke like episodes: A distinctive clinical syndrome. *Ann Neurol* 1984;16: 481–488.
45. Poulton J, Deadman ME, Ramacharan S, Gardiner RM. Germ-line deletions of mtDNA in mitochondrial myopathy. *Am J Hum Genet* 1991;48:649–653.
46. Poulton J, Morten KJ, Weber K et al. Are duplications of mitochondrial DNA characteristic of Kearns-Sayre syndrome? *Hum Mol Genet* 1994;3:947–951.
47. Robertson WC Jr, Viseskul C, Lee YE, Lloyd RV. Basal ganglia calcification in Kearns-Sayre syndrome. *Arch Neurol* 1979;361:711–713.
48. Rose FC, Bowden AN, Bowden PMA. The heart in Leber's optic atrophy. *Br J Ophthalmol* 1970;54:388–393.
49. Smith JL, Hoyt WF, Susac JO. Ocular fundus in acute Leber optic neuropathy. *Arch Ophthalmol* 1973;90:349–354.
50. Stone EM, Newman NJ, Miller NR, Johns DR, Lott MT, Wallace DC. Visual recovery in patients with Leber's hereditary optic neuropathy and the 11778 mutation. *J Clin Neuro-ophthalmol* 1992;12:10–14.
51. Van Senus AHC. Leber's disease in the Netherlands. *Doc Ophthalmol* 1963;17:1–162.
52. Vilkki J, Ott J, Savontaus ML, Aula P, Nikoskelainen E. Optic atrophy in Leber hereditary optic neuroretinopathy is probably determined by an X-chromosomal gene closely linked to DXS7. *Am J Hum Genet* 1991; 48:486–491.
53. Von Graefe A. Ein ungewohnlicher Fall von hereditarer Amaurose. *Graefe's Arch Ophthalmol* 1858;4(2):266–268.
54. Wallace DC, Singh G, Lott MT et al. Mitochondrial DNA mutation associated with Leber's hereditary optic neuropathy. *Science* 1988;242:1427–1430.
55. Wallace DC. Mitochondrial genetics: A paradigm for aging and degenerative diseases? *Science* 1992;256:628–632.

36

The Phakomatoses

NICOLA K. RAGGE
ELIAS I. TRABOULSI

In 1923 J. Van der Hoeve introduced the term *phakomatosis* (from the Greek *phakos,* meaning *birthmark*) to include a group of hereditary disorders united by distinctive dermatologic manifestations and including tuberous sclerosis and neurofibromatosis (NF).[357] In his Doyne Memorial Lecture he states:

> So you see that it is not an idle whim of mine to talk and write so often about these phakomatoses, but that the study of them can be of great advantage for our patients and of great value for our knowledge.[358]

The phakomatoses came to include other diseases, such as von Hippel-Lindau disease, Sturge-Weber syndrome, ataxia-telangiectasia (Louis-Bar syndrome), and Wyburn-Mason syndrome. Overlapping clinical features, such as pheochromocytoma in neurofibromatosis type 1 and von Hippel-Lindau disease persuaded the medical world initially to unite these diseases. Other articles presented families with coincidental occurrence of more than one phakomatosis (e.g., tuberous sclerosis with Sturge-Weber or von Hippel-Lindau with NF1), suggesting that these diseases were possibly derived from a single gene.[106,347] However, modern molecular genetics has correctly redivided them into distinct genetic disorders.

THE NEUROFIBROMATOSES

The neurofibromatoses are a group of at least two genetically distinct diseases that have in common multiple tumor types, including neurofibromas, central nervous system tumors, and dermatological features. Developmental abnormalities such as hamartomas also occur, illustrating a need to define the role of the *normal* NF genes in development. Genetic mapping has confirmed the separation of neurofibromatosis type 1 (NF1) from 2 (NF2) in the last decade. The gene products for NF1 (neurofibromin) and NF2 (merlin or schwannomin) have been isolated and characterized in the last 5 to 7 years.

Neurofibromatosis Type 1

Introduction and History

Neurofibromatosis type 1 (NF1) or von Recklinghausen neurofibromatosis is an autosomal dominant condition characterized by the development of multiple specific types of tumors in affected individuals. It is one of the most common inherited diseases in humans and has an incidence of 1 in 2000 to 1 in 4000.[66,100,154,156,286] Although the gene is almost 100% penetrant, the disease has extremely variable expressivity.[44,287] The principal external features of NF1 are café-au-lait (CAL) patches, freckling, multiple cutaneous and subcutaneous neurofibromas, and iris hamartomas. The main complications are caused by the development of central nervous system tumors, including gliomas, ependymomas, and neurofibromas.

The first convincing descriptions of NF1 were in the eighteenth century by Akenside[4] and Tilesius von Tilenau.[348] Akenside describes a man with a "constant succession of wens that shot out in several places; on his head, trunk, arms, and legs: which indisposition he inherited from his father." The man shaved the lesions off with a razor! The description that follows is very convincing for NF1, and this appears to be the first mention of an inherited case.[4] Tilesius von Tilenau describes a man he had seen in Professor Ludwig's class in a manuscript titled "Case History of Extraordinarily Unsightly Skin." The man, referred to as the "Wart Man" by Professor Ludwig, had multiple cutaneous fibrous growths, pigmented patches, an enlarged head, elevation of one shoulder, and pruritus.[242,348]

Other possible early portrayals of NF1 are a Hellenistic statue,[281] a beautiful illustrative plate by de Bakker in Buffon's *Histoire Naturelle*,[141,185] and cited works including "Monstrorum Historia" by Aldrovandi, a sixteenth-century naturalist, physician, and philosopher[5,141,214,388]; Conrad von Megenberg's "Buch der Natur,"[388] a thirteenth-century Austrian medieval monastic manuscript[215]; and the Tiberius B V manuscript on "Marvels of the East," dating around the fourth century C.E.[388]

Von Recklinghausen produced a classic monograph on NF1 in 1882 and deservedly had the disease named after him (Fig. 36.1).[365] He gave one of the finest descriptions of this disease and is credited as the first person to recognize a neural origin of the tumors, a fact that was disputed at the time.[50] However, an earlier treatise in 1849 by Smith from Dublin,[329] which shows beautiful illustrations of the gross appearance of the disease and of dissected neurofibromas clearly originating from nerves, receives little of the credit that it deserves. Other notable works around this time included those by Virchow[146,359] and Hitchcock.[144]

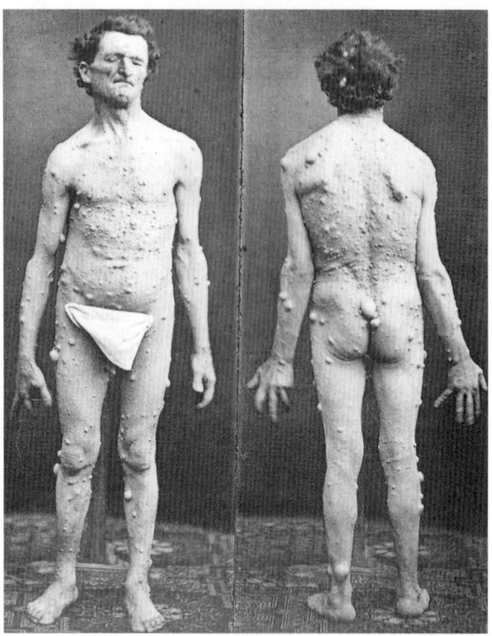

Figure 36.1. Original illustration from Von Recklinghausen's treatise on neurofibromatosis 1.[365]

Following von Recklinghausen's description of neurofibromatosis, an overwhelming number of case reports has appeared in the literature. However, it was not until the advent of several large surveys that the prevalence and full spectrum of complications began to emerge.[31,39,44,66,157,288,305]

Non-Ocular Clinical Features

Neurofibromatosis type 1 is defined clinically by major features—peripheral neurofibromas, multiple CAL patches with or without axillary freckling, and iris hamartomas (Sakurai-Lisch nodules)—and minor features—macrocephaly and short stature. Particular clinical features are critical for establishing the diagnosis of NF1 in any individual, whereas a multitude of other features are commonly and variably present. According to the National Institutes of Health (NIH) criteria, the disease is defined by an individual having two or more of the following: six or more CALs, measuring at least 1.5 cm in diameter in adults[66] or 0.5 cm in diameter in children; multiple neurofibromas of any type

Table 36.1. Complications of Neurofibromatosis Type 1

Nervous System	***Genitourinary Tract***
Plexiform neurofibromas	Neurofibromas
Spinal neurofibromas	Pelvic rhabdomyosarcoma
Gliomas	***Eye***
Optic pathway gliomas	Iris hamartoma (Sakurai-Lisch nodules)
Other orbit tumors	Prominent corneal nerves
Neurofibrosarcoma	Glaucoma
Aqueductal stenosis	***Endocrine System***
Cerebrovascular abnormalities	Pheochromocytoma
Intellectual handicap	Duodenal carcinoid
Seizures	Premature or delayed puberty
Coordination problem	***Cardiovascular System***
Electroencephalogram abnormality	Renal artery stenosis
Skeleton	Cerebrovascular disease
Scoliosis	Angiomas
Pseudarthrosis of distal long bone	***Respiratory System***
Lateral thoracic meningocoele	Neurofibromas of oral cavity, larynx, mediastinum
Lambdoidal suture defects	***Gastrointestinal System***
Sphenoid wing dysplasia	Visceral neurofibromas
Pectus excavatum	Colon ganglioneuromatosis
Genu valgum/varum	Abdominal pain
Skin	***Hematopoietic System***
Café-au-lait patches	Atypical forms of childhood leukemia[312]
Hyperpigmentation overlying plexiform neurofibromas	Increased risk of acute lymphoblastic leukemia and Hodgkins lymphoma[339]
Other hyperpigmentation	
Hypopigmentation	
Axillary or inguinal freckling	
Other freckling	
Neurofibromas, cutaneous or subcutaneous	
Juvenile xanthogranuloma	

Table adapted from VM Riccardi[288] and S Huson.[154]

or one plexiform neurofibroma; axillary or inguinal freckling: two or more iris hamartomas (Sakurai-Lisch nodules); optic glioma; distinctive osseous lesions, such as sphenoid dysplasia or twinning of long-bone cortex, with or without pseudoartharoses, and a first-degree relative with NF1.[243]

Every system in the body appears to be affected by complications arising from NF1 (Table 36.1). No figures are available for life expectancy because of variability of the disease and ascertainment bias.[288] Patients are, however, at higher risk for malignancies and NF1-related complications.[157,331]

Skin Hyperpigmentation. The skin hyperpigmentation in NF1 occurs in several forms, notably CALs, freckling, and diffuse hyperpigmentation.

Café-au-lait Patches. Crowe and Schull in 1953 stated that any person with more than six CALs greater than 1.5 cm must be presumed to have neurofibromatosis until proved otherwise, as none of their normal controls had this many CALs.[65] Their paper is the basis for inclusion of CALs in the NIH criteria today. In children, the equivalent diameter of the CALs is 0.5 cm.[376]

Multiple CALs are present in over 99% of individuals with NF1, and can range in size from a few millimetres to over 50 cm in diameter.[288] They tend to be present at birth or develop within the first year of life and are usually the presenting feature of the disease.[156] Larger areas of hyperpigmentation may be either a typical flat CAL or may outline an underlying plexiform neurofibroma. When the hyperpigmentation overlying a plexiform neurofibroma extends to the midline, it may signify underlying spinal cord involvement. In a large proportion of white adults with NF1, biopsies of CALs demonstrate a high density of cellular giant pigment markers called melanin macroglobules (or macromelanosomes) and an increased number of dihydroxyphenylalanine (DOPA)-positive melanocytes.[224,288]

Freckling. Freckling is present in 70%–80% of individuals with NF1 by adulthood.[156] Axillary freckling occurs only in the presence of other hyperpigmentation, such as CALs or diffuse duskiness, and can also be seen in dark-skinned ethnic groups.[64]

Neurofibromas. There are four types of neurofibromas.[288] The classical skin neurofibromas of NF1 are cutaneous and may be few or multiple in number. These discrete, soft, fleshy tumors develop toward the end of the first decade, in early puberty, during pregnancy, or after trauma to the skin when they may be preceded by itching. They are initially sessile but later often become pedunculated. The three other types of neurofibromas are subcutaneous neurofibromas, nodular plexiform neurofibromas, which involves major nerve plexuses, and the diffuse plexiform neurofibromas that encompass all the other types and insinuate into the tissue planes.

Malignant transformation can occur in all types of neurofibromas but is much more common in those with a deeper somatic location. The overall risk of neurofibrosarcoma to the NF1 patient is about 5%.[288,290] The cardinal signs of malignant transformation are pain, increasing tumor size, and focal neurological deficit.[287]

Neurologic Complications. Mild mental retardation and/or learning difficulties appear to affect about 30%–45% of individuals with NF1, independent of the severity of disease, although these symptoms may correlate with the number of brain lesions on magnetic resonance imaging.[86,148,306] Ventriculomegaly or hydrocephalus are pesent in about 2%–5% of NF1 patients and are secondary to gliomas, aqueductal stenosis, irradiation, cerebral atrophy, Chiari type 1 malformations, and partial absence of the corpus callosum.[288]

Other clinical features of NF1 include seizures, headaches, abdominal pain (intestinal neurofibromas, idiopathic), skin itching, early or delayed puberty, hypertension (due to pheochromocytoma or renal artery abnormalities),[288] vasculopathy,[202] and possibly reduced platelet function.[283] Some patients with NF1 have a phenotype overlapping with the Noonan syndrome.[288] Also, Watson syndrome, a disease characterized by CAL patches, mental retardation, and pulmonary stenosis, is thought to be allelic to NF1.[7,196]

Another distinctive feature of NF1 is the occurrence of bright foci in the brain parenchyma on T2-weighted MRI scans. These "bright spots" are much more prevalent in children. Typically located in the basal ganglia and internal capsule, they are also seen in the midbrain, pons, cerebellar peduncles and subcortical white matter.[79,164] They may correspond to areas of dysplastic glial proliferation and aberrant myelination. One group has correlated the bright spots pathologically with fluid-filled vacuoles.[80] The possible association of bright spots with intellectual impairment is controversial.[98,257]

Ophthalmic Features

Iris hamartomas (Sakurai-Lisch nodules) are one of the cardinal features of NF1 and are present in the majority of adults with NF1. Other anterior segment manifestations of NF1 include prominent corneal conjunctival and ciliary nerves,[155] congenital ectropion uveae,[43]

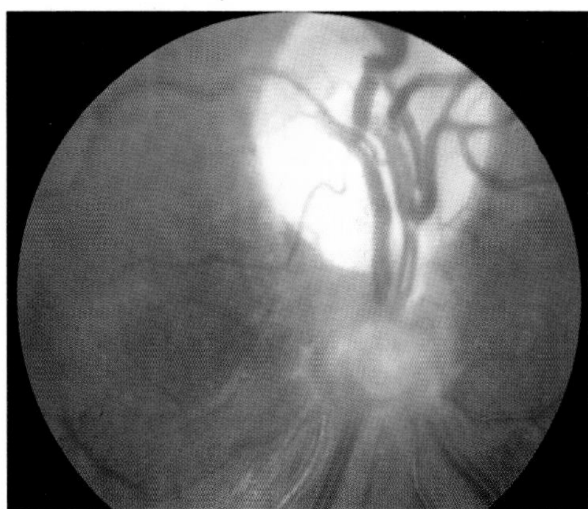

Figure 36.2. Retinal hamartoma in a patient with neurofibromatosis 1.

angle anomalies, posterior embryotoxon, buphthalmos or later onset glaucoma, especially in association with an ipsilateral plexiform neurofibroma of the eyelid,[41,308] heterochromia iridis, iris mammillations,[155,278] neurofibromas of conjunctival and ciliary nerves,[41,59] and anterior subcapsular cataract.[41]

Posterior segment manifestations include hamartomas of the optic disc, retina, and choroid (Fig. 36.2), retinal hemangioma, congenital hypertrophy of the retinal pigment epithelium, myelinated nerve fibers, sectoral retinitis pigmentosa, and cone–rod dystrophy.[41,78,155,189,333] Multiple choroidal hamartomas, which appear as multiple, small pigmented, circumscribed lesions, together with hypopigmented areas probably corresponding to pigment epithelial defects, have been described.[309,381] The histology reveals a diffusely thickened choroid with many ganglion cells, nerve fibers, and ovoid bodies consisting of hyperplastic Schwann cells.[43,186,381] Choroidal nevi and melanoma have been described in increased numbers in NF1, although these may be coincidental findings.[17,61,115,189,256] Combined pigment epithelial and retinal hamartomas, which are sometimes associated with retinal tear and detachment, have been described mainly in association with NF2. However, patients in at least two cases may have had NF1.[117,264]

Gliomas of the Optic Pathway. Gliomas of the optic pathway can occur as isolated findings or in association with NF1. Michel reported the first case of subclinical glial hyperplasia of the chiasm and optic nerve in a boy with NF1.[237] The occurrence of gliomas of the anterior visual pathway in NF1 has been well established.[153,161,204,288] Although the quoted frequency of this complication varies from 10%–70% depending on the study, a retrospective analysis of reported cases[222] and three recent prospective studies have shown the frequency to be about 15%–19%.[145,204,209] However, only 5% of NF1 patients appear to be symptomatic from their gliomas, regardless of location in the optic nerve or chiasm.[204] Neither absence of optic atrophy nor normality of size of optic foramen reliably excludes the presence of optic nerve gliomas.[204] Although flash visual evoked potentials are not a useful screening test for young children with optic gliomas, pattern visual evoked potentials may be more helpful.[297]

Bilateral optic nerve gliomas or 'multicentric' gliomas make up between 30% and 80% of the lesions, depending on whether or not minor optic nerve thickening is included.[204] The recent use of MR scanning demonstrates a higher incidence of subclinical lesions not detected on computed tomography (CT) scan, especially in the optic nerves. Some short-term follow-up studies have recently been published,[136,184] but only long-term studies will demonstrate the significance of these lesions and their relationship to the full spectrum of optic nerve gliomas (OPG). A recent study of children with NF1 suggests that out of 176 who underwent cranial magnetic resonance imaging (MRI), 33 (19%) had optic pathway gliomas of whom 21 (64%) had normal ophthalmic examinations.[209] Although these authors concluded that screening by imaging had a limited use, they had detected 25 cases with OPG who were asymptomatic, 6 of these with undetected decreased visual acuity. Overall, only 3 patients' tumors progressed in their relatively short follow-up period (maximum 8.1 years, median 2.4 and 3.4 years for MRI and eye examinations, respectively). There were no specific features (e.g., site, size, and so on) that could predict which tumor would progress in these cases. OPGs involving the chiasm are often complicated by precocious puberty.[136]

Optic pathway gliomas can display features

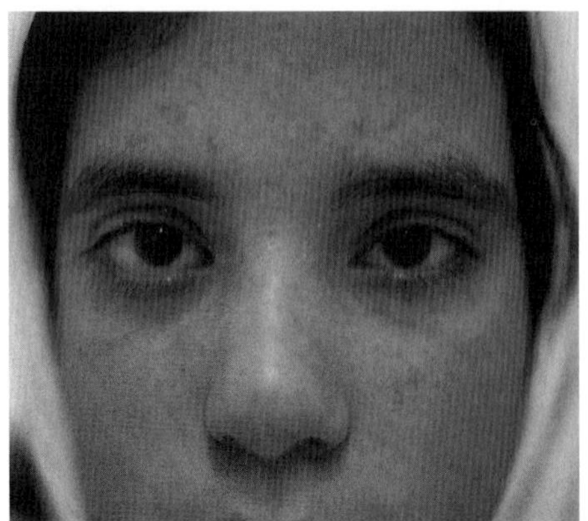

Figure 36.3. Eight-year-old girl with neurofibromatosis 1, unilateral proptosis and visual acuity of 20/70.

that are deemed to be diagnostic or highly suggestive of NF1. Bilateral OPGs are felt to be pathognomonic of NF1.[153,161] Tubular expansion of one or both optic nerves, often with lengthening and kinking and extension to include the chiasm and even optic tracts, are highly characteristic of NF1 gliomas. Computed tomography (Figs. 36.3 and 36.4), and now MRI scans demonstrate another hallmark of NF1 optic gliomas—the double-density tubular thickening of fusiform tumors of the optic nerve. On T2-weighted MRIs, a zone of high intensity surrounds a central low-density core, representing the optic nerve.[153,161] The high-

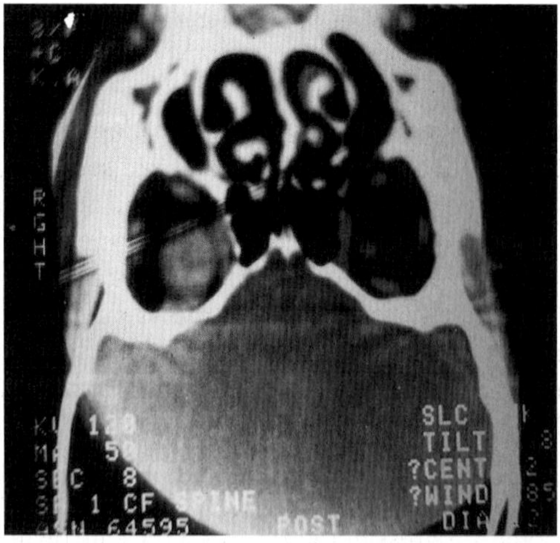

Figure 36.4. Coronal computed tomography scan of the orbits of patient shown in Figure 36.3 shows cross section of optic nerve glioma.

intensity area appears to correspond to the pathological finding of perineural arachnoidal gliomatosis.[153,161,314,337] This perineural pattern of arachnoidal proliferation is a characteristic feature of NF1 optic gliomas,[337] as compared with intraneural astrocytic proliferation seen more in isolated orbital optic gliomas.

There is a controversy as to whether gliomas of the optic pathways represent truly invasive astrocytomas or whether they are hamartomas.[152] Invasiveness and prognosis are related to position of the tumor and histological grade. In general, anterior gliomas, that is those located in the optic nerves alone, tend to have a more benign histology and are less invasive.[337] This type tends to predominate in NF1. An abundance of confounding factors prevent easy segregation between optic gliomas in NF1 and non-NF1 patients.[263] Many authors, however, claim that OPGs in NF1 patients are relatively benign, with the exception of large hypothalamic tumors, and that patients are more likely to succumb to second tumors.[153,160,301]

Iris Hamartomas. Although iris hamartomas have been described since the early part of the twentieth century,[56,58,102,107,330,367] the classic descriptions were made by Sakurai and Lisch[208,280,304] and as a result they have come to be known eponymously as Sakurai-Lisch nodules.[108,111,127,187,358] Lewis and Riccardi described the high prevalence of these nodules in NF1 and focused medical attention on their diagnostic importance.[205]

Iris hamartomas vary widely in appearance, depending on the background color of the iris.[280] In blue and green irides, they appear as pale-to-medium brown, somewhat fluffy elevations, and in dark brown irides they are cream-colored, dome-shaped, and well-defined (Fig. 36.5). They vary in size and number from a single lesion on one iris alone, barely visible by slit-lamp examination, to numerous or large nodules up to 2 mm in diameter. The nodules are distributed in a random fashion on the anterior surface of the iris and occasionally just in the angle, where they can be viewed by gonioscopy. In most adults, except in those with very dark irides, the nodules can be seen with the naked eye or with the aid of an illuminated magnifying glass. On the other hand, declaring

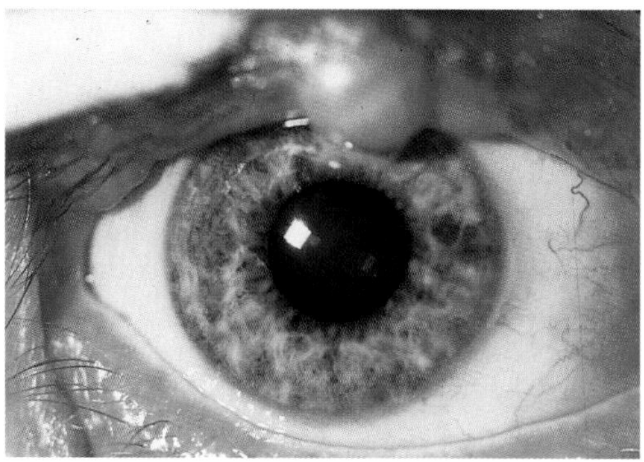

Figure 36.5. Numerous iris hamartomas on a lightly colored iris and neurofibromas of the lid of a middle-aged man with neurofibromatosis 1.

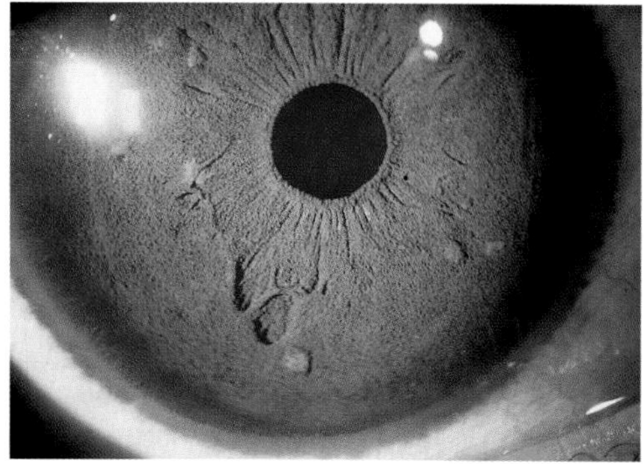

Figure 36.6. Iris hamartomas on a dark iris in a black teenager with neurofibromatosis 1.

their absence requires slit-lamp examination. Although iris hamartomas have a highly characteristic appearance, there are a few iris lesions that may be confused with them (Table 36.2).

Iris mammillations have been mistaken for the iris hamartomas of NF1, even in Lisch's original paper.[121,208,278] The two types of lesions are quite distinct, however. The nodules of NF1 are fluffier in appearance, tend to be more irregularly placed on the iris, do not overlie areas of hyperpigmented iris, are more variable in size and number, and tend to be a medium brown color in blue or green eyes, and pale or medium brown in brown eyes (Fig. 36.6). In contrast, iris mammillations are usually of the same color as the underlying iris in brown eyes and medium brown in blue or green eyes (Fig. 36.7) and have an even distribution over the iris.[278]

Histologically, iris hamartomas consist of a condensation of spindle cells on the anterior iris surface. They are of melanocytic origin. When they are pigmented, an underlying stromal nevus is often present.[271,379]

Iris hamartomas increase in prevalence with age in a semilogarithmic fashion.[280] They are present in approximately 33% of NF1 patients age 2.5 years, almost 50% of 5-year-olds, approximately 75% of 15-year-olds and 90% of 25-year-olds. Over the age of 30, between 95% and 100% of adults with NF1 have iris hamarto-

Table 36.2. Differential Diagnosis of Iris Hamartoma (Sakurai-Lisch Nodules)

Iris Nevi
Multiple
Iridocorneal endothelial syndromes
Iris Mammillations
Inflammatory Nodules
Granulomatous uveitis (e.g., sarcoidosis [Koeppe and Busacca nodules]), tuberculosis
Roseolae and gummae in syphilis
Iris pearls in leprosy
Tumors
Iris cysts
Iris melanoma
Tapioca melanoma
Retinoblastoma

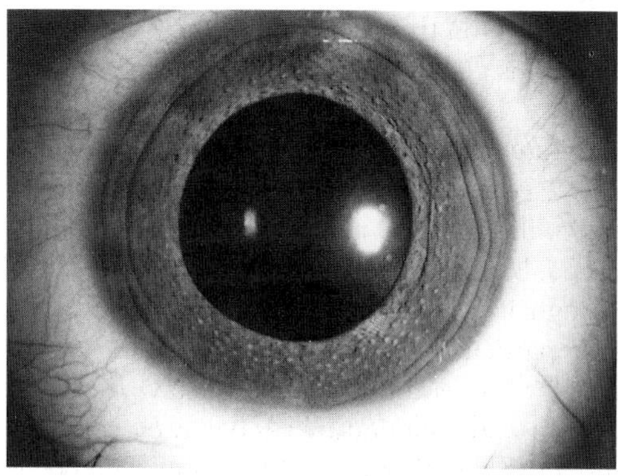

Figure 36.7. Iris mammillations in a patient with melanosis of the iris. (Reproduced with permission from EI Traboulsi and IH Maumenee. Bilateral melanosis of the iris. *Am J Ophthalmol* 1987;103:115–116.)[351a]

mas.[280] This is in general agreement with a recent study of over 500 patients by Rainey and colleagues.[282] These authors found the probability of NF1 patients having iris hamartomas to be <12% under 5 years of age, >80% in 6- to 10-year-olds, >90% of over 40-year-olds, and approaching 100% by age 65 years. Unlike neurofibromas, there is no acceleration in the rate of appearance of these nodules associated with puberty.[205]

In the presence of other diagnostic features of NF1 or a positive family history, iris hamartomas confirm the diagnosis. In the absence of other signs of NF1, their presence is highly suggestive of NF1. Iris hamartomas are not, however, exclusive to NF1 and have also been reported in Cushing disease,[37,141,185] NF2,[49,114,141,185,279] and in normal individuals, with a frequency of 0.28%.[129] Although the NIH diagnostic criteria include two or more iris hamartomas, a single nodule in only one eye can contribute to the diagnosis in the presence of other signs or family history of NF1. In the pediatric population where café-au-lait patches are the most common sign, iris hamartomas, if present, are highly specific for the disease (more than axillary freckling or neurofibromas) and may rarely be the only sign of NF1[289] or occur in relatives of patients with NF1 who have no other signs of the disease.[350] Furthermore, patients with Watson syndrome (an allelic variant of NF1 characterized by café-au-lait patches, mental retardation and pulmonary stenosis), have these nodules.[7] In patients with segmental neurofibromatosis, iris hamartomas may occur on the same side as the other manifestations.[373]

Orbitotemporal Involvement. Orbital involvement, generally referred to as orbitotemporal neurofibromatosis, may occur as part of generalized NF1 or as a separate syndrome.[166] Although it is a relatively rare finding in NF1, this particular manifestation is often familial.[42,166,276] A neurofibroma may involve the orbit, eyelids, and temporal area and may even extend intracranially. Proptosis of the globe can occur and there may be associated buphthalmos and optic nerve compression. The skeletal changes include partial or total absence of the greater wing of the sphenoid, resulting in prolapse of the temporal lobe into the orbit. This increases the proptosis and causes pulsation of the globe. The orbit is enlarged and egg shaped with hypoplastic supra- and infraorbital rims. There may be an associated temporal lobe arachnoid cyst.[166] Alternatively, there may be enophthalmos associated with an increase in size of the bony orbit and enlargement of superior and inferior orbital fissures.[109] Pulsating enophthalmos is uncommon and occurs in about 1%–2% of cases.[309] Van der Hoeve mentions a case of NF1 where pulsatile exophthalmos could be easily converted to pulsatile enophthalmos by pressure on the eye.[358] It is not clear whether the superior orbital fissure enlargement is always due to a developmental abnormality of the mesoderm or is related to pressure effects by neurofibromas of the orbit.[109] The management options of orbitotemporal neurofibromatosis have been well described by Jackson and associates.[166] These authors have adopted an aggressive management approach to this condition on the basis that conservative management often leads to tumor recurrence.[166] Their radical surgical techniques are likely to be associated with a higher intraoperative complication rate, but their long-term results in a selected group of patients is encouraging. They have divided this condition into three groups:

1. Orbital soft tissue involvement with a seeing eye
2. Orbital soft tissue involvement and significant bony involvement with a seeing eye
3. Orbital soft tissue involvement and significant bony involvement with a blind or absent eye

Group 1 is managed by local resection of the upper (or lower) lid neurofibroma with or without closure of the posterior orbital defect with a bone graft. Later, the levator aponeurotic defect can be addressed. In group 2, a lid and orbital resection of the extensive tumor with reconstruction of the bony orbit and levator shortening is performed. Group 3 has an extensive soft tissue mass and orbital involvement with a blind eye and pulsating exophthalmos. Extensive resection of the neurofibroma and orbital contents is carried out, followed by reconstruction with a total eye and eyelid prosthesis. If the lids are less extensively involved and can be preserved, an ocular prosthesis with orbital reconstruction is used.

Genetics

In 1987 the gene for NF1 was mapped to 17q11.2 by linkage analysis and the analysis of two translocations between chromosomes 1 and 17 and 17 and 22 in NF1 patients.[105,197,232,261] Further work on these translocations and the technique of reverse genetics led to the cloning and isolation of the NF1 gene.[46,360,369] In 1991, the complete sequence of the NF1 gene product was published[221] and its cellular expression and function were further characterized.[75,135] The NF1 gene product has been named "neurofibromin."

About 30%–50% of cases of NF1 are considered to result from new mutations, the majority on the individual's paternally derived chromosome 17.[168,286,336] This is an extremely high mutation rate, due in part to the large size of the gene and transcript or possibly to the presence of sequences within the gene that are highly susceptible to mutation.

The NF1 Gene. The NF1 gene is one of the largest genes in which mutations lead to disease in humans, spanning 300 kb of genomic DNA (Fig. 36.8).[46,75,135,221,360,361,369] The NF1 promoter region consists of a CpG-rich region characteristic of housekeeping genes. The NF1 gene contains at least 56 exons (coding portions) which, after transcription, form a messenger

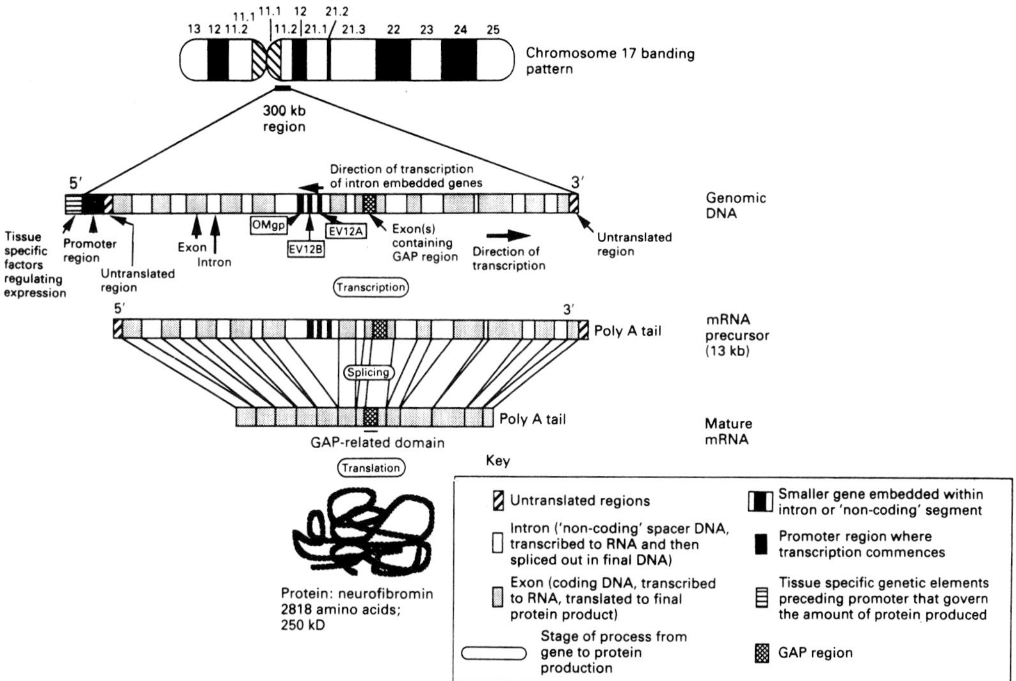

Figure 36.8. Schematic representation of the neurofibromatosis (NF) 1 gene showing its position in the 11.2 region of the long arm of chromosome 17. When expanded (second level), the layout of genomic DNA can be seen with the 5′ end to the left and 3′ end to the right. The genomic DNA is transcribed to RNA in the direction left to right. The 5′ end of the gene contains the promoter and trone specifications upstream of the NF1 gene itself, that regulates the transcription of the gene. The exons, which are coding regions of the gene eventually spliced to be contiguous, are separated by introns in the genomic DNA. The guanosine triphosphate (GTPase) activating protein or GAP region is shown with cross hatching. There are three embedded minigenes: OMgp, EV12A, and EV12B which are transcribed in the opposite direction to the rest of the gene. After being transcribed to the messenger RNA precursor, which is shown in the third level, the exons are spliced to become contiguous in the mature RNA. The mature RNA is translated to form the protein neurofibromin. (Reproduced with permission from NK Ragge. Clinical and genetic patterns of neurofibromatosis 1 and 2. *Br J Ophthalmol* 1993;77:662–672.)

RNA of 13 kb with a coding region of 9 kb. The 8454 nucleotides in this open reading frame produce a protein product of 2818 amino acids (Fig. 36.8).[132] Expression of the gene product neurofibromin appears to be ubiquitous, but it is in highest abundance in neurons, Schwann cells, and oligodendrocytes.[70] In neurons, neurofibromin is equally abundant regardless of its location in the brain or neurotransmitter. It is highly concentrated in the dendritic processes, the site for input messages. It has been found to colocalize with microtubules and is presumably related to the cytoskeleton.[132]

Rather curiously, three genes (OMgp, EV12A, EV12B) that read in the opposite direction to the rest of the gene, were found to be located within one intron (a "noncoding" region) of the NF1 gene. These genes may play a role in NF1: the OMgp (oligodendrocyte myelin glycoprotein) gene because of its role in cell–cell communication in the central nervous system,[132] and the EV12A and EV12B genes because of their mouse homologues playing a role in murine leukemia. It has been suggested that the coexistence of multiple sclerosis and NF1 in the same patients may be related to mutations in OMgp.[99] Alternatively, these introns could merely be remnants of phylogenetically older genes.[313]

Function of the Gene Product Neurofibromin. The main functions of neurofibromin appear to be related to growth and cell cycle regulation, with possible additional roles in signal transduction and differentiation. The NF1 gene product has striking sequence homology with the catalytic domain of mammalian GAP (guanosine triphosphatase activating) protein and yeast equivalent proteins IRA 1 and 2.[19a,383a] GAP is an important cell cycle regulatory protein that interacts with the cellular oncogene *ras*, catalyzing the conversion of the active GTP-bound form of ras to its inactive GDP-bound form. Cellular oncogenes or protooncogenes code for a group of proteins that are important in cell cycle regulation, but when transformed under certain circumstances are potentially capable of inducing tumor formation by releasing normal controls on cellular proliferation. Tumor or growth suppressor genes, such as the retinoblastoma, NF2, Wilms' tumor, and probably NF1 genes, act as the controller to the cell cycle.

Neurofibromin may have three specific functions: the regulation of cellular oncogenes (*ras*) that are important in growth and differentiation, microtubular function,[9] and involvement in phosphorylation-mediated signal transduction pathways.[133] The mammalian GAP protein and the GAP-related domain of the NF1 protein have been shown to interact with the wild-type (normal) *ras* protein and may act as cell cycle controllers.[223] Neurofibromin is known to inactivate p21ras via its GTPase activity. However, if the ras gene is mutated, the *ras* protein appears to lose its ability to bind to GAP and may continue to activate the cell, thus losing an important control mechanism. What is not known is whether GAP regulates *ras*, converting it from active to inactive form via GTP hydrolysis, or if GAP activates *ras* by binding to it.[137]

Neurofibromin is associated with microtubules. This physical association may regulate neurofibromin availability and activity with *ras*. Alternatively neurofibromin might have further actions involving the regulation of microtubular functions via tubulin.[133] Perhaps the intronic regions of the gene also play a role in tumorigenesis.[258] Neurofibromin may play various roles depending on the stage of development and tissue involved.[69] There is some evidence that *ras* is important in embryonic development; it has been shown to be part of a signal transduction path controlling development of a differentiated photoreceptor cell in *Drosophila*.[104,326]

Three isoforms of neurofibromin have now been characterized.[9,47] Types 1 and 2 differ by 21 amino acids.[9,133] Type 1 tends to have stronger GAP properties than type 2 and is also expressed more prominently in fetal human brain, with a switch to type 2 after week 22.[133] This is supported by another study that found that the type 1 is predominantly expressed in undifferentiated cells, with type 2 transcript predominating in differentiated cells.[255] Type 1 tends to be expressed more in certain tumors, such as pheochromocytomas, whereas type 2 is expressed more in other neural crest–derived tissues such as adrenal gland and Schwann cells.[134] Another study found that type 1 is expressed predominantly in normal brain tissue, whereas type 2 predominates in brain tumors.[343]

The alternative splicing of neurofibromin is highly conserved, suggesting that the isoforms of neurofibromin may mediate important biological functions.[9] The size and complexity of neurofibromin suggests the presence of several active domains and therefore the potential for more than one function. The inclusion or exclusion of a particular exon enables one gene to be used for multiple functions. For instance, they may differ in their GAP activity or in their biological function or their predilection for different members of the ras family of oncogenes.

The evidence suggests that the development of tumors in NF1 appears to be dependent on the up-regulation of ras activity by release of the negative control by neurofibromin-GAP. Early treatment approaches to prevent tumor development in NF1 are being developed based on the use of farnesyl transferase inhibitors, which prevent the farnesyl transferase-mediated membrane association of ras.[385] This would, in theory, inhibit the malignant potential of ras-activated cells and is a potentially exciting development.

Germline Mutations in the NF1 Gene. Several types of germline mutations in the NF1 gene have been characterized so far in individuals with NF1. These include megadeletions, which may lead to NF1 associated with other characteristics (e.g., mental retardation), microdeletions, point mutations, and splice-site errors responsible for exon skipping, insertions, or translocations.[2,46,91,105,139,175,200,206,261,277,334,354,360,368] Many of the mutations lie in CpG dinucleotides.[46,91,147,296,355,383] Mutations that can affect the expression of the affected NF1 allele are not necessarily those that induce stop mutations in nonterminal exons. Instead, they may affect RNA processing or stability or production via regulatory sequences.[147] In keeping with other tumor suppressor genes, there is a lack of mutational "hot spots" in the NF1 gene. However, one "warm spot" for mutation has been found in exon 31.[3,46,91] Common clinical features include the presence of dermal neurofibromas and scoliosis.[3]

Other Genetic Influences in NF1-Genomic Imprinting. Can imprinting affect the expression of disease type and severity in NF1? The variability in expression of disease phenotypes in different members of a family who clearly have the same type of NF1 gene mutation suggests that other genetic influences are at play. Miller and Hall[239] suggested that the disease was more severe when the mutation was maternally derived. However, further studies failed to confirm this.[45,291,295] Certain specific disease manifestations of NF1 may be affected by imprinting. These may include the association of juvenile chronic myelogenous leukemia in NF1 with bone marrow monosomy 7, maternal inheritance and predilection for boys,[320] and paraganglioma.[143] Otherwise, the sex of the individual patient does not appear to affect the expression of disease with the exception of pregnancy effects. Tumors appear to grow under the effects of pregnancy hormones and pregnancy can sometimes be the first time the disease is expressed.

The Role of the p53 Gene in Tumor Formation in NF1. Mutations have been found in p53 in malignant tumors in NF1, including neurofibrosarcomas.[199,231,254] The body of recent evidence suggests that initiation of tumor formation in NF1 is by the somatic inactivation of the second NF1 allele. Tumor progression occurs by accumulation of further genetic abnormalities, such as the inactivation of p53.

Phenotype–Genotype Correlation in NF1. Phenotype–genotype correlation has begun in earnest following the cloning of the NF1 gene. It is more likely that the type of manifestation, rather than the degree of severity, will be determined by specific mutations. There are many reported cases of similar manifestations in first-degree affected relatives with NF1. These clinical features include a similar distribution of neurofibromas, familial occurrence of orbital neurofibromatosis, and possibly a tendency of the neurofibromas to undergo malignant change.[13,42,120,245,276]

The clinical symptoms of NF1 show extremely variable expressivity, raising the possibility that the expression of the NF1 mutation may be modulated by other genetic or epigenetic factors. The importance of epigenetic factors is suggested by a twin study in NF1, where it was found that concordance was far greater between monozygotic twins with NF1 than between siblings with NF1.[274]

Tumor Formation

Neurofibromatosis type 1 (NF1) is associated with the formation of multiple tumor types including neurofibromas, plexiform neurofibromas, optic gliomas, neurofibrosarcomas, astrocytomas, meningiomas, and pheochromocytomas. Patients with NF1 may also be at increased risk of developing other more common malignancies, for example, acute nonlymphocytic leukemia, Wilms' tumor, and rhabdomyosarcoma.[331]

Evidence is now growing that the NF1 gene acts as a classical tumor suppressor gene similar to retinoblastoma.[23,76,131,201,244,344] Mutations occur in both alleles of the NF1 gene in tumors in NF1 patients. However, neurofibromin may also play an important role in the genesis of tumors in non-NF1 patients. Loss of NF1 gene expression has been found in malignant melanoma and in neuroblastoma, both of which are not commonly found in NF1. Loss of NF1 gene expression has also been found in sporadic instances of pheochromocytomas.[134] This is similar to loss of other growth suppressor genes such as the retinoblastoma gene in tumors not especially associated with hereditary retinoblastoma, for example, breast carcinoma.[346]

Management

The management of NF1 is mainly concerned with the early detection and treatment of complications of the disease and advice regarding presymptomatic screening of relatives. The patient and their family are best managed by a multidisciplinary team involving a geneticist, surgical specialist, ophthalmologist, and genetics counselor as appropriate to the complications.

Medical therapy includes anticonvulsant medications for seizures, analgesics for headache, abdominal and other pain that may or may not be related to neurofibromas, and antihypertensive agents. Radiotherapy can be used for selected tumors, but there may be a risk of increasing tumorigenesis. Neurofibromas are never treated with radiotherapy. Chemotherapy is generally not of benefit but has been considered in the context of optic gliomas.[288] Preliminary studies have shown that ketotifen may be effective in treating the itching and pain in association with neurofibromas.[288] Surgical therapy forms a large part of the treatment of tumors in NF1 but is rarely needed for optic gliomas.

Individuals with NF1 and their families need a great deal of supportive care as they encounter new and added complications of NF1. Depression and anxiety are common and compounded by misinformation. It is of vital importance that they have access to adequate counseling in addition to correct medical and surgical strategies.

Prenatal Diagnosis

It is possible to perform prenatal diagnosis in families with at least three affected individuals in at least two generations using closely linked or intragenic markers for the NF1 gene.[89] Although the intragenic markers are more accurate, they are not always informative.[235] Screening and mutational analysis on a large scale is not feasible as yet, although methods for rapid screening of affected families are being developed.[85,195] There is a huge variation between centres on the availability and use of prenatal testing.[148]

Neurofibromatosis Type 2

Introduction and History

Neurofibromatosis type 2 (NF2) is a dominantly inherited disorder characterized by the development of bilateral vestibular schwannomas (acoustic neuromas) and multiple central nervous system tumors including meningiomas, gliomas, ependymomas, and schwannomas.[243,288] In 1917, Cushing rightly pointed out that the eighth nerve tumors arose in the internal auditory canal on the vestibular nerve, rather than the acoustic nerve,[68] although the misnomer "acoustic neuroma" has persisted to the present day.

The first documented case of NF2 was by Wishart who described a case of bilateral acoustic tumors with multiple meningeal tumors.[380] Several other early cases of bilateral acoustic tumors in association with neurofibromatosis were described.[22,26,28,68,180,284,285] Some reports correctly emphasized the association of acoustic tumors with a particular form of NF, with few skin findings or meningiomas present.[68,142]

NF2 has only been defined as an entity distinct from NF1 in the last 15 years following mounting clinical and genetic evidence.[87,171,243,299] The genes responsible for these diseases were mapped to separate chromosomes in 1987—the NF1 gene to chromosome 17 and the NF2 gene to chromosome 22.[20,299] Since this division, a clearer, but also continuously evolving, clinical picture of NF2 is emerging. NF2 is a much rarer disease than NF1, with a prevalence of 1 in 33,000–40,000.[96] About 50% of all cases and 75% of index cases appear to represent new mutations. Like NF1, there is an extremely high penetrance, over 95% in one study.[171]

Clinical Features

The hallmark of NF2 is the presence of bilateral vestibular schwannomas that occur in 85% of patients.[93] However, according to the National Institutes of Health criteria (Table 36.3),[243,266] the diagnosis can also be made if there is a first-degree relative with NF2 and there is either a unilateral eighth nerve mass or any two of the following: neurofibroma, meningioma, glioma, schwannoma, or posterior capsular cataract or lens opacity at a young age. Spinal tumors are a frequent manifestation of NF2.[228] These are often multiple and of different pathological types.[228] Patients with NF2 tend to develop tumors of the neural coverings or linings, such as meningiomas, optic nerve sheath meningiomas, schwannomas, and ependymomas, whereas those with NF1 tend to develop neural or astrocytic tumors (astrocytomas, gliomas, and optic nerve gliomas). Bilateral vestibular schwannomas do not appear to occur in NF1,[225] despite claims to the contrary.[12,22,238]

Although NF1 and NF2 are separate diseases genetically, some clinical features overlap, which has led to much of the confusion over the years (Table 36.4). Overall, the skin manifestations of NF2 tend to be less prolific than NF1. For example, it is rare to find an NF2 patient with more than five CAL spots,[113,171,387] although there may be larger and atypical CAL patches. There are exceptional cases of NF2 described with multiple CAL spots, and occasional cases with axillary freckling[158,275] or iris hamartomas.[49,279]

Cutaneous and subcutaneous neurofibromas are found in NF2 but not usually in florid abundance as in NF1. Cutaneous and subcutaneous schwannomas (Fig. 36.9) are found in NF2 but not NF1. The problem is that some patients with NF2 can fulfill the current criteria for the diagnosis of both NF2 and NF1 if they have two of the following: cutaneous neurofibromas, six CAL patches, more than two iris hamartomas, or a CNS glioma.[238] Definitive genetic studies will clarify this group of individuals with overlapping features. The presumed occurrence of both NF1 and NF2 in the same individual has also been described due to inheritance of NF1 from the father and NF2 from the mother.[303] In this case there was extremely early onset and rapid progression of the disease.

As in NF1, there is huge variability in expression of the disease phenotype between individuals with NF2, both in terms of tumor type and location and the clinical severity of disease.[229] There does not appear to be any difference in

Table 36.3. Diagnostic Criteria for Neurofibromatosis 2[243,266]

The diagnostic criteria are met if a person has either of the following:

1. Bilateral eighth nerve masses seen with appropriate imaging technique (e.g., computerized tomographic or magnetic resonance imaging)
2. A first-degree relative with neurofibromatosis 2 and either unilateral eighth nerve mass or two of the following:
   - Neurofibroma
   - Meningioma
   - Glioma
   - Schwannoma
   - Posterior capsular cataract or lens opacity at a young age

Table 36.4. Comparison of Clinical Features of NF1 and NF2

Feature	NF1	NF2
Skin		
Café-au-lait patches	++	+
Subcutaneous, cutaneous, or plexiform neurofibromas	++	+[a]
Schwannomas[b]	−	+
Central Nervous System		
Spinal neurofibromas	+	(+)
Spinal schwannomas	?	++
Meningiomas	+	++
Gliomas	+	++
Ependymomas	(+)	+
Ophthalmic		
Optic nerve glioma	++	?
Optic nerve sheath meningioma	−	+
Iris hamartomas	++	(+)
Cataracts	−	++
Retinal hamartomas	+	+
Myelinated nerve fibers	(+)	?
Choroidal hamartoma	+	?
Choroidal nevus	+	?
Uveal melanoma	(+)	(+)
Choroidal hemangioma	+	?
Epiretinal membrane	−	+
Combined pigment epithelial and retinal hamartoma	(+)	+

[a] Special locations—palmar, nasolabial fold.
[b] Cutaneous or subcutaneous.
++ = profuse or common; + = present; (+) = rare; − = absent; ? = unknown.

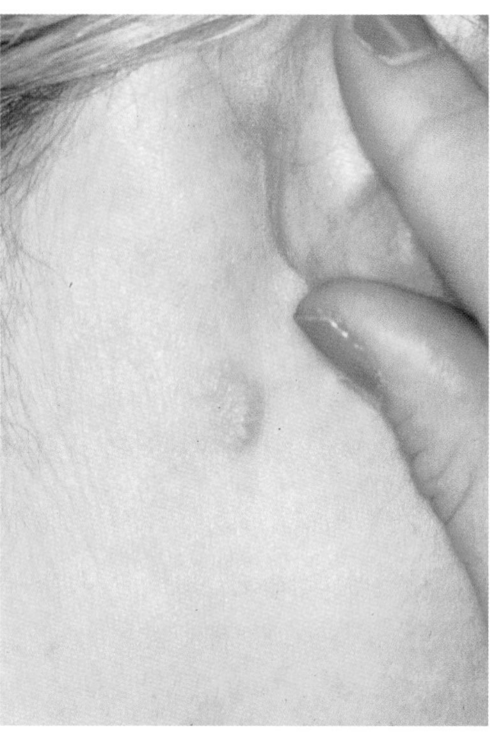

Figure 36.9. Cutaneous schwannoma behind the ear of a patient with neurofibromatosis 2.

severity of disease between men and women.[325] The phenotypic manifestations of NF2 show high intrafamilial variability.[93] However, it has been suggested that within the clinical spectrum of NF2, there may be certain disease phenotypes that breed true within families as follows.[88,267,382]

1. Wishart phenotype, characterized by early onset, rapid progression of hearing loss, and multiple associated tumors.[380]
2. Feiling-Gardner phenotype, which has a late onset of manifestations, slow progression of hearing loss, and few associated tumors.[97,113]
3. Lee-Abbott phenotype, which has a more variable age of onset and clinical progression of hearing loss, multiple associated spinal cord tumors, cerebellopontine angle meningiomas, and meningiomatosis en plaque of the falx.[198]

These phenotypes have now been merged into two groups, mild and severe, that occur with similar frequency.[8,88,96,268] The mild and severe types differ with respect to age of onset, clinical course, and the occurrence of spinal tumors and cranial meningiomas.[96,229,268]

Individuals with NF2 most commonly present with hearing loss, unilateral or bilateral, sometimes with concomitant tinnitus or unsteadiness.[96,171,225,249] There is often a delay in the diagnosis of NF2. In one study, the mean age of onset of symptoms (unspecified) was 27.9 years (range 11–42 years) with a mean age at diagnosis of 35.9 years (range 18–66 years).[249] In a second study, the ages at onset and diagnosis were 21.8 years and 27.8 years, respectively.[95] The average age of onset of hearing loss in NF2 is in the teens or twenties, however it is possible to present as early as the first or as late as the seventh decade.[95,225] In another study, the mean age of onset of symptoms from vestibular schwannomas was 20.4 years.[171] Deafness does not always correlate with the size of the tumor; the side with the smaller tumor may have worse deafness.[28] Surgery on large tumors is associated with low chance of hearing preservation. However, occasional surgical successes are described, with recovery from deafness after surgical removal of a 4 cm tumor using an intracapsular technique.[173]

Schwann cell tumors of the central nervous system are the commonest type of tumor in NF2. In addition to vestibular schwannomas, these include other cranial nerves—mainly the fifth, ninth, and tenth—the spinal root, and intramedullary schwannomas. Other tumors include multiple meningiomas, optic nerve sheath meningiomas (Fig. 36.10), and gliomas, which, although of low histological grade, can cause devastating disease if located in the brain stem or spinal cord. Deep plexiform neurofibromas occur as in NF1 and can lead to neurological dysfunction and malignant degeneration. Patients with NF2 also show calcified subependymal deposits, probably sited within glial hamartomas, and bilateral choroid plexus calcification.[14,55,366,374]

Dermatological signs tend to be less profuse and are less often the presenting feature of NF2 than in NF1. The skin signs that overlap with NF1 include typical CAL patches, atypical areas of hyperpigmentation with indistinct borders, which if they extend to the midline on the back can overlie spinal tumors, hypopigmented macules, hairy nevi, and cutaneous neurofibromas (usually fewer than in NF1). However, more specific signs of NF2 include cutaneous schwannomas, which are harder than the more fleshy neurofibromas and have a roughened surface (Fig. 36.9), subcutaneous schwannomas, sometimes in the spinal region, and neurofibromas in special locations such as the nasolabial folds and the palms.

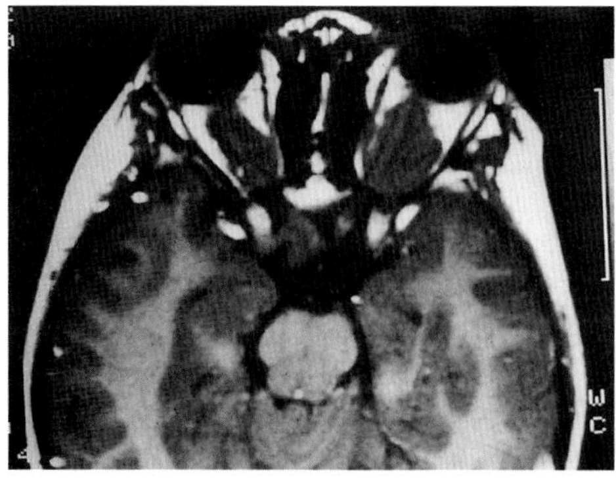

Figure 36.10. Bilateral optic nerve sheath meningiomas in a patient with neurofibromatosis 2. The patient had multiple spinal cord meningiomas, including one at the foramen magnum. He also had a sectoral cortical unilateral cataract. (Courtesy of Dr. John F. O'Neill.)

Ophthalmic Findings

The importance of ocular signs in NF2 has only been appreciated recently, although many of the older case reports mention eye problems. Indeed, Wishart's original patient was blind in one eye from birth[380] and other reports mention congenital cataract, optic nerve sheath meningiomas, third nerve palsies and probably retinal hamartomas.[321,358,382]

In 1969, Lee and Abbott, in their classic paper describing a large pedigree with NF2, described early onset lenticular opacities, mostly posterior polar, in 7 of 16 members.[198] However, it was not until 1986 that medical attention was drawn toward the rarity of iris hamartomas and the high frequency of juvenile-onset posterior subcapsular or capsular cataract (PSCC) in NF2.[269] Larger studies have corroborated this initial finding and established that early onset cortical cataract is also seen in NF2.[36,170,174,279]

Following the separation of NF2 from NF1, further unusual ocular findings started to be reported in NF2. These included isolated[128,191,327] and familial[38] cases of combined pigment epithelial and retinal hamartomas (also in retrospect reported earlier),[61] optic disc gliomas[82,192] (also reported earlier),[126,307] epiretinal membrane formation,[174,192] iris hamartomas,[49,114,174] hypertrophied corneal nerves,[114] and conjunctival neurofibroma.[270] Other previously reported findings include retinal hemangioblastomas,[106] medullated nerve fibers,[126] choroidal nevi,[61] uveal melanoma, and choroidal hamartomas.[114] Optic nerve sheath meningiomas are also a well-described association with NF2 and can lead to progressive visual loss (Fig. 36.10).[67,174,321]

A very high proportion of NF2 patients have ocular abnormalities: 86% in a recent large survey.[279] Other findings in this study were early onset lens opacities in 69% of cases, characteristically PSCC and cortical cataract, retinal hamartomas (23%), juvenile-onset ocular motor pareses (12%), and vitreoretinal degeneration (6%).[279] There was an age-related increase in the prevalence of cataract, indicating that although there was a genetic predisposition to develop early onset lens opacities, they were not congenital. PSCC and cortical cataract were each present in 41% of individuals, although PSCC were more likely to be bilateral. Another large study found PSCC in 80% of NF2 patients, although different methods were used to view the lens opacities in the two studies.[36,170,279]

The lens opacities in NF2 have a variable visual morbidity, low in one study[279] and high in another,[170] and are often undetectable unless the pupil is dilated. Plaque-like capsular opacities and dense posterior, central cortical cataract cause most visual loss. There are also reports of Mittendorf dot (a remnant of the hyaloid system), embryonal cataract, and persistent hyperplastic primary vitreous,[96,279] suggesting that there may be a spectrum of changes of a developmental nature at the posterior lens pole in NF2. Moderately severe visual loss in NF2 is more commonly due to intracranial and optic nerve sheath meningioma than to cataracts. Other causes of visual loss include retinal abnormalities, such as combined pigment epithelial and retinal hamartomas (CPERH) and epiretinal membranes, chronic papilledema, amblyopia secondary to childhood ocular motor paresis or strabismus, and corneal scarring.[279]

Retinal astrocytic hamartomas are rare developmental anomalies often described in patients with tuberous sclerosis or NF1. They are also common in NF2, where they are found in a peripapillary, macular, peripheral retinal location (Fig. 36.11), often over blood vessels. Macular hamartomas may be part of a spectrum of CPERH, which has been well described in NF2.[38,247,279] Retinal scars of similar size to small retinal hamartomas are seen in NF2 patients and may represent involuted hamartomas.[279]

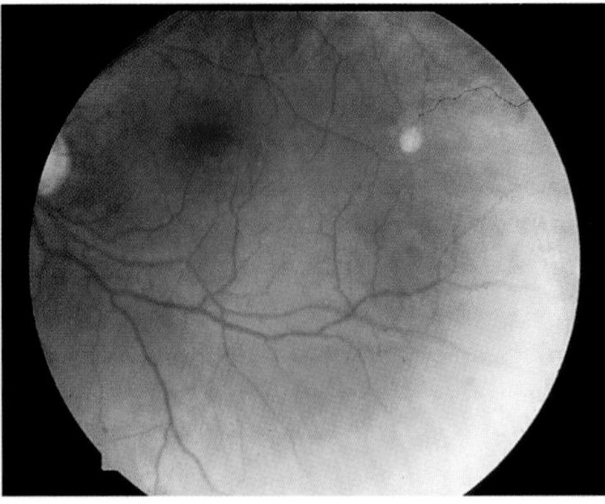

Figure 36.11. Retinal hamartoma in neurofibromatosis 2.

Retinal hamartomas also occur on the disc and in a subpapillary location when they may be indistinguishable from optic disc drusen.[71,279]

Juvenile-onset vitreoretinal degeneration with retinal detachment is a newly described complication in NF2.[279] Idiopathic epiretinal membranes may form.[174,192,279,349] It has been suggested that epiretinal membranes are also part of the spectrum of CPERH.[103,192,310]

Ocular motor pareses occur in over 10% of children with NF2 and strabismus is common.[279] Out of 16 individuals in Lee and Abbott's pedigree, 2 had juvenile-onset palsies and 4 had secondary exotropia or extraocular movement abnormality associated with lens opacity.[198] There are other descriptions of childhood third nerve palsies and anisocoria.[226,349]

Genetics

There are many parallels that can be drawn between the tumor formation in retinoblastoma and in NF2.[112,181] In the inherited form of both diseases, retinoblastoma or vestibular schwannomas occur bilaterally and earlier, and other tumor types may develop. The NF2 gene was mapped by observing that deletions of chromosome 22 occurred in sporadic meningiomas and vestibular schwannomas.[315–317,389] Until recently it was observed that entire chromosome copies were lost, but when partial losses were detected, this led to the mapping of the NF2 gene to chromosome 22q band 11.2.[229,248,299,315–317,374] In 1992, 12 families with NF2 were found to map to the same region on the long arm of chromosome 22 nearest to the marker D22S32, between the markers D22S1 and D22S28.[248] In 1993, the gene for NF2 was cloned and the gene product—merlin or schwannomin—was characterized as a 595 amino acid protein.[298,352] The term "merlin" was used by Trofatter and others[352] to denote the NF2 gene product as a moesin-, ezrin-, radixin-like protein (*vide infra*) that may play a role in mediating interactions between the cell membrane and the cytoskeleton.[211] The term "schwannomin" was used by Rouleau and others[298] to denote its role in the production of schwannomas (similar to 'neurofibromin' in NF1).

Structure of Merlin. In keeping with other members of the moesin, ezrin, and radixin family of proteins, merlin has two different domains.[233] The N-terminal domain, which shares the greatest homology with other members of the family of proteins, may be involved in membrane binding. The C-terminal domain may interact with cytoskeletal elements. This part of the protein consists of two alphahelical regions bounded by residues 304–474 and 509–559 separated by a small peptide sequence containing proline residues. The C-terminal end appears to be critical for normal functioning of the NF2 protein, since even quite distal disruptions lead to loss of function.[233] Several isoforms of merlin have been detected, both in mouse and human cell lines, which diverge in the C-terminal end.[159] At least in the mouse, there is differential expression in various tissues and at different stages of embryogenesis.[159] This suggests that there may be distinct functional roles of different isoforms of merlin.

Phenotype–Genotype Correlation. A wealth of germline mutations have now been described.[27,33,34,167,203,212,353] The majority of these are predicted to lead to synthesis of a truncated protein. The remainder of mutations are missense[34,212,298] or in frame deletions.[27,203] Early studies of phenotype–genotype correlations suggested that mild manifestations of the disease are associated with mutations that preserve the C-terminal of merlin,[233] with the exception of a family described by Evans and colleagues with a mild type of NF2 associated with a missense mutation at the C-terminal end.[92] One mutational hot spot in exon 2 with a C to T transition at codon 57 has been associated with severe phenotype, except for one individual who was a somatic mosaic for the mutations.[33,34,233]

Germline mutations in the NF2 gene have been found in tumors from patients with schwannomatosis, suggesting that this disease may be identical with NF2.[149] Schwannomatosis (neurilemmomatosis) is characterized by multiple schwannomas of the spine and skin, without any other features of NF2.

Presymptomatic Diagnosis

Ocular examination is valuable in the presymptomatic diagnosis of NF2. Macular hamartoma, juvenile-onset retinal detachment, and juvenile-onset ocular motor nerve pareses were the first presenting feature of NF2 in 10% of the patients in one study.[279] Furthermore, many NF2 patients have asymptomatic lens opacities in the first two decades of life. Ocular findings in NF2 can assist with early diagnosis when other signs are absent. This is important because removal of small vestibular tumors may allow preservation of hearing and a reduced complication rate from surgery.[101,123,318] In one study, 13 of 120 patients were known to have a cataract as the first manifestation of NF2.[94] Mautner and colleagues reported four further pediatric cases of NF2 with cataract; the youngest patient was 10 years old.[227] There are some reports of congenital cataract in NF2.[158,279,374,382] Epiretinal membranes can also occur in youth.[55,279]

Tightly linked DNA markers can now be used for presymptomatic diagnosis of NF2 in large pedigrees with at least three affected individuals.[212,248,302] Eleven percent of cases have been found to be asymptomatic at the time of screening.[96] However, sporadic cases comprise one third to one half of all NF2 patients.[93] As a result, segregation analysis is not possible for many at-risk individuals, and at present direct mutation screening cannot detect all mutations.[213,233] Thus clinical examinations continue to be important in diagnosis. Audiological testing may detect an early sensorineural hearing loss, but MRI with gadolinium diethylenetriamine pentaacetic acid (Gd-DTPA) enhancement is required for definitive diagnosis or exclusion of small vestibular schwannomas.[273] Current recommendations for at-risk relatives (before the availability of a genetic diagnostic test) are that subjects should be seen every two years from 10 to 16 years of age and then on a yearly basis until 50 years, when screening may be ceased if the subjects remain asymptomatic.[249] Phenotypic differences in genetically identical twins suggest that mutational analysis will be of limited value in predicting specific disease features.[21] However, molecular testing using linked genetic markers or direct mutation analysis can eliminate unnecessary clinical testing for at risk individuals who do not carry the disease mutation and lead to early detection and improved treatment.[40,266]

Other Forms of Neurofibromatosis

There may be additional forms of neurofibromatosis, including NF3, NF4, NF5, multiple meningiomatosis, and spinal schwannomatosis, that do not fit precisely into current diagnostic classifications. These disorders may eventually map to different genes. Some parents may have only single manifestations of the disease, such as iris hamartomas, and have offspring with a full expression of the disorder. The explanation for this intrafamilial variability is still unclear, although it may just reflect the variable expressivity of dominantly inherited disorders.

Segmental NF (NF5) is characterized by cutaneous neurofibromas and CAL patches limited to a circumscribed area in a lateral and dermatomal distribution that does not cross the midline.[163,286]

Von Hippel-Lindau Disease

Von Hippel-Lindau disease (VHL) is a classical inherited tumor suppressor gene syndrome predisposing affected individuals to hemangioblastomas of the retina and central nervous system, renal cell carcinoma, pheochromocytoma, and renal, pancreatic, and epididymal cysts.[52,62,151,218,220,251] The incidence is 3 per 100,000.[218] There is almost complete penetrance (97%) by the age of 60 years.[218] The mutation rate is 4.4×10^{-6}—similar to the same order as retinoblastoma.[218] Renal cell carcinoma is the most common cause of death, and median survival is reduced to 49 years.[220]

History

Treacher Collins and von Hippel were the first to describe familial retinal hemangioblastomas.[57,363,364] However, Lindau recognized the association between retinal hemangioblastomas and cerebellar hemangioblastoma and described the development of renal cell carcinoma and pancreatic cysts.[207]

Clinical Features

The diagnostic criteria and clinical features of VHL disease are summarized in Tables 36.5 and 36.6. The most common presenting features of VHL disease are retinal, followed by cerebellar hemangioblastomas; renal cell carcinoma and pheochromocytoma are the initial complications in 10% and 5% of patients, respectively. CNS hemangioblastomas are often asymptomatic and need to be detected by gadolinium-enhanced MRI.[100] The cumulative risk of an individual with VHL disease developing a retinal hemangioblastoma, cerebellar hemangioblastoma, and renal cell carcinoma at age 30 years are 44%, 38%, and 5%, respectively. This increases to 84%, 70%, and 69%, respectively, by age 60 years.[220]

Patients with VHL disease develop cerebellar hemangioblastomas and renal cancers at an earlier age than those who develop sporadic forms of these tumors (29 versus 48 years and 44 versus 62 years, respectively).[220] The earliest age at which renal cell carcinoma has been detected was 16 years.[176] Renal cell carcinomas are bilateral or multicentric in 50% of pa-

Table 36.5. Criteria for Diagnosis of von Hippel-Lindau Disease

Isolated Cases
Two or more hemangioblastomas (retinal or CNS) or a single hemangioblastoma in association with a visceral manifestation (e.g., pancreatic, renal, epididymal cysts, or renal carcinoma)
Familial Cases
Single hemangioblastoma or visceral complication

Table 36.6. Incidence of Clinical Features of von Hippel-Lindau Disease as Reported in Three Studies

Disease	Study Findings (%)			
	Lamiell et al.[190] (n = 554)	Maher et al.[220] (n = 152)	Neumann et al.[253] (Freiburg Study)	Mean Age at Diagnosis (years)[220]
Retinal hemangioblastoma	57	50	52	25
Cerebellar hemangioblastoma	55	50	43[a]	29
Spinal cord hemangioblastoma	14	13	—	34
Renal cell carcinoma	24	28	25[b]	44
Pheochromocytoma	19	7	35	20
Epididymal cystadenoma	—	—	3	—

[a] Includes all central nervous system hemangioblastoma.
[b] Includes renal cysts and cancer.
Adapted from Maher.[217]

tients.[220] Small localized tumors may be treated by nephron-sparing surgery, whereas larger or multicentric lesions may need radical nephrectomy and transplantation.[335]

Pheochromocytomas in VHL also occur at an earlier age than in nonfamilial cases and are frequently multifocal.[252] Pancreatic tumors in VHL disease are usually islet cell adenomas or carcinomas, which are frequently asymptomatic and detected on routine screening.[151] Other tumors that have been detected in these patients include visceral hemangioblastoma, meningioma, cerebellar primitive neuroectodermal tumor,[24] choroid plexus papilloma,[29] paraganglioma, testicular tumor,[48] spermatic cord mesenchymal hamartoma,[169] and germ cell teratoma (unpublished observation). A recently recognized complication of VHL disease that may produce hearing loss is a low-grade papillary adenocarcinoma of the endolymphatic sac.[77] Polycythemia may be associated with cerebellar hemangioblastomas due to release of erythropoietin.[150]

Ophthalmic Features

Retinal hemangioblastomas are the most common presenting findings in patients with VHL disease.[138] The mean age at diagnosis of retinal hemangioblastoma in VHL disease is 25 years. Between 25% and 80% of patients with retinal hemangioblastomas will have VHL disease.[219] All patients with a retinal hemangioblastoma and their first-degree relatives should be screened for VHL. The younger the age at presentation with a retinal hemangioblastoma, the greater the likelihood of VHL. Multiple retinal hemangioblastomas are diagnostic of VHL, as are a single retinal hemangioblastoma and a first-degree family member with any of the manifestations of VHL.

Clinically, there are two types of retinal and optic nerve head hemangioblastomas of VHL: endophytic and exophytic. Endophytic lesions are elevated red vascular tumors arising from the superficial retina or optic disc and growing into the vitreous (Fig. 36.12).[25,240] Larger peripheral tumors often have a feeding arteriole and draining venule (Fig. 36.13). Smaller tumors consist of a net of dilated capillaries and can be harder to diagnose on ophthalmoscopy. However, fluorescein angiography or angios-

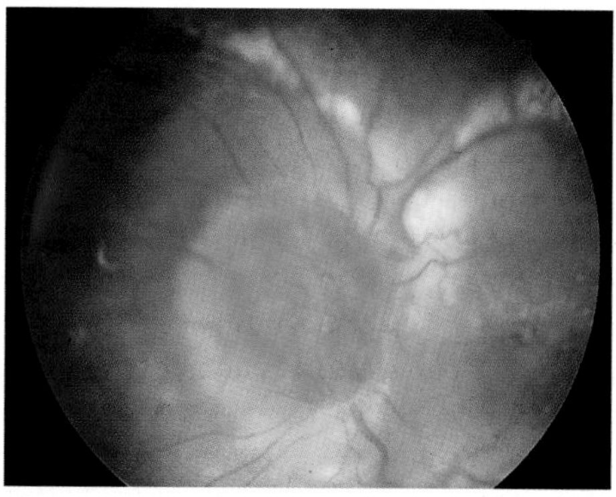

Figure 36.12. Endophytic optic nerve head hemangioblastoma in a patient with von Hippel-Lindau disease.

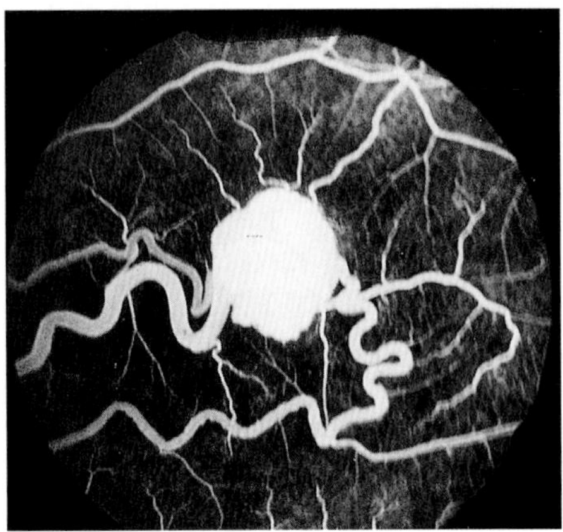

Figure 36.13. Peripheral hemangioblastoma in von Hippel-Lindau disease with a large feeding arteriole and a draining venule. (Courtesy of Dr. Irene H. Maumenee.)

copy will readily demonstrate them.[124,240] Visual loss results from exudative or traction retinal detachment, vitreous hemorrhage, macular edema, epiretinal membrane formation, or macular holes.[210] Vascular hamartomas, which are characterized by small moss fiberlike, minimally elevated vascular lesions in the superficial retina usually adjacent to a retinal vein have also been described.[311] Exophytic hemangioblastomas are less common and arise from the outer retinal layers, often in the peripapillary area;[118,386] they should be differentiated from peripapillary neovascularization, juxtapapillary choroiditis, and papilledema. More posterior optic nerve hemangioblastomas may present as a progressive optic neuropathy or a chiasmal syndrome.[19,122,162,177,250] These latter lesions should be differentiated from optic nerve sheath meningioma or optic neuritis.[300]

The retinal, optic nerve, and central nervous system vascular tumors are indistinguishable in histologic appearance and are best classified as hemangioblastomas.[122,130] They consist of vascular endothelial-lined channels separated by vacuolated "foam" cells. The tumors consist of three main cell types: endothelial cells, pericytes, and lipid-laden interstitial stromal cells—the foam cells. In contrast to the normal situation, the tumor endothelial cells are fenestrated, explaining the high prevalence of exudation from these vascular tumors.

The management of retinal hemangioblastomas depends on their location and size. They are often not symptomatic until serious damage occurs due to complications such as hemorrhage, retinal detachment, or macular edema. Spontaneous regression of retinal hemangioblastomas has been described but is exceptional.[378] Generally, hemangioblastomas progressively enlarge, hence the advantage of early detection and prophylactic treatment. Several treatment modalities have been used, including cryotherapy, xenon arc photocoagulation, diathermy, laser photocoagulation, radiotherapy, and local resection.[10,18,182,293] Small peripheral tumors are best treated with argon laser photocoagulation sometimes enhanced by fluorescein to improve uptake.[11,124,193,293] Cryotherapy can be applied to larger peripheral tumors.[293]

Genetics

The gene for VHL disease was identified in 1993, 5 years after its localization to the short arm of chromosome 3p25-p26.[194,216] The cDNA consists of three exons that encode 284 amino acids. There is also 0.3 kb of 5′ sequence that does not appear to contribute additional exons. There is a long 3′ sequence that is not translated. The promoter region has recently been characterized.[188] There is some evidence that the VHL protein is a nuclear protein, possibly with some capability of moving between the nucleus and cytosol. It may function by forming specific multiprotein complexes in the cytoplasm.[83] Furthermore, it may act as a controller of a cellular transcription factor, elongin (SIII), which is a heterotrimer that activates transcription elongation by RNA polymerase II.[84]

Phenotype–Genotype Correlation. Von Hippel-Lindau disease has been broadly divided into two phenotypes:

- Type 1: VHL without pheochromocytoma
- Type 2: VHL with pheochromocytoma
  - Without renal cell carcinoma or pancreatic cysts
  - With renal cell carcinoma or pancreatic cysts

Almost half of the VHL intragenic mutations are missense mutations. Missense mutations at codon 238 account for 9% of patients with VHL disease—reflecting the deamination of 5-methyl cytosine at a CpG dinucleotide. There are no phenotypic differences between patients with nonoverlapping 5′ and 3′ gene deletions. However, whereas pheochromocytoma is uncommon in patients with germline deletions, insertions, or nonsense mutations, most patients with pheochromocytoma have missense mutations.[51,63] In particular, the substitution of an arginine residue at codon 238 is associated with a high risk of pheochromocytoma.[51,63] Furthermore, there were no differences in the incidence of renal cell carcinoma or retinal or cerebellar hemangioblastomas between families with large deletions, missense mutations, and frameshift or nonsense mutations.

Screening and Presymptomatic Diagnosis

The early diagnosis of complications in VHL such as retinal hemangioblastomas and renal cell carcinoma reduces morbidity and mortality.[172,217] The Cambridge screening protocol is given in Table 36.7. One should be cautious in using epididymal, pancreatic, or renal cysts as diagnostic criteria (Table 36.5), as they are common in the general population. Gadolinium-enhanced MRI in two separate sessions is the most useful way of screening for brain and spinal cord hemangioblastomas.

Mutation analysis is possible in about 75% of families.[253] Patients with large germline deletions and nonsense and frameshift mutations have a lower risk of pheochromocytoma than patients with missense mutations. The availability of linkage studies enables us to perform presymptomatic diagnosis and appropriate screening in selected families.

Table 36.7. Recommended Cambridge Screening Protocol for von Hippel-Lindau Disease[220]

Affected Patient

1. Annual physical examination and urine testing
2. Annual direct and indirect ophthalmoscopy with fluorescein angioscopy or angiography
3. Magnetic resonance imaging (MRI) or computed tomography (CT) of brain every 3 years to age 50 and every 5 years thereafter
4. Annual renal ultrasound
5. 24-hour urine collection for vanilyl mandelic acids (VMAs)

Relatives at Risk

1. Annual physical examination and urine testing.
2. Annual direct and indirect ophthalmoscopy from age 5. Annual fluorescein angioscopy or angiography from age 10 until age 60.
3. MRI or CT of brain every 3 years from age 15 to 40 years and then every 5 years until age 60.
4. Annual renal ultrasound scan with abdominal CT scan every 3 years from age 20 to 65 years.
5. 24-hour urine collection for VMAs.

Tuberous Sclerosis (Bourneville Disease)

Introduction and History

Bourneville used the adjective "tuberous" in his original description of the disease because the protuberances from the gyri of patients were reminiscent of tubers.[35] The term "sclerosis" was added later to reflect the firmness of these tumors. The classic Vogt triad of seizures, mental retardation, and facial angiofibromas[362] is only present in a minority of patients but is diagnostic when present. The term "tuberous sclerosis complex" (TSC) is also used now to describe the disease. Diagnostic criteria have been revised a number of times, lastly by Roach and co-workers[294] who divided clinical and radiographic findings into primary, secondary, and tertiary diagnostic features (Table 36.8). Patients will be given a definite diagnosis of tuberous sclerosis if they either have one primary feature, two secondary features, or one secondary plus two tertiary features. Probable tuberous sclerosis is diagnosed in the presence of either one secondary plus one tertiary feature or three tertiary features. Patients are tuberous sclerosis suspects if they have either one secondary feature or two tertiary features. TSC has an incidence of 1 in 10,000 and is characterized by the development of benign tumors in multiple organ systems from all primary germ layers. The majority of lesions are classified as hamartomas.

Clinical Features

The most common, yet not specific, skin lesion is the hypopigmented ashleaf spot. Eighty-six percent of patients have these 1 to 2 cm hypomelanotic macules, best detected with Wood's

Table 36.8. Diagnostic Criteria for Tuberous Sclerosis Complex[294]

Diagnostic Features	Confirmation
Primary Features	
Facial angiofibromas (adenoma sebaceum)	Clinical
Multiple ungual fibromas	Clinical
Cortical tuber	Histological
Subependymal nodule or giant cell astrocytoma	Histological
Multiple calcified subependymal nodules protruding into the ventricle	Radiographic
Multiple retinal astrocytomas	Clinical
Secondary Features	
Affected first-degree relative	—
Cardiac rhabdomyoma	Histological or radiographic
Other retinal hamartoma or achromic patch	Clinical
Cerebral tubers	Radiographic
Noncalcified subependymal nodules	Radiographic
Shagreen patch	Clinical
Forehead plaque	Clinical
Pulmonary lymphangiomatosis	Histological
Renal angiomyolipoma	Histological or radiographic
Renal cysts	Histological
Tertiary Features	
Hypomelanotic macules	Clinical
"Confetti" skin lesions	Clinical
Renal cysts	Radiographic
Randomly distributed enamel pits in deciduous and/or permanent teeth	Clinical
Hamartomatous rectal polyps	Histological
Bone cysts	Radiographic
Pulmonary lymphangiomatosis	Radiographic
Cerebral white-matter "migration tracts" or heterotopias	Radiographic
Gingival fibroma	Clinical
Hamartoma of other organs	Histological
Infantile spasms	Clinical

lamp. Diagnostic cutaneous lesions include facial angiofibromas in 47% of patients and subungual fibromas. First noted when patients are between 3 and 5 years of age, facial angiofibromas progress until young adulthood (Fig. 36.14). They are small, often confluent, red, raised nodules and may be treated by repeated dermabrasion. Typical locations are the nasolabial folds, the malar areas, and on the chin. Individual tumors are composed of hyperplastic connective and vascular tissue. Fibrous forehead plaques and shagreen patches are considered secondary diagnostic criteria. Shagreen patches are confluent areas of skin tumor with a waxy, yellowish brown or flesh-colored appearance and are most often present on the forehead, back, or legs. Ashleaf spots and confetti skin lesions are considered tertiary diagnostic criteria. Secondary features that support a diagnosis of the TSC include cardiac rhabdomyomas in 43% of patients, mostly in the interventricular septum or in the ventricular wall, pulmonary lymphangiomatosis, renal angiomyolipomas in 50%–80% of patients, and renal cysts. Renal tumors and cysts are usually asymptomatic, but patients may have hematuria and pain and may develop renal failure with hypertension. Tertiary diagnostic features of TSC include hamartomatous rectal polyps, bone cysts, gingival fibromas, and hamartomas of other organs. Seventy-one percent of patients with TSC have pits of the tooth enamel usually located on the outer surfaces of the teeth and away from the gingiva.

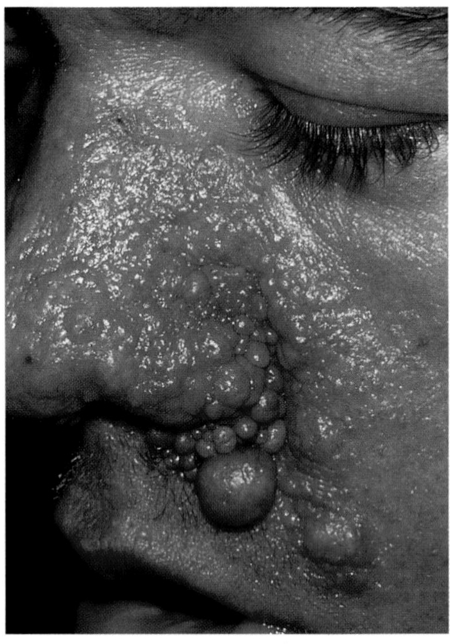

Figure 36.14. Characteristic facial angiofibromatous rash on the nose of an adult with tuberous sclerosis.

All patients with TSC have central nervous system involvement, but the extent and severity of symptoms varies widely among patients, among families, and within families. The cerebellum is involved in less than 15% of patients and the spinal cord is rarely affected. The most typical MRI abnormality on neuroimaging is a high signal lesion involving the cerebral cortex that corresponds to the cortical hamartoma (tuber). T2-weighted images are helpful in detecting cortical tubers, whereas subependymal nodules are better demonstrated with T1-weighted images. Giant cell astrocytomas of the brain occur in 2% of patients. The tubers of TSC occur predominantly at the gray-white matter interface. They are characterized by loss of normal cortical cytoarchitecture and the presence of abnormal neurons and glial cells.[292] The subependymal nodules usually line the third ventricle. They are composed of densely aggregated and uniformly appearing large irregular cells. The nodules may grow to a size of 3 cm or more and are then termed subependymal giant cell astrocytomas.

About 40% of patients with TS are mentally subnormal. Sixty percent of patients have seizures.[370] The severity of seizures correlates with the degree of mental retardation. Patients who have seizures in the first year of life are usually more severely affected. In infancy patients may have myoclonus, infantile spasms, and hypsarrhythmias on electroencephalography. Tonic seizures are most common after age 1 year. Other types of seizures may coexist. Some patients are autistic. Hyperactivity, screaming, and self-injurious behavior are other neuropsychiatric manifestations of TSC and are not necessarily correlated with mental retardation. Patients with TSC have a small decrease in overall survival compared with the general population; this is a result of excess mortality from status epilepticus, obstructive hydrocephalus, renal failure, renal carcinoma, and pulmonary complications such as pneumonia and recurrent pneumothorax.[322]

Ophthalmic Features

The optic nerve and retinal tumors of TSC were first described by Van der Hoeve in 1920.[356] Forty-eight percent of 116 patients from the Mayo Clinic had retinal or optic nerve lesions.[259] Two morphologic types of retinal hamartomata have been recognized: (1) a more common, relatively flat and translucent, soft-appearing lesion usually located in the peripheral fundus and (2) an elevated, nodular, calcific mulberrylike lesion (Fig. 36.15). The mulberry lesions are typically located in the posterior pole adjacent to the optic nerve but may be found anywhere in the fundus. An intermediate type of lesion with features of the translucent and the mulberry types may also be encountered. Most retinal tumors are static in size and appearance. Some, however, grow and become calcific with time.[183,259,390] Zimmer-Galler and Robertson reported on photographic follow-up of 37 retinal lesions in 16 patients with TSC over an average of 16 years.[390] They found that hamartomas in three patients showed progressive or new calcification; one patient developed a new hamartoma in a site that was previously documented to be normal; the rest of the hamartomas appeared unchanged over the follow-up period. These authors concluded that most astrocytic hamartomas remain stable and change little with time, that translucent lesions do not necessarily develop into mulberry lesions, that calcification occurs in utero or early in life, and that lesions generally do not increase in number with time except rarely when new translucent tumors arise in older individuals. Shami et al.[319] studied several translucent lesions in a 7-day-old baby, documenting the intrauterine development of these lesions. Centrally located tumors have been postulated to become large, multinodular, and calcific and

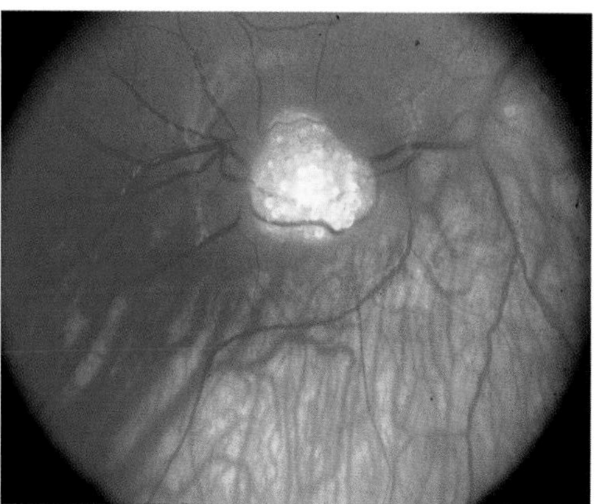

Figure 36.15. Astrocytic hamartoma of the retina in a patient with tuberous sclerosis.

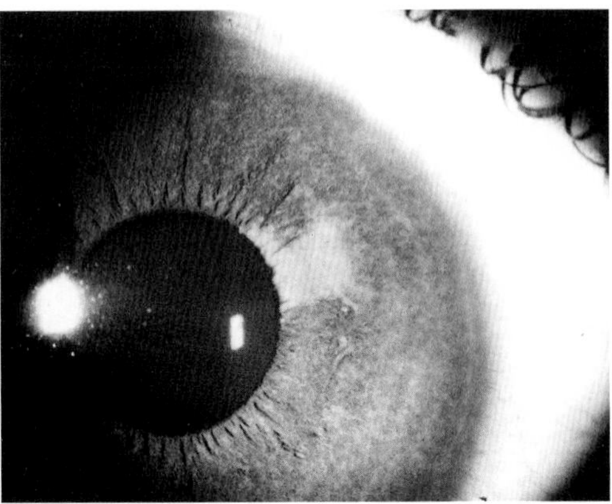

Figure 36.16. Ash-leaf lesion of iris of patient with confirmed tuberous sclerosis.

resemble hyaline bodies or giant drusen.[230] Mulberry tumors are rarely complicated by vitreous hemorrhage[16,183,356] or glaucoma. They never undergo malignant degeneration. Tumors are composed of astrocytes with small oval nuclei and long processes. They contain large blood vessels and calcific deposits.

Other ocular findings include peripheral depigmented or hyperpigmented RPE lesions, atypical colobomata, optic atrophy, eyelid angiofibromas, white patches of the iris (Fig. 36.16) or eyelashes, and strabismus. Van der Hoeve[356] and de Juan et al.[74] have described release of tumor granules into the vitreous. Papilledema and sixth nerve palsy may result from hydrocephalus secondary to brain tumors.

Genetics

Tuberous sclerosis (TS) is inherited in an autosomal dominant fashion with a rate of about 60% new mutations. The trait is highly penetrant with a moderate variability in symptoms within families[328] and no evidence of anticipation. Nonpenetrance is rare but has been documented.[6,371] The first TSC gene was mapped in 1987 to the long arm of chromosome 9 near the ABO blood group locus. Evidence for genetic heterogeneity soon followed when the disease in some families did not map to the TSC1 locus on 9q34. A consortium of researchers finally mapped another locus TSC2 to 16p13.3, near the autosomal dominant polycystic kidney gene ADPKD. The gene was cloned in 1993[60] and several deletion mutations have been identified. The gene encodes a 5.5-kb transcript expressed in a wide range of tissues. The protein product was named tuberin and has a region of homology to the Rap1 activator Rap 1-GAP. The 16p gene is presumed to function as a tumor suppressor gene. It is now estimated that TSC1 and TSC2 each account for about 50% of cases of TSC.

Genetic counseling may be difficult in some families with TSC where some relatives have soft clinical signs of the disease but do not fulfill the minimal diagnostic criteria. In the absence of DNA testing, an extensive screening protocol with cutaneous, neuroradiological, cardiac, renal and ophthalmological evaluations should be used to screen first-degree relatives before counseling is given. Even if extensive screening of parents is negative, a recurrence risk of 2% in subsequent pregnancies should be given. Prenatal diagnosis is now possible using mutation analysis of the *TSC2* gene. Fetal ultrasonography and MRI studies have also been used to detect cardiac and brain tumors, but their sensitivity and specificity are suboptimal.

Sturge-Weber Syndrome (Encephalotrigeminal Angiomatosis)

Diagnosis

The condition is characterized by the classic triad of nevus flammeus (port-wine stain) of the face, leptomeningeal angiomatosis with cerebral gyriform calcifications, and choroidal hemangioma with or without glaucoma; these signs were first described by Sturge in 1897[340] (Weber described the radiological findings in 1922[372]). It is important to note that between 85% and 92% of patients with port-wine facial nevi do not have brain or eye problems.[90,345] The presence of the hemangioma, however, prompts the investigation for ocular or brain pathology. Not all patients have all three components of the syndrome, but two are required for the diagnosis. There are no patients with neurologic and ocular disease without a cutaneous hemangioma.

Clinical Features

The facial angioma occurs along the distribution of the ophthalmic, maxillary and, rarely,

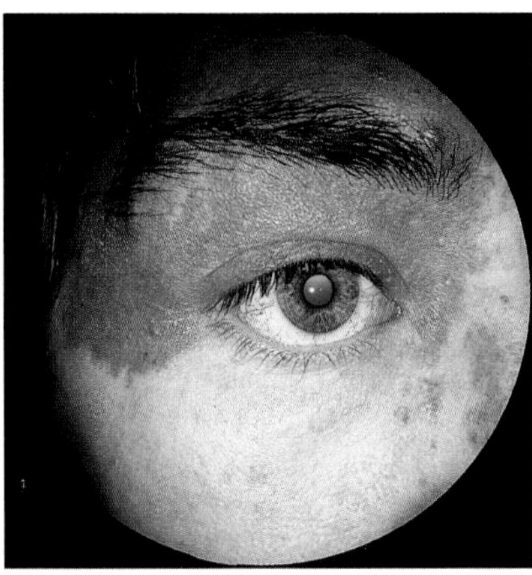

Figure 36.17. Nevus flammeus of the face in an adult with Sturge-Weber syndrome.

mandibular divisions of the trigeminal nerve (Fig. 36.17). It may extend into the region of the upper cervical nerves. The lesion usually stops along the facial midline but may cross it. The flat angioma, which consists of dermal ectatic capillary to venular-sized blood vessels, may become nodular or verrucous with age. The port-wine stain does not regress and does not respond to sclerosing agents or topical steroids but is currently treated successfully with the carbon dioxide laser.

The central nervous system vascular malformations are most often confined to the pial vessels of the occipitoparietal area. The slow flow of blood through these vessels leads to hypoxia, encephalomalacia, cortical atrophy, and subsequent calcification. Fifty-four percent of patients are developmentally delayed and 31% have contralateral hemiplegia. The majority of patients have intracranial calcifications with a characteristic "tram-line" pattern. The affected hemisphere may be smaller in size and there usually is a variety of vascular anomalies of circulation and perfusion.

About 80% of patients with the Sturge-Weber syndrome develop focal or generalized seizures because of CNS involvement.[15,341] The presence of seizure activity in the first year of life is a poor prognostic factor and, in one series,[260] all patients who had seizures in the first year of life were not able to live independently and none of those with early neurologic symptomatology was able to maintain gainful employment or was married. In another series of 52 adults with Sturge-Weber syndrome, Sujansky and Conradi compared the prevalence of developmental delay, emotional and behavioral problems, special education requirements, and employability between patients with seizures and those without; the percentages were 43% versus 0% for delay, 85% versus 58% for emotional and behavioral problems, 71% versus 0% for special education requirements and 46% versus 78% for employability.[341] Thirty-nine percent of patients in their series were financially self-sufficient, 55% were or could be married, and 10 patients produced a total of 20 liveborn offspring, the majority of whom were healthy and had no signs of the syndrome. In a series of 23 children with Sturge-Weber syndrome and seizures, Arzimanoglou and Aicardi found seizure activity to be the only neurologic symptom in 6 patients; seizures were associated with developmental delay in 13 patients, with permanent hemiplegia in 10 and with hemianopsia in 15.[15] Late onset of seizures was associated with better functional outcome but with more resistance to control of activity with medications. Nine of the 23 patients required surgery for seizure control.[15] These authors recommend initial management of seizures with antiepileptic medications, with vigorous management of emergent episodes of status epilepticus to prevent postconvulsive hemiplegia. When medications fail, surgery is considered after neuroimaging assures monohemispheric involvement.[15]

Medical therapy for the seizures is usually disappointing and a number of medications may be used concurrently without success. Excision of the involved cortical areas, or even a hemispherectomy have been used with encouraging results in patients in whom seizures are refractory to medical treatment.[262]

Ophthalmic Features

Thirty percent of patients with Sturge-Weber syndrome develop glaucoma, 60% before age 2 years with buphthalmos (Fig. 36.18), and 40% in late childhood or young adulthood.[54] In a series of 51 patients examined at the Hospital for Sick Children, Toronto as part of their systemic evaluation, Sullivan et al.[342] found 36 (71%) with glaucoma and commented that this percentage is a more accurate estimate of the

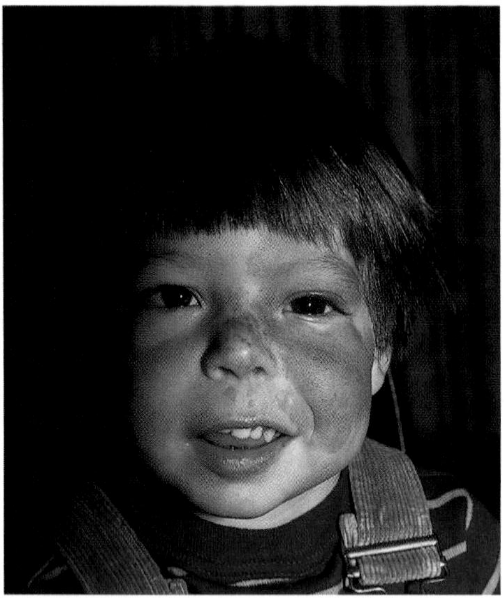

Figure 36.18. Two-year-old boy with Sturge-Weber syndrome and ipsilateral glaucoma. Intraocular pressure was well controlled by administration of a topical beta-blocking agent. (Courtesy of Dr. John F. O'Neill.)

prevalence of glaucoma in this syndrome. Twenty-one patients had unilateral and 15 had bilateral disease. Two-thirds of these patients had onset of their glaucoma before the age of 2 years and the rest after age 5. Episcleral hemangiomas were present in 69% of patients (Fig. 36.19) and choroidal hemangiomas in 55%. Sixty-seven percent of glaucomatous eyes had visual acuity of 20/40 or better or maintained central and steady fixation in both eyes. Congenital glaucoma in the Sturge-Weber syndrome is almost always associated with involvement of both lids and the areas of distribution V1 and V2 branches of the trigeminal nerve by the port-wine stain.[342] In general, the more extensive the hemangioma, the more severe the glaucoma and the earlier its presentation. Glaucoma can be associated with hemangiomas of the lid without intracranial involvement. Eyes with raised intraocular pressure all have episcleral hemangiomas, whereas not all eyes with choroidal hemangiomas have increased intraocular pressure. The proposed mechanisms for the development of glaucoma include *(1)* outflow obstruction because of abnormal angle development and vascularization of the iris, *(2)* elevated episcleral pressure with reduced outflow,[272] *(3)* secondary angle closure in older patients with choroidal hemangioma, retinal detachment, and neovascular glaucoma, *(4)* hypersecretion of aqueous humor, *(5)* hyperpermeability of blood vessel walls of choroidal hemangioma, and *(6)* adult open-angle glaucoma mechanisms.

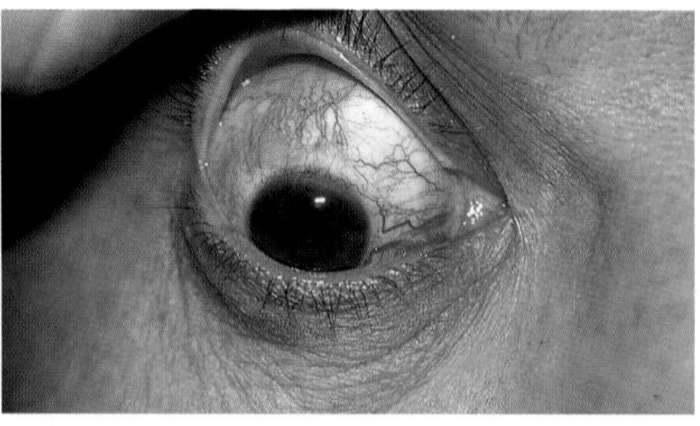

Figure 36.19. Dilated episcleral vessels in a patient with Sturge-Weber syndrome. (Courtesy of Dr. John F. Gillis.)

Although the corneal diameter is enlarged, there are usually no horizontal breaks in Descemet's membrane.[342] Gonioscopy and histopathologic studies reveal an angle pattern suggestive of goniodysgenesis in infantile cases; the uveal meshwork is thick, the scleral spur is poorly developed, the iris insertion may be high, and there may be a Barkan's membrane.[53,54,342] There may also be vascularization of the angle and trabecular meshwork.[246] The histopathologic changes of the anterior chamber angle in older patients are similar to those of simple open-angle glaucoma.[54,165,272,338]

Glaucoma generally does not respond well to topical medical treatment. However, 8 of the 36 patients reported by Sullivan et al.[342] did not require surgery; their intraocular pressure was controlled on medications alone. Furthermore, medications are useful in maintaining good control of the intraocular pressure after surgery.[165] Goniotomy or trabeculotomy in infants,[165] and trabeculotomy with or without trabeculectomy[1,30] in older children and adults, have been used in patients with Sturge-Weber syndrome with varying degrees of success. Surgery may be complicated by intraoperative serous choroidal detachment and occasionally by suprachoroidal hemorrhage. Four of 17 patients reported by Iwach et al. developed uveal effusions and choroidal detachments following trabeculectomy.[165] Sullivan et al.[342] gave details of surgical complications in 101 procedures in

41 eyes. Shihab et al. advocated the use of prophylactic posterior sclerostomies that are left open before the anterior chamber is entered in a filtering procedure.[323] The tightness of the scleral flap of a trabeculectomy should be adjusted to avoid over filtration. The problem of fibrosis of the scleral fistula is the same as in other young patients and there may be a role for the adjunctive use of antimetabolite.[241,377] Thus, it is reasonable to start patients with Sturge-Weber syndrome on topical beta-blockers and carbonic anhydrase inhibitors as soon as their glaucoma is diagnosed. If the intraocular pressure is controlled, surgery may be avoided or delayed. If the pressure remains elevated, a goniotomy or a trabeculotomy are most likely the initial procedures of choice. Filtering procedures with or without antimetabolites could be performed next.

Choroidal cavernous hemangiomas occur in about 40% of patients and may be isolated or diffuse. They are most often located temporal to the optic disc and are most elevated in the macular area. Hemangiomas do not cause any visual disturbances early in life but may lead to the late development of overlying retinal cystoid changes or exudative retinal detachment.

Other ocular findings in Sturge-Weber syndrome include heterochromia irides, conjunctival angioma, dilatation of episcleral vessels, and retinal aneurysms associated with an arteriovenous angioma of the thalamus and midbrain. Visual field defects may be present in patients with occipital lobe meningeal involvement and cortical atrophy. Shin and Demer[324] described retinal arteriovenous communicating vessels in a 7-year-old patient with ipsilateral episcleral dilated vessels, and glaucoma but no choroidal hemangioma. The arteriovenous communicating channels were direct without the interposition of capillary or arteriolar elements and with a hyperdynamic flow pattern in the involved vessels.

Genetics and Pathogenesis

There are no reports of familial occurrence of Sturge-Weber syndrome. The condition may be more prevalent in Caucasians than in other races.[342] The only reported chromosomal abnormalities are a fragile site on 10q24 in a young boy with the syndrome[351] and a supernumerary bisatellited chromosome in a patient and several unaffected family members.[72]

It is hypothesized that the primary lesion in Sturge-Weber is a defective structural differentiation of the vascular wall and persistence of the sinusoid embryonal character of the vascular bed in the region of angiomatosis. This leads to fibrosis, hyaline degeneration, dilatation and calcification of the vascular walls with venous stasis, obliteration of the lumen, recurrent thrombotic events, and transient ischemic attacks and gradual neurologic deterioration. Another possible embryological basis for the syndrome is a defective migration and differentiation of the pro- and mesencephalic neural crest leading to abnormal proliferation of blood vessels and goniodysgenesis.

OTHER SYNDROMES WITH HEMANGIOMATOUS OR VASCULAR LESIONS

Klippel-Trenaunay-Weber syndrome is comprised of nevus flammeus of the face and extremities associated with hypertrophy of the underlying soft tissues and bone.[179]

In cutis marmorata telangiectatica, there is widespread reticulated marbleization of the skin from prominent veins and capillaries.[332] Patients may also have a nevus flammeus and congenital glaucoma.

Cavernous Hemangioma Syndrome

Clinical Features

Weskamp and Cotlier[375] were the first to report the association of cavernous hemangioma of the retina with similar lesions of the skin and brain (Figs. 36.20–36.22). Since then a number of families have been reported with this neuro-oculo-cutaneous syndrome.[81,116,125,140,265] The inheritance is autosomal dominant with high penetrance and variable expressivity.

Central nervous system tumors may lead to headaches, seizures, and strokes that may be fatal; but lesions can be asymptomatic and may

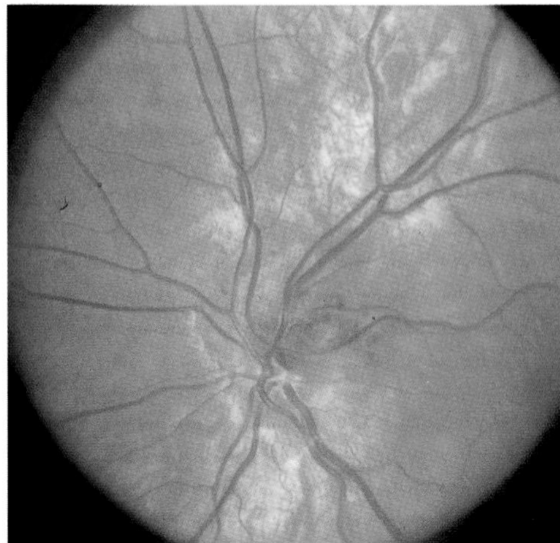

Figure 36.20. Optic nerve head cavernous hemangioma misdiagnosed as papilledema. (Courtesy of Dr. John F. Gillis.)

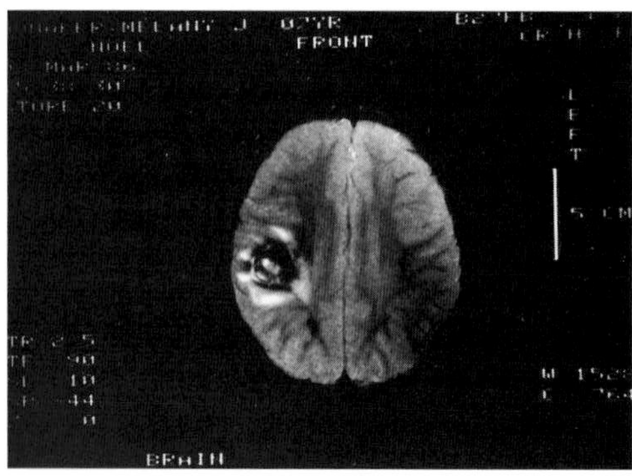

Figure 36.22. Magnetic resonance imaging scan of the head in same patient shows cavernous hemangioma (documented histopathologically after excision). (Courtesy of Dr. John F. Gillis.)

only be detected by brain imaging studies. The prevalence of intracranial hemorrhage varies from 12%–48%.[81] Hayman and colleagues[140] recommended neuroimaging of all first-degree relatives of patients with intracranial cavernous hemangiomas. CNS hemangiomas may be excised depending on their location and on symptomatology.

Cutaneous lesions are the least common component of the syndrome and are absent in certain families.[81] Retinal cavernous hemangiomas have also been associated with angioma serpiginosum in which there is progressive widespread dilation of the subpapillary venous plexuses.[119]

Retinal Tumors

Retinal hemangiomas are usually single at the disc or in the fundus periphery but may be bilateral.[32,125] Ten percent of lesions occur in the macular area.[32,234] The hemangioma arises from the inner retinal layers and consists of thin-walled saccular aneurysms filled with dark blood; it appears like a cluster of grapes and may be covered with a fibroglial membrane (Fig. 36.23).[234] The tumors do not enlarge, but

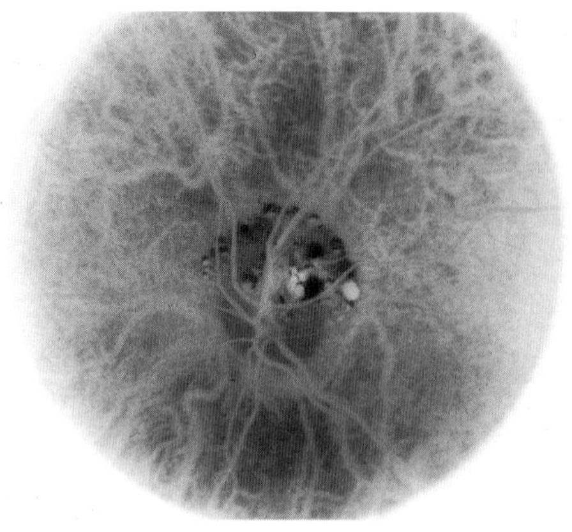

Figure 36.21. Fluorescein angiogram of lesion shown in Figure 36.20, delineating vascular spaces, some of which have a red blood cell–serum interface. (Courtesy of Dr. John F. Gillis.)

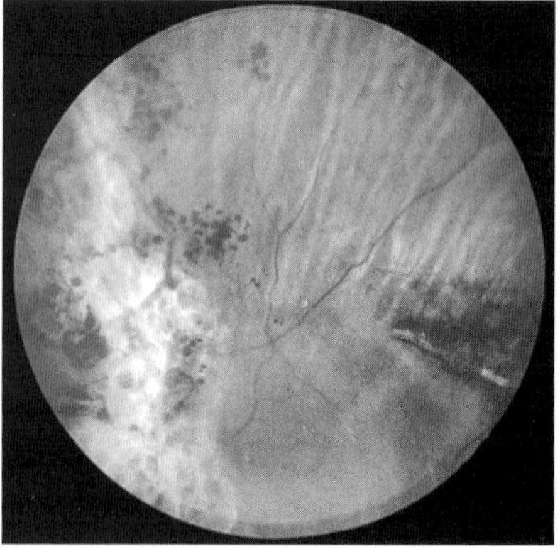

Figure 36.23. Cavernous hemangioma of the retina. The vascular malformation looks like clusters of grapes. There is associated fibrosis and some pigment migration. The patient also had a central nervous system hemangioma.

the vascular saccules may thrombose. Fluorescein angiography is diagnostic and shows a red blood cell–plasma level in each saccule; there is no leakage of dye from the lesion. Ocular complications are rare, but patients may present with a vitreous hemorrhage.[116] When the hemorrhage occurs in a child, strabismus and amblyopia may develop.[384] Messmer and co-workers[236] reported the ocular histopathological findings in the eye of a 6-month-old girl who presented with total retinal detachment and a widespread cavernous hemangioma of the retina. Twin vessels, defined as paired retinal arterioles and venules, separated by less than one venule width, located at least two disk diameter from the disk and extending for a distance of more than one disk diameter, have been reported in four of six affected members of a family with cavernous hemangioma syndrome.[32] The same type of vessels has been reported in von Hippel-Lindau disease, and may represent an early diagnostic sign of the disease.[73] De Jong and co-workers[73] found twin vessels in 5.5% of normal individuals and in 64% of patients with von Hippel-Lindau syndrome.

No treatment is necessary for the retinal angiomas in the vast majority of patients. Laser photocoagulation may be used to ablate the tumor in case of vitreous hemorrhage.[178]

REFERENCES

1. Agarwal HC, Sandramouli S, Sihota R, Sood NN. Sturge-Weber syndrome: management of glaucoma with combined trabeculotomy-trabeculectomy. *Ophthalmic Surg* 1993;24: 399–402.
2. Ainsworth P, Rodenhiser D, Stuart A, Jung J. Characterization of an intron 31 splice junction mutation in the neurofibromatosis type 1 (NF1) gene. *Hum Mol Genet* 1994;3:1179–1181.
3. Ainsworth PJ, Rodenhiser DI, Costa MT. Identification and characterization of sporadic and inherited mutations in exon 31 of the neurofibromatosis (NF1) gene. *Hum Genet* 1993;91:151–156.
4. Akenside M. Observations on cancers. *Med Trans* 1768; 1:64–92.
5. Aldrovandi U. *Monstrorum historia. Cum paralipomenis historiae omnium animalium. Bononiae, typis nicolai tibaldini,* Bologna, 1642, cited in reference 388.
6. Al-Gazali L, Arthur R, Lamb J, Hammer H, Coker T, Hirschmann P, et al. Diagnostic and counseling difficulties using a fully comprehensive screening protocol for families at risk for tuberous sclerosis. *J Med Genet* 1989;26: 694–703.
7. Allanson JE, Upadhyaya M, Watson GH, Partington M, MacKenzie A, Lahey D, et al. Watson syndrome—Is it a subtype of type 1 neurofibromatosis? *J Med Genet* 1991;28: 752–756.
8. Alliez J, Masse J-L, Alliez B. Tumeurs bilatérles de l'acoustique et maladie de Recklinghausen observées dans plusieurs générations. *Rev Neurol* 1975;131:545–558.
9. Andersen LB, Ballester R, Marchuk DA, Chang E, Gutmann DH, Saulino M, et al. A conserved alternative splice in the von Recklinghausen neurofibromatosis (NF1) gene produces two neurofibromin isoforms, both of which have GTPase protein activity. *Mol Cell Biol* 1993;13:487–495.
10. Annesley WH, Leonard BC, Shields JA, Tasman WS. Fifteen year review of treated cases of retinal angiomatosis. *Trans Am Acad Ophthalmol Otolaryngol* 1977;83:446–453.
11. Apple DJ, Goldberg MF, Wyhinny GJ. Argon laser treatment of von Hippel-Lindau retinal angiomas. II. Histopathology of treated lesions. *Arch Ophthalmol* 1974;92:126–130.
12. Argenyi ZB, Thieberg MD, Hayes CM, Whitaker DC. Primary cutaneous meningioma associated with von Recklinghausen's disease. *J Cutan Pathol* 1994;21:549–556.
13. Arnozan X, Prioleau L. Sur les dermatofibromes congénitaux généralisés. *Ann Dermatol Syphil* 1883;2 s, iv:689–698.
14. Arts WFM, Dongen KJV. Intracranial calcified deposits in neurofibromatosis. *J Neurol Neurosurg Psychiatry* 1986;49:1317–1320.
15. Arzimanoglou A, Aicardi J. The epilepsy of Sturge-Weber syndrome clinical features and treatment in 23 patients. *Acta Neurol Scand* 1992(Suppl);140:18–22.
16. Atkinson A, Sanders M, Wong V. Vitreous hemorrhage in tuberous sclerosis: report of two cases. *Br J Ophthalmol* 1973;57:773–779.
17. Bacin F, Kemeny JL, D'Hermies F, Rozan R, Decroix P, Dalens H, et al. Mélanome malin de la choroïde associé à une neurofibromatose. *J Fr Ophthalmol* 1993;16: 184–190.

18. Balazs E, Berta A, Rozsa L, Kolozsvari L, Rigo G. Hemodynamic changes after ruthenium irradiation of Hippel's angiomatosis. *Ophthalmologica* 1990;200:128–132.
19. Balcer LJ, Galetta SL, Curtis M, Maguire A, Judy K. Von Hippel-Lindau disease manifesting as a chiasmal syndrome. *Surv Ophthalmol* 1995;39:302–306.
19a. Ballester R, Marchuk D, Boguski M, Saulino A, Letcher R, Wigler M, Collins F. The NF1 locus encodes a protein functionally related to mammalian GAP and yeast IRA proteins. *Cell* 1990;63:851–859.
20. Barker D, Wright E, Nguyen K, Cannon L, Fain P, Goldgar D, et al. Gene for von Recklinghausen neurofibromatosis is in the pericentromeric region of chromosome 17. *Science* 1987;236:1100–1102.
21. Baser ME, Mautner V-F, Sainz J, Ragge NK, Nechiporuk A, Klein J, et al. Presymptomatic diagnosis in neurofibromatosis 2 using linked genetic markers, neuroimaging, and ocular examinations. *Neurology* 1996;47:1269–1277.
22. Basoe P, Nuzum F. Report of a case of central and peripheral neurofibromatosis. *J Nerv Ment Dis* 1915;42:785–796.
23. Basu TN, Gutmann DH, Fletcher JA, Glover TW, Collins FS, Downward J. Aberrant regulation of ras proteins in malignant tumor cells from type 1 neurofibromatosis patients. *Nature* 1992;356:713–715.
24. Becker R, Bauer BL, Mennel HD, Plate KH. Cerebellar primitive neuroectodermal tumor with multipotent differentiation in a family with von Hippel-Lindau disease. *Clin Neuropathol* 1993;12:107–111.
25. Benson M, Mody C, Rennie I, Talbot J. Haemangioma of the optic disc. *Graefes Arch Clin Exp Ophthalmol* 1990;228:332–334.
26. Berggrün E. Ein Fall von allgemeiner Neurofibromatose bei einem 11-jährigen Knaben. *Arch Kinderheilkd* 1897;21:89–113.
27. Bianchi AB, Hara T, Ramesh V, Gao J, Klein-Szanto AJP, Morin F, et al. Mutations in transcript isoforms of the neurofibromatosis 2 gene in multiple human tumor types. *Nature Genet* 1994;6:185–193.
28. Biggs GN. A case of multiple intracranial tumours with involvement of both auditory nerves. *Lancet* 1909;2:14–15.
29. Blamires TL, Maher ER. Choroid plexus papilloma: a new presentation of von Hippel-Lindau (VHL) disease. *Eye* 1992;6:90–92.
30. Board J, Shields M. Combined trabeculotomy-trabeculectomy for the management of glaucoma associated with Sturge-Weber syndrome. *Ophthalmic Surg* 1981;12:813–817.
31. Borberg A. Clinical and genetic investigations into tuberous sclerosis and Recklinghausen's neurofibromatosis. *Acta Psychiatr Neurol Scand* 1951;71:1–239.
32. Bottoni F, Canevini M, Canger R, Orzalesi N. Twin vessels in familial retinal cavernous hemangioma. *Am J Ophthalmol* 1990;109:285–289.
33. Bourn D, Carter SA, Evans DGR, Goodship J, Coakham H, Strachan T. A mutation in the neurofibromatosis type 2 tumor suppressor gene, giving rise to widely different clinical phenotypes in two unrelated individuals. *Am J Hum Genet* 1994;55:69–73.
34. Bourn D, Carter SA, Mason S, Evans DGR, Strachan T. Germ-line mutations in the neurofibromatosis 2 gene in multiple tumor types. *Hum Mol Genet* 1994;3:813–816.
35. Bourneville D. Sclérose tubéreuse des circonvolutions cérébrales idiotie et épilepsie hémiplegique. *Arch Neurol* 1880:181–191.
36. Bouzas EA, Freidlin V, Parry DM, Eldridge R, Kaiser-Kupfer MI. Lens opacities in neurofibromatosis 2: further significant correlations. *Br J Ophthalmol* 1993;77:354–357.
37. Bouzas EA, Mastorakos G, Chrousos GP, Kaiser-Kupfer MI. Lisch nodules in Cushing's disease. *Arch Ophthalmol* 1993;111:439–440.
38. Bouzas EA, Parry DM, Eldridge R, Kaiser-Kupfer MI. Familial occurrence of combined pigment epithelial and retinal hamartomas associated with neurofibromatosis 2. *Retina* 1992;12:103–107.
39. Brasfield RD, Gupta TKD. Von Recklinghausen's disease: a clinicopathological study. *Ann Surg* 1972;175:86–104.
40. Briggs RJ, Brackmann DE, Baser ME, Hitselberger WE. Comprehensive management of bilateral acoustic neuromas: current perspectives. *Arch Otolaryngol Head Neck Surg* 1994;120:1307–1314.
41. Brownstein S, Little J. Ocular neurofibromatosis. *Ophthalmology* 1983;90:1595–1599.
42. Bruns P. Das Ranken-Neurom. *Virchows Arch* 1870;1:80–112.
43. Burke JP, Leitch RJ, Talbot JF, Parsons MA. Choroidal neurofibromatosis with congenital iris ectropion and buphthalmos: relationship and significance. *J Pediatr Ophthalmol Strabismus* 1991;28:265–267.
44. Carey JC, Laub JM, Hall BD. Penetrance and variability in neurofibromatosis: A genetic study of 60 families. *Birth Defects Orig Art Ser* 1979;15(5B):271–281.
45. Carnevale A, Santillan Y. Effect of the sex of the progenitor on the clinical manifestations

of neurofibromatosis. *Rev Invest Clin* 1991;43:359–363.

46. Cawthon R, Weiss R, Xu G, Viskochil D, Culver M, Stephens J, et al. A major segment of the neurofibromatosis type 1 gene: cDNA sequence, genomic structure, and point mutations. *Cell* 1990;62:193–201.
47. Cawthon RM, O'Connell P, Buchberg AM, Viskochil D, Weiss RB, Culver M, et al. Identification and characterization of transcripts from the neurofibromatosis 1 region: the sequence and genomic structure of EV12 and mapping of other transcripts. *Genomics* 1990;7:555–565.
48. Cendron M, Wein AJ, Schwartz SS, Murtagh F, Livoli VA, Tomaszewski JE. Germ cell tumor of testis in a patient with von Hippel-Lindau disease. *Urology* 1991;37:69–71.
49. Charles SJ, Moore AT, Yates JRW, Ferguson-Smith MA. Lisch nodules in neurofibromatosis type 2. *Arch Ophthalmol* 1989;107:1571–1572.
50. Chauffard MA. Dermo-fibromatose pigmentaire (ou neuro-fibromatose généralisée) Mort par adénome des capsules surrénales et du pancréas. *Bull Mem Soc Med Hop Paris* 1896;13:777–784.
51. Chen F, Kishida T, Yao M, Hustad T, Glavac D, Dean M, et al. Germline mutations in the von Hippel-Lindau disease tumor suppressor gene: correlations with phenotype. *Hum Mutat* 1995;5:66–75.
52. Choyke PL, Glenn GM, Walther MM, Zbar B, Weiss GH, Alexander RB, et al. The natural history of renal lesions in von Hippel-Lindau disease: a serial CT study in 28 patients. *Am J Roentgenol* 1992;159:1229–1234.
53. Christensen G, Records E. Glaucoma and expulsive hemorrhage mechanisms in the Sturge-Weber syndrome. *Ophthalmology* 1979;86:1360–1366.
54. Cibis G, Tripathi R, Tripathi B. Glaucoma in Sturge-Weber syndrome. *Ophthalmology* 1984;91:1061–1071.
55. Clarke A, Church W, Gardner-Medwin D, Sengupta R. Intracranial calcification and seizures: A case of central neurofibromatosis. *Dev Med Child Neurol* 1990;32:729–732.
56. Coats G. Unilateral diffuse melanosis of the uvea, with small elevations on the surface of the iris. *Trans Ophthalmol Soc UK* 1912;32:164–171.
57. Collins ET. Two cases, brother and sister, with peculiar vascular new growth, probably primarily retinal, affecting both eyes. *Trans Ophthalmol Soc UK* 1894;14:141–149.
58. Collins ET. Unilateral melanosis of the uvea and sclera, with numerous small elevations on the surface of the iris. *Trans Ophthalmol Soc UK* 1912;32:171–173.
59. Collins ET, Batten RD. Neuro-fibroma of the eyeball and its appendages. *Trans Ophthalmol Soc UK* 1905;25:248–257.
60. Consortium ECTS. Identification and characterization of the tuberous sclerosis gene on chromosome 16. *Cell.* 1993;75:1305–1315.
61. Cotlier E. Café-au-lait spots of the fundus in neurofibromatosis. *Arch Ophthalmol* 1977;95:1990–1993.
62. Crossey PA, Foster K, Richards FM, Phipps ME, Latif F, Tory K, et al. Molecular genetic investigations of the mechanism of tumourigenesis in von Hippel-Lindau disease: analysis of allele loss in VHL tumours. *Hum Genet* 1994;93:53–58.
63. Crossey PA, Richards FM, Foster K, Green JS, Prowse A, Latif F, et al. Identification of intragenic mutations in the von Hippel-Lindau disease tumour suppressor gene and correlation with disease phenotype. *Hum Mol Genet* 1994;3:1303–1308.
64. Crowe FW. Axillary freckling as a diagnostic aid in neurofibromatosis. *Ann Intern Med* 1964;61:1142–1143.
65. Crowe FW, Schull WJ. Diagnostic importance of café-au-lait spot in neurofibromatosis. *Arch Intern Med* 1953;91:758–766.
66. Crowe FW, Schull WJ, Neel JV. *A Clinical, Pathological, and Genetic Study of Multiple Neurofibromatosis.* Springfield, IL: Charles C Thomas, 1956.
67. Cunliffe IA, Moffat DA, Hardy DG, Moore AT. Bilateral optic nerve sheath meningiomas in a patient with neurofibromatosis type 2. *Br J Ophthalmol* 1992;76:310–312.
68. Cushing H. *Tumours of the Nervus Acusticus and the Syndrome of the Cerebello-Pontile Angle.* Philadelphia: W.B. Saunders, 1917.
69. Danglot G, Regnier V, Fauvet D, Vassal G, Kujas M, Bernheim A. Neurofibromatosis 1 (NF1) mRNAs expressed in the central nervous system are differentially spliced in the 5′ part of the gene. *Hum Mol Genet* 1995;4:915–920.
70. Daston MM, Scrable H, Nordlund M, Sturbaum AK, Nissen LM, Ratner N. The protein product of the neurofibromatosis type 1 gene is expressed in highest abundance in neurons, Schwann cells, and oligodendrocytes. *Neuron* 1992;8:415–428.
71. De Bustros S, Miller NR, Finkelstein D, Massof R. Bilateral astrocytic hamartomas of the optic nerve head in retinitis pigmentosa. *Retina* 1983;3:21–23.

72. De Guttierrez A, Salamanca F, Lisker R, Segovia A. Supernumerary bisatellited chromosome in a family ascertained through a patient with Sturge-Weber syndrome. *Ann Genet* 1975;18:45–49.
73. De Jong P, Verkaart R, Van de Vooren M, Majoor-Krakauer D, Wiegel A. Twin vessels in von Hippel-Lindau disease. *Am J Ophthalmol* 1988;105:165.
74. de Juan E Jr, Green W, Gupta P, Baranano E. Vitreous seeding by retinal astrocytic hamartoma in a patient with tuberous sclerosis. *Retina* 1984;4:100–102.
75. DeClue JE, Cohen BD, Lowy DR. Identification and characterization of the neurofibromatosis type 1 protein product. *Proc Natl Acad Sci USA* 1991;88:9914–9918.
76. DeClue JE, Papageorge AG, Fletcher JA, Diehl SR, Ratner N, Vass WC, et al. Abnormal regulation of mammalian p21ras contributes to malignant tumor growth in von Recklinghausen (type 1) neurofibromatosis. *Cell* 1992; 69:265–273.
77. Delisle MB, Uro E, Rouquette I, Yardeni E, Rumeau JL. Papillary neoplasm of the endolymphatic sac in a patient with von Hippel-Lindau disease. *J Clin Pathol* 1994;47: 959–961.
78. Destro M, D'Amico DJ, Gragoudas ES, Brockhurst RJ, Pinnolis MK, Albert DM, et al. Retinal manifestations of neurofibromatosis Diagnosis and management. *Arch Ophthalmol* 1991;109:662–666.
79. DiMario Jr FJ, Ramsby G, Greenstein R, Langshur S, Dunham B. Neurofibromatosis type 1 magnetic resonance imaging. *J Child Neurol* 1993;8:32–39.
80. DiPaolo DP, Zimmerman RA, Rorke LB, Zackai EH, Bilaniuk LT, Yachnis AT. Neurofibromatosis type 1: Pathologic substrate of high-signal-intensity foci in the brain. *Radiology* 1995;195:721–724.
81. Dobyns W, Michels V, Groover R, Mokri B, Trautmann J, Forbes G, et al. Familial cavernous malformations of the central nervous system and retina. *Ann Neurol* 1987;21:578–583.
82. Dossetor FM, Landau K, Hoyt WF. Optic disk glioma in neurofibromatosis type 2. *Am J Ophthalmol* 1989;108:602–603.
83. Duan DR, Humphrey JS, Chen DY, Weng Y, Sukegawa J, Lee S, et al. Characterization of the VHL tumor suppressor gene product localization, complex formation, and the effect of natural inactivating mutations. *Proc Natl Acad Sci USA* 1995;92:6459–6463.
84. Duan DR, Pause A, Burgess WH, Aso T, Chen DY, Garrett KP, et al. Inhibition of transcription elongation by the VHL tumor suppressor protein. *Science* 1995;269:1402–1406.
85. Dublin S, Riccardi VM, Stephens K. Methods for rapid detection of a recurrent nonsense mutation and documentation of phenotypic features in neurofibromatosis type 1. *Hum Mutat* 1995;5:81–85.
86. Dunn DW, Roos KL. Magnetic resonance imaging evaluation of learning difficulties and incoordination in neurofibromatosis. *Neurofibromatosis* 1989;2:1–5.
87. Eldridge R. Central neurofibromatosis with bilateral acoustic neuroma. *Adv Neurol* 1981; 29:57–65.
88. Eldridge R, Parry D. Neurofibromatosis 2: Evidence for Clinical Heterogeneity Based on 54 Affected Individuals Studied by MRI with Gadolinium, 1987–1991. Conference Proceedings, First International Conference on Acoustic Neuroma, Copenhagen, Denmark. Amsterdam: Kugler Publications, 1992.
89. Elyakim S, Lerer I, Zlotogora J, Sagi M, Gelman-Kohan Z, Merin S, Tos M, Thomsen J. Neurofibromatosis type 1 (NF1) in Israeli families: Linkage analysis as a diagnostic tool. *Am J Med Genet* 1994;53:325–334.
90. Enjolras O, Riche M, Merland J. Facial portwine stains and Sturge-Weber syndrome. *Pediatrics* 1985;76:48.
91. Estivill X, Lazaro C, Casals T, Ravella A. Recurrence of a nonsense mutation in the NF1 gene causing classical neurofibromatosis type 1. *Hum Genet* 1991;88:185–188.
92. Evans DG, Bourn D, Wallace A, Ramsden RT, Mitchell JD, Strachan T. Diagnostic issues in a family with late onset type 2 neurofibromatosis. *J Med Genet* 1995;32:470–474.
93. Evans DGR, Huson SM, Donnai D, Neary W, Blair V, Teare D, et al. A genetic study of type 2 neurofibromatosis in the United Kingdom I: Prevalence, mutation rate, fitness and confirmation of maternal transmission effect on severity. *J Med Genet* 1992;29: 841–846.
94. Evans DGR, Huson SM, Neary W, Blair V, Newton V, Strachan T, et al. A genetic study of type 2 neurofibromatosis in the United Kingdom. II. Guidelines for genetic counselling. *J Med Genet* 1992;29:847–852.
95. Evans DGR, Ramsden R, Huson SM, Harris R, Lye R, King TT. Type 2 neurofibromatosis: The need for supraregional care? *J Laryngol Otol* 1993;107:401–406.

96. Evans DRG, Huson SM, Donnai D, Neary W, Blair V, Newton V, et al. A clincial study of type 2 neurofibromatosis. *Q J Med* 1992;84: 603–618.
97. Feiling A, Ward E. A familial form of acoustic tumor. *Br Med J* 1920;1:496–497.
98. Ferner RE, Chaudhuri R, Bingham J, Cox T, Hughes RAC. MRI in neurofibromatosis 1: the nature and evolution of increased intensity T2 weighted lesions and their relationship to intellectual impairment. *J Neurol Neurosurg Psychiatry* 1993;56:492–495.
99. Ferner RE, Hughes RA, Johnson MR. Neurofibromatosis 1 and multiple sclerosis. *J Neurol Neurosurg Psychiatry* 1995;58:582–585.
100. Filling Katz MR, Choyke PL, Oldfield E, Charnas L, Patronas NJ, Glenn GM, et al. Central nervous system involvement in von Hippel-Lindau disease. *Neurology* 1991;41: 41–46.
101. Fischer G, Fischer C, Remond J. Hearing preservation in acoustic neurinoma surgery. *J Neurosurg* 1992;76:910–917.
102. Fleischer B. Zwei Fälle von einseitiger Melanosis der Sklera, der Iria und des Augenhintergrundes mit warzenförmigen, kleinen Erhebungen an der Iris vorderfläche. *Klin Monatsbl Augenheilkd* 1913;51:170–174.
103. Font RL, Moura RA, Shetlar DJ, Martinez JA, McPherson AR. Combined hamartoma of sensory retina and retinal pigment epithelium. *Retina* 1989;9:302–311.
104. Fortini ME, Simon MA, Rubin GM. Signalling by the sevenless protein tyrosine kinase is mimicked by Ras1 activation. *Nature* 1992;355:559–561.
105. Fountain JW, Wallace MR, Bruce MA, Seizinger BR, Menon AG, Gusella JF, et al. Physical mapping of a translocation breakpoint in neurofibromatosis. *Science* 1989;244:1085–1087.
106. Frenkel M. Retinal angiomatosis in a patient with neurofibromatosis. *Am J Ophthalmol* 1967;63:804–808.
107. Friedenwald H, Friedenwald JS. Melanosis of the lids, conjunctiva, and sclera, with wartlike growths on the iris. *Arch Ophthalmol* 1925; 54:51–54.
108. Fuchs E. Naevus pigmentosus und Naevus vasculosus der Iris. *Albrecht von Graefe's Arch Ophthalmol* 1913;86:155–169.
109. Fukuta K, Jackson IT. Orbital neurofibromatosis with enophthalmos. *Br J Plast Surg* 1993;46:36–38.
110. Fuller LC, Cox B, Gardner RJM. Prevalence of von Recklinghausen neurofibromatosis in Dunedin, New Zealand. *Neurofibromatosis* 1989;2:278–283.
111. Gabriélidès C. Fibroneurome orbito-temporo-palpébral (maladie de Recklinghausen). *Ann Ocul* 1931;168:187–206.
112. Gallie B, Dunn J, Hamel P, Muncaster M, Cohen B, Phillips R. How do retinoblastoma tumours form? *Eye* 1992;6:226–231.
113. Gardner WJ, Frazier CH. Bilateral acoustic neurofibromas. A clinical study and field survey of a family of five generations with bilateral deafness in thirty-eight members. *Arch Neurol Psychiatry* 1930;23:266–302.
114. Garretto NS, Ameriso S, Molina HA, Arberas C, Salvat J, Monteverde D, et al. Type 2 neurofibromatosis with Lisch nodules. *Neurofibromatosis* 1989;2:315–321.
115. Gartner S. Malignant melanoma of the choroid in von Recklinghausen's disease. *Am J Ophthalmol* 1940;23:73–78.
116. Gass J. Cavernous hemangioma of the retina. A neuro-oculo-cutaneous syndrome. *Am J Ophthalmol* 1971;71:799–814.
117. Gass J. An unusual hamartoma of the pigment epithelium and retina simulating choroidal melanoma and retinoblastoma. *Trans Am Ophthalmol Soc* 1973;71:171–185.
118. Gass JDM, Braunstein R. Sessile and exophytic capillary angiomas of the juxtapapillary retina and optic nerve head. *Arch Ophthalmol* 1980;98:1790–1797.
119. Gauter-Smith P, Sanders M, Sanders M, Sanderson K. Ocular and nervous system involvement in angioma serpiginosum. *Br J Ophthalmol* 1971;55:433–443.
120. Gilchrist TC. Two cases (including one in the negro) of molluscum fibrosum, with the pathology. *Johns Hopkins Hosp Rep* 1896; 1:349–362.
121. Gilliam AC, Ragge NK, Perez MI, Bolognia JL. Phakomatosis pigmentovascularis type IIb with iris mammillations. *Arch Dermatol* 1993;129:340–342.
122. Ginzburg BM, Montanera WJ, Tyndel FJ, Griesman JA, McLennan MD, Terbrugge KG, et al. Diagnosis of von Hippel-Lindau disease in a patient with blindness resulting from bilateral optic nerve hemangioblastomas. *Am J Roentgenol* 1992;159:403–405.
123. Glasscock MEI, Hays JW, Minor LB, Haynes DS, Carrasco VN. Preservation of hearing in surgery for acoustic neuromas. *J Neurosurg* 1993;78:864–870.
124. Goldberg MF, Koenig S. Argon laser treatment of von Hippel-Lindau retinal angiomas.

I. Clinical and angiographic findings. *Arch Ophthalmol* 1974;92:121–125.
125. Goldberg R, Pheasant T, Shields J. Cavernous hemangioma of the retina. A four generation pedigree with neurocutaneous manifestations and an example of bilateral retinal involvement. *Arch Ophthalmol* 1979;97:2321–2324.
126. Goldsmith J. Neurofibromatosis associated with tumors of the optic papilla. *Arch Ophthalmol* 1949;41:718–729.
127. Goldstein I, Wexler D. Melanosis uveae and melanoma of the iris in neurofibromatosis (Recklinghausen). *Arch Ophthalmol* 1930;30:288–296.
128. Good W, Brodsky M, Edwards M, Hoyt W. Bilateral retinal hamartomas in neurofibromatosis type 2. *Br J Ophthalmol* 1991;75:190.
129. Greene C, Male W, Orlick M, Gordon R. Lisch nodules prevalence and specificity for neurofibromatosis. *Am J Hum Genet* 1987;41:A189.
130. Grossniklaus HE, Thomas JW, Vigneswaran N, Jarrett WH. Retinal hemangioblastoma. A histologic, immunohistochemical, and ultrastructural evaluation. *Ophthalmology* 1992;99:140–145.
131. Gutmann DH, Cole JL, Stone WJ, Ponder BA, Collins FS. Loss of neurofibromin in adrenal gland tumors from patients with neurofibromatosis type 1. *Genes Chromosom Cancer* 1994;10:55–58.
132. Gutmann DH, Collins FS. Recent progress toward understanding the molecular biology of von Recklinghausen neurofibromatosis. *Ann Neurol* 1992;31:555–561.
133. Gutmann DH, Collins FS. The neurofibromatosis type 1 gene review and its protein product. *Neuron* 1993;10:335–343.
134. Gutmann DH, Geist RT, Rose K, Wallin G, Moley JF. Loss of neurofibromatosis type 1 (NF1) gene expression in pheochromocytomas from patients without NF1. *Genes Chromosom Cancer* 1995;13:104–109.
135. Gutmann DH, Wood DL, Collins FS. Identification of the neurofibromatosis type 1 gene product. *Proc Natl Acad Sci USA* 1991;88:9658–9662.
136. Habiby R, Silverman B, Listernick R, Charrow J. Precocious puberty in children with neurofibromatosis type 1. *J Pediatr* 1995;126:364–367.
137. Hall A. Ras and GAPb. Who's controlling whom? *Cell* 1990;61:921–923.
138. Hardwig P, Robertson DM. Von Hippel-Lindau disease: A familial, often lethal, multisystem phakomatosis. *Ophthalmology* 1984;91:263–270.
139. Hatta N, Horiuchi T, Watanabe I, Kobayashi Y, Shirakata Y, Ohtsuka H, et al. NF1 gene mutations in Japanese with neurofibromatosis 1 (NF1). *Biochem Biophys Res Commun* 1995;212:697–704.
140. Hayman L, Evans R, Ferrell R. Familial cavernous angiomas. Natural history and genetic study over a 5-year period. *Am J Med Genet* 1982;11:147.
141. Hecht F. Recognition of neurofibromatosis before von Recklinghausen. *Neurofibromatosis* 1989;2:180–184.
142. Henneberg, Koch M. Ueber centrale neurofibromatose und die Geschwulste des Kleinhirnbrhckenwinkels (Acusticusneurome). *Arch Psychiatry* 1902;36:251–304.
143. Heutink P, van der Mey AGL, Sandkuijl LA, van Gils APG, Bardoel A, Breedveld GJ, et al. A gene subject to genomic imprinting and responsible for hereditary paragangliomas maps to chromosome 11q23-qter. *Hum Mol Genet* 1992;1:7–10.
144. Hitchcock A. Some remarks on neuroma, with a brief account of three cases of anomalous cutaneous tumours in one family. *Am J Med Sci* 1862;93:320–328.
145. Hochstrasser H, Boltshauser E, Valavanis A. Brain tumors in children with von Recklinghausen neurofibromatosis. *Neurofibromatosis* 1988;1:233–239.
146. Hoffman E. Rudolf Virchow und die Recklinghausenche Krankheit. *Dtsch Med Wochenschr* 1955;80:293–295.
147. Hoffmeyer S, Assum G, Kaufmann D, Krone W. Unequal expression of NF1 alleles. *Nature Genet* 1994;6:331.
148. Hofman KJ. Diffusion of information about neurofibromatosis type 1 DNA testing. *Am J Med Genet* 1994;49:299–301.
149. Honda M, Arai E, Sawada S, Ohta A, Niimura M. Neurofibromatosis 2 and neurilemmomatosis gene are identical. *J Invest Dermatol* 1995;104:74–77.
150. Horton JC, Harsh GR4th, Fisher JW, Hoyt WF. Von Hippel-Lindau disease and erythrocytosis: radioimmunoassay of erythropoietin in cyst fluid from a brainstem hemangioblastoma. *Neurology* 1991;41:753–754.
151. Hough DM, Stephens DH, Johnson CD, Binkovitz LA. Pancreatic lesions in von Hippel-Lindau disease: prevalence, clinical significance, and CT findings. *Am J Roentgenol* 1994;162:1091–1094.

152. Housepian EM, Chi TL. Neurofibromatosis and optic pathway gliomas. *J Neuro-Oncol* 1993;15:51–55.
153. Hoyt WF, Imes RK. Optic gliomas of neurofibromatosis-1 (NF-1): Contemporary perspectives, chapter 22. In *Tuberous Sclerosis and Neurofibromatosis: Epidemiology, Pathophysiology, Biology, and Management.* Editors J. Ishibashi and Y. Hori. Amsterdam: Elsevier Science Publishers, B. V., 1990: 239–246.
154. Huson S. *Clinical and Genetic Studies of von Recklinghausen Neurofibromatosis.* MD Thesis, Edinburgh University, 1989.
155. Huson S, Jones D, Beck L. Ophthalmic manifestations of neurofibromatosis. *Br J Ophthalmol* 1987;71:235–238.
156. Huson SM, Compston DAS, Clark P, Harper PS. A genetic study of von Recklinghausen neurofibromatosis in south east Wales. I. Prevalence, fitness, mutation rate, and effect of parental transmission on severity. *J Med Genet* 1989;26:704–711.
157. Huson SM, Harper PS, Compston DA. Von Recklinghausen neurofibromatosis. A clinical and population study in south-east Wales. *Brain* 1988;111:1355–1381.
158. Huson SM, Thrush DC. Central neurofibromatosis. *Q J Med* 1985;55:213–224.
159. Huynh DP, Nechiporuk A, Pulst SM. Alternative transcripts in the mouse neurofibromatosis type 2 (NF2) gene are conserved and code for schwannomins with distinct C-terminal domains. *Hum Mol Genet* 1994;3:1075–1079.
160. Imes RK, Hoyt WF. Childhood chiasmal gliomas: update on the fate of patients in the 1969 San Francisco study. *Br J Ophthalmol* 1986; 70:179–182.
161. Imes RK, Hoyt WF. Magnetic resonance imaging signs of optic nerve gliomas in neurofibromatosis 1. *Am J Ophthalmol* 1991;111: 729–734.
162. Imes RK, Monteiro ML, Hoyt WF. Incipient hemangioblastoma of the optic disk. *Am J Ophthalmol* 1984;98:116.
163. Ingordo V, D'Andria G, Mendicini S, Grecucci M. Segmental neurofibromatosis: is it uncommon or underdiagnosed? *Arch Dermatol* 1995;131:959–960.
164. Itoh T, Magnaldi S, White RM, Denckla MB, Hofman K, Naidu S, et al. Neurofibromatosis 1: The evolution of deep gray and white matter MR abnormalities. *Am J Neuroradiol* 1994;15:1513–1519.
165. Iwach A, Hoskins D, Hetherington J, Shaffer R. Analysis of surgical and medical management of glaucoma in Sturge-Weber syndrome. *Ophthalmology* 1990;97:904–909.
166. Jackson IT, Carbonnel A, Potparic Z, Shaw K. Orbitotemporal neurofibromatosis classification and treatment. *Plast Reconstruct Surg* 1993;92:1–11.
167. Jacoby LB, MacCollin MM, Louis DN, Mohney T, Rubio M-P, Pulaski K, et al. Exon scanning for mutation of the NF2 gene in schwannomas. *Hum Mol Genet* 1994;3: 413–419.
168. Jayadel D, Fain P, Upadhyaya M, Ponder MA, Huson SM, Carey J, et al. Paternal origin of new mutations in von Recklinghausen neurofibromatosis. *Nature* 1990;343:558–559.
169. Jennings AM, Smith C, Cole DR, Jennings C, Shortland JR, Williams JL, et al. Von Hippel-Lindau disease in a large British family: clinicopathological features and recommendations for screening and follow-up. *Q J Med* 1988;66:233–249.
170. Kaiser-Kupfer M, Freidlin V, Datiles M, Edwards P, Sherman J, Parry D, et al. The association of posterior capsular lens opacities with bilateral acoustic neuromas in patients with neurofibromatosis type 2. *Arch Ophthalmol* 1989;107:541–545.
171. Kanter WR, Eldridge R, Fabricant R, Allen JC, Koerber T. Central neurofibromatosis with bilateral acoustic neuroma: genetic, clinical and biochemical distinctions from peripheral neurofibromatosis. *Neurology* 1980; 30:851–859.
172. Karsdorp N, Elderson A, Post DW, Hene RJ, Vos J, Feldberg MA, et al. Von Hippel-Lindau disease new strategies in early detection and treatment. *Am J Med* 1994;97:158–168.
173. Kawaguchi T, Tanaka R, Kameyama S, Yamazaki H. Full recovery from deafness after removal of a large acoustic neurinoma associated with neurofibromatosis 2 case report. *Surg Neurol* 1994;42:326–329.
174. Kaye L, Rothner A, Beauchamp G, Meyers S, Estes M. Ocular findings associated with neurofibromatosis type 2. *Ophthalmology* 1992;99:1424–1429.
175. Kayes LM, Riccardi VM, Burke W, Dennett RL, Stephens K. Large de novo deletions in a patient with sporadic neurofibromatosis type 1, mental retardation, and dysmorphism. *J Med Genet* 1992;29:686–690.
176. Keeler LL, Klauber GT. Von Hippel-Lindau disease and renal cell carcinoma in a 16-year-old boy. *J Urol* 1992;147:1588–1591.

177. Kerr DJ, Scheithauer BW, Miller GM, Ebersold MJ, McPhee TJ. Hemangioblastoma of the optic nerve: case report. *Neurosurgery* 1995;36:573–580.
178. Klein M, Goldberg M, Cotlier E. Cavernous hemangioma of the retina report of four cases. *Ann Ophthalmol* 1975;7:1213–1221.
179. Klippel M, Trenaunay P. Du noevus variqueux osteo-hypertrophique. *Arch Gen Med* 1900;3:642–672.
180. Knoblauch (1843). *De neuromate et gangliis accessoriis Inaug. Dissert. liked by Adrian C, Beiträge zur Klin Chirurgie* 1901;31:1–98.
181. Knudson AGJ. Mutation and cancer: statistical study of retinoblastoma. *Proc Natl Acad Sci USA* 1971;68:820–823.
182. Kremer I, Gilad E, Sira IB. Juxtapapillary exophytic retinal capillary hemangioma treated by yellow krypton (568 nm) laser photocoagulation. *Ophthalmic Surg* 1988;19:743–747.
183. Kroll, AJ, Ricker DP, Robb RM, Albert DM. Vitreous hemorrhage complicating retinal astrocytic hamartoma. *Surv Ophthalmol* 1981;26:31–38.
184. Kuenzle C, Weissert M, Roulet E, Bode H, Schefer S, Huisman T, et al. Follow-up of optic pathway gliomas in children with neurofibromatosis type 1. *Neuropediatrics* 1994;25: 295–300.
185. Kunze J, Nippert I. *Genetics and Malformations in Art.* Berlin: Grosse, 1986.
186. Kurosawa A, Kurosawa H. Ovoid bodies in choroidal neurofibromatosis. *Arch Ophthalmol* 1982;100:1939–1941.
187. Kurz J. Tumorbefund in der Iris bei Neurofibromatose. *Ofthalm Sborn* [Abstract in *Zentralbl Gesamte Ophthalmol* 28, 566] 1932; 7:294–295.
188. Kuzmin I, Kuh FM, Latif F, Geil L, Zbar B, Lerman MI. Identification of the promoter of the human von Hippel-Lindau disease tumor suppressor gene. *Oncogene* 1995;10:2185–2194.
189. Kylstra JA, Aylsworth AS. Cone-rod retinal dystrophy in a patient with neurofibromatosis type 1. *Can J Ophthalmol* 1993;28:79–80.
190. Lamiell JM, Salazar FG, Hsia YE. Von Hippel-Lindau disease affecting 43 members of a single kindred. *Medicine* 1989;68:1–29.
191. Landau K, Dossetor FM, Hoyt WF, Muci-Mendoza R. Retinal hamartoma in neurofibromatosis type 2. *Arch Ophthalmol* 1990; 108:328–329.
192. Landau K, Yasargil GM. Ocular fundus in neurofibromatosis type 2. *Br J Ophthalmol* 1993;77:646–649.
193. Lane CM, Turner G, Gregor ZJ, Bird AC. Laser treatment of retinal angiomatosis. *Eye* 1989;3:33–38.
194. Latif F, Tory K, Gnarra J, Yao M, Duh F-M, Orcutt ML, et al. Identification of the von Hippel-Lindau disease tumor suppressor gene. *Science* 1993;260:1317–1320.
195. Lázaro C, Gaona A, Ravella A, Volpini V, Estivill X. Prenatal diagnosis of neurofibromatosis type 1 from flanking RFLPs to intragenic microsatellite markers. *Prenat Diagn* 1995;15:129–134.
196. Leao M, da Silva ML. Evidence of central nervous system involvement in Watson syndrome. *Pediatr Neurol* 1995;12:252–254.
197. Ledbetter DH, Rich DC, O'Connell P, Leppert M, Carey JC. Precise localization of NF1 to 17q112 by balanced translocation. *Am J Hum Genet* 1989;44:20–24.
198. Lee KD, Abbott ML. Familial central nervous system neoplasia. *Arch Neurol* 1969;20:154–160.
199. Legius E, Dierick H, Wu R, Hall BK, Marynen P, Cassiman JJ, et al. TP53 mutations are frequent in malignant NF1 tumors. *Genes Chromosom Cancer* 1994;10:250–255.
200. Legius E, Hall BK, Wallace MR, Collins FS, Glover TW. Ten base pair duplication in exon 38 of the NF1 gene. *Hum Mol Genet* 1995; 3:829–830.
201. Legius E, Marchuk DA, Collins FS, Glover TW. Somatic deletion of the neurofibromatosis type 1 gene in a neurofibrosarcoma supports a tumour suppressor gene hypothesis. *Nature Genet* 1993;3:122–126.
202. Lehrnbecher T, Gassel AM, Rauh V, Kirchner T, Huppertz HI. Neurofibromatosis presenting as a severe systemic vasculopathy. *Eur J Pediatr* 1994;153:107–109.
203. Lekanne Deprez RH, Bianchi AB, Groen NA, Seizinger BR, Hagemeijer A, van Drunen E, et al. Frequent NF2 gene transcript mutations in sporadic meningiomas and vestibular schwannomas. *Am J Hum Genet* 1994;54: 1022–1029.
204. Lewis RA, Gerson LP, Axelson KA, Riccardi VM, Whitford RP. Von Recklinghausen neurofibromatosis. II. Incidence of optic gliomata. *Ophthalmology* 1984;91:929–935.
205. Lewis RA, Riccardi VM. Von Recklinghausen Neurofibromatosis. Incidence of iris hamartomata. *Ophthalmology* 1981;88:348–354.
206. Li Y, Bollag G, Clark R, Stevens J, Conroy L, Fults D, et al. Somatic mutations in the neurofibromatosis 1 gene in human tumors. *Cell* 1992;69:275–281.

207. Lindau A. Studien über Kleinhirncysten. Bau, Pathogenese und Beziehungen zur Angiomatosis Retinae. *Acta Pathol Microbiol Scand* 1926(Suppl);1:1–128.
208. Lisch K. Ueber Beteiligung der Augen, insbesondere das Vorkommen von Irisknötchen bei der Neurofibromatose (Recklinghausen). *Z Augenheilkd* 1937;93:137–143.
209. Listernick R, Charrow J, Greenwald M, Mets M. Natural history of optic pathway tumors in children with neurofibromatosis type 1. *J Pediatr* 1994;125:63–66.
210. Loewenstein JI. Bilateral macular holes in von Hippel-Lindau disease. *Arch Ophthalmol* 1995;113:143–144.
211. Luna EJ, Hitt AL. Cytoskeleton-plasma membrane interactions. *Science* 1992;258:955–964.
212. MacCollin M, Mohney T, Trofatter J, Wertelecki W, Ramesh V, Gusella J. DNA diagnosis of neurofibromatosis 2. Altered coding sequence of the merlin tumor suppressor gene in an extended pedigree. *JAMA* 1993;270:2316–2320.
213. MacCollin M, Ramesh V, Jacoby LB, Louis DN, Rubio M-P, Pulaski K, et al. Mutational analysis of patients with neurofibromatosis 2. *Am J Hum Genet* 1994;55:314–320.
214. Madigan P, Masello M. Report of a neurofibromatosis-like case Monstrorum Historia, 1642. *Neurofibromatosis* 1989;2:53–56.
215. Madigan P, Shaw RV. Neurofibromatosis in thirteenth century Austria. *Neurofibromatosis* 1988;1:339–341.
216. Maher ER, Bentley E, Yates JRW, Barton D, Jennings A, Fellows IW, et al. Mapping of von Hippel-Lindau disease to chromosome 3P confirmed by genetic linkage analysis. *J Neurol Sci* 1990;100:27–30.
217. Maher ER. Von Hippel-Lindau disease. *Eur J Cancer* 1994;30A:1987–1990.
218. Maher ER, Iselius L, Yates JRW, Littler M, Benjamin C, Harris R, et al. Von Hippel-Lindau disease a genetic study. *J Med Genet* 1991;28:443–447.
219. Maher ER, Moore AT. Von Hippel-Lindau disease. *Br J Ophthalmol* 1992;76:743–745.
220. Maher ER, Yates JR, Harries R, et al. Clinical features and natural history of von Hippel-Lindau disease. *Q J Med* 1990;77:1151–1163.
221. Marchuk DA, Saulino AM, Tavakkol R, Swaroop M, Wallace MR, Anderson LB, et al. cDNA cloning of the type 1 neurofibromatosis gene: complete sequence of the NF1 gene product. *Genomics* 1991;11:931–940.
222. Marshall D. Glioma of the optic nerve as a manifestation of von Recklinghausen's disease. *Am J Ophthalmol* 1954;37:15–36.
223. Martin GA, Viskochil D, Bollag G, McCabe PC, Crosler WJ, Haubruck H, et al. The GAP-related domain of the neurofibromatosis type 1 gene product interacts with ras p21. *Cell* 1990;63:843–849.
224. Martuza R, Philippe I, Fitzpatrick T, Zwaan J, Seki Y, Lederman J. Melanin macroglobules as a cellular marker of neurofibromatosis a quantitative study. *J Invest Dermatol* 1985; 85:347–350.
225. Martuza RL, Eldridge R. Neurofibromatosis 2 (bilateral acoustic neurofibromatosis). *N Engl J Med* 1988;318:684–688.
226. Martuza RL, Ojemann RG. Bilateral acoustic neuromas: clinical aspects, pathogenesis and treatment. *Neurosurgery* 1982;10:1–12.
227. Mautner VF, Tatagiba M, Guthoff R, Sanii M, Pulst SM. Neurofibromatosis in the pediatric age group. *Neurosurgery* 1993;33:92–96.
228. Mautner VF, Tatagiba M, Lindenau M, Funsterer C, Pulst S-M, Kluwe L, et al. Spinal tumors in patients with neurofibromatosis type 2: MR imaging study of frequency, multiplicity, and variety. *Am J Roentgenol* 1995;165:951–955.
229. Mayfrank L, Wullich B, Wolff G, Finke J, Gouzoulis E, Gilsbach JM. Neurofibromatosis 2: A clinically and genetically heterogeneous disease? Report on 10 sporadic cases. *Clin Genet* 1990;38:362–370.
230. McLean J. Glial tumors of the retina in relation to tuberous sclerosis. *Trans Am Ophthalmol Soc* 1955;53:209–215.
231. Menon AG, Anderson KM, Riccardi VM, Chung RY, Whaley JM, Yandell DW, et al. Chromosome 17p deletions and p53 gene mutations associated with the formation of malignant neurofibrosarcomas in von Recklinghausen neurofibromatosis. *Proc Natl Acad Sci USA* 1990;87:5435–5439.
232. Menon AG, Ledbetter DH, Rich DC, Seizinger BR, Rouleau GA, Michels VF, et al. Characterization of a translocation within the von Recklinghausen neurofibromatosis region of Chromosome 17. *Genomics* 1989;5:245–249.
233. Mérel P, Hoang-Xuan K, Sanson M, Bijlsma E, Rouleau G, Laurent-Puig P, et al. Screening for germ-line mutations in the NF2 gene. *Genes Chromosom Cancer* 1995;12:117–127.
234. Mesmer E, Laqua H, Wessing A, Spitznas M, Weidle E, Ruprecht K, et al. Nine cases of

cavernous hemangioma of the retina. *Am J Ophthalmol* 1983;95:383–390.

235. Messiaen L, Bie SD, Moens T, Van den Enden A, Leroy J. Lack of independence between five DNA polymorphisms in the NF1 gene. *Hum Mol Genet* 1993;2:485.
236. Messmer E, Font R, Laqua H, Hopping W, Naumann G. Cavernous hemangioma of the retina Immunohistochemical and ultrastructural observations. *Arch Ophthalmol* 1984; 102:413–418.
237. Michel J. Ueber eine Hyperplasie des Chiasma und des rechten Nervus opticus bei Elephantiasis. *Albrecht von Graefes Arch Ophthalmol* 1873;19:145–163.
238. Michels VV, Whisnant JP, Garrity JA, Miller GM. Neurofibromatosis type 1 with bilateral acoustic neuromas. *Neurofibromatosis* 1989; 2:213–217.
239. Miller M, Hall JG. Possible maternal effect on severity of neurofibromatosis. *Lancet* 1978;2: 1071–1074.
240. Moore AT, Maher ER, Rosen P, Gregor Z, Bird AC. Ophthalmological screening for von Hippel-Lindau disease. *Eye* 1991;5:723–728.
241. Morlet N, Goldberg I. Sturge-Weber syndrome and secondary glaucoma. *Aust N Z J Ophthalmol* 1993;21:271–272.
242. Mulvihill JJ. Neurofibromatosis history, nomenclature, and natural history. *Neurofibromatosis* 1988;1:124–131.
243. Mulvihill JJ, Parry DM, Sherman JL, Pikus A, Kaiser-Kupfer MI, Eldridge R. Neurofibromatosis 1 (Recklinghausen disease) and neurofibromatosis 2 (bilateral acoustic neurofibromatosis): An update (NIH conference). *Ann Intern Med* 1990;113:39–52.
244. Murphree AL, Munier FL. Retinoblastoma, Chapter 27. In *Retina,* vol 1. Editor: S. Ryan. Mosby, St. Louis 1994;1:571–626.
245. Murray J. On three cases of a peculiar form of molluscum fibrosum in children. *Lancet* 1873;1:410–411.
246. Mwinula J, Sagawa T, Tawara A, Inomata H. Anterior chamber angle vascularization in Sturge-Weber syndrome. *Graefes Arch Clin Exp Ophthalmol* 1994;232:387–391.
247. Nager GT. Association of bilateral eighth nerve tumors with meningiomas in von Recklinghausen's disease. *Laryngoscope* 1964;74:1220–1261.
248. Narod S, Parry D, Parboosingh J, Lenoir G, Ruttledge M, Fischer G, et al. Neurofibromatosis type 2 appears to be a genetically homogeneous disease. *Am J Hum Genet* 1992; 51:486–496.
249. Neary WJ, Newton VE, Vidler M, Ramsden RT, Lye RH, Dutton JEM, et al. A clinical, genetic and audiological study of patients and families with bilateral acoustic neurofibromatosis. *J Laryngol Otol* 1993;107:6–11.
250. Nerad JA, Kersten RC, Anderson RL. Hemangioblastoma of the optic nerve. Report of a case and review of literature. *Ophthalmology* 1988;95:398–402.
251. Neumann HP, Eggert HR, Scheremet R, Schumacher M, Mohadjer M, Wakhloo AK, et al. Central nervous system lesions in von Hippel-Lindau syndrome. *J Neurol Neurosurg Psychiatry* 1992;55:898–901.
252. Neumann HPH, Berger DP, Sigmund G, Blum U, Schmidt D, Parmer RJ, et al. Pheochromocytomas, multiple endocrine neoplasia type 2 and von Hippel-Lindau disease. *N Engl J Med* 1993;329:1531–1538.
253. Neumann HPH, Lips CJM, Hsia YE, Zbar B. Von Hippel-Lindau syndrome. *Brain Pathol* 1995;5:181–193.
254. Nigro JM, Baker SJ, Preisinger AC, Jessup JM, Hostetter R, Cleary K, et al. Mutations in the p53 gene occur in diverse human tumour types. *Nature* 1989;342:705–708.
255. Nishi T, Lee PSY, Oka K, Levin VA, Tanase S, Morino Y, et al. Differential expression of two types of the neurofibromatosis type 1 (NF1) gene transcripts related to neuronal differentiation. *Oncogene* 1991;6:1555–1559.
256. Nordmann J, Brini A. Von Recklinghausen's disease and melanoma of the uvea. *Br J Ophthalmol* 1970;54:641–648.
257. North K, Hoy P, Yuille D, Cocks N, Mobbs E, Hutchins P, et al. Specific learning disability in children with neurofibromatosis type 1: Significance of MRI abnormalities. *Neurology* 1994;44:878–883.
258. Nowak R. Mining treasures from "junk DNA." *Science* 1994;263:608–610.
259. Nyboer J, Robertson D, Gomez M. Retinal lesions in tuberous sclerosis. *Arch Ophthalmol* 1976;94:1277–1280.
260. Oakes W. The natural history of patients with the Sturge-Weber syndrome. *Pediatr Neurosurg* 1992;18:287–290.
261. O'Connell P, Leach R, Cawthon RM, Culver M, Stevens J, Viskochil D, et al. Two NF1 translocations map within a 600-kilobase segment of 17q112. *Science* 1989;244:1087–1088.
262. Ogunmekan A, Hwang P, Hoffman H. Sturge-Weber-Dimitri disease. Role of hemispherectomy in prognosis. *Can J Neurol Sci* 1989;16:78.

263. Packer RJ, Bilaniuk LT, Cohen BH, Braffman BH, Obringer AC, Zimmerman RA, et al. Intracranial visual pathway glioma in children in neurofibromatosis. *Neurofibromatosis* 1988;1: 212–222.
264. Palmer M, Carney M, Combs J. Combined hamartomas of the retinal pigment epithelium and retina. *Retina* 1990;10:33–36.
265. Pancurak J, Goldberg M, Frenkel M, Crowell R. Cavernous hemangioma of the retina: Genetic and central nervous system involvement. *Retina* 1985;5:215–220.
266. Consensus Development Panel. National Institutes of Health Consensus Development Conference Statement on Acoustic Neuroma, December 11–13, 1991. *Arch Neurol* 1994; 51:201–207.
267. Parry DM, Eldridge R. Acoustic neuromas: Clinical characteristics of heritable bilateral tumors. *National Institutes of Health* Consensus Statement 1991 Dec. 11–13, 9:1–24. Available from the Office of Medical Applications of Research, National Institutes of Health. Federal Building Room 618, Bethesda, MD 20892.
268. Parry DM, Eldridge R, Kaiser-Kupfer MI, Bouzas EA, Pikus A, Patronas N. Neurofibromatosis 2 (NF2): Clinical characteristics of 63 affected individuals and clinical evidence for heterogeneity. *Am J Med Genet* 1994;52:450–461.
269. Pearson-Webb M, Kaiser-Kupfer M, Eldridge R. Eye findings in bilateral acoustic (central) neurofibromatosis: Association with presenile lens opacities and cataracts but absence of Lisch nodules. *N Engl J Med* 1986;315:1553–1554.
270. Perry H. Isolated neurofibromas of the conjunctiva. *Am J Ophthalmol* 1992;89:112–113.
271. Perry HD, Font RL. Iris nodules in von Recklinghausen's neurofibromatosis: Electron microscopic confirmation of their melanocytic origin. *Arch Ophthalmol* 1982; 100:1635–1640.
272. Phelps C. The pathogenesis of glaucoma in Sturge-Weber syndrome. *Trans Am Acad Ophthalmol Otolaryngol* 1978;85:276–286.
273. Pikus AT. Pediatric audiologic profile in type 1 and type 2 neurofibromatosis. *J Am Acad Audiol* 1995;6:54–62.
274. Ponder M, Easton D, Huson S, Ponder B. Variation in expression in NF1: A twin study. Proceedings of the 8th International Congress of Human Genetics. *Am J Hum Genet* 1991; 49:3.
275. Pool JL, Pave AA, Greenfield EC. *Acoustic Nerve Tumors: Early Diagnosis and Treatment.* Springfield, IL: Charles C Thomas, 1970.
276. Preiser SA, Davenport CB. Multiple neurofibromatosis (von Recklinghausen's disease) and its inheritance with description of a case. *Am J Med Sci* 1918;156:507–540.
277. Purandare SM, Lanyon WG, Conner JM. Characterisation of inherited and sporadic mutations in neurofibromatosis type 1. *Hum Mol Genet* 1994;3:1109–1115.
278. Ragge NK, Acheson J, Murphree AL. Iris mammillations: Significance and associations. *Eye* 1996;10:86–91.
279. Ragge NK, Baser ME, Klein J, Nechiporuk A, Sainz J, Pulst SM, et al. Ocular abnormalities in neurofibromatosis 2. *Am J Ophthalmol* 1995;120:634–641.
280. Ragge NK, Falk RE, Cohen WE, Murphree AL. Images of Lisch nodules across the spectrum. *Eye* 1993;7:95–101.
281. Ragge NK, Munier F. Ancient neurofibromatosis. *Nature* 1994;368:815.
282. Rainey M, Lewis RA, Moye LA. Probability of Lisch nodules in neurofibromatosis type 1 by age (abstract). *Invest Ophthalmol Vis Sci* 1994;36:S1057.
283. Rasko JE, North KN, Favaloro EJ, Grispo L, Berndt MC. Attenuated platelet sensitivity to collagen in patients with neurofibromatosis type 1. *Br J Haematol* 1995;89:582–588.
284. Raymond F. Leçons sur les maladies du système nerveux. Series 3, Clinic 6, Pan's. 1898: 229.
285. Raymond F. Sur un cas de tumeur de cervelet. N Iconog de la Salpêtrière 1898;11:213–229.
286. Riccardi V. Type 1 neurofibromatosis and the pediatric patient. *Curr Prob Pediatr* 1992; 22:66–106.
287. Riccardi VM. Von Recklinghausen neurofibromatosis. *N Engl J Med* 1981;305:1617–1627.
288. Riccardi VM. *Neurofibromatosis: Phenotype, Natural History, and Pathogenesis.* Baltimore: Johns Hopkins University Press, 1992.
289. Riccardi VM, Lewis RA. Penetrance of von Recklinghausen neurofibromatosis: A distinction between predecessors and descendants. *Am J Hum Genet* 1988;42:284–289.
290. Riccardi VM, Powell PP. Neurofibrosarcoma as a complication of von Recklinghausen neurofibromatosis. *Neurofibromatosis* 1989;2: 152–165.
291. Riccardi VM, Wald JS. Discounting an adverse maternal effect on neurofibromatosis severity. *Pediatrics* 1987;79:386–393.

292. Richardson E. Pathology of tuberous sclerosis: Neuropathologic aspects. *Ann NY Acad Sci* 1991;615:128–139.
293. Ridley M, Green J, Johnson G. Retinal angiomatosis: The ocular manifestations of von Hippel-Lindau disease. *Can J Ophthalmol* 1986;21:276–283.
294. Roach E, Smith M, Huttenlocher P, Bhat M, Alcorn D, Hawley L. Diagnostic criteria tuberous sclerosis complex. *J Child Neurol* 1992;7:221–224.
295. Rodenhiser DI, Coulter-Mackie MB, Jung JH, Singh SM. A genetic study of neurofibromatosis 1 in south-western Ontario. Population, familial segregation of phenotype, and molecular linkage. *J Med Genet* 1991; 28:746–751.
296. Rodenhiser DI, Coulter-Mackie MB, Singh SM. Evidence of DNA methylation in the neurofibromatosis type 1 (NF1) gene region of 17q112. *Hum Mol Genet* 1993;2:439–444.
297. Rossi LN, Pastorino G, Scotti G, Gazocchi M, Maninetti MM, Zanolini C, et al. Early diagnosis of optic glioma in children with neurofibromatosis type 1. *Child Nerv Syst* 1994; 10:426–429.
298. Rouleau GA, Merel P, Lutchman M, Sanson M, Zucman J, Marineau C, et al. Alteration in a new gene encoding a putative membrane-organizing protein causes neurofibromatosis type 2. *Nature* 1993;363:515–521.
299. Rouleau GA, Wertelecki W, Haines JA, Hobbs WJ, Trofatter JA, Seizinger BR, et al. Genetic linkage of bilateral acoustic neurofibromatosis to a DNA marker on chromosome 22. *Nature* 1987;329:246–248.
300. Rubio A, Meyers SP, Powers JM, Nelson CN, de Papp EW. Hemangioblastoma of the optic nerve. *Hum Pathol* 1994;25:1249–1251.
301. Rush JA, Younge BR, Campbell RJ, MacCarthy CS. Optic glioma: Long-term follow-up of 85 histopathologically verified cases. *Ophthalmology* 1982;89:1213–1219.
302. Ruttledge MH, Narod SA, Dumanski JP, Parry DM, Eldridge R, Wertelecki W, et al. Presymptomatic diagnosis for neurofibromatosis 2 with chromosome 22 markers. *Neurology* 1993;43:1753–1760.
303. Sadeh M, Marinovits G, Goldhammer Y. Occurrence of both neurofibromatoses 1 and 2 in the same individual with a rapidly progressive course. *Neurology* 1989;39:282–283.
304. Sakurai T. Eigenartige Fleckchen an der Irisvorderfläche und Neurofibromatosis Recklinghausen. *Acta Soc Ophthalmol Jpn* 1935; 39:87–93.
305. Samuelsson B, Axelsson R. Neurofibromatosis. A clinical and genetic study of 96 cases in Gothenburg, Sweden. *Acta Dermato Venereal* Suppl (*Stockh*) 1981;95:67–71.
306. Samuelsson B, Riccardi VM. Neurofibromatosis in Gothenburg, Sweden II: Intellectual compromise. *Neurofibromatosis* 1989; 2:78–83.
307. Saran N, Winter FC. Bilateral gliomas of the optic discs associated with neurofibromatosis. *Am J Ophthalmol* 1967;64:89–94.
308. Satran L, Letson RD, Seljeskob EL. Neurofibromatosis with congenital glaucoma and buphthalmos in a newborn. *Am J Dis Child* 1980;134:182–183.
309. Savino PJ, Glaser JS, Luxenberg MN. Pulsating enophthalmos and choroidal hamartomas: Two rare stigmata of neurofibromatosis. *Br J Ophthalmol* 1977;61:483–488.
310. Schachat AP, Shields JA, Fine SL, Sanborn GE, Weingeist TA, Valenzuela RE, et al. Combined hamartomas of the retina and retinal pigment epithelium. *Ophthalmology* 1984;91:1609–1615.
311. Schmidt D, Neumann HP. Retinal vascular hamartoma in von Hippel-Lindau disease. *Arch Ophthalmol* 1995;113:1163–1167.
312. Schmidt MA, Michels VV, Dewald GW. Cases of neurofibromatosis with rearrangements of chromosome 17 involving band 17q112. *Am J Med Genet* 1987;28:771–777.
313. Seidel H, Pompliano D, Knowles J. Exons as microgenes. *Science* 1992;257:1489–1490.
314. Seiff SR, Brodsky MC, MacDonald G, Berg BO, Howes ELJ, Hoyt WF. Orbital optic glioma in neurofibromatosis. Magnetic resonance diagnosis of perineural arachnoidal gliomatosis. *Arch Ophthalmol* 1987;105: 1689–1692.
315. Seizinger BR, Martuza RL, Gusella JF. Loss of genes on chromosome 22 in tumorigenesis of human acoustic neuroma. *Nature* 1986; 322:644–647.
316. Seizinger BR, de la Monte S, Atkins L, Gusella JF, Martuza RL. Molecular genetic approach to human meningioma: Loss of genes on chromosome 22. *Proc Natl Acad Sci USA* 1987;84:5419–5423.
317. Seizinger BR, Rouleau G, Ozelius LJ, Lane AH, George-Hyslop PS, Huson S, et al. Common pathogenetic mechanism for three tumor types in bilateral acoustic neurofibromatosis. *Science* 1987;236:317–319.
318. Selesnick SH, Jackler RK, Pitts LW. The changing clinical presentation of acoustic tu-

mors in the MRI era. *Laryngoscope* 1993; 103:431–436.

319. Shami M, Benedict W, Myers M. Early manifestations of retinal hamartomas in tuberous sclerosis. *Am J Ophthalmol* 1993;115: 539–540.
320. Shannon KM, Watterson J, Johnson P, O'Connell P, Lange B, Shah N, et al. Monosomy 7 myeloproliferative disease in children with neurofibromatosis type 1: epidemiology and molecular analysis. *Blood* 1992;79:1311–1318.
321. Shapland CD, Greenfield JG. A case of neurofibromatosis with meningeal tumour involving the left optic nerve. *Trans Ophthalmol Soc UK* 1935;55:257–279.
322. Shepherd C, Gomez M, Lie J, Crowson C. Causes of death in patients with tuberous sclerosis. *Mayo Clin Proc* 1991;66:792–796.
323. Shihab ZM, Kristan RW. Recurrent intraoperative choroidal effusion in Sturge-Weber syndrome. *J Pediatr Ophthalmol Strabismus* 1983;20:250–252.
324. Shin GS, Demer JL. Retinal arteriovenous communications associated with features of the Sturge-Weber syndrome. *Am J Ophthalmol* 1994;117:115–117.
325. Short MP, Bove C, MacCollin M, Mohney T, Ramesh V, Terenzio A, et al. Gender differences in neurofibromatosis type 2. *Neurology* 1994;44(suppl 2):A159.
326. Simon MA, Bowtell DDD, Dodson GS, Laverty TR, Rubin GM. Ras1 and a putative guanine nucleotide exchange factor perform crucial steps in signaling by the sevenless protein tyrosine kinase. *Cell* 1991;67:701–716.
327. Sivalingam A, Augsburger J, Perlongo G, Zimmerman R, Barabas G. Combined hamartoma of the retina and retinal pigment epithelium in a patient with neurofibromatosis type 2. *J Pediatr Ophthalmol Strabismus* 1991;28: 320–322.
328. Smalley S, Burger F, Smith M. Phenotypic variation of tuberous sclerosis in a single extended kindred. *J Med Genet* 1994;31; 761–765.
329. Smith RW. *A Treatise on the Pathology, Diagnosis and Treatment of Neuroma.* Dubin: Hodges and Smith, 1849.
330. Snell S. Plexiform neuroma (elephantiasis neuromatosis) of temporal region, orbit, eyelid, and eyeball. Notes of three cases. *Trans Ophthalmol Soc UK* 1903;23:157–177.
331. Sørensen SA, Mulvihill JJ, Nielsen A. Long-term follow-up of von Recklinghausen neurofibromatosis: survival and malignant neoplasms. *N Engl J Med* 1986;314:1010–1015.
332. South D, Jacobs A. Cutis marmorata telangiectatica congenita (congenital generalized phlebectasia). *J Pediatr* 1978;93:944–949.
333. Spencer WH. *Ophthalmic Pathology: An Atlas and Textbook.* Philadelphia: W.B. Saunders, 1985.
334. Stark M, Assum G, Krone W. A small deletion and an adjacent base exchange in a potential stem-loop region of the neurofibromatosis 1 gene. *Human Genet* 1991;87:685–687.
335. Steinbach F, Novick AC, Zincke H, Miller DP, Williams RD, et al. Treatment of renal cell carcinoma in von Hippel-Lindau disease: A multicenter study. *J Urol* 1995;153:1812–1816.
336. Stephens D, Kayes L, Riccardi VM, Rising M, Sybert VP, Pagon RA. Preferential mutation of the neurofibromatosis type 1 gene in paternally derived chromosomes. *Hum Genet* 1992;88:279–282.
337. Stern J, Jakobiec FA, Housepian EM. The architecture of optic nerve gliomas with and without neurofibromatosis. *Arch Ophthalmol* 1980;98:505–511.
338. Stevenson R, Morin J. Ocular finding in nevus flammeus. *Can J Ophthalmol* 1975;10: 136–139.
339. Stiller CA, Chessells JM, Fitchett M. Neurofibromatosis and childhood leukaemia/lymphoma a population based UKCCSG study. *Br J Cancer* 1994;70:969–972.
340. Sturge W. A case of partial epilepsy apparently due to a lesion of one of the vasomotor centers of the brain. *Trans Clin Soc London* 1879; 12:162.
341. Sujansky E, Conrad S. Outcome of Sturge-Weber syndrome in 52 adults. *Am J Med Genet* 1995;57:35–45.
342. Sullivan T, Clarke M, Morin J. The ocular manifestations of the Sturge-Weber syndrome. *J Pediatr Ophthalmol Strabismus* 1992;29:349–356.
343. Suzuki Y, Suzuki H, Kayama T, Shibahara S. Brain tumors predominantly express the neurofibromatosis type 1 gene transcript containing the 63 base insert in the region coding for GTPase activating protein-related domain. *Biochem Biophys Res Commun* 1991;181: 955–961.
344. Takahashi K, Suzuki H, Hatori M, Abe Y, Kokubun S, Sakurai M, et al. Reduced expression of neurofibromin in the soft tissue tumours obtained from patients with neurofi-

bromatosis type 1. *Clin Sci (Colch)* 1995; 88:581–585.

345. Tallman B, Tan O, Morelli J, Piepenbrink J, Stafford T, Trainor S, et al. Location of port-wine stains and the likelihood of ophthalmic and/or central nervous system complications. *Pediatrics* 1991;87:323–327.
346. T'Ang A, Varley JM, Chakraborty S, Murphree AL, Fung Y-KT. Structural rearrangement of the retinoblastoma gene in human breast carcinoma. *Science* 1988; 242:263–266.
347. Thomas JV, Schwartz PL, Gragoudas ES. Von Hippel's disease in association with von Recklinghausen's neurofibromatosis. *Br J Ophthalmol* 1978;62:604–608.
348. Tilesius von Tilenau WG. *Historia Pathologica Singularis Cutis Turpitudinis Jo Godofredi Rheinhardi Viri 50 Annorum.* Leipzig: S.L. Crusius. Index Cat Surgeon General (1893) 1793;14.
349. Tonsgard JH, Oesterle CS. The ophthalmologic presentation of NF2 in childhood. *J Pediatr Ophthalmol Strabismus* 1993;30:327–330.
350. Toonstra J, Dandrieu MR, Ippel PF, Delleman JW, Rupert PHJM Jr, Huitema HB. Are Lisch nodules an ocular marker of the neurofibromatosis gene in otherwise unaffected family members? *Dermatologica* 1987;174: 232–235.
351. Traboulsi E, Dudin G, To'mey K, Bashow A, Solh H. The association of a fragile site on chromosome 10 with the Sturge-Weber syndrome and congenital glaucoma. *Ophthalmic Paediatr Genet* 1983;3:135–140.
351a. Traboulsi EI, Maumenee IH. Bilateral melanosis of the iris. *Am J Ophthalmol* 1987; 103;115–116.
352. Trofatter JA, MacCollin MM, Rutter JL, Murrell JR, Duyao MP, Parry DM, et al. A novel moesin-, ezrin-, radixin-like gene is a candidate for the neurofibromatosis 2 tumor suppressor. *Cell* 1993;72:791–800.
353. Twist EC, Ruttledge M, Rousseau M, Sanson M, Papi L, Merel P, et al. The neurofibromatosis type 2 gene is inactivated in schwannomas. *Hum Mol Genet* 1994;3: 147–151.
354. Upadhyaya M, Chreyson A, Broadhead W, Fryer A, Shaw DJ, Huson S, et al. A 90 kb deletion associated with neurofibromatosis type 1. *J Med Genet* 1990;27:738–741.
355. Valero MC, Velasco E, Moreno F, Hernandez-Chico C. Characterization of four mutations in the neurofibromatosis type 1 gene by denaturing gradient gel electrophoresis (DGGE). *Hum Mol Genet* 1994;3:639–641.
356. Van der Hoeve J. Eye symptoms in tuberous sclerosis of the brain. *Trans Ophthalmol Soc UK* 1920;40:329–340.
357. Van der Hoeve J. Eye diseases in tuberous sclerosis of the brain and in Recklinghausen's disease. *Trans Ophthalmol Soc UK* 1923; 43:524–541.
358. Van der Hoeve J. The Doyne Memorial Lecture. Eye symptoms in phakomatoses. *Trans Ophthalmol Soc UK* 1932;52:380–401.
359. Virchow R. Ueber Die Reform der pathologischen und therapeutischen Anschauungen durch die mikroskopischen Untersuchen. *Virchows Arch Pathol Anat Physiol Klin Med* 1847;1:207–255.
360. Viskochil D, Buchberg AM, Xu G, Cawthorn RM, Stevens J, Wolff RK, et al. Deletions and a translocation interrupt a cloned gene at the neurofibromatosis type 1 locus. *Cell* 1990; 62:187–192.
361. Viskochil D, White R, Cawthon R. The neurofibromatosis type 1 gene. *Annu Rev Neurosci* 1993;16:183–205.
362. Vogt H. Zur Diagnostik der tuberosen Sclerose Z Erforsch Behandl. *Jugendl Schwachsinns* 1908;2:1–16.
363. Von Hippel E. Uber eine sehr seltene Erkrankung der Netzhaut. *Arch Ophthalmol* 1904; 59:83–106.
364. Von Hippel E. Die anatomische Grundlage der von mir beschriebenen sehr seltenen Erkrankung der Netzhaut. *Albrecht von Graefes Arch Ophthalmol* 1911;59:83–86.
365. von Recklinghausen F. *Ueber die multiplen Fibrome der Haut und ihre Beziehung zu den multiplen Neuromen.* Berlin: Hirschwald, 1882.
366. Vouge M, Pasquini U, Salvolini U. CT findings of atypical forms of phakomatosis. *Neuroradiology* 1980;20:99–101.
367. Waardenburg PJ. Heterochromie en melanosis. *Ned Tijdschr Geneeskd* 1918;62:1453–1455.
368. Wallace MR, Andersen LB, Saulino AM, Gregory PE, Glover TW, Collins FS. A de novo Alu insertion results in neurofibromatosis type 1. *Nature* 1991;353:864–866.
369. Wallace MR, Marchuk DA, Andersen LB, Letcher R, Odeh HM, Saulino AM, et al. Type 1 neurofibromatosis gene identification of a large transcript disrupted in three NF1 patients. *Science* 1990;249:181–186.
370. Webb D, Fryer A, Osborne J. On the inci-

dence of fits and mental retardation in tuberous sclerosis. *J Med Genet* 1991;28:395–397.
371. Webb D, Osborne J. Non-penetrance in tuberous sclerosis. *J Med Genet* 1991; 28:417–419.
372. Weber F. Right-sided hemi-hypotrophy resulting from right-sided congenital spastic hemiplegia; with a morbid condition of the left side of the brain; revealed by radiograms. *Proc R Soc Med* 1922;3:134–139.
373. Weleber RG, Zonana J. Iris hamartoma (Lisch nodules) in a case of segmental neurofibromatosis. *Am J Ophthalmol* 1983;96:740–743.
374. Wertelecki W, Rouleau GA, Superneau DW, Forehand LW, Williams JP, Haines JL, et al. Neurofibromatosis 2 clinical and DNA linkage studies of a large kindred. *N Engl J Med* 1988;319:278–283.
375. Weskamp C, Cotlier E. Angioma del cerebro y de la retina con malformaciones capilares de la piel. *Arch Oftal Buenos Aires* 1940;15:1–10.
376. Whitehouse D. Diagnostic value of the café-au-lait spot in children. *Arch Dis Child* 1966;41:316–319.
377. Whiteside-Michel J, Liebmann J, Ritch R. Initial 5FU trabeculectomy in young patients. *Ophthalmology* 1992;99:7–13.
378. Whitson JT, Welch RB, Green WR. Von Hippel-Lindau disease: Case report of a patient with spontaneous regression of a retinal angioma. *Retina* 1986;6:253–259.
379. Williamson TH, Garner A, Moore AT. Structure of Lisch nodules in neurofibromatosis type 1. *Ophthalmic Paediatr Genet* 1991;12: 11–17.
380. Wishart JH. Case of tumours in the skull, dura mater, and brain. *Edinburgh Med Surg J* 1822;18:393–397.
381. Wolter JR, Gonzales-Sirit R. Neurofibromatosis of the choroid. *Am J Ophthalmol* 1962;54:217–225.
382. Worster-Drought C, Dickson WEC, McMenemey WH. Multiple meningeal and perineural tumours with analogous changes in the glia and ependyma (neurofibroblastomatosis). *Brain* 1937;60:85–117.
383. Xavier E, Lázaro C, Casals T, Ravella A. Recurrence of a nonsense mutation in the NF1 gene causing classical neurofibromatosis type 1. *Hum Genet* 1991;88:185–188.
383a. Xu GF, Lin B, Tanaka K, Dunn D, Wood D, Gesteland R, White R, Weiss R, Tamanoi F. The catalytic domain of the neurofibromatosis type 1 gene product stimulates ras GTPase and complements ira mutants of S. cerevisiae. *Cell* 1990;63:835–841.
384. Yamaguchi K, Yamaguchi K, Tamai M. Cavernous hemangioma of the retina in a pediatric patient. *Ophthalmologica* 1988;197: 127–129.
385. Yan N, Ricca C, Fletcher J, Glover T, Seizinger BR, Manne V. Farnesyltransferase inhibitors block the neurofibromatosis type 1 (NF1) phenotype. *Cancer Res* 1995;55:3569–3575.
386. Yimoyines DM, Topilow HW, Abedin S, McMeel JW. Bilateral peripapillary exophytic retinal haemangioblastoma. *Ophthalmology* 1982;89:1388–1392.
387. Young DF, Eldridge R, Nager GT, Deland FH, McNew J. Hereditary bilateral acoustic neuroma (central neurofibromatosis). *Birth Defects Orig Art Ser* 1971;7:73–86.
388. Zanca A, Zanca A. Antique illustrations of neurofibromatosis. *Int J Dermatol* 1980;19: 55–58.
389. Zang KD, Singer H. Chromosomal constitution of meningiomas. *Nature* 1967;216:84–85.
390. Zimmer-Galler I, Robertson D. Long-term observation of retinal lesions in tuberous sclerosis. *Am J Ophthalmol* 1995;119:318–324.

37

Syndromes with Craniofacial Anomalies

AMY FELDMAN LEWANDA
ELIAS I. TRABOULSI
ETHYLIN WANG JABS

Craniosynostosis, or the premature fusion of one or more cranial sutures, occurs in approximately 1 in 3000 births and may lead to derangements of craniofacial development. In mild cases, the result may only be a slight asymmetry of the face and cranium without significant sequelae; in severe cases, however, medical and surgical intervention may be required to prevent substantial morbidity.

CRANIOSYNOSTOSIS SYNDROMES

Although it is clear that the premature closure of a single suture can alter the development of the entire craniofacial region, there is debate surrounding the actual sequence in which these events occur. Craniosynostosis, especially when it is unilateral, is often associated with abnormalities of the skull base, and various authors have explored the relation between the two. For example, a theory proposed in the 1970s by Moss[80,81] states that it is the skull base abnormality that is the primary defect, with craniosynostosis occurring as a secondary event. However, several more recent studies reviewed by Cohen[25] find instead that cranio-synostosis is the cardinal event, with skull base abnormalities and midface hypoplasia occurring as secondary and tertiary effects.

Craniosynostosis can affect the development of any structure in the craniofacial region.[26] The shape of the head is usually abnormal and depends on the suture or sutures involved. Dolichocephaly (a long and narrow cranium) results from sagittal suture synostosis, and brachycephaly (a broad cranium), from bilateral coronal synostosis. More complex patterns of plagiocephaly (asymmetric skull shape) are evident when synostosis is unilateral, or when there is a combination of sutures involved. The most severe malformation, a *kleeblattschadel*, or cloverleaf skull deformity, arises when there is early synostosis of the coronal and lambdoid sutures. Intracranial pressure may be elevated and can lead to vision or hearing loss from cranial nerve compression, respiratory depression, neurologic compromise, and death.

The altered skull shape affects the facial landscape as well. The forehead may appear prominent or receding, depending on the specific sutures involved. There may be ocular and orbital involvement with hypertelorism, proptosis, strabismus, abnormal angulation of the palpebral fissures, or ptosis. The midface is often depressed, which can lead to a narrowed airway and respiratory difficulties. Dental anomalies (especially malocclusion) are frequent. The ears may be displaced or placed asymmetrically.

Cases of craniosynostosis may be sporadic or familial.[23] As the expression of the craniosynostosis genes is highly variable, the parents of an affected child should always be examined for subtle abnormalities of cranial shape to rule out mild expression of the genetic defect. The majority of familial craniosynostosis is inherited in an autosomal dominant pattern, so an affected parent would have a 50% chance of having additional children with the disease. Although much less common, autosomal recessive forms also occur and should be suspected if the proband has affected siblings with unaffected parents.

Most commonly, craniosynostosis occurs as an isolated finding, without associated defects. However, over 70 genetic syndromes have been described in which craniosynostosis is a feature. In syndromic cases, the most frequent concomitant anomalies involve the limbs, ears, and cardiovascular system.[22,24]

Ophthalmic features are common in craniosynostotic syndromes. In a survey conducted by Dufier and colleagues[37] in a series of 244 craniosynostotic patients, 36.5% had strabismus and 45% had hypertelorism. Optic discs were pale or atrophic in 50% of patients with Crouzon syndrome and 24% with Apert syndrome. Disc swelling was present in 31% of Crouzon syndrome patients and 9.5% of Apert syndrome patients.

Recently, the genetic basis of several well-known craniosynostoses (Crouzon, Apert, Pfeiffer, and Jackson-Weiss syndromes) was found to be mutations in the family of fibroblast growth factor receptor (FGFR) genes.[68] At present, the FGFR family is known to have four genes, designated FGFR1–FGFR4[14,45,50,57] and located on chromosomes 8p11(FGFR1), 10q25-q26(FGFR2), 4p16(FGFR3), and 5q35 (FGFR4). These genes share a common basic structure, and their proteins have significant amino acid homology. The extracellular region of the FGFR includes a signal peptide, an "acid box" (8–10 consecutive acidic amino acid residues), and three immunoglobulin-like domains (designated IgI, IgII, and IgIII). There is also a transmembrane domain and an intracellular split tyrosine kinase domain. When these receptors are bound to ligands (fibroblast growth factors) and dimerized, they are activated to stimulate differentiation, chemotaxis, angiogenesis, mitogenesis and cell survival, and to regulate key functions of growth and development. There are numerous isoforms of the FGFR genes formed by alternative splicing and fifteen known fibroblast growth factors, leading to great functional diversity. Alterations in the genetic information that forms these ligand–receptor complexes would be expected to have a variety of phenotypic effects and explain the variability of expression that occurs within and between the resulting syndromes. However, it is now known that all four of the craniosynostotic syndromes are allelic and result from mutations in the FGFR2 gene. In fact, identical mutations have been identified in patients diagnosed with different craniosynostotic syndromes,[105] suggesting the effect of modifying genes elsewhere in the genome.

CRANIOSYNOSTOSIS SYNDROMES CAUSED BY FIBROBLAST GROWTH FACTOR RECEPTOR DEFECTS

The craniosynostotic syndromes caused by FGFR mutations have a similar facial appearance and are usually distinguished by the presence or absence of associated limb defects (Fig. 37.1; Table 37.1). These conditions have tremendous variability in expression, and mild cases may go undiagnosed until the birth of an affected child with more characteristic features.

With the exception of Apert syndrome, all of these craniosynostotic conditions are caused by many different mutations. A significant proportion of these mutations involves a loss or gain of a cysteine residue, affecting the formation of disulfide bonds responsible for the tertiary structure of the Ig-like domain. Such mutations are thought to change the ligand binding affinity to the Ig-like domain. Identical mutations have been described in Crouzon, Pfeiffer, and Jackson-Weiss syndromes, raising the possibility that they repre-

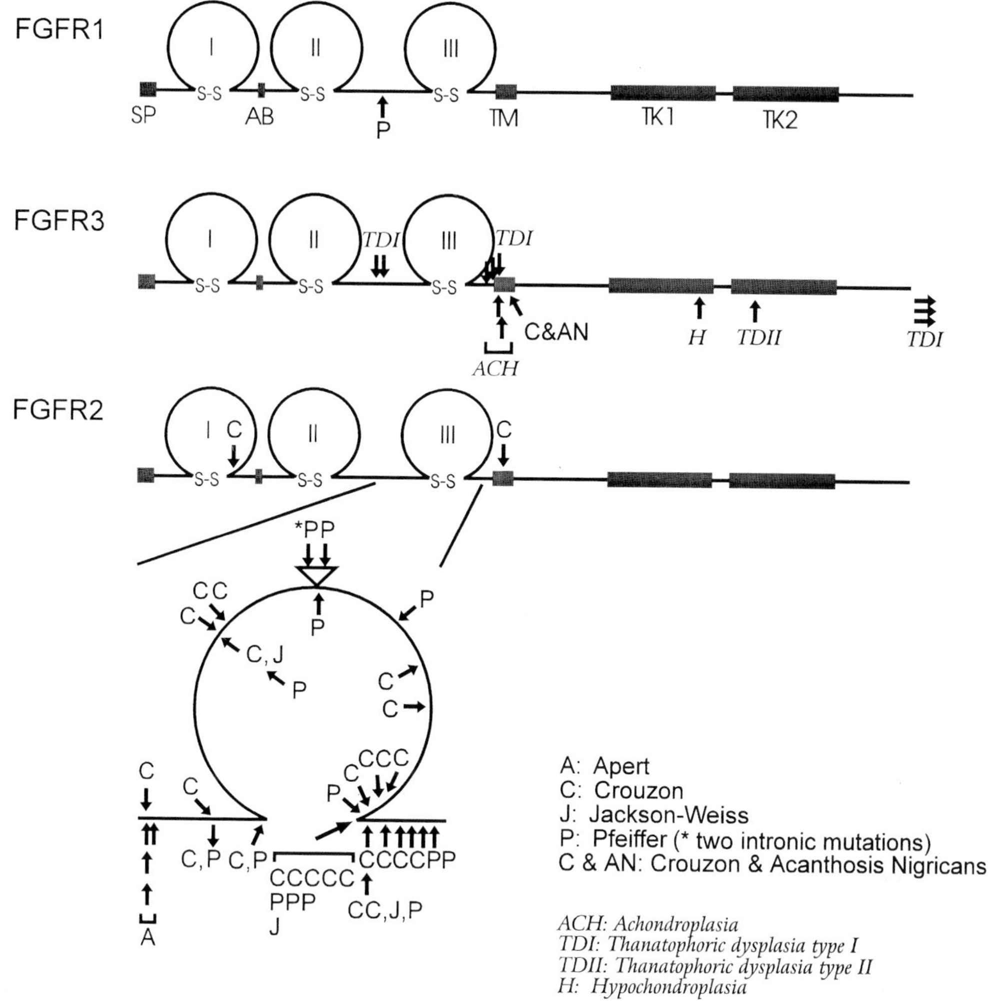

Figure 37.1. Human mutations in fibroblast growth factor receptor genes (FGFR). The structure of human FGFRs, with the location of mutations, is shown for each disorder. Each mutation site is indicated by one arrow, and the number of disease symbols at the same location indicates the number of different amino acid changes at the same residue. SP = signal peptide; AB = acidic box; I, II, and III = immunoglobulinlike domains; S-S = the disulfide bond; TM = transmembrane domain; TK1 and TK2 = tyrosine kinase domain; ACH, TDI, TDII, and HCH are dwarfing conditions mentioned only in comparison to the craniofacial disorders. (Adapted with permission from W-J Park et al. Analysis of phenotypic features and FGFR2 mutations in Apert syndrome. *Am J Hum Genet* 1995;57:321–328, published by The University of Chicago Press.)[90]

sent a single disorder with a wide spectrum of phenotypic expression.

Crouzon Syndrome

Crouzon syndrome, initially described in 1912,[32] involves craniosynostosis, midface hypoplasia, and ocular proptosis (Fig. 37.2). It occurs in approximately 1 in 25,000 births.[26] It is inherited in an autosomal dominant fashion, with a significant percentage (estimated at 33%–56%)[5,63] of cases resulting from spontaneous mutations. In a study by Kreiborg,[63] advanced paternal age was associated with the occurrence of such mutations. In addition, several cases of germinal mosaicism have been

Table 37.1. Craniofacial Syndromes: Clinical Features and Causative Genes

Syndrome	Gene	Digital Features	Ocular Features	Internal Organ Involvement
Crouzon	*FGFR2/FGFR3*	None	Proptosis, exotropia, optic atrophy, extraocular muscle abnormalities	None
Apert	*FGFR2*	Symmetric mitten-type syndactyly of hands and feet	Proptosis, hypertelorism, downslanting palpebral fissures, exotropia, extraocular muscle abnormalities	Cardiovascular (10%) Genitourinary (10%) Respiratory (1.5%) Gastrointestinal (1.5%) Intellectual impairment (great majority)
Pfeiffer	*FGFR1/FGFR2*	Broad, medially deviated thumbs and great toes, brachydactyly	Proptosis, downslanting palpebral fissures, hypertelorism, strabismus	Various anomalies reported; more frequent in subtypes 2 and 3
Jackson-Weiss	*FGFR2*	Broad first metatarsal, abnormally shaped tarsal bones, calcaneo-cuboid fusion; hands are unaffected	Proptosis, strabismus	None
Saethre-Chotzen	*TWIST*	Soft tissue syndactyly (usually digits 2–3) of hands and feet	Ptosis, hypertelorism, strabismus	None
Boston Type	*MSX2*	Single individual with triphalangeal thumb	Myopia, hyperopia, visual field defects	Single individual with cleft soft palate
Carpenter	?	Brachydactyly, soft tissue syndactyly, preaxial polydactyly of feet, decreased number of phalanges	Laterally displaced inner canthi, epicanthal folds	Cardiovascular (approx 33%), structural brain defects, and intellectual impairment
Baller-Gerold	?	Thumb aplasia or hypoplasia, radial aplasia or hypoplasia, shortened and bowed ulnae. Lower limb anomalies in a small percentage of patients	Downslanting palpebral fissures, epicanthal folds Exotropia, nystagmus, ectropion and severe myopia described	Anal, renal, genital, cardiac, central nervous system defects, vertebral anomalies
Treacher Collins	(Treacle) *TCOF1*	None	Downslanting palpebral fissures, lower eyelid coloboma	None
Miller	?	Preaxial upper limb defects	Downslanting palpebral fissures, lower eyelid coloboma	None
Nager	?	Postaxial upper limb defects	Downslanting palpebral fissures, lower eyelid coloboma	None
Oculoauriculovertebral spectrum	?	None	Asymmetry of eyes, epibulbar dermoid, microphthalmia	Cervical vertebral anomalies, cardiac defects, renal defects

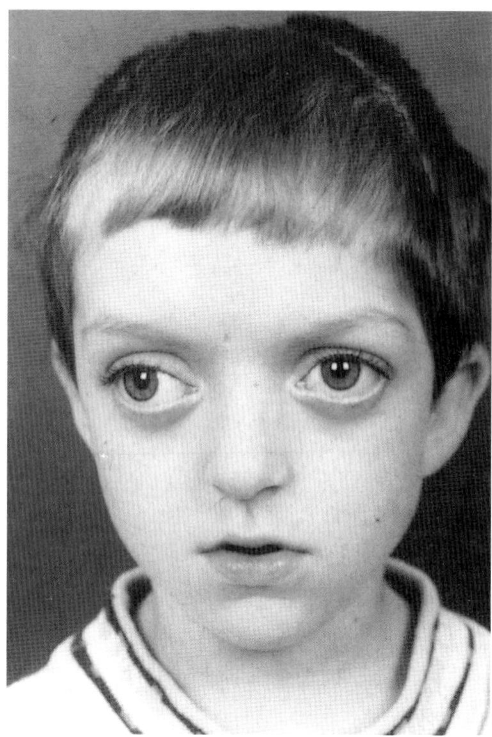

Figure 37.2. Crouzon syndrome. Note exotropia, proptosis, hypertelorism, and midface hypoplasia. This patient is status postcraniectomy for sutural synostosis, which had caused increased intracranial pressure and visual deficits. (From X. Li et al. Two craniosynastotic syndrome loci, Crouzon and Jackson-Weiss, Map to chromosome 10q23-q26. *Genomics* 1994;22:418–424, with permission.)

reported,[85,103] including one of an unaffected mother having two affected children with different fathers.[61] Because this report was published before the availability of molecular testing for Crouzon syndrome, it is possible that the mother was actually affected, but had very mild phenotypic expression.

The head is most commonly brachycephalic, secondary to synostosis of the coronal sutures. However, this feature is quite variable and may range from almost no sutural involvement to severe multisutural involvement and a cloverleaf skull. The striking clinical variability is best illustrated by the report of Shiller,[110] who found individuals at both ends of the spectrum within the same family. Conductive hearing loss is common, and intelligence is generally normal, with only 3% of patients having marked mental deficiency.[63]

Other characteristic facial features of Crouzon syndrome include midfacial hypoplasia, a "beaked" nose, and relative prognathism. The hypoplastic maxilla can create significant dental problems such as malocclusion and crowding of teeth. Lateral palatal swellings are common. Other frequent anomalies noted in Kreiborg's study[63] included calcification of the stylohyoid ligament in 88% of patients and cervical spine anomalies (most frequently C2–C3 fusion) in 30%. Limb defects are *not* typical of Crouzon syndrome; their presence should prompt consideration of other related craniosynostotic syndromes as a clinical diagnosis. Acanthosis nigricans, a dermatologic disorder involving hyperpigmentation and hyperkeratosis, is also associated with Crouzon syndrome.[88]

Ophthalmic Features

There is significant orbital and ocular involvement in Crouzon syndrome. The presence of proptosis (secondary to shallow bony orbits) and hypertelorism are important diagnostic criteria for this condition. The proptosis may lead to exposure keratitis, and, in extreme cases, spontaneous subluxation of the globe.[10,38]

Exotropia is also common, occuring in 77% of patients in Kreiborg's series.[63] The typical V-pattern exotropia is due to overaction of the inferior oblique extraocular muscles and underaction of the superior oblique ones. Limon de Brown[70] proposed that the superior oblique weakness is due to the interplay of musculature around the foreshortened orbit. Others have proposed that the weakness of the superior oblique muscles in Crouzon syndrome is of a primary nature.[51] Diamond et al.[35] reported absence of various extraocular muscles in patients with Crouzon syndrome with strabismus.

Bertelson reported that 80% of patients with Crouzon syndrome had some degree of optic nerve involvement.[8] Optic atrophy was found in 22% of the patients in Kreiborg's series and may have been the result of prolonged papilledema from elevated intracranial pressure. Visual loss and blindness are found in a smaller percentage of cases. Infrequent ocular abnormalities include nystagmus, iris coloboma, aniridia, anisocoria, corectopia, micro- or megalocornea, keratoconus with acute hydrops, cataract, ectopia lentis, blue sclerae, and glaucoma.[12,63,125]

Genetics

The FGFR2 gene mutations in Crouzon syndrome were first described by Reardon et al.[98] To date, causative mutations have been found in approximately 65% of patients studied. Over 25 mutations have been identified and are located predominantly in the IgIII domain and its adjacent linker regions of the extracellular domain.[49,54,77,87,91,98,108] Mutations may be single nucleotide substitutions (missense), small deletions, or insertions. Some of the changes alter RNA splicing, creating mutant isoforms.[69]

A mutation in the transmembrane domain of a different FGFR gene (FGFR3) has been identified in the subset of Crouzon patients who have acanthosis nigricans.[78] Allelic mutations of FGFR3 had previously been determined to be responsible for three dwarfing syndromes: achondroplasia, thanatophoric dysplasia, and hypochondroplasia.[68] The Crouzon patients in whom FGFR3 mutations were found did not have radiographic features consistent with these syndromes, nor did they have concomitant FGFR2 mutations.

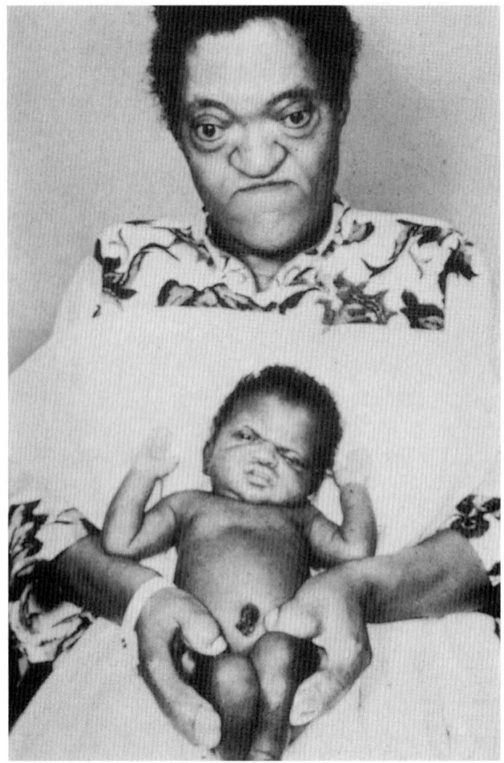

Figure 37.3. Mother and child with Apert syndrome. Both exhibit hypertelorism, proptosis, midface hypoplasia, and typical symmetric syndactylyl. The mother's nails are continuous over syndactylous digits. (From K. B. Roberts and J. G. Hall, in D Bergsma, ed. *Birth Defects: Original Article Series*, Vol. VII, No. 7. Baltimore: Williams and Wilkins for the National Foundation—March of Dimes, with permission.) Apert's acrocephalosyndactyly in mother and daughter: cleft palate in the mother. 1971:262–263.

Apert Syndrome

Apert syndrome is characterized by craniosynostosis, ocular proptosis, and midface hypoplasia. In addition, a distinctive, symmetric "mitten-type" syndactyly of the hands and feet make this syndrome the most easily recognizable of the acrocephalosyndactylies (Fig. 37.3). Since Apert's first report of this condition in 1906,[3] large series of affected patients have been extensively reviewed by Cohen,[26] and Cohen and Kreiborg.[19,20,29]

Apert syndrome has a birth prevalence of 1/160,000.[9] Because of the decreased reproductive fitness of affected individuals, the vast majority of cases are sporadic and have been associated with advanced paternal age.[39] However, this condition is known to be inherited in an autosomal dominant fashion, and 11 cases of familial inheritance have been documented.[65] Furthermore, Allanson[1] reported a case of germinal mosaicism.

The pathogenesis of the cranial anomaly in Apert syndrome is distinct from the other craniosynostoses. Instead of having normal cranial sutures that fuse prematurely, patients with this condition are born with a wide midline calvarial defect where the metopic and sagittal sutures would normally be found.[62] In the 2 to 4 years after birth, this defect is gradually filled by islands of bone that gradually coalesce until the gap is obliterated. No true sagittal or metopic sutures are ever formed. The coronal sutures are generally fused at birth.

The unusual pattern of skull development may help to explain some of the central nervous system abnormalities seen in this condition.[29] The brain of patients with Apert syndrome is typically megalencephalic. The brain is forced to grow upward and laterally because of the fusion of the coronal suture and the constricted cranial base; this process maintains the midline calvarial defect and can also lead to gross distortions of brain shape. The shortened cranial base can cause growing brain tissue to extend through the open metopic area, resulting in an anterior encephalocele. A significant proportion of patients with Apert syndrome are mentally retarded, possibly as a result of malformations of the central nervous system rather than increased intracranial pressure. Cohen and Kreiborg[29] documented numerous abnormalities, including an absent or abnormal corpus callosum, limbic structure defects, gyral abnormalities, white matter hypoplasia, and heterotopic gray matter. The wide midline calvarial defect allows adequate decompression of the skull, avoiding elevation of the intracranial pressure in the first 2 years of life.[62] There is no significant difference in the prevalence of mental retardation between patients who undergo a craniectomy during the first year of life and those who do not, suggesting that factors other than increased pressure are involved in the pathogenesis of the mental defect.[93]

In patients with Apert syndrome the forehead is typically high, with a horizontal groove above the supraorbital ridges in some affected infants; a finding that tends to disappear with age.[48] The nasal bridge is depressed and the nose is beaked. The midface is hypoplastic, resulting in relative prognathism. Oral abnormalities are common. The palate is narrow and high arched, often with a median furrow, giving the appearance of a Byzantine arch.[48] There are lateral palatal swellings, and clefting of the soft palate (or its forme fruste, a bifid uvula) occurs in 30%. The teeth are crowded because of the constricted dental arch, and malocclusion is common.

Abnormalities of the hands and feet are the true hallmarks of Apert syndrome. There is consistent syndactyly of the second, third, and fourth digits; the first and fifth are involved to a variable degree. Nails may be separated or continuous over two or more digits. In addition to syndactyly, the digits exhibit a number of other abnormalities, including brachydactyly, and misshapen and/or fused bones. The proximal interphalangeal joints become fused by 4–6 years, and progressive calcification and fusion of the bones in the hands, feet, and cervical spine occurs with age.[52,107]

Apert syndrome is the only FGFR2 craniosynostosis thus far known to be significantly associated with internal malformations. Cardiovascular and genitourinary anomalies were each found in approximately 10% of the 136 patients reported by Cohen and Kreiborg.[20] Respiratory tract and gastrointestinal abnormalities occurred in 1.5% of cases. As autopsies were performed on only 12 of the 136 study subjects, the authors caution that these frequencies should be considered a minimum estimate, as minor anomalies or anatomic variations could have been missed in the remaining subjects.

The same authors examined the cutaneous manifestations of Apert syndrome.[19] Hyperhidrosis was found in all patients. Beginning in adolescence, the skin becomes oily, and the majority of patients develop significant acneiform lesions of the face, chest, back, and upper arms. Other unusual cutaneous findings include an interruption of the continuity of the eyebrow and excessive wrinkling of the skin of the forehead, both attributable to underlying bony abnormalities.

Ophthalmic Features

The bony orbits are shallow, leading to significant ocular proptosis. Hypertelorism and downslating palpebral fissues are frequent. Also common is a V-pattern exotropia similar to that which occurs in Crouzon syndrome. Extraocular muscle abnormalities have been reported,[75] as has absence of the superior rectus muscle.[33,122]

Features of ocular albinism have been described in Apert syndrome, including depigmentation of the fundus and absence of foveal reflexes. However, in contrast to oculocutaneous albinism, vision is not markedly impaired, and pendular nystagmus is absent.[48]

Other ocular features occasionally seen in Apert syndrome include optic atrophy, keratoconus, glaucoma, and subluxation of the globe.[31]

Genetics

The FGFR2 gene defects responsible for the Apert syndrome were first elucidated by Wilkie et al.[123] To date, over 100 patients have been studied, and one of two mutations (located in adjacent amino acid residues) have been identified in all but two cases. A C → G transversion occurred either at position 934 (causing a serine → tryptophan substitution at amino acid 252) or at position 937 (causing a proline → arginine substitution at amino acid 253). These amino acids lie within the linker region between IgII and IgIII. Although the two mutations have not shown a significant difference in phenotypic expression, oral clefting appears to be more frequent with the Ser252Trp mutation and syndactyly more severe with the Pro253Arg mutation.[90,123]

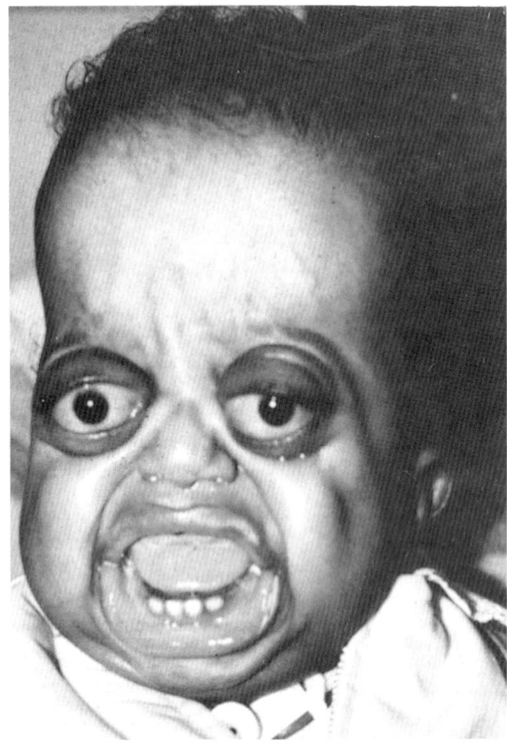

Figure 37.4. Pfeiffer syndrome. Severely affected patient with craniosynostosis, midface hypoplasia, proptosis, and hypertelorism.

Pfeiffer Syndrome

Pfeiffer syndrome is an autosomal dominant condition that was first described by Pfeiffer in 1964.[95] It is characterized by craniosynostosis and a high broad skull with a shortened anteroposterior diameter (Fig. 37.4). The thumbs and great toes are broad and there is variable soft tissue syndactyly (Figs. 37.5 and 37.6). Expressivity is quite variable, and a cloverleaf skull deformity has been reported with Pfeiffer syndrome in several instances.[21] Patients with this severe cranial deformity are more likely to have other abnormalities not typically present in Pfeiffer syndrome.[30] Individuals with the cloverleaf skull have thus far all been sporadic cases, with no family history of Pfeiffer syndrome. Mental development is generally poor in severely affected individuals but is usually normal in familial cases.

The differences among patients with Pfeiffer syndrome led Cohen[30] to propose three clinical subtypes of the disorder. Although this is the only formal classification of Pfeiffer syndrome subtypes clinical experience has shown that

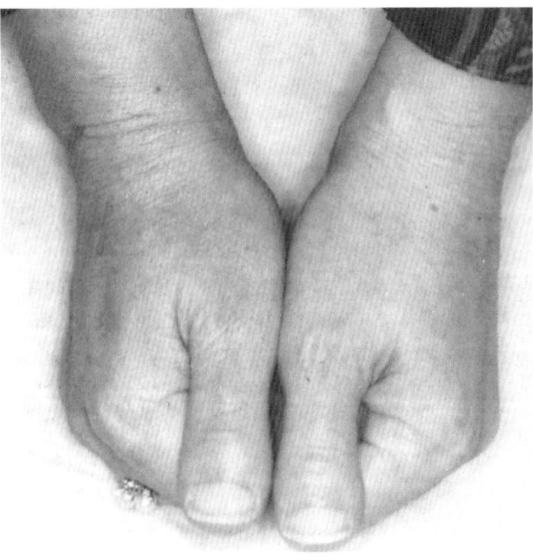

Figure 37.5. Pfeiffer syndrome showing broad thumbs.

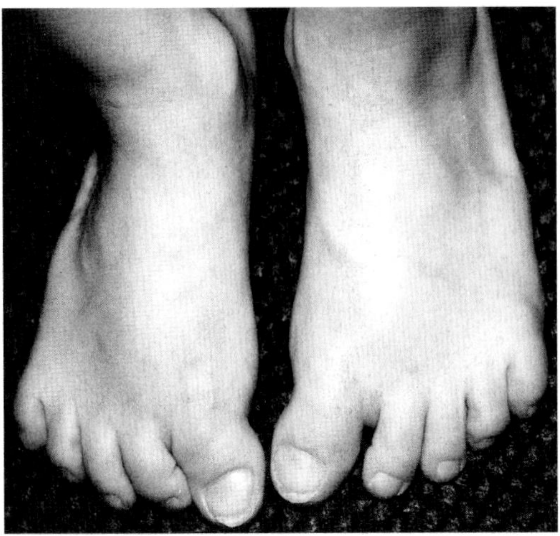

Figure 37.6. Pfeiffer syndrome showing broad great toes.

more than one subtype may occur in the same family, showing variable phenotypic expression of the same mutation. The distinction is based on both cranial and extracranial manifestations. It does not depend on the appearance of the hands and feet; brachydactyly, broad thumbs and great toes (often with a delta-shaped phalanx), and variable soft tissue syndactyly are presented in all three subtypes. The delta phalanx is typical but not pathognomonic for this disorder.[73]

Classic Pfeiffer syndrome is designated type 1, with craniosynostosis, midface hypoplasia, relative prognathism, a high arched palate, and dental crowding. Other anomalies are found at a low frequency. This form is autosomal dominant and is sometimes inherited from an affected parent.

Type 2 Pfeiffer syndrome is marked by the presence of a cloverleaf skull and severe ocular proptosis. The central nervous system is frequently involved with abnormalities such as hydrocephalus, and patients have elbow ankylosis/synostosis. Type 2 Pfeiffer syndrome is more often associated with clusters of unusual anatomic anomalies, although the specific anomalies vary from patient to patient. All cases reported to date have been sporadic.

Type 3 Pfeiffer syndrome is similar to type 2 but lacks the cloverleaf skull. Anomalies reported with this condition include intestinal malrotation and prune belly syndrome.[7] As in type 2, all reported cases have been sporadic.

The separation of Pfeiffer syndrome patients into one of these three categories is not absolute. Features such as elbow ankylosis may be found in any category, although more so in types 2 and 3. The classification is important to determine prognosis, with type 1 patients usually having normal intelligence and a generally good outcome,[30] whereas patients with types 2 and 3 often have neurologic involvement and a shortened life expectancy. A second purpose of this classification system is to avoid misdiagnosing patients with type 3 craniosynostosis and various internal anomalies as having an unknown or unique syndrome.[28,30,124]

Ophthalmic Features

The ocular features are similar to those of Crouzon and Apert syndromes and include proptosis, downslanting palpebral fissures, hypertelorism, and strabismus. Jones et al.[60] reported atypical, bilateral superior iris coloboma in an affected patient. Other findings include ptosis, scleralization of the cornea, and optic nerve hypoplasia.[48] There are a few reported cases of anterior chamber defects, including Peters' anomaly.[115a]

Genetics

Pfeiffer syndrome was mapped to the FGFR1 region on chromosome 8 by Robin et al.[100] However, linkage was established in only 5/11 families studied, and was excluded in the other six families, proving genetic heterogeneity. A single mutation in the FGFR1 gene causing the substitution of a proline by an arginine residue at codon 252 was found in three of the linked families. This mutation was located in the linker region between IgII and IgIII and has now been found in seven unrelated patients.[77,82] A second locus for the Pfeiffer syndrome gene was reported to be FGFR2 on chromosome 10q.[64,105,108] To date, over fifteen different FGFR2 mutations have been identified.[64,77,105,108] Five of these mutations have also been reported in patients with Crouzon syndrome.

Jackson-Weiss Syndrome

This syndrome of craniofacial and foot abnormalities was first described by Jackson et al.[56] in a very large Amish kindred, in which 88 affected individuals were observed, and another 50 were reliably reported to be affected. As craniofacial abnormalities were noted in conjunction with broad great toes, the kindred was initially thought to exhibit Pfeiffer syndrome. However, no individual in this extensive group possessed the thumb abnormalities characteristic of Pfeiffer syndrome. The authors were struck by the variable expressivity of this new syndrome and prophetically noted that "the entire spectrum of dominantly inherited craniofacial dysostoses-acrocephalosyndactylies (except the typical Apert syndrome) was seen in this kindred.[56]

The syndrome described by Jackson and Weiss is characterized by craniosynostosis, midface hypoplasia, and bony abnormalities of the feet. However, none of the 138 affected people exhibited broad thumbs, helping to distinguish it from Pfeiffer syndrome. The cranium was generally acrocephalic (Fig. 37.7) although at least one affected individual with premature sutural synostosis documented by radiographs was described as having a normal cranial shape. Intelligence was generally normal with no correlation to the severity of cranial deformity. Common facial features include a prominent forehead and maxillary hypoplasia.

The only common feature shared by all affected members of this extended family was a clinical or radiographic abnormality of the feet. Minimal manifestations included short, broad first metatarsal, abnormally shaped tarsal bones, and calcaneocuboid fusion.[48] The most severely affected individual required bilateral toe amputation secondary to the extreme deformity, including medial deviation of the great toes of almost 90° (Fig. 37.8).[56]

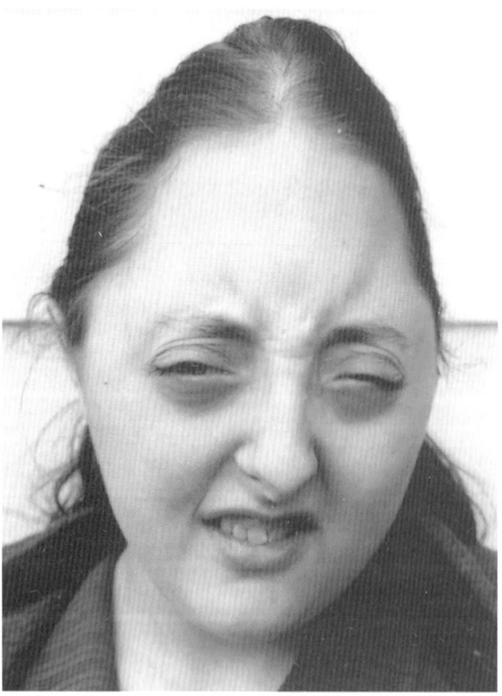

Figure 37.7. Jackson-Weiss syndrome. Affected individual with striking acrocephaly. (From C. E. Jackson et al., Craniosynostosis, midfacial hypoplasia, and foot abnormalities: An autosomal dominant phenotype in a large Amish kindred. *J Pediatr* 1976;88:963–968, with permission.[56])

Ophthalmic Features

Common features include ocular proptosis, hypertelorism, and strabismus.

Genetics

The FGFR2 mutation responsible for Jackson-Weiss syndrome was reported by Jabs et al.[54] using patient samples from the family in which the condition was initially described. An argi-

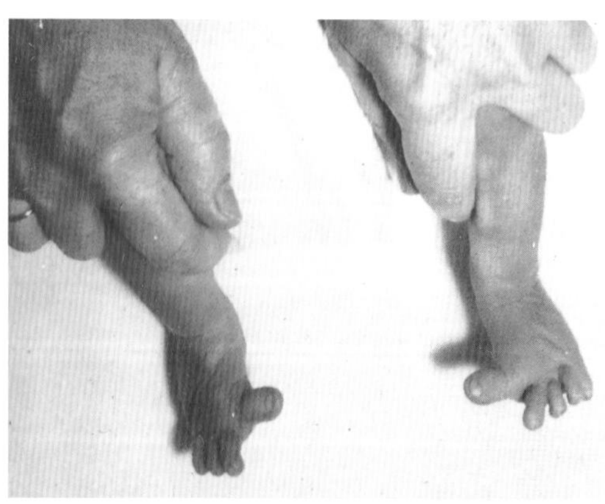

Figure 37.8. Jackson-Weiss syndrome. The great toes are broad and severely medially deviated. (Courtesy of Dr. Charles E. Jackson.)

nine → glycine mutation at position 344 was identified in all affected, and none of the unaffected individuals. This mutation is located in the C-terminal half of the third Ig domain. Two additional mutations have been identified in the same Ig domain in sporadic cases of Jackson-Weiss syndrome.

OTHER CRANIOSYNOSTOSIS SYNDROMES

Saethre-Chotzen Syndrome

Saethre-Chotzen syndrome, which involves craniosynostosis, facial asymmetry, and partial soft tissue syndactyly, was reported independently by both Saethre[106] and Chotzen.[17] It is inherited in an autosomal dominant fashion with high variability of expression. Because of this high degree of variability, neither craniosynostosis nor syndactyly is an obligate feature for the diagnosis. Although this syndrome may occur more frequently than other syndromic craniosynostoses, its actual prevalence at birth is unknown. It is most likely underdiagnosed, as mild cases may never come to medical attention, and sporadic cases that exhibit only craniosynostosis or syndactyly are often misdiagnosed.[26]

Synostosis of the coronal suture is frequent and leads to a brachycephalic or acrocephalic head. As the synostosis is often asymmetric, plagiocephaly with facial asymmetry is also a common finding (Fig. 37.9). The frontal hairline is usually low-set. The ears may be dysmorphic with a prominent helical crus. Intelligence is usually normal.[89]

There may be various degrees of soft tissue syndactyly of the hands and feet, most commonly between the second and third digits, but these may involve the fourth digit as well. The hands and feet often show brachydactyly.[27]

Ophthalmic Features

Although hyperterlorism occurs frequently, hypotelorism has been reported in conjunction with metopic suture synostosis.[48] Ptosis of the eyelids is usually unilateral or asymmetric, and strabismus is common. Blepharophimosis and dacryostenosis have been reported in some cases. Less common features include epicanthal folds, optic atrophy, downslanting palpebral fissues, and anomalies of the eyelids and brows.

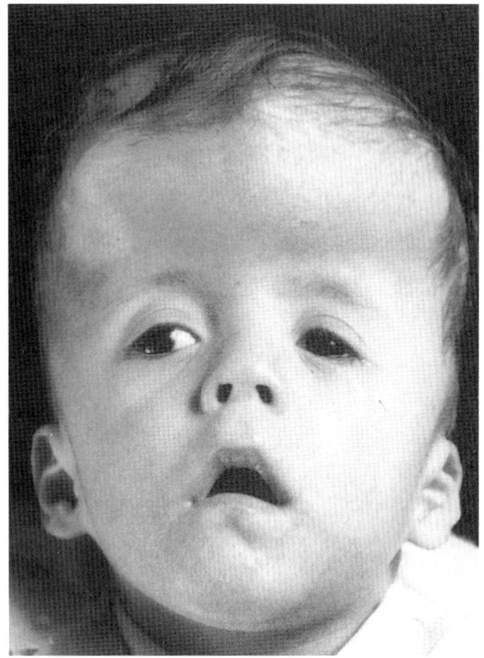

Figure 37.9. Saethre-Chotzen syndrome. Note abnormal head shape, facial asymmetry, ptosis, and prominent helical ears. (From Saethre-Chotzen syndrome with familial translocation at chromosome 7p22, C. S. Reid, *Am J Med Genet*, Copyright © (1993). Reprinted by permission of John Wiley & Sons, Inc.[99])

Genetics

The gene responsible for the Saethre-Chotzen syndrome has been identified to be the *TWIST* gene on distal chromosome 7p.[13,52a,66,67] Over 25 distinct mutations have already been identified in this transcription factor with a helix-loop-helix domain. Several affected individuals with chromosomal translocations of this region have been reported, implicating 7p21.2-7p22 as the gene site.[97,99,104] As these translocations do not appear to disrupt the gene itself, they may instead affect an associated regulatory region. Because of the highly variable phenotype, more than one gene locus may be involved.

Boston-Type Craniosynostosis

Boston-type craniosynostosis, an autosomal dominant syndrome, was initially described in a large three-generation family from Boston.[120] The range of expressivity in the 19 affected family members was wide enough to identify four general phenotypes of cranial malformation. These phenotypes were frontoorbital recession, frontal bossing, turribrachycephaly, and cloverleaf skull. This disorder is distinct from the more common craniosynostosis syndromes because other characteristic features such as the proptosis, hypertelorism, malocclusion, and midface hypoplasia of Crouzon syndrome, the broad thumbs and great toes seen in Pfeiffer syndrome, the foot anomalies of the Jackson-Weiss syndrome, and the ptosis, soft tissue syndactyly, and ear anomalies of Saethre-Chotzen syndrome, are all absent. Intelligence is normal. Three of the four affected adults on whom foot radiographs were obtained had short, but not broad, first metatarsals. Other malformations identified in this kindred were a cleft soft palate and a triphalangeal thumb, each found in only one individual.

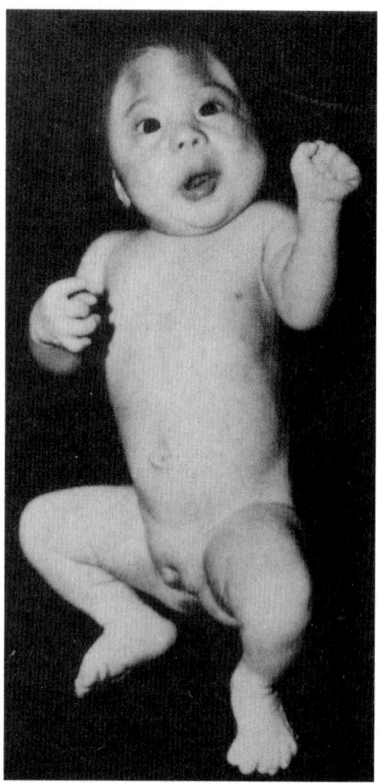

Figure 37.10. Carpenter syndrome. This patient has bifrontal narrowing of the skull and preaxial polydactyly of the feet. (From *SYNDROMES OF THE HEAD AND NECK*, edited by R. J. Gorlin et al. Copyright © 1990 by Robert J. Gorlin, M. Michael Cohen, Jr., and L. Stefan Levin. Used by permission of Oxford University Press, Inc.[48])

Ophthalmic Features

Almost all affected individuals in this kindred had myopia or hyperopia, and two had visual field defects.

Genetics

This condition was mapped to the long arm of chromosome 5,[83] the same region known to contain the *MSX2* homeobox gene. This gene is one of a class of transcription regulators known to play an important role in morphogenesis and development.[76,109] A C → A transversion, causing substitution of a histidine for a proline residue at amino acid position 7 of the homeodomain was found in all affected, and no unaffected individuals.[55] This discovery made *MSX2* the first homeobox gene known to cause a malformation syndrome in humans.

Carpenter Syndrome

Carpenter syndrome, originally reported in 1901,[16] is characterized by craniosynostosis, polydactyly, cutaneous syndactyly, and cardiac defects (Fig. 37.10). It is one of the few craniosynostosis syndromes inherited in an autosomal recessive fashion. The causative gene has not yet been identified.

Multiple cranial sutures are usually involved, often beginning with the sagittal and lambdoid sutures.[48] The multisutural involvement can lead to very dramatic alterations of cranial shape with marked asymmetry and acrocephaly. A cloverleaf skull deformity has been reported in Carpenter syndrome.[21,27] Intellectual impairment is present in approximately three-fourths of affected individuals.[18] Taravath and Tonsgard[112] used computed tomography and magnetic resonance imaging to search for structural brain defects in a patient with profound developmental delay. They found widespread atrophy of the cortex, right frontal and parietal lobes, and cerebellar vermis. In addition, the lateral ventricles were abnormal in appearance and orientation, and there was partial agenesis of the corpus callosum and bilateral decrease in white matter.

The fingers are typically short, with varying degree of soft tissue syndactyly. The feet often have preaxial polydactyly, and each toe has only two phalanges. Approximately one-third of patients have congenital heart defects, including atrial and ventricular septal defects, patent ductus arteriosus, pulmonic stenosis, and tetralogy of Fallot.[48]

Ophthalmic Features

The inner canthi are usually laterally displaced, and there may be epicanthal folds present. Infrequent ophthalmologic findings include microcornea, corneal opacity, slight optic atrophy, and blurring of the disc margins.[48] Conjugate downward movements alternating with horizontal and vertical nystagmus, foveal hypoplasia, and posterior embryotoxon have also been reported.[115] The ears are low-set and may have minor abnormalities such as preauricular pits.[58]

Baller-Gerold Syndrome

Baller[6] and Gerold[47] independently described an autosomal recessive malformation syndrome of craniosynostosis and preaxial upper limb abnormalities (Fig. 37.11). A wide variety of internal malformations have been identified in the 23 patients reported to date; most frequently these defects affect the anus, urogenital system, heart, and central nervous system.[43,71]

A minority of the reported cases exhibit only the cardinal manifestations without visceral anomalies, or growth or psychomotor retardation.[43] This led Galea and Tolmie[44] to suggest that patients with Baller-Gerold syndrome are divisible into two groups, and to propose genetic heterogeneity. Others, however,[34,43] feel that intrafamilial variability and the small number of reported cases make this theory unlikely. Artlich and colleagues[4] describe a girl with a phenotype reminiscent of Baller-Gerold syndrome whose mother had been treated for acute myelocytic leukemia prior to the recognition of pregnancy. She received cytarabine, daunorubicin, and doxorubicin around the time of conception and cytarabine and thioguanine approximately 35–37 days postconception, suggesting a possible teratogenic etiology for the phenotype in this case.

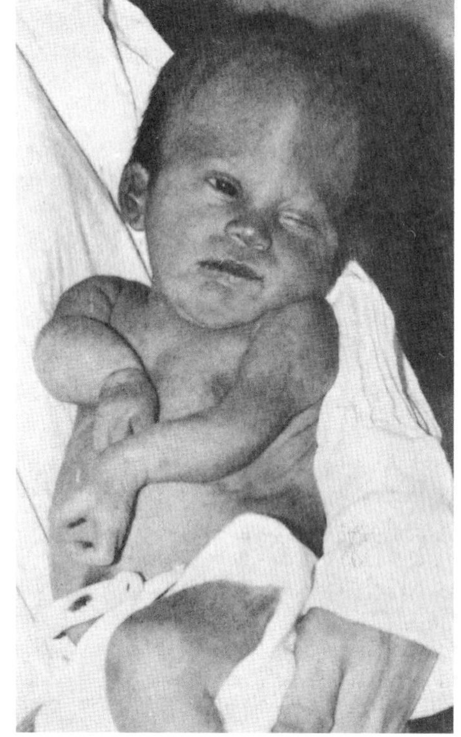

Figure 37.11. Baller-Gerold syndrome. Craniosynostosis with metopic ridge and radial aplasia with shortened forearms. (From *SYNDROMES OF THE HEAD AND NECK*, edited by R. J. Gorlin et al. Copyright © 1990 by Robert J. Gorlin, M. Michael Cohen, Jr., and L. Stefan Levin. Used by permission of Oxford University Press, Inc.[48])

Craniosynostosis is a major diagnostic criterion for Baller-Gerold syndrome. Any of the cranial sutures may be affected. A detailed review by Fuentes et al.[43] showed that the coronal suture is most commonly affected (64% of cases), followed by the metopic (36%), lambdoid (27%), and sagittal (9%). Approximately one-third of patients have involvement of multiple sutures. Extensive agenesis of the frontal and parietal bones has been reported.[118] Because of variable sutural involvement, there is no head shape typical of Baller-Gerold syndrome. Similarly, dysmorphic facial features are common but do not produce a distinctive and recognizable phenotype.[43] Frequent craniofacial features include low-set, posteriorly rotated ears; micrognathia; microstomia; midline facial hemangiomas; prominent nasal bridge; and high arched palate.[11,43]

Preaxial upper limb defects are the second cardinal feature of Baller-Gerold syndrome. This most often involves aplasia or hypoplasia of the thumb(s), followed by aplasia or hypoplasia of the radius. These defects are bilateral in over 90% of cases.[43] As a result of radial aplasia, the ulna bears an increased mechanical load due to radial muscular traction, which leads to shortening and bowing.[34] Metacarpal abnormalities are also common. The lower limbs are generally normal, although minor abnormalities of the femora, fibulae, and toes[34,43] have been described.

A wide variety of internal organ defects have been associated with this condition. Anal anomalies are the most frequent, and include anal malposition and imperforate anus with perineal or rectovaginal fistula.[2,34,118]

Abnormalities of the kidneys (renal ectopia, agenesis, or hypoplasia) or genitals (common cloaca, hypoplastic labia majora, absent vaginal orifice[71]) are described. Almost one-quarter of reported patients have had cardiac defects[43] including ventriculoseptal defects and tetralogy of Fallot. A number of central nervous system abnormalities occur. A detailed postmortem examination of the patient reported by Lin et al.[71] showed polymicrogyria (which has been noted in other cases), a thin corpus callosum, poor inward folding of the hippocampi, hypoplasia of the olfactory bulbs and tracts, and leptomeningeal glioneuronal heterotopias at the base of the hypothalamus.[86] Skeletal anomalies other than those affecting the skull and upper arms are also common. Approximately one-third of patients will have vertebral anomalies, including spina bifida occulta, scoliosis, platyspondyly, absent vertebrae, or cervical lordosis.[43] A smaller percentage have bony abnormalities of the feet and toes such as tarsal coalition, proximally placed great toes, brachyclinodactyly, and phalangeal aplasia or hypoplasia.[34] The first report of malignancy in this condition was of an osteosarcoma of the distal femur in a 16-year-old male.[96]

Of the first 20 reported cases of Baller-Gerold syndrome, 5 patients died unexpectedly in the first year of life.[71] Because pancreatic islet cell hypertrophy was noted on one patient at autopsy, abnormal glucose homeostasis has been suggested as a possible explanation.[118] The diagnosis of Baller-Gerold syndrome may be missed if patients die before craniosynostosis becomes apparent.[71]

Ophthalmic Features

Ophthalmologic anomalies were found in 32% of patients,[43] most frequently downslanting palpebral fissures and epicanthal folds. The patient described by Dallapiccola et al.[34] had these features in addition to exotropia, ectropion, nystagmus, and severe nonfamilial myopia (9 D in the right eye and 3 D in the left).

MANDIBULOFACIAL DYSOSTOSES

Treacher Collins Syndrome

Treacher Collins syndrome is the most common condition involving abnormal development of branchial arch derivatives, occurring in 1/25,000–1/50,000 births. It is inherited in an autosomal dominant manner. New mutations account for approximately 60% of cases, and are often associated with advanced paternal age.[48,59] The syndrome was characterized in 1960 by the ophthalmologist Treacher Collins, although patients with this condition had been described as early as the mid-1800s.[113,114,116]

The primary features of this syndrome are downslanting palpebral fissures, lower eyelid colobomas, malar and mandibular hypoplasia, and malformed external ears (Fig. 37.12).[101] Conductive deafness and cleft palate occur in approximately 50% and 30% of patients, respectively. The hair growth patterns are unusual, often showing tonguelike extension of hair onto the cheeks.

Ophthalmic Features

The ophthalmic features are among the most consistent and diagnostic in this syndrome.

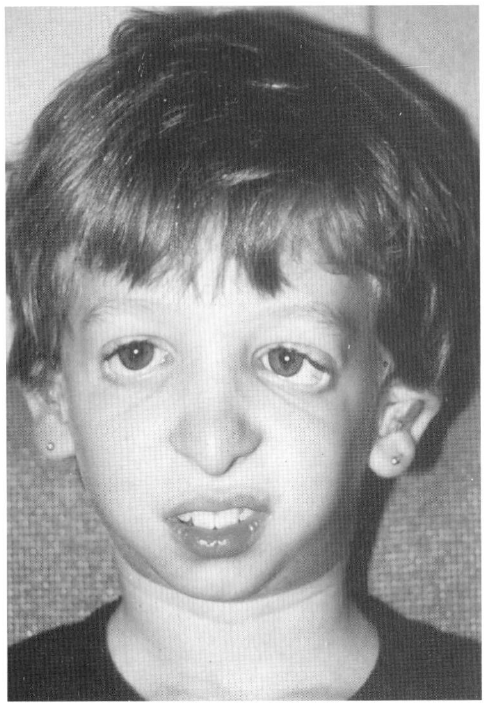

Figure 37.12. Treacher Collins syndrome. Note downslanting palpebral fissure, lower eyelid coloboma, malar hypoplasia, and ear abnormalities. (From M. Sharma et al. Molecular aspects of mandibulofacial dysostosis, in M. M. Cohen, Jr., ed., *Studies in Stomatology and Craniofacial Biology on the Threshold of the 21st Century*, IOS Press, Amsterdam, in press.)

They include downslanting palpebral fissures, colobomas of the lateral third of the lower lid in 75% of cases, with partial to total absence of the lower eyelashes in about half. Colobomas of the iris may be present, as well as absence of the lacrimal puncta and Meibomian glands.[42,48,74]

Genetics

The gene for Treacher Collins syndrome was mapped to the long arm of chromosome 5 by linkage analysis.[36,53] The *TCOF1* (treacle) gene has been implicated in this condition, although its function is unknown at this time.[117,124a] Mutations have been identified in the portion of the gene isolated to date. These mutations cause premature termination of the protein. There may be additional gene(s) causing similar phenotypes and related conditions.

Miller Syndrome

Miller syndrome is characterized by Treacher Collins–like facial features in addition to postaxial abnormalities of the ulnae and fibulae. It was defined as a distinct clinical entity by Miller et al. in 1979,[79] although it was reported by Genee 10 years earlier.[46] Miller syndrome generally results in hypoplasia or aplasia of the fifth digital ray. Abnormalities may extend to the radius and ulna, which can be shortened or even fused.[78] The mode of inheritance is not established, as most cases have been sporadic. An autosomal recessive mode of inheritance has been suggested, however, by two pairs of affected siblings with distantly consanguineous parents.[41]

Nager Syndrome

Patients with Nager syndrome have facial features similar to those of Treacher Collins syndrome, but they also have preaxial upper limb defects.[84,119] The occurrence of this condition is usually sporadic, but both autosomal dominant[72,121] and recessive[15,94] inheritance has been suggested.

The Oculoauriculovertebral Spectrum

The oculoauriculovertebral spectrum is characterized by hemifacial microsomia affecting the development of the ear, mouth, and mandible in addition to vertebral defects. Unlike Treacher Collins syndrome, in which abnormalities are bilateral and symmetric, this condition generally affects one side of the face. When there is bilateral involvement, it is usually asymmetric, with the right side being affected in over 60% of patients.[102] The oculoauriculovertebral spectrum is generally sporadic, although 1%–2% of cases have a positive family history. Goldenhar syndrome, which is characterized by the additional feature of epibulbar dermoids, is also considered part of this spectrum.[40]

REFERENCES

1. Allanson JE. Germinal mosaicism in Apert syndrome. *Clin Genet* 1986;29:429–433.

2. Anyane-Yeboa K, Gunning L, Bloom AD. Baller-Gerold syndrome: Craniosynostosis-radial aplasia syndrome. *Clin Genet* 1980; 17:161–166.
3. Apert ME. De l'acrocephalosyndactylie. *Bull Mem Soc Hop Paris* 1906;23:1310–1330.
4. Artlich A, Moller J, Tschakaloff A, Schwinger E, Kruse K, Gortner L. Teratogenic effects in a case of maternal treatment for acute myelocytic leukemia—Neonatal and infantile course. *Eur J Pediatr* 1994;153(7):488–491.
5. Atkinson FRB. Hereditary craniofacial dysostosis, or Crouzon's disease. *Med Press Circular* 1937;195:118–124.
6. Baller F. Radiusaplasie und inzucht. *Z meschl vereb-Konstit-Lehre* 1950;29:782–790.
7. Barone CM, Marion R, Shanske A, Argamaso RV, Shprintzen RJ. Craniofacial, limb, and abdominal anomalies in a distinct syndrome: Relation to the spectrum of Pfeiffer syndrome type 3. *Am J Med Genet* 1993;45:745–750.
8. Bertelson TI. The premature synostosis of the cranial sutures. *Acta Ophthalmol* 1958;51 (Suppl):1–176.
9. Blank CE. Apert's syndrome (a type of acrocephalosyndactyly): Observations on a British series of thirty-nine cases. *Ann Hum Genet* 1960;24:151–164.
10. Blodi FC. Developmental abnormalities of the skull affecting the eye. *Arch Ophthalmol* 1957;57:593–610.
11. Boudreaux JM, Colon MA, Lorusso GD, Parro EA, Pelias MZ. Baller-Gerold syndrome: An 11th case of craniosynostosis and radial aplasia. *Am J Med Genet* 1990;37: 447–450.
12. Brazier J. Craniofacial abnormalities. In *Pediatric Ophthalmology*, D. Taylor, ed. Cambridge, MA: Blackwell Scientific Publications, Inc., 1990:213–222.
13. Brueton LA, van Herwerden L, Chotai KA, Winter RM. The mapping of a gene for craniosynostosis: Evidence for linkage of the Saethre-Chotzen syndrome to distal chromosome 7p. *J Med Genet* 1992;29:681–685.
14. Burgess WH, Maciag T. The heparin-binding (fibroblast) growth factor family of proteins. *Annu Rev Biochem* 1989;58:575–606.
15. Burton BK, Nadler HL. Nager acrofacial dysostosis: Report of a case. *J Pediatr* 1977;91: 84–86.
16. Carpenter G. Two sisters showing malformations of the skull and other congenital abnormalities. *Rep Soc Study Dis Child (Lond)* 1901;1:110–118.
17. Chotzen F. Eine eigenartige familiare Entwicklungsstorung. (Akcrocephalosyndaktylie, Dysostosis craniofacialis und Telorismus.) *Monatschr Kinderheilkd* 1932;55:97–122.
18. Cohen DM, Green JG, Miller J, Gorlin RJ, Reed JA. Acrocephalopolysyndactyly type II—Carpenter syndrome: Clinical spectrum and an attempt at unification with Goodman and Summit syndromes. *Am J Med Genet* 1987;28:311–324.
19. Cohen MM Jr, Kreiborg S. Cutaneous manifestation of the Apert syndrome. *Am J Med Genet* 1995;58:94–96.
20. Cohen MM Jr, Kreiborg S. Visceral anomalies in the Apert syndrome. *Am J Med Genet* 1993;45:758–760.
21. Cohen MM Jr. An etiologic and nosologic overview of the craniosynostosis syndromes. In *Malformation Syndromes,* D. Bergsma, ed. *Birth Defects Orig Art Ser* XI (2), Amsterdam, 1975. Excerpta Medica for the National Foundation—March of Dimes, pp. 137–189.
22. Cohen MM Jr. Craniosynostosis and syndromes with craniosynostosis: Incidence, genetics, penetrance, variability, and new syndrome updating. *Birth Defects Orig Art Ser* 1979;15(5B):13–63.
23. Cohen MM Jr. Craniosynostosis update 1987. *Am J Med Genet* 1988;4:99–148.
24. Cohen MM Jr. Perspectives on craniosynostosis. *West J Med* 1980;132:507–553.
25. Cohen MM Jr. Sutural biology and the correlates of craniosynostosis. *Am J Med Genet* 1993;47:581–616.
26. Cohen MM Jr (ed.). *Craniosynostosis: Diagnosis, Evaluation and Management.* New York: Raven Press, 1986:467–471.
27. Cohen MM Jr. An etiologic and nosolgic overview of craniosynostosis syndromes. *Birth Defects Orig Art Ser* 1975;11(2):137–189.
28. Cohen MM Jr, Barone CM. Reply to Dr. Winter (letter). *Am J Med Genet* 1994;49: 358–359.
29. Cohen MM Jr, Kreiborg S. The central nervous system in the Apert syndrome. *Am J Med Genet* 1990;35:36–45.
30. Cohen MM Jr. Pfeiffer syndrome update, clinical subtypes, and guidelines for differential diagnosis. *Am J Med Genet* 1993;45: 300–307.
31. Collin R. The craniofacial dysostoses. In *Pediatric Ophthalmology: Current Aspects,* K. Wybar, D. Taylor (eds.). New York: Marcel Dekker, 1983.
32. Crouzon O. Dystose cranio-faciale hereditaire. *Bull Mem Soc Hop Paris* 1912;33: 545–555.

33. Cuttone JM, Brazis P, Miller M, Folk S. Absence of superior rectus muscle in Apert's syndrome. *J Pediatr Ophthalmol* 1980;16: 349–354.
34. Dallapiccola B, Zelante L, Mingarelli R, Pellegrino M, Bertozzi V. Baller-Gerold syndrome: Case report and radiological review. *Am J Med Genet* 1992;42:365–368.
35. Diamond GR, Katowitz JA, Whitaker LA, Quin GE, Schafer DB. Variations in extraocular muscle number and structure in craniofacial dysostosis. *Am J Ophthalmol* 1980;90:416.
36. Dixon MJ, Read AP, Donnai D, Colley A, Dixon J, Williamson R. The gene for Treacher Collins syndrome maps to the long arm of chromosome 5. *Am J Hum Genet* 1991; 49:17–22.
37. Dufier JL, Vinurel MC, Renier D, Marcharc D. Les complications ophthalmologiques des craniofaciostenoses. A propos de 244 observations. *J Fr Ophthalmol* 1986;9:273–280.
38. Duke-Elder S. Normal and abnormal development. Congenital deformities. In *System of Ophthalmology*, Vol. III, Part 2, S. Duke-Elder, ed. London: Henry Kimpton, 1964, pp. 1037–1057.
38a. El Ghouzzi V, Le Merrer M, Perrin-Schmitt F, Lajeunie E, Benit P, Reinier D, Bourgeois P, Bolcato-Bellemin A-L, Munnich A, Bonaventure J. Mutations of the *TWIST* gene in the Saethre-Chotzen syndrome. *Nature Gent* 1997;15:42–46.
39. Erickson JD, Cohen MM Jr. A study of parental age effects on the occurrence of fresh mutations for the Apert syndrome. *Ann Hum Genet (Lond)* 1974;38:89–96.
40. Feingold M, Baum J. Goldenhar's syndrome. *Am J Dis Child* 1978;132:136–138.
41. Fineman RM. Recurrence of the postaxial acrofacial dysostosis syndrome in a sibship: Implications for genetic counseling. *J Pediatr* 1981;98:87–88.
42. Franceschetti A, Klein D. Mandibulo-facial dysostosis: New hereditary syndrome. *Acta Ophthalmol (Copenh)* 1949;27:143–224.
43. Fuentes FJR, Nicholson L, Scotte CI Jr. Phenotypic variability in the Baller-Gerold syndrome: Report of a mildly affected patient and review of the literature. *Eur J Pediatr* 1994;153:483–487.
44. Galea P, Tolmie JL. Normal growth and development in a child with Baller-Gerold syndrome (craniosynostosis and radial aplasia). *J Med Genet* 1990;27:784–787.
45. Gavel D, Yayon A. Complexity of FGF receptors: Genetic basis for structural diversity and functional specificity. *FASEB J* 1992;6:3362–3369.
46. Genee E. Une forme extensive de dysostose mandibulo-faciale. *J Genet Hum* 1969;17: 45–52.
47. Gerold M. Frakturheilung bei einem seitenen Fall kongenitaler Anomalie der oberen Gliedmassen *Z Chir* 1959;84:831–834.
48. Gorlin RJ, Cohen MM Jr, Levin LS. Syndromes with craniosynostosis: General aspects and well known syndromes. In *Syndromes of The Head and Neck*, 3rd ed., R. J. Gorlin et al. (eds.). New York: Oxford University Press, 1990:521.
49. Gorry MC, Preston RA, White GJ et al. Crouzon syndrome: Mutations in two spliceoforms of FGFR2 and a common point mutation shared with Jackson-Weiss syndrome. *Hum Mol Genet* 1995;4(8):1387–1390.
50. Gospodarowicz D. Fibroblast growth factor and its involvement in developmental processes. *Curr Top Dev Biol* 1990;24:57–93.
51. Greaves B, Walker J, Wybar K. Disorders of ocular motility in craniofacial dysostosis. *J R Soc Med* 1979;72:21–24.
52. Hoover GH. The hand and Apert's syndrome. *J Bone Joint Surg* 1970;52A:878–895.
52a. Howard TD, Paznekas WA, Green ED, Chiang LC, Ma N, Ortiz DeLuna RI, Delgado CG, Gonzalez-Ramos M, Kline AD, Jabs EW. Mutations in TWIST, a basic helix-loop-helix transcription factor, in Saethre-Chotzen syndrome. *Nature Genet* 1997;15:36–41.
53. Jabs EW, Li X, Coss CA, Taylor EW, Meyers DA, Weber JL. Mapping the Treacher Collins syndrome locus to 5q31.3-5q33.3. *Genomics* 1991;11:193–198.
54. Jabs EW, Li X, Scott AF, Meyers G, Chen W, Eccles M, Mao J. Jackson-Weiss and Crouzon syndromes are allelic with mutations in fibroblast growth factor receptor 2. *Nature Genet* 1994;8:275–279.
55. Jabs EW, Muller U, Li X, Ma L, Luo W, Haworth IS, Klisak I, Sparkes R, Warman ML, Mulliken JB, Snead ML, Maxon R. A mutation in the homeodomain of the human *MSX2* gene in a family affected with autosomal dominant craniosynostosis. *Cell* 1993; 75(5):443–450.
56. Jackson CE, Weiss L, Reynolds WA, Formar TF, Peterson JA. Craniosynostosis, midfacial hypoplasia, and foot abnormalities: An autosomal dominant phenotype in a large Amish kindred. *J Pediatr* 1976;88(6):963–968.

57. Johnson DE, Williams LT. Structural and functional diversity in the FGF receptor multigene family. *Adv Cancer Res* 1993;60: 1–41.
58. Jones KL. *Smith's Recognizable Patterns of Human Malformation*, 4th ed. Philadelphia: W.B. Saunders, 1988:370.
59. Jones KL, Smith D, Harvey MAS, Hall BD, Quan L. Older paternal age and fresh gene mutations: Data on additional disorders. *J Pediatr* 1975;86:84–88.
60. Jones MR, de Sa LCF, Good WV. Atypical iris colobomata and Pfeiffer syndrome. *J Pediatr Ophthalmol Strabismus* 1993;30:266–267.
61. Kreiborg S, Cohen MM Jr. Germinal mosaicism in Crouzon syndrome. *Hum Genet* 1990; 84:487–488.
62. Kreiborg S, Cohen MM Jr. The infant Apert skull. *Neurosurg Clin North Am* 1991;2(3): 551–554.
63. Kreiborg S. Crouzon syndrome. *Scand J Plast Reconstr Surg Suppl* 1981;18:1–198.
64. Lajeunie E, Ma HW, Bonaventure J, Munnich A, Le Merrer M, Renier D. FGFR2 mutations in Pfeiffer syndrome. *Nature Genet* 1995;9:173–176.
65. Lewanda AF, Cohen MM Jr, Hood J, Morsey S, Walters M, Kennedy JL Jr, Jabs EW. Cytogenetic survey of Apert syndrome. Reevaluation of a translocation (2;9)p11.2; q34.2) in a patient suggests the breakpoints are not related to the disorder. *Am J Dis Child* 1993; 147:1306–1308.
66. Lewanda AF, Cohen MM Jr, Jackson CE, Taylor EW, Li X, Beloff M, Day D. Genetic heterogeneity among craniosynostosis syndromes: Mapping the Saethre-Chotzen syndrome locus betwen D7S513 and D7S516 and exclusion of Jackson-Weiss and Crouzon syndrome loci from 7p. *Genomics* 1994;19: 115–119.
67. Lewanda AF, Green ED, Weissenback J, Jerald H, Taylor E, Summar ML, Phillips JA. Evidence that the Saethre-Chotzen syndrome locus lies between D7S664 and D7S507 by genetic analysis and detection of a microdeletion in a patient. *Am J Hum Genet* 1994; 55:1195–1201.
68. Lewanda AF, Meyers GA, Jabs EW. Craniosynostosis and skeletal dysplasias: Fibroblast growth factor receptor defects. *Proc Assoc Am Physicians* 1996;1:19–24.
69. Li X, Park W-J, Pyeritz RE, Jabs EW. Effect on splicing of a silent FGFR2 mutation in Crouzon syndrome (letter). *Nature Genet* 1995;9:232–233.
70. Limon de Brown E. Proceedings of the 2nd International Strabismological Association. Diffusion Generale de Librarie, Paris, 1974: 371.
71. Lin AE, McPherson E, Nwokoro NA, Clemens M, Losken HW, Mulvihill JJ. Further delineation of the Baller-Gerold syndrome. *Am J Med Genet* 1993;45:519–524.
72. Lowry RB. Case reports. A. The Nager syndrome (acrofacial dysostosis): Evidence for autosomal dominant inheritance. In *Natural History of Specific Birth Defects,* D. Bergsma, R. B. Lowry, eds. New York: Alan R. Liss, *Birth Defects Orig Art Ser* 1977; XIII(3C):195–202.
73. Lyon JR, Burgess RC. Pfeiffer's syndrome family tree. Review of the literature. *Clin Orthop* 1993;294:294–298.
74. Mann I, Kilner TP. Deficiency of the malar bones with defect of the lower lids. *Br J Ophthalmol* 1943;27:13–20.
75. Margolis S, Pachter BR, Breinin GM. Structural alterations of extraocular muscle associated with Apert syndrome. *Br J Ophthalmol* 1977;61:683–689.
76. McGinnis W, Krumlauf R. Homeobox genes and axial patterning. *Cell* 1992;68:283–302.
77. Meyers GA, Day D, Goldberg R, Daentl D, Przylepa KA, Abrams LJ, Graham JM Jr. FGFR2 exon IIIa and IIIc mutations in Crouzon, Jackson-Weiss, and Pfeiffer syndromes: Evidence for missense changes, insertions, and a deletion due to alternative RNA splicing. *Am J Hum Genet* 1996;58:491–498.
78. Meyers GA, Orlow SJ, Munro IR, Przylepa KA, Jabs EW. Fibroblast growth factor receptor 3 (FGFR3) transmembrane mutation in Crouzon syndrome with acanthosis nigricans. *Nature Genet* 1995;11:462–464.
79. Miller M, Fineman R, Smith DW. Postaxial acrofacial dysostosis syndrome. *J Pediatr* 1979;95:970–975.
80. Moss ML. Functional anatomy of cranial synostosis. *Childs Brain* 1975;1:22–33.
81. Moss ML. The pathogenesis of premature cranial synostosis in Man. *Acta Anat (Basel)* 1959;37:351–370.
82. Muenke M, Schell U, Hehr A, Robin NH, Losken HW, Schinzel A, Pulleyn LJ. A common mutation in the fibroblast growth factor receptor 1 gene in Pfeiffer syndrome. *Nature Genet* 1994;8:269–274.
83. Muller U, Warman ML, Mulliken JB, Weber JL. Assignment of a gene locus involved in craniosynostosis to chromosome 5qter. *Hum Mol Genet* 1993;2(2):119–122.

84. Nager FR, de Reynier JP. Das Gehororgan bei den angeborenen Kopfmissbildungen. *Prac Oto-Rhino-Laryngol (Basel)* 1948;10: 1–128.
85. Navarete C, Pena R, Penaloza R, Salamanca F. Germinal mosaicism in Crouzon syndrome. A family with three affected siblings of normal parents. *Clin Genet* 1991;40:29–34.
86. Nwokoro NA, Jaffe R, Barmada M. Baller-Gerold syndrome: A postmortem examination (letter). *Am J Med Genet* 1993;47:1233.
87. Oldridge M, Wilkie AOM, Slaney SF, Poole MD, Pulleyn LJ, Rutland P, Hockley AD. Mutations in the third immunoglobulin domain of the fibroblast growth factor receptor-2 gene in Crouzon syndrome. *Hum Mol Genet* 1995;4(6):1077–1082.
88. Orlow SJ. Cutaneous findings in craniofacial malformation syndromes. *Arch Dermatol* 1992;128:1379–1386.
89. Pantke OA, Cohen MM Jr, Witkop CJ, Feingold M, Shaumann B, Pantke HC, Gorlin RJ. The Saethre-Chotzen syndrome. In *Malformation Syndromes,* D. Bergsma, ed. New York: Elsevier, for the National Foundation—March of Dimes, *Birth Defects Orig Art Ser,* 1975;11(2):190–225.
90. Park W-J, Theda C, Maestri NE, Meyers GA, Fryburg J, Dufresne C, Cohen MM Jr, Jabs EW. Analysis of phenotypic features and FGFR2 mutations in Apert syndrome. *Am J Hum Genet* 1995;57:321–328.
91. Park W-J, Meyers GA, Li X, Theda C, Day D, Orlow SJ, Jones MC, Jabs EW. Novel FGFR2 mutations in Crouzon and Jackson-Weiss syndromes show allelic heterogeneity and phenotypic variability. *Hum Mol Genet* 1995;4:1229–1233.
92. Park W-J, Bellus GA, Jabs EW. Mutations in fibroblast growth factor receptors: Phenotypic consequences during eukaryotic development. *Am J Hum Genet* 1995;57:748–754.
93. Patton MA. Intellectual development in Apert syndrome: A long term follow up of 29 patients. *J Med Genet* 1988;25:164–167.
94. Pfeiffer RA, Stoess H. Acrofacial dysostosis (Nager syndrome): Synopsis and short review of a new case. *Am J Med Genet* 1983; 15:255–260.
95. Pfeiffer RA. Dominant erbliche Akrocephalosyndaktylie. *Z Kinderheilkd* 1964;90:301–320.
96. Preis S, Majewski F, Korholz D, Gobel U. Osteosarcoma in a 16-year-old boy with Baller-Gerold syndrome. *Clin Dysmorphol* 1995;4(2):161–168.
97. Reardon W, McManus SP, Summers D, Winter RM. Cytogenetic evidence that the Saethre-Chotzen Gene maps to 7p21.2. *Am J Med Genet* 1993;47:633–636.
98. Reardon W, Winter RM, Rutland P, Pulleyn LJ, Jones BM, Malcolm S. Mutations in the fibroblast growth factor receptor 2 gene cause Crouzon syndrome. *Nature Genet* 1994;8: 98–103.
99. Reid CS, McMorrow, LE, McDonald-McGinn DM, Grance KJ, Ramos FJ, Zackai EH, Cohen MM Jr. Saethre-Chotzen syndrome with familial translocation at chromosome 7p22. *Am J Med Genet* 1993;47: 637–639.
100. Robin NH, Feldman GJ, Mitchell HF, Lorenz P, Wilroy RS, Zackai EH, Allanson JE. Linkage of Pfeiffer syndrome to chromosome 8 centromerey and evidence for genetic heterogeneity. *Hum Mol Genet* 1994;3(12):2153–2158.
101. Rogers BO. Berry-Treacher Collins syndrome: A review of 200 cases. *Br J Plast Surg* 1964;17:109–137.
102. Rollnick BR, Kaye CI, Nagatoshi K, Hauck W, Martin AO. Oculoauriculovertebral dysplasia and variants: Phenotypic characteristics of 294 patients. *Am J Med Genet* 1987;26:361–375.
103. Rollnick BR. Germinal mosaicism in Crouzon syndrome. *Clin Genet* 1988;33:145–150.
104. Rose CSP, King AAJ, Summers D, Palmer R, Yang S, Wilkie AOM, Reardon W. Localization of the genetic locus for Saethre-Chotzen syndrome to a 6 cM region of chromosome 7 using four cases with apparently balanced translocations at 7p21.2. *Hum Mol Genet* 1994;3:1405–1408.
105. Rutland P, Pulleyn LJ, Reardon W, Baraitser M, Hayward R, Jones B, Malcolm S. Identical mutations in the FGFR2 gene cause both Pfeiffer and Crouzon syndrome phenotypes. *Nature Genet* 1995;9:173–176.
106. Saethre H. Ein eitrag zum turmschadelproblem (pathogenese, erbuchkeit und symptomologie). *Dtsch Z Nervheil* 1931;117: 533–555.
107. Schauerte EW, St. Aubin PM. Progressive synosteosis in Apert's syndrome (acrocephalosyndactyly) with a description of roentgenographic changes in the feet. *Am J Roentgenol* 1966;97:67–73.
108. Schell U, Hehr A, Feldman GJ, Robin NH, Zackai EH, de Die Smulders C, Viskochil DH. Mutations in FGFR1 and FGFR2 cause familial and sporadic Pfeiffer syndrome. *Hum Mol Genet* 1995;4(3):323–328.
109. Scott MP, Tamkun JW, Hartzell GW III. The

structure and function of the homeodomain. *Biochem Biophys Acta* 1989;989:25–48.

110. Shiller JG. Craniofacial dysostosis of Crouzon: A case report and pedigree with emphasis on heredity. *Pediatrics* 1959;23:107–112.

111. Steinberger D, Mulliken JB, Muller U. Predisposition for cysteine substitutions in the immunoglobulin-like chain of FGFR2 in Crouzon syndrome. *Hum Genet* 1995;96: 113–115.

112. Taravath S, Tonsgard JH. Cerebral malformations in Carpenter syndrome. *Pediatr Neurol* 1993;9:230–234.

113. Thomson A. Notice of several cases of malformations of the external ear, together with experiments on the state of hearing in such persons. *Mon J Med Sci* 1953;42:1846–1847.

114. Toynbee J. Description of a congenital malformation in the ears of a child. *Mon J Med Sci* 1847;1:738–739.

115. Traboulsi EI, Kattan HM. Skeletal and connective tissue disorders with corneal manifestations. In *Cornea,* J. H. Krachmer, M. J. Mannis, E. J. Holland, eds. St. Louis: C. V. Mosby, 1997:925–942.

115a. Traboulsi EI, Maumenee IH. Peters' anomaly and associated congenital malformations. *Arch Ophthalmol* 1992;110:1739–1742.

116. Treacher Collins E. Cases with symmetrical congenital notches in the outer part of each lid and defective development of the malar bones. *Trans Ophthalmol Soc UK* 1960;20: 190–192.

117. Treacher Collins Syndrome Collaborative Group. Positional cloning of a gene involved in the pathogenesis of Treacher Collins syndrome. *Nature Genet* 1996;12:130–136.

118. Van Maldergem L, Verbes A, Lejeune L, Gillerot Y. The Baller-Gerold syndrome. *J Med Genet* 1992;29:266–268.

119. Vatre J-L. Etude genetique et classification clinique de 154 cas de dysostose mandibulofaciale (syndrome de Franceschetti), avec description de leurs associations malformatives. *J Med Genet* 1971;22:408–410.

120. Warman ML, Mulliken JB, Hayward PG, Muller U. Newly recognized autosomal dominant disorder with craniosynostosis. *Am J Med Genet* 1993;46:444–449.

121. Weinbaum M, Tussell L, Bixler D. Autosomal dominant transmission of Nager acrofacial dysostosis. *Am J Hum Genet* (abstract) 1981; 33:93A.

122. Weinstock FJ, Hardesty HH. Absence of superior recti in craniofacial dysostosis. *Arch Ophthalmol* 1965;74:152–153.

123. Wilkie AOM, Slaney SF, Oldridge M, Poole MD, Ashworth GJ, Hockley AD, Hayward RD. Apert syndrome results from localized mutations of FGFR2 and is allelic with Crouzon syndrome. *Nature Genet* 1995;9: 165–172.

124. Winter RM. Pfeiffer syndrome (letter). *Am J Med Genet* 1994;49:357.

124a. Wise CA, Chiang LC, Paznekas WA, Sharma M, Musy MM, Ashley JA, Lovett M, Jabs EW. *TCOF1* gene encodes a putative nucleolarphosphoprotein that exhibits mutations in Treacher Collins syndrome throughout its coding region. *Proc Natl Acad Sci USA* 1997;94:3110–3115.

125. Wolter JR. Bilateral keratoconus in Crouzon syndrome with unilateral acute hydrops. *J Pediatr Ophthalmol Strabismus* 1977;14:141.

38

Norrie Disease

ELIAS I. TRABOULSI

Warburg gave the first detailed description of the clinical features of Norrie disease in a paper read before the Danish Ophthalmological Society in 1960.[32,33] She had reviewed the records of all patients enrolled in the Institute for the Blind and had identified eight boys with X-linked inherited congenital blindness. She named the condition Norrie disease (ND) after Gordon Norrie, a former consulting ophthalmologist to the Institute for the Blind in Copenhagen, the institution to which she had recently been appointed in the same capacity. Warburg acknowledged Norrie's interest in these cases and his identification of their condition as one that did not fit with known clinical entities. Norrie had mentioned in a report on the causes of blindness in Denmark two families from which seven of these patients had originated.[22] The central nervous system aspects of the disease, however, had not been appreciated by Norrie but were covered in detail by Warburg.

The earliest description of what might have been Norrie disease is attributed to Fernandez, who, in 1905 reported two brothers from Cuba with congenital bilateral retinal detachment and blindness.[12] Warburg reviewed the literature up to 1966 on families and patients who may have had Norrie disease. She found 106 individuals in 16 families from England, Germany, Czechoslovakia, Canada, Spain, and Cyprus. It has become apparent since then that the disease had a worldwide distribution and shows no founder effect or racial predilection. Its impact on certain communities is reflected by the fact that it is called "Episkopi blindness" in Cyprus, where numerous members of one large family in the village of Episkopi are blind from this condition.

CLINICAL MANIFESTATIONS AND DIFFERENTIAL DIAGNOSIS

Patients with Norrie disease classically present very early in life with bilateral retrolental masses, bilateral retinal folds, or retinal detachment. There is usually no perception of light. The globe may be initially of normal size but usually becomes phthisical in older patients.

Mental retardation becomes apparent at an early age in some patients and is frequently significant and progressive. In a review of 35 patients from six families, Warburg commented that 20 patients were moderately or severely retarded, while only 3 had intelligence levels above normal.[33] Psychosis, manifested by dementia, aggressive behavior, and rarely, hallucinations, occurs in over 25% of patients. In a few patients, the dementia appears late and is not severe. Some patients have grand mal seizures. Female carriers of the Norrie disease gene do not generally have neurological problems that are attributable to the abnormal gene. One woman with a microdeletion of Xp11.3 that included the Norrie disease and the monoamine oxidase genes met diagnostic criteria for "chronic hypomania and schizotypal features."[10] Whether her psychiatric disorder was coincidental, or whether it was a manifestation of a heterozygote status for microdeletion of the Norrie disease gene, remains undetermined.

Auditory impairment may be severe and occurs in about 25% of patients.[1,25,32] The hearing loss is progressive, sensorineural, affects the high tones, and has its onset in the second or third decade of life.

The clinical diagnosis of Norrie disease is based on the pattern of inheritance, ocular findings, and on associated hearing loss, dementia, or psychosis. Although ocular signs are present at birth in virtually all reported patients, the other features are not congenital and may not appear until later in life.

The differential diagnosis of this disorder includes bilateral retinoblastoma, retinopathy of prematurity, X-linked juvenile retinoschisis, Coats' disease, bilateral retinal falciform folds, familial exudative vitreoretinopathy, bilateral persistent hyperplastic primary vitreous (PHPV), incontinentia pigmenti and congenital toxoplasmosis. In older patients who present with phthisis, the differential diagnosis includes X-linked microphthalmia and X-linked cataract. A diagnosis of Norrie disease should be considered very highly in male patients with presumed bilateral PHPV, bilateral falciform retinal folds, and in those with so-called X-linked familial exudative vitreoretinopathy. Some families with X-linked microphthalmia and mental retardation, or with X-linked cataracts and mental retardation, may indeed have Norrie disease. With the cloning of the Norrie disease gene and the availability of mutation analysis, the clinical diagnosis can be confirmed at the molecular level.

OCULAR FINDINGS

The bilateral congenital retrolental masses formed by the dysplastic detached retina may not be appreciated for a few months. Warburg described a localized cystic retinal detachment characterized by hemorrhages that soon involved the entire retina.[33] So there seems to be progression from retinal dysplasia and traction to a hemorrhagic retinal detachment very early in infancy or late in gestation. The globes usually become phthisical, although normal appearing, and even buphthalmic eyes have been observed.[35] The anterior chamber is usually shallow and the pupils are frequently dilated. The iris is hypoplastic with posterior synechiae and ectropion uveae. The vitreous opacities appear as a gray membrane or a gray-yellow-pink mass. The ciliary processes are elongated and often visible through the pupil. If the fundus can be visualized, retinal folds or retinal detachment are frequently observed (Fig. 38.1).

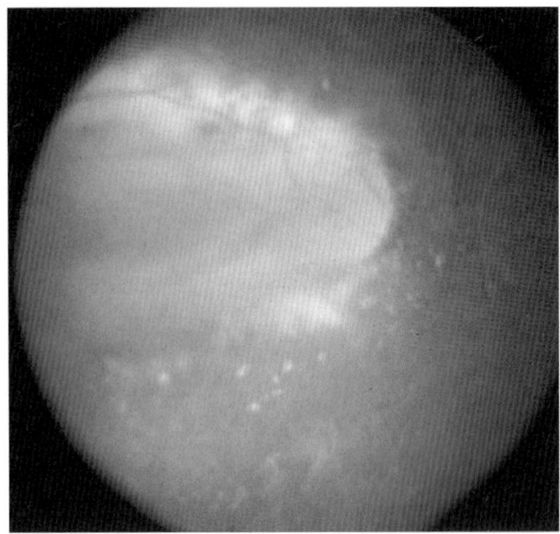

Figure 38.1. Retinal fold from the optic disc to the temporal periphery in a patient with Norrie disease.

OCULAR FINDINGS IN FEMALES

Although this X-linked disease has been reported predominantly in males, a few recent reports have described retinal abnormalities in female carriers of the abnormal gene. One patient with normal ophthalmoscopic findings at birth developed retinal detachment at the age of 2 years. She had a C69S mutation.[9,34] One woman with an unbalanced translocation 46,XX, t(X;10) had ocular abnormalities compatible with Norrie disease in addition to other systemic abnormalities.[23] A likely mechanism for the expression of disease in female carriers of Norrie disease mutations is nonrandom or unfavorable X inactivation.

HISTOPATHOLOGY

Warburg reported the ocular pathology of an 8-month-old baby with Norrie disease.[33] Photoreceptors and ganglion cells were absent. Vascular abnormalities are present in eyes of patients with Norrie disease and may simulate Coats disease, another cause of a white pupillary reflex in infants (Fig. 38.2).[2,5] The two conditions, however, can be distinguished on histopathological grounds by the absence of intraretinal exudation, periodic acid–Schiff positive material, cholesterol deposits in areas without organizing hemorrhage, and retinal telangiectasias in Norrie disease, as opposed to Coats disease, where all these changes are common and characteristic.[2] Pigmentary changes and retinal pigment epithelial proliferation are commonly present in Norrie disease but are not characteristic.[1,5,18]

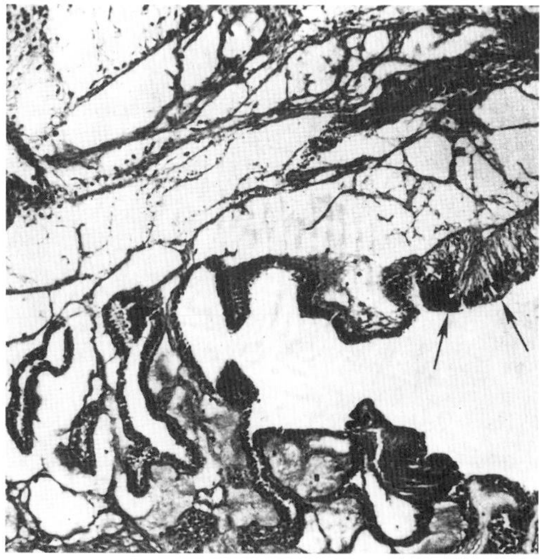

Figure 38.2. Preretinal mass in a patient with Norrie disease. Cords or rows of cuboidal epithelium are seen in the preretinal mass. The convoluted cords (lower left) are low cuboidal and resemble embryonic neuroepithelium. Arrows indicate elongation of cells and attempts to form primitive sensory retina. (Courtesy of Dr. Morton F. Goldberg, produced with permission from D. Apple et al., ref. 2.)

Parsons et al. studied the eyes of a fetus with Norrie disease who was aborted at 11 weeks gestation following prenatal diagnosis using linkage analysis.[24] The eyes were histologically normal. The authors postulate that the retinal and other ocular manifestations of Norrie disease occur after 14 weeks of gestation as a result of genetically determined angiogenic or neurodevelopmental abnormalities.

GENETICS

The Norrie gene was mapped to Xp11.4-p11.3[14,31] and later cloned.[3,8] Schroeder and coworkers found marked hypoplasia of the inner retinal cell layers and fibrovascular proliferation in the vitreous cavity of a 6-month-old boy with a 1-base pair insertion (544/545msA) in the Norrie disease gene.[29a] The gene that spans 28 kb, consists of three exons and two introns; the first exon is entirely contained within the 5′ untranslated region.[3] The Norrie disease gene product, norrin, is a 133 amino acid extracellular protein and resembles the C-terminal domain of mucins.[19] Norrin has a tertiary structure similar to a group of cysteine-rich proteins that include transforming growth factor, nerve growth factor-β, platelet-derived growth factor, and glial cell-derived growth factor.[21] These proteins have in common a central cystine knot motif that consists of three disulfide bridges connecting cysteine residues. Because some of these proteins play an important role in the development of the central nervous system, it was postulated that norrin plays a role in the development of the retina and the brain.[21] Chen et al. proposed that the Norrie disease gene is involved in neural cell differentiation and proliferation.[7]

Mutational analysis studies have identified numerous deletions as well as mutations in coding and noncoding regions of the gene. Although most mutations have been found in patients with the classic phenotype of bilateral congenital retinal detachment and phthisis, some have been in patients with a slightly milder ocular phenotype unaccompanied by mental retardation or hearing loss, previously described as X-linked retinal dysplasia.[20] Other mutations have been in patients who had received a clinical diagnosis of familial exudative vitreoretinopathy.[6] It seems most appropriate to consider all three diagnoses as variable expressions of the same genetic disorder, and it is the preference of this author to refer to all of them as Norrie disease.

X-LINKED EXUDATIVE VITREORETINOPATHY

Some families previously diagnosed with X-linked exudative vitreoretinopathy such as the one reported by Plager et al.[26] were found to have mutations in the Norrie disease gene.[6,13,17,20,30] Patients with X-linked exudative vitreoretinopathy do not have mental retardation or hearing loss. The retina may be detached, or there may be peripheral areas of retinal avascularity. A diagnosis of X-linked vitreoretinopathy should always be reevaluated, and all such patients should be presumed to have mutations in the Norrie gene until proven otherwise.

X-LINKED PRIMARY RETINAL DYSPLASIA

This condition is characterized by congenital retinal folds and severe reduction of vision in males, and peripheral retinal traction or retinal detachment in some female carriers.[15] Mental retardation and hearing loss are absent. The family previously reported by Godel and Goodman to have primary X-linked retinal dysplasia[16] was found to be linked to the Norrie disease locus,[27] and an R121G mutation was identified in the Norrie gene.[20,35] Two female carriers in that family had retinal abnormalities.

PHENOTYPE–GENOTYPE CORRELATION

Shuback et al. reviewed their experience in mutation identification in 26 kindreds with Norrie disease.[29] Using single strand conformation polymorphism (SSCP) analysis of all coding exons, noncoding regions of exons 1 and 2636 nucleotides in the noncoding region of exon 3 and 197 nucleotides of 5′ flanking sequence, these investigators were able to identify disease-causing mutations in 92% of instances. Mutations varied from submicroscopic deletions involving the whole gene (3), to intragenic deletions (6), missense mutations (8), nonsense mutations (6), and one 10 bp insertion. Except for two mutations, each found in two families, all other sequence changes were unique to the individual pedigrees. Most point mutations were at, or near, cysteine residues that are presumed to be critical to the tertiary structure of norrin.[21] Shuback et al. were unable to draw conclusions about phenotype–genotype correlation in their patients, except that large submicroscopic deletions were possibly associated with more severe neurologic symptoms.[29] Meindl and co-workers reported missense mutations that were associated with a less severe course of the disease, with some patients retaining vision in one eye, and absence of hearing loss and mental retardation.[20]

MOUSE MODEL

Using gene targeting mutagenesis, Berger and co-workers generated mice with an ocular phenotype very reminiscent of Norrie disease.[4] The polypeptide coded by the murine gene shares 94% of the amino acid sequence with human norrin. The mouse gene was expressed in the brain, retina, and olfactory bulb and epithelium. Hemizygous mutant mice with a mutation in exon 2 developed vitreous masses and had a disorganized retinal ganglion cell layer with outer segment photoreceptor atrophy in areas of ganglion cell abnormalities.

TREATMENT AND PRENATAL DIAGNOSIS

There is no specific therapy for Norrie disease. Prenatal diagnosis is available using mutation analysis or linkage analysis on chorionic villus samples or amniocytes.[36] Obstetrical ultrasonography detected bilateral retinal detachments in a third-trimester fetus at risk for Norrie disease, and postnatal examination confirmed the diagnosis.[11,28]

REFERENCES

1. Anderson S, Warburg M. Norrie's disease. Congenital bilateral pseudotumor of the retina with recessive X chromosomal inheritance. *Arch Ophthalmol* 1961;66:614–618.
2. Apple D, Fishman G, Goldberg M. Ocular histopathology of Norrie's disease. *Am J Ophthalmol* 1974;78:196–203.
3. Berger W, Meindl A, van de Pol TJ, Cremers FP, Ropers HH, Doerner C, et al. Isolation of a candidate gene for Norrie disease by positional cloning [published erratum appears in *Nature Genet* 1992 Sept;2(1):84]. *Nature Genet* 1992;1(3):199–203.
4. Berger W, van de Pol DDB, Oerlemans F, Winkens H, Hameister H, et al. An animal model for Norrie disease (ND): Gene targeting of the mouse ND gene. *Hum Mol Genet* 1996;5:51–59.
5. Blodi F, Hunter W. Norrie's disease in North America. *Doc Ophthalmol* 1969;26:434–450.
6. Chen ZY, Battinelli EM, Fielder A, Bundey S, Sims K, Breakefield XO, et al. A mutation in the Norrie disease gene (NDP) associated with X-linked familial exudative vitreoretinopathy. *Nature Genet* 1993;5(2):180–183.
7. Chen ZY, Battinelli EM, Hendriks RW, Powell JF, Middleton-Price H, Sims KB, et al. Norrie disease gene: Characterization of deletions and possible function. *Genomics* 1993;16(2):533-535.
8. Chen ZY, Hendriks RW, Jobling MA, Powell JF, Breakefield XO, Sims KB, et al. Isolation and characterization of a candidate gene for Norrie disease. *Nature Genet* 1992;1(3):204–208.
9. Chen Z-Y, Battineli E, Woodruff G, et al. Characterization of a mutation within the NDP gene in a family with a manifesting carrier. *Hum Mol Genet* 1993;2:1727–1729.
10. Collins FA, Murphy DL, Reiss AL, Sims KB, Lewis JG, Freund L, et al. Clinical, biochemical, and neuropsychiatric evaluation of a patient with a contiguous gene syndrome due to a microdeletion Xp11.3 including the Norrie disease locus and monoamine oxidase (MAOA and MAOB) genes. *Am J Med Genet* 1992;42(1):127–134.
11. De la Chapelle A, Sankila EM, Lindlof M, Aula P, Norio R. Norrie disease caused by a gene deletion allowing carrier detection and prenatal diagnosis. *Clin Genet* 1985;28(4):317–320.
12. Fernandez S. Total congenital detachment of the retina in two brothers. *Arch Ophthalmol* 1905;34:338.
13. Fuchs S, Kellner U, Wedemann H, Gal A. Missense mutation (Arg121Trp) in the Norrie disease gene associated with X-linked exudative vitreoretinopathy. *Hum Mutat* 1995;6:257–259.
14. Gal A, Bleeker-Wagemakers L, Wienker T, Warburg M, Ropers H. Localization of the gene for Norrie disease by linkage to DXS7 locus. *Cytogenet Cell Genet* 1985;40, 633.
15. Godel V, Goodman R. X-linked recessive primary retinal dysplasia: Clinical findings in affected males and carrier females. *Clin Genet* 1981;20:260–266.
16. Godel V, Goodman R. X-linked recessive primary retinal dysplasia: clinical findings in affected males and carrier females. *Clin Genet* 1981;20:260–266.
17. Johnson K, Mintz-Hittner H, Perry Y, Ferrell R. X-linked familial exudative vitreoretinopathy caused by an arginine to leucine substitution in exon 3 of the Norrie gene. *Am J Hum Genet* 1994;55(suppl):A1309.
18. Liberfarb R, Eavey R, De Long G, Albert D, Dieckert J, Hirose T. Norrie's disease: A study of two families. *Ophthalmology* 1985;92:1445–1451.
19. Meindl A, Berger W, Meitinger T, van de Pol D, Achatz H, Dorner C, et al. Norrie disease is caused by mutations in an extracellular protein resembling C-terminal globular domain of mucins. *Nature Genet* 1992;2(2):139–143.
20. Meindl A, Lorenz B, Achatz H, Hellebrand H, Schmitz-Valckenberg P, Meitinger T. Missense mutations in the NDP gene in patients with a less severe course of Norrie disease. *Hum Mol Genet* 1995;4(3):489–490.
21. Meitinger T, Meindl A, Bork P, Rost B, Sander C, Haasemann M, et al. Molecular modelling of the Norrie disease protein predicts a cysteine knot growth factor tertiary structure. *Nature Genet* 1993;5(4):376–380.
22. Norrie G. Causes of blindness in children. *Acta Ophthalmol (Copenh)* 1927;5:357–386.

23. Ohba N, Yamashita T. Primary vitreoretinal dysplasia resembling Norrie's disease in a female: Association with X autosome translocation. *Br J Ophthalmol* 1986;70:64–71.
24. Parsons MA, Curtis D, Blank CE, Hughes HN, McCartney AC. The ocular pathology of Norrie disease in a fetus of 11 weeks' gestational age. *Graefe's Arch Clin Exp Ophthalmol* 1992; 230(3):248–251.
25. Parving A, Warburg M. Audiologic findings in Norrie's disease. *Audiology* 1977;16:124–131.
26. Plager D, Orgel I, Ellis F, et al. X-linked recessive familial exudative vitreoretinopathy. *Am J Ophthalmol* 1992;114:145–148.
27. Ravia Y, Braier-Goldstein O, Bat-Miriam KM, Erlich S, Barkai G, Goldman B. X-linked recessive primary retinal dysplasia is linked to the Norrie disease locus. *Hum Mol Genet* 1993; 2(8):1295–1297.
28. Redmond RM, Vaughan JI, Jay M, Jay B. In-utero diagnosis of Norrie disease by ultrasonography. *Opthalmic Paediatr Genet* 1993;14(1): 1–3.
29. Schuback DE, Chen ZY, Craig IW, Breakefield XO, Sims KB. Mutations in the Norrie disease gene. *Hum Mutat* 1995;5(4):285–292.
29a. Schroeder B, Hesse L, Bruck W, Gal A. Histopathological and immunohistochemical findings associated with a null mutation in the Norrie disease gene. *Ophthal Genet* 1997;18: 71–77.
30. Shastry BS, Hejtmancik JF, Plager DA, Hartzer MK, Trese MT. Linkage and candidate gene analysis of X-linked familial exudative vitreoretinopathy. *Genomics* 1995;27(2):341–344.
31. Sims KB, Lebo RV, Benson, G, Shalish C, Schuback D, Chen ZY, et al. The Norrie disease gene maps to a 150 kb region on chromosome Xp11.3. *Hum Mol Genet* 1992;1(2):83–89.
32. Warburg M. Norrie's disease. A new hereditary bilateral pseudotumor of the retina. *Acta Ophthalmol (Copenh)* 1961;39:757.
33. Warburg M. Norrie's disease: A congenital progressive ocular-acoustico-cerebral degeneration. *Acta Ophthalmol (Copenh)* 1966;89: 1–147.
34. Woodruff G, Newbury-Ecob R, Plaha D, Young I. Manifesting heterozygosity in Norrie's disease? *Br J Ophthalmol* 1993;77:813–814.
35. Zhu D, Maumenee I. Mutation analysis of the Norrie gene in eleven families. *Invest Ophthalmol Vis Sci* 1994;35(suppl):1265.
36. Zhu DP, Antonarakis SE, Schmeckpeper BJ, Diergaarde PJ, Greb AE, Maumenee IH. Microdeletion in the X-chromosome and prenatal diagnosis in a family with Norrie disease. *Am J Med Genet* 1989;33(4):485–488.

VI.

Tumors

39

Genetic Aspects of Uveal Melanoma

ARUN D. SINGH

Uveal melanoma usually occurs sporadically without obvious genetic or environmental predisposing factors. However, in rare instances, when it affects more than one family member, there is a suggestion of poorly understood genetic factors. Over 100 years ago Silcock first reported the occurrence of uveal melanoma in a mother and her two daughters.[54] Since then, many reports have discussed the role of genetic factors in uveal melanoma. This chapter presents a comprehensive review of clinical genetics, cytogenetics, and molecular genetics related to uveal melanoma.

CONDITIONS PREDISPOSING TO UVEAL MELANOMA

Oculodermal Melanocytosis

Oculodermal melanocytosis represents congenital hyperpigmentation of the skin, episclera, uvea, orbit, and meninges.[44] It is estimated to occur about 35 times more often in patients with uveal melanoma than in the general Caucasian population.[17] Melanoma can also arise from other hyperpigmented sites such as the orbit and meninges. In most cases, oculodermal melanocytosis is unilateral and uveal melanoma develops on the same side as the hyperpigmentation. Less often, oculodermal melanocytosis is bilateral, and a rare case of bilateral uveal melanoma in association with bilateral oculodermal melanocytosis has been reported.[55] Although oculodermal melanocytosis is known to occur in families, it has not been reported with familial uveal melanoma.[69] It is recommended that patients with oculodermal melanocytosis be examined on a regular basis for the early detection of melanoma.

Familial Atypical Mole and Melanoma Syndrome (FAM-M Syndrome)

The syndrome of autosomal dominant predisposition to cutaneous melanoma has been previously described by various names such as the B-K mole syndrome, and the dysplastic nevus syndrome.[11,18] The term "FAM-M syndrome" is now preferred.[38] According to a National Institutes of Health (NIH) consensus panel, FAM-M is characterized by the occurrence of a large number of atypical (often more than 50) irregular and multicolored cutaneous nevi, cutaneous melanoma in one or more first- or second-degree relatives, and by the presence of certain distinct histologic features such as melanocytic nuclear pleomorphism, hyperchromatism, melanocytic hyperplasia, architectural disorder with asymmetry, subepidermal fibroplasia, and frequent dermal lymphocytic infiltration.[38]

Several cases of uveal melanoma in patients with FAM-M syndrome have been reported.[56] The lifetime chance of coexistence of primary uveal melanoma and primary cutaneous melanoma is remote (estimated to be 1 in 160,000) and therefore, such an occurrence is thought to represent true association between the two entities.[45,56] This hypothesis is appealing because cutaneous and uveal melanocytes share similar embryologic, morphologic, and antigenic properties. Increased number of uveal nevi in patients with the FAM-M syndrome and the occurrence of cutaneous melanoma and uveal melanoma in different members of a family with FAM-M syndrome supports an association between FAM-M syndrome and uveal melanoma.[28,32,46] In a prospective study of 207 consecutive patients with ocular melanoma (uveal, conjunctival, and eyelid melanoma) there was a greater than expected prevalence of cutaneous melanoma (5 patients). Two of these 5 patients had features of the FAM-M syndrome. The authors concluded that FAM-M syndrome predisposes to both cutaneous and ocular melanoma.[4] Other reports, however, suggest that the coexistence of uveal melanoma and FAM-M syndrome is coincidental.[19,67] The Connecticut Tumor Registry Data revealed only one case of uveal melanoma (representing the expected prevalence) in a population of 13,841 individuals with cutaneous melanoma.[20] Some of the discrepancy between the different studies could be attributed to the lack of uniform criteria used for the diagnosis of the FAM-M syndrome. With the use of a uniform definition as proposed by the NIH consensus panel, this will be eliminated in the future. Long-term prospective studies are necessary to investigate the relationship between FAM-M syndrome and uveal melanoma because the interval between the diagnosis of these two entities may be as long as 10 years.[56] With increased awareness, we may realize a stronger association between FAM-M syndrome and primary uveal melanoma.

Neurofibromatosis Type 1

An autosomal dominant, multisystem disorder with characteristic ophthalmic findings, neurofibromatosis type 1 (NF) is primarily a disorder of neural crest–derived cells.[6] Cutaneous and uveal melanocytes are both derived from the neural crest. NF patients have an excess of melanocytes in the skin (café-au-lait spots). There is probably an excess of uveal melanocytes as well. This is seen in the iris as Lisch's nodules. Increased numbers of uveal nevi in patients with NF have also been reported.[22] NF is also associated with neural crest–derived cell malignancies such as malignant schwannoma and pheochromocytoma. Rarely has uveal melanoma been documented in patients with NF type 1.[64]

FAMILIAL UVEAL MELANOMA

Incidence

Familial uveal melanoma (FUM) is a rare entity. In addition to Silcock's original family, only 51 families with FUM have been reported.[9,57,73] In a recent report it was estimated that 0.6% of all uveal melanoma patients have familial involvement.[57] All families with FUM that have been reported so far are Caucasian.

Pedigree Structure

Based on the two large published series of FUM,[57,73] certain characteristic features of families with FUM become apparent: *(1)* usually only one other member in the family has uveal melanoma, *(2)* the other affected family member is most often (63%) a first-degree relative, and *(3)* extensive involvement of kindreds over many generations is extremely rare.

Coincidence or Inheritance

Consider the low incidence of uveal melanoma; the likelihood of FUM by chance alone is very remote. Because of the small number of families with FUM and the incidence of only a few members in a given family with FUM, formal methods of genetic analysis such as segregation analysis cannot be applied to ascertain the likelihood of coincidence versus inheritance in FUM. However, on the basis of available limited data, an autosomal dominant mode of inheritance has been postulated.[33]

Inherited Cancer Predisposition Syndrome

In general, patients with a cancer predisposition syndrome tend to develop cancer at an earlier age and have bilateral involvement of paired organs, multiple primary tumors, familial occurrence of cancer, and phenotypic associations.[41] There are only two studies that have explored the possibility that FUM is part of a generalized inherited cancer predisposition syndrome.[27,33,41,57] It was hypothesized that FAM-M syndrome may form a basis for FUM.[14] So far this has not been substantiated. To the contrary, recent studies have suggested a lack of correlation between occurrence of FUM and FAM-M syndrome.[56,57]

Presence of breast cancer in a family with FUM led Jay and McCartney to speculate on the presence of the Li–Fraumeni syndrome.[27] Li–Fraumeni syndrome is an autosomal dominant trait that predisposes to soft tissue sarcoma, brain tumors, leukemia, breast cancer, and other cancers in many members of a family.[5,16,31] Patients with familial uveal melanoma have been calculated to have a four times greater likelihood of developing a second primary malignancy than the general population.[57] Association of FUM with a generalized inherited predisposition to cancer remains to be firmly established.

Constitutional Cytogenetic Studies

In the setting of familial cancer syndromes such as retinoblastoma and neurofibromatosis type 1, demonstration of a constitutional cytogenetic abnormality has been critical in the identification of the gene. A search for such constitutional cytogenetic abnormality was negative in 14 probands with FUM. Submicroscopic chromosomal changes such as single base-pair mutations are not detectable by cytogenetic techniques. Therefore, the absence of constitutional cytogenetic abnormality does not exclude the presence of an inherited genetic defect.[37]

Germline Mutations

Linkage analysis of some familial cutaneous melanoma kindreds has strongly implicated a locus in chromosomal region 9p21.[10] The cyclin dependent kinase-4 inhibitor gene (*CDKN2* gene) also known as $p16^{INK4}$ or multiple tumor suppressor gene 1 (*MTS1*) was recently mapped to the 9p21 region.[29,39] Because of location and frequent mutations in cutaneous melanoma cell lines, involving the *CDKN2* gene, it is proposed as a candidate cutaneous melanoma tumor suppressor gene. *CDKN2* germline mutations in familial cutaneous melanoma kindreds have been described.[26] However, absence of *CDKN2* gene germline mutations in familial uveal melanoma patients has also been reported.[59] Although a study by Singh et al. eliminated the *CDKN2* gene as a familial uveal melanoma predisposition gene in most cases, the presence of another tumor suppressor gene in the 9p21 region was suggested.[59]

Uveal Melanoma in Young Individuals

Approximately 1% of all uveal melanomas occur in patients less than 20 years of age.[2,51] Most pediatric uveal melanomas occur around puberty, although they can even be present at birth.[2,21,51] The clinical features of pediatric uveal melanoma are similar to those of adult uveal melanoma.[2,51] Uveal melanomas in young patients have been successfully treated with the same modalities used to treat uveal melanoma in adults[51]: enucleation, local resection, episcleral radioactive plaque application, and photocoagulation. The data regarding systemic prognosis suggest that the long-term prognosis (15 years survival) is no worse than in adults (30% mortality) and the short-term prognosis (up to 5 years survival) may be even better than in adults.[2,51]

Occurrence of a tumor at an early age, among other features, suggests an inherited cancer predisposition. Verdaguer reported the presence of ocular melanocytosis, a condition predisposing to uveal melanoma in 4 of 7 young patients with choroidal melanoma.[71] In a case report of a congenital uveal melanoma, Greer noted "numerous pigmented cutaneous nevi in infant and mother."[21] A case of iris melanoma in a 10-year-old boy with features suggestive of familial atypical mole and melanoma (FAM-M) syndrome has also been reported.[60] Children with either uveal melanoma or cutaneous melanoma provide a unique opportunity to investigate presence of genetic or nongenetic predisposing conditions.

Bilateral Uveal Melanoma

Primary uveal melanoma is rarely bilateral.[52] Since the report of Shine in 1930, approximately 44 well-documented cases of bilateral primary uveal melanoma have been reported worldwide.[53,55] Bilateral primary uveal melanoma should be distinguished from BDUMP syndrome (benign diffuse uveal melanocytic proliferation syndrome), which is characterized by a benign paraneoplastic proliferation of uveal melanocytes in association with a systemic malignancy.[3] Shammas and Watzke estimated that only one case of bilateral uveal melanoma will occur every 18 years in the United States.[50] In the absence of identifiable predisposing factors, the occurrence of bilateral primary uveal melanoma has been assumed to be a rare random event.

In a series of bilateral primary uveal melanoma, patients who were evaluated for the role of genetic predisposition were found to have no apparent clinical evidence of inherited predisposition to cancer.[55] Bilateral ocular melanocytosis was thought to be contributory in two patients. No association between bilateral primary uveal melanoma with FAM-M syndrome, FUM, neurofibromatosis type 1, or Li–Fraumeni syndrome was observed. Occurrence of bilateral primary uveal melanoma is probably not a random event and unidentified germline mutations may be important in its pathogenesis.[55]

CYTOGENETIC STUDIES

Few reports have characterized cytogenetic changes in uveal melanoma. Nonrandom changes have included monosomy 3, trisomy 8, and structural or numerical abnormalities of chromosome 6.[23,24,42,61] These observations have been confirmed by restriction fragment length polymorphism analysis.[25] Loss of chromosome 3 alleles and multiplication of chromosome 8 alleles suggest the presence of a tumor suppressor gene on chromosome 3 and an oncogene on chromosome 8 in the formation of uveal melanoma. The numerical and structural changes of chromosome 8 all resulted in gain of material, the smallest region of common gain being 8q13-qter. C-myc, a nuclear oncogene involved in cellular proliferation is located in the region 8q24. Mukai and Dryja had previously reported loss of alleles at polymorphic loci on chromosome 2 in 2 of the 15 cases studied.[37]

The absence of monosomy 3 and 8q trisomy in several cases suggests that there is more than one pathway for malignant transformation. This concept is supported by the distinct cytogenetic changes observed in iris melanoma (one reported case).[72] Alterations of chromosome 9p are less frequently observed cytogenetic changes. Loss of 9pter-p22 as a cytogenetic abnormality in cutaneous nevi and cutaneous melanoma has implicated the interferon gene (located on 9p13-p22 and 9p22-pter) as an initial step of malignant transformation of cutaneous melanocytes.[12] This is a very significant finding as a locus for familial cutaneous melanoma has been assigned to chromosome region 9p13-p22.[10]

Cytogenetic abnormalities have been used as markers for prognosis in conditions such as chronic myeloid leukemia.[49] Similar prognostic significance of cytogenetic changes in uveal melanoma has also been suggested.[43] Cytogenetic dissimilarities between ciliary body and choroidal melanoma offers a genetic basis for the observed difference in prognosis between ciliary body and choroidal melanomas. However, worse prognosis associated with ciliary body melanoma may be an epiphenomenon explainable by size, cytology, or vascular pattern[34,48] and the cytogenetic differences noted between ciliary body melanoma and choroidal melanoma may correlate with these prognostic parameters.

MOLECULAR GENETICS

The Ras Oncogene

The ras family of protooncogenes (c-Ha-*ras* 1, c-Ki-*ras* 2, and N-*ras*) frequently show mutations in a wide variety of human malignancies.[7] In cutaneous melanoma, mutations of the N-*ras* (codons 13 and 61) are near dipyrimidine sites which implicates ultraviolet radiation in pathogenesis.[70] Human choroidal melanomas lack mutations in codons 12, 13, and 61 (commonly mutated sites).[63] Specifically, absence of mutations in the N-*ras* protooncogene raises doubts about the role of ultraviolet radiation in the pathogenesis of choroidal melanoma.[63]

The c-myc Oncogene

C-myc is a nuclear oncogene located on chromosome 8q24.[13] Immunohistochemical staining for C-myc with monoclonal antibodies have indicated a role of the myc protein in cellular proliferation that can be correlated with other prognostic markers.[47]

p53

Mutations of the p53 suppressor gene are some of the commonest abnormalities found in human cancers.[30] In a comparative study of choroidal melanoma and choroidal nevi, mutations in exon 7 were detected in choroidal melanomas but were lacking in choroidal nevi. These findings suggest a role of p53 mutations in the pathogenesis of uveal melanoma.[68]

Cyclin-Dependent Kinase-4 Inhibitor *(CDKN2)* Gene

The *CDKN2* gene, a putative tumor suppressor gene located on chromosomal region 9p21, is mutated in cell lines of many cancers affecting lung, breast, brain, kidney, ovary, and cutaneous melanoma.[29,39] More than 90% of the reported mutations have involved exon 2 of the *CDKN2* gene.[65] Loss of heterozygosity studies on uncultured uveal melanoma samples have shown loss of markers from the CDKN2 locus.[40] However, sequence analysis of all 3 exons of the *CDKN2* gene did not reveal mutations in any of the uveal melanoma samples analyzed.[40] These findings suggest the presence of another tumor suppressor gene in the 9p21 region that is involved in pathogenesis of uveal melanoma.

TRANSGENIC MOUSE MODELS

Transgenic mouse models provide a powerful tool for the study of molecular mechanisms of carcinogenesis.[13] Transgenic mice developed using tyrosinase promoter tagged with mutated ras gene or SV40-Tag oncoprotein have melanocytic tumors that mimic uveal melanoma.[1,8,35,66] The tumors arise from the retinal pigment epithelium and have morphologic features consistent with retinal pigment epithelium carcinoma.[1]

CONCLUSIONS

The genetic aspects of uveal melanoma remain to be investigated further. All cases of FUM, bilateral primary uveal melanomas, or uveal melanomas occurring in presence of a clinical syndrome such as FAM-M or Li–Fraumeni should be documented with complete family history and evaluated for a second primary malignancy. At the time of enucleation, samples from the tumor should be frozen for molecular genetic studies. Development of transgenic models offers many exciting opportunities for the future.

REFERENCES

1. Anand R, Ma D, Alizadeh H et al. Characterization of intraocular tumors arising in transgenic mice. *Invest Ophthalmol Vis Sci* 1994;35:3533–3539.
2. Barr CC, McLean IW, Zimmerman LE. Uveal melanoma in children and adolescents. *Arch Ophthalmol* 1981;99:2133–2136.
3. Barr CC, Zimmerman LE, Curtin VT, Front RL. Bilateral diffuse melanocytic uveal tumors associated with systemic malignant neoplasms. A recently recognized syndrome. *Arch Ophthalmol* 1982;100:249–255.

4. Bataille V, Pinney E, Hungerford JL et al. Five cases of coexistent primary ocular and cutaneous melanoma. *Arch Dermatol* 1993;129: 198–201.
5. Birch JM, Hartley AL, Blair V et al. Cancer in the families of children with soft tissue sarcoma. *Cancer* 1990;66:2239–2248.
6. Bolande RP. Neurofibromatosis—the quintessential neurocristopathy: Pathogenetic concepts and relationships. *Adv Neurol* 1981;29:67–75.
7. Bos JL. *Ras* oncogenes in human cancer. A review. *Cancer Res* 1989;49:4682–4689.
8. Bradl M, Klein-Szanto AJP, Porter S, Mintz M. Malignant melanoma in transgenic mice. *Proc Natl Acad Sci USA* 1992;88;164–168.
9. Canning CR, Hungerford J. Familial uveal melanoma. *Br J Ophthalmol* 1988;72:241–243
10. Cannon-Albright LA, Goldgar DE, Meyer LJ et al. Assignment of a locus for familial melanoma, MLM, to chromosome 9p13-p22. *Science* 1992;258:1148–1151.
11. Clark WH, Reimer RR, Greene M et al. Origin of familial malignant melanomas from heritable melanocytic lesions: "The B-K Mole syndrome." *Arch Dermatol* 1978;114;732–738.
12. Cowan JM, Halaban R, Francke U. Cytogenetic analysis of melanocytes from premalignant nevi and melanomas. *J Natl Cancer Inst* 1988; 80:1159–1164.
13. Dalla-Favera R, Bregni M, Erikson J et al. Human *c-myc onc* gene is located on the region of chromosome 8 that is translocated in Burkitt's lymphoma cells. *Proc Natl Acad Sci USA* 1982;79:7824–7827.
14. Egan KM, Seddon JM Glynn RJ Gragoudas ES, Albert DM. Epidemiologic aspects of uveal melanoma. *Surv Ophthalmol* 1988;32:239–251.
15. Fowlis DJ, Balmain A. Oncogenes and tumor suppressor genes in transgenic mouse models of neoplasia. *Eur J Cancer* 1993;29:A:638–645.
16. Garber JE, Goldstein AM, Kantor AF, Dreyfus MG, Fraumeni JF Jr, Li FP. Follow-up study of twenty-four families with Li-Fraumeni syndrome. *Cancer Res* 1991;51:6094–6097.
17. Gonder JR, Ezell PC, Shields JA, Augsburger JJ. Ocular melanocytosis. A study to determine the prevalence rate of ocular melanocytosis. *Ophthalmology* 1982;89:950–952.
18. Greene MH, Clark WH, Tucker MA et al. Precursor nevi in cutaneous malignant melanoma: A proposed nomenclature. *Lancet* 1980;2:1024.
19. Greene MH, Sanders RJ, Chu FC et al. The familial occurrence of cutaneous melanoma, intraocular melanoma, and the dysplastic nevus syndrome. *Am J Ophthalmol* 1983;96:238–245.
20. Greene MH, Sanders RJ, Chu FC et al. The familial occurrence of cutaneous melanoma, intraocular melanoma, and the dysplastic nevus syndrome. *Am J Ophthalmol* 1984;97:115–117.
21. Greer CH. Congenital melanoma of the anterior uvea. *Arch Ophthalmol* 1966;76:77–78.
22. Hope DG, Mulvihill JJ. Malignancy in neurofibromatosis. *Adv Neurol* 1981;29:33–56.
23. Horsman DE, Sroka H, Rootman J, White VA. Monosomy 3 and isochromosome 8q in a uveal melanoma. *Cancer Genet Cytogenet* 1990; 45:249–253.
24. Horsman DE, White VA. Cytogenetic analysis of uveal melanoma: Consistent occurrence of monosomy 3 and trisomy 8q. *Cancer* 1993; 71:811–819.
25. Horsthemke B, Precher G, Bornfeld N, Becher R. Loss of chromosome 3 alleles and multiplication of chromosome 8 alleles in uveal melanoma: *Genes Chromosomes Cancer* 1992;4:217–221.
26. Hussussian CJ, Struewing JP, Goldstein AM et al. Germline p16 mutations in familial melanoma. *Nature Genet* 1994;8:15–21.
27. Jay M, McCartney A. Familial malignant melanoma of the uvea and p53: A Victorian detective story. *Surv Ophthalmol* 1993;37:457–462.
28. Jensen OA, Movin M, Muller J. Malignant melanoma of the choroid in an infant with the dysplastic nevus syndrome. *Acta Ophthalmol* 1987;65:91–100.
29. Kamb A, Gruis NA, Weaver-Feldhaus J et al. A cell regulator potentially involved in genesis of many tumor types. *Science* 1994;264:436–440.
30. Levine AL, Momand J, Finlay CA. The p53 tumor suppressor gene. *Nature* 1991;351: 453–456.
31. Li FP, Fraumeni JF. Soft tissue sarcomas, breast cancer and other neoplasms: A familial syndrome? *Ann Intern Med* 1969;71:747–752.
32. Lynch HT, Fusaro RM, Pester J et al. Tumor spectrum in the FAMM-M syndrome. *Br J Cancer* 1981;44:553–560.
33. Lynch HT, Anderson DE, Krush AJ. Heredity and intraocular melanomas. *Cancer* 1968; 21:119–125.
34. McLean IW, Ainbinder AJ, Gamel JW, McCurdy JB. Choroidal-ciliary body melanoma: A multivariate survival analysis of tumor location. *Ophthalmology* 1995;102:1060–1064.
35. Mintz B, Klein-Szanto AJP. Malignancy of eye melanomas originating in the retinal pigment epithelium of transgenic mice after genetic ablation of choroidal melanocytes. *Proc Natl Acad Sci USA* 1992;89:11421–11425.
36. Mooy CM, Van der Helm MJ, Van der Kwast

Th H et al. No N-*ras* mutations in human uveal melanoma: The role of ultraviolet light revisited. *Br J Cancer* 1991;64:411–413.

37. Mukai S, Dryja T. Loss of alleles at polymorphic loci on chromosome 2 in uveal melanoma. *Cancer Genet Cytogenet* 1986;22:45–53.
38. NIH Consensus conference. Diagnosis and treatment of early melanoma. *JAMA* 1992; 268:1314–1319.
39. Nobori T, Miura K, Wu DJ et al. Deletion of the cyclin dependent kinase-4 inhibitor gene in multiple human cancers. *Nature* 1994;368: 753–756.
40. Ohta M, Nagai H, Shimizu M et al. Rarity of somatic and germline mutations of the cyclin dependent kinase-4 inhibitor gene in melanoma. *Cancer Res* 1994;84:5269–5272.
41. Ponder BAJ. Inherited cancer syndromes. In *Genes and Cancer,* D. Carney, K. Sikora, eds. New York: Wiley, 1990:99–106.
42. Prescher G, Bornfeld N, Becher R. Nonrandom chromosomal abnormalities in primary uveal melanoma. *J Natl Cancer Inst* 1990;82:1765–1769.
43. Prescher G, Bornfeld N, Horsthemke B, Becher R. Chromosomal aberrations defining uveal melanoma of poor prognosis. *Lancet* 1992;339:691–692.
44. Reese AB. *Tumors of the Eye.* New York: Hoeber, 1976:174.
45. Rodriguez-Sains RS. The familial occurrence of cutaneous melanoma, intraocular melanoma, and the dysplastic nevus syndrome. *Am J Ophthalmol* 1984;97:114–115.
46. Rodriguez-Sains RS. Ocular findings in patients with dysplastic nevus syndrome. *Ophthalmology* 1986;93:661–665.
47. Royds JA, Sharrad RM, Parsons MA et al. C-*myc* oncogene expression in ocular melanomas. *Graefe's Arch Clin Exp Ophthalmol* 1992; 230:366–371.
48. Rummelt V, Folberg R, Woolsen RF, Hwang T, Pe'er J. Relation between the microcirculation architecture and the aggressive behavior of ciliary body melanomas. *Ophthalmology* 1995; 102:844–851.
49. Sandberg AA. The chromosomes in human leukemia. *Semin Hematol* 1986;23:201–217.
50. Shammas HF, Watzke RC. Bilateral choroidal melanomas. Case report and incidence. *Arch Ophthalmol* 1977;95:617–623.
51. Shields CL, Shields JA, Milite J, De Potter P, Sabbagh R, Menduke H. Uveal melanoma in teenagers and children: A report of 40 cases. *Ophthalmology* 1991;98:1662–1666.
52. Shields JA, Shields CL. *Intraocular Tumors: A Text and Atlas.* Philadelphia: W.B. Saunders, 1992:156.
53. Shine FW. Report of a case of bilateral sarcoma of the uveal tract. *NY Eye Ear Infirm Clin Rep* 1930;1:31–33.
54. Silcock AQ. Hereditary sarcoma of the eyeball. *Trans Pathol Soc Lond* 1892;43:140–141.
55. Singh AD, Shields CL, Shields JA, De Potter P. Bilateral primary uveal melanoma: Bad luck or bad genes? *Ophthalmology* 1996;103: 256–262.
56. Singh AD, Shields CL, Shields JA, Eagle RC, De Potter P. Uveal melanoma and familial atypical mole and melanoma (FAM-M) syndrome. *Ophthalmic Genet* 1995;16:53–61.
57. Singh AD, Shields CL, De Potter P, Shields JA, Trock B, Cater J, Pastore D. Familial uveal melanoma—Clinical observations on 56 patients. *Arch Ophthalmol* 1996;114:392–399.
58. Singh AD, Donoso LA, Jackson L, Shields CL, De Potter P, Shields JA. Familial uveal melanoma—Absence of constitutional cytogenetic abnormalities in 14 cases. *Arch Ophthalmol* 1996;114:502–503.
59. Singh AD, Croce CM, Wary KK et al. Familial uveal melanoma: Absence of germline mutations involving the cyclin dependent kinase-4 inhibitor gene (p16). *Ophthalmic Genet* 1996;17:39–40.
60. Singh AD, Shields JA, Eagle RC, Shields CL, Marmor M, De Potter P. Iris melanoma in a ten-year-old boy with familial atypical mole-melanoma (FAM-M) syndrome. *Ophthalmic Genet* 1994;15:145–149.
61. Singh AD, Boghosian-Sell L, Wary KK et al. Cytogenetic findings in primary uveal melanoma. *Cancer Genet Cytogenet* 1994;72: 109–115.
62. Sisley K, Rennie IG, Cottam DW, Potter AM, Potter CW, Rees RC. Cytogenetic findings in six posterior uveal melanomas: Involvement of chromosome 3,6 and 8. *Genes Chromosomes Cancer* 1990;82:1765–1769.
63. Soparker CN, O'Brien JM, Albert DM. Investigation of the role of the *ras* protooncogene point mutation in human uveal melanomas. *Invest Ophthalmol Vis Sci* 1993;34:2203–2209.
64. Specht CS, Smith TW. Uveal malignant melanoma and von Recklinghausen's neurofibromatosis. *Cancer* 1988;62:812–817.
65. Spruck CH, Gonzalez-Zulueta M, Shibata A et al. p16 Gene in uncultured tumors. *Nature* 1994;370:183–184.
66. Syed NA, Windle JJ, Darjatmoko SR, Lokken

JM, Albert DM. Natural history of a transgenic murine model of intraocular melanoma. *Invest Ophthalmol Vis Sci* 1995;36(Suppl):770.

67. Taylor MR, Guerry D, Bondi EE et al. Lack of association between intraocular melanoma and cutaneous dysplastic nevi. *Am J Ophthalmol* 1984;98:478–482.
68. Tobal K, Warren W, Cooper CS et al. Increased expression and mutation of p53 in choroidal melanoma. *Br J Cancer* 1992;66:900–904.
69. Trese MT, Pettit TH, Foos RY et al. Familial nevus of Ota. *Ann Ophthalmol* 1981;13: 855–857.
70. van't Veer LJ, Burgering BM, Beersteeg R et al. N-*ras* mutations in human cutaneous melanoma from sun exposed body sites. *Mol Cell Biol* 1989;9:3114–3116.
71. Verdaguer J Jr. Prepuberal and puberal melanomas in Ophthalmology. *Am J Ophthalmol* 1965;60:1002–1011.
72. White VA, Horsman DE, Rootman J. Cytogenetic characterization of an iris melanoma. *Cancer Genet Cytogenet* 1995;82:85–87.
73. Young LHY, Egan KM, Walsh SM, Gragoudas ES. Familial uveal melanoma. *Am J Ophthalmol* 1994;117:516–520.

40

Retinoblastoma

A. LINN MURPHREE

THE BASIS OF HUMAN CANCER

Our current understanding of the etiology of cancer in general owes a great debt to retinoblastoma (Rb). It was in this disease that suppressor tumor genes were first defined. The first human cancer gene to be cloned was the RB1 gene.[59,60] Errors at mitosis (mitotic recombination) were described for the first time as tumorigenic events in human cancer by researchers working on retinoblastoma.[29]

Retinoblastoma (Rb), an embryonal small-cell malignancy of the retina, arises from retinal precursor cells and presents clinically most commonly a leucocoria (Fig. 40.1). Virtually, all retinoblasts are terminally differentiated by age $2\frac{1}{2}$ years. The diagnosis of Rb is rare after that age. Rb is the classic example of the dominant cancer predisposition that is also observed with other solid childhood neoplasms.[90–94]

Genetic (bilateral or multifocal) (Fig. 40.2) and nongenetic (unilateral, unifocal) (Fig. 40.1) forms of retinoblastoma are both caused by loss of function (LOF) mutations in both copies[29] of the growth suppressor gene RB1.[117] Spontaneous reduction to homozygosity of a loss of function mutant allele is a common and powerful tumorigenic event.

Two distinct families of "cancer" genes have been identified: oncogenes or protooncogenes (growth factors), which promote cell proliferation, and antioncogenes (suppressor genes), which inhibit it.[92,168] Cancer-promoting mutations result in either activation of a protooncogene or inactivation of an antioncogene. Protooncogenes code for both extra- and intracellular factors involved in transmitting signals for cell growth and differentiation from receptors in the cell membrane to genetic material in the nucleus. A protooncogene that is activated by a mutational event may lead to malignant transformation by enhancing this last pathway (a "gain-of-function" mutation). A transformed cell is one reprogrammed to divide continuously.

Inheritance of the predisposition to retinoblastoma is an autosomal dominant trait because the presence of a single mutant allele renders the cell susceptible to tumorigenesis. Tumor formation, however, is a recessive trait and requires the additional loss or inactivation of the remaining wild-type, or normal, allele. Data from retinoblastoma, as well as other childhood cancers including neuroblastoma, osteosarcoma, Wilms' tumor, fibrosarcoma, and adult cancers such as breast, lung, and colon cancer among others, indicate that inactivation of tumor suppressor genes plays a major role in the etiology or progression of many human malignancies.[75,102,152,168] These comprehensive reports review the data that antioncogenes are sequences of DNA that suppress cell growth and negatively regulate or inhibit cell proliferation. The retinoblastoma gene is the prototype of this entire class of genes. The default mode in all of these genes is prevention of cell growth. It would be expected, and indeed is the case, that the RB1 gene product must be temporarily inactivated for cells to initiate DNA synthesis. The RB1 protein pRB is ubiquitously expressed in normal tissues.[36]

Other antioncogenes described after RB1 include p53 on chromosome 17,[82] the Wilms' tumor gene, and the gene for neurofibroma, NF1.[108,167] More "candidate" antioncogenes may eventually be placed in this category because there are at least 50 forms of hereditary cancer.[92] To date, only three dominantly inherited forms of cancer are not associated with antioncogene mutation.[16,94]

Cancer arises when there is a dysregulation, or an imbalance, between the activating and inhibiting factors that regulate cell growth and differentiation. A major component of cell growth: initiation of DNA synthesis is negatively regulated by the RB1 locus. In addition, in *Drosophila melanogaster,* and likely in humans, genes such as RB1 are instrumental in the establishment and maintenance of the differentiated state.

A

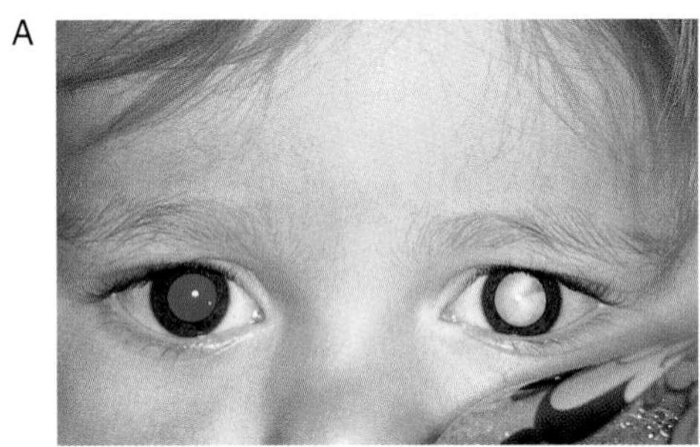

B

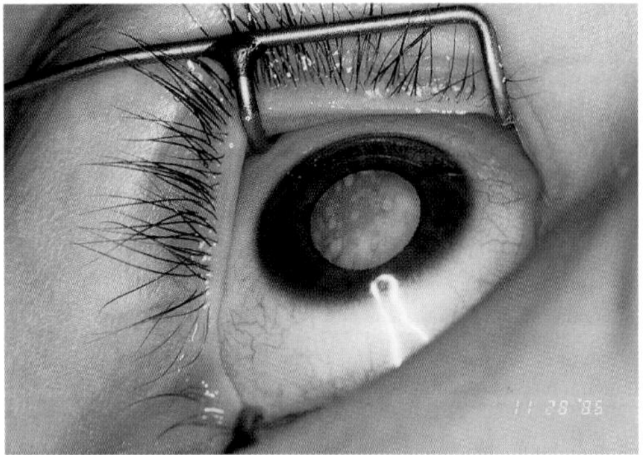

Figure 40.1. (**A**) Unilateral retinoblastoma. Leucocoria in the left eye and a normal red reflex in the right eye of a child with newly diagnosed unilateral nongenetic retinoblastoma. The left eye is virtually filled with tumor. The leucocoria is strikingly obvious here because of the dilated pupil and the flash photography. (**B**) Note the dispersion or seeding of the tumor in this eye filled with retinoblastoma.

A

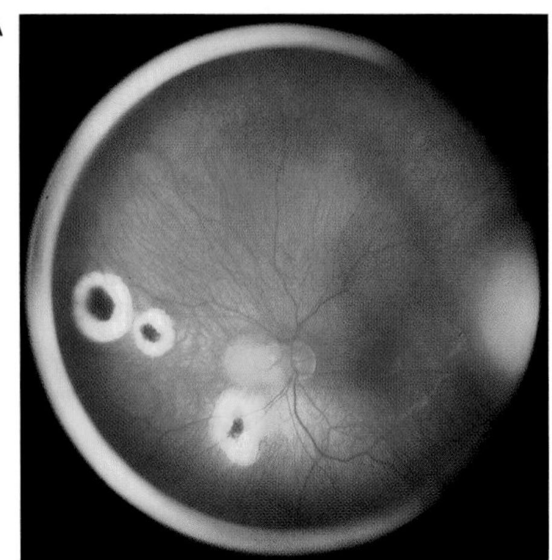

B

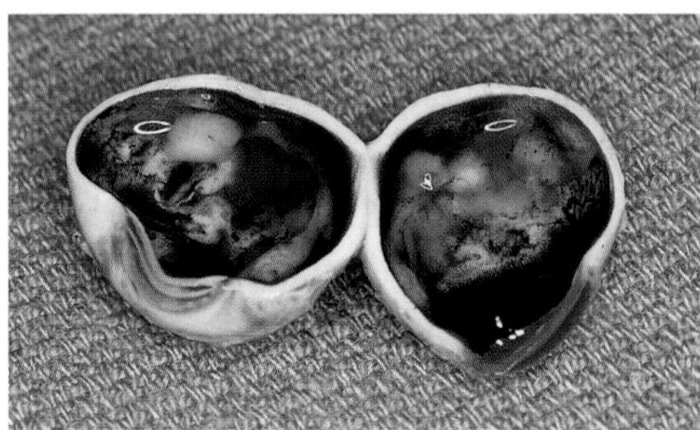

Figure 40.2. (**A**) Bilateral retinoblastoma. Wide-field image of multifocal retinoblastoma in the second eye of a child who had lost the fellow eye to enucleation because of advanced disease at the time of diagnosis. One active tumor is present immediately nasal to the optic nerve. Type 4 flat regression scars following laser SALT treatment of other independently arising tumors are seen inferiorly and nasal to this tumor. (**B**) Multifocal creamy active tumors are present. The RPE disturbance in this eye opened at the time of enucleation represents chorioretinal scars from previous laser treatment.

MITOTIC RECOMBINATION AND REDUCTION TO HOMOZYGOSITY

A germline loss of function (LOF) mutation at the RB1 locus (RB1+/RB1−) can be heritable or spontaneous, but it always results in a genetic predisposition to retinoblastoma because of its presence in every cell in the body. A spontaneous LOF mutation of the second wild-type allele (RB1+/RB1− → RB1−/RB1−) is necessary for tumorigenesis. Loss of heterozygosity (LOH) at the RB1 locus demonstrated for the first time that the tumorigenic event in Rb was recessive at the cellular level.[29] The dominantly inherited trait is the predisposition to cancer. Pedigrees of patients with retinoblastoma are compatible with dominant inheritance of the tumor because there are so many "primed" retinoblasts at risk for the second spontaneous LOF mutation that, on average, several independently arising tumors will develop in each eye (Fig. 40.2). The clinical result of a germline LOF mutation is bilateral retinoblastoma. The spontaneous second mutation occurs at least once in each eye in 90% of children with germline mutations. These patients also have an extremely strong predisposition to develop second malignant neoplasms such as osteosarcoma. The heterozygote is highly susceptible to the oncogenic effects of environmental agents such as radiation and chemical carcinogens. Because of this, there has been a dramatic shift away from primary external beam radiotherapy in the treatment of retinoblastoma. Several articles and an editorial in the November 1996 issue of the *Archives of Ophthalmology* discuss these issues.[51,62,121]

Somatic or nongenetic Rb, caused by two spontaneous LOF mutations in the same retinoblast, is a rare event. Statistically, such a rare double hit in one single cell would never occur more than once in a single individual. The requirement for two spontaneous rare genetic events accounts for both the unilateral, unifocal nature of nongenetic retinoblastoma (Fig. 40.1) and for the older age of onset of these tumors (average 24 months for somatic Rb, versus 12 months for genetic Rb).

Occasionally, patients with unilateral tumors (Fig. 40.1) and patients who are unaffected carriers of the predisposing germinal mutations are observed in pedigrees of hereditary retinoblastoma. It is possible that these individuals, although genetically predisposed, did not receive the second LOF mutation in one or both eyes by chance alone. Such individuals are usually easily identified. However, the issue of low penetrance,[37a,103a] versus pseudo-low penetrance sporadic unilateral disease[116a] induces difficult problems in genetic counseling. Approximately 15% of sporadic unilaterally affected individuals (Fig. 40.1) are heterozygous at the RB1 allele (RB1+/RB1−).[117]

THE NATURE OF THE DOMINANTLY INHERITED PREDISPOSING MUTATION

Of all germinal RB1 mutations, only 3%–5% can be recognized by advanced cytogenetic techniques, including high-resolution karyograms. These mutations are either large microscopic interstitial deletions or translocations of the long arm of chromosome 13.[113] The remainder, approximately 95%, of the predisposing germinal mutations are submicroscopic. Of these, 15%–20% are macromolecular deletions and major structural rearrangements and are detectable by Southern blot hybridization techniques.[18,77,84] The remaining 75%–80% of germinal RB1 mutations are point mutations or other minute deletions and mutations that are generally undetectable. Direct sequencing of polymerase chain reaction (PCR)-amplified genomic DNA[170] and ribonuclease (RNAse) protection assay have been employed successfully to detect the presence of these point mutations. Although these techniques are effective in detecting very small changes in DNA sequence, they are of little routine clinical use. Newer available methods to prescreen amplified fragments of DNA include denaturing gradient gel electrophoresis (DGGE), electrophoresis of heteroduplex DNA, and chemical cleavage mismatch methods such as single-strand conformation polymorphism (SSCP).[125] SSCP is the most frequently used clinical detection method at the present time.

THE SECOND TUMORIGENIC MUTATION

Advanced intraocular retinoblastoma has been detected at 21 weeks gestation,[104] in a premature infant born at 28 weeks gestation (personal observation), in a term infant,[130] or as late as 5 to 7 years of age. Classically, most cases are brought to medical attention before the age of

3 years. Once the retina is terminally differentiated, usually by age $2\frac{1}{2}$ years, the risk for new retinal tumors is practically nil, but patients with the genetic form of retinoblastoma are still at high risk of developing second malignant nonocular neoplasms.

In general, cancer is rarely found in the newborn and is seldom the cause of neonatal death and spontaneous abortion. Strong evidence exists for the inhibition of cancerous growth during embryonic development.[48] Attempts to induce cancer in early-stage embryos have been unsuccessful; however, the embryos become susceptible to carcinogenesis after the period of major organogenesis,[48] sometimes referred to as the "oncogenic grace period."[20]

It is of more than passing interest that the most common embryonic tumors in humans arise in tissues that have an unusually late date of completion of embryogenesis, and are still partially immature at birth, such as the kidney (Wilms' tumor), brain (neuroblastoma), and retina (retinoblastoma). The human retina is far from having completed its maturation at the end of gestation.[73] Studies have shown that the primate retina differentiates and matures in waves that begin in the posterior pole and extend to the ora serrata.[137] In one species of fish, the superior and nasal retina complete the process of differentiation before the inferior and temporal retina.[74] There is evidence[116] that the topography of human retinoblastoma follows the horizontal visual streak, supporting a cone cell lineage for retinoblastoma.[19,81] New tumors virtually never develop in the macula after the diagnosis of retinoblastoma in an infant, suggesting that the macula completes terminal differentiation shortly after birth.

In 75% of hereditary and nonhereditary retinoblastomas, the second or tumorigenic mutation is chromosomal in nature. Loss of heterozygosity (LOH) (i.e., reduction of the cell to homozygosity or hemizygosity) is characteristic. The most common mechanism appears to be mitotic recombination (50%), followed by nondisjunction, with or without subsequent reduplication (approximately 40%).[174] Small deletions, and possibly gene conversion, account for some of the remaining 10% of second events. The second hit occurs at much higher frequency (10-3 versus 10-7) than the first.[167] Furthermore, the second event is more sensitive to environmental factors, especially those that create chromosomal rearrangements. For example, exposure to ionizing radiation clearly increases the risk of death from second malignant neoplasms (SMNs) in genetically predisposed patients.

Once transformed, retinoblastomas accumulate additional chromosomal aberrations and randomly conferred growth advantages (usually by loss or inactivation of growth suppressor genes). As a result, tumor subpopulations emerge and rapidly dominate the proliferating tumor mass. The consistent presence of three or four copies of a portion of the genome associated with retinoblastoma, such as trisomy of the long arm of chromosome 1 (1q+) and tetrasomy of the short arm of chromosome 6 (iso6p) likely are examples of extra copies of oncogenes or growth factors, the other class of human cancer genes.

RETINOBLASTOMA'S CONTRIBUTION TO THE "ORIGIN OF CANCER" STORY

In the second decade of the twentieth century, Theodore Boveri defined a chromosomal basis for the origin of cancer for the first time.[21,22,109] Over the past two decades, research into the genetic basis of tumorigenesis has led to the confirmation of Boveri's remarkable prediction more than 80 years ago. In 1957, Vogel[164] proposed and elaborated on a "unified gene theory," suggesting that mutations in a single gene caused both hereditary and nonhereditary retinoblastoma.

Knudson's "two-hit" theory sought to explain the origin of retinoblastoma.[90,91] His work was based on a comparison of the age at diagnosis in unilateral and bilateral cases. When the curves were plotted, unilateral disease (Fig. 40.1) fit a pattern consistent with two separate events, whereas bilateral disease could be explained by a single genetic event. Although, at the time, Knudson did not know that the two events inactivated the two alleles at the same locus, it is now clear that, in the case of bilateral disease (where one of the mutations has been inherited and each retinoblast is "primed"), the child develops an average of three tumors in each eye as a result of the second LOF genetic event (Fig. 40.2). The shorter time required to accumulate one genetic event compared to two (in the case of somatic, nongenetic disease) accounts, at least in part, for the difference in the average age of diagnosis of bilateral disease (12 months) and unilateral disease (24 months).

In 1973, Comings described a general theory of carcinogenesis.[34] His concept that cancer could result from loss of both alleles of a single gene was proven with the identification and characterization of tumor suppressor genes in general, and the retinoblastoma gene in particular. A viral cause of human retinoblastoma was proposed[164] but has never had scientific support. The description of a microscopic deletion of a portion of the long arm of chromosome 13 (13q−) in approximately 5% of patients with retinoblastoma was the first clue to the location of the gene. Chromosome banding techniques allowed the demonstration that chromosome 13 carried the retinoblastoma-associated deletion.[55] The location of the gene was narrowed to the region of bands 13q14.1–13q14.3 by defining the region of least common overlap in a series of patients with retinoblastoma.[171]

Further refinement of the gene locus was achieved by measuring levels of the enzyme esterase D (ESD), the only known gene mapped to chromosome 13.[155] Sparkes and coworkers demonstrated that each of 5 subjects with retinoblastoma and 13q− syndrome had a 50% reduction of esterase D activity compared to normal individuals. The tight linkage between the esterase D and the retinoblastoma genes was confirmed.[156] Clinical testing for the retinoblastoma deletion by measurement of esterase D activity became possible. The test has been occasionally used in lieu of chromosomal analysis,[30,114] and it is arguably more sensitive than high-resolution banding in detecting small deletions.

In 1983, incontrovertible proof of the recessive nature of the retinoblastoma mutations was presented by Cavenee et al.[29] Mitotic recombination, a previously unrecognized event, was demonstrated to be the genetic mechanism responsible for the majority of inactivating second mutations. In 1984, a review of the available data suggested that a single locus accounted for all forms of retinoblastoma.[117] The evidence that sporadic unilateral retinoblastoma (Fig. 40.1) resulted from mutations at this locus came from analysis of genetic material from tumors of patients with bilateral and unilateral disease. In unilateral nongenetic tumor material, loss of both copies of the RB1 gene at 13q14 could be demonstrated.[9] The fact that a single genetic defect resulted in a tumor that was, in both sporadic and hereditary forms, histologically and biologically indistinguishable was further strong support that a single locus—RB1—was responsible for all forms of retinoblastoma.

EPIDEMIOLOGY, MORBIDITY, AND MORTALITY

Prevalence of Retinoblastoma

In the United States, the prevalence of retinoblastoma (total number of cases of a disease in a given population at a given period of time) is 11 cases for every million children under the age of 5 years.[40] Worldwide, the incidence of retinoblastoma is estimated to range from 1/15,000 to 1/20,000 live births.[95,159] Prevalence figures are a more accurate reflection of the frequency of Rb as children remain at risk of developing the disease until approximately 5 years of age.[127] Incidence figures, however, provide a degree of uniformity that allows for comparison of the disease among various populations.

The prevalence of retinoblastoma among the various populations of the world is remarkably constant. This constancy strongly implies that environmental factors play little role in the etiology of the tumor. Further evidence against environmental influence was provided by Buckley in his review of the epidemiology of cancer in the very young.[25] The lack of environmental influence on the prevalence of retinoblastoma is further supported by the lack of an increase in the number of cases of retinoblastoma in Nagasaki and Hiroshima after the atomic bombs.[6] These data imply that endogenous mutations are required in the genesis of retinoblastoma.

There have been reports of an increase in the prevalence of retinoblastoma over the past few decades. As part of a World Health Organization (WHO) study on cancer of the eye in children, a negative correlation between the prevalence of retinoblastoma and infant mortality rate was found, suggesting that the quality of medical care and, ultimately, survival, will affect the prevalence of retinoblastoma. François and colleagues concurred with that concept and proposed that a lowering of infant mortality rate and improvement in the quality of diagnosis and management of patients with retinoblastoma provide a better explanation for the apparent increase in the number of children with retinoblastoma in a given population than a proposed increase in the RB1 mutation rate.[56]

Because of early detection and good medical and surgical treatment, the overall survival of retinoblastoma may surpass 90% in developed countries.[2] Where access to medical care is limited, survival of patients with this tumor is rare. Retinoblastoma expands locally by filling the eye and extending into the optic nerve, orbit, sinuses, and brain. Blood-borne distant metastases appear most commonly in bone marrow, bone, and brain.

Factors Influencing Visual Outcome

Presently, the size and location of the tumor(s) and the presence or absence of intraocular tumor dispersion are the most important factors that determine visual outcome. There exists the possibility that vision may ultimately be better than one would expect from the initial presentation, especially in the case of macular tumors where eccentrically arising tumors may "mushroom" over the fovea.[98] In one report of 17 patients with large macular tumors, vision ranged from 5/200 to 20/50[25]; in another, 2 of 11 patients regained 20/20 vision despite the presence of fluid in the macula at the time of diagnosis.[98] We have treated one patient whose macular tumor initially filled the space between the temporal arcades; the patient regained excellent vision and central fixation after treatment. In this case, as in a number of others, the tumor "mushroomed" over a large area of the retina while destroying only the smaller site of tumor origin.

Factors Influencing Survival

Extraocular tumor extension, a significant delay in diagnosis, and persistently recurrent intraocular disease are the strongest predictors of death from retinoblastoma. A delay commonly occurs between the observation of the first sign by the family and a visit to the primary care physician where they report observation of that sign. Once informed of the family's observation of a white pupil (Fig. 40.1) or strabismus, the most common presenting signs of Rb, the primary care physician is obligated to confirm the diagnosis with a red reflex exam using a direct ophthalmoscope, and/or immediately refer the patient to a pediatric ophthalmologist. In the absence of a family history, a pediatrician will rarely make the initial diagnosis. A posterior location and large tumor size increase the likelihood of an abnormal red reflex (Fig. 40.1).

In developing countries, the overall survival rate is directly related to the delay in receiving medical attention. For example, in one report, only 6 of 20 patients survived; all had advanced disease (Fig. 40.3).[151] African countries have reported similar high mortality rates.[96] In contrast, only 26 (8%) of 317 patients seen at Moorfields and St. Bartholomew's hospitals in London developed metastatic disease.[87]

The overall survival from retinoblastoma in the United States is 92%. However, this num-

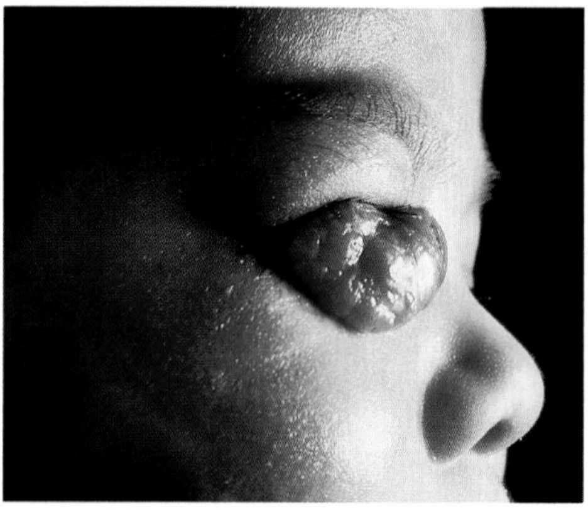

Figure 40.3. Extraocular retinoblastoma in a 4-year-old child who had not received medical attention in a developing country. This retinoblastoma had ruptured the globe at the inferior limbus and grown only anteriorly. There was no extension of disease into the orbit. No metastatic disease was present. This lesion disappeared with 3 three cycles of triple drug systemic chemotherapy. The eye was enucleated successfully. The child is now disease free with a good cosmetic prosthesis 10 years later. He did lose his left arm at age 6 years to an aggressive osteosarcoma (second malignant neoplasm).

ber can be misleading and should not be used in a discussion with parents about any individual case. For example, the New York group reported that only 86% of bilateral cases survive 15 years.[2] A second confounding factor is that survival rates are reported by large referral centers, where the more difficult or advanced cases are treated.[85] Overall survival after diagnosis was 93%, 82%, and 66% at 5, 10, and 20 years, respectively, in one report.[137] Thus, after 20 years, one third of patients had died. These figures include deaths from second malignant neoplasms as well as from retinoblastoma.

Second Malignant Neoplasms

The overall survival rate in retinoblastoma is complicated by the high risk of second malignant neoplasms (SMNs) in survivors of hereditary disease. A major controversy exists regarding the percentage of patients who will develop an SMN. Abramson and colleagues initially reported that 89 (13%) of 693 cases of bilateral retinoblastoma developed SMNs.[1] Sixty-two of the 89 who had received radiation developed the SMN in the field of radiation. In that report, the most common SMN both within and outside the field of radiation was osteosarcoma (Fig. 40.4). The life-table incidence of second tumors, according to the 1984 report, increased with time: 20% at 10 years, 50% at 20 years, and 90% at 30 years; the mean latency was 10.4 years. Questions were raised about the high (90%) death rates at 30 years after diagnosis. The increased risk of SMNs with external beam radiotherapy (EBR) was refined in a more recent report of nearly 1000 patients with essentially complete follow-up.[50] Forty years after diagnosis of bilateral disease, 35% of patients treated with EBR developed SMNs, versus 6% of those treated without it. The increased risk of SMN in the field of EBR has been confirmed by others.[5,27,57,58,72,154]

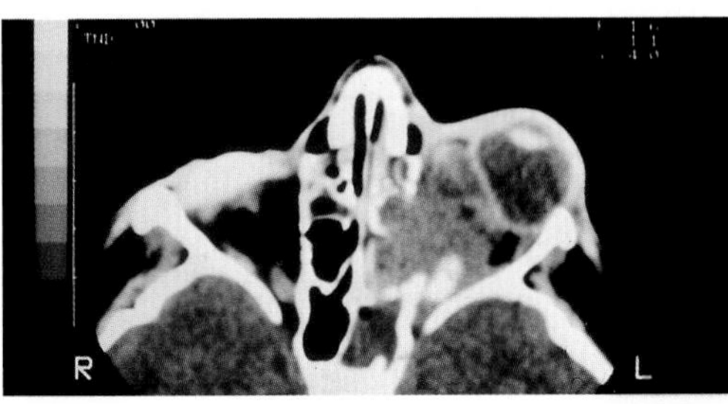

Figure 40.4. A radiogenic osteosarcoma arising in the radiated field in a child treated with external beam radiotherapy for bilateral retinoblastoma. The tumor is pushing the globe temporally.

Treatment with radiotherapy and, to a lesser extent, alkylating agents, increases the risk for SMNs.[163] The most common histologic type of SMN is osteogenic sarcoma (58% of cases), (Fig. 40.4) followed by fibrosarcoma (21%) and various other tumors (21%).[32,39,44,50,53,54,110,135,141,162] Management of these SMNs must be aggressive to be successful.[111,153]

GENETICS OF RETINOBLASTOMA

Why Genetic Counseling Is Important

Genetic counseling is very important for the family of a child with retinoblastoma. When there is a well-established family history of the disease, the genetics and genetic counseling are straightforward.[43] For sporadic bilateral cases, however, the news of a possible genetic component to this horrendous diagnosis often comes as a blow to the family. Although the issue may arise at the time of diagnosis of the affected child, we usually prefer to delay formal counseling until the initial treatment is underway. If therapy is anticipated to require some considerable period of time, we advise the parents to avoid pregnancy until after counseling.

Ideally, the genotype at the RB1 locus would be determined prior to instituting therapy in a child with retinoblastoma. The increased incidence of SMNs in retinoblastoma patients with a RB1 genotype of RB1+/RB1−, especially in the field of radiation, highlights the importance of the genotype in these patients. Unfortunately, at the present time, such screening is not logistically or financially possible. If both RB1 alleles are normal everywhere in the body except in the tumor, and the retinoblastoma arose from the chance occurrence of two RB1 mutations in a single retinal cell, then radiation and alkylating agents pose little additional risk of SMN. If, on the other hand, one of the two mutations is present in the germline, either as an "old" mutation (inherited from a parent) or "new" (arising in sperm, ovum, or de novo in the child's germline), then every cell in the body contains one mutated "retinoblastoma gene." Such a child would have a 95% chance of developing a tumor before the age of 5 years. If the mutation occurred after fertilization, at the two-, four-, or eight-cell-stage embryo, only that portion of the individual descended from the mutated embryonal cell will be heterozygous at the RB1 locus. Such "mutational mosaicism" may confound genetic predictions as only part of the body is heterozygous at the RB1 locus.

Recurrence Risk for Eye Disease

Because all patients with bilateral or multifocal disease, as well as all patients with a positive family history of retinoblastoma, are known heterozygotes at the RB1 locus, pretreatment screening in these cases is unnecessary. It is in the unilaterally affected child who presents with either a large tumor or a single smaller tumor that pretreatment screening would be most helpful. Based on chance alone, 15% of individuals who carry germinal mutations will not develop a second retinoblastoma in the second eye. If external beam radiotherapy is being considered in a child with unilateral retinoblastoma, it is justifiable to request a high-resolution banded karyotype or quantitative esterase D (ESD) analysis prior to treatment to determine whether the child carries a gene deletion.

Individuals with germline retinoblastoma or those likely to have germline retinoblastoma (sporadic bilaterally affected patients or those in a pedigree of retinoblastoma) are appropriate candidates for DNA testing. Retinoblastoma arises from functional loss of both maternal and paternal copies of the RB1 gene. If both mutations occur in a somatic (retinal) cell, the germline is uninvolved and there is no risk of retinoblastoma occurring in siblings or offspring. Somatic retinoblastoma is always manifested as a single tumor in only one eye (unilateral disease). In general, in the absence of a fresh tumor sample, unilaterally affected patients can only be screened for deletions. Efforts at molecular diagnosis are directed at detecting any germline mutation in RB1 manifested in cells more easily biopsied than those comprising the retina (e.g., leukocytes, fibroblasts, or amniotic cells). RB1 mutations in these cells would most likely result from a germline mutation, possibly inherited from a parent, but more likely occurring spontaneously at or about the time of conception.

Why Chromosome or Esterase D Analysis Alone Is Insufficient

Unfortunately, only 3% of sporadic retinoblastoma patients have a deletion of 13q14 that is large enough to be detected by either high-resolution banding chromosomal analysis or esterase D measurements. Half normal levels of esterase D may be a more accurate marker of 13q deletion than chromosome analysis, and this test is definitely more cost effective.[37] Neither test will detect submicroscopic mutations, which account for more than 70% of RB1 changes associated with an increased likelihood that retinoblastoma will develop.

CLINICAL DNA TESTING OF RETINOBLASTOMA PATIENTS

Commercial Laboratories Offering DNA Testing

In the fall of 1996, one of the two laboratories offering commercial clinical DNA testing for retinoblastoma, the Ophthalmic Genetics Laboratory in Boston, discontinued the service. In Toronto, Canada, the service previously offered by Visible Genetics, Inc. was moved back into the Eye Department at the Hospital for Sick Children. The Toronto team, headed by Brenda Gallie, M.D., can be reached at 416-813-7822. Always call ahead and talk with the laboratory prior to collecting a specimen for testing. The Toronto laboratory accepts samples for prenatal diagnosis in addition to mutation screening in affected and at-risk individuals. Their mutation analysis begins with qualitative and quantitative sizing of all RB gene exons. Abnormal-sized fragments are then sequenced using an automated sequencer. These mutations account for approximately 30% of RB1 mutations. If all fragments appear normal, the 27 exons and the promoter region of RB1 are sequenced. FISH (fluorescent in situ hybridization) is applied to detect chromosomal rearrangements when tests 1 and 2 are normal.

IN WHAT SETTINGS ARE DNA STUDIES APPROPRIATE?

Familial Retinoblastoma

All affected family members with familial retinoblastoma (more than one family member affected with unilateral or bilateral retinoblastoma) and all of their first-degree relatives (i.e., parents, siblings, and offspring) are appropriate candidates for DNA testing. Spouses of affected family members should also be included. The presence of a retinoma or osteosarcoma in a member of a retinoblastoma family should be considered as evidence that that individual is "affected" and carries a mutant RB1 allele.

Sporadic Bilateral Retinoblastoma

Sporadic bilateral retinoblastoma (no family history of retinoblastoma, retinoma, or osteosarcoma), the new or first time appearance of retinoblastoma in a family, is appropriately studied for germline DNA changes. By definition, bilateral disease indicates the presence of a germline mutation, even when there is no family history of retinoblastoma. Submission of a fresh tumor sample following enucleation helps the laboratory determine which RB1 allele is the predisposing allele by first determining which allele is homozygous in the tumor.

Sporadic Unilateral Retinoblastoma

In the absence of a family history, there is only a 15% chance that unilateral retinoblastoma patients (Fig. 40.1) carry a germline mutation. The Toronto group will accept blood alone for testing in these patients but only to screen for exon size change. If there are no changes in the initial screen, the risk of that patient being heterozygous for the RB1 gene decreases to 10% from 15%. If a fresh tumor specimen is submitted along with the blood, the laboratory will perform DNA sequencing studies.

GENETIC COUNSELING INFORMATION PROVIDED

Linkage Analysis in Familial Retinoblastoma

Tracking the mutant gene carriers through a pedigree can now be achieved by linkage analysis in virtually all retinoblastoma families.[120] Application of these techniques has allowed the prediction of the carrier status of individuals at risk.

Linkage Analysis in Sporadic Bilateral Retinoblastoma

In sporadic bilateral cases, the same linkage analysis diagnostic approach can be applied, provided that tumor material is available at the time of enucleation (freshly frozen tumor fragment—paraffin embedded material does not provide enough DNA for sequence analysis). In 70% of cases, the tumor will retain the germline mutated allele as a result of loss of heterozygosity (LOH). This information can be used to identify noncarriers among the unaffected probands' siblings. In the absence of tumor material, detection of the germline mutated allele can still be achieved by linkage analysis, if advantage is taken of the fact that in over 90% of the cases, new germline mutations are paternal in origin.[47,115,173] The confidence level of molecular diagnosis is lower (90%), however.

In the absence of linkage analysis information (a cold search), molecular diagnosis depends on the direct detection of the causative mutation. As a first step, Southern blot analysis is performed using a combination of DNA and genomic probes for the RB1 gene. If this fails to reveal gross structural rearrangement, single strand conformation polymorphism (SSCP) prescreening for mutations is undertaken in the coding sequence, flanking introns and the proximal promoter region. Each detectable variant is then further analyzed by direct genomic sequencing. Once the mutation is identified, other family members at risk can be screened for the presence or absence of the mutation.

Considering the genomic dispersion of the RB1 locus, the cold search is an intense and time-consuming effort. In addition, the sensitivity of SSCP, which approximates 90%, does not allow the identification of all mutants. Altogether, positive results can be expected for 80% of bilateral cases in the absence of the availability of tumor specimens. The rest of the mutations are possibly lying in introns far from the surveyed DNA sequences or, alternatively, are missed because of lack of sensitivity of current techniques.

Typically, DNA testing requires venous blood samples from the affected proband and his or her immediate relatives (5–10 mL in a heparinized tube; EDTA should not be used). As a prerequisite to any molecular diagnosis, however, we recommend an ophthalmoscopic screening of all first-degree relatives. We have detected a significant number of asymptomatic retinomas in family members of the propositus by this type of screening examination.

Until DNA technology is refined enough to make a reliable, rapid, relatively inexpensive RB1 DNA analysis available for pretreatment RB1 screening, ophthalmologists will have to rely primarily on clinical clues to identify carriers of RB mutations in order to make the initial selection of treatment modalities. A positive family history is the strongest predictor of a carrier state. Multiple first- and second-degree relatives with retinoblastoma makes the diagnosis almost certain in a child with an intraocular white mass. Bilateral disease and early diagnosis (before 6 months of age) of unilateral disease are the next most reliable indicators of genetic predisposition. The pretreatment screening information is useful solely as a guide in selecting the initial treatment modalities. Formal genetic counseling is usually done after treatment.

EMPIRIC RECURRENCE RISKS

Prior to the isolation, cloning, and sequencing of the RB1 gene, evidence of genetic predisposition relied almost entirely on the clinical phenotype of the tumor and the associated empiric risk data.[120] In order for somatic, non-germline Rb to be bilateral or multifocal, both the priming or predisposing first mutation (frequency rate of 10^{-6} or 1 : 1,000,000) and the tumorigenic mutation (frequency of 10^{-3} or 1 : 1,000) would be required to occur in the same cell by chance alone more than once in a single individual. The likelihood of that happening could be calculated at 1×10^{-9} for each cell at risk or 1 : 1,000,000,000 (1 in 1 billion). This chance occurrence is so unlikely that, virtually without exception, patients with nonhereditary (somatic) retinoblastoma have a single tumor in only one eye.

In the genetic form of retinoblastoma, the retinoblastoma predisposing mutation is already present in the germline, and most or all cells in the body. Because the second tumorigenic event occurs spontaneously at a relatively frequent rate of 1 : 1,000, and almost always as a result of mitotic recombination errors, and since there are several thousand susceptible retinoblasts in each retina, multiple tumors in both eyes are expected, and, in fact, occur.

If unilateral retinoblastoma (Fig. 40.1) were always somatic, and never arose from a germline mutation as bilateral disease does, the phenotype (bilateral versus unilateral) would predict the genotype. Unfortunately, that is not the case. In the group of patients with germline mutations, and because of the normal distribution of the spontaneous tumor-causing second mutation, some patients develop retinoblastoma only in one eye. These patients account for approximately 15% of unilaterally affected individuals. In these patients, the germline mutation (RB1+/RB1−) is present but, by chance alone, tumor developed in only one eye. As a result, 15% of sporadic unilateral Rb patients will, in fact, have germline Rb but clinically cannot be distinguished from the true somatic, unilateral, nongenetic retinoblastoma patients. Because of this impurity in clinical discrimination, the empiric risk for recurrence in offspring of unilaterally affected sporadic Rb patients is not zero. This blend gives the <1% risk for siblings and the 1%–5% risk for offspring of sporadical unilaterally affected individuals.

A 1992 report of 916 cases listed in the British National Registry is the basis for the empiric risk figures.[45] Forty percent of the patients had bilateral tumors, and 44% were hereditary. The 44% figure includes unilateral cases with a positive family history of retinoblastoma but does not include the 15% of unilateral sporadic retinoblastoma cases who have new germline mutations. The empirical risk for siblings of patients with sporadic bilateral retinoblastoma for developing Rb is approximately 2%. Children with unilaterally affected siblings not known to be carriers of germinal mutations have a risk of developing retinoblastoma of about 1%.[45] If there are other unaffected siblings, the risk is less. The 1992 review confirmed the fact that for individuals with the germline mutation (gene carriers), the probability of developing tumors is close to 90%.

Empirical risks relate to probabilities within large populations. The new molecular diagnostic approach determines the genotype, and predictive power of this analysis will therefore approach the real risks of 0% or 90% probability of developing tumors. For accurate genetic counseling it is very important that retinal examination of first-degree relatives be a part of the workup of any child with sporadic Rb. This effort is essential in order to ascertain the presence of retinomas that are as significant as retinoblastoma in determining whether unifocal or multifocal retinoblastoma is present.[10,61]

THE RB1 GENE

The retinoblastoma gene, RB1, is located on the long arm of chromosome 13 in region 13q14. The RB1 genomic locus consists of 27 exons distributed over 180 kilobases (kb). The largest exon (#27) contains 1889 base pairs (bp) and the smallest (#5) is composed of only 31. The 27 exons are grouped in four clusters, A (exons 1 and 2), B (exons 3–6), C (exons 7–17), and D (exons 18–27). The 26 intervening introns range in size from 80 bp–71,712 bp. The 5′ end of the gene is oriented toward the centromere.

The genomic organization and function of the RB1 gene have been fully characterized and recently reviewed with extensive references elsewhere.[119] The entire sequence of the 180-kb locus is known. The 5′ end is oriented toward the centromere and contains an unmethylated CpG-rich sequence characteristic of "housekeeping" gene promoters. There is no typical TATA box. The role of RB1 in the cancer pathway came from studies of transforming DNA tumor viruses. These viruses, specifically human adenovirus (HAdV), simian virus 40 (SV40), and human papilloma virus (HPV), specify oncoproteins (E1A, large T antigen, and E7, respectively) that complex with the active underphosphorylated p110-RB1. These transforming proteins bind to and inactivate the active form, thereby releasing the cell growth constraints. The phosphoprotein p110-RB1 is a cell-cycle regulated growth suppressor that acts, at least partly, through the repression of transcription. In normal cells, the activity of p110-RB1 is closely regulated at the posttranslational level by a cell cycle-dependent cdc2-related kinase. In quiescent cells, as well as those in the G1 stage of the cell cycle, terminal differentiation, and senescence, p110-RB1 is in its active hypophosphorylated state. As the cell progresses to the late G1 and S phase, p110-RB1 is inactivated by hyperphosphorylation at serine–threonine residues. In late mitosis, p110-RB1 returns to its active hypophosphorylated state.

RB1 has a clear role in embryogenesis. Transgenic mice that are either RB1 deficient[31,83,99] or overexpress the RB1 gene product have been created.[14] At least one functional copy of RB1 gene is required for normal embryogenesis. Overexpression leads to dwarfism.[14] Homozygous mutant deficient RB1 mice all died between 12 and 15 days of gestation from defective neurogenesis and hepatic erythropoiesis that was characterized by increased mitotic activity and failure to differentiate. Heterozygous mice were not prone to retinoblastoma, but, rather, to pituitary tumors similar to the pinealblastomas seen in the so-called trilateral retinoblastoma. Mice containing extra copies of a human RB1 complementary DNA (cDNA) transgene demonstrate generalized growth suppression as dwarfism.[14] The degree of dwarfism correlated with the dose of RB1 expression. All transgenic mice that express the SV40 T antigen oncogene specifically in photoreceptors, develop retinal and/or intracranial tumors by 2 weeks of age.[79]

In summary, the retinoblastoma gene product, p100-RB1, is a nuclear protein that arrests the cell's progression through the G1 phase of the cell cycle.[78] It appears to act as a transducer of afferent (cdc2 kinase/phosphatase PP1) and efferent signals (transcription factors) in the pathway controlling cell cycle progression, most likely by blocking the exit from G1. To retain its activity, p100-RB1 relies on intact binding domains. It has been clearly demonstrated that RB1 sequences coding for kinase recognition and E2F binding (a domain that extends far beyond that of the so-called binding pocket) are also essential for activity.[133,134] Mutations in these domains may result in complete or only partial diminution of biologic activity.

The RB1 Gene Product

The retinoblastoma gene generates a 4.7-kb messenger RNA transcript. The translated product of the RB1 locus is a 110-kd nuclear phosphoprotein of 928 amino acids. The protein product of RB1 is abbreviated as "$p110^{RB1}$." The normal function of $p110^{RB1}$ is to suppress cell growth via the ability of the active (underphosphorylated) form of the protein to repress DNA transcription.[71] The "off-on" switch for $p110^{RB1}$ is a phosphate group. When the protein is phosphorylated, it is in its inactive form. Once the phosphate group is cleaved, the protein is active.

Tumor-Associated Mutations in RB1

In human cellular growth and differentiation, mutagenesis may be spontaneous (endogenous) or induced (exogenous). The spectrum of endogenous genetic disorders has been ascribed to two major spontaneous mechanisms of mutagenesis: slipped mispairing at the replication fork, and 5-methylcytosine deamination at CpG pairs.[35] Exogenous agents that induce DNA damage have been strongly linked to the development of a number of cancers in adults. These cancers are typically those that occur at rates in excess of those that would be expected in a population. For instance, G–T transversions have been demonstrated in the p53 gene in patients with hepatocellular carcinoma exposed to aflatoxin.[24,80] Other examples include single- or double-base C–T changes induced by exposure to ultraviolet light,[112] and G–T transversions caused by benzo(*a*)pyrene in lung carcinoma.[28] Recognition of an (induced) pattern of mutagenesis is particularly important because it can lead to the identification of an environmental mutagen.[158]

Murphree and Munier have reviewed the evidence that the majority of mutations found in retinoblastoma are consistent with endogenous rather than induced mutagenesis.[119] It is possible that the overwhelming preference for the paternal origin of new germline mutations in retinoblastoma[47,173] may be explained by the spontaneous mutagenic mechanism, deamination of methylated CpG pairs. The female germline is highly unmethylated when compared to the male.[46] A similar strong preference for the paternal origin of new germline mutations has been demonstrated in hemophilia B.[86]

Point Mutations

Systematic screening has revealed that besides exon mutations, noncoding regions of RB1, such as the promoter or introns at splice junctions, are also commonly mutated. Most frequent are single base substitutions (>50%), followed, in descending order of frequency, by transitions, small deletions or duplications (<103 bp), and transversions. This spectrum applies to both germinal and somatic mutations. The vast majority are functionally null mutations. The fact that LOF alleles in RB1 are frequently functional nulls likely reflects the frequency of new nonsense mutations (new stop codon or frameshift), or ones that affect a splice junction. (Missense mutations and base substitutions in the promoter region rarely occur.)

Recent data imply that CpG dinucleotides are mutation "hot spots" within the RB1 locus. Of all known human germline disease-related point mutations, 30%–40% are spontaneous deamination of methylated CpG sites,[35] despite the underrepresentation of this dinucleotide in human DNA, the strong CpG suppression in coding sequences, the inherent resistance to methylation of mammalian promoter CpG islands, and the existence of efficient repair mechanisms. Interestingly, spontaneous deamination occurs at a higher rate in single-stranded DNA, especially during transcription in the nontranscribed strand (which is repaired less efficiently than the transcribed strand). Similar findings have been reported in other tumor suppressor genes, including p53.[28] Additionally, hypermethylation of the RB1–CpG island appears to be a significant mutational event in nonhereditary unilateral retinoblastoma.[67,78,139] It has been observed in 9 of 69 (13%) unilateral tumors and in none of 57 bilateral tumors.[78]

DIAGNOSIS AND STAGING

In the absence of a known family history of retinoblastoma, the early months of retinoblastoma growth in a child's eye usually go undetected by both family and primary care physician. Even if the pediatrician or family practitioner performs a red reflex test or examines the optic nerve with a direct ophthalmoscope in the first year of life, he or she may well miss seeing the tumor because of a small pupil and not suspect its presence, unless a member of the family has observed leukocoria, (a white reflection in the pupil; Fig. 40.5) or strabismus (misaligned eyes) and alerted the pediatrician. The earliest sign of retinoblastoma is almost always noted first by the family.

Intraocular retinoblastoma does not cause pain or discomfort as it enlarges, and virtually never causes a red or inflamed eye until late in the course of the disease. If central vision is interfered with by the tumor in one eye, strabismus (misalignment of the eyes) may occur, but the unilateral visual loss caused by the tumor will not be apparent clinically to the child or the parents because of the normal vision in the other eye. Early detection does not always equate with good treatment outcome. Advanced intraocular retinoblastoma has been diagnosed by prenatal ultrasound at 21 weeks gestation.[104] When all patients who were diagnosed by 3 months of age were evaluated for extent of disease, the percentage with advanced disease was similar to that for patients who were diagnosed at 1 year of age.[4]

The presence of intraocular calcium demonstrated on CT scan (Fig. 40.6*A*) or ultrasound (Fig. 40.6*B*) is a classic feature of retinoblastoma but is not required for the diagnosis. There is no predisposition for either sex. The tumor occurs with equal incidence in right and left eyes.

A

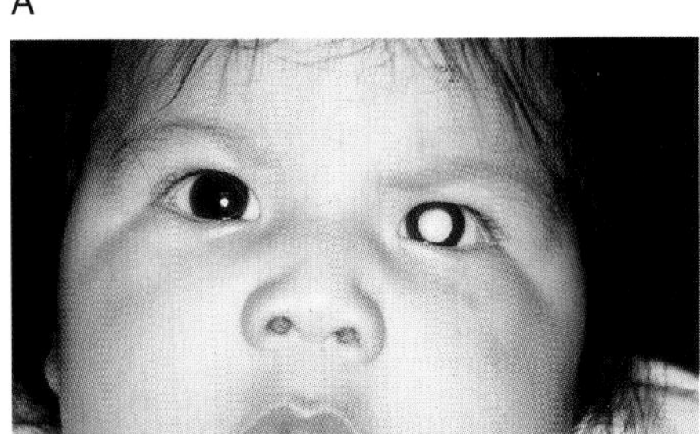

B

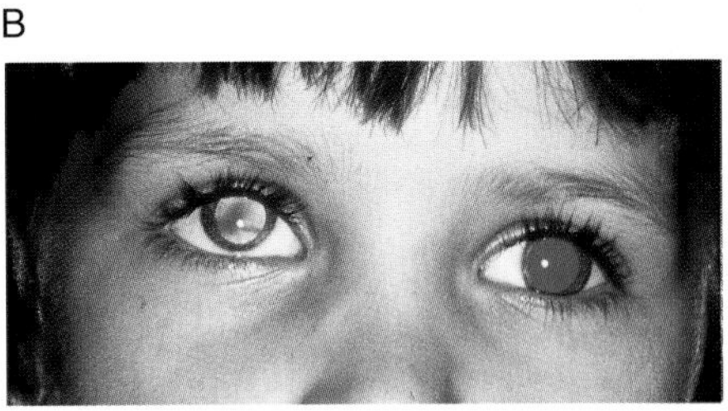

Figure 40.5. (**A**) Leucocoria or white pupil on the left is easily seen because of wide pupil dilation and flash photography. Parents or family members would see this white "glow" at dusk or in dim illumination when the pupil naturally dilates. (**B**) The leucocoria in the right is more subtle than that in Figure 5*A*. It is only seen when this child's intermittent DVD (vertical strabismus) is obvious as it is in this photograph. As the right eye drifts upward, the tumor which in superior retina moves down into position to reflect light coming in through the pupil. When the eye is straight or the pupil not dilated the leucocoria is not seen.

Once the signs of retinoblastoma have been detected, its presence must be confirmed or ruled out without delay. Retinoblastoma is best managed by an ocular oncology center team with considerable experience in the diagnosis and treatment of this rare tumor. Unless referral is logistically impossible, no general ophthalmologist, pediatric ophthalmologist, or retinal specialist who lacks training and experience in managing patients with intraocular tumors should undertake a course of treatment. Numerous studies indicate that in addition to being more cost efficient, treatment in an ocular oncology center results in an improved outcome and survival. In a study from Great Britain of factors associated with salvage of the eye with retinoblastoma, the choice of the treating center was second only to stage of the tumor at diagnosis in significance.[101]

A diagnostic evaluation of the child with sus-

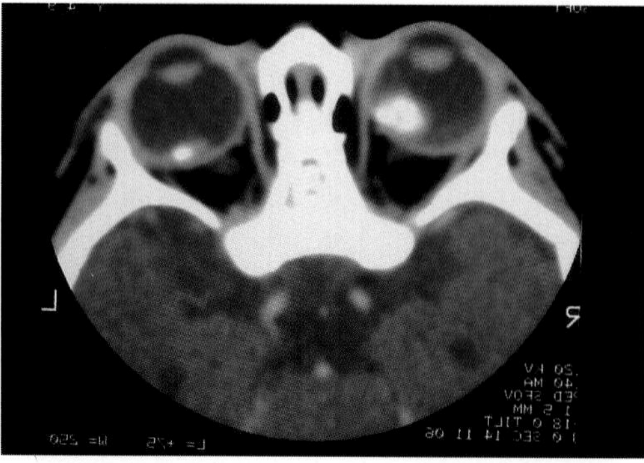

A

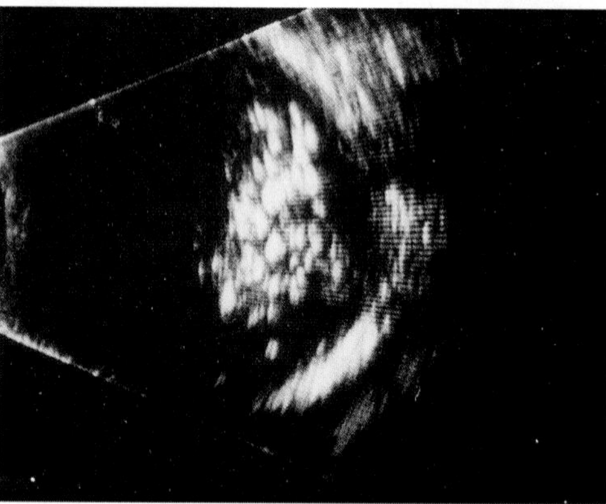

B

Figure 40.6. (**A**) Intraocular calcium demonstrated in both eyes of a child with bilateral retinoblastoma on CT scan. (**B**) Intraocular calcium in an eye with suspected retinoblastoma. The signal has been attenuated to demonstrate persistence of the echoes from intraocular calcium. Note the shadowing (absence of echoes from the posterior globe because of blockage by the intraocular calcium).

pected retinoblastoma has two purposes: first, to confirm the diagnosis, and second, to ensure that the tumor is confined to the eye. At the Clayton Ocular Oncology Center at Childrens Hospital Los Angeles, the child referred with a diagnosis of possible retinoblastoma is always seen initially in the office with his or her family for a complete history, including detailed pedigree and examination of family photographs. Assessment of vision and optic nerve function and a dilated retinal examination, with as much a look at the intraocular mass(es) as an awake child will allow, is essential to confirm the referring diagnosis. Infants under 3–4 months of age can be examined in a papoose with depression of peripheral retina using only topical anesthesia. Older children will often allow a surprisingly good examination of the more involved eye because of relatively poor vision, especially if the intensity of the light is lowered and the examiner does not touch the child. Occasionally at this stage, retinoblastoma can be ruled out with such certainty that an unnecessary exam under anesthesia (EUA) can be avoided.

AGE AT DIAGNOSIS

Bilateral retinoblastoma is most often asymmetric and is usually diagnosed at an earlier age than unilateral disease. The average age at diagnosis in unilateral cases is 24 months; in bilateral disease, it is 12 months. The tumor can be present at birth as noted above but may appear initially after birth as well. In the United States, nearly 90% of cases are diagnosed before 5 years of age.[139] In 400 consecutive cases, 34 (8.5%) were 5 years of age or older at the time of diagnosis.[144] Twenty-six of the 34 had active tumor; the remaining 8 had retinomas or retinocytomas. All 26 had sporadic, unilateral disease; their average age was 6 years. A small number of cases have been reported in older children and adolescents and in two adults.[12,15,23,97,123,143,160,172] The persistence of a rare embryonal retinal cell has been offered as one explanation for the occurrence of the tumor at an advanced age.[160]

PRESENTING SIGNS

Leukocoria

Over half of all cases are discovered following the observation of a white pupillary reflex (leukocoria; Figs. 40.1 and 40.5), usually by a parent or family member. Examples of descriptive terms used by parents to describe the observation of leukocoria include "cat's eye," "animal eye," "gleam," "glint," "glow," "eye looks strange," "something is wrong with my child's eye," "film over the eye."

Parents frequently take flash photographs of young children. If a flash is used and the tumor is either large or located in the posterior pole, leukocoria may be documented in a family photograph. In our experience, however, there is often a delay of several months after such photos are taken before the parents examine the photograph, note the white pupillary reflex, and alert the pediatrician. Parents should bring the photograph with them to see the pediatrician.

Extremely well-lit examination rooms in most medical offices and clinics can delay the detection of retinoblastoma by primary care physicians by inducing pupillary constriction and limiting light entry for the red reflex test. Parents or other family members who observe the child in low lighting, when the pupil is relatively more dilated (e.g., a dimly lit room, outside at dusk), are far more likely to observe asymmetry in the normally red pupillary light reflex (Fig. 40.5*B*). It is not uncommon for leukocoria to be recorded in a family snapshot, often at holidays or birthdays. The flash of a camera floods the face with a great amount of illumination quickly before the child's pupils have a chance to constrict. Asymmetry of the red reflex (i.e., one eye red, the other white) is, by definition, a positive red reflex test (Fig. 40.5*B*). It is not uncommon for the pediatrician's red reflex exam to be interpreted as normal even after such family photos have been taken. This discrepancy is due to the fact that the direct ophthalmoscope used for the red reflex test allows light into the eye, and the pupil constricts before the observer can make a diagnosis. In a review of 254 cases with documented delayed diagnosis, delays could be assigned to one of three time periods: *(1)* from birth to first sign, *(2)* from first sign to examination by the primary care physician, and *(3)* from the examination by the primary physician to examination by the specialist.[69] Haik et al.[69] found that 50% of primary care physicians made a referral within one week in the absence of a family history of retinoblastoma, and 75% within a week in the presence of a family history. However, 47% of patients without a family history, and 25% of those with a family history experienced a delay in referral to a specialist averaging 4 to 5 months.

For reasons cited earlier, we recommend that pediatricians either use routine dilation with 0.5% tropicamide at the 6 week well baby exam for all infants 15–20 minutes prior to the red reflex test. An alternative is an instant flash photograph, after the baby has been in a darkened room for 2–5 minutes, that may document leukocoria if it exists. We advise full retinal examination in the first 1–2 weeks after birth and then every 2 months thereafter for all babies in families with a history of retinoblastoma.

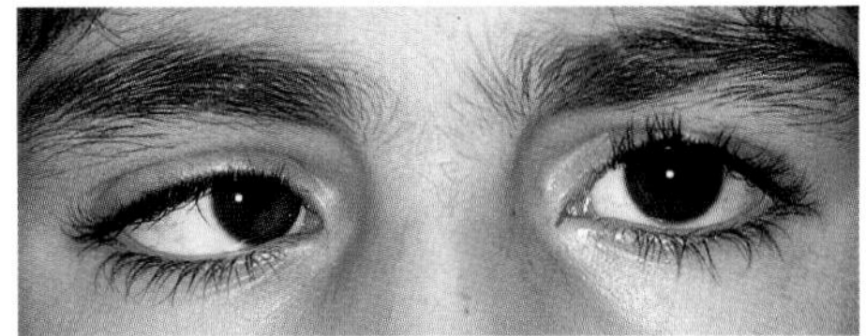

Figure 40.7. Strabismus in a child with bilateral retinoblastoma. The lesion on the right arises in the macula and has destroyed central vision. The tumors in the left do not affect the macula. This child's right eye turns in (esotropia). Turning out (exotropia) can also be seen but is less common in a young child with a sensory strabismus secondary to a macular tumor.

Strabismus

Strabismus is the second most common presenting sign of retinoblastoma (Fig. 40.7). Parents will report variable amounts and frequency of turning in (esotropia) or turning out (exotropia) of one or both eyes. Almost without exception in the patient with retinoblastoma, the eye that turns in or out will have a tumor in the posterior pole, causing decreased vision. The poor vision is the direct cause of the strabismus. The gradual loss of the ability to locate or identify familiar objects or faces or, in the case of toddlers, to negotiate familiar surroundings, may result from tumors obstructing vision in both eyes. Unilateral or asymmetrical Rb is rarely detected as a result of vision loss, because one eye always retains good vision.

ATYPICAL PRESENTATION

Although most patients with retinoblastoma present with leukocoria or strabismus, unusual presenting signs can occur. Often these signs confuse or delay the diagnosis. Intraocular Rb may present as glaucoma, orbital cellulitis, uveitis, hyphema, or vitreous hemorrhage.[11]

WORK-UP

CT and MRI Scanning

If the office exam is compatible with retinoblastoma, or if it is inconclusive, the one indispensable imaging study is computerized tomography (CT).[68,166,175] The presence of intraocular calcium in a mass lesion with the clinical appearance of retinoblastoma can help confirm the diagnosis (Fig. 40.6*A*).[26] Although useful in detecting extraocular tumor spread, the CT is not sensitive enough to detect microscopic nerve involvement. Although magnetic resonance imaging (MRI) is not as specific as CT because it lacks sensitivity in detecting calcification, MRI done with a surface coil and using both gadolinium enhancement and fat suppression may demonstrate tumor invasion of the optic nerve before the nerve is grossly enlarged by central enhancement. In our center both CT scan and MRI studies are usually obtained if there is a significant amount of tumor in the eye and the optic nerve head is obscured.

When extraocular extension into the brain is present, MRI can demonstrate infiltrative spread along the intracanalicular and cisternal portions of the optic nerve, subarachnoid seeding, and involvement of the brain.[140] Also it is especially useful if there is central invasion of the proximal optic nerve.

The value of CT scanning was convincingly reported in a review of 80 cases of retinoblastoma with retinal detachment.[68] In exophytic tumors, all cases demonstrated calcification in either solitary or multifocal location(s). In addition, soft tissue components of retinoblastoma were demonstrated with contrast. In cases where retinoblastoma-stimulating lesions produced calcium (i.e., severe ocular disruption, or phthisis, and rarely in other disorders such as Coats disease), secondary calcification was usually deposited along the planes of normal structures rather than grouped inside a mass lesion.

In cases where retinoblastoma presents as orbital cellulitis, perineural edema may lead to a misdiagnosis of optic nerve invasion on CT scan because of an apparently enlarged optic nerve (personal observation). In such cases, further workup should be delayed a few days while the child is treated with systemic steroids. Repeating the CT scan after this treatment will provide a more accurate assessment of optic nerve size. In addition to their diagnostic value, neuroimaging studies can detect several important features which will alter the treatment approach: (*1*) trilateral retinoblastoma, (*2*) extraocular orbital disease, and (*3*) gross invasion of the optic nerve.

Ultrasonography

After neuroimaging ultrasonography is the next most useful test to confirm the diagnosis of retinoblastoma (Fig. 40.6*B*).[33] It can be used to detect tumors as small as 2 mm in diameter. It is particularly useful in cases of opaque ocular media (e.g., vitreous hemorrhage or dense vitreous seeding). In experienced hands ultrasonography may be useful in differentiating and defining the extent of tumors and contiguous retinal detachments. In this latter instance, it is usually superior to CT. Ultrasonography has its limitations in retinoblastoma, however, and, when it is used in the absence of CT, may lead to misdiagnosis. Murphree et al. use ultrasonography to confirm the presence of intraocular calcium and to record the height and basal diameter of each tumor at the staging exam under anesthesia.[121]

LEGAL CONSIDERATIONS

Failure to Diagnose for Primary Care Physicians

Retinoblastoma is a rare disease. Most pediatricians will have only one patient with a new primary retinoblastoma in a typical practice stretching over a 30-year period. It is not necessarily malpractice for pediatricians or other primary care physician to fail to suspect or make the diagnosis of retinoblastoma in a child in the absence of signs or symptoms of the disease and when the family has not reported anything unusual about the eyes. The red reflex test used by most pediatricians to screen for serious pathology in the eye is useful and reliable in direct proportion to the diameter of the pupil. It is not currently the standard of care for pediatricians to dilate a child's pupils in the office. Both the overhead lights and the light from the direct ophthalmoscope used in the red reflex test ensure that the pupils are small and the likelihood of detecting an unequivocally abnormal red reflex test is small. Primary care providers are at legal risk, if they fail to refer a child to an ophthalmologist when the parents report the presence of leucocoria or abnormal flash photograph, even when there are no evident abnormal ocular signs or symptoms on the physician's exam.

An abnormal red reflex is the result of light that enters the eye being reflected back out of the eye by the white tumor to be seen by an observer as a white pupil or leucocoria. Unfortunately daylight, overhead room light, and light from a direct ophthalmoscope all cause the pupil to constrict, severely limiting the opening for light to exit the eye for observation. As a result in a child with retinoblastoma, leucocoria is most commonly seen first by a family member at dusk or in a slightly darkened room with a dim illuminating source when the pupil dilates normally to allow sufficient exiting light to be seen. It is for this reason that the pediatrician or primary care physician may not observe an abnormal red reflex in a brightly lit office or even in a dimly lit office using the light from the ophthalmoscope.

Just as a pet's eyes are observed to glow only at night when the pupil is naturally large and never in the daytime when it is constricted, the observation of a abnormal red reflex in the pupil of an eye with retinoblastoma varies with the level of ambient light and pupillary size.

The appearance of a white pupil in a flash photograph is a special case. A flash is necessary for a photograph taken indoors and when ambient light is relatively low. Under those circumstances the child's pupils would be expected to be moderately dilated. The flash puts a tremendous amount of light through the pupil quickly, and the film instantly records the reflected exiting light before reflex pupillary constriction has a chance to occur. Normally "red eye" results from the light being reflected from the blood in choroid. Expensive cameras avoid "red eye" by the use of a preflash, which causes the pupils to constrict and eliminate the exiting reflex.

Parents should take flash photographs of their new infants frequently and look for the "red eye." Any asymmetry in the pupillary reflex or white reflex should be called to the attention of the pediatrician. It should be borne in mind that the degree of redness in the normal red pupillary reflex reflects the degree of background pigmentation of the individual tested. In darkly pigmented individuals the reflex may appear gray.

Failure to Diagnose by Pediatric Ophthalmologists

For ophthalmologists, it is the atypical presentation of retinoblastoma (e.g., tumors presenting in older children), those growing along the surface of the retina, and those associated with pseudohypopyon, hyphema, or vitreous hemorrhage that are the most common cause of delayed diagnosis or misdiagnosis. Unfortunately, the risk of death is higher with atypical presentations.[141,157] Perhaps the most misleading presentation is orbital cellulitis.[122] Ophthalmologists who see this tumor only rarely may misdiagnose the orbital swelling and treat it as an inflammatory process.[157] Diffuse infiltrating retinoblastoma may be initially indistinguishable from uveitis.[52,107] The disorders most commonly confused with retinoblastoma are persistent hyperplastic primary vitreous (PHPV; Fig. 40.8) and Coats disease.

Staging Exam under Anesthesia

A staging examination under anesthesia (EUA) is essential in virtually all patients for a detailed retinal examination, retinal drawings, ultrasound examination, and retinal imaging. A recently introduced digital, handheld, wide-angle retinal camera, the RetCam® marketed by Massie Research Laboratories (Pleasanton, CA), holds promise for much improved retinal imaging in the management of these patients. It is helpful for an ocular oncology team member from Heme/onc and/or radiotherapy to be present for the EUA or for an emergency meeting to customize the treatment approach for the individual patient. An E-mail message to team members with details of the EUA findings is an effective way of communicating the result. Accurate measurement and localization of each

A

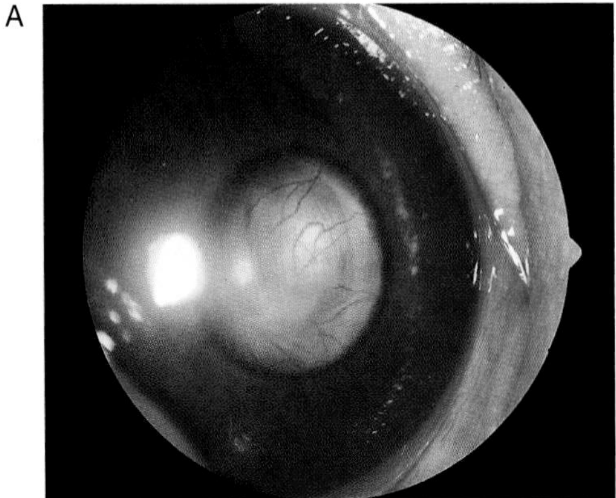

B

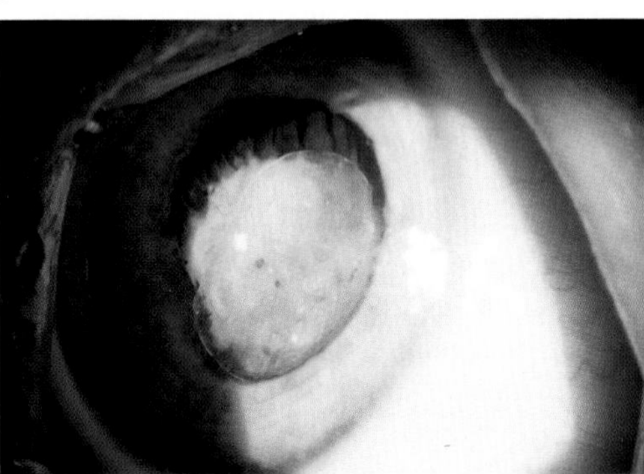

Figure 40.8. (**A**) Persistent Hyperplastic Primary Vitreous (PHPV) in a two-week-old baby. The retrolenticular membrane is vascularized and in this case fairly smooth. Ultrasound will demonstrate a transvitreal stalk connecting the center of this membrane to the optic nerve head. (**B**) A different appearance to the PHPV membrane than seen in Figure 8*A*. Ciliary processes are dragged centrally in both cases. The leucocoria in both 8*A* and 8*B* could be misinterpreted as representing retinoblastoma.

focus of tumor will be important if brachytherapy is contemplated. We have found that RetCam images presented to the parents at the postexamination discussion are a powerful tool for conveying the nature and extent of the disease and for obtaining understanding and consent for treatment.

Discussion of treatment options begun with the family at the functional office exam can be expanded after the staging EUA. As soon as removal of one or both eyes is a viable treatment option, a thorough discussion with the family is necessary. A social worker or other person with experience in working with the families of visually impaired childen is invaluable, especially if enucleation is imminent.[106]

The number of tumors may vary from none to more than 10 in each of the eyes of a genetically predisposed child. Only a single tumor in one eye will be present in the somatic nongenetic form of the disease (Fig. 40.9*A*). In the patient with multifocal disease, in the early stage, each of the separate round lesions has

A

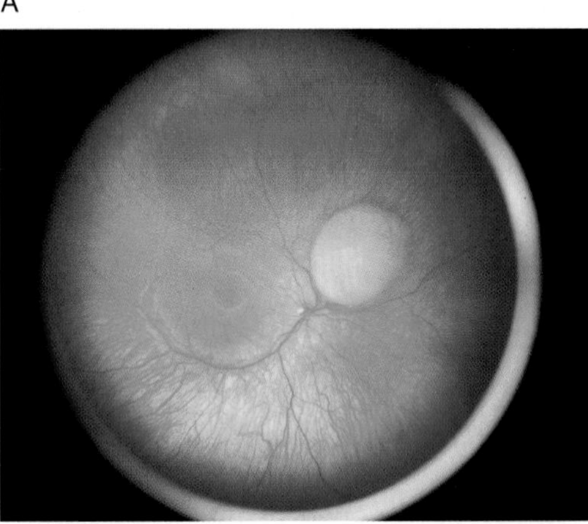

B

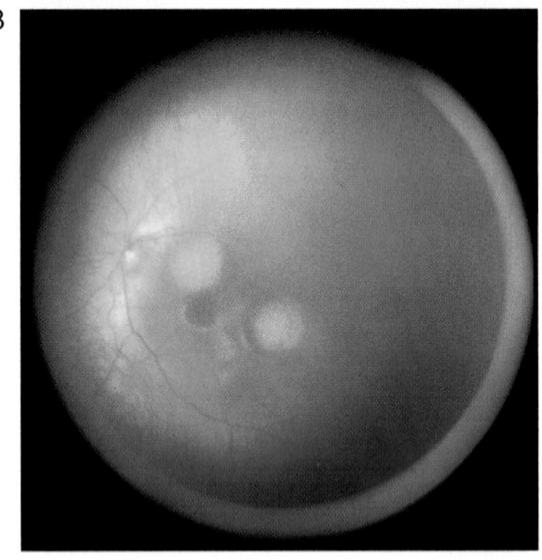

Figure 40.9. (**A**) Small, unilateral, unifocal retinoblastoma. Small lesions are always round. As they grow one cell in the mass will, likely through an error at mitosis, lose all or part of a chromosome containing a growth suppresser gene. The absence of that growth restraint defines a new clone of daughter cells which have a growth advantage. The clinical result is a part of the mass which grows faster changing the round appearance of the mass. (**B**) Multifocal retinoblastoma in the second eye of a child with the germline mutation in the RB1 gene. Retinoblastoma is most commonly asymmetrical as in this case where the other eye was almost half full of tumor. These two tumors are clearly independently arising since both are round and of similar size.

arisen independently of the others (Fig. 40.9*B*), a result of the spontaneous occurrence of the second genetic event, usually an error at mitosis leading to loss of all or part of the 13 chromosome carrying the wild-type RB1 allele. Incontrovertible proof that each arose independently would require tumor karyotyping from each tumor to demonstrate the lack of a shared marker chromosome (Fig. 40.9*B*).

Most retinoblastomas have a consistency similar to toothpaste. Fresh tumors containing considerable necrosis can be so liquid as to make their being lifted by forceps from an opened globe virtually impossible (Fig. 40.10*A*). Because of the lack of cellular adherence, there is a tendency of retinoblastoma to shed small clumps of tumor cells into the vitreous from endophytic tumors (Fig. 40.10*B*) and into the subretinal space from exophytic ones. This "seeding" of the vitreous or subretinal space may eventually lead to tumor implants that are clones of previously existing lesions. Implanted subretinal tumors can generally be distinguished from new tumors by their location and pattern of distribution.

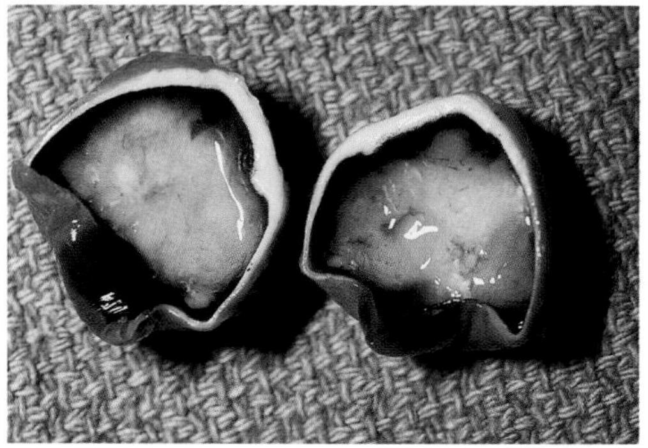

A

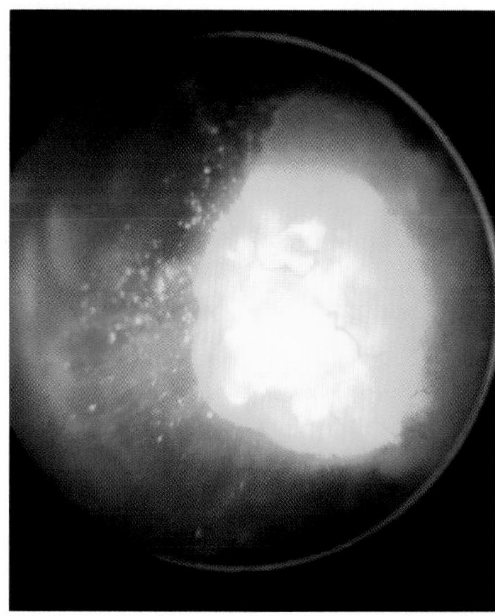

B

Figure 40.10. (**A**) An enucleated opened globe. The consistency of large partially necrotic retinoblastoma can vary from firm to soupy. (**B**) Dispersion of retinoblastoma cells from this large tumor into the vitreous is occurring from virtually all surfaces of the tumor. Vitreous seeding occurs in endophytic tumors and causes this eye to be classified as Intraocular Group D disease. Group D is easy to remember in the newly proposed classification since it represents diffuse or disseminated intraocular tumor.

CLINICAL FEATURES

Tumor-Associated Retinal Detachment

Massive retinal detachment, frequently found in eyes with large tumors, is more common with exophytic than endophytic trumor growth patterns (Fig. 40.11). Yellow-white infiltrates, often present beneath the detached portion of the retina, consist of foamy-appearing macrophages. These "foam cells" contain abundant lipid droplets, lysosomes, and glycogen particles. The presence of retinal detachment in an eye with retinoblastoma was formerly considered an absolute indication for enucleation; however, Murphree et al. have treated a number of these eyes with systemic carboplatin, etoposide, and vincristine, and have achieved remarkable involution of the tumor and resolution of the detachment.[121] In some eyes, retinal reattachment has been accompanied by the return of useful vision. Retinal detachment may be local and insignificant. The extent of the detachment may be marked by subretinal spread of tumor debris and calcium (Fig. 40.12).

A long-standing retinal detachment secondary to a large retinoblastoma can lead to retinal ischemia and secondary neovascularization of the iris (rubeosis). Initially, this may lead to darkening of the iris and asymmetric iris color (heterochromia). Over time, these vessels can bleed spontaneously into the anterior chamber (hyphema) or block the outflow of aqueous from the anterior chamber (neovascular glau-

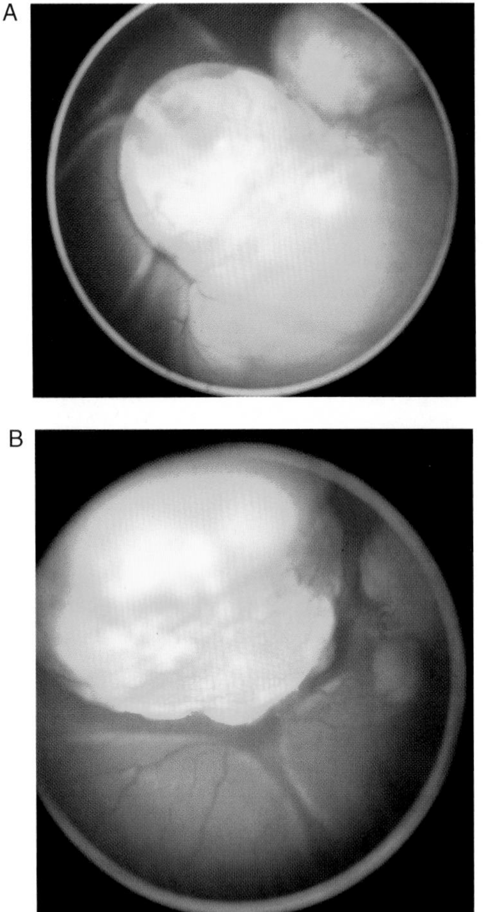

Figure 40.11. (**A**) Endophytic retinoblastoma with a tumor associated total retinal detachment. Subretinal fluid in these eyes nearly always contains a suspension of retinoblastoma cells, which, when the retinal detachment resolves with treatment, have the potential to develop into new foci of implanted tumor. In some eye tens to hundreds of new tumor colonies can be generated once systemic chemotherapy is discontinued. Consolidation with whole eye external beam radiotherapy following the completion of chemotherapy may prevent or treat these recurrent tumors. (**B**) Two daughter subretinal implants are seen in this eye. Initially subretinal fluid is mostly dependent to the tumor.

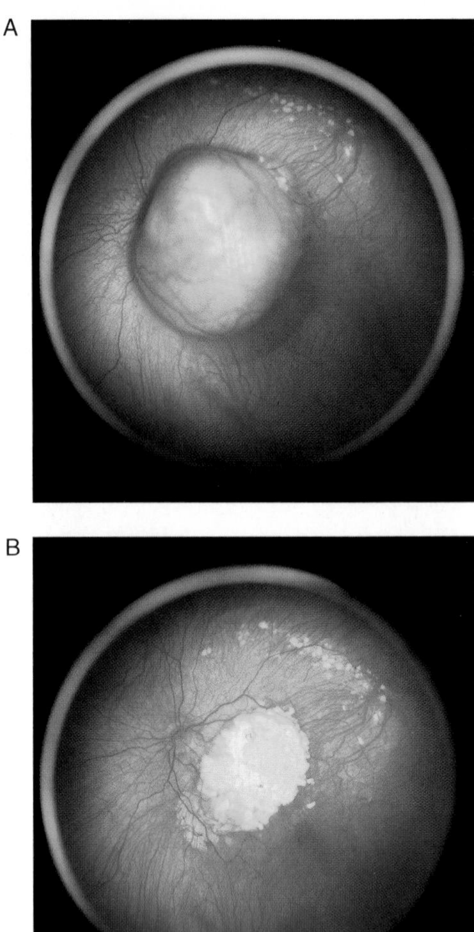

Figure 40.12. (**A**) Solitary sporadic unifocal, unilateral retinoblastoma arising in the macula and overhanging the optic disc. Note the dependent tumor debris and calcium defining the extent of local tumor associated subretinal fluid. If the area of subretinal fluid is less than the retinal area occupied by the tumor the detachment is considered insignificant. This tumor was treated with chemoreduction (3 cycles of 3 drug chemotherapy). (**B**) The tumor in Figure 12A following chemoreduction therapy and laser SALT consolidation. It now displays a stable type 1 regression pattern. The extent of the local retinal detachment accompanying the untreated tumor can easily be appreciated in this photograph.

coma). The resulting high intraocular pressure will result in a cloudy cornea and a red, painful eye.

Tumor Extension into the Anterior Segment

Involvement of the anterior segment of the eye with tumor can lead to layering of white cells in the anterior chamber as one would see with endophthalmitis, or may result in a white, fluffy iris mass. Survival of the eye is unlikely once tumor has extended into the anterior chamber.[71] Murphree has recently had one patient whose anterior segment tumor extension regressed with systemic carboplatin, etoposide, and vincristine, but regrowth occurred.[121a] In contrast to infectious endophthalmitis, most commonly seen after intraocular surgery or penetrating trauma to the globe, these tumor pseudohypopyons generally are not associated with other signs of ocular inflammation but rather with massive intraocular tumors or tumor recurrences in the peripheral retina.

Large and small deposits of retinoblastoma cells may collect on the corneal endothelium in uninflamed eyes with tumor in the anterior segment (Fig. 40.13). Corneal edema and clouding can occur in the setting of neovascular or inflammatory glaucoma.

Pseudoorbital Cellulitis

The presentation of retinoblastoma as an "orbital cellulitislike" condition is well described.[150] Extraocular extension should be suspected in such cases, although signs mimicking extraocular extension can be the result of massive intraocular tumor necrosis alone. The periocular edema is presumably due to a diffusible molecule originating in the necrotic tumor.

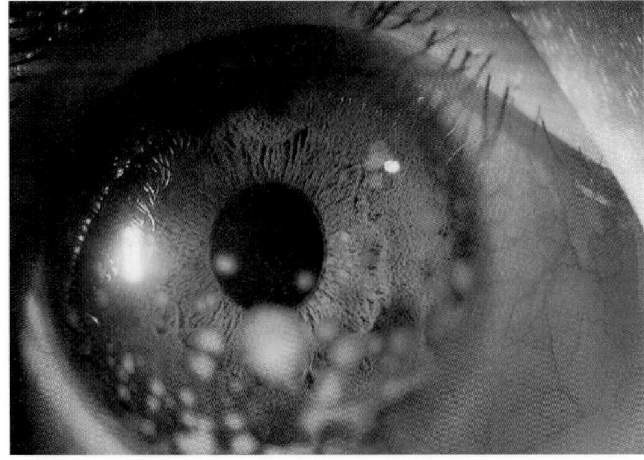

Figure 40.13. Extraretinal extension of intraocular retinoblastoma into the anterior chamber. In this eye colonies of implanted retinoblastoma are growing on the endothelial surface of the cornea, on the surface of the iris and in the anterior chamber angle. Other eyes may show tumor implants on the iris only. Extraretinal disease such as this causes this eye to be classified as Intraocular Group E disease in which enucleation is the treatment of choice.

Extraocular Retinoblastoma

Although rarely seen in Western countries, massive extraocular retinoblastoma is not an infrequent presentation in developing countries (Fig. 40.3). As the tumor mass in the orbit increases, the globe may be pushed forward (proptosis). If the mass ruptures the integrity of the globe anteriorly, the tumor may enlarge between the lids. We treated one 3-year-old boy from a developing country with a lemon-sized mass protruding between the lids of one eye (Fig. 40.3).[121a] In this case, chemotherapy was employed to shrink the tumor and facilitate enucleation. The child is alive 5 years later and is tumor free. His left arm was amputated for an osteosarcoma, an Rb-associated second malignant neoplasm.

Trilateral Retinoblastoma

This term refers to the rare finding of a midline intracranial neoplasm in individuals carrying the predisposing mutation in RB1 (Fig. 40.14). Such a third focus of malignant disease occurs in approximately 1%–3% of all retinoblastoma patients[38] but in as many as 6% of bilateral Rb patients and 10% of those with a family history.[17] Because of tissue similarity between the pineal gland and the retina, pineal neoplasms are not categorized as second malignant neoplasms. Pinealoblastomas are usually diagnosed in patients found to have retinoblastoma at an early age (average 3 months) and have been almost uniformly fatal.[17] In the series of Blach et al.,[17] 12 trilateral Rb patients died after a mean period of 11 months from diagnosis. The midline tumor may be diagnosed before or after the retinoblastoma. All newly diagnosed Rb patients should have CT scans that image the region of the pineal. CT scans every 3 to 4 months after diagnosis of the genetic form of Rb have been proposed to screen for trilateral disease. Such frequent scanning is difficult to support until the treatment of these midline lesions improves.

Directions or Patterns of Tumor Growth

From its origins in the neural retina, retinoblastoma may grow primarily (*1*) toward the center of the eye into the vitreous cavity (endophytic growth) (Figs. 40.9 and 40.12) (*2*) beneath the

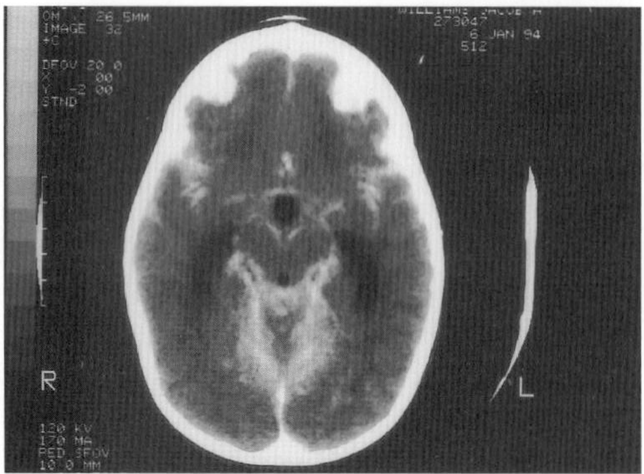
A

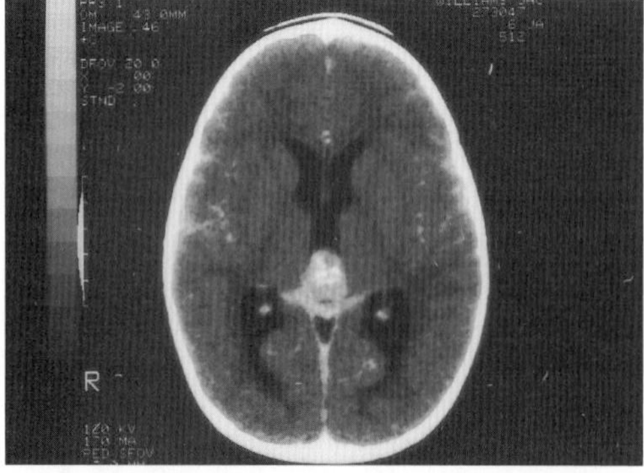
B

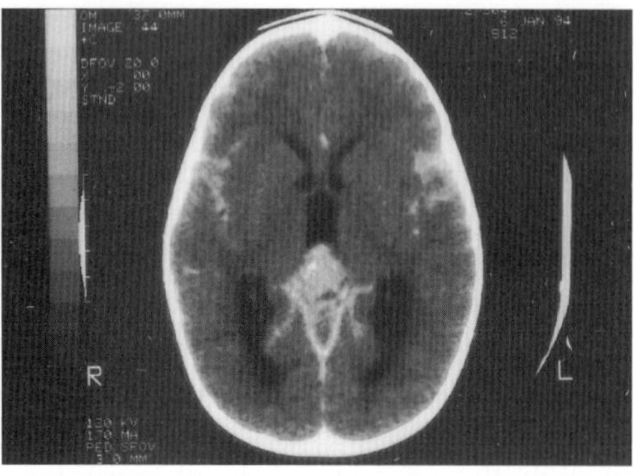
C

Figure 40.14. (**A**, **B**, **C**) Trilateral retinoblastoma. A pinealoblastoma shown here in three sections. These mid-line malignancies arise from the cells of the pineal gland which share a common ancestor with retinal precursors. Pinealoblastomas can be diagnosed both before and after bilateral retinoblastoma. They are almost invariably fatal.

retina away from the center of the eye and toward the choroid (exophytic growth) (Fig. 40.11A). Endophytic growth is more common. Retinal detachment and choroidal and optic nerve invasion are more likely in exophytic tumors (Fig. 40.11). In one study of 297 unilateral cases, the two growth patterns were analyzed for prognostic significance.[126] The endophytic tumors were more frequently associated with positive family histories; the exophytic tumors were more commonly associated with glaucoma and had a greater tendency to invade the choroid. In a recent study, large exophytic retinoblastoma was found to have the highest risk for invading the optic nerve, a feature that increases the chance of metastatic disease.[105] The same study confirmed previously published data that tumors must invade the optic nerve past the lamina cribrosa to confer an increased metastatic potential sufficient to require prophylactic treatment.[145]

A rare type of growth pattern is the diffuse infiltrating type, in which no mass forms but the tumor diffusely infiltrates the retina in a pagetoid fashion. Calcification is rare in this form. In a review of 28 published cases, histologic evidence of calcification was present in only 4.[13] Additionally, in some cases in that review, CT scanning and ultrasonography revealed only thickened retina and failed to demonstrate an intraocular mass.[13] Eyes with this type of retinoblastoma typically have symptoms of inflammation (redness, irritation), and signs of anterior segment involvement. The vitreous is often hazy and the retina may appear gray and thickened. The physical appearance and lack of calcification leads to frequent misdiagnosis. Fortunately, diffuse infiltrating retinoblastoma has only been seen in unilateral cases, and the prognosis after enucleation is usually good.[63] As tumors grow, retinal vessels are recruited to provide the necessary nourishment. These vessels, seen disappearing into the mass, provide diagnostic assistance.

Fine-Needle Biopsy

Fine-needle aspiration biopsy (FNAB) is not recommended in suspected retinoblastoma. In a report of FNAB in suspected choroidal melanomas and retinoblastomas, retinoblastoma cells were noted to be dragged across the vitreous during the procedure.[7] These authors consider their indication for FNAB in suspected retinoblastoma only in the rare situation where parents refuse treatment until pathologic verification is obtained. The eye in Figure 40.13

had a FNAB in Mexico. In an ocular oncology center, the clinical appearance would have been diagnostic.

Metastatic Work-up

Until the late 1980s it was general practice in ocular oncology centers to examine the bone marrow and spinal fluid on all new retinoblastoma patients for tumor cells. Pratt and colleagues[131] described bone marrow aspirations (115) and lumbar punctures (114) in 115 newly diagnosed retinoblastoma patients. Three marrows and three spinal fluids were positive for tumor cells. Five of the six positives were in patients with known extraocular disease. Although individual centers still perform these tests because of a concern about legal consequences, an international consensus has emerged among retinoblastoma specialists that routine bone marrow aspiration and lumbar puncture are not necessary at the time of initial diagnosis unless there is evidence of extraocular disease. These tests add considerably to the expense and discomfort of the patient. Routine clinical laboratory evaluation such as complete blood count and serum chemistries are also typically negative except in the rare case of advanced metastatic disease. Radiographic surveys of long bones and bone scans are not necessary in the vast majority of newly diagnosed cases.

The one exception to the above rule of withholding ancillary testing is when treatment with chemotherapy is considered; oncologists generally request bone marrow and cerebrospinal fluid evaluation prior to the administration of the first cycle of drugs. Following enucleation, histologic evidence of tumor past the lamina cribrosa is an indication to search for metastatic disease and begin prophylactic chemotherapy. Tumor at the cut end of the optic nerve requires the addition of radiation to the orbit.

MANAGEMENT OF RETINOBLASTOMA

Clinical Classification

At present, the most widely utilized staging of retinoblastoma remains the Reese-Ellsworth classification, which was initially devised in the 1950s to predict the survivability of the eye after external beam radiotherapy (EBR). Despite its widespread usage, Ellsworth himself believed that it should be revised (R. M. Ellsworth, personal communication, 1987). Any new classification should be (*1*) simple and easy to use, (*2*) reliable and reproducible, and (*3*) capable of predicting both the likelihood of successful treatment and relative morbidity of the treatment. Anterior lesions, now easily recognized and treated, assign the patient to a more advanced stage under the Reese-Ellsworth classification system. Second, most cases fall into groups 4 or 5, and there is very little discrimination between the two groups. Third, any amount of vitreous seeding places the eye in group 5b and suggests the worst possible prognosis. Today, local vitreous seeding may be treated successfully with brachytherapy. Many ocular oncology centers do not currently use the Reese-Ellsworth or any other standard classification system.

Planning is in its final stage following the National Cancer Center's approval for a multicenter clinical trial evaluating the recently published chemoreduction approaches to the management of intraocular retinoblastoma.[62,121] For the planned Retinoblastoma Study (RBS), a simplified classification of intraocular retinoblastoma has been proposed.[121b] It consists of five groups that are designated with the letters A through E (Table 40.1).

Both Group A and B retinoblastoma eyes can be managed primarily with local treatment modalities. Group A is the classification of an eye containing single or multiple tumors none of which are closer than 1DD to either the disc or the fovea and none is larger than 3 mm. Such tumors can easily be treated with local modalities alone without need to resort to chemotherapy or radiotherapy. Group B disease is the rare special case in which the tumors in an eye can be treated with primary *brachytherapy* alone. Visual outcome in Group A and B eyes should be excellent.

Both Group C and D eyes require systemic chemotherapy. Group C eyes have *confined* tumors which have not yet become dispersed within the eye and require a relatively shorter course of chemotherapy followed by local consolidation. Group D eyes contain *dispersed* dis-

Table 40.1. Classification of Intraocular Retinoblastoma[121b]

Group A	One or more intraretinal tumors 3 mm in size or less; all 1DD or more from the optic nerve or fovea. **No** vitreous seeding or subretinal fluid.
Group B	*Brachytherapy* eligible disease. Solitary retinoblastoma outside the posterior pole no larger than 10 mm or multiple closely spaced smaller tumors confined to a retinal area no greater than 10 mm in diameter. **No** diffuse vitreous seeding or significant retinal detachment.[1]
Group C	*Confined* disease. One or more intraretinal or endophytic tumors none exceeding 15 mm in size. **No** vitreous seeding or significant retinal detachment.[1]
Group D	*Dispersed* disease. Vitreous seeding and/or significant retinal detachment[1] is present. The total volume of the tumor does not exceed half the volume of the eye. **No** detectable extraretinal disease except for vitreous involvement.
Group E	*Extraretinal*[2] retinoblastoma or the presence of intraocular tumor volume > half the volume of the eye. Anterior segment disease; glaucoma; hyphema; extraocular extension

[1] Significant retinal detachment (SRD) is defined as an area of detachment equal to or greater than the retinal area occupied by the tumor.
[2] Extraretinal defines disease extending beyond the retina and vitreous.

ease, require longer more intensive chemotherapy and consolidation of the vitreous and/or potential subretinal space in order to salvage the eye. Visual outcome is guarded in both Groups. Morbidity of treatment is increased and the likelihood of salvaging Group D eyes in decreased significantly. For these reasons unilateral Group D disease is usually managed like Group E eyes.

Group E is used to describe those eyes for which enucleation is the only viable primary treatment. These eyes have either extraretinal or extraocular disease. In the presence of extraocular disease, treatment with chemotherapy may precede enucleation.

Since each patient has two eyes, treatment for each child is driven by the more advanced eye. When one eye is either group C or D and the other is either A or B, then systemic chemotherapy given to the child would also shrink the tumors in the Group A or B eye. Often tumors in Group A eyes have minimal response to systemic chemoreduction primarily because tumors less than 3 mm in size have little blood supply. Local treatment in Group A eyes can begin concurrently with systemic chemotherapy. Brachytherapy in Group B eyes should precede systemic chemotherapy. When brachytherapy in the usual dose (40 Gy) follows carboplatin containing chemotherapy, radiation retinopathy is virtually certain to follow. If it must follow the chemotherapy the total dose of brachytherapy should be reduced by $\frac{1}{3}$ to $\frac{1}{2}$.

Treatments Available

Enucleation of the eye containing the tumor is the treatment of choice for Group E disease and perhaps the most definitive treatment option. It is indicated when there is little or no possibility of salvage of usable vision. It should be performed only by surgeons who have extensive experience in treating retinoblastoma. Some ophthalmologists may be tempted to enucleate an involved eye before referring the patient to an oncology center. This should be discouraged. Fresh tumor harvested at the time of enucleation may be key for accurate DNA diagnosis (Fig. 40.15*A*). An inadequate amount of optic nerve obtained at enucleation can significantly increase the risk for metastatic disease. Tumor in the optic nerve requires pre-enucleation chemotherapy.

The most important goals in enucleation are obtaining a long section of optic nerve and delivering the globe intact (Fig. 40.15*B*). In a report of 40 enucleated eyes, obtaining less than 5 mm of optic nerve at the time of enucleation was an independent risk for extraocular spread of disease.[137] At least 10 mm of optic nerve should be obtained.[49] There is a high risk of orbital recurrence of retinoblastoma if the globe is perforated during the course of the

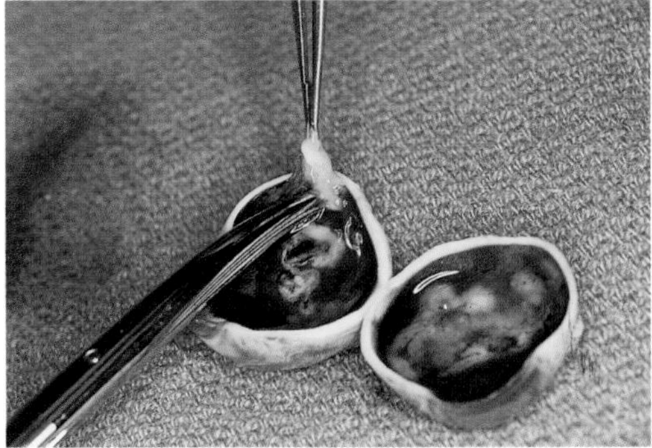

A

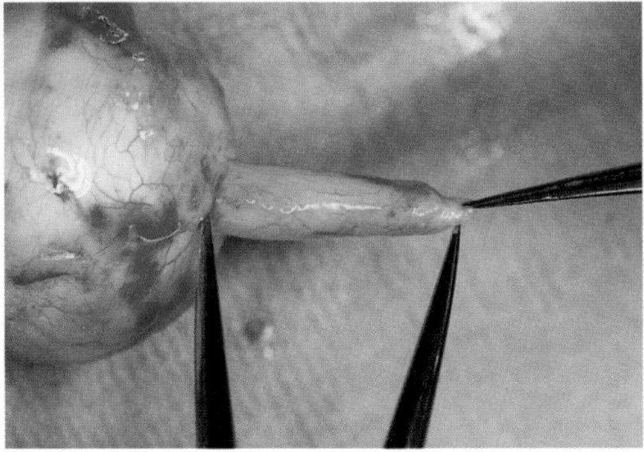

B

Figure 40.15. (**A**) After the optic nerve has been removed flush with the globe in the enucleated eye, with the consent of the pathologist, the globe can be safely bisected with a sterile, hand-held 2″ single edge razor blade and as much tumor as necessary removed from the calotte not containing the optic nerve. (**B**) At least 10 mm of optic nerve can be assured by using straight scissors passed along the nasal wall of the orbit. Note on Figure 6*A* how nasal the optic nerve travels after it leaves the back of the globe. Curved enucleation scissors only assure one of transecting the nerve near its exit from the eye.

procedure. In an effort to eliminate any possibility of perforation, the use of retrobulbar injections and intra scleral sutures for traction during the enucleation procedure should be avoided.

Enucleation Technique

Attention to other details of enucleation is extremely important. Dilated ophthalmoscopic examination as a first step of the procedure is mandatory as a final check of eye to be enucleated. The nerve should not be clamped prior to enucleation, and sectioning should be performed with long, *straight* scissors passed posteriorly along the medial orbital wall. The straight scissors maximize the possibility that a long section of nerve will be obtained (Fig. 40.15*B*).

We have employed several modifications of the basic procedure that we find particularly useful.[119] As mentioned above, to avoid any possibility of eye perforation, we never use retrobulbar injection. Instead, after the peritomy is made, the Tenon's capsule is opened and the muscles are removed, we irrigate with 10 cc of an anesthetic solution containing epinephrine (1 : 1 mixture of 2% Lidocaine with 1 : 100,000 epinephrine and 0.5% bipuvicaine, to which a vial of Wydase is added) into the retrobulbar space via a blunt irrigating cannula passed around the globe. We leave the solution in place for 10 min. We have found that this maneuver has three beneficial effects: (*1*) effective control of bleeding once the optic nerve is cut, (*2*) slight prolapse of the globe and straightening of the optic nerve, and (*3*) postoperative pain control. In many instances, we have seen virtually no bleeding following sectioning of the nerve using this technique.

Whether a silicone ball or integrated implant is used, a meticulous and complete closure is essential to prevent implant extrusion.[119] A careful search for defects in the tissue layers should follow the closure of each layer. At the end of the procedure, a plastic conformer is fit into the fornices. Ideally, the lids should close only halfway over the conformer. On postoperative day 1, there is typically edema that results in additional closure, but after this resolves, the lids should move over the conformer without restriction. Copious amounts of antibiotic ointment are placed between the conformer and the conjunctival surface. We do not inject antibiotic(s) into the orbit; rather, we administer a broad spectrum cephalosporin intravenously during the course of the procedure.

All of our enucleations are performed on an outpatient basis. We have not found postoperative intravenous or oral antibiotics to be necessary in most cases but have a low threshold for employing them if there is an increase in swelling or erythema in the early postoperative course. If subsequent chemotherapy or radiation is planned, at least a week should pass from the enucleation to the initiation of such treatment to avoid problems with wound healing.

Tumor Harvesting

Immediately following the enucleation, the globe is removed to a separate area for sectioning and tumor harvesting (Fig. 40.15A).[119] If DNA screening for RB1 mutations is desired, freshly harvested and frozen tumor is required. The globe can be inspected for obvious extraocular extension and photographed. Loose fibrovascular and connective tissue should be removed from the posterior surface of the globe with gentle dissection. The nerve is measured from its insertion to its cut end with surgical calipers, and then cut at its insertion flush with the globe with a straight razor blade. To avoid contaminating the nerve specimen with intraocular tumor, the globe is never opened before the nerve is placed in a sealed container of formalin. Thereafter, the globe is opened in an anteroposterior fashion with a straight razor blade. Once the globe has been cut and begins to collapse, firm back-and-forth motions continue until the bisection is complete. The section should traverse the cornea and, most importantly, avoid the optic nerve.

Tumor cells are harvested with blunt forceps from the calotte without the optic nerve attached (Fig. 40.15A). They are then handled as suggested by the laboratory for DNA diagnosis or snap frozen for storage. Scissors can be used if the tumor is sufficiently firm. The calottes are then placed in containers with formalin and sent for pathology. If there is to be a delay in the processing of tumor cells for DNA diagnosis, they should be quickly frozen to −70° Celsius in a sterile container without culture media or formalin.

Choice of Surgical Implant

The traditional implant used is a solid silicone ball. The largest size that can fit into the orbit is chosen from a sterilized inventory. It is rinsed in antibiotic solution for a few minutes before being placed in the orbit. Thereafter, Tenon's capsule is closed in two layers with a long-absorbing suture before the conjunctival layer is closed with a 6-0 plain or gut suture. One variation, which adds some cost to the procedure, involves wrapping the ball in a layer of eyebank donor sclera and sewing the four recti muscles to the corresponding anterior aspect of the sclera-encased implant. This will theoretically give improved motility. Without the sclera, the recti muscles are usually left to retract into the orbit. Although we are aware of some surgeons who sew the recti muscles directly to the ball without sclera, we have not had success with this approach.

Recently, both hydroxyapatite (HA)[129] and Medpore have been approved for use as orbital implants. The HA material is derived from sea coral heated to very high temperatures. The result is a chemical change that produces hydroxyapatite. The finished product, which was introduced into ophthalmic practice in 1990, contains large and small porous spaces that permit the ingrowth of fibrovascular tissue in the orbit and thus provides better integration and lessens the risk of extrusion. Medpore is a plastic material with properties similar to hydroxyapatite. After sterilization, the integrated implant is immersed in an antibiotic solution, then covered with eyebank sclera. Four windows corresponding to the insertion of the four recti are cut into the anterior surface of the sclera, and each of the four rectus muscles is secured to the anterior edge of one window. The anterior Tenon's capsule and conjunctiva are then closed over the implant as described above. The suturing of the extraocular muscles to the scleral wrapping provides better motility and secures the implant in the orbit. Over time, fibrovascular elements originating from the muscles will grow into the substance of the implant. To further facilitate motility, 6 months or more after the enucleation a hole may be drilled into the center of the HA implant or a titanium screw inserted into the Medpore implant. The prosthesis is attached to the implant via a peg in the HA material or the screw in the Medpore material, resulting in integrated movement of the prosthesis and implant. To date we have not connected any of our young patients' integrated implants with their prostheses. Presumably, the cosmetic effects of enucleation that would prompt the second procedure are not of much importance until the child reaches the teenage years.

CHEMOTHERAPY

Historical Issues

Historically, there has been a great deal of controversy regarding the use of chemotherapy for retinoblastoma.[169] Traditionally, chemotherapy has been most effective for treating orbital recurrence and extraocular tumor. The original regimens and doses of chemotherapeutic agents did not prevent the occurrence of new tumors in predisposed retina. Drugs were chosen because they were known to be effective in other tumors similar to retinoblastoma (e.g., neuroblastoma). Cyclophosphamide was the most commonly used agent, but relapses were invariable when it was used to treat metastatic disease. It had little effect on intraocular tumor at the doses used.

In the St. Jude experience with chemotherapy for extraocular retinoblastoma between 1962 and 1984, 11 of 114 patients received chemotherapy for extraocular disease that was either present at diagnosis (7/11) or subsequently developed (4/11).[130] There was initial response to cyclophosphamide, ifosfamide, vincristine, doxorubicin, cisplatin, and VM-26, both alone and in combination. Only two patients, who had orbital but no other metastases, survived. Both were, however, treated with a combined chemotherapy–radiotherapy protocol.

In 1994, the St. Jude group updated their experience with chemotherapy in the treatment of extraretinal retinoblastoma.[132] Pratt et al. found that, in four patients, two chemotherapy combinations, cyclophosphamide/doxorubicin and cisplatin/etoposide, were effective when given before radiotherapy.[132] We have found that both combinations treat extraocular retinoblastoma effectively. The platinum/etoposide combination, however, is more effective for intraocular disease.

The Children's Cancer Study Group Protocol 962, a randomized trial of adjunctive chemotherapy in patients with Reese-Ellsworth group 5 disease, was designed to evaluate the value of prophylactic chemotherapy in patients at risk for metastatic retinoblastoma. The protocol was unfortunately discontinued in 1980 because of insufficient recruitment and not published.

Background of Current Chemotherapy Protocols

In 1992, Judith Kingston and John Hungerford, from St. Bartholomew's Hospital in London, reported their efforts to salvage eyes with group 5b disease using carboplatin, etoposide (VP-16) and vincristine given prior to, and following, external beam radiotherapy.[87a] Their protocol consisted of a triple drug regimen (VP-16 100 mg/m2 day 1,2,3; carboplatin 560 mg/m2 day 1; vincristine 1.5 mg/m2 day 1) given for 2 months, at which time external beam radiotherapy was given over a 1-month period. This was followed by two additional monthly cycles of chemotherapy.

In the fall of 1992, Murphree et al. modified the London protocol for use with other Reese–Ellsworth stages but with a slightly different goal. We set out to reduce the volume of intraocular disease with short-term chemotherapy (chemoreduction) in order to allow definitive treatment with local modalities and avoid the use of external beam radiotherapy, an attractive and potentially rewarding approach to large intraocular retinoblastoma (Fig. 40.12). We have recently reported the results of our 6-year experience with chemotherapy for intraocular disease,[121] as have others.[62,88]

Sequential Additional Local Therapy

The term "SALT" (sequential additional local therapy) was coined to call attention to the need for local consolidation treatment that was vigilant, frequent, and proactive following chemoreduction.[121] Originally the term "aggressive" was suggested but was replaced by the less provocative term "additional."

Thermochemotherapy

In order to develop an alternative to external beam radiotherapy (EBR) for the treatment of small posterior pole tumors in the second eye of infants under the age of 6 months with bilateral disease; Murphree et al. examined the combination of systemic platinum chemotherapy (carboplatin) combined with local transpupillary laser hyperthermia.[121] Gentle heat is synergistic with the chemotherapy and increases carboplatin uptake in the tumor.[121] Thermochemotherapy (TCT) is effective in Reese-Ellsworth groups 1 and 2 and in Group C eyes that are receiving 3 drug chemoreduction. In tumors over 4 DD or 6 mm in size TCT is better replaced with chemoreduction and SALT.

Chemoreduction

Triple chemotherapy for tumor reduction or chemoreduction, as we prefer to call this approach, is highly effective in reducing the volume of intraocular tumors (Fig. 40.16). When combined with SALT it cures Group C retinoblastoma eyes (Reese-Ellsworth groups 2–4).[121] Murphree et al.[121] have had remarkable success using chemoreduction to treat eyes with total retinal detachment, if imaging studies such as CT scan and ultrasonography reveal that less than half the globe is involved with tumor. In these cases, resolution of the detachment occurs after one or two cycles of therapy (Fig. 40.16). Similarly, the use of chemoreduction in treating large tumors that initially obscure the optic nerve and fovea can reveal an eccentric origin and present the possibility of restoring useful vision. Smaller tumors are also effectively treated with chemoreduction plus SALT (Fig. 40.12).

Cyclosporin A

Gallie and colleagues have reported an encouraging salvage rate in Group D retinoblastoma eyes (Reese-Ellsworth groups 5a and 5b) with the addition of high doses of cyclosporin A (CsA). 9–12 cycles of CsA, commonly used in postcardiac transplant patients, is given concurrently with the chemotherapy in high doses with the presumption that it competitively inhibits the multiple drug resistance (mdr) membrane pump. These authors also employed pretreatment cryotherapy to increase chemotherapy concentration in the eye. Our experience with this protocol has shown recurrence of vitreous or subretinal disease 1–6 months following cessation of the chemotherapy. Consolidation of the dispersed disease must be added to the protocol.

A

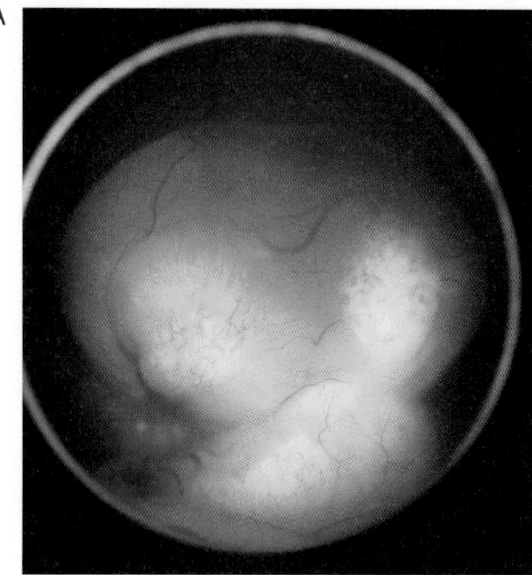

B

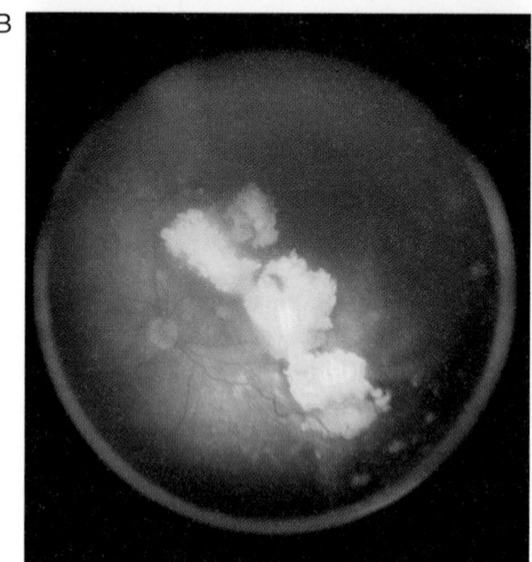

Figure 40.16. (**A**) Large volume retinoblastoma surrounding the optic nerve. (**B**) The same eye as in Figure 16A after three 3-week cycles of carboplatin, etoposide and vincristine (chemoreduction). Regrowth will occur along the edge of the calcified type I regression unless the residual mass is consolidated with SALT which would consist of direct gentle photocoagulation because of the posterior position of this tumor.

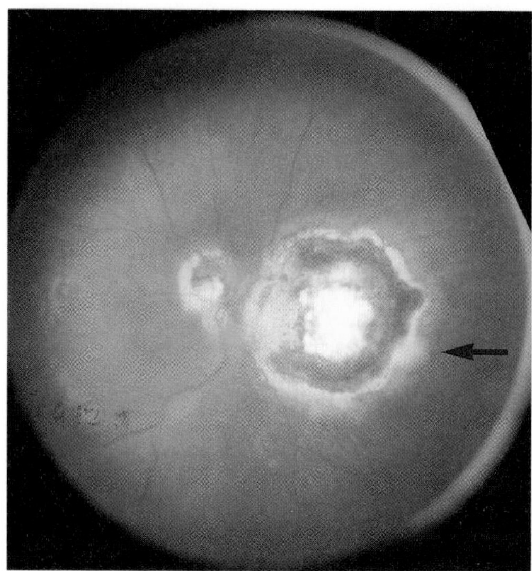

Figure 40.17. An edge recurrence following chemoreduction is indicated by the arrow. It appears clinically as a soft white round area at the edge of the Type IV regression scar. The recurrence would be treated with gentle direct photocoagulation using the diode laser in this case. This frequent surveillance for edge recurrence is a major component of SALT (sequential additional local therapy).

Planned Multicenter Clinical Trial

Based on the encouraging pilot data published from several ocular oncology centers[63,89,122] on the positive benefits of chemoreduction, ±CsA, +SALT for the treatment of intraocular retinoblastoma, a multicenter trial is being currently planned to evlauate in a randomized way the benefits of cyclosporin A in the management of Group D retinoblastoma eyes (groups 5a and 5b). A second hypothesis testing arm will document the efficacy of three cycles of chemoreduction plus SALT (without CsA) for Group C eyes (Reese–Ellsworth groups 2–4) retinoblastomas. Group A and B retinoblastoma eyes will not be included in the trial.

Cryotherapy

Transcleral cryotherapy is an effective procedure for destroying small anterior tumors that are confined to the sensory retina,[146,161] as part of SALT, or as primary treatment of Group A disease. Ice crystals formed in the substance of the tumor rupture cellular membranes. It is not useful when vitreous seeding is present.

A standard retinal cryoprobe used transconjunctivally will generally reach tumors as far posterior as the equator. There are rare indications for treating lesions posterior to the equator. In such cases, a conjunctival incision at the limbus and blunt dissection of Tenon's capsule will provide access to the posterior aspects of the globe (cutting cryo). We have successfully treated small local recurrences at the edge of previously radiated posterior lesions to avoid exceeding the threshold for radiation-associated retinopathy. One possible severe complication of treating posterior lesions in this fashion is the incorporation of the optic nerve in the ice ball. Inadvertent freezing of the larger posterior vessels can precipitate intraocular and orbital hemorrhages.

Cryotherapy is successful in treating lesions that are no greater than 2.5 mm in diameter and 1.0 mm high.[148] Lesions up to 3.5 mm in diameter and 2.0 mm thick can be successfully treated but may require several treatment sessions.[147] Using binocular indirect ophthalmoscopy, the lesion is localized with the tip of the cryoprobe. Freezing is begun and continued until the tumor mass is completely encased in the ice ball. The ice ball is allowed to thaw and the freezing cycle is repeated two more times (the "triple freeze-thaw" technique). Cryotherapy generally destroys contiguous areas of normal retina. Other complications include subretinal and vitreous hemorrhage, the accumulation of subretinal fluid, and the formation of retinal breaks with the development of a rhegmatogenous retinal detachment. Cryotherapy results in strong adhesions at the margins of scars and vitreous contraction.[103] The latter may result in retinal detachment, especially if accompanied by a break (hole) in the retina. One should avoid extensive (more than 4 sites) cryotherapy, which can result in acute serous retinal detachment and atrophy fo the sclera, with formation of a pseudocoloboma.

Cryodisruption

Cryodisruption is a newly coined term describing the use of single freeze-thaw applications to disrupt the blood–ocular barrier and facilitate entry of chemotherapy into the vitreous. It is a part of the chemotherapy protocol for Group D disease.

Traditional "Surround" Photocoagulation

Traditional "surround" photocoagulation can be effectively used to treat small posterior retinoblastomas.[8,76,149] Photocoagulation deprives the tumor of its blood supply. Traditional "surround" photocoagulation is used relatively infrequently today because of the required destruction of normal retina surrounding the lesion. Lesions amenable to "surround" photocoagulation are those equal to or smaller than 3.5 mm in diameter and 1.5 mm thick that are confined to the sensory retina and do not extend into the vitreous. Sharp margins on fluorescein angiography can confirm the latter.[146]

Xenon arc photocoagulators were employed in the past but have been replaced by argon,[8] frequency-doubled YAG (yttrium-argon-garnet), dye, or diode laser systems. The laser is used with a fundus contact lens, and the power is adjusted to produce a white retinal burn and to close retinal vessels. The tumor is treated by surrounding it with one or two rows of confluent burns. The tumor is not treated directly in this approach. A tumor cannot be considered completely cured until the site is completely flat for at least 3 years.[3] Any residual mass requires treatment.

Recently, the indirect ophthalmoscope delivery system has been used successfully to deliver argon laser surround photocoagulation to small retinoblastomas anywhere in the retina.[8] Augsburger and Faulkner used the "continuous" setting on the indirect laser to create a confluent white burn around the tumor.[8]

Direct "Gentle" Photocoagulation

With the development of chemoreduction,[121] the need for more effective local therapy was clear. Following reduction in volume of the tumor with chemotherapy, there is less concern with exploding a "tense" Rb lesion by direct photocoagulation. Also, the introduction of the Iris Medical, Inc. (Menlo Park, CA) diode laser-through-the-microscope delivery system allows the use of larger spot sizes, significantly reducing the concentration of laser energy and the likelihood of disrupting directly treated tumors. Murphree et al. have now treated more than 100 individual tumors directly with both the diode (810 nm) and green (532 nm). The spot sizes with the diode laser vary from 0.8 mm, 1.2 mm, to 2.0 mm. Power output ranges from 350 mW to 700 mW. The end point is a slight "blanching" or whitening of the tumor. The entire tumor is covered with a small overlap onto normal retina (approximately one quarter spot). Hemorrhage is to be avoided. Tumor vessel closure is not required. This treatment is aimed at direct coagulation of tumor cell proteins.[121] Gentle direct photocoagulation can safely be used to treat lesions 3 mm in diameter or less in Group A eyes.

EXPERIMENTAL TREATMENTS UNDER EVALUATION

Photodynamic Therapy

In the past decade, a great deal of interest has been generated among ocular oncologists regarding the use of photosensitizing agents to treat posterior pole Reese-Ellsworth groups 1–3 tumors (see Thermochemotherapy above). These agents, such as porphyrin derivatives, offer the potential advantage of avoiding the side effects of both radiotherapy and chemotherapy. They transfer energy from specific wavelengths of light to tissue oxygen, creating highly active singlet oxygen radicals. In sufficient concentrations, these radicals will disrupt cellular membranes. Photodynamic therapy (PDT) consists of the systemic administration of a selected agent and the application of light energy, as with a laser, when adequate tissue concentrations have been achieved.

Dougherty and colleagues have advanced the use of PDT in oncology,[41,42] and our experimental therapeutics group have done the basic research on the ocular pharmacology, pharmacokinetics, and ocular toxicity of porphyrins.[64–66] In 1987, we reported the results of using PDT to treat nine retinoblastomas in six patients. Each received subthermal thresholds of red light (631 nm) after the administration of hematoporphyrin derivative (HpP).[118] Good results using PDT with suprathermal thresholds of continuous-wave green light from an argon laser have also been reported.[124] Based on their findings, Ohnishi et al. recommended instituting phototherapy 3 days after the intravenous administration of 2.5 mg/kg of a hematoporphyrin derivative.[125] They treat with argon green light at 200 mW for 20 minutes. If the tumor remains viable, they recommend that the procedure be repeated after 1 month.

Our initial experiences were severely limited by the long-acting nature of the available agents, and the resultant skin phototoxicity (sunburn). Currently, the interest in PDT is revived because newer agents, such as benzoporphyrin derivative (BPD) and others based on the chlorophyll molecule, are rapidly excreted from the body and pose little such risk. Once these newer agents become readily available, we foresee that they may replace carboplatin in the TCT protocol for the treatment of smaller posterior tumors.

REFERENCES

1. Abramson DH, Ellsworth RM, Kitchin FD, Tung G. Second nonocular tumors in retinoblastoma survivors—Are they radiation induced? *Ophthalmology* 1984;91:1351–1355.
2. Abramson DH, Ellsworth RM, Grumbach N, Kitchin FD. Retinoblastoma: Survival, age at detection and comparison 1914–1958, 1958–1983. *J Pediatr Ophthalmol Strabismus* 1985; 22:246–250.
3. Abramson DH. The focal treatment of retinoblastoma with emphasis on xenon arc photocoagulation. *Acta Ophthalmol Suppl (Copenh)* 1989;194:3–63.
4. Abramson DH, Servodidio CA. Retinoblastoma in the first year of life. *Ophthalmic Paediatr Genet* 1992;13:191–203.
5. Albert DM, McGhee CNJ, Seddon JM, Weichselbaum RR. Development of additional primary tumors after 62 years in the first patient with retinoblastoma cured by radiation therapy. *Am J Ophthalmol* 1984;97: 189–196.
6. Amemiya T, Takano J, Choshi K. Did atomic bomb radiation influence the incidence of retinoblastoma in Nagasaki and Hiroshima? *Ophthalmic Paediatr Genet* 1993;14:75–79.
7. Augsburger JJ, Shields JA, Folberg R et al. Fine needle aspiration biopsy in the diagnosis of intraocular cancer. *Ophthalmology* 1985; 92:39–49.
8. Augsburger JJ, Faulkner CB. Indirect ophthalmoscope argon laser treatment of retinoblastoma. *Ophthalmic Surg* 1992;23:591–593.
9. Balaban-Malenbaum G, Gilbert F, Nichols W. Abnormalities in chromosome 13 in direct preparations from human retinoblastoma (abstract). *Am J Hum Genet* 1980;32:62a.
10. Balmer A, Munier F, Gailloud C. Retinoma case studies. *Ophthalmic Paediatr Genet* 1991;12:131–137.
11. Balmer A, Gailloud C, Munier F, Uffer S, Guex-Crosier Y. Retinoblastoma: Unusual warning and clinical signs. *Ophthalmic Paediatr Genet* 1993;14:33–38.
12. Berkeley JS, Kalita BC. Letter to the editor. *Lancet* 1977;2:508–509.
13. Bhatnagar R, Vine AK. Diffuse infiltrating retinoblastoma. *Ophthalmology* 1991;98:1657–1661.
14. Bignon YJ, Chen Y, Windle J et al. Overexpression of the retinoblastoma gene in transgenic mice results in dwarfism (abstract). *Ann Oncol* 1992;3(suppl) 5:30.
15. Binder PS. Unusual manifestations of retinoblastoma. *Am J Ophthalmol* 1974;77:674–679.
16. Bishop JM. Molecular themes in oncogenesis. *Cell* 1991;64:235–248.
17. Blach LE, McCormick B, Abramson DH, Ellsworth RM. Trilateral retinoblastoma—Incidence and outcome: A decade of experience. *Int J Radiat Oncol Biol Phys* 1994; 29:729–733.
18. Blanquet V, Creau-Goldberg N, de Grouchy J, Turleau C. Molecular detection of constitutional deletions in patients with retinoblastoma. *Am J Med Genet* 1991;39:355–361.
19. Bogenmann E, Lochine MA, Simon MI. Cone cell-specific genes expressed in retinoblastoma. *Science* 1988;240:76–78.
20. Bolande RP. Spontaneous regression and cytodifferentiation of cancer in early life: The oncogenic grace period. *Surv Synthesis Pathol Res* 1985;4:296–311.
21. Boveri, T. Zür frage der entstehung maligner tumoren Jena: Verlag, von Gustave Fisher,

1914. In McKusick VA, Marcella O'Grady Boveri (1865–1950) and the chromosome theory of cancer. *J Med Genet* 1985;22: 431–440.
22. Boveri, T. The origin of malignant tumors (translated by M. Boveri). Baltimore: Williams & Wilkins, 1929:26–27.
23. Bremner MH. Retinoblastoma in the anterior chamber of the eye. *Aust J Ophthalmol* 1983; 11:123–126.
24. Bressac B, Kew M, Wands J, Ozturk M. Selective G to T mutation of p53 gene in hepatocellular carcinoma from Southern Africa. *Nature* 1991;350:429–431.
25. Buckley JD. The aetiology of cancer in the very young. *Br J Cancer* 1992;18:32.
26. Bullock JD, Campbell RJ, Waller RR. Calcification in retinoblastoma. *Invest Ophthalmol Vis Sci* 1977;16:252–255.
27. Cade S. Radiation induced cancer in man. *Br J Radiol* 1957;30:393.
28. Caron de Fromentel C, Soussi T. TP53 tumor suppressor gene: A model investigating human mutagenesis. *Genes Chromsomes Cancer* 1992;4:1–15.
29. Cavenee WK, Dryja TP, Phillips RA et al. Expression of recessive alleles by chromosomal mechanisms in retinoblastoma. *Nature* 1983;305:779–784.
30. Cavenee WK, Murphree AL, Shull MM et al. Prediction of familial predisposition to retinoblastoma. *N Engl J Med* 1986;314:1201–1207.
31. Clarke AR, Maandag ER, van Roon M et al. Requirement for functional Rb-1 gene in murine development. *Nature* 1992;359:328–330.
32. Cole CH, Magee JF, Gianoulis M, Rogers PC. Malignant fibrous histiocytoma in childhood. *Cancer* 1993;71:4077–4083.
33. Coleman DJ. Reliability of ocular tumor diagnosis with ultrasounds. *Trans Am Acad Ophthalmol Otolaryngol* 1973;77:677–686.
34. Comings DE. A general theory of carcinogenesis. *Proc Natl Acad Sci USA* 1973;70:3324–3328.
35. Cooper DN, Krawaczak M. The mutational spectrum of single base-pair substitutions causing human genetic disease: Patterns and predictions. *Hum Genet* 1990;85:55–74.
36. Cordon-Cardo C, Richon VM. Expression of the retinoblastoma protein is regulated in normal human tissues. *Am J Pathol* 1994;144; 500–510.
37. Cowell JK, Hungerford J, Rutland P, Jay M. Genetic and cytogenetic analysis of patients showing reduced esterase-D levels and mental retardation from a survey of 500 individuals with retinoblastoma. *Ophthalmic Paediatr Genet* 1989;10:117–127.
37a. Cowell JK, Bia B, Akoulitchev A. A novel mutation in the promoter region in a family with a mild form of retinoblastoma indicates the location of a new regulatory domain for the RB1 gene. *Oncogene* 1996;12(2):431–436.
38. De Potter P, Shields CL, Shields JA. Clinical variations of trilateral retinoblastoma: A report of 13 cases. *J Pediatr Ophthalmol Strabismus* 1994;31:26–31.
39. Desjardins L, Haye C, Schlienger P et al. Second non-ocular tumors in survivors of bilateral retinoblastoma. A 30-year follow-up. *Ophthalmic Paediatr Genet* 1991;12:145–148.
40. Devesa SS. The incidence of retinoblastoma. *Am J Ophthalmol* 1975;80:263–265.
41. Dougherty TJ. Activated dyes as antitumor agents. *J Nat Cancer Inst* 1974;52:1333–1336.
42. Dougherty TJ. The future of photoradiation therapy in the treatment of cancer. *Laser Focus* 1983;19:55–57.
43. Draper GJ, Heaf MM, Kinnier Wilson LM. Occurrence of childhood cancers among sibs and estimation of familial risks. *J Med Genet* 1977;14:81–90.
44. Draper GJ, Sanders BM, Kingston JE. Second primary neoplasms in patients with retinoblastoma. *Br J Cancer* 1986;53:661–671.
45. Draper GJ, Sanders BM, Brownbill PA, Hawkins MM. Patterns of risk of hereditary retinoblastoma and applications to genetic counselling. *Br J Cancer* 1992;66:211–219.
46. Driscoll DJ, Migeon BR. Sex difference in methylation of single-copy genes in human meiotic germ cells: Implications for X inactivation, parental imprinting, and origin of CpG mutations. *Somatic Cell Mol Genet* 1990;16:267–282.
47. Dryja TP, Mukai S, Petersen R et al. Parental origin of mutations of the retinoblastoma gene. *Nature* 1989;339:556–558.
48. Einhorn L. Are there factors preventing cancer development during embryonic life? *Oncodev Biol Med* 1983;4:219–229.
49. Ellsworth RM. Orbital retinoblastoma. *Trans Am Ophthalmol Soc* 1974;72:79–88.
50. Eng C, Lin FP, Abramson DH et al. Mortality from second tumors among long term survivors of retinoblastoma. *J Nat Cancer Inst* 1993;85:1121–1128.
51. Ferris III FL, Chew EY. A new era for the

treatment of retinoblastoma (editorial). *Arch Ophthalmol* 1996;114:1412.

52. Flick H, Schwab B. Infiltrating retinoblastoma—A difficult differential diagnosis. *Klin Monatsbl Augenheilkd* 1980;177:220–224.
53. Folberg R, Cleasby G, Flanagan JA et al. Orbital leiomyosarcoma after radiation therapy for bilateral retinoblastoma. *Arch Ophthalmol* 1983;101:1562–1565.
54. Font SL, Jurco III S, Brechner RJ. Postradiation leiomyosarcoma of the orbit complicating bilateral retinoblastoma. *Arch Ophthalmol* 1983;101:1557–1561.
55. Francke U. Retinoblastoma and chromosome 13. *Cytogenet Cell Genet* 1976;16:131–134.
56. François J, Matton MD, De Bie S et al. Genesis and genetics of retinoblastoma. *Ophthalmologica* 1975;170:405–425.
57. François J. Retinoblastoma and osteogenic sarcoma. *Ophthalmologica* 1977;175:185–191.
58. François J, de Sutter E, Coppieters R, de Bie S. Late extraocular tumors in retinoblastoma survivors. *Ophthalmologica* 1980;181:93–99.
59. Friend SH, Bernards R, Rogelj S. A human DNA segment with properties of the gene that predisposes to retinoblastoma and osteosarcoma. *Nature* 1986;323:643–646.
60. Fung YKT, Murphree AL, Tang A et al. Structural evidence for the authenticity of the human retinoblastoma gene. *Science* 1987;236: 1657–1661.
61. Gallie BL, Ellsworth RM, Abramsom DH, Phillips RA. Retinoblastoma: Spontaneous regression of retinoblastoma or benign manifestation of the mutation? *Br J Cancer* 1982;45: 513–521.
62. Gallie BL, Budning A, DeBoer G, Thiessen JJ, Koren G, Verjee Z, Ling V, Chang HSL. Chemotherapy with focal therapy can cure intraocular retinoblastoma without radiotherapy. *Arch Ophthalmol* 1996;114:1321–1328.
63. Girard B, LeHoang P, D'Hermies F, Quere MA, Rousselie F. Diffuse infiltrating retinoblastoma [in French]. *J Fr Ophthalmol* 1989; 12:369–381.
64. Gomer CJ. DNA damage and repair in CHO cells following hematoporphyrin photoradition. *Cancer Lett* 1980;11:161–167.
65. Gomer CJ, Doiron DR, Jester JV et al. Hematoporphyrin derivation photoradiation therapy for the treatment of intraocular tumors: Examination of acute normal ocular tissue toxicity. *Cancer Res* 1983;43:721–727.
66. Gomer CJ, Doiron DW, White L et al. Hematoporphyrin derivative photoradiation induced damage to normal and tumor tissue of the pigmented rabbit eye. *Curr Eye Res* 1984;3:229–237.
67. Greger V, Passarge E, Hopping W et al. Epigenetic changes may contribute to the formation and regression of retinoblastoma. *Hum Genet* 1989;83:155–158.
68. Haik BG, Saint Louis L, Smith ME et al. Computed tomography of the nonrhegmatogenous retinal detachment in the pediatric patient. *Ophthalmology* 1985a;92:1133–1142.
69. Haik BG, Siedlecki A, Ellsworth RM et al. Documented delays in the diagnosis of retinoblastoma. *Ann Ophthalmol* 1985b;17:731–732.
70. Haik BG, Dunleavy SA, Cooke C et al. Retinoblastoma with anterior chamber extension. *Ophthalmology* 1987;94:367–370.
71. Hamel PA, Gill RM, Phillips RA, Gallie BL. Transcriptional repression of the E2-containing promoters EIIaE, c-myc, and RB1 by the RB1 gene. *Mol Cell Biol* 1992;12:3431–3438.
72. Hawkins MM, Draper GJ, Kingston JE. Incidence of second primary tumours among childhood cancer survivors. *Br J Cancer* 1987; 56:339–347.
73. Hollenberg MJ, Spira AW. Early development of the human retina. *Can J Ophthalmol* 1972;7:472–491.
74. Hollyfield JG. Histiogenesis of the retina in the killifisch, Fundulus heteroclitus. *J Comp Neurol* 1972;144:373–380.
75. Hoppe-Seyler F, Butz K. Tumor suppressor genes in molecular medicine. *Clin Investig (Germany)* 1994;72:619–630.
76. Hopping W, Meyer-Schwickerath G. Light coagulation treatment in retinoblastoma. In *Ocular and Adnexal Tumors*, M. Boniuk, ed. St. Louis: Mosby-Year Book, 1964.
77. Horsthemke B, Greger V, Barnert HJ et al. Detection of submicroscopic deletions and a DNA polymorphism at the retinoblastoma locus. *Hum Genet* 1987;76:257–261.
78. Horsthemke B. Genetics and cytogenetics of retinoblastoma. *Cancer Genet Cytogenet* 1992;63:1–7.
79. Howes KA, Ransom N, Papermaster DS, Lasudry JG, Albert DM, Windle JJ. Apoptosis or retinoblastoma: Alternative fates of photoreceptors expressing the HPV-16 E7 gene in the presence or absence of p53. *Genes Dev* 1994;8:1300–1310.

80. Hsu IC, Metcalf RA, Sun T et al. Mutational hotspot in the p53 gene in human hepatocellular carcinoma. *Nature* 1991;350:427–428.
81. Hurwitz RL, Bogenmann E, Font RL et al. Expression of the functional cone phosphotransduction cascade in retinoblastoma. *J Clin Invest* 1990;85:1872–1878.
82. Isobe M, Emanuel BS, Givol D, Oren M, Croce CM. Localization of gene for human p53 tumour antigen to band 17p13. *Nature* 1986;320:84–85.
83. Jacks T, Fazseli A, Schmitt EM et al. Effects of Rb mutation in the mouse. *Nature* 1992;359:295–300.
84. Janson M, Kock E, Nordensjkjold M. Constitutional deletions predisposing to retinoblastoma. *Hum Genet* 1990;85:21–24.
85. Jay M, Cowell JK, Kingston JE, Hungerford J. Demonstration of bias in series of retinoblastoma. *Ophthalmic Paediatr Genet* 1989; 10:89–92.
86. Ketterling RP, Vielhaber E, Bottema CDK et al. Germ-line origins of mutation in families with hemophilia B: The sex ratio varies with the type of mutation. *Am J Hum Genet* 1993;52:152–166.
87. Kingston JE, Hungerford JL, Plowman PN. Chemotherapy in metastatic retinoblastoma. *Ophthalmic Paediatr Genet* 1987;8:69–72.
87a. Kingston JE, Hungerford JL. Chemotherapy and Radiotherapy for Group 5b Retinoblastoma. Presented at the Retinoblastoma Symposium, Nyon, France, May 1992.
88. Kingston JE, Hungerford JL, Madreperla SA, Plowman PN. Results of combined chemotherapy and radiotherapy for advanced intraocular retinoblastoma. *Arch Ophthalmol* 1996;114:1339–1343.
89. Knudson AG. Mutation and cancer: Statistical study on retinoblastoma. *Proc Nat Acad Sci USA* 1971;68:820–823.
90. Knudson AG. The genetics of childhood cancer. *Cancer* 1975;35:1022–1026.
91. Knudson AG. Genetics and the etiology of childhood cancer. *Pediatr Res* 1976;10:513–517.
92. Knudson AG. Hereditary cancer, oncogenes, and antioncogenes. *Cancer Res* 1985;45: 1437–1443.
93. Knudson AG. Hereditary Cancer: two hits revisited. *J Cancer Res Clin Oncol* 1996;122(3): 135–140.
94. Knudson AG. Antioncogenes and human cancer. *Proc Nat Acad Sci USA* 1993;90:109–121.
95. Kock E, Naeser P. Retinoblastoma in Sweden 1958–1971: A clinical and histopathological study. *Acta Ophthalmol (Copenh)* 1979;57: 344–350.
96. Kodilinye HC. Retinoblastoma in Nigeria: Problems of treatment. *Am J Ophthalmol* 1967;63:469–481.
97. Labib MAM, El Gammal Y, El Aguizy H. Retinoblastoma: Unusual presentation. *Bull Ophthalmol Soc Egypt* 1975;68:385–389.
98. Lam BL, Judisch GF, Sobol WM, Blodi CF. Visual prognosis in macular retinoblastomas. *Am J Ophthalmol* 1990;110:229–232.
99. Lee EYHP, Chang CY, Hu N et al. Mice deficient for Rb are nonviable and show defects in neurogenesis and hematopoiesis. *Nature* 1992;359:288–294.
100. Lees JA, Buchovich KJ, Marshak DR et al. The retinoblastoma protein is phosphorylated on multiple sites by human cdc1. *EMBO J* 1991;10:4279–4290.
101. Lennox EL, Draper GJ, Sanders BM. Retinoblastoma: A study of natural history and prognosis of 268 cases. *Br Med J* 1975;3:731–734.
102. Levine AJ. The tumor suppressor genes. *Annu Rev Biochem* 1993;62:623–651.
103. Lincoff HA, McLean JM. Cryosurgical treatment of retinal detachment, part II. *Trans Am Acad Ophthalmol Otolaryngol* 1966;70: 202–211.
103a. Lohmann DR, Brandt B, Hopping W et al. Distinct RB1 gene mutations with low penetrance in hereditary retinoblastoma. *Hum Genet* 1994;94(4):349–354.
104. Maat-Kievit JA, Oepkes D, Hartwig NG, Vermeij-Keers C, van Kamp IL, van de Kamp JJ. A large retinoblastoma detected in a fetus at 21 weeks of gestation. *Prenat Diagn* 1993; 13:377–384.
105. Magramm I, Abramson DH, Ellsworth RM. Optic nerve involvement in retinoblastoma. *Ophthalmology* 1989;96:217–222.
106. Mansfield NC, Horn M. *My Fake Eye*. The Institute for Families of Blind Children, Los Angeles CA, 1993.
107. Mansour AM, Greenwald MJ, O'Grady R. Diffuse infiltrating retinoblastoma. *J Pediatr Ophthalmol Strabismus* 1989;26:152–154.
108. Marshall CJ. Tumor suppressor genes. *Cell* 1991;64:313–326.
109. McKusick VA. Marcella O'Grady Boveri (1865–1950) and the chromosome theory of cancer. *J Med Genet* 1985;22:431–440.
110. Meadows AT, Baum E, Fossati-Bellani F et

al. Second malignant neoplasms in children: An update from the Late Effects Study Group. *J Clin Oncol* 1985;3:532–538.

111. Mizuno M, Yoshida J, Shimosawa S, Kuchiwaki H. Intracranial fibrosarcoma fifteen years after radiotherapy in bilateral retinoblastomas: Effect of combined chemotherapy with cisplatin and VP-16 [in Japanese] No Shinkei Geka. *Neurol Surg (Jpn)* 1989;17:653–657.
112. Moles JP, Moyret C, Guillot B et al. p53 Gene mutations in human epithelial skin cancers. *Oncogene* 1993;8:583–588.
113. Munier F, Pescia G, Jotterand-Bellomo M et al. Constitutional karyotype in retinoblastoma: Case report and review of the literature. *Ophthalmic Paediatr Genet* 1989;10:129–150.
114. Munier F, Balmer A, Moos C von et al. Lausanne study of retinoblastoma, 1986–1990: Deletion of esterase D locus in a collective of 128 patients. *Klin Monatsbl Augenheilkd* 1991;198:419–424.
115. Munier F, Spence AM, Pescia G et al. Paternal selection favoring mutant alleles of the retinoblastoma susceptibility gene. *Hum Genet* 1992;89:508–512.
116. Munier FL, Balmer A, Van Melle G, Gailloud C. Radial asymmetry in the topography of retinoblastoma. *Ophthalmic Genet* 1994;15:101–106.
116a. Munier FL, Wang MX, Spence MA et al. Pseudo low penetrance in retinoblastoma. Fortuitous familial aggregation of sporadic cases caused by independently derived mutations in two large pedigrees. *Arch Ophthalmol* 1993;111(11):1507–1511.
117. Murphree AL, Benedict WF. Retinoblastoma: Clues to human oncogenesis. *Science* 1984;223:1028–1033.
118. Murphree AL, Cote M, Gomer CJ. The evolution of photodynamic therapy techniques in the treatment of intraocular tumors. *Photochem Photobiol* 1987;46:919–923.
119. Murphree AL, Munier F. Retinoblastoma. In *Retina,* S. J. Ryan, ed. St. Louis: Mosby, 1994:571–626.
120. Murphree AL. Molecular genetics of retinoblastoma. In *Ophthalmology Clinics of North America,* H. Grossniklaus, ed. Philadelphia: W.B. Saunders, 1995.
121. Murphree AL, Villablanca JG, Deegan III WF et al. Chemotherapy plus local treatment in the management of intraocular retinoblastoma. *Arch Ophthalmol* 1996;114:1348–1356.
121a. Murphree AL. Personal observation, 1996.
121b. Murphree AL. A New Classification for Intraocular Retinoblastoma. *Archives Ophthalmol* (submitted) 1998.
122. Nadol Jr JB. Pseudocellulitis of the orbit—A case report of retinoblastoma masquerading as orbital cellulitis. *Ann Otol* 1977;86:86–88.
123. Ohnishi Y, Yamana Y, Minei M, Yoshitomi F. Snowball opacity in retinoblastoma. *Jpn J Ophthalmol* 1982;26:159–165.
124. Ohnishi Y, Yamana Y, Minei M. Photoradiation therapy using argon laser and a hematoporphyrin derivative for retinoblastoma—A preliminary report. *Jpn J Ophthalmol* 1986;30:409–419.
125. Orita M, Susuki Y, Sekiya T, Hayashi K. Rapid and sensitive detection of point mutations and DNA polymorphism using the polymerase chain reaction. *Genomics* 1989;5:874–879.
126. Palazzi M, Abramson DH, Ellsworth RM. Endophytic vs exophytic unilateral retinoblastoma: Is there any real difference? *J Pediatr Ophthalmol Strabismus* 1990;27:255–258.
127. Pendergrass TW, Davis S. Incidence of retinoblastoma in the United States. *Arch Ophthalmol* 1980;98:1204–1210.
128. Perry AC. Integrated orbital implants. *Adv Ophthalmic Plast Reconstr Surg* 1990;8:75–81.
129. Plotsky D, Quinn G, Eagle Jr R, Shields J, Granowetter L. Congenital retinoblastoma: A case report. *J Pediatr Ophthalmol Strabismus* 1987;24:120–123.
130. Pratt CB, Crom DB, Howarth C. The use of chemotherapy for extraocular retinoblastoma. *Med Pediatr Oncol* 1985;13:330–333.
131. Pratt CB, Meyer D, Chenaille P, Crom DB. The use of bone marrow aspirations and lumbar punctures at the time of diagnosis of retinoblastoma. *J Clin Oncol* 1989;7:140–143.
132. Pratt CB, Fontanesi J, Chenaille P et al. Chemotherapy for extraocular retinoblastoma. *Pediatr Hematol Oncol* 1994;11:301–309.
133. Qian Y, Luckey C, Horton L et al. Biological function of the retinoblastoma protein requires distinct domains for hyperphosphorylation and transcription factor binding. *Mol Cell Biol* 1992;12:5363–5372.
134. Qin XQ, Chittenden T, Livingston DM, Kaelin WG. Identification of a growth suppression domain within the retinoblastoma gene product. *Genes Devel* 1992;6:953–964.
135. Roarty JD, McLean JW, Zimmerman LE. Incidence of second neoplasms in patients with

bilateral retinoblastoma. *Ophthalmology* 1988;95:1583–1587.

136. Rubenfeld M, Abramson DH, Ellsworth RM, Kitchin FD. Unilateral vs bilateral retinoblastoma—Correlations between age at diagnosis and stage of ocular disease. *Ophthalmology* 1986;93:1016–1019.
137. Rubin CM, Robison LL, Cameron JD et al. Intraocular retinoblastoma group v—An analysis of prognostic factors. *J Clin Oncol* 1985; 3:680–685.
138. Rugh R. X-rays and the retina of the primate foetus. *Arch Ophthalmol* 1973;89:221–227.
139. Sakai T, Toguchida J, Ohtani N et al. Allele-specific hypermethylation of the retinoblastoma tumor-suppressor gene. *Am J Hum Genet* 1991;48:880–888.
140. Schulman JA, Peyman GA, Mafee MF et al. The use of magnetic resonance imaging in the evaluation of retinoblastoma. *J Pediatr Ophthalmol Strabismus* 1986;23:144–147.
141. Schuster SAD, Ferguson III EC. Unusual presentations of retinoblastoma. *South Med J* 1970;63:4–8.
142. Schwarz MB, Burgess LP, Fee Jr WE, Donaldson SS. Postirradiation sarcoma in retinoblastoma. Induction or predisposition? *Arch Otolaryngol Head Neck Surg* 1988;114: 640–644.
143. Sheta A. Some aspects on the different clinical characteristics of retinoblastoma. *Bull Ophthalmol Soc Egypt* 1971;64:413–424.
144. Shields CL, Shields JA, Shah P. Retinoblastoma in older children. *Ophthalmology* 1991;98:395–399.
145. Shields CL, Shields JA, Baez K, Cater JR, de Potter P. Optic nerve invasion of retinoblastoma. Metastatic potential and clinical risk factors. *Cancer* 1994;73:692–698.
146. Shields JA. *Diagnosis and management of intraocular tumors.* St. Louis: Mosby Year-Book, 1983.
147. Shields JA, Parsons H, Shields CL, Giblin ME. The role of cryotherapy in the management of retinoblastoma. *Am J Ophthalmol* 1989;108:260–264.
148. Shields JA, Shields CL. Treatment of retinoblastoma with cryotherapy. *Trans Pa Acad Ophthalmol Otolaryngol* 1990;42:977–980.
149. Shields JA, Shields CL, Parsons H, Giblin ME. The role of photocoagulation in the management of retinoblastoma. *Arch Ophthalmol* 1989;108:205–208.
150. Shields JA, Shields CL, Suvarnamani C et al. Retinoblastoma manifesting as orbital cellulitis. *Am J Ophthalmol* 1991;112:442–449.
151. Sinniah D, Narasimha G, Prathap K. Advanced retinoblastoma in Malaysian children. *Acta Ophthalmol (Copenh)* 1980;58:819–824.
152. Skuse GR, Ludlow JW. Tumor suppressor genes in disease and therapy. *Lancet* 1995; 345:902–906.
153. Smith LM, Donaldson SS. Incidence and management of secondary malignancies in patients with retinoblastoma and Ewing's sarcoma. *Oncology* 1991;5:135–141; discussion 142, 147–148.
154. Soloway HB. Radiation-induced neoplasms following curative therapy for retinoblastoma. *Cancer* 1966;19:1984–1988.
155. Sparkes RS, Sparkes MC, Wilson MG et al. Regional assignment of genes for human esterase D and retinoblastoma to chromosome band 13q14. *Science* 1980;208:1042–1044.
156. Sparkes RS, Murphree AL, Lingua RW et al. Gene for hereditary retinoblastoma assigned to human chromosome 13 by linkage to esterase D. *Science* 1983;219:971–973.
157. Stafford WR, Yanoff M, Parnell BL. Retinoblastomas initially misdiagnosed as primary ocular inflammations. *Arch Ophthalmol* 1969; 82:771–773.
158. Strauss BS. The origin of point mutations in human tumor cells. *Cancer Res* 1992;52: 249–253.
159. Suckling RD, Fitzgerald PH, Stewart J, Wells E. The incidence and epidemiology of retinoblastoma in New Zealand: A 30 year survey. *Br J Cancer* 1982;46:729–736.
160. Takahashi T, Tamura S, Inoue M et al. Retinoblastoma in a 26-year-old adult. *Ophthalmology* 1983;90:179–183.
161. Tolentino FI, Tablante RT. Cryotherapy of retinoblastoma. *Arch Ophthalmol* 1972;87: 52–55.
162. Traboulsi EI, Zimmerman LE, Manz H. Cutaneous malignant melanoma in survivors of heritable retinoblastoma. *Arch Ophthalmol* 1988;106:1059–1061.
163. Tucker MA, D'Angio GJ, Boice Jr JD et al. Bone sarcomas linked to radiotherapy and chemotherapy in children. *N Engl J Med* 1987;317:588–593.
164. Vogel F. Beratung beim retinoblastom. *Acta Genet* 1957;7:565.
165. Vogel F. Genetics of retinoblastoma. *Hum Genet* 1979;52:1–54.
166. Wackenheim A, van Damme W, Kosmann

P, Bittighoffer B. Computed tomography in ophthalmology. *Neuroradiology* 1977;13: 135–138.

167. Weinberg RA. Tumor suppressor genes. *Science* 1991;254:1138–1146.
168. Weinberg RA. Oncogenes and tumor suppressor genes. *Cancer J Clin* 1994;44:160–170.
169. White L. The role of chemotherapy in the treatment of retinoblastoma. *Retina* 1983; 3:194–199.
170. Yandell DW, Dryja TP. Detection of DNA sequence polymorphisms by enzymatic amplification and direct genomic sequencing. *Am J Hum Genet* 1989;45:547–555.
171. Yunis JJ, Ramsey N. Retinoblastoma and subband deletion of chromosome 13. *Am J Dis Child* 1978;132:161–163.
172. Zakka KA, Yee RD, Foos RY. Retinoblastoma in a 12-year-old girl. *Ann Ophthalmol* 1983; 15:88–91.
173. Zhu XP, Dunn JM, Phillips RA et al. Preferential germline mutation of the paternal allele in retinoblastoma. *Nature* 1989;340:312–313.
174. Zhu X, Dunn JM, Goddard AD et al. Mechanisms of loss of heterozygosity in retinoblastoma. *Cytogenet Cell Genet* 1992;59:248–252.
175. Zimmerman RA, Bilaniuk LT. Computed tomography in the evaluation of patients with bilateral retinoblastoma. *J Comput Assisted Tomogr* 1979;3:251–257.

VII.

Management

41

Vision Rehabilitation of the Patient with Genetic Eye Disease

JOSEPH L. DeROSE

Like everyone else, visually impaired people want to lead full, productive lives, and any intervention that may help them reach their goals should be considered. Low-vision rehabilitation services are scarce,[11] and most patients with low vision are left in the hands of eyecare practitioners who often do not attend to their rehabilitative needs.[7] This is not to say that these patients are poorly managed from a medical perspective; indeed, many receive the finest care possible. However, while their medical care may be flawless, their functional needs are not addressed. The thorough clinician should question patients about their functional problems and offer assistance accordingly. Rehabilitation should be thought of as the next logical step in patient management.

Working with patients with low vision should be thought of as a rehabilitation effort, not a procedural one. This is a critical distinction. Refractions, for example, are not always included in a low-vision evaluation and may be done only as needed to help determine the patient's visual abilities or for incorporation into an enhancement device. While many patients would benefit from a refraction, which is often overlooked during months or years of otherwise careful management, it should not be left for the low-vision rehabilitation team to conduct. Further, the goal of the low-vision evaluation should not be simply to prescribe devices. The specialist must address mobility, psychosocial issues, educational and occupational concerns, comorbidities, family support, and financial concerns, among others.

As low-vision rehabilitation evolves and matures, it behooves the eyecare professions to think of it as medical intervention. One desired benefit of this change in attitude may be better third-party funding for low-vision care, devices, and other services. Unfortunately, patients often are not referred for care because the practitioner believes that they cannot afford the services. Decisions about services and assistive devices should be based on medical necessity, efficacy, and cost-effectiveness of the desired outcome. Better funding may allow all patients to receive the rehabilitative care that they need.

THE STRUCTURE OF REHABILITATION

The World Health Organization has developed a hierarchical list of health problems.[30] Health care providers use this list to help define the flow of patient care, level of intervention, and providers' roles.[15]

Patients enter the medical system with a *disease* that is defined in terms of pathology and etiology. The dysfunction caused by the disease results in an *impairment* that depends on the severity and chronicity of the disease. Severe and chronic impairments cause *disabilities*. Disability is the inability to perform a necessary or desired function. Again, depending on their severity and chronicity, disabilities may turn into *handicaps*. Handicaps are barriers to functioning normally in society because of the interaction of disabilities with social and environmental constraints.[15] The aim of rehabilitation medicine is to diagnose and treat disabilities, with the objective of eliminating or limiting handicaps.

In treating visual disorders, ophthalmologists see patients at the start of this hierarchy. Visual disorders may eventually lead to disabilities and then handicaps. At every step, there should be intervention aimed at improving the patient's quality of life. If the clinician cannot resolve the disorder and a disability results, the patient should be transferred for low-vision rehabilitation. Although not every patient will want to take advantage of all the assistive devices and services offered, the decision should be the patient's, based on information and education.

NEW MODEL FOR DELIVERY OF LOW-VISION CARE

Vision rehabilitation has many parallels with rehabilitation medicine. However, one strength of rehabilitation medicine that vision rehabilitation could better emulate is a comprehensive team approach that exploits each member's specialty.[15]

The rehabilitation medicine team is led by the physiatrist, who evaluates the patient, diagnoses disabilities, and coordinates the rehabilitation effort. The other members of the team are the occupational therapist, physical therapist, and social worker. The low-vision research team at the Johns Hopkins Wilmer Eye Institute in Baltimore has proposed that vision rehabilitation provide a cohesive, coordinated service drawing on the traditional rehabilitation model, with members analogous to those on the rehabilitation medicine team. The analog to the physiatrist is the optometrist or ophthalmologist involved in the rehabilitation program (not necessarily the physician diagnosing and treating the visual disorder). The analog to the occupational therapist is the vision rehabilitation teacher. The analog to the physical therapist is the orientation and mobility instructor. The social worker performs in an identical crossover role. The ultimate goal of creating the interdisciplinary team is to provide better patient care, standardize low-vision services, and integrate low-vision rehabilitation into mainstream medicine.

SYSTEMS APPROACH TO LOW-VISION REHABILITATION

Patients are considered to have low vision when they are unable to perform desired or required tasks because of visual disability. Employed persons typically seek low-vision care sooner than retired persons because of the visual demands of maintaining job performance. Patient's attitude toward their vision loss may also contribute to their functional state. People differ in their ability to deal with an impairment and to keep it from becoming a disability or handicap.

Patients should qualify for low-vision rehabilitation when they experience difficulty performing important tasks or activities. Because of patients' individual temperaments and requirements, it is difficult if not impossible to quantify criteria numerically, as by visual acuity, contrast sensitivity function, visual field loss, etc. For this reason, the low-vision rehabilitation effort is often goal oriented, helping patients achieve stated goals such as writing checks, reading food labels or the newspaper, using low-vision aids, skills training, or modification of the environment. Rehabilitation can also be function or attitude oriented. A functional goal would be to help restore lost function, such as improving visual acuity and contrast and increasing visual field awareness. The aim of attitude-oriented rehabilitation is to help patients adjust psychologically to their visual loss and resulting impairment.

What most patients need is help in achieving specific goals. One way of defining these goals is by exploring the patient's life state. The life state is "a complex dynamic construct that encompasses a complete description of all aspects of the individual's life including emotional, psychological, and physical qualities."[14] The rehabilitation team determines the patient's life state through the following:

- Comprehensive intake questionnaires
- Thorough history
- Examination of the visual and other pertinent systems
- Functional assessment of impairments
- Performance of the visual and other pertinent systems

The rehabilitation team and the patient use the information they have gathered to develop a hierarchy of rehabilitation objectives, goals, and tasks. They might determine that the patient's objectives are education, career, and recreation. Then for each objective, they list goals. For example, for an objective of completing college, the goals might be traveling to and around the college, attending classes, taking part in extracurricular activities, and keeping up with coursework. Finally, for each goal, they list necessary tasks. For example, for the goal of attending classes, the tasks might be seeing the chalkboard, taking notes, reading in-class exercises, and taking exams. It is at this task level that most low-vision rehabilitation concentrates.

Clearly, patients should receive early and proper rehabilitation to improve their quality of life, enable them to meet as many of their objectives as possible, and enhance their medical management. As rehabilitation succeeds and patients' life state improves, their need for intervention lessens.

HISTORY TAKING IN PATIENTS WITH LOW VISION

In contrast to medical history taking, which seeks information about the disease process, low-vision history taking seeks to determine how the disease is affecting the patient's lifestyle and function. If possible, the questioner should minimize queries about the pathology (important as that is), recording only the basics of past and current treatments and other pertinent medical information. Instead, the discussion should explore lost visual functions and which functions patients consider most important to meeting their objectives. As a common example, a patient may present complaining of difficulty reading. The interviewer should ask follow-up questions aimed at identifying what types of material the patient reads and the settings in which it is read. Her answers help define the main goals of the intervention. Other goals and training strategies may evolve as the program proceeds.

With some patients, the questioner cannot help being drawn into a prolonged discussion about the disease and its prognosis. Patients should understand their visual prognosis and why they need low-vision rehabilitation. Those who lack this understanding face a hurdle to the rehabilitation process. If they falsely believe that their vision will improve, they may not be fully receptive to intervention. Alternatively, if they falsely believe that they are about to go totally blind, they may think that rehabilitation is useless. Patients must be disabused of these misconceptions if they are to understand their true situation and benefit from rehabilitation. But if total blindness is truly a possibility, it is advisable to get the rehabilitation process started and then introduce the concept of services for the blind. All states have agencies for the blind, and there are national organizations as well.

Duration of vision loss is very important. If the disability is long standing, patients have probably adapted to some extent. They may also have had prior low-vision evaluations and may have experience with assistive devices and services. Newly impaired individuals still have psychosocial hurdles to overcome, and this will have an impact on their rehabilitation.

Patients should be questioned carefully about the effects of lighting conditions and weather, both of which can significantly affect visual function. Improving illumination is one of the simplest yet most effective modifications a patient can make. Reading almost always improves with bright direct lighting, such as halogen desk lamps. Many people also find that their visual performance changes with the weather. Sunny days may cause too much glare, but cloudy ones may be tolerable. Patients with diseased peripheral retinal tissue may experience glare on sunny days but may not have enough illumination at night. Glare and sunlight problems can often be alleviated with light-absorbing filters (see "Absorptive Filters" below). The rehabilitation specialist must individualize recommendations for each patient.

Other critical areas to discuss include family support and the availability of help with tasks such as reading and writing. Most patients who live alone wish to be more autonomous than those who live with others and have more support. Transportation must be addressed; in particular, many visually impaired individuals want to be able to drive (see "Concerns About Driving" below).

The interviewer must also review patients' visual needs at school and work. Students require resources that will enable them to do significant amounts of reading and writing. They should be considered for magnifiers, closed-circuit television (CCTV), text enlargement, text-to-speech devices, and volunteer readers. Although many students can read the chalkboard if they sit close to it, some students need distance devices such as telescopes or the Low Vision Enhancement System (LVES) (developed at the Lions Vision Rehabilitation Center of the Johns Hopkins University School of Medicine). Most office workers need some form of magnification for reading, such as prismatic or aspheric spectacles (referred to as microscopes). They may also need bright desk lighting for their paperwork or text-enlargement software for their computers.

Recording the initial history can be one of the most valuable parts of the evaluation, as it sets the tone for the remaining intervention and helps establish the service provider's relationship with the patient.

VISION ASSESSMENT

Visual acuity and contrast sensitivity measure specific components of visual capabilities but do not always predict functional visual performance. The physician should determine patients' color vision, stereo acuity, the effect of varying illumination and glare, and the effects of scotomas and distortion. Patients need this information, for example, for obtaining financial assistance, driving licenses (restricted or unrestricted), status of legal blindness, handicap-designated license tags, income tax deductions, job disability determination, free 411 phone service, and special mass transportation privileges.

It is preferable to avoid "counting fingers" and "hand motion" recordings of acuity; they often translate into a real measurement of 20/300 to 20/1000. Record and tell patients their actual acuity measurements. This may be the first time in years that their vision has had a number attached to it. Knowing their true vision can help them accept their visual loss and make them more receptive to rehabilitation. Acuity measurements also let the physician monitor how the underlying disease is affecting the patient's visual function and how the rehabilitation program may need to be adjusted.

The ETDRS (Early Treatment Diabetic Retinopathy Study) high-contrast illuminated chart (Fig. 41.1) is a better choice for low-vision patients than the standard Snellen chart. The ETDRS chart permits acuity measurement of all but the most profoundly impaired individuals. This chart uses Sloan optotypes[25] with the optotype size decreasing geometrically from line to line. This format more closely follows the functioning of the visual system and has been adopted by National Eye Institute-sponsored studies.

Start the acuity measurement using a close working distance. Twenty feet is too far for patients with an acuity worse than 20/100.[5] The ETDRS chart is placed at a distance of 1–3 m. This lets patients begin by succeeding at reading the chart and demonstrating their capability. Low-vision assessments are more concerned with determining a patient's capability than loss. Early success helps keep patients motivated, and motivation is one of the most important factors in a successful rehabilitation program. Handheld flip charts, such as the Feinbloom Distance Test Chart, can be held very close to the patient and is good for bedridden individuals. Because this chart is not illuminated, ambient lighting conditions affect acuity measurements and should be taken into consideration.

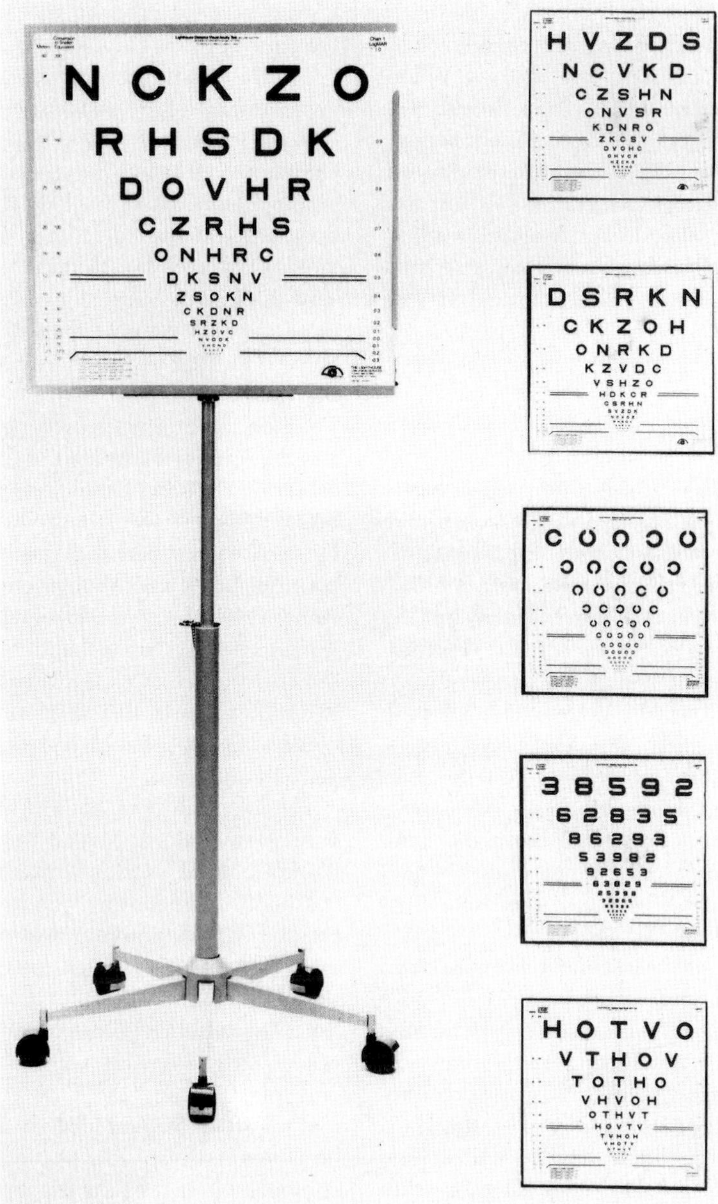

Figure 41.1. The Ferris-Bailey Early Treatment Diabetic Retinopathy Study (ETDRS) Distance Visual Acuity Test. (Courtesty of Lighthouse Low Vision Products.)

Near vision is best tested with charts or cards that use metric or "M" notation. An example of these cards are the MNREAD cards developed at the University of Minnesota.[13] In this system, the height of the print is expressed, in meters, as the distance at which the letters subtend 5 minutes of arch (Snellen equivalent of 20/20). Therefore, 1 M text is equivalent to 20/20 acuity when viewed at 1 m. Similarly, 0.4 M print is equivalent to 20/20 when held at 40 cm. The M system allows the physician to quickly compute the equivalent reading add (see "Magnifiers for Near Use" below). When testing near acuity, the physician should give attention to proper illumination and patient posture. Because reading is the most desired near task, cards that have continuous text are preferred over single-letter designs. Reading speed can be plotted against letter size; this helps determine the print size that yields fastest reading speed.

CONTRAST TESTING

Contrast is defined as the difference in luminance between an object and its background relative to the luminance of the background. *Contrast threshold* is the minimum contrast needed to distinguish a target; the reciprocal of this value is *contrast sensitivity*. Contrast sensitivity varies with spatial frequency (i.e., fineness of detail). These values can be plotted as a *contrast sensitivity function*. Small targets and fine detail test high spatial frequency, but most daily activities require lower frequency. Contrast sensitivity falls off at the higher and lower frequencies, with a maximum value roughly at the spatial frequency corresponding to a visual acuity of 20/100.

The contrast sensitivity function can become distorted in four ways[21]: loss of contrast sensitivity at higher spatial frequencies, a general loss at all frequencies, a loss mainly at the intermediate and low frequencies, or loss restricted to the intermediate frequencies. A loss at higher frequencies may begin to show up at an acuity level of about 20/40, but may not cause the patient significant problems. Loss at lower and intermediate frequencies can cause problems with mobility and face recognition because facial features, like most details of natural objects, have very low contrast.

Reasons for testing contrast include gathering baseline data other than visual acuity; determining the need for increased magnification, lighting, and contrast control; and predicting the better functioning eye. Some patients prefer using the eye with poorer visual acuity; this apparent paradox is often solved when contrast testing reveals better sensitivity in the preferred eye.

Contrast testing can be done with printed low-contrast letter charts such as the Pelli-Robson (distributed by Clement Clark, Inc., Columbus, OH) and Regan charts,[21] sine wave grating charts, which include the Vision Contrast Test System (VCTS by Vistech Consultants, Dayton, OH), the Sine-Wave Contrast Test (SWCT by Stereo Optical, Chicago), and the Functional Acuity Contrast Test (FACT by Stereo Optical); and electronic systems such as the Mentor (Santa Barbara, CA) BVAT unit. The electronic units are used mostly in research and the printed charts are usually used in clinical settings.[3] Rubin found that test–retest reliability is highest with the Pelli–Robson chart. He also determined that grating charts have poor reliability.[22] Ginsburg found that the Pelli-Robson chart tests very low spatial frequencies (target sizes are larger than the region of peak sensitivity at 3–6 cycles per degree), compared to grating charts that test an approximately equal range of spatial frequencies around the peak frequencies.[9]

Patients with poor contrast sensitivity have only a few options. Magnifying a target shifts it into a more sensitive area of the contrast sensitivity curve putting it above threshold. Increased illumination improves reading by lowering the patient's contrast threshold and allows the object to fall within the curve. Contrast is not easy to enhance, but it can be done with optoelectronic devices such as the closed circuit television and the Low Vision Enhancement System. Several of these approaches can be combined. Probably the most widely used combination in clinical practice is increased illumination and magnification.

VISUAL FIELD ASSESSMENT

Mapping of central and peripheral scotomas is useful in the management of visually impaired individuals, especially those with genetic eye diseases. Documenting visual field loss helps the physician monitor progression of the underlying disease. It helps the rehabilitation team provide mobility and visual skills training and evaluate the potential benefit of assistive devices. Visual field measurements are used in the determination of legal blindness status and driving privileges.

Patients with macular dystrophies may have intact peripheral visual fields allowing automated perimetry. Testing of the central 10° permits close scrutiny of scotomas and monitoring of disease. Peripheral field testing requires kinetic testing. This type of study identifies islands of vision and blindness in the far periphery, such as that seen in retinitis pigmentosa, and is important for mobility concerns.

There is some controversy over whether patients with central scotomata should use their parafoveal fixation point during visual field testing or should "look into the scotoma" and try to place the fixation target in the foveal area even though they cannot see it. The latter technique is often recommended in low-vision textbooks, but there are good clinical arguments for testing the visual field relative to the patient's true locus of fixation rather than the macula. Eccentric fixation training, mobility training, and the fitting of assistive devices all benefit from knowledge of the relative position of scotomas with respect to true fixation.

COLOR VISION

Color capabilities can be determined with an enlarged version of the Farnsworth D-15 test (Munsell Color, New Windsor, NY). Knowing patients' color vision may help the clinician counsel them about career choice and job training, and will also aid in making remedial suggestions (see "Reduced Central Vision with Intact Peripheral Function" below). Color perception can be used diagnostically to differentiate the inherited macular dystrophies and optic neuropathies.

ECCENTRIC VIEWING

Most low-vision patients with central scotomas tend to use off-foveal retinal locations for fixation.[4] These locations are commonly called *preferred retinal loci,* or PRL, and this visual behavior is called *eccentric fixation.*[23] Eccentric fixation allows patients to maintain a relatively steady state of fixation despite their poor acuity. The PRL develops spontaneously and tends to be very close to the edge of the scotoma. Development of the PRL most likely is related to a reorganization of the primary visual cortex in response to the scotoma.[10]

Patients with scotomas are not readily aware of the resultant blind spots, but they are aware of their effects. They usually complain of distortion or report that their visual targets flash in and out of view as they try to fixate on them. Work by Sunness et al.[29] and Guez et al.[8] shows that patients prefer to put the scotoma above or to the right of fixation in visual field space. Placing the scotoma superiorly in visual space makes sense because it leaves the inferior field available for locomotion and reading. But research on normal eyes shows that the field to the right of the fovea is important for word recognition.[19,20] Reading with the scotoma projected to the right is believed to cut off words and can reduce reading speed.

Sunness et al.[29] also compared off-foveal fixation patterns in patients with geographic atrophy to those with Stargardt disease. She found that 63% of the eyes with geographic atrophy placed the fixation point to the left of the scotoma, whereas 90% of the eyes with Stargardt disease preferred to fixate with the scotoma projected superiorly. Sunness also found that eyes with geographic atrophy fixated immediately adjacent to the atrophy, but most eyes with Stargardt's placed the PRL as much as 2° from the edge of the atrophy. The authors postulated that this latter fixation pattern results from disease in the intervening tissue.

Neuromuscular Re-education

While all patients with a central scotoma demonstrate some type of PRL, some do not maintain a steady state of fixation and are constantly searching for the best off-foveal location. Anecdotal clinical evidence supports the notion that when these individuals are trained to find and use the optimal retinal locus, they improve their reading rate and overall visual performance.

Thus, they should be offered training for eccentric viewing. Finding the best PRL can be guided by visual field data, but is done largely by trial and error. Once patients find the best PRL, they are instructed to use it consistently and not search for other locations. With time, patients should learn to use the same eccentric viewing position almost automatically. Reading tests can be used to determine their increase in reading speed and efficiency, and to monitor their progress. While eccentric viewing certainly has limitations, it is one of the most valuable visual skills that the rehabilitation team can offer.

DETERMINATION OF ASSISTIVE DEVICES

The best assistive device for a particular task is often determined experimentally. Success with low-vision devices is very subjective. Similarly impaired patients have varied responses to the same aid. Many physical and mental factors influence the outcome. However, the rehabilitation team should direct the device selection process and not allow nonproductive preference testing.

Types of Magnification

There are four types of magnification:

1. *Relative distance magnification* is simple—moving the target closer to the patient. The retinal images become larger and hence easier to see. The relationship is linear, so the magnification is directly related to how much the viewing distance changes. Decreasing the distance to one third of the original results in 3× magnification. Patients are often told to sit closer to their television set.
2. *Relative size magnification* is also simple—enlarging the target. This is the principle used by large-print reading material, large screen TVs, large-print phone dials, etc.
3. *Angular magnification* is used when neither target size nor viewing distance can be modified. The angular size of the image at the eye is enlarged through the use of lenses. This type of enlargement is provided by telescopes.
4. *Optoelectronic magnification* is provided by electronic systems such as CCTV and LVES.

Telescopes

Determination of required magnification depends on the goals of the patient. A simple illustration is a man who needs to see 20/40 at distance. If his best corrected acuity is 20/200, then he needs 5× magnification to achieve his goal (reference size/goal size = 200/400 = 5). Telescopes are *afocal* systems, that is, light rays are parallel both entering and leaving the device (Fig. 41.2). The targets are at optical infinity and the light rays are changed only in the angular magnification of the target's image. Because the light rays leaving the telescope are parallel, the patient needs to wear his distance corrective lenses, but an add is not needed because additional focusing is not required. Clinically, the telescope's focusing system can compensate, within limts, for uncorrected refractive error, so patients may not always have to wear their distance correction.

Two types of telescope are used for low-vision patients:

Kepler (astronomical) telescopes use plus lenses for both the ocular and the objective. This creates an inverted image, so a prism is used to make the image erect. The disadvantage is that the prism makes the telescope larger and heavier. The advantage is that the image is brighter and larger.

Galilean (terrestrial) telescopes use a minus lens for the ocular. This creates an erect image. The image is smaller and not quite as bright as with the Kepler telescope. However, the Galilean telescope is usually preferred because of its simpler optics, lighter weight, and smaller size.

Telescopes can be used in several ways:

A *hand-held spotting device* is the simplest. In this capacity, the telescope is used for only brief periods to view a specific target, much like binoculars. Hand and arm motion can cause blurring of the image, especially at the higher powers (above 6×).

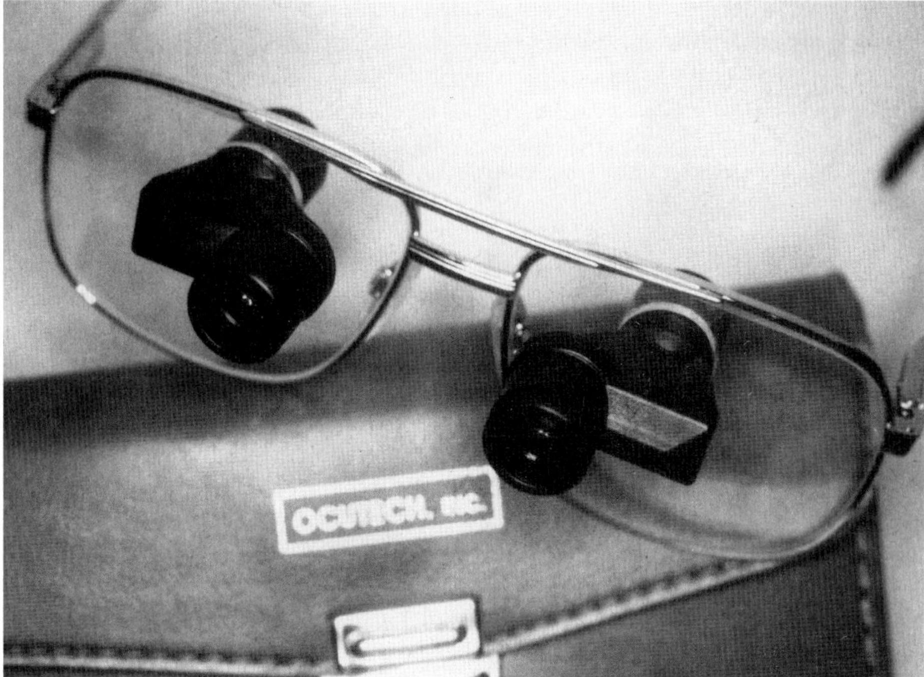

A

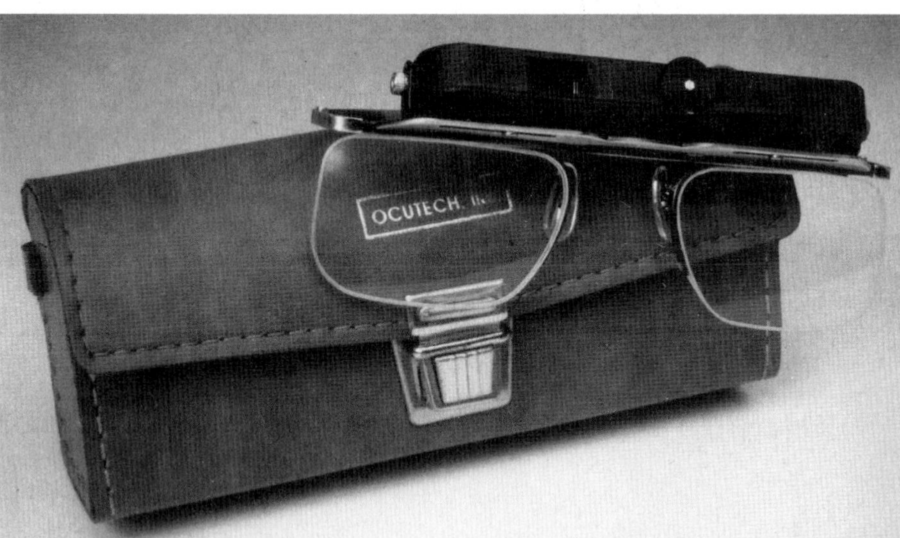

B

Figure 41.2. Bioptic mounted telescopic systems by Ocutech, Inc. **A:** The Vision Enhancement System (VES) minibinocular device. A single telescope may be used if acuities are unequal. **B:** The VES II. This is a monocular system; the telescope may be placed above the frame as shown, or mounted flush with the top of the frame. (Courtesy of Ocutech, Inc., Chapel Hill, NC.)

Bioptic position: This is a permanently mounted telescope. If the patient requires unmagnified as well as magnified vision, the telescope is mounted on the superior part of the lens, above the visual axis. In this bioptic position, it stays out of the way until it is needed. The patient uses the telescope by tilting her head down to align her visual axis with the telescope's exit pupil. This type of mounting is good for driving, walking, and other distance viewing tasks.

Full-diameter position: The telescope is permanently mounted at the optical center of the carrier lens. This central positioning is appropriate for prolonged viewing such as watching television and sporting events, and allows an unobstructed alignment of the person's visual axis with the telescope's exit pupil. Because of the more correct alignment, the image tends to be largest and brightest in this position.

Reading mount: The telescope is permanently mounted low in the lens, requiring users to lower their eyes for proper alignment. This position is useful for reading, occupational tasks, and hobbies. Because these targets are not at optical infinity (less than 20 ft), the device is technically operating as a microscope, and the optics are designed accordingly.

Monocular versus binocular systems: Some patients may require only one telescope, especially if one eye has particularly poor acuity. In a monocular system, the scope is mounted in front of the better eye, and the other eye can still be used for mobility. Binocular systems can be used when acuity is reasonably equivalent in the two eyes and the patient's desired use would benefit from binocularity, such as watching television, sporting events, or theater. Drawbacks of a binocular system include heavier weight and extra cost.

Temporary versus permanent mounting: Telescopes can be clipped on as needed, or mounted permanently (e.g., glued into the carrier lens). Students especially like temporary mounting, as they would rather not walk around school with a telescope protruding from their spectacles.

Telemicroscope: This is a telescope capable of focusing on close targets (e.g., having microscopic capability). It is usually hand-held or a monocular mount. Although telemicroscopes offer flexibility by providing two functions, the trade-off is that they tend to be larger and heavier. There is no sense using telemicroscopes in binocular systems because the convergence angle cannot be changed and the viewing distance is necessarily fixed.

Magnifiers for Near Use

Prescribing devices for near use can be confusing because of differences in labeling techniques and reference distance. The important point is to select these aids according to the dioptric power needed to achieve the required magnification at the initial testing (reference) distance. For example, a patient with a +2.50 add who can read 4 M print at 40 cm would need 4× to read a print size of 1 M at 40 cm (i.e., reference size/goal size = 4 M/1 M = 4). What power lens would be needed to provide this magnification? We can determine the required *equivalent add* by multiplying the add on the patient's distance correction by the print size she reads (using M notation). In this example, the equivalent add = 2.50 × 4 = 10.00 diopters. The equivalent add is the dioptric power of a lens required to magnify 1 M print to the same retinal image size as the unmagnified reference print.

American manufacturers use the specification that 4 diopters equals 1×. Four diopters is the add required for a reference distance of 25 cm. A 6× magnifier would have a lens of 24 diopters (6 × 4 diopters = 24). If we return to the example in the previous paragraph, the amount of magnification yielded by the 10 diopter lens was 4×, but using the specification of 1× = 4 diopters, we see that the calculated amount of magnification is 10/4 = 2.5×, and not the 4× we actually obtained. This discrepancy is explained by the fact that we used a different reference distance (40 cm) from the manufacturers' (25 cm).

European manufacturers make things even more complicated. Their specification is the manufacturer's magnification minus 1 times 4 (e.g., [10 − 1] × 4 = 36 diopters for a 10× device). The best way to avoid this confusion is to determine the equivalent add needed as per the discussion above, and then select a magnifier based on its dioptric value, rather than its labeled magnification power.

Near aids come in spectacle, hand-held, and stand versions. Some are illuminated and can be powered by batteries or plug-in alternating

Table 41.1. Advantages and Disadvantages of Near Magnification Devices

Type of Device	Advantages	Disadvantages	Primary Use
Spectacle	Hands free	Close reading distance	Reading
Handheld magnifier	Small, light	Hard to maintain focal distance	Brief spotting
Stand magnifier	Fixed focal distance	Bulkier	Reading
Closed-circuit television	Very powerful	Large, not portable	Prolonged reading

current. Choice of an aid depends on its advantages and disadvantages (Table 41.1) in relation to the patient's resources and ability.

Spectacles have the considerable advantage of leaving the patient's hands free. This is particularly helpful for patients who have weak muscle strength, motor tremors, paralysis or paresis, or other conditions that would make it difficult for them to hold a device properly. Because spectacles allow for relative distance magnification, increasing power requires decreasing distance from the object to the patient's eyes. This working distance can sometimes be very small and uncomfortable to the patient. A 20 diopter lens (5×) has a focal point of 5 cm. For this reason, given a choice, many individuals select a stand magnifier.

Stand magnifiers also use relative distance magnification, but the distance between the device (which rests on the target object) and the patient's eyes does not affect the amount of magnification, so the patient can hold the device farther away, at a more comfortable working distance. The disadvantages of stand magnifiers are that they must rest on a flat, stable surface, and the patient usually must be hunched over to some degree to view through them. Conditions such as arthritis can make this a less desirable option.

Hand-held magnifiers are smaller, lighter, and more portable. This makes them the device of choice for traveling, shopping, and brief spotting (such as appliance dials, price-tags, and food labels). Although handheld magnifiers are good for brief reading tasks, they are usually unsuitable for prolonged use as they need to be held at a fixed distance from the target to maintain the proper focal distance. This can be quite burdensome, especially for patients with problems like hand tremors, poor grip strength, peripheral neuropathies, or paresis.

Illuminated versions of stand and hand-held devices are available. Illumination can be critical for the majority of low-vision patients who have reduced contrast sensitivity. A major advantage of illuminated magnifiers is that they can be used without regard to the ambient lighting. Small illuminated hand-held devices are excellent choices for shopping, theater, restaurant dining, etc. Larger stand units are good for reading at a desk or table and are particularly good for low-contrast material such as newspapers.

The most powerful device available for near use is CCTV (Fig. 41.3). A video camera captures a signal and feeds it to the viewing monitor. Magnification can range from 3× to over 60×. Units are available in color and black and white. Users place a document on a movable table and view its image projected onto the screen. At first, some people find it awkward to look in a direction different from the target material. Becoming proficient requires some practice and adaptability, but the payoff is tremendous. No other device is as effective as CCTV. It is particularly useful for patients like students and business people who must read for long periods. Because the screen is illuminated and has controls for contrast, brightness, and color, CCTV is well suited to people with poor contrast sensitivity.

SPECIALIZED DEVICES

The Low Vision Enhancement System

The Low Vision Enhancement System (Fig. 41.4) uses electronic processing to create an enhanced image. The LVES provides contrast enhancement, automatic focus, and variable zoom magnification. Automatic gain control ad-

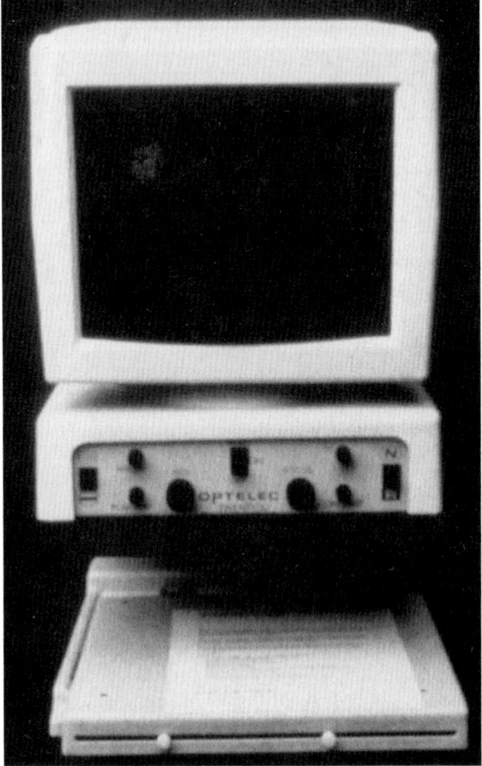

Figure 41.3. The Spectrum 2020 closed-circuit television by Optelec, Inc. (Courtesy of Optelec, Inc., Westford, MA.)

justs for varying levels of environmental illumination to maintain relatively constant image brightness. Future features will include text manipulation and image remapping around scotomas. Advantages of the LVES include the ability to improve both distance and near vision as well as contrast; operation in dim illumination; variable magnification; and automatic focus. Disadvantages include cost, size, weight, and necessary training.

Text Enlargement Software

Software programs such as Zoomtext (Ai Squared, Manchester Center, VT) LP-DOS (Optelec US, Inc., Westford, MA), and Magic (Microsystems Software, Framingham, MA) enlarge the text on personal computer displays. This software is particularly helpful to patients whose jobs require using personal computers.

Speech Output Devices

Although we tend to think of low-vision rehabilitation as vision oriented, we should consider any device that helps patients achieve their goals. Speech output (also called "text-to-speech") units can be very beneficial because they bypass the eyes and use the ears. Once patients adapt to using a different sense for familiar tasks, they can reach levels of efficiency and speed not possible by their vision alone. Two systems currently available are The Reading Edge by Xerox Corporation (Stamford, CT) and the Arkenstone (Arkenstone, Sunnyvale, CA) system. Printed text is scanned in then read back through speech synthesis algorithms (text-to-speech conversion). Current versions of these systems can quite accurately recognize text in different fonts and cases, the output rate can be varied, and they offer various voices representing both genders. The Reading Edge is a standalone system but can be connected to a personal computer for additional capabilities. The Arkenstone unit requires a personal computer that has at least an 80486 processor. Patients can save money if they already own an appropriate computer to which they can attach the unit (Fig. 41.5).

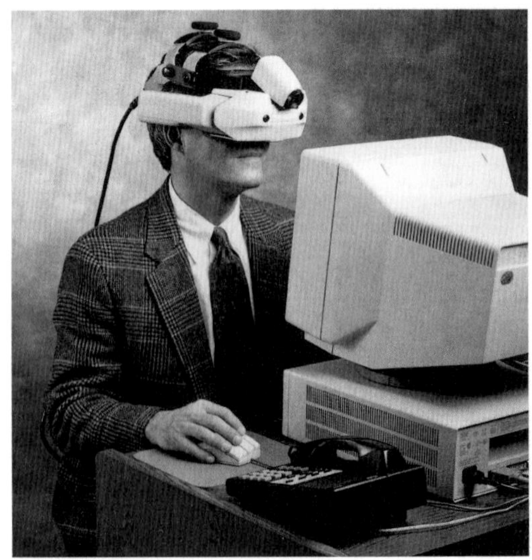

Figure 41.4. The Low Vision Enhancement System, manufactured by Visionics Corporation. (Courtesy of Visionics Corp.)

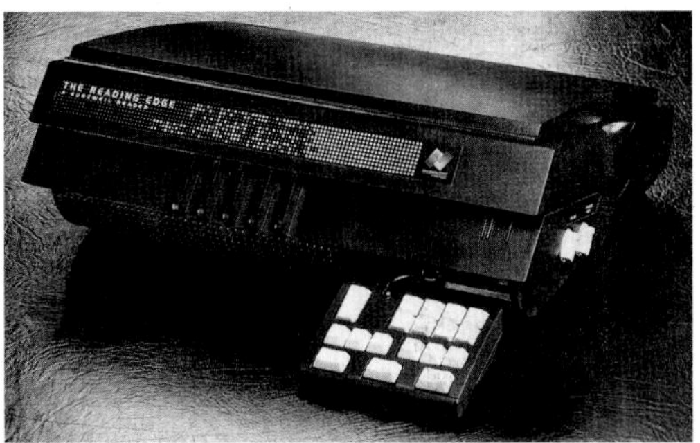

Figure 41.5. The Reading Edge by Xerox Corporation, Stamford, CT. Documents are placed on the scanning bed and the text is converted to synthesized speech. (Courtesy of Xerox Corp.)

Other systems can be used in conjunction with personal computers to convert text to speech as it scrolls on the monitor. These systems are paticularly useful for totally blind patients who need to operate a personal computer. For patients who have some vision, combining large-print software with speech output can increase reading speed more than either system can alone. As technology produces more powerful processors and as software becomes more capable of using this additional power, we can only expect even more benefits for people with impairments. Text enlargement and speech output, combined with easier access to the Internet, offer unprecedented opportunities.

IMPORTANT NONOPTICAL CONSIDERATIONS

Illumination

As we have been stressing, most low-vision patients require strong illumination. Sheedy et al. reported that acuity in normally sighted people increases with increasing luminance, up to about 600 cd/m^2.[24] Sloan found that patients with macular degeneration benefit greatly from increased illumination[26] and suggested that high-intensity lamps be used routinely in evaluating low-vision patients.[27] Small high-intensity lamps, particularly halogen, are often recommended as an adjunct to optical devices, and are the only enhancement that some patients need.

The visual system is not equally sensitive to the entire visible spectrum. Sensitivity is greatest between 500 nm and 600 nm. Sunlight energy is fairly constant in all areas of the spectrum because the light is produced by the sun's very high temperature. Most patients see best with natural sunlight. Artificial light sources do not produce equal energy levels across the spectrum. Fluorescent emission is high in the shorter wavelengths (blue–violet) that scatter more and cause glare. Incandescent lamps emit higher energy in the longer wavelengths (red–orange–yellow) and tend to be better tolerated by low-vision patients. Halogen lamps are incandescent bulbs that burn hotter and therefore produce a whiter light, more closely resembling sunlight.

Some patients cannot tolerate bright or even modest levels of illumination. Photosensitivity may be found with rod monochromatism, achromatopsia, cone–rod dystrophies, some variants of retinitis pigmentosa, and diabetic retinopathy. However, there is great variation among patients, even those with the same pathology. Thus, subjective responses are essential in selecting lighting.

Overhead lights are typically poor sources since the light is diffuse by the time it reaches the target. The patient may block the light when leaning over to read, especially when using a magnifier. Flexible neck lamps with a reflector shade are preferred because they can direct the light onto the reading material and can be aligned to prevent glare and reflections. Placing the light source behind the patient so that the light comes over the shoulder is a popular position that directs reflected light away from the patient's eyes. When patients cannot control their lighting, as in restaurants and theaters, illuminated magnifiers can be particularly useful.

Absorptive Filters

Patients who are photosensitive to sunlight, or even to normal levels of indoor illumination, can be helped by sunglasses or special absorptive filters. Selection is largely by trial and error, but filters that absorb the shorter wavelengths are generally more effective. Photoreceptors are most sensitive to green light.[17] This means that less energy in the green area is needed to produce a given luminance intensity than the other colors. Therefore, wavelengths shorter than green (blue–violet–ultraviolet) can be filtered out to reduce glare and internal scatter, but without significantly reducing brightness.

A widely used series of lenses that have been thoroughly researched and designed to filter specific wavelengths are the Corning Photochromic Filters (CPF) (Corning, Inc., Corning, NY). They are available with spectral cutoffs of 450 nm, 511 nm, 527 nm, and 550 nm. The lenses absorb almost all light falling below the cutoffs. The 550 nm filter, the first one produced, was designed for and has proven popular among patients with retinitis pigmentosa. The lighter CPF 527 and CPF 511 filters are more often used for persons who are less photosensitive; because these filters leave more visible spectrum unattenuated, they produce a brighter image. All the CPF lenses are photochromic, darkening when exposed to sunlight. They are made of glass, so they are heavier than plastic lenses, although lighter clip-on lenses are available. Another popular series is the plastic NoIR filters (NoIR Medical Technologies, South Lyon, MI), which come in a variety of spectral cutoffs and densities.

Daily Living Aids

Reduced peripheral fields and central scotomas make it difficult to localize on a page and maintain line position. Writing guides are helpful in maintaining position on the paper. Reading guides, commonly referred to as *typoscopes,* are small pieces of black cardboard or plastic with windows cut out to help maintain position on the line. Other useful devices are large-print phone dialers, needle threaders, talking clocks, bold-lined writing paper, and dark felt-tipped pens.

Large-print reading materials use relative-size magnification. Religious materials and several periodicals, including *Reader's Digest,* are available in large print. There are even large-print versions of income tax preparation packages. Most larger cities have libraries that handle large-print books and periodicals as well as "talking books" (audiocassette tapes). Also available in many larger cities are radio reading services, in which on-air volunteers read magazine articles, portions of books, newspapers, religious materials, etc., according to a daily schedule. The signals, carried as a subband on frequencies usually used by public radio stations, require special decoding receivers. These receivers are usually loaned to users, and voluntary donations solicited.

ORIENTATION AND MOBILITY TRAINING

Many people with total or partial visual loss, especially those with reduced peripheral fields, can benefit from orientation and mobility (O&M) instruction. This training is provided by specialists who have a master's degree in O&M and vision rehabilitation. Patients learn to be more aware of their position in the environment and to move about in that environment more safely and independently. Training can be intensive, taking several weeks or months. Patients may use visual aids such as telescopes and prisms, and nonvisual assistance such as sighted guides, canes, and guide dogs. Training is usually offered through state rehabilitation or educational systems, or on a fee-for-service basis.

MANAGEMENT OF SPECIFIC PATTERNS OF VISION LOSS

Hereditary eye diseases affect vision in one of three ways: (*1*) reduced central vision with intact peripheral function, (*2*) intact central acuity with abnormal peripheral function, and (*3*) reduced central and peripheral function. Determining the type of vision loss a given pathology produces allows the visual rehabilitation specialist to design an intervention strategy.

Reduced Central Vision with Intact Peripheral Function

The hereditary macular dystrophies fall into this category. Magnification is generally very useful in these cases since enlargement of the retinal image places some of it onto the healthier peripheral tissue. The early age of onset of disease in affected patients allows the development of good eccentric viewing techniques, and as a result, many have good reading speed. Central visual fields (e.g., Humphrey central 10°) help determine the size and depth of the scotoma.

Devices for near are helpful with reading. Spectacle-mounted lenses permit hands-free reading. Lower-powered prismatic spectacles in the +6.00 diopter to +12.00 diopter range are sufficient for individuals with moderate loss. Higher powered aspheric lenses are needed by patients with more severe loss. Stand magnifiers are useful at the patient's desk or workstation, and more portable hand-held magnifiers are useful for reading labels, tags, menus, short memos, and the like. Increased lighting at the patient's desk or reading area improves reading speed. Incandescent lamps may be sufficient, but halogen sources usually help patients with more severe functional loss.

Patients who use computers may benefit from text-enlarging software. However, with the decreasing costs of computer hardware, some users would do better to obtain a larger monitor (17 inches or more), which is only slightly more expensive than some software programs. New hardware and operating systems let users adjust text size, font, color, contrast, and brightness. Those with severe loss can add text-to-speech programs to their systems, or use a stand-alone speech output machine such as The Reading Edge by Xerox. Some employers fund part or all of the purchase of these systems. Closed-circuit television systems are very useful, especially for those who do a lot of reading. Some newer CCTV models may be interfaced with personal computers. The Reading Edge can also be interfaced with a personal computer and store large quantities of text. Entire articles and books may be scanned, stored, and then read back at the patient's discretion.

Because most patients in this category have good peripheral retinal function, few have serious problems with orientation and mobility. Handheld telescopes can be prescribed to help spot landmarks, bus numbers, signs, etc. Mounted bioptic telescopes are useful for seeing television, movies, blackboards, theater, and driving (see "Concerns about Driving," below). These patients do well to have several devices, each suited to a different type of task.

Most patients' color vision is impaired by their disease. They may need to be counseled about this. Young patients should be told that they may not qualify for certain careers because of their loss of acuity and color vision. Increasing color contrast helps compensate for loss of color vision. Patients should experiment to find the optimal color choices, but generally they are helped by maximizing the contrast between foreground and background colors.[1] For example, black on white (and vice versa) gives the most contrast, but any light color should also contrast well against black. Patients should be helped to apply this advice to modifying their home and workplace.

Intact Central Acuity with Abnormal Peripheral Function

The hereditary disorder that usually causes this pattern is retinitis pigmentosa. Central vision may be preserved for many years. If patients have a small central visual field, they may be helped by field expanders—devices that work like reverse telescopes to "minify" the image, allowing more of it to fit in the visual field. However, not all patients like field expanders because they can distort the image. Visual field testing shows the extent of field loss, but since it is rarely central, patients do not need to learn eccentric viewing. Those who have reduced central acuity may be helped with some magnification if their central visual field is sufficiently large. They should try modestly powered spectacle magnifiers, but they may prefer stand and hand magnifiers. They can manipulate the field area on stand magnifiers by moving the device away from their eyes. Similarly, they can alter the position of hand-held devices to change the size of the image.

Photophobia and glare control are important concerns for these patients since their rod function is most affected. Patients with extreme photophobia will require lenses with very low light transmission, such as the CPF 550 XD (Extra Dark, for outdoor use), and may need filters indoors. Absorptive filters can also help patients with slow light and dark adaptation. Unfortunately, little can be done to correct reduced night vision. Patients can be advised to carry a bright flashlight when walking in the dark. Other solutions include image intensifiers such as nightscopes. Increasing contrast helps some patients. Patients who use a computer can adjust the brightness, colors, contrast, and size of the text using software and the computer television monitor's own controls. Closed-circuit TV is also a good option, but it must be used at low magnification if the patient has small visual fields. The Low Vision Enhancement System can be helpful because of its ability to enhance contrast. Text-to-speech systems may be advisable for those with greatly reduced reading speeds.

Mobility is often a problem for people with reduced peripheral fields. Orientation and mobility training can be helpful, especially cane travel training. Goldmann fields should be done to determine the extent of field loss and determine if the patient has peripheral islands of vision that can help with mobility. Fresnel prisms can sometimes help compensate for the visual field constriction; they are placed base out on one or both spectacle lenses to shift the image closer to the central area of seeing. Telescopes are often counterproductive due to the effects of magnification with field loss; nevertheless, some patients have enough central field to benefit from low-powered magnifiers. Pharmacological mydriasis may help patients with posterior subcapsular cataracts. The specialist may need to talk with patients about driving limitations.

Because patients lose their vision slowly, they have time to adjust to the loss (both physically and psychologically) and develop their own compensations as the disorder progresses. Many patients have specific needs that can be addressed directly, with minimal attention to areas that are not of concern. For example, a patient may begin by asking for help with mobility and help with glare on sunny days. Orientation and mobility training will help with travel, and a CPF 527 or 550 filter can help with the sunlight glare. The patient may not be having problems with reading and therefore needs no intervention in this area.

A special case is the patient who has both vision loss and hearing loss, as in Usher syndrome. Patients born with hearing loss who learn to sign or read lips can lose this ability when they lose much of their visual acuity. However, patients who are blind first and then lose hearing may do better, especially if they know Braille and cane travel. Whenever patients present with Usher syndrome or another disorder that can impair both sight and hearing, it is good to recommend Braille training as early as possible. These patients will require orientation and mobility training, but it may not be completely effective since they will have difficulty listening for environmental cues like traffic noise. Early counseling and referral will give them time to secure proper training and rehabilitation.

Reduction in Both Central and Peripheral Vision

Patients with reduced central and peripheral vision are the most difficult to manage because of abnormal function of the entire field of vision. This group includes people with advanced retinitis pigmentosa, other retinal dystrophies, microphthalmia, glaucoma and macular degeneration combined, and aniridia with advanced glaucoma. These diseases have great variability in nature and severity, so each patient must be evaluated individually. Patients should be allowed to try many types of magnifiers to see which they prefer.

Telescopes are helpful for distance use and may be hand-held or spectacle-mounted. Patients with photophobia or reduced contrast sensitivity should try absorptive filters. The Low Vision Enhancement System is also valuable for patients with visual acuity down to about 20/800, particularly if they need contrast enhancement. Orientation and mobility training should be considered. If patients do a lot of reading, CCTV is an excellent option. Text-to-speech programs and text-enlarging software can help patients who use computers.

Young people should be given educational and career counseling. They need to be advised of their prognosis and of factors like color vision loss that may keep them from certain careers.

Table 41.2. The Main Rehabilitation Effort of Selected Pathologies

Pathology	Visual Consequences	Main Rehabilitation Effort
Achromotopsia	Reduced central vision and color perception	Magnification; light filters; contrast enhancement
Albinism	Photophobia, reduced central vision	Magnification; light filters
Aniridia	Photophobia, reduced central vision	Magnification; light filters
Cone–rod dystrophy	Reduced central vision and color perception; photophobia	Magnification; light filters
Fundus flavimaculatus	Reduced central vision	Magnification; contrast enhancement
Leber's congenital amaurosis	Reduced central and/or peripheral vision; nyctalopia	Magnification; contrast enhancement; orientation and mobility training
Stargardt disease	Reduced central vision and color perception	Magnification; light filters; contrast enhancement
Retinitis pigmentosa	Reduced peripheral vision; nyctalopia	Field expanders; illumination at night; contrast enhancement; orientation and mobility training
Usher syndrome	Reduced peripheral vision; hearing loss	Orientation and mobility training; Braille training; magnification when indicated; contrast enhancement

A social worker can help patients address psychosocial issues. Some may need referral to local community services or state agencies such as the Division of Rehabilitation Services. Technology access centers may help those who are interested in working with computers (Table 41.2).

THE YOUNG PATIENT

Vision in babies and preschool children is tested objectively by electrophysiological techniques such as visual evoked potentials, electroretinograms, and electrooculograms. Subjective testing such as preferential looking is also widely used. Another way to get some indication of visual function is to test the ability to see bright lights, balls, optokinetic drums, matching letter charts, and flashcards. It is also important to have an infant's cognitive status assessed, as visual function does not exceed cognitive development.[2] Many children with visual impairments have other deficits that may need to be addressed.

If a child is found to be visually impaired, the parents should be referred for counseling, as the diagnosis will place the family in crisis.[6] Children who are expected to go totally or near-totally blind may need to learn Braille. Infants who are not totally blind require both active and passive visual stimulation. Visual targets can be brightly colored mobiles and toys as well as contrasting colors in the nursery. Paper cutouts of animals, toys, and people can be taped onto windows to create a silhouette. With multiply impaired children, the practitioner must assess other systems (vestibular, tactile, auditory, and olfactory) to determine the best plan for sensory integration and active visual stimulation. With proper attention to system integration and the appropriate level of stimulation for the child's threshold level, the child may be more receptive to visual stimulation.[28] For example, a child may be most receptive to your intervention when she is engaged in slow rocking, the lights are dim, quiet music is played, and light touching is avoided. Occupational and physical therapists will be needed to assist with this effort.

Because macular dystrophies manifest during the first and second decades of life, educational endeavors are affected. Students need telescopic devices to help them see the chalkboard. Near devices are less often prescribed because most children's amount of accommodation allows for a very close reading distance, providing relative distance magnification. Children with more serious vision loss (20/200 or worse) may need large print or magnification devices, or even a closed-circuit television. Other helpful services include taped lectures, volunteer readers, and large-print textbooks. Adolescents are concerned about their appearance. The specialist must discuss honestly with young people how noticeable assistive devices are, to help them be reasonably satisfied with and likely to use their prescribed device. All the professionals involved in young patients' care must help them learn to deal effectively with peer pressure.

It is important for ophthalmologists to work with young patients' educators and provide meaningful reports to the school. Physician reports should explain the student's diagnosis, level of visual function, and recommendations. Some teachers may not be accustomed to dealing with visually impaired children and will appreciate any help. They can be confused by students who appear to play satisfactorily on the playground, but complain of difficulty seeing the chalkboard, which requires better acuity. Teachers should be made aware of visual field losses that may affect a child's mobility, as well as color vision loss, contrast sensitivity loss, binocularity factors, and other problems that may affect school activities. Most schools have vision teachers who advocate for students and can give them assistance. Parents, too, may need information about their child's disease and visual function. They are often unsure of the child's current and future capabilities for education and career. If a child loses vision quickly, the family needs time to adjust, and the rehabilitation team needs to be able to respond appropriately.

Teenagers worry about how their vision will affect driving and dating. Driving is covered in the next section. Social concerns can be discussed with a social worker, and marriage and inheritance patterns can be addressed by a genetic counselor.

CONCERNS ABOUT DRIVING

Patients' concerns about driving often become a major rehabilitative issue. All states have laws specifying visual criteria for driving. The main factor is acuity, but most states also consider visual fields. Visual acuity and peripheral visual fields must be tested carefully to determine whether state requirements are met. More than half of states allow for a restricted telescopic license,[18] but regulations about driving with bioptics vary among states. In Maryland, for example, drivers must have 20/100 or better acuity in at least one eye with conventional correction and must be able to achieve 20/70 through the telescope; they must also have had the device for several months and be able to demonstrate proficiency in its use. Most states require training, proficiency, and experience before granting driving privileges. Check with each state's Division of Motor Vehicles for exact specifications.

When patients' vision becomes impaired to the degree that they will be permitted to drive only with a telescopic license, they seek a bioptic fitting from a low-vision practitioner. A bioptic system simply contains the patient's regular spectacle prescription in the carrier lens, and a telescopic device permanently mounted in a superior position. Patients look through the regular spectacle correction while driving, and use the telescope only for brief spotting.

Although most studies show higher accident rates for drivers with bioptics than for normally sighted control groups, bioptics drivers' accident rates may be lower than those of drivers with other impairments such as heart and neurological disorders.[12] However, there is more to driver safety than vision. Cognition, attitude, experience, road and weather conditions, and personal values regarding safety, are also important factors. The decision to allow a visually impaired person to drive often rests with the low-vision practitioner.

REFERENCES

1. Arditi A, Knoblauch K. Effective color contrast and low vision. In *Functional Assessment of Low Vision*, B. P. Rosenthal, R. G. Cole, eds. St. Louis: Mosby-Year Book, 1996:129–135.
2. Barraga NC, Collins ME. Development of efficiency in visual functioning: Rationale for a comprehensive program. *J Vis Impairm Blindn* 1979;73:121–126.
3. Cohen JM. Illumination, contrast, and glare:

Problems in poor vision. *Prac Optom* 1993;4(2): 60–66.
4. Cummings RW, Whittaker SG, Watson GR, Budd JM. Scanning characters and reading with a central scotoma. *Am J Optom Physiol Opt* 1985;62:833–843.
5. Faye EE. Refraction for conventional and prism spectacles. In *Clinical Low Vision,* 2nd ed. E. E. Faye, ed. Boston: Little, Brown and Company, 1984:27–44.
6. Gardner L. Understanding and helping parents of blind children. *J Vis Impairm Blindn* 1982; 76:81–85.
7. Greenblatt SL. Physicians and chronic impairment: A study of ophthalmologists' interactions with visually impaired and blind patients. *Soc Sci Med* 1988;26:393–399.
8. Guez J-E, Le Gargasson JF, Rigaudiere F, O'Regan JK. Is there a systematic location for the pseudo-fovea in patients with central scotoma? *Vis Res* 1993;33:1271–1279.
9. Ginsburg AP. Next generation contrast sensitivity testing. In *Functional Assessment of Low Vision,* B. P. Rosenthal, R. G. Cole, eds. St. Louis: Mosby-Year Book, 1996:77–88.
10. Heinen SJ, Skavenski AA. Adaptation of saccades and fixation to bilateral foveal lesions in adult monkey. *Vis Res* 1992;32:365–373.
11. Kirchner C, Phillips B. Report of a survey of U.S. low vision services. *J Vis Impairm Blindn* 1980;74:122–124.
12. Lippman O, Corn AL, Lewis, MC. Bioptic telescope spectacles and driving performance: A study in Texas. *J Vis Impairm Blindn* 1988; 82:182–187.
13. Mansfield JS, Ahn SJ, Legge GE, Leubker A. A new reading-acuity chart for normal and low vision. *Ophthalmic Vis Opt/Noninvasive Assess Vis Syst Tech Dig* (Optical Society of America, Washington, DC) 1993;3:232–235.
14. Massof RW. A systems model for low vision rehabilitation. 1. Basic concepts. *Optom Vis Sci* 1995;72:725–736.
15. Massof RW, Dagnelie G, Deremeik JT, DeRose JL, Alibhai SS, Glasser NM. Low vision rehabilitation in the U.S. health care system. *J Vis Rehab* 1995;9(3):1–31.
16. Massof RW, Rickman DL, Lalle PA. Low vision enhancement system. *APL Tech Dig* (Applied Physics Laboratory, The Johns Hopkins University, Laurel, MD) 1994;15:120–125.
17. Moses RA. Energy relationships. In *Adler's Physiology of the Eye,* 7th ed., R. A. Moses, ed. St. Louis: C.V. Mosby, 1981:357–369.
18. Nowakowski RW. Driving with impaired vision. In *Primary Low Vision Care,* R. W. Nowakowski, ed. Norwalk, CT: Appleton and Lange, 1994: 275–284.
19. O'Regan JK, Jacobs AM. Optimal viewing position effect in word recognition: A challenge to current theory. *J Exp Psychol: Hum Percept Perform* 1992;18(1):185–197.
20. Rayner K, Well AD, Pollatsek A, Bertera, JH. The availability of useful information to the right of fixation in reading. *Percept Psychophys* 1982; 31:537–550.
21. Regan D, Neima D. Low-contrast letter charts as a test of visual function. *Ophthalmology* 1983;90:1192–1200.
22. Rubin GS. Reliability and sensitivity of clinical contrast sensitivity tests. *Clin Vis Sci* 1989;2: 169–177.
23. Schuchard RA, Raasch TW. Retinal locus for fixation: Pericentral fixation targets. *Clin Vis Sci* 1992;7:511–520.
24. Sheedy JE, Bailey IL, Raasch TW. Visual acuity and chart luminance. *Am J Optom Physiol Opt* 1984;61:595–600.
25. Sloan LL. New test charts for the measurement of visual acuity at far and near distances. *Am J Ophthalmol* 1959;48:807–813.
26. Sloan LL. Variation of acuity with luminance in ocular diseases and anomalies. *Doc Ophthalmol* 1969;26:384–393.
27. Sloan LL, Habel A, Feiock K. High illumination as an auxilliary reading aid in diseases of the macula. *Am J Ophthalmol* 1973;76:745–757.
28. Smith AU, Cote KS. Sensory integration. In *Look at Me,* A. U. Smith, K. S. Cote, eds. Philadelphia: Pennsylvania College of Optometry Press, 1982:43–57.
29. Sunness JS, Applegate CA, Haselwood D, Rubin GS. Fixation patterns and reading rates in eyes with central scotomas from advanced atrophic age-related macular degeneration and Stargardt's disease. *Ophthalmology* 1996;103:1458–1466.
30. World Health Assembly. *International Classification of Impairments, Disabilities, and Handicaps: A Manual of Classification Relating to the Consequences of Disease.* Geneva: World Health Organization, 1980.

42

Organizations Serving the Visually Impaired and Individuals with Genetic Diseases

LARA PALINCSAR

From the initial suspicions of potential problems in a person born with a genetically inherited disorder, the affected individual and the family may experience a sense of isolation. Upon confirmation of the diagnosis at any age, these feelings may intensify as the potential lifelong impact of the condition is gradually appreciated. Parents may mourn the loss of the "perfect child" even as they initiate the process of acquiring needed services. Newly diagnosed older children or adults may experience a loss of self-esteem.[1] At this vulnerable time and in subsequent contacts, sensitivity on the part of the professional in recognizing the needs of patients and their families is critical. One means by which this recognition may be demonstrated is through knowledge of resources and appropriate referrals to service providers and self-help groups.

Voluntary self-help groups and private foundations vary in objectives. Some organizations focus on legislative advocacy or procuring funds for research; others mainly provide a forum for social support and networking. Organizations may also provide medical information in lay terms, literature for professionals and family members, tips for addressing changing emotional and physical needs, equipment banks, and referral services. Through database listings, groups may also facilitate voluntary participation in research protocols. Regardless of stated goals, most afford individuals an opportunity to interact with a community of peers, share common concerns and coping strategies, and encourage self-advocacy and active participation in health care and social issues.

Numerous organizations exist to serve the needs of the visually impaired (Table 42.1). Referral to condition-specific support groups may also be beneficial (Table 42.2). National organizations have been listed. Information on regional chapters can be obtained from the national offices. Information on organizations for conditions not listed may be obtained from the Alliance of Genetic Support Groups[2] and the National Organization for Rare Disorders.

Alliance of Genetic Support Groups
35 Wisconsin Circle, Suite 440
Chevy Chase, MD 20815
(301) 652-5553
1-800-336-4363

National Organization for Rare Disorders (NORD)
P.O. Box 8923
New Fairfield, CT 06812
(203) 746-6518
1-800-999-6673

Table 42.1. National Organizations Serving the Visually Impaired°

Purpose	Educational Materials	Referrals	Research Support	Other Services
		American Council of the Blind 1155 15th St., N.W. Suite 720, Washington DC 20005 (202) 467-5081; 1-800-424-8666		
Legislative advocacy, national convention, peer support	Newsletters (local)	Adaptive products, local chapters	—	Scholarships for blind students, national convention, special-interest subgroups
		American Foundation for the Blind (AFB) 15 West 16th St., New York, NY 10011 (212) 620-2000; 1-800-AFB-LINE		
Direct assistance, legislative advocacy, education and outreach, research	Booklets, *Journal of Visual Impairment and Blindness*, newsletter, public education programs	Community agencies, adaptive products	National Technology Center, independent research efforts, thesis incentives	Mogul Memorial Library and Information Center; identification card; local, regional, national conferences; scholarships for blind students
		National Association for the Parents of the Visually Impaired, Inc. P.O. Box 317, Watertown, MA 02272-0317 1-800-562-7444		
Peer support; advocacy; education and outreach	Newsletter, publications for families and professionals	Local chapters, nonmedical services	Registry of affected individuals	Parent/individual matching service
		National Association for the Visually Handicapped 22 West 21st. St., New York, NY 10010 (212) 889-3141		
Advocacy; education and outreach for the partially sighted	Newsletters, books, large-print publications including textbooks	Sources of optical aids		Loaning library of large-print books
		National Federation for the Blind 1800 Johnson St., Baltimore, MD 21230 (410) 659-9314		
Legislative advocacy; national convention; peer support	Newsletters (local), national magazine, public education programs	Local/regional groups		Scholarships for blind students, local conventions, training programs

° All organizations have regional chapters.

In addition to information on, and referral to, support groups and voluntary organizations, both of the groups advocate on a national level for the needs of those affected by genetic conditions and rare disorders. Both also offer technical assistance for the formation of new support groups and training in advocacy.

Visual impairment can significantly affect all aspects of life, including education, access to information, and mobility. Most states within the United States offer services for the legally

Table 42.2. Selected Condition-Specific Voluntary Support Organizations

Local/Regional Chapters	Services	Educational Material	Research Support
	ALBINISM National Organization for Albinism and Hypopigmentation 1530 Locust St., Box 29, Philadelphia, PA 19102 (215) 545-2322; 1-800-473-2310		
Yes	Information for professionals, families, public, media telephone "helpline"; information and referral for medical and nonmedical services peer support	Fact sheets; pamphlets; newsletter; computer bulletin board; videos	Linking families and researchers
	GALACTOSEMIA Parents of Galactosemic Children 11470 Southern Lites Dr., Clackamas, OR 97015 (503) 698-7722		
Matching service	Information for professionals, families, public, media telephone "helpline"; referral for medical services; peer support	Pamplets; newsletter; bibliography	Linking families and researchers
	MACULAR DISEASE Association for Macular Diseases (AMD) 210 East 64th St., New York, NY 10021 (212) 605-3719		
	Information for professionals, families, public, media; referral for medical services; peer support	Booklets; newsletter; audiotapes; videos	Registry of affected individuals
	Macular Degeneration International 2968 West Ina Rd., #106 Tuscon, AZ 85741 (602) 797-2525		
Yes	Information for professionals, families, public, media; referral for medical services; peer support	Fact sheets; booklets; newsletter; membership directory; resource guide; audiotapes	Registry of affected individuals; linking families and researchers
	MARFAN SYNDROME National Marfan Foundation 382 Main St., Port Washington, NY 11050 (516) 883-8712; 1-800-MARFAN		
Yes	Information for professionals, families, public, media; referral for medical services; peer support; information and referral for medical and nonmedical services	Fact sheets; booklets; newsletter; pamphlets; bibliography; video	Research grants
	MICROPHTHALMIA/ANOPHTHALMIA International Children's Anophthalmia Network (ICAN) Developmental Medicine and Genetics Albert Einstein Medical Center 5501 Old York Road, Philadelphia, PA 19141 (215) 456-8722; 1-800-580-4226		
Yes	Information for professionals, families, public, media; referral for medical services; peer support	Fact sheets; newsletter; resource guide	Registry of affected individuals

(continued)

Table 42.2. Continued

Local/Regional Chapters	Services	Educational Material	Research Support
	RETINITIS PIGMENTOSA The Foundation Fighting Blindness 1401 Mount Royal Ave., 4th Floor, Baltimore, MD 21217-4245 (410) 225-9400; 1-800-683-5555		
Yes	Information for professionals, families, public, media; referral for medical services; peer support	Fact sheets; pamphlets; newsletter; audiotapes	Registry of affected individuals; linking families and researchers; research grants
	Laurence Moon Bardet-Biedl Support Network 124 Lincoln Ave., Purchase, NY 10577 (914) 251-1163		
Yes	Information for professionals, families, public, media	Fact sheets; newsletter; membership directory; resource guide	Registry of affected individuals; linking families and researchers
	RETINOBLASTOMA (New England) Retinoblastoma Support Group 110 Allen Rd., Bow, NH 03304 (603) 224-4085; 1-800-562-6265		
Yes Matching service	Information for professionals, families, public, media; information and referral for medical and nonmedical services; telephone "helpline"	Fact sheets; newsletter	Registry of affected individuals; linking families and researchers
	USHER'S SYNDROME Usher Family Support 4918 42nd Ave., South, Minneapolis, MN 55417 (612) 724-6982		
Yes Matching service		Newsletter	Registry of affected individuals

blind including schools for the blind; however, many affected individuals are able to be included in regular school programming. Local departments of education can provide information about available services. Departments of vocational rehabilitation offer training to facilitate a return to the workforce and may be able to direct clients to appropriate services or provide local resource guides.

The National Library Service for the Blind and Physically Handicapped provides reading material to individuals who can document their inability to utilize printed material because of physical or visual limitations. Individuals seeking information on this service should be directed to:

National Library Service for the Blind and Physically Handicapped
1291 Taylor Street, NW
Washington, D.C. 20542
1-800-424-8567

REFERENCES

1. Burns J. Self-help and life-cycle needs. March of Dimes Birth Defects Foundation. *Birth Defects Orig. Art Ser* 1986;22(2):103.
2. Alliance of Genetic Support Groups. *Directory of National Voluntary Organizations and Related Resources,* 2nd ed. Chevy Chase, MD: Alliance of Genetic Support Groups, 1995.

APPENDIX
Gene Map of Heritable Ocular Disorders

IAN M. MacDONALD

Gene Map of Heritable Ocular Disorders

Condition	MIM#	Gene (MIM#)	Map Location
Anterior Segment Conditions			
Aniridia	106210	*PAX6*	11p13
Avellino dystrophy (ACD)		*βig-h3* (601692)	5q31
Axenfeld-Rieger anomaly	601631		6p25
Cornea plana congenita (CNA1)			12q21
Cornea plana congenita (CNA2)	121400		12q21
Corneal dystrophy, granular (CDGG1)	217300	*βig-h3* (601692)	5q31
Corneal dystrophy, Meesmann	121900 122100	K3 (148043) K12 (601687)	12q12-q13 17q12-q21
Iridogoniodysgenesis anomaly (IRID1)	601631		6p25
Iridogoniodysgenesis syndrome (iris hypoplasia) (IRID2)	137600	*RIEG1* (601542)	4q25
Lattice corneal dystrophy (LCDI)	122200	*βig-h3* (601692)	5q31
Macular corneal dystrophy	217800		16q22
Megalocornea (X-linked)	309300		Xq12-q26
Peters' anomaly	106210	*PAX6*	11p13
Posterior polymorphous dystrophy	122000		20q11
Reis-Bücklers (CDRB)	121900	*βig-h3* (601692)	5q31
Rieger syndrome, Type 1	180500	*RIEG1* (601542)	4q25
Rieger syndrome, Type 2	601499		13q14
Schnyder crystalline corneal dystrophy	121800		1p36-p34.1
Lens Disorders			
Cataract, anterior polar 1 (CTAA1)	115650		14q24-qter
Cataract, anterior polar 2 (CTAA2)	601202		17p13
Cataract, Cerulean Type (CCA1)	115660		17q24
Cataract, Cerulean Type II (CCA2)	601547	*CRYBB2* (123620)	22q11.2-q12.2
Cataract, congenital total	302200		Xp
Cataract, dominant, congenital		*CRYAA* (123580)	21q22.3
Cataract, Coppock-like (CCL)		*CRYGA* (123660)	2q33-q35
Cataract, Marner Type (CAM)	116800		16q22.1
Cataract, posterior polar (CPP)	116600		1pter-p36.1
Cataract, Volkmann Type	115665		1p36
Cataract, dominant, zonular pulverulant (CZP)	601885		13q11-q12
Cataract, lamellar, zonular pulverulant, Coppock (CAE), Duffy-linked	116200	Connexin50 (600897)	1q21-q25
Cataract, zonular with sutural opacities (CCZS)	600881		17q11-q12
Ectopia lentis, simple	129600	Fibrillin (134797)	15q21.1
Glaucoma as Primary Disorder			
Glaucoma, open angle, juvenille onset (GLC1A)	137750	Myocilin (601652)	1q23-q25
Glaucoma, adult onset POAG (GLC1B)	137760		2cen-q13

(continued)

Gene Map of Heritable Ocular Disorders—Continued

Condition	MIM#	Gene (MIM#)	Map Location
Glaucoma, adult onset POAG (GLC1C)	601682		3q21-q24
Glaucoma, adult onset POAG (GLC1D)	602429		8q23
Glaucoma, adult onset POAG (GLC1E)	602432		10p15-p14
Glaucoma, primary infantile (GLC3A)	231300	Cytochrome p4501B1 (CYP1B1) (601771)	2p21
Glaucoma, primary infantile (GLC3B)	600975		1p36
Glaucoma, pigment dispersion type	600510		7q35-q36
Vitreo-retinal Disorders			
Familial exudative vitreoretinopathy (EVR1)	133780		11q13-q23
Familial exudative vitreoretinopathy (EVR2) (X-linked)	305390	Norrin	Xp11.4-p11.23
Myopia, Bornholm eye disease (X-linked)	310460		Xq28
Norrie disease	310600	Norrin	Xp11.4-p11.23
Neovascular inflammatory vitreoretinopathy (VRNI)	193235		11q13
Primary retinal dysplasia (PRD) (X-linked)	312550	Norrin	Xp11.4-p11.23
Retinoschisis (RS)	312700		Xp22.2-p22.1
Wagner syndrome Type 1 (WGN1)	143200		5p13-q14
Wagner syndrome Type 2 (WGN2)		COL2A1 (120140)	12q13.11-q13.2
Tapeto-retinal Disorders			
Achromatopsia	200930		2p11-q12
Albinism			
OCA1-A (tyrosinase −)	203100	Tyrosinase	11q14-q21
OCA1-B (yellow)	203100	Tyrosinase	11q14-q21
OCA2 (tyrosinase +)	203200	*P*	15q11.2-q12
OCA3 (Brown)	203290	TRP-1 (115501)	9p23-p22
Chediak-Higashi syndrome (CHS1)	214500	*LYST*	1q42.1-q42.2
HPS (Hermansky-Pudlak syndrome)	203300	Novel transmembrane protein	10q23.1-q23.3
OA1 (Nettleship-Falls)	300500	*OA1*	Xp22.3
OA2 (Åland island eye disease/ Forsius-Eriksson)	300600		Xp11
Ocular albinism with late-onset sensorineural deafness (OASD)	300650		Xp22.3
Atrophia areata (helicoid chorioretinal degeneration)	108985		11p15
Bardet-Biedl syndrome			
BBS1	209901		11q13
BBS2	209900		16q21
BBS3	600151		3p13-p12
BBS4	600374		15q22.2-q23
Doyne honeycomb retinal dystrophy	126600		2p16
Central areolar choroidal dystrophy	215500		17p
Choroideremia	303100	REP1	Xp21.1-q21.3

Gene Map of Heritable Ocular Disorders—Continued

Condition	MIM#	Gene (MIM#)	Map Location
Color vision defects			
Blue cone monochromacy (CBBM)	303700	Red, green color genes	Xq28
Deuteranopia	303800	Green color genes	Xq28
Dominant tritanopia	190900	Blue color genes	7q31.3-q32
Protanopia	303900	Red color genes	Xq28
Cone dystrophy, dominant (COD3)	602093	GUCA1A (600364)	6p21.1
Retinal cone dystrophy 1 (RCD1)	180020		6q25-q26
Retinal cone dystrophy 2 (RCD2)	601251		17p13.1
XL progressive cone dystrophy (COD1)	304020		Xp11.4
XL progressive cone dystrophy 2 (COD2)	300085		Xq27
Cone rod dystrophy			
CORD1	600624		18q21.1-q21.3
CORD2	120970	*CRX* (602225)	19q13.1-q13.4
CORD5	600977		17p13-p12
CORD6	601777		17p13-p12
Congenital stationary night blindness			
Oguchi disease, RHOK-related	258100	RHOK (180381)	13q34
Oguchi disease, SAG-related	258100	arrestin (SAG) (181031)	2q37.1
CSNB1	310500		Xp11
CSNB2	300071	*CSNB2*	Xp21.1
CSNB3, PDE6B-related	163500	PDE6B (180072)	4p16.3
CSNB, RHO-related (CSNB4)	163500	RHO (180380)	3q21-q24
CSNB, Nougaret	163500	GNATI (139330)	3p21
Gyrate atrophy	258870	OAT	10q26
Leber congenital amaurosis			
LCA1	204000	retinal guanylate cyclase (60179)	17p13
LCA2	204100	RPE65	1p31
LCA3		*CRX* (602225)	19q13.3
Macular dystrophy			
Macular dystrophy, age-related	153800	*ABCR* (601691)	1p21-p13
Macular dystrophy, peripherin-related		*RDS/* peripherin (179605)	6p21.2-p11.2
Macular dystrophy, dominant cystoid	153880		7p21-p15
North Carolina macular dystrophy (MCDR1)	136550		6q14-q16.2
Progressive bifocal chorioretinal atrophy (CRAPB)	600790		6q14-q16.2
Sorsby fundus dystrophy	136900	TIMP3 (188826)	22q13-qter
Stargardt disease			
STGD1	248200	*ABCR* (601691)	1p21-p13
STGD2	153900		13q34
STGD3	600110		6cen-q14
Vitelliform macular dystrophy (Best)	153700		11q13
Retinitis punctata albescens	136880	*RDS/* peripherin (179605)	6p21.2-p11.2
		RHO (180380)	3q21-q24

(continued)

Gene Map of Heritable Ocular Disorders—Continued

Condition	MIM#	Gene (MIM#)	Map Location
Retinoblastoma	180200	$p100^{RBI}$	13q14
Retinitis pigmentosa			
Digenic RP (*ROM/RDS*)		*RDS*/ peripherin (179605)	6p21.2-p11.2
		ROM1 (180721)	11q13
Autosomal recessive RP			
RP with preserved paraarteriole retinal pigment epithelium	268030		1q
unassigned			2q31-q33
unassigned		PDE6B (180072)	4p16.3
unassigned		CNCG1 (123825)	4p12-cen
unassigned		PDE6A (cGMP-specific) (180071)	5q31.2-q34
unassigned		*ROM1* (180721)	11q13
RP4		RHO (180380)	3q21-q24
RP12	600105		1q31-q32.1
RP14	600132		6p
RP16			14
RP19	601718	ABCR (601691)	1p21-p13
RP22	602594		16p12.3-p12.1
Autosomal dominant RP			
RP1	180100		8q11-q13
RP4		RHO (180380)	3q21-q24
RP7		*RDS*/ peripherin (179605)	6p21.2-p11.2
RP8	180103		unlinked
RP9	180104		7p15-p13
RP10	180105		7q31
RP11	600138		19q13.4
RP13	600059		17p13.3
RP17	600852		17q25
RP18	601414		1p13-q23
X-linked RP			
RP2	312600		Xp11.3
RP3	312610	RPGR	Xp21
RP6	312612		Xp11.4-p11.23
RP15	300029		Xp22.13-p22.11
Usher Syndrome			
USH1A	276900		14q32
USH1B	276903	myosin VIIA	11q13.5
USH1C	276904		11p15.1
USH1D	601067		10q
USH1E			21q21
USH2A	276901		1q41
USH2B	276905		not 1q
USH3	276902		3q21-q25
Optic Nerve Disorders			
Coloboma of optic nerve with renal disease (ONCR)	120330	*PAX2* (167409)	10q24.3-q25.1
Dominant optic atrophy, Kjer type (OPA1)	165500		3q27-q28
X-linked optic atrophy (OPA2)	311050		Xp11.4-Xp11.2
Leber hereditary optic neuropathy	535000		mtDNA

Gene Map of Heritable Ocular Disorders—Continued

Condition	MIM#	Gene (MIM#)	Map Location
Lid Disorders			
Bleopharophimosis syndrome			
BPES	110100		3q22-q23
BPES2	601649		7p21-p13
Congenital ptosis, dominant	178300		1p34.1-p32
Eye Movement Disorders			
Congenital fibrosis of extraocular muscles	135700		12q13.2-q24.1
Chronic progressive external ophthalmoplegia (Kearns-Sayre syndrome)	530000		mtDNA
Nystagmus, dominant congenital	164100		6p12
Ocular Development Disorders			
Microphthalmia with linear skin defects (MLS)	309801		Xp22
Microphthalmia-Cataract	156850		16p13.3
Anophthalmos, X-linked	301590		Xq27-q28

Abbreviations: ABCR = ATP-binding cassette transporter; GNATI = alpha-subunit of rod transducin; GUCA1A = guanylate cyclase activator 1A; GUC2D = retinal duanylate cyclase; MIM# = Mendelian Inheritance in Man # (McKusick); OAT = ornithine amino-transferase; PDE = cGMP phosphodiesterase; REP1 = Rab escort protein-1; TIMP-3 = tissue inhibitor of metalloproteinase-3; TRP-1 = tyrosinase-related protein-1.

Index